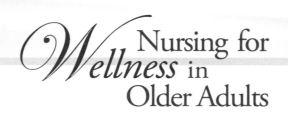

Brief Contents

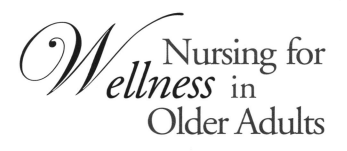

Nursing for Wellness in Older Adults

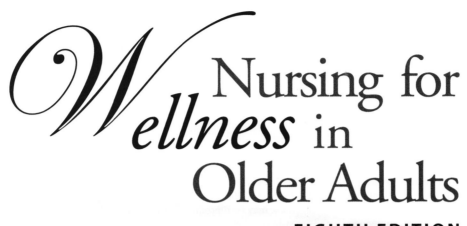

Nursing for Wellness in Older Adults

EIGHTH EDITION

Carol A Miller, MSN, RN-BC

Gerontological Clinical Nurse Specialist and Nurse Case Manager
Care & Counseling, Miller/Wetzler Associates
Cleveland, Ohio

Faculty
Frances Payne Bolton School of Nursing
Case Western Reserve University
Cleveland, Ohio

Wolters Kluwer

Philadelphia • Baltimore • New York • London
Buenos Aires • Hong Kong • Sydney • Tokyo

Vice President and Publisher: Julie K. Stegman
Acquisitions Editor: Natasha McIntyre
Director of Product Development: Jennifer K. Forestieri
Senior Development Editor: Meredith L. Brittain
Marketing Manager: Katie Schlesinger
Editorial Coordinator: Lindsay Ries
Editorial Assistant: Leo Gray
Design Coordinator: Holly Reid McLaughlin
Art Director, Illustration: Jennifer Clements
Production Project Manager: Marian Bellus
Manufacturing Coordinator: Karin Duffield
Prepress Vendor: Aptara

Eighth Edition

NANDA International, Inc.: Nursing Diagnoses - Definitions and Classification 2018-2020 © 2017 NANDA International, ISBN 978-1-62623-929-6. Used by arrangement with the Thieme Group, Stuttgart/New York.

Library of Congress Cataloging-in-Publication Data

Names: Miller, Carol A., author.
Title: Nursing for wellness in older adults / Carol A. Miller.
Description: Eighth edition. | Philadelphia : Wolters Kluwer, [2019] |
    Includes bibliographical references and index.
Identifiers: LCCN 2017046468 | ISBN 9781496368287
Subjects: | MESH: Geriatric Nursing | Aged–psychology | Health Promotion |
    Nursing Theory | Case Reports
Classification: LCC RC954 | NLM WY 152 | DDC 618.97/0231–dc23
LC record available at https://lccn.loc.gov/2017046468

LWW.com

Dedications

I lovingly dedicate this book to my parents,
Margaret 'n' Bob Miller, who have always given
me boundless support, encouragement, and inspiration.
They have been shining examples of living long and full lives.
This book also is dedicated to the many older adults and their
families who teach invaluable lessons about successfully
navigating the challenges of older adulthood.

Contributors

Contributor to the Eighth Edition

Georgia J. Anetzberger, PhD, ACSW
Adjunct Assistant Professor of Medicine
Case Western Reserve University
Cleveland, Ohio
Past President, National Committee for the Prevention
    of Elder Abuse
Washington, DC

For a list of the contributors to the Student and Instructor
Resources accompanying this book, please visit http://the point.
lww.com/Miller8e.

Contributor to the Seventh Edition

Georgia J. Anetzberger, PhD, ACSW
Adjunct Assistant Professor of Medicine
Case Western Reserve University
Cleveland, Ohio
Past President, National Committee for the Prevention
    of Elder Abuse
Washington, DC

A Student's Perspective Contributors for the Eighth and Seventh Editions

*These features were contributed by students from the
following programs:*

Brigham Young University
Provo, Utah

Western Michigan University
Kalamazoo, Michigan

Angelo State University
San Angelo, Texas

Reviewers

Catherine Bevil, RN, EdD
Professor and Director
University of Nebraska Medical Center College of Nursing
Omaha, Nebraska

Edith Claros, PhD, MSN, RN
Assistant Dean and Associate Professor
MCPHS University
Boston, Massachusetts

Kathy J. Fabiszewski, PhD, MSN
Assistant Professor
Salem State University
Salem, Massachusetts

Catherine C. Kenney, DNP
Assistant Clinical Professor
University of Wisconsin Eau Claire
Eau Claire, Wisconsin

Teresa Page, DNP, MSN, RN, EdS, FNP-BC
Assistant Professor
Liberty University
Lynchburg, Virginia

LoriAnn Pajalich, DNP, MSN
Assistant Professor
Wilkes University
Avoca, Pennsylvania

VaLinda Pearson, PhD
Professor of Nursing
St. Catherine University
St. Paul, Minnesota

Karen Reynolds, DNP, MSN, BSN
Adjunct Professor
State College of Florida
Sarasota, Florida

Gina M. Severino, DNP, MSN
Associate Lecturer/Clinical Instructor
Kent State University, Trumbull Campus
Warren, Ohio

Gladdi Tomlinson, MSN, RN
Adjunct Professor
Harrisburg Area Community College
Harrisburg, Pennsylvania

Mary Ellen Yonushonis, MS, RN, CNE
Senior Lecturer
The Pennsylvania State University
University Park, Pennsylvania

Preface

When I began my nursing career in 1970, I chose to work in a visiting nurse program that addressed the needs of older adults in home settings. When friends and family expressed surprise about my choice of "geriatric nursing," I told them that I was excited about the opportunity to care for older adults whose health care needs were not being addressed. At that time, "geriatrics" and "gerontology" were new topics in health care, and health care professionals knew little about the unique needs of older adults. It would be 4 years before gerontological nursing would be an approved specialization and 5 years before the first gerontological nursing journal would be published. By the late 1970s, I was practicing as a gerontological nurse practitioner, and I found great satisfaction when an older adult told me that the complete physical examination I had provided was the first one he or she had ever received.

In my clinical practice, I frequently encountered older adults who would attribute their symptoms to "old age," and I wondered if at least some of these problems were due to treatable conditions. I began delving into the information that was emerging because of the unprecedented increases in the older adult population, and I found much science-based evidence that many of the problems attributed to aging were indeed caused by other factors. By the late 1980s, I had formulated the Functional Consequences Theory to help nurses identify and address the many interacting factors that affect the level of functioning and quality of life of older adults. This theory provided the framework for the first edition of this textbook.

During the early 2000s, the concept of "wellness" emerged as a major focus of health care; however, the concept was generally associated with physical fitness and "preventing aging." I wondered why the concept seemed to exclude older adults. Further research and clinical practice enabled me to connect the concepts of aging and wellness and broaden the framework for my textbook to the Functional Consequences Theory for Promoting Wellness in Older Adults. This expanded framework is based on the following premises: (1) achieving wellness is not limited by age; (2) nurses have a vital role in promoting wellness for older adults; and (3) nurses promote wellness for older adults through interventions that support their optimal level of functioning and quality of life.

After the seventh edition of *Nursing for Wellness in Older Adults* won first place in the gerontological nursing category as an *American Journal of Nursing* Book of the Year, I continued to explore evidence-based information related to wellness for older adults. I found an ongoing emphasis on the essential roles of nurses in teaching older adults about nutrition, physical activity, stress reduction, and other self-care interventions that are effective for health promotion. While working on this eighth edition, one of my biggest challenges has been setting boundaries on what is included in this text, because research on all aspects of aging and older adulthood is constantly expanding. In keeping with the focus on promoting wellness for older adults, this text emphasizes the evidence-based information that is most pertinent to helping nurses work proactively with older adults to promote high levels of functioning and quality of life, despite the limitations associated with aging, disease, and other conditions.

Evidence-based information is widely cited throughout the text and is also summarized in boxes in clinically oriented chapters. Assessment and intervention guidelines help nurses identify and address factors that affect the functioning and quality of life of older adults. Nursing interventions focus on teaching older adults and their caregivers about actions they can take to promote wellness. Chapters also include information about applicable nursing diagnoses and wellness outcomes. Unfolding case examples illustrate common experiences of older adults as they progress from young-old to old-old and are affected by combinations of age-related changes and risk factors. Consistent with the current emphasis on safety and quality concerns related to care of older adults, competencies of Quality and Safety Education in Nursing (QSEN) are applied in many of the case examples. Theory illustrations at the beginning of chapters illustrate how the Functional Consequences Theory for Promoting Wellness in Older Adults is integrated with the nursing process with regard to specific aspects of functioning.

This eighth edition includes enhanced coverage of two topics that have been discussed in previous editions: interprofessional collaboration and transitional care. Interprofessional collaboration is particularly important when nurses care for older adults with complex needs, such as those related to medication management, elder abuse, fall prevention, cognitive impairment, and legal and ethical concerns. When nurses care for older adults who are relatively healthy and independent, interprofessional collaboration often involves working and communicating with community-based care providers. Chapter 6 provides an overview of interprofessional collaboration, and the clinical chapters address the topic in multiple contexts.

Transitional care is increasingly recognized as a major concern when older adults receive care across different settings. This topic is discussed in Chapter 6 and applied to a Transitional Care Unfolding Case Study in Chapters 27 through 29.

This edition highlights the new topic of gerontechnology, which refers to the increasing development of technology-based interventions that are available for improving functioning and quality of life in the daily lives of older adults. Nurses have key roles in developing and implementing care plans that may include the use of technology. This topic is presented in Chapter 5, and examples of technology to promote wellness in older adults are incorporated in boxes throughout the text.

ORGANIZATION

Nursing for Wellness in Older Adults has 29 chapters, organized into five parts. Chapters in Parts 1 and 2 introduce topics relevant to aging, wellness, diversity, older adults, and the role of nurses in promoting wellness in older adults. Chapters in Parts 3 and 4 are organized around the Functional Consequences Theory for Promoting Wellness in Older Adults, so each facet of physiologic or psychosocial function is presented according to age-related changes, risk factors, functional consequences, nursing assessment, nursing diagnosis, wellness outcomes, nursing interventions, and evaluation of nursing care. Chapters in Part 5 help nurses apply a wellness perspective as they care for older adults who are ill, experiencing pain, or at the end of life.

The intent of Part 1 (Chapters 1 through 4), *Older Adults and Wellness*, is to help nurses apply a wellness philosophy to their care of older adults. Chapters 1 and 2 integrate the concepts of wellness and aging and provide an overview of characteristics and diversity of older adults, with emphasis on the uniqueness of each older adult. Chapter 3 explicates the Functional Consequences Theory for Promoting Wellness in Older Adults, which is applied throughout this text as a framework for wellness-oriented nursing care of older adults. Chapter 4 provides an overview of theories that are pertinent to aging well.

Part 2 (Chapters 5 through 10), *Nursing Considerations for Older Adults*, addresses the unique challenges of caring for older adults. Chapter 5 discusses nursing care of older adults as a specialization and as a responsibility for all nurses. This chapter also addresses health promotion, with emphasis on ways in which nurses can apply evidence-based guidelines to help older adults develop health-promoting behaviors. Chapter 6 helps nurses identify the many types of community-based services and health care programs that address the complex needs of older adults. This chapter also includes information about QSEN, interprofessional collaboration, and transitional care. Chapters 7 through 9 cover the multifaceted topics of assessment, medications, and legal and ethical concerns because nurses commonly address these aspects of care when they care for older adults. The important topic of elder abuse and neglect is addressed in Chapter 10, with emphasis on the roles of nurses in preventing, identifying, and addressing this serious—and all too common—issue.

Part 3 (Chapters 11 through 15), *Promoting Wellness in Psychosocial Function*, extensively reviews cognitive and psychosocial function and provides guidelines for a comprehensive nursing assessment of psychosocial function, with emphasis on healthy older adults. In addition, this part covers delirium, dementia, and depression, which are three of the most commonly occurring pathologic conditions that have serious psychosocial consequences for older adults.

Part 4 (Chapters 16 through 26), *Promoting Wellness in Physical Function*, includes chapters that address each of the following specific aspects of functioning in older adults: hearing, vision, digestion and nutrition, urinary function, cardiovascular function, respiratory function, safe mobility, integumentary function, sleep and rest, thermoregulation, and sexual function. Selected common pathologic conditions are also addressed in these chapters when these conditions affect a particular aspect of functioning in older adults.

Part 5 (Chapters 27 through 29), *Promoting Wellness During Illness and Transitions in Care*, addresses topics of caring for older adults during illness and when they are experiencing pain or are at the end of life. Each chapter includes a new section, Spotlight on Transitional Care, which includes a Transitional Care Unfolding Case Study.

SPECIAL FEATURES OF THE EIGHTH EDITION

Special features from past editions have been retained in this edition, and several new features have been added.

New Features

- *NEW!* **Technology to Promote Wellness in Older Adults** boxes describe examples of technology-based interventions that can be effective for promoting wellness for older adults.
- *NEW!* **Interprofessional Collaboration (IPC)** material, which is found in boxes or is highlighted with orange bars in the margins, indicates the responsibilities and opportunities of nurses to collaborate with other professionals and paraprofessionals in health care and community-based settings when caring for older adults.
- *NEW!* **Global Perspective** boxes provide examples of the various ways in which health care professionals in other countries provide care for older adults.
- *NEW!* **Unfolding Patient Stories**, written by the National League for Nursing, are an engaging way to begin meaningful conversations in the classroom. These vignettes, which open each unit, feature patients from Wolters Kluwer's *vSim for Nursing | Gerontology* (codeveloped with Laerdal Medical) and DocuCare products; however, each Unfolding Patient Story in the book stands alone, not requiring purchase of these products. For your convenience, a list

of these case studies, along with their location in the book, appears in the "Case Studies in This Book" section later in this frontmatter.

- *NEW!* **A Transitional Care Unfolding Case Study,** which unfolds across Chapters 27 through 29, illustrates ways in which nurses can provide effective transitional care to an older adult whose progressively worsening condition requires that her needs be met in several settings. For your convenience, a list of the parts of this case study, along with their location in the book, appears in the "Case Studies in This Book" section later in this frontmatter.

Features Retained From Previous Editions

- Multipart **Unfolding Case Studies** within the chapters provide real-life examples of the cumulative effects of age-related changes and risk factors, beginning in young-old adulthood and continuing through all the stages of later adulthood. **Thinking Points** after each segment and **Nursing Care Plans** after the concluding segments assist the student in applying the content of the chapter to the case example. For your convenience, a list of these case studies, along with their location in the book, appears in the "Case Studies in This Book" section later in this frontmatter.
- **QSEN examples** of application of knowledge, skills, and attitudes for care plans relate to unfolding case examples.
- Single-part **Case Studies** in some chapters illustrate application of content to clinical settings. For your convenience, a list of these case studies, along with their location in the book, appears in the "Case Studies in This Book" section later in this frontmatter.
- **Online Learning Activities** cited throughout every chapter point readers to the book's companion web page, where readers can access enhanced information related to the topic, including resources, articles, and evidence-based guidelines.
- **Icons** identify the five major components of the Functional Consequences Theory for Promoting Wellness in Older Adults:

 Age-related changes

 Risk factors

 Functional consequences

 Nursing assessment

 Nursing interventions

- **Wellness Opportunities** are sprinkled throughout the clinically oriented chapters to draw attention to ways in which nurses can promote wellness during the usual course of their care activities.

- **Diversity Notes** give brief information about differences among specific groups (e.g., men and women, whites and African Americans).
- **Figures** to illustrate important points, including timelines to illustrate major trends pertinent to the care of older adults.
- Chapter-opening features:
  - **Learning Objectives** help readers identify important chapter content and focus their reading.
  - **Key Terms** listed at the beginning of each chapter and bolded in the text highlight important vocabulary.
  - **Theory Illustrations** at the beginning of each chapter on specific aspects of functioning present an overview of the Functional Consequences Theory for Promoting Wellness in Older Adults in the context of the nursing process.
- Special boxes:
  - **Assessment** boxes provide the reader with specific approaches for nursing assessment. Commonly used assessment tools are described (and, in many cases, illustrated).
  - **Interventions** boxes provide succinct guides for nursing interventions, with a strong focus on health promotion. Guides for "best practices" in nursing interventions are given. Many of the interventions boxes can be used as tools for teaching older adults and their caregivers about how to improve functional abilities. All Interventions boxes can be downloaded from this book's companion web page at http://thepoint.lww.com/Miller8e.
  - **Evidence-Based Practice** boxes are included in clinically oriented chapters to summarize guidelines for research-based care of older adults.
  - **Cultural Considerations** boxes help readers appreciate cultural differences that may influence their approach to a patient, resident, or client.
  - **A Student's Perspective** boxes provide reality-based stories written by nursing students that illustrate the application of wellness concepts in clinical practice.
  - **Caregiver Wellness** boxes provide caregivers with information that the reader can use to address concerns of caregivers related to specific aspects of functioning for older adults.
- Chapter-ending features:
  - **Chapter Highlights** facilitate review of the material.
  - **Critical Thinking Exercises** at the end of each chapter help readers to gain insight and develop problem-solving skills through purposeful, goal-directed thinking.
  - **References** give readers additional information about the most up-to-date research that supports evidence-based practice.

A COMPREHENSIVE PACKAGE FOR TEACHING AND LEARNING

To further facilitate teaching and learning, a carefully designed ancillary package has been developed to assist faculty and students.

Instructor Resources

The following tools to assist you with teaching your course are available upon adoption of this text at http://thepoint. lww.com/Miller8e:

- An **eBook** allows access to the book's full text and images online.
- The **Test Generator** lets you generate new tests from a bank of NCLEX-style questions to help you assess your students' understanding of the course material.
- **PowerPoint Presentations** provide an easy way for you to integrate the textbook with your students' classroom experience, via either slide shows or handouts. Multiple-choice and True/False questions are integrated into the presentations to promote class participation and allow you to use i-clicker technology.
- **Case Studies** with answers can be used as a class activity or group assignment.
- **Assignments** (and suggested answers) include group, written, clinical, and Web assignments to engage students in varied activities and assess their learning.
- A sample **Syllabus** provides guidance for structuring your course.
- A **Curriculum Integration Guide** shows how book content relates to other nursing courses.
- An **Interprofessional Collaboration (IPC) Guide** describes the IPC content that appears in the book and indicates where it can be found.
- A **QSEN Map** shows how book content integrates QSEN concepts.
- An **AACN/HIGN Guide** shows how book content integrates American Association of Colleges of Nursing and Hartford Institute for Geriatric Nursing competencies.
- An **Image Bank** contains all the illustrations and tables from the book in formats suitable for printing and incorporating into PowerPoint presentations and Internet sites.
- **Strategies for Effective Teaching** offer creative approaches.
- **Learning Management System Cartridges.**
- Access to all **Student Resources** is provided so that you can understand the student experience and use these resources in your course as well.

Student Resources

Students can visit http://thepoint.lww.com/Miller8e and access the following tools and resources using the codes printed in the front of their textbooks:

- **Online Learning Activities** direct readers to websites that provide enhanced information related to the topic, including resources, articles, and evidence-based guidelines.
- **Journal Articles** corresponding to book chapters offer access to current research available in Wolters Kluwer journals.
- Plus a **Spanish–English audio glossary, Nursing Professional Roles and Responsibilities, Learning Objectives**, and **Interventions Boxes** from the textbook.

Adaptive Learning Powered by prepU

Lippincott's Adaptive Learning Powered by prepU helps every student learn more, while giving instructors the data they need to monitor each student's progress, strengths, and weaknesses. The adaptive learning system allows instructors to assign quizzes or students to take quizzes on their own that adapt to each student's individual mastery level. Visit http://thepoint.lww.com/prepU to learn more.

vSim for Nursing

vSim for Nursing, jointly developed by Laerdal Medical and Wolters Kluwer, offers innovative scenario-based learning modules consisting of Web-based virtual simulations, course learning materials, and curriculum tools designed to develop critical thinking skills and promote clinical confidence and competence. *vSim for Nursing | Gerontology* includes 12 virtual simulations based on the National League for Nursing Advancing Care Excellence for Seniors (ACES) Unfolding Cases. Students can progress through suggested readings, pre- and post-simulation assessments, documentation assignments, and guided reflection questions, and will receive an individualized feedback log immediately upon completion of the simulation. Throughout the student learning experience, the product offers remediation back to trusted Lippincott resources, including Lippincott Nursing Advisor and Lippincott Nursing Procedures—two online, evidence-based, clinical information solutions used in health care facilities throughout the United States. This innovative product provides a comprehensive patient-focused solution for learning and integrating simulation into the classroom.

Contact your Wolters Kluwer sales representative or visit http://thepoint.lww.com/vsim for options to enhance your medical-surgical nursing course with *vSim for Nursing*.

Lippincott DocuCare

Lippincott DocuCare combines web-based academic EHR simulation software with clinical case scenarios, allowing students to learn how to use an EHR in a safe, true-to-life setting, while enabling instructors to measure their progress. Lippincott DocuCare's nonlinear solution works well in the classroom, simulation lab, and clinical practice.

Contact your Wolters Kluwer sales representative or visit http://thepoint.lww.com/DocuCare for options to enhance your medical-surgical nursing course with DocuCare.

A Comprehensive, Digital, Integrated Course Solution

Lippincott CoursePoint+ is an integrated digital learning solution designed for the way students learn. It is the only nursing education solution that integrates:

- **Leading content in context:** Content provided in the context of the student learning path engages students and encourages interaction and learning on a deeper level.

- **Powerful tools to maximize class performance:** Course-specific tools, such as adaptive learning powered by prepU, provide a personalized learning experience for every student.
- **Real-time data to measure students' progress:** Student performance data provided in an intuitive display lets you quickly spot which students are having difficulty or which concepts the class as a whole is struggling to grasp.
- **Preparation for practice:** Integrated virtual simulation and evidence-based resources improve student competence, confidence, and success in transitioning to practice.
  - *vSim for Nursing:* Codeveloped by Laerdal Medical and Wolters Kluwer, *vSim for Nursing* simulates real nursing scenarios and allows students to interact with virtual patients in a safe, online environment.
  - *Lippincott Advisor for Education:* With over 8500 entries covering the latest evidence-based content and drug information, *Lippincott Advisor for Education* provides students with the most up-to-date information possible, while giving them valuable experience with the same point-of-care content they will encounter in practice.
- **Training services and personalized support:** To ensure your success, our dedicated educational consultants and training coaches will provide expert guidance every step of the way.

Carol A. Miller, MSN, RN-BC

Acknowledgments

I am deeply grateful to my family, friends, and colleagues who have supported me on my journey as this book has grown from a dream to a reality and now into its eighth edition. Pat Rehm, in particular, promotes my wellness as I pursue my goals as a nurse and author. My work with older adults and their families provides valuable lessons that have become part of this text. These experiences, which cannot be learned in books, have taught me to care deeply about, and to care sensitively for, older adults. I thank these older adults and their families and appreciate their contributions to my life and my writings.

I appreciate and acknowledge the many people who helped bring this text to fruition. I especially extend my deepest appreciation to all those at Wolters Kluwer who assisted with all phases of development and production. I also thank Sharyn Hunter, author of the Australia/New Zealand edition of this textbook, for allowing me to use design elements and some additional text for the theory illustrations. I thank all these people, and many unnamed people, for advice, guidance, support, assistance, and encouragement on my journey through all eight editions of *Nursing for Wellness in Older Adults*.

Contents

chapter 7

Assessment of Health and Functioning   99

chapter 8

Medications and Other Bioactive Substances   117

chapter 14
Impaired Cognitive Function: Delirium and Dementia   260

chapter 15
Impaired Affective Function: Depression   291

part **4**

Promoting Wellness in Physical Function   313

chapter **16**

Hearing   314

chapter 19
Urinary Function   392

chapter 20
Cardiovascular Function   418

Assessment, Interventions, and Evidence-Based Practice Boxes

 ASSESSMENT BOXES

INTERVENTIONS BOXES

E-B-P EVIDENCE-BASED PRACTICE BOXES

Case Studies in This Book

part **1**

Older Adults and Wellness

Unfolding Patient Stories: Millie Larsen · Part 1

Millie Larsen is an 84-year-old female who lives alone. Her husband passed away a year ago, and she now depends on her daughter, Dina, who lives nearby. Her current medical problems include hypertension, glaucoma, osteoarthritis of the knee, stress incontinence, osteoporosis, and hypercholesterolemia. She takes several medications to treat hypertension and pain. How can ageism influence the nurse's view of Millie's health care needs? How can the nurse identify Millie's attitudes toward her own aging that might be influencing her self-care behaviors? What options for caregiving support should the nurse be prepared to discuss if Millie's wellness and function decline? (Millie Larsen's story continues in Part 3.)

Care for Millie and other patients in a realistic virtual environment: **vSim** _for Nursing_ (thepoint.lww.com/vSimGerontology). Practice documenting these patients' care in DocuCare (thepoint.lww.com/DocuCareEHR).

Unfolding Patient Stories: Julia Morales and Lucy Grey · Part 1

Julia Morales, age 65, and Lucy Grey, age 73, are partners who have been together for more than 25 years. Julia's son, Neil, age 54, also provides support. Julia is undergoing treatment for lung cancer. What strengths and challenges should the nurse consider for an older, retired couple whose sexual orientation is not heterosexual? How can the nurse identify the unique needs of this couple to provide holistic and culturally competent care? What culturally specific resources would be available to address the unique needs of Julia and Lucy? (The story of Julia Morales and Lucy Grey continues in Part 2.)

Care for Julia, Lucy, and other patients in a realistic virtual environment: **vSim** _for Nursing_ (thepoint.lww.com/vSimGerontology). Practice documenting these patients' care in DocuCare (thepoint.lww.com/DocuCareEHR).

chapter 1

Seeing Older Adults Through the Eyes of Wellness

This perspective is consistent with the broadening base of knowledge about ways in which older adults can achieve what gerontologists call "healthy aging" or "successful aging." It is also consistent with a biopsychosocial–emotional–spiritual perspective on aging, which focuses on the increasing diversity of older adults as a group and respect for the unique characteristics of each older person. Although knowledge about all aspects of aging—ranging from healthy aging to frail elders— is evolving rapidly, many gaps still exist. Because many challenges of older adulthood involve health and functioning, older adults need accurate information, not only about normal aging but also about interventions to promote wellness during all stages of health and illness. Nurses are in ideal positions to teach older adults about health and aging and empower them to implement problem-solving strategies directed toward achieving and maintaining a high level of functioning and a good quality of life.

The intent of this gerontological nursing text is to provide comprehensive and research-based information so that nurses can distinguish between the changes associated with normal aging and those that result from risk factors. In addition, the text provides tools and guides for nursing assessment, interventions, and health education in relation to all aspects of physical and psychosocial functioning. Nurses can use this information to promote wellness—which includes improved health, functioning, and quality of life—for the older adults for whom they provide care.

This chapter provides an overview of concepts related to wellness and aging and presents information about myths and realities. It also presents information about older adults in the United States in terms of demographic, health, and socioeconomic characteristics. Last, it presents a brief overview of aging worldwide to provide a broader perspective.

THE RELATIONSHIP BETWEEN WELLNESS AND AGING

The concept of wellness in relation to aging was first brought to public attention more than a half century ago

Despite the common perception that older adulthood is an extended period of declining health and functioning, conceptualizations of aging are broadening. Currently, most gerontologists and many older adults themselves view aging as a complex process that includes both losses and gains.

by Halbert L. Dunn, MD, PhD, who developed a series of radio talks about high-level wellness, which he defined as an "integrated method of functioning that is oriented toward maximizing each person's potential, while maintaining a continuum of balance and purposeful direction within the person's environment" (Dunn, 1961, pp. 4–5). In one radio program, Dunn addressed stereotypes about aging and emphasized that "healthy maturity" is characterized not only by physical decline but also by wisdom. Moreover, he discussed the relationship between mind, body, and spirit and stressed the importance of older adults having a purpose in life, communicating with others, maintaining personal dignity, and contributing to society (Dunn, 1961). Today, the concept of wellness in relation to aging is closely associated with the increasing attention to successful aging, as discussed in the section on Descriptions of Successful Aging.

If asked to define *wellness* and *aging*, most people associate wellness with peak achievement in younger adulthood, and they associate aging with declining health that eventually leads to death. Although somewhat accurate with regard to biologic aging, this description of wellness does not address well-being of the body, mind, and spirit. Similarly, many definitions of human aging focus narrowly on physical health and functioning rather than holistically—and more accurately—on humans as complex biopsychosocial–spiritual individuals. Thus, the apparent disconnect between definitions of wellness and aging results not only from misunderstandings about aging but also from a narrow focus on physical health and functioning.

Promoting wellness in older adults is an ideal; however, nurses may not believe it is achievable in practice because of barriers such as the following:

- Older adults may be pessimistic about their ability to improve their health and functioning.
- Survival needs and a multitude of health problems may take precedence over the "luxury" of being able to focus on wellness and quality of life.
- Despite the increasing emphasis on wellness and health promotion, health care environments focus more on treating diseases than on preventing illness and addressing whole-person needs.
- Often older adults and health care providers mistakenly attribute symptoms to aging rather than identify and address the contributing factors that are reversible and treatable.
- Health care providers may not believe that older adults are capable of learning and implementing health-promoting behaviors that are inherent in wellness-oriented care.

Because many of these barriers arise from myths, misperceptions, and lack of knowledge, accurate information about older adults and the relationship between aging and wellness is an indispensable tool for addressing these barriers.

WELLNESS AND NURSING CARE OF OLDER ADULTS

Nurses have many opportunities to promote wellness for older adults through actions that are integral to holistic nursing. A major focus of a "wellness approach" to older adult health care is addressing the body–mind–spirit interconnectedness of each older adult as a unique and respected individual. This requires that nurses assess each older adult in the full context of his or her personal history and current situation. Based on this holistic assessment, nurses identify realistic wellness outcomes and plan interventions directed toward improved health, functioning, and quality of life. This approach may seem challenging—or even impossible—for older adults who are seriously or terminally ill or for those who have overwhelming chronic conditions. Even when caring for someone who is seriously ill or dying, however, nurses can implement interventions directed toward improved physical comfort and psychological and spiritual growth. Some nursing actions that promote wellness for older adults are as follows:

- Addressing the body–mind–spirit interrelatedness of each older adult
- Identifying and challenging ageist attitudes (including their own), especially those that interfere with optimal health care
- Assessing each older adult from a whole-person perspective
- Incorporating wellness nursing diagnoses as a routine part of care
- Planning for wellness outcomes, which are directed toward improved health, functioning, and quality of life
- Using nursing interventions to address conditions that interfere with optimal functioning (including lack of accurate information about aging)
- Recognizing each older adult's potential for improved health and functioning as well as psychological and spiritual growth
- Teaching about self-care behaviors to improve health and functioning (or teaching caregivers of dependent older adults)
- Promoting wellness for caregivers and other people who provide care for older adults (including self-care for nurses)

McMahon and Fleury published a concept analysis of wellness related to nursing care of older adults and stated (2012, p. 49):

Wellness coexists across all functional and health statuses.... In its current state of development within geriatric nursing, wellness has the potential to provide geriatric nurses with tools to foster being well and living values among older adults by addressing their strengths and promoting growth while simultaneously addressing their changing and diverse needs.

 See **ONLINE LEARNING ACTIVITY 1-1: ARTICLE ABOUT APPLYING THE CONCEPT OF WELLNESS TO NURSING CARE OF OLDER ADULTS** at http://thepoint.lww.com/Miller8e.

DEFINITIONS OF AGING

Gerontologists and lay people define aging from many perspectives. Objectively, aging is a universal process that begins at birth; in this context, it applies equally to young and old people. Subjectively, however, aging is typically associated with being "old" or reaching "older adulthood," and people define aging in terms of personal meaning and experience. Children usually do not view themselves as aging, but they delight in announcing how old they are, and they anticipate birthdays with great enthusiasm. They view their birthdays as positive events that will permit them to enjoy additional opportunities and responsibilities. Adolescents, likewise, view aging as the mechanism that allows them to participate legally in important activities, such as driving and voting. In contrast, adults tend to view "old age" as something to be avoided and they are likely to define the onset of older adulthood as a decade beyond their current age.

The term subjective age (also referred to as *feel* age or *age identity*) describes a person's perception of his or her age. Studies of subjective age identification examine how old a person feels, how the person categorizes himself or herself in age groups, and how one sees oneself relative to one's younger self and relative to other people (Settersten & Godlewski, 2016). Nurses often observe this phenomenon when they hear people whose chronologic age is 75 years, 80 years, or older refer to "old people" as if they were a group older than and distinct from themselves. Studies show that most older adults feel significantly younger than their chronologic age and that this perception positively influences an older adult's health, functioning, and sense of well-being (Agogo, Haijat, Milne, et al., 2017; Morelock, Stokes, & Moorman, 2017).

Objectively, people define chronologic age as the length of time that has passed since birth. Society is particularly fascinated by numbers, quantities, and relative values that can be measured. Among the questions frequently asked and answered are *How much? How far? How often?* and *How old?* Our fascination with age is particularly evident in media newspaper articles, which invariably state the age of the subjects, regardless of the relevance of age to the topic. In addition to being easily measured, another advantage of chronologic age is that it serves as an objective basis for social organization. For example, societies establish chronologic age criteria for certain activities, such as education, voting, driving, marriage, employment, alcohol consumption, military service, and the collection of retirement benefits. To participate legally in these activities, people must provide documentation of a certain chronologic age.

With the passage of the 1935 Social Security Act and the 1965 amendment that created Medicare, the age of 65 years was established as the standard age criterion for eligibility for retirement and health care benefits in the United States. Although 65 years continues to be the age criterion for Medicare, the age for full retirement benefits under Social Security has been increasing slightly and gradually for people born in or after 1938. The change in age-based criteria for full Social Security retirement benefits is based on socioeconomic trends and health-related statistics, such as increased longevity and improved health status. Even this chronologic age criterion, however, varies across different government-sponsored programs, such as the Older Americans Act (OAA). For example, the qualifying age for Native Americans' participation in OAA-funded programs is 45 years in Montana, but it is 55 years in all other states.

During the 1960s, gerontologists tended to view 65 years of age as an acceptable chronologic criterion at which aging processes begin to occur. However, as information about aging evolved, gerontologists recognized that from both scientific and humanistic perspectives, one's chronologic age is relatively insignificant because there is no biologic measurement that applies to everyone at a specific age. During the 1970s, gerontologists proposed that older adults be categorized as young-old, middle-old, old-old, and oldest-old. The trend in gerontology to divide old age into chronologic subcategories is an improvement over the categorization of all people older than 65 years as one homogeneous group, but it has the disadvantage of creating additional stereotypes and age biases. A recent review of concepts related to age and aging emphasized that chronologic age itself is generally not the mechanism that underlies changes; however, it is a variable that may cause age-related differences (Settersten & Godlewski, 2016). Currently, geriatricians emphasize that decisions about preventive care and treatment of disease should consider chronologic age as only one of the many factors that affect the person's health, functioning, and quality of life.

For health care providers whose practice focuses on older adults, as well as for most older adults, the important indicators of age are physiologic health, psychological well-being, socioeconomic factors, and the ability to function and participate in desirable activities. Based on this understanding of aging, gerontologists have used the term functional age for several decades. This concept is associated with a shift in emphasis from chronologic factors to factors such as whether individuals can contribute to society and experience personal quality of life. Functional age is a concept that is used worldwide, but its definition varies according to different cultural contexts. A qualitative study of how older adults describe optimal functionality identified the following components:

- Body-related factors: health, activity, autonomy, physical ability
- Self-related factors: psychological aspects, capability aspects
- External factors: social interactions, environmental aspects

(Algilani, Ostlund-Lagerstrom, Schoultz, et al., 2016). One advantage of functional definitions of age over chronologic definitions is that the former are associated with higher levels of well-being and with more positive attitudes about aging. From a holistic perspective, the concept of functional age provides a more rational basis for care than the measurement of how many years have passed since the person was born. Thus, the question *How functional?* is more relevant than *How old?* Even more relevant for promoting wellness in older adults are questions such as the following:

- How well do you feel?
- What goals do you have for improving your level of wellness?
- Is there anything that you would like to do that you cannot do?
- What goals do you have for improving your quality of life?

In this text, the term *older adult* applies to individuals experiencing the cumulative effects of age-related changes and risk factors that affect their health and functioning. As discussed in Chapter 3, a person does not automatically reach "old age" at a particular point in time. Rather, from a holistic perspective, this conceptualization addresses all aspects of biopsychosocial–spiritual health and functioning, as discussed in the next section.

DESCRIPTIONS OF SUCCESSFUL AGING

The 1987 publication of landmark studies of the MacArthur Research Network on Successful Aging transformed the study of aging from a discipline focused on disease and decline to one emphasizing health and growth (Pruchno & Carr, 2017). In recent decades thousands of studies have been published internationally describing components of successful aging, with input from interprofessional collaboration and conversations (Rowe & Kahn, 2015). Components of successful aging that are identified in the original and recent studies include the following:

- Low probability of disease and disability
- High physical and cognitive functional capacity
- Active engagement with life (e.g., caring engagement, productive engagement, social activities, and solitary activities)
- Psychological dimensions (e.g., optimism, positive attitudes, spirituality, religiosity, self-efficacy)

(Carver & Buchanan, 2016; Huijg, van Delden, van der Ouderaa, et al., 2017; Mejia, Ryan, Gonzalez, et al., 2017).

Two emerging foci of successful aging models are resilience and cultural inclusiveness. Resilience as an aspect of successful aging focuses on the ability of older adults to adapt to challenges and find meaning and productivity when experiencing chronic conditions or disablement (Freedman, Kasper, & Spillman, 2017; Kail & Carr, 2017; Tkatch, Musich, MacLeod, et al., 2017). For example, when an older adult experiences a transition to frailty, theories related to caring and nursing suggest that successful aging can encompass a joint endeavor of the care receiver and the care

provider striving to maintain self-determination and quality of life for the older adult with care needs (Tesch-Romer & Wahl, 2017). Focus groups of middle-aged and older adults growing older with a physical disability identified the following key components of successful aging: resilience and adaptation, autonomy, social connectedness, maintenance of current physical health, and access to appropriate health care (Molton & Yorkston, 2017). An example of an inclusive model of successful aging is a focus on the interrelationship between wellness, empowerment, and engagement, and the importance of family, community, and environment (Pace & Grenier, 2017).

Gerontologists have applied the concept of successful aging to people who have overcome disabilities and disease to achieve success during later adulthood, as illustrated by the following examples of well-known people:

- Grandma Moses (Anna Maria Robertson) became a famous painter after arthritis interfered with her ability to make quilts.
- Monet developed the painting technique known as modern impressionism after his eyesight was clouded by cataracts.
- Renoir painted with a clenched fist after he developed arthritis.
- Pablo Casals played his cello each day in his 90s.
- Maurice Ravel composed the famous *Bolero* after he was affected with dementia.

(Morley, 2009).

GLOBAL PERSPECTIVE

Conceptualizations of successful aging in non-Western cultures may include an additional component related to strong family support in older age (Feng & Straughan, 2017).

A Student's Perspective

I personally have aging anxiety. After working at an assisted living facility for the past year and a half, I have seen some pretty tragic and depressing events happen in the lives of these residents. Many of these residents tell me they do not know why God has kept them around this long. But listening to the stories of others has given me hope. I found it very encouraging to see the elderly people taking classes and enjoying the discussions they were a part of. I would imagine that it would be tempting to give up when the mental or physical functioning is not what it used to be, but some of the people gave me hope for aging. They make me want to be a stronger person even now at the age of 19 years. They seem to have so much passion and intensity to their lives. Not only can they serve to encourage people in their younger years to continually embrace life, but I hope other elderly people can be encouraged that they do not have to let go of their dreams just because they are aging. You can age successfully as these people have by living life to its fullest and persevering to keep your individuality and talents alive.

Jessica S.

ATTITUDES TOWARD AGING

Images of and attitudes toward aging arise from long-term patterns of falsely attributing pathologic conditions and undesirable characteristics to normal aging. In reality, most older adults function independently and report high levels of satisfaction with their health and quality of life, even with their high prevalence of chronic conditions. Historically, societal attitudes toward aging have ranged from respect and veneration to fear of aging and idealization of youth. As indicated in Figure 1-1, the pendulum is slowly swinging again toward positive attitudes toward aging and older adulthood. This shift is attributable to the increasing emphasis on successful aging and the emergence of accurate information about the difference between aging and disease. Despite this focus on successful aging, however, health care professionals are likely to be influenced by long-standing negative attitudes toward aging that are embedded in society. Thus, an important part of gerontological nursing is to recognize the effects of ageism and address attitudes that can interfere with holistic care of older adults.

Age Stereotypes

Age stereotypes exist in all cultures with varying degrees of negative attributes (e.g., decreased attractiveness, limited functional ability, and diminished ability to learn new things) and positive attributes (e.g., increased levels of wisdom, knowledge, and respect). Age stereotypes differ across cultural groups; however, studies indicate that most cultures view aging in a negative light (Meisner & Levy, 2016). A potentially positive outcome of the increasing cultural diversity in the United States is that the more positive views of aging held by some cultural groups may influence the dominant negative societal views. Box 1-1 identifies cultural perspectives on elders and family caregiving relationships.

 GLOBAL PERSPECTIVE

Analysis of cross-cultural studies has found the strongest negative age stereotypes in Argentina, Czech Republic, Serbia, and the United Kingdom. Countries with more neutral or positive age stereotypes included India, Mainland China, Malaysia, New Zealand, and Russia (Meisner & Levy, 2016).

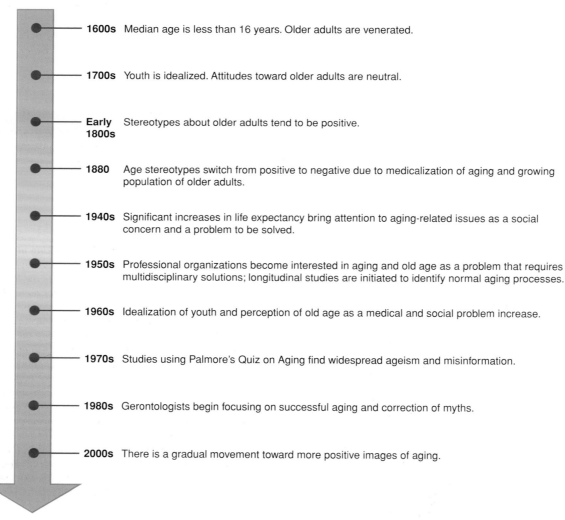

1600s   Median age is less than 16 years. Older adults are venerated.

1700s   Youth is idealized. Attitudes toward older adults are neutral.

Early 1800s   Stereotypes about older adults tend to be positive.

1880   Age stereotypes switch from positive to negative due to medicalization of aging and growing population of older adults.

1940s   Significant increases in life expectancy bring attention to aging-related issues as a social concern and a problem to be solved.

1950s   Professional organizations become interested in aging and old age as a problem that requires multidisciplinary solutions; longitudinal studies are initiated to identify normal aging processes.

1960s   Idealization of youth and perception of old age as a medical and social problem increase.

1970s   Studies using Palmore's Quiz on Aging find widespread ageism and misinformation.

1980s   Gerontologists begin focusing on successful aging and correction of myths.

2000s   There is a gradual movement toward more positive images of aging.

FIGURE 1-1 Historic trends in views on aging in the United States.

Box 1-1 Cultural Considerations: Cultural Perspectives on Elders and Family Caregiving Relationships

African Americans

- Elders are a source of wisdom and deserve respect.
- Grandparents are often involved with caring for grandchildren and may live in the same household.

American Indians/Alaskan Natives

- Elder status is characterized by health status and roles as counselors, teachers, or grandparents.
- Grandparents often care for grandchildren, who then are expected to care for the elders; grandmother may be called mother.

Chinese

- Traditional Chinese values place family and society above the individual.
- Elders are highly respected and honored.
- Multigenerational households are common.

Filipinos

- Respect for elders is a cornerstone of Filipino values, demonstrated by deference in verbal and nonverbal communication.
- Children (especially the oldest daughter) are expected to care for parents to repay their debt of gratitude (utang na loob).

Germans

- Close intergenerational relationships are maintained by first- and second-generation German Americans, but family mobility may affect this.
- Children are expected to help their parents stay in their own homes as long as possible.
- Because Amish and German Baptists view family relationships as reciprocal throughout life, grandparents usually live with their children or move from child to child.

Greek

- Elderly women have higher status and more power within the family than younger women do and are expected to live with or near adult children, especially daughters.

Haitians

- Elders assume roles as family advisers, babysitters, historians, and consultants.
- Children are expected to care for elders at home.

Japanese

- Elders are highly respected and those who are able, help in caring for children and grandchildren.
- Elders commonly maintain separate households; when they need help, the eldest son's family is expected to care for them at home.

Koreans

- Caring for elderly kin is a family duty that is associated with respect for elders and family bonds inherent in Confucianism.
- Grandparents frequently provide care for grandchildren; elders are welcome to live with family during times of need.

Mexican Americans

- Elders are revered, but acculturation reduces the sense of obligation to provide care.
- *Marianismo* (i.e., the traditional role of women in the Mexican family) is a cultural value that socializes women to the role of caregiving beginning in early childhood.

Puerto Ricans

- *La abuela(o)* (elder or grandparent) is a Figure of respect, wisdom, and admiration.
- Both men and women care for elders and share caregiving responsibilities with family members and a close family network.

Russians

- Elders are highly respected and remain close to their children.
- Even if elders do not live with their children, they are expected help raise grandchildren and participate in decision making.

Vietnamese

- The more one respects the elderly, the greater one's chance is of reaching old age.
- Young adults are expected to assume full responsibility for caring for elders at home.

Source: Lipson, J. G., & Dibble, L. (2005). *Culture and clinical care*. San Francisco: UCSF Nursing Press.

Ageism

Robert Butler coined the term *ageism* in 1968, and with the publication of his Pulitzer Prize-winning book *Why Survive? Being Old in America* (Butler, 1975), the term became an accepted new word in the English language. **Ageism** is "the prejudices and stereotypes that are applied to older people sheerly on the basis of their age.... Ageism, like racism and sexism, is a way of pigeonholing people and not allowing them to be individuals with unique ways of living their lives" (Butler, Lewis, & Sunderland, 1991, p. 243). Common manifestations of ageism include negative stereotypes of older adults as frail, vulnerable, asexual, stubborn, socially isolated, and burdensome to families and society. The Ageism Survey (Figure 1-2) has consistently

found that older adults experience numerous instances of ageism.

Ageism is similar to racism, sexism, and heterosexism in that it leads to bigotry and discrimination. However, it is unique in that it is a fluid social construct, and everyone who lives long enough eventually becomes a member of this "out-group" and is vulnerable to ageism (Palmore, 2015; Sargent-Cox, 2017). Also in contrast to other forms of discrimination, ageism is pervasive, socially condoned, strongly institutionalized, often undetected or unnoticed, and largely unchallenged (Gendron, Welleford, Inker, et al., 2016; Nelson, 2016; Officer, Schneiders, Wu, et al., 2016). In North America, ageism has developed and grown as a result of dominant cultural beliefs and trends, such

---

The Ageism Survey

Please put a number in the blank that shows how often you have experienced that event: Never = 0; Once = 1; More than once = 2.
("Age" means older age.)

_____ 1. I was told a joke that pokes fun at old people.

_____ 2. I was sent a birthday card that pokes fun at old people.

_____ 3. I was ignored or not taken seriously because of my age.

_____ 4. I was called an insulting name related to my age.

_____ 5. I was patronized or "talked down to" because of my age.

_____ 6. I was refused rental housing because of my age.

_____ 7. I had difficulty getting a loan because of my age.

_____ 8. I was denied a position of leadership because of my age.

_____ 9. I was rejected as unattractive because of my age.

_____ 10. I was treated with less dignity and respect because of my age.

_____ 11. A waiter or waitress ignored me because of my age.

_____ 12. A doctor or nurse assumed my ailments were caused by my age.

_____ 13. I was denied medical treatment because of my age.

_____ 14. I was denied employment because of my age.

_____ 15. I was denied promotion because of my age.

_____ 16. Someone assumed I could not hear well because of my age.

_____ 17. Someone assumed I could not understand because of my age.

_____ 18. Someone told me, " You're too old for that."

_____ 19. My house was vandalized because of my age.

_____ 20. I was victimized by a criminal because of my age.

Please write in your age: _____

Please check: Male _____ Female _____

What is the highest grade in school that you completed? _____

Survey © Copyright 2000 by Erdman Palmore.

FIGURE 1-2 The Ageism Survey is being used to measure the prevalence and identify types of ageism. (Used with permission from Palmore, E. (2000). *The ageism survey*. Durham, NC: Duke Center for the Study of Aging.)

---

as the glorification of youth, the valuing of independence over interdependence, and the equating of human worth with economic worth. For example, although addressing an older woman as "young lady" may be well intentioned, this ageist viewpoint perpetuates the notion that being young is better than being old (Gendron, Welleford, Inker, et al., 2016).

Effects of Ageism and Age Stereotypes

Gerontologists are currently focusing on the effects of ageism and age stereotypes on the health of older adults, with increasing concern about the detrimental effects of negative age stereotypes (Meisner & Levy, 2016; Phibbs & Hooker, 2017). Increasingly, gerontologists are discussing the negative effects of ageism and negative age stereotypes as a serious threat and chronic stressor for older adults that "warrants greater recognition, social condemnation, and scientific study as a possible social determinant of chronic disease" (Allen, 2016, p. 610; Scheidt, 2017).

In recent years, gerontologists have identified some of the specific effects of ageism and negative age stereotypes on older adults, including the following:

- Poor health outcomes
- Increased cardiovascular stress
- Poorer performance on cognitive performance tests
- Increased risk for depression and anxiety
- Competition between generations for limited public resources related to health, housing, and social welfare
- Discrimination in employment opportunities
- Increased mortality

(Fernandez-Ballesteros, Olmos, Santacreu, et al., 2017; Freeman, Santini, Tyrovolas, et al., 2016; Jopp, Jung, Damarin, et al., 2017). By contrast, studies consistently link more positive views on aging with improved physical functioning and self-rated health (Hicks & Siedlecki, 2017).

Another outcome of ageism is aging anxiety, which is defined as fears and excess concern about detrimental effects associated with older adulthood (e.g., social losses, financial insecurity, changes in appearance, and declines in health and functioning). Aging anxiety can occur in people of any age and is reinforced by negative stereotypes of older adults and the associated fear that these problems are likely to occur in one's own later life. Aging anxiety is more common among women than men and is associated with poor health, social relationships, and societal perceptions of female physical attractiveness (Barrett & Toothman, 2017).

A concept that is closely related to ageism and age stereotypes is age attribution, which is the tendency to attribute problems to the aging process rather than to pathologic and potentially treatable conditions. For example, the phrase *senior moment* has been used since the mid-1990s to describe a lapse in memory. When older adults or health care professionals falsely attribute symptoms of pathologic conditions to normal aging, they are likely to overlook treatable conditions, and significant harm can result from this negligence. An important responsibility of gerontological nurses is to be knowledgeable about the differences between age-related changes and pathologic conditions, so appropriate nursing interventions can be initiated. An essential first step in planning interventions, especially health promotion interventions, is to identify those factors that are not inherent consequences of aging. Throughout this text, emphasis is placed on differentiating between age-related changes, which cannot be modified, and those factors that can be addressed through interventions. Chapter 3 describes a nursing model for this approach to promoting wellness for older adults.

Another consequence of ageism is the emergence of the anti-aging movement, which has been promoted by the American Academy of Anti-Aging Medicine since the early 1990s. This movement views aging as an enemy to be conquered and a process that can be reversed so the life span can be extended. Anti-aging interventions include lifestyle modifications, but there also is much emphasis on dietary supplements and other products that have not been proved effective. Mainstream gerontologists view the anti-aging movement as an enterprise that is directed more toward selling products than toward the advancement of sound scientific evidence (Samuel, 2017).

Roles of Nurses in Addressing Ageism and Age Stereotypes

Negative attitudes about aging that are held by health care workers can negatively affect the care older adults receive. Nurses and all health care workers are likely to be influenced not only by ageism and negative age stereotypes in society but also by their own experiences in health care, which often are with those older adults who are the most impaired and in need of interventions. It is important, therefore, that health care workers in all clinical settings recognize that most older adults are healthy and functional and strive toward improved levels of wellness and functioning.

Attitudes are changed through education, but changing attitudes requires first recognizing their existence. Because ageism is subtle but pervasive in American society, nurses first need to become aware of the attitudes they hold toward older adults. The first critical thinking exercise at the end of this chapter suggests ways of becoming aware of one's own attitudes about older adults. Another way of improving negative age stereotypes is to ask older adults about their beliefs, values, hopes, and experiences that contribute to their self-identities (Levy, 2016). Nurses have daily opportunities to learn about aging and older adulthood simply by listening to the older adults for whom they provide care. In addition, nurses can equip themselves with accurate information about the older adult population. Accurate information may be the most effective antidote to negative attitudes resulting from misunderstandings or myths (Cherry, Brigman, Lyon, et al., 2016). The next sections address myths about aging by providing an accurate snapshot of older adults in the United States.

A Student's Perspective

My interview with Mr. H. was an enlightening experience. I was able to learn a great deal about the time period in which this man grew up. Also, it was eye-opening to see how healthy a man of 84 years could be. His health reinforced what we are learning. He does have a chronic illness, diabetes (like 80% of those aged 65+), but he still is independent and free of any noticeable cognitive impairments. He can still drive and get around, which also defeats a lot of ageist attitudes. Negative attitudes that I have heard about elders were defeated by this man. Reading about aging in a book is one thing, but actually interacting with elders and learning first hand are much more influential. Mr. H. really taught me not to hold ageist attitudes.

Jordan S.

DEBUNKING MYTHS: UNDERSTANDING REALITIES ABOUT OLDER ADULTS IN THE UNITED STATES

As a consequence of ageism and negative attitudes about aging, many myths and negative stereotypes about older adults have been perpetuated, especially with regard to aspects of health and functioning. These myths and stereotypes can be particularly detrimental when health care providers lack accurate information on which to base their decisions or actions about older adults because misconceptions lead to suboptimal goals for care. At best, older adults do not experience the benefits of wellness-focused care; at worst, they experience unnecessary decline. A leading gerontologist stated that "Innovative ways to effectively negate or reduce the damaging effects on health brought about by negative age stereotypes must be discovered, while simultaneously finding ways to support the health-promoting properties of positive age stereotypes" (Meisner & Levy, 2016, p. 271).

This chapter provides information about characteristics of the older adult population, and Chapter 2 extends this overview by addressing cultural diversity of older adults. Chapters in Parts 3 and 4 of this text address aspects of functioning that can be significantly affected by myths and misunderstandings about aging. Table 1-1 lists some of the myths and misperceptions about aging that are commonly held by older adults and health care professionals. The related realities about each aspect of health and functioning also are identified, along with a reference to the chapter that provides accurate information to dispel the myths.

The characteristics of the older adult population in the United States summarized in this chapter are based on census data and other reliable sources; however, this information can only reflect trends and grouped data. The intent is to provide an overview of population demographics and characteristics of older adults that are most pertinent to holistically caring for older adults. Nurses need to keep in

TABLE 1-1 Myths and Realities of Aging

Myth	Reality
Older adulthood is something to be dreaded because it represents disability and death.	Most older adults live independently, have high levels of self-reported health, and are aging successfully (*Chapter 1*).
People consider themselves "old" on their 65th birthday.	People usually feel old based on their health and function, rather than on their chronologic age (*Chapter 1*).
Gerontologists have discovered that, by the age of 75 years, people are quite homogeneous as a group.	The more gerontologists learn about aging, the more they realize that, with increased age, people become more diverse and individuals become less like their age peers (*Chapters 1, 2, and 4*).
Ageism is a natural part of all societies.	Ageism is more common in industrialized societies and is highly influenced by stereotypes and cultural values (*Chapter 1*).
Gerontologists have recently discovered a theory that explains biologic aging.	Theories about biologic aging continue to evolve, and there is little agreement on any one theory (*Chapter 4*).
In today's society, families no longer care for older people.	In the United States, 80% of the care of older adults is provided by their families (*Chapter 1*).
As people grow older, it is natural for them to want to withdraw from society.	Because older people are unique individuals, each of them responds differently to society (*Chapter 4*).
By the age of 70 years, an individual's psychological growth is complete.	People never lose their capacity for psychological growth (*Chapters 4 and 12*).
Increased disability in older people is attributable to age-related changes alone.	Although age-related changes increase one's vulnerability to functional impairments, the disabilities are attributable to risk factors, such as diseases and adverse medication effects (*Chapter 3*).
Health promotion efforts are not beneficial to older adults who have two or more chronic conditions.	Research has debunked the myths that prevention is not effective after onset of chronic illness (*Chapter 5*).
About 20% of people aged 65 years and older live in nursing homes as long-term residents.	Between 4% and 5% of older adults live in a nursing home at any time (*Chapters 1 and 6*).
Widowhood and other life events have been found to have a consistently negative impact on older people.	No one life event affects all older people negatively. The most important consideration governing the impact of an event is its unique meaning for the individual (*Chapter 12*).
In old age, there is an inevitable decline in all intellectual abilities.	A few areas of cognitive ability decline in healthy older adults but other areas show improvement (*Chapter 11*).
Older adults cannot learn complex new skills.	Older adults are capable of learning new things, but the speed with which they process information slows down with age (*Chapter 11*).
Constipation develops primarily because of age-related changes.	Constipation is attributable primarily to risk factors, such as restricted activity and poor dietary habits (*Chapter 18*).
Urinary incontinence is a normal consequence of aging that is best managed by using incontinence products.	In most cases, underlying causes of urinary incontinence can be addressed and a variety of self-care methods can be initiated (*Chapter 19*).
Skin wrinkles can be prevented by using oils and lotions.	The best way to prevent skin wrinkles is to avoid exposure to ultraviolet light (*Chapter 23*).
Older people are less sexually active primarily because they lose the ability to enjoy sex.	Declines in sexual activity in older people are primarily because of risk factors, such as diseases, adverse medication effects, and loss of partner (*Chapter 26*).
Health care professionals readily recognize adverse medication effects in older adults.	Adverse medication effects are often overlooked in older adults because they are mistakenly attributed to aging or pathologic conditions (*Chapter 8*).
Some degree of "senility" is normal in very old people.	"Senility" is an inaccurate term used to refer to dementing conditions, which are always caused by pathologic changes (*Chapter 14*).
Most old people are depressed and should be allowed to withdraw from society.	About one-third of older people exhibit depressive symptoms; however, depression is a very treatable condition at any age (*Chapter 15*).

mind that older adults are a highly diverse group and this general information does not necessarily apply to every older individual.

Demographics of Aging

Discussions of current demographic trends in the United States inevitably focus on the so-called baby boomers, which is the very large group of people born between 1946 and 1964. Although baby boomers were all born during one 18-year period, this period was characterized by dramatic changes in socioeconomic and political trends. As with other socially labeled groups, the baby boomer generation is extremely heterogeneous, and each person in this group has a unique life story. The influence of this and other population trends, such as greater cultural diversity (see Chapter 2) and increased life expectancy (see Chapter 4), is reflected in the statistics summarized in Box 1-2 and Figure 1-3.

Health Characteristics

A major focus of health characteristics of older adults is on chronic conditions and levels of functioning. During the past few decades, the prevalence of disability among older adults has been gradually decreasing, and the majority of older adults report good to excellent health, as illustrated in Figure 1-4. At the same time, many older adults live with chronic health conditions, as illustrated in Figure 1-5. Thus, a major

Box 1-2 Stats in Brief: Changing Demographics of Aging in the United States	
Median Age	
● 1900	23 years
● 2000	35 years
● 2035	39 years
Average Life Expectancy at Age 65 Years	
● 1900	11.9 years
● 1960	14.4 years
● 2007	18.6 years
● 2014	19.3 years
Actual and Projected Percentage of People Aged 65+ Years	
● 1900	4.1%
● 2010	12.8%
● 2050	20.6%
Actual and Estimated Number and Percentage of People Aged 85+ Years	
● 1900	100,000 (0.2%)
● 2006	5.3 million (1.8%)
● 2050	21 million (5%)
Approximate or Estimated Number of Centenarians	
● 1990	37,300
● 2009	104,000
● 2050	1.5 million

Source: U.S. Census Bureau, American Fact Finder (2010); Health United States, 2015. Available at www.census.gov

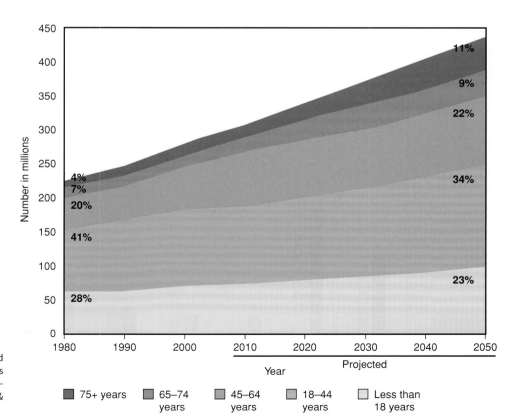

FIGURE 1-3 Actual and projected total population of the United States by age, 1980–2050. (*Source:* U.S. Census Bureau, Population Estimates & Projections.)

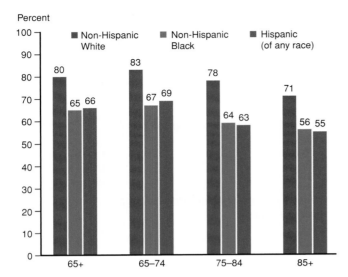

Note: Data are based on a 3-year average from 2012 to 2014. See data sources for the definition of race and Hispanic origin in the National Health Interview Survey.
Reference population: These data refer to the civilian noninstitutionalized population.

FIGURE 1-4 Percentage of people aged 65+ years reporting good to excellent health, by age, race, and Hispanic origin, 2012–2014. (Adapted from Federal Interagency Forum on Aging-Related Statistics, *Older Americans 2016,* at http://www.agingstats.gov.)

focus of health care is on interventions to prevent and manage chronic diseases so older adults can maintain optimal levels of functioning, as discussed in detail in Chapters 5 and 6. In recent years, increasing attention has been paid to the negative consequences of health disparities among groups of older blacks and other minorities, as discussed in more detail in Chapter 2 (see Chapter 4 for more information on life expectancy and race).

Socioeconomic Characteristics

Socioeconomic characteristics that are most strongly correlated with healthy aging are poverty and lower educational level. Although census data predict gradual and continuing increases in level of education for older adults—with associated better health and higher incomes—many older adults will remain socioeconomically disadvantaged. Limited English proficiency and poor health literacy skills are two variables that are common among older adults and have a negative impact on health and functioning, as discussed in Chapter 2. Figure 1-6 illustrates educational levels of older adults by race and Hispanic origin.

In recent decades, the overall poverty rate for older adults has been declining, but this does not mean that all older people are economically better off today than they were 40 years ago. For example, economic conditions of older adults vary considerably as indicated by the following information from the Federal Interagency Forum on Aging (2016):

● Older women are more likely to live in poverty than older men (12% for women vs. 7% for men).
● Older adults over age 75 were more likely to live in poverty than those aged 65 to 74 years (12% vs. 9%).
● Rates of poverty for older men vary by race and Hispanic origin: white, 5%; Asian, 13%; black, 17%; Hispanic, 16%.
● Rates of poverty for older women vary by race and Hispanic origin: white, 10%; Asian, 16%; black, 21%; Hispanic, 20%.

Marital status affects other aspects of older adults' lives in many ways, including economic resources, living arrangements, and availability of a caregiver for those who are dependent. Marital status varies significantly by sex and age, as illustrated in Figure 1-7.

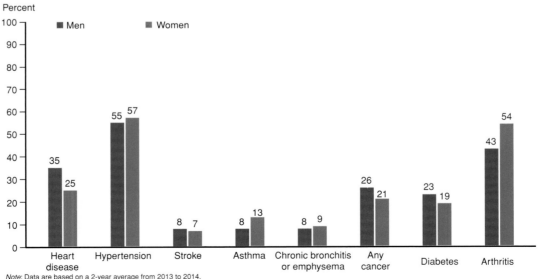

Note: Data are based on a 2-year average from 2013 to 2014.
Reference population: These data refer to the civilian noninstitutionalized population.

FIGURE 1-5 Percentage of people aged 65 years and over who reported having selected chronic health conditions, by sex, 2013–2014. (Adapted from Federal Interagency Forum on Aging-Related Statistics, *Older Americans 2016,* at http://www.agingstats.gov.)

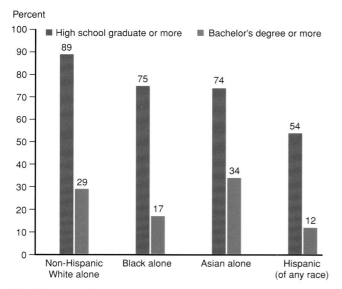

Note: The term "non-Hispanic White alone" is used to refer to people who reported being White and no other race and who are not Hispanic. The term "Black alone" is used to refer to people who reported being Black or African American and no other race, and the term "Asian alone" is used to refer to people who reported only Asian as their race. The use of single-race populations in this report does not imply that this is the preferred method of presenting or analyzing data. The U.S. Census Bureau uses a variety of approaches. Reference population: These data refer to the civilian noninstitutionalized population.

FIGURE 1-6 Educational levels of older adults, by race and Hispanic origin, 2015. (Adapted from Federal Interagency Forum on Aging-Related Statistics, *Older Americans 2016,* at http://www.agingstats.gov.)

Living Arrangements of Older Adults

Living arrangements for older adults are influenced by factors such as health, marital status, family relationships, and socioeconomic conditions, as indicated in the following statistics from the Federal Interagency Forum on Aging-Related Statistics (2016):

- Older women were more than twice as likely as men to live alone (37% vs. 20%).
- Older black and non-Hispanic white women were more likely than women of other races to live alone.
- Older black men were more likely than men of other races to live alone.
- Older black, Asian, and Hispanic women were more likely than non-Hispanic white women to live with relatives other than a spouse.
- Older Hispanic men were more likely than men of other races to live with relatives other than a spouse.

Figure 1-8 provides additional details about living arrangements of older adults by sex, race, and Hispanic origin.

The statistic that is most relevant for nurses is that overall, about 93% of the older adult population lives in independent housing settings in the community, with the remaining 7% about equally divided between nursing facilities and settings that provide some assistance with daily needs (e.g., assisted living) (Federal Interagency Forum on Aging-Related Statistics, 2016). Many older adults who live in independent settings receive significant levels of assistance from family members as discussed in the following sections on caregiving. Many also receive significant levels of support from the broad range of community-based services and agencies that increasingly are available (discussed in Chapter 6).

Older adults also have an increasingly wide range of housing options that address the needs of the growing number of older adults who require daily assistance but not full-time care. For example, assisted living residences are now

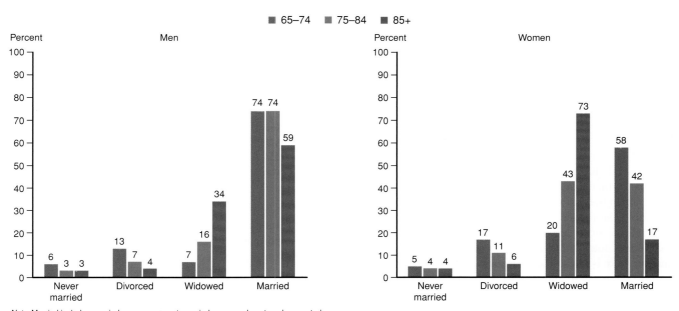

Note: Married includes married, spouse present; married, spouse absent; and separated.
Reference population: These data refer to the civilian noninstitionalized population.

FIGURE 1-7 Marital status of adults 65+ years, by sex and age groups, 2015. (Adapted from Federal Interagency Forum on Aging-Related Statistics, *Older Americans 2016,* at http://www.agingstats.gov.)

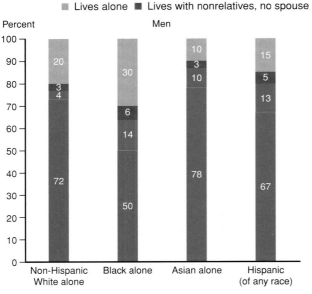
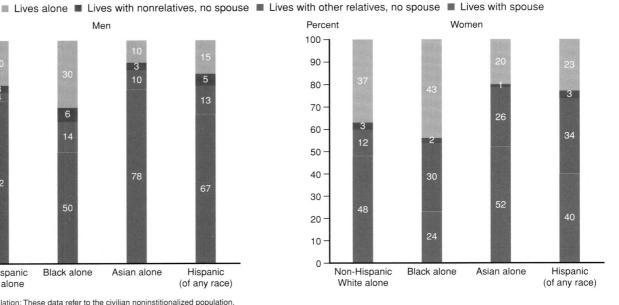

Reference population: These data refer to the civilian noninstitionalized population.

FIGURE 1-8 Living arrangements of noninstitutionalized people aged 65+ years, by sex and race and Hispanic origin, 2015. (Adapted from Federal Interagency Forum on Aging-Related Statistics, *Older Americans 2016*, at http://www.agingstats.gov.)

available in most areas of the country. Although the services provided by these facilities vary widely, basic services generally include a single residential unit, at least one daily meal, and 24-hour availability of assistance. People who live in assisted living facilities usually need help with three or more daily activities and these services are provided either as part of the care agreement or through other arrangements.

Because the range of housing options and community-based services is rapidly increasing, decisions about staying in one's own home or moving to another type of living facility are becoming more complex. Although terms, such as continuing care and aging in place, have been widely used in recent decades, definitions vary significantly. For example, some aging-in-place or continuing care programs require that residents move to a new location within a larger group of facilities when their needs change. Because these moves require that older adults adjust to new staff and a different environment, they can be as disruptive as a move that is not defined as continuing care.

Although nurses may not be familiar with all the housing options in their communities, at a minimum, they need to know about the various types of facilities that are commonly available. Moreover, nurses are responsible for suggesting referrals to social service agencies and offices on aging so that older adults and their families can find additional information. Box 1-3 describes various housing options for older adults that are available in most parts of the United States.

Assisted Living Facilities

Assisted living facilities and continuing care retirement communities vary widely in the types and amounts of services

provided. Although assisted living facilities developed during the 1980s as settings for independent living, the focus has gradually shifted toward addressing the needs of older adults with complex medical needs. Because of this trend, some assisted living facilities are integrally associated with and physically connected to nursing homes and provide a high level of care for residents who no longer meet qualifications for Medicare-covered services. Another recent development is that some assisted living facilities provide specialized dementia care, as discussed in Chapter 6. End-of-life care is another issue being addressed in assisted living facilities because residents express the desire to die at home. Because of this, many assisted living facilities are now working closely with hospice organizations to provide end-of-life care.

 See ONLINE LEARNING ACTIVITY 1-2: ADDITIONAL INFORMATION ABOUT OLDER ADULTS IN THE UNITED STATES at http://thepoint.lww.com/Miller7e.

Older Adults as Givers and Recipients of Care

Major demographic trends in the United States have brought about important changes in many aspects of family and societal relationships in recent decades. Trends toward improved health and increased longevity for older adults have occurred in parallel with trends toward increased diversity of family constellations among all generations. Concurrent with these trends, the prevalence of dementia and other chronic conditions that lead to functional decline has led to increased demands for family caregiving. On the other side of the coin,

---

Box 1-3 Housing Options for Older Adults

Homecare Suite or **In-Law Suite:** A fully functional and accessible modular apartment built as an addition, remodeled in basements, or installed in attached garages.

Shared Housing: A house or apartment shared by two or more unrelated people, with each occupant having a private or semi-private bedroom. Occupants share expenses and responsibilities, and offices on aging may provide services and coordinate these programs.

Retirement Community: A specially designed residential development occupied by self-sufficient older adults. Recreational programs and support services are usually available.

Cohousing Communities: A residential development of 15 to 25 individually owned houses and commonly owned land and buildings designed to encourage community interaction. These communities typically emphasize individual privacy, resident involvement in planning, and collaborative community management. Intergenerational cohousing communities began in the United States in the 1990s, and in recent years, some communities have been developed for adults older than 50 or 55 years as senior cohousing communities.

The Village: An organized approach, governed by a nonprofit agency, to coordinating and delivering services within a neighborhood to older adults who live in their own homes. These organizations are funded through annual membership fees, and services are provided by volunteers or formal service providers at prenegotiated rates.

Life Care or **Continuing Care Retirement Community:** A residential complex designed to provide a wide range of services and accommodations to meet each resident's needs as they change. The development includes independent housing, congregate housing, assisted living, and nursing home care.

Congregate Housing: Individual apartments within a specially designed, multiunit dwelling. Supportive services typically include meals, laundry, housekeeping, limited transportation, and social and recreational activities.

Foster Care or **Board-and-Care Home:** A privately owned group home or small facility, which usually is licensed and regulated by a state agency. Each resident has a private or shared bedroom and use of common space. Services typically include the same ones as in congregate housing, plus assistance with daily care and some type of 24-hour emergency services. Public funding is available for older adults who meet income and health criteria.

Assisted Living Facility: A residential facility with individual apartments, which typically consist of one to three rooms and a bathroom, and shared space for meals and social activities. Services, licensing, regulation, and funding are similar to those described for foster care homes.

---

societal changes have led to increased demands for grandparents to assume roles of caregiving for dependent younger generations. This section discusses implications of these shifting demographics in relation to older adults as both receivers and givers of care.

Family Caregiver

A rapidly increasing population of adults aged 80 and older (i.e., the group most likely to be physically or cognitively impaired) has led to an increasing need for family members to provide many types of assistance. The term **family caregiver** (also referred to as informal caregiver) includes all those support people who have a helping relationship with an older adult, regardless of the nature of the relationship (e.g., spousal, kinship, friendship, partnership).

Since the preindustrial period, nuclear family living arrangements have been predominant in Western Europe and the United States. Typically, younger family members establish separate households after marriage, and older family members attempt to maintain independent households for as long as possible. For much of American history, the "ideal" relationship between older and younger generations in families has been to be far enough away to preserve independent lifestyles but close enough for social support and emotional connectedness. Moreover, this kind of family relationship provides for meeting occasional caregiving needs of family members while allowing for the maintenance of differing lifestyles for both younger and older generations. These family relationships are based on the principle of reciprocity across generations, characterized by mutual assistance and extensive exchanges among kin.

In recent years, increased rates of divorce and remarriage among younger generations have resulted in the proliferation of varieties of blended families across several generations. In addition, increased rates of remarriage among older adults who are widowed or divorced have led to increasing numbers of later-life blended families. One consequence of these trends is that family dynamics can become quite complex, particularly when adult stepchildren assume new roles as caregivers or decision makers for dependent older adults. For example, adult children may share caregiving and decision-making responsibilities regarding their impaired parent with a parent's spouse whom they hardly know. Similarly, adult children may assist their parent with caregiving or decision making about a stepparent whom they are just getting to know. In addition, concerns among members of blended families regarding assets and financial resources often complicate decisions about caregiving responsibilities and plans for care.

Expectations and attitudes about caregiving practices also have changed due to societal trends that affect relationships between older adults and their families. In the early 1900s, for example, the tradition of deep involvement in generational assistance, reinforced by strong family and ethnic values, was dominant in American culture. By the mid-1960s, trends were shifting toward individualistic values and lifestyles, due in part to the proliferation of public support and services for older Americans. Another major influence has been the increasing numbers of women who have careers independent of their roles in families, which can lead to conflict between the younger generation of adult children and older family members who expect care.

Spousal and filial responsibilities are traditions that have directed family caregiving in the United States for centuries, and this continues even though the specific dynamics of the care are changing. A national study found that the percentage of caregiving hours provided by informal caregivers was as follows:

- Daughters: 31%
- Spouses: 31%
- Sons: 18%

- Other relatives: 16%
- Nonrelatives: 4%

(Federal Interagency Forum on Aging-Related Statistics, 2016).

Grandparents Raising Grandchildren

A phenomenon that gerontologists, the federal government, and many national organizations (e.g., AARP) are currently

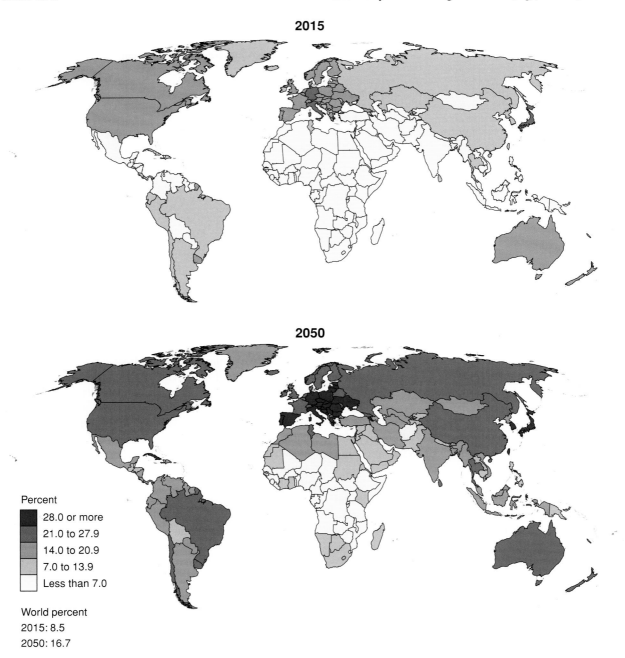

2015

2050

Percent

■	28.0 or more
■	21.0 to 27.9
■	14.0 to 20.9
■	7.0 to 13.9
□	Less than 7.0

World percent
2015: 8.5
2050: 16.7

Sources: U.S. Census Bureau, 2013, 2014; International Data Base, U.S. population projections.

FIGURE 1-9 Percentage of population aged 65 and over: 2015 and 2050. (Adapted from U. S. Census Bureau International Population Reports (2016). *An Aging World: 2015*. Washington, DC: U. S. Government Publishing Office.)

addressing is the dramatic increase in the number of children younger than 18 years living in households maintained by a custodial grandparent with no parent present. These households are referred to as **grandfamilies** (also called *skipped-generation households).* Households in which children are being raised by both their parents and grandparents are called three-generation, shared-care households. Although the overall percentage of older adults and children in these situations is small, the number has been increasing rapidly and significantly in recent decades, particularly among ethnic minority groups in the United States (Choi, Sprang, & Eslinger, 2016). Common reasons for grandparent custody include child abuse; teen pregnancy; parental abuse of drugs or alcohol; and death, disability, mental illness, or incarceration of adult parents. Rewards of grandparent caregiving include role enhancement, sense of purpose in life, motivation to keep physically active, close relationships with younger generations, and satisfaction with maintaining family well-being. Negative consequences include significant stresses, role overload, social isolation, detrimental effects on health, and increased likelihood of being poor.

OLDER ADULTS IN THE WORLD

This chapter has presented characteristics of older adults in the United States that are pertinent to gerontological nursing, but it would be incomplete without a brief perspective on global aspects of aging because the world's population is now aging at an unprecedented rate. The combination of declines in fertility rates and improvements in health and life expectancy that occurred during the 20th century is resulting in significant increases in the number and proportion of older adults in most parts of the world. The World Health Organization estimates that between 2015 and 2050 the proportion of the world's population over 60 years will nearly double from 12% to 22% (World Health Organization, 2015). Figure 1-9 illustrates the percentage of populations aged 65 and over in 2015 and 2050.

Chapter Highlights

The Relationship Between Wellness and Aging

- Since the late 1960s, health care professionals have recognized the importance of incorporating wellness goals in their care of older adults; however, there are many conceptual and practical barriers.
- Barriers to promoting wellness in older adults include older adults' negative attitudes about being able to improve, the existence of more serious or pressing health concerns, the focus of health care environments on disease treatment rather than prevention or health promotion, the false attribution of symptoms of pathologic conditions to normal aging processes, and the belief that older adults are not capable of learning and implementing health-promoting behaviors inherent in wellness-oriented care.

Wellness and Nursing Care of Older Adults

- Rather than having a narrow focus on physical health and functioning, wellness-focused nursing considers the older adult's physical, mental, social, and spiritual well-being.

Definitions of Aging

- Aging is defined in many ways (e.g., subjectively, chronologically, functionally).
- Concepts related to functional age are most appropriate in wellness-oriented nursing care.

Descriptions of Successful Aging

- The current emphasis on successful aging involves optimal physical, mental, emotional, spiritual, and social well-being and quality of life.
- Two emerging foci of successful aging models are resilience and cultural inclusiveness.

Attitudes Toward Aging

- Negative images of aging and ageism are pervasive in modern societies (Figure 1-1) and can have a negative impact on care provided to older adults, especially when health care providers—including nurses—base their care on myths and inaccurate information.
- Age stereotypes exist in all cultures with varying degrees of negative and positive attributes (Box 1-1).
- Ageism is pervasive in American society and is associated with negative consequences on older adults.
- Nurses need to identify myths about older adults (Figure 1-2), examine attitudes toward aging (including their own), and use accurate information as an antidote so they can provide wellness-oriented care for older adults.
- Cultural perspectives have a significant influence on attitudes about aging, older adults, and family caregiving relationships (Box 1-1).

Debunking Myths: Understanding Realities About Older Adults in the United States

- Nurses need to be aware of myths related to health of older adults and provide accurate information about realities (Table 1-1).
- The older adult population in the United States has been increasing and will continue to increase at a rapid pace (Figure 1-3; Box 1-2).
- Despite a high prevalence of chronic illnesses, most older adults report good to excellent health (Figures 1-4 and 1-5).
- Socioeconomic characteristics and living arrangements of older adults vary significantly among subgroups (Figures 1-6, 1-7, and 1-8).
- Older adults have many choices of community-based housing options (Box 1-3).

Older Adults as Givers and Recipients of Care

- The current trend in the United States is that caregiving needs of elders are met primarily by spouses and secondarily by adult children, especially daughters and unmarried children.
- Older adults may be responsible for raising grandchildren in skipped-generation households.

Older Adults in the World

- Declines in fertility rates and improvements in health and life expectancy have led to an aging population worldwide (Figure 1-9).

Critical Thinking Exercises

1. Increase your awareness of attitudes toward aging and older adults through the following exercises:
   - During the next 2 weeks, as you go about your usual activities, keep a small notebook handy and jot down examples of images of older adults that you see or hear in the following media: newspapers, magazines, Internet, television, greeting cards, and social conversations. Note whether the images convey a neutral, positive, or negative image.
   - During the next 2 weeks, pay attention to your thoughts and conversations about older adults and identify the perceptions you hold, the terms you use, and the images you convey.
   - Rephrase each of the 20 questions in the Ageism Survey (Figure 1-2) and ask yourself how often you have done any of those activities in the past few months (e.g., "How often did I tell a joke that pokes fun at old people?").
   - Ask an older relative, friend, or acquaintance to fill out the Ageism Survey and discuss his or her experiences.
2. Carefully review the cultural perspectives on elders and family caregiving relationships (Box 1-1) and think about how you have formed your attitudes about aging.
3. Review the myths and realities of aging listed in Table 1-1 and think about times in your personal or professional experiences when you might have "bought into" a myth.
4. On the Internet, use the key words about types of housing options in Box 1-3 to find information about residential settings for older adults in your community. Consider which of these are most appropriate for independent older adults who are interested in social contacts and which would be most appropriate for older adults who have cognitive or functional limitations.

 For more information about the topics discussed in this chapter, be sure to check out the interactive Online Learning Activities and other helpful resources at http://thepoint.lww.com/Miller7e.

REFERENCES

Agogo, D., Haijat, F., Milne, G. R., et al. (2017). An empirical examination of subjective age in older adults. *Health Marketing Quarterly, 34,* 62–79.

Algilani, S., Ostlund-Lagerstrom, L., Schoultz, I., et al. (2016). Increasing the qualitative understanding of optimal functionality in older adults: A focus group based study. *BioMed Central Geriatrics,* doi: 10.1186/s12877–016–0244-z.

Allen, J. O. (2016). Ageism as a risk factor for chronic disease. *Gerontologist, 56,* 610–614.

Barrett, A., & Toothman, E. (2017). Multiple "old ages": The influence of social context on women's aging anxiety. *Journals of Gerontology: Psychological Sciences and Social Sciences,* [Epub] doi: 10.1093/geronb/gbx027.

Butler, R. N. (1975). *Why survive? Being old in America.* New York: Harper & Row.

Butler, R. N., Lewis, M. I., & Sunderland, T. (1991). *Aging and mental health* (4th ed.). New York: Merrill/Macmillan.

Carver, L., & Buchanan, D. (2016). Successful aging: Considering non-biomedical constructs. *Clinical Interventions in Aging, 11,* 1623–1630.

Cherry, K. E., Brigman, S., Lyon, B. A., et al. (2016). Self-reported ageism across the lifespan: Role of aging knowledge. *International Journal of Aging and Human Development, 83,* 366–380.

Choi, M., Sprang, G., & Eslinger, J. (2016). Grandparents raising grandchildren. *Family and Community Health, 39,* 120–127.

Dunn, H. L. (1961). *High-level wellness.* Arlington, VA: R.W. Beatty.

Federal Interagency Forum on Aging-Related Statistics. (2016). *Older Americans 2016: Key indicators of well-being.* Washington, DC: U.S. Government Printing Office.

Feng, Q., & Straughan, P. T. (2017). What does successful aging mean? Lay perception of successful aging among elderly Singaporeans. *Journals of Gerontology Psychological Sciences and Social Sciences, 72,* 204–213.

Fernandez-Ballesteros, R., Olmos, R., Santacreu, M., et al. (2017). The role of perceived discrimination on active aging. *Archives of Gerontology and Geriatrics, 71,* 14–20.

Freedman, V., Kasper, J., & Spillman, B. (2017). Successful aging through successful accommodation with assistive devices. *Journals of Gerontology Psychological Sciences and Social Sciences, 72,* 300–308.

Freeman, A., Santini, Z., Tyrovolas, S., et al. (2016). Negative perceptions of ageing predict the onset and persistence of depression and anxiety. *Journal of Affective Disorders, 199,* 132–138.

Gendron, T. L., Inker, J., & Welleford, E. A. (2017). A theory of relational ageism: A discourse analysis of the 2015 White House Conference on Aging. *Gerontologist,* [Epub] doi: 10.1093/geront/gnw155.

Gendron, T. L., Welleford, E. A., Inker, J., et al. (2016). The language of ageism: Why we need to use words carefully. *Gerontologist, 56,* 997–1006.

Hicks, S. A., & Sielecki, K. L. (2017). Leisure activity engagement and positive affect partially mediate the relationship between positive views on aging and physical health. *Journals of Gerontology: Psychological Sciences and Social Sciences, 72,* 259–267.

Huijg, J., van Delden, A., van der Ouderaa, F., et al. (2017). Being active, engaged, and healthy: Older persons' plans and wishes to age successfully. *Journals of Gerontology: Psychological Sciences and Social Sciences, 72,* 228–236.

Jopp, D., Jung, S., Damarin, A., et al. (2017). Who is your successful aging role model? *Journals of Gerontology: Psychological Sciences and Social Sciences, 72,* 237–247.

Kail, B., & Carr, D. (2017). Successful aging in the context of the disablement process: Working and volunteering as moderators on the association between chronic conditions and subsequent functional limitations. *Journals of Gerontology: Psychological Sciences and Social Sciences, 72,* 340–350.

Levy, S. (2016). Toward reducing ageism: PEACE (Positive Education about Aging and Contact Experiences) Model. *Gerontologist*, [Epub] doi: 10.1093/geront/gnw116.

McMahon, S., & Fleury, J. (2012). Wellness in older adults: A concept analysis. *Nursing Forum, 47*(1), 39–49.

Meisner, B. A., & Levy, B. R. (2016). Age stereotypes' influence on health: Stereotype Embodiment Theory. In V. L. Bengston & R. A. Settersten (Eds.). *Handbook of theories of aging* (3rd ed., pp. 259–275). New York: Springer Publishing Company.

Mejia, S., Ryan, L., Gonzalex, R., et al. (2017). Successful aging as the intersection of individual resources, age, environment, and experiences of well-being in daily activities. *Journals of Gerontology, 72,* 279–289.

Molton, I., & Yorkston, K. (2017). Growing older with a physical disability: A special application of the Successful Aging Paradigm. *Journals of Gerontology, 72,* 290–299.

Morelock, J. C., Stokes, J. E., & Moorman, S. M. (2017). Rewriting age to overcome misaligned age and gender norms in later life. *Journal of Aging Studies, 40,* 16–22.

Morley, J. E. (2009). Successful aging or aging successfully. *Journal of the American Medical Directors Association, 10*(2), 85–86.

Nelson, T. (2016). The age of ageism. *Journal of Social Issues, 72,* 191–198.

Ng, R., Allore, H., Trentalange, M., et al. (2015). Increasing negativity of age stereotypes across 200 years: Evidence from a database of 400 million words. *PLOS ONE,* doi: 10.1371/journal.pone.0117086.

Officer, A., Schneiders, M. L., Wu, D., et al. (2016). Valuing older people: Time for a global campaign to combat ageism. *Bulletin of the World Health Organization, 94,* 710–710A.

Pace, J., & Grenier, A. (2017). Expanding the circle of knowledge: Reconceptualizing successful aging among North American older indigenous peoples. *Journals of Gerontology: Psychological Sciences and Social Sciences, 72,* 248–258.

Palmore, E. (2015). Ageism comes of age. *Journals of Gerontology: Psychological Sciences and Social Sciences, 70,* 873–875.

Phibbs, S., & Hooker, K. (2017). An exploration of factors associated with ageism stereotype threat in a medical setting. *Journals of Gerontology,* [Epub] doi: 10.1093/geronb/gbx034.

Pruchno, R., & Carr, D. (2017). Successful aging 2.0: Resilience and beyond. *Journals of Gerontology, 72,* 201–203.

Rowe, J. W., & Kahn, R. L. (2015). Successful aging 2.0: Conceptual expansions for the 21st century. *Journals of Gerontology, 70,* 593–596.

Samuel, L. R. (2017). *Aging in America.* Philadelphia, PA: The University of Pennsylvania Press.

Sargent-Cox, K. (2017). Ageism: We are our own worst enemy. *International psychogeriatrics, 29,* 1–8.

Scheidt, R. (2017). The defense of my aging self: A report from the field. *Gerontologist, 57,* 110–115.

Settersten, R., & Godlewski, B. (2016). Concepts and theories of age and aging. In V. L. Bengston & R. A. Settersten (Eds.). *Handbook of theories of aging* (3rd ed., pp. 9–25). New York: Springer Publishing Company.

Tesch-Romer, C., & Wahl, H. W. (2017). Toward a more comprehensive concept of successful aging: Disability and care needs. *Journals of Gerontology, 72,* 310–318.

Tkatch, R., Musich, S., MacLeod, S., et al. (2017). A qualitative study to examine older adults' perceptions of health: Keys to aging successfully. *Geriatric Nursing,* [Epub] doi: 10.1016/gerinurse.2017.02.009.

World Health Organization. (2015). *Ageing and health: Fact Sheet 404.* Available at www.who.int

chapter 2

Addressing Diversity of Older Adults

LEARNING OBJECTIVES

After reading this chapter, you will be able to:

1. Discuss the importance of providing linguistically and culturally competent care for older adults.
2. Perform a cultural self-assessment.
3. Describe three major health belief systems that influence cultural perspectives on health and wellness.
4. Describe health disparities that affect older adults of different cultural groups.
5. Identify sources of information that nurses can use to improve their cultural competence.
6. Describe characteristics of the cultural groups of older adults in the United States.

KEY TERMS

cultural competence
cultural self-assessment
ethnogeriatrics
health belief system
health disparities
health literacy
linguistic competence

The increasing diversity of all age groups in the United States affects almost every facet of health care because cultural background significantly influences values, communication, health beliefs and health-related behaviors, and many other aspects of daily life. Older adults' cultural heritage and lived experiences significantly affect their health beliefs and behaviors as well as their relationships with health care providers and their receptivity to interventions. Although it is beyond the scope of this text to discuss all the implications related to cultural diversity of older adults, this chapter provides overviews of diverse groups of older adults in the United States. It also addresses the topics of health disparities and health literacy, because these are closely related to cultural diversity and are especially pertinent to health promotion for older adults. As with any information related to cultural diversity, it is imperative to recognize that although the overviews provide general information about particular groups, each group is made up of many individuals, and each individual has some characteristics that are common to the group but many that are not. Because overviews do not apply to individuals within the group, nurses need to avoid stereotypes and generalizations as they care for individual older adults.

CULTURAL DIVERSITY IN THE UNITED STATES

As discussed in Chapter 1, remarkable changes have occurred in the demographic characteristics of all countries because of increased life expectancy among most groups and decreased fertility rates among many groups. While the trend toward population aging has been occurring worldwide, a trend toward increasing racial and ethnic diversity has been occurring in the United States. Major changes in immigration patterns over the past 50 years combined with high fertility rates among immigrant groups have led to a gradual shift from African Americans being the largest minority group to Hispanics becoming the largest minority group. By 2044, minority groups (i.e., any group other than non-Hispanic white) will make up more than half of the U.S. population. Between 2014 and 2060 the percentage of Americans who are foreign born will increase among all groups; however, the greatest increase will be among older adults, with the percentage doubling from 13% in 2014 to 26% in 2060 (Colby & Ortman, 2015). Figure 2-1 illustrates changes in the racial and ethnic composition of the older adult population that are projected between 2014 and 2060.

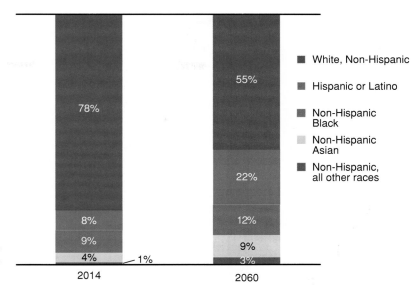

FIGURE 2-1 Actual and projected distribution of U.S. population age 65 and over by race and Hispanic origin, 2014 and 2060. Note: Totals do not necessarily add up to 100% due to rounding. *(Source: U. S. Census. (2014). Annual Estimates and Projected Population Sex, Age, Race, and Hispanic Origin for the United States 2014 to 2060.)*

Race, ethnicity, and gender are the characteristics most often addressed in census data and research; however, there is increasing attention to additional variables that affect health. The current emphasis of gerontologists is on identifying the relationship between health and minority status, whether that is based on gender, ethnicity, citizenship, religion, sexual orientation, geographic location, socioeconomic status, or other factors.

It is important to recognize that any defined group also includes many subgroups. To further complicate the issue, the 2010 census added subgroups and allowed for more combinations of race and ethnicity. Thus, definitions of groups and subgroups vary depending on the census definitions and other classifications available when data were collected or cited in research. Again, it is imperative to keep in mind that even the best evidence-based information does not address individual differences and that each person has unique characteristics that are not representative of any particular cultural group.

The increasing diversity that is characteristic of the general U.S. population also is reflected in the health care workforce and is especially noticeable in nursing staff, including nursing assistants, who provide care for older adults in community and long-term care settings. In urban home care settings, care is often provided by caregivers who have recently come to the United States and have not learned to speak English fluently. In these situations, communication barriers between care providers and care recipients are a challenge that needs to be addressed. Thus, it is important to recognize that cultural diversity in health care settings encompasses a wide range of situations, and each situation requires a high degree of cultural competence on the part of the health care provider.

HEALTH DISPARITIES

One of the ways in which cultural characteristics affect individuals is through the effect of minority status on health. In recent years, there has been increasing awareness of major health disparities, with much data pointing toward lower levels of health and functioning in groups of non-white older adults. Health disparities are defined as significant differences with regard to the rates of disease incidence, prevalence, morbidity, mortality, or life expectancy between one population and another. Until the 1970s, research on health disparities was limited to African Americans, but as the percentage of other groups has increased, these groups are increasingly being included in research. Currently, the concept of health disparities refers to different health outcomes based on greater obstacles to health due to any of the following: age, race, ethnicity, gender, gender identity, sexual orientation, religion, socioeconomic status, geographic location, mental health, or any form of disability. For example, despite improvements in the overall health of the U.S. population, older adults in a racial or ethnic minority, older adults living in rural areas, and those with low socioeconomic status experience a disproportionate burden of illness and premature death (American Geriatrics Society, 2016). Figure 2-2 illustrates health disparities for heart disease, hypertension, cancer, diabetes, and heart disease for three groups of Americans aged 65 years and over.

Although some health disparities arise from biocultural factors, such as a genetic predisposition to certain cancers, most are associated with sociocultural factors, such as low income and education. Some health disparities are associated with access to care, health care delivery, and acceptability of health care (e.g., culturally and linguistically appropriate). Another common theme is that health disparities are especially pronounced for diseases that can be prevented through health promotion interventions, such as preventive care and patient teaching. The Centers for Medicare and Medicaid and the Centers for Disease Control and Prevention have emphasized that all physicians, nurses, and allied health professionals must be aware of health care disparities and eliminate

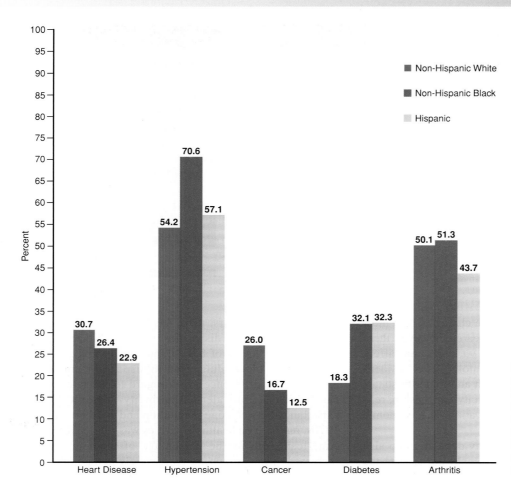

FIGURE 2-2 Percentage of adults aged 65 years and over who reported having heart disease, hypertension, cancer, diabetes, or heart disease, by race and Hispanic origin, 2013–2014. (Adapted from Federal Interagency Forum on Aging-Related Statistics, *Older Americans 2016,* at http://www.agingstats.gov.)

them at the patient level. Box 2-1 lists some of the most widely identified health disparities that are pertinent to promoting wellness for older adults. Information about health disparities is not intended to reinforce stereotypes; rather, a major purpose is to be aware of risk factors based on race or ethnicity. Another major clinical implication is that health promotion interventions, such as teaching about prevention and early detection of certain conditions, are particularly important when caring for older adults who are members of a minority group. In addition to race and ethnic factors, a lower level of health literacy is a major risk for health disparities, as discussed in the following section.

HEALTH LITERACY

Health literacy is increasingly recognized by health care practitioners and policy makers as a major determinant of health outcomes and a measure of quality of care. Definitions that have been widely used during the past three decades all include the straightforward idea "that health literacy involves the need for people to understand information that helps them maintain good health" (Institute of Medicine, 2013, p. 1). The Centers for Medicare and Medicaid (2017) estimates that 8% of Medicare beneficiaries have limited English proficiency,

which is one of the conditions that is strongly associated with health literacy. Additional factors that increase the risk for low health literacy are poverty, less education, and minority group membership. Low health literacy is associated with the following negative outcomes related to individual health and increased health care costs (Kobayashi, Wardle, Wolf, et al., 2016; Kopera-Frye, 2017; MacLeod, Musich, Gulyas, et al., 2017):

- Increased hospitalizations, visits to emergency rooms, and readmissions within 30 days of discharge
- Decreased use of preventive services, such as immunizations and cancer screenings
- Shorter life expectancy
- Increased prevalence of multiple chronic diseases
- Poor access to health care
- Decreased adherence to prescribed medication regimen
- Lower levels of self-reported functional status and physical and mental health
- Decreased ability to self-manage chronic conditions

National initiatives addressing health literacy include the 2010 National Action Plan to Improve Health Literacy, the Plain Writing Act of 2010, and the Agency for Healthcare Research and Quality Universal Precautions Toolkit. Online Learning Activity 2-1 provides links to resources

Box 2-1 Examples of Health Disparities Affecting Older Adults, Based on National Data and Reviews of Studies

Life Expectancy and Levels of Functional Impairment (Hummer, Melvin, Sheehan, et al., 2014; Mathews, Croft, Liu, et al., 2017)

- Among adults age 45 years and older, blacks and American Indians have a 30% higher risk of mortality compared with whites.
- Native Americans and blacks have the highest levels of functional impairment.
- People who live in rural areas experience poorer health and shorter life expectancy compared with those who live in urban areas.
- Hispanic subgroups vary in rates of disability, with older Puerto Rican men and women experiencing highest rates of disability and those of Spanish origin experiencing the lowest rate of disability.
- Asian subgroups vary in rates of disability, with Hawaiians, Pacific Islanders, and Vietnamese having the highest rates and Chinese and Japanese reporting the lowest rates.

Disparities Related to Preventive Care (Huff, Kline, & Peterson, 2015)

- Groups of older adults that are least likely to receive an influenza vaccination are blacks, Hispanics, and poor or low-income people.
- American Indian/Alaska Natives age 50 years and older are less likely to be screened for colorectal cancer.
- Hispanic and black adults with diabetes are less likely to receive recommended care. Adults age 65 years and over and men at any age with doctor-diagnosed arthritis are less likely to receive education about exercise compared with younger adults and women.

Disparities Related to Access to Care

- Percentage of ethnic/racial groups experiencing poorest access to care, compared with whites: Asian (39%), American Indian/Alaska Native (38%), black (21%), and Hispanic (16%) (Rose, 2017).

- American Indian/Alaska Native on reservations have limited access to even minimal health services (National Rural Health Association, 2016).

Disparities Related to Chronic Diseases

- Hypertension and cardiovascular disease occur at an earlier age and are associated with worse health outcomes in African Americans (Rooks & Thorpe, 2014).
- Blacks and Mexican Americans with hypertension are less likely to have controlled blood pressure (Go, Mozaffarian, Roger, et al., 2014).
- Depression is likely to be undiagnosed and undertreated in all ethnic minority groups (Mezuk & Gallo, 2014).
- Asian Americans are more likely to develop end-stage renal disease due to diabetes (Agency for Healthcare Research and Quality, 2013).

The Six Leading Causes of Death, in Order of Prevalence, by Race and Hispanic Origin (National Center for Health Statistics, 2016)

- White: (1) heart disease, (2) cancer, (3) chronic lower respiratory disease, (4) unintentional injuries, (5) cerebrovascular disease, (6) Alzheimer's disease
- Black: (1) heart disease, (2) cancer, (3) cerebrovascular disease, (4) diabetes, (5) unintentional injuries, (6) chronic lower respiratory disease
- Hispanic: (1) heart disease, (2) cancer, (3) cerebrovascular disease, (4) unintentional injuries, (5) diabetes, (6) Alzheimer's disease
- Asian or Pacific Islander: (1) cancer, (2) heart disease, (3) cerebrovascular disease, (4) unintentional injuries, (5) diabetes, (6) influenza and pneumonia
- American Indian or Alaska Native: (1) heart disease, (2) cancer, (3) unintentional injuries, (4) diabetes, (5) chronic lower respiratory disease, (6) cerebrovascular disease

---

about health disparities and health literacy, including an article about communication tips for nurses.

 See ONLINE LEARNING ACTIVITY 2-1: ARTICLE ABOUT HEALTH LITERACY AND NURSING at http://thepoint.lww.com/Miller8e.

CULTURAL COMPETENCE

During the 1950s, transcultural nursing (i.e., the provision of nursing care across cultural boundaries) focused on the comparative study of different cultural groups. Although transcultural nursing is an important specialization, the demographic trend toward ever expanding diversity requires that *all* health care professionals are culturally competent. Every nurse–client encounter involves some degree of cultural differences because of the distinctive values and characteristics of each individual. Even when two people have ostensibly similar cultural backgrounds, each one experiences and expresses cultural factors in a unique way. Consequently, nurses, nursing organizations, and schools of nursing are among the groups that are taking action to ensure the provision of culturally competent care.

Many professional organizations, such as the Gerontological Society of America and the American Society on Aging, are emphasizing the need to address cultural diversity in the aging population. Since 1987, the Stanford Geriatric Education Center has been a national resource center for **ethnogeriatrics**, which is the component of geriatrics that integrates the influence of race, ethnicity, and culture on health and well-being of older adults.

When using any sources of information, however, it is imperative to recognize that these resources can describe general characteristics of a particular group, but they cannot describe the unique way in which each individual is a member of the group. These generalizations can be detrimental if they lead to stereotypical perceptions rather than provide a compilation of information that may be applicable to individuals within the group. As already stated, all health care providers need to recognize that the culture of each individual is based on his or her membership in many groups and is internalized in a unique and personal way. Thus, nurses need to be knowledgeable about different cultural groups, but they need to use this information as a backdrop for exploring the ways in which individuals identify with the characteristics of the various cultural groups to which they belong. This is achieved by communicating a nonjudgmental attitude and asking open-ended questions to elicit information about each person's life experiences and cultural influences, as discussed in Chapter 13.

In this text, culturally specific information pertinent to nursing care of older adults is discussed in the following sections of this chapter and highlighted in other chapters in featured Cultural Considerations boxes and Diversity Notes. Nurses are encouraged to supplement this information by reading journals and other references and by exploring the resources in Online Learning Activities in this chapter. In addition, many of the organizations listed at the end of other chapters provide culturally appropriate educational materials and resources in languages other than English. These materials can be important resources for health promotion interventions and are usually available at little or no cost. In addition, all health care professionals are encouraged to contact local organizations to obtain culturally specific information about groups that reside in their locale.

See **ONLINE LEARNING ACTIVITY 2-2: RESOURCES FOR INFORMATION ABOUT CULTURAL AND LINGUISTIC COMPETENCY** at http://thepoint.lww.com/Miller8e.

Performing a Cultural Self-Assessment

Nursing texts emphasize that individual cultural competence is a fluid, dynamic, and ongoing process, rather than an end point, in which the nurse continuously strives to work effectively within the cultural context of the individual, family, or community (Andrews, 2016a; Giger, 2017). This process is often described as a progression from judgmental attitudes and practices to positive approaches. For example, Purnell (2013) describes a continuum that begins with being *unconsciously incompetent*, which is being unaware that one is lacking knowledge about another culture. When the person becomes aware of this knowledge gap, he or she is *consciously incompetent* and takes actions to learn about the cultural group. The next stage of being *consciously* competent involves learning about the other culture, verifying generalizations, and providing culturally specific interventions. In the final stage, the care provider is *unconsciously competent* and automatically provides culturally congruent care to clients of diverse cultures.

Although health care professionals rarely achieve high levels of cultural competency in relation to a broad spectrum of different ethnic/cultural groups, they are expected to achieve cultural competency in relation to the specific cultural groups for whom they provide care. Moreover, they are expected to be nonjudgmental and avoid stereotyping by recognizing the extent to which cultural views and practices influence their own attitudes and perceptions, as well as the care they provide. This can be achieved through a cultural self-assessment, which is an awareness-raising tool for gaining insight into the health-related values, beliefs, attitudes, and practices that one holds (Andrews, 2016a). Box 2-2 describes a cultural self-assessment that is particularly applicable for nurses caring for older adults. It is important to recognize that people can internalize social stigma and prejudices that apply to members of one's own groups. Thus, the self-assessment includes questions to increase one's awareness of internalized stigma.

 Box 2-2 Cultural Self-Assessment for Nurses Working With Older Adults

What Self-Identity Influences My World View?

- With what sociocultural and religious groups do I most closely identify?
- What does it mean to belong to these groups?
- Is there any stigma associated with any of these groups?
- What negative and positive images are associated with these groups?
- What do I like and dislike about these groups and my sociocultural identity?

How has My Cultural Background Influenced Me?

- How has (does) the society in which I grew up (currently live in) influenced the dominant values that I now hold?
- What is my perception of concepts such as time, work, leisure, health, family, and relationships?
- How do my perceptions differ from those of people who come from different cultural backgrounds?

What is My Attitude Toward People, Especially Older Adults Who

- Are immigrants?
- Have difficulty with the English language?
- Have difficulty communicating?
- Have a cultural background different from my own?
- Look or act like the stereotype of people who are gay, lesbian, or transgender?

What are My Attitudes About and Experiences With Health Practices That Differ From My Own?

- Do (did) members of my family have health care practices that differ(ed) from conventional Western medicine practices (e.g., herbs, poultices, folk remedies)?
- Do (did) they consult with folk, indigenous, religious, or spiritual healers?
- How do I feel about alternative or complementary health care practices for myself and for older adults?

How Well do I Communicate and Understand?

- What do I do and how do I feel when I have difficulty understanding people whose accents and primary language are different from my own?
- What have I learned about myself because of this self-assessment?

A Student's Perspective

After completing the cultural assessment, I learned that I do not have a thorough grasp on my own culture. We learned in class that nurses must be aware and knowledgeable about their own culture before they can relate to their clients. I have not gotten that one under wraps yet. I do not know, for example, what religious group that I best fit in with. I know that it is necessary to firmly understand your own beliefs and background before you can help a client be comfortable with theirs, yet I obviously do not! Doing the cultural assessment does make me aware of biases. I do feel uncomfortable thinking about immigrants, in that, I do not know who I define as immigrants or where I believe they come from. I also tend to imagine "we are all the same." When in reality all cultures are very different in positive ways, and to generalize is to say that the things that make cultures different are unimportant, when that is not true.

It is definitely the time to answer these questions about culture. Not only is it important for me to identify with my culture, but I also need help in developing an understanding of other people's cultures. Doing this assessment is only the first step; I must continue to question what I believe, where I come from, and who I relate to. Then I can help my clients.

Erin H.

Linguistic Competence in Care of Older Adults

Linguistic competence, which refers to health care services that are respectful of and responsive to a person's linguistic needs, is one small part of cultural competence. This concept is important for gerontological nurses because they frequently work with older adults whose primary language differs from their own. Immigrants who come to the United States as adults may be particularly disadvantaged because they may not have the same opportunities to learn English as do school age children. The challenge of communicating with people who do not speak the same language or dialect is magnified when the person also has dementia or sensory impairments, as is often the case in long-term care settings.

Because the Civil Rights Act of 1964 upholds the rights of individuals with limited English proficiency to have equal access to health and social service programs, health care providers must ensure effective use of interpretation services. In 2001, the U.S. Office of Minority Health published *National Standards for Culturally and Linguistically Appropriate Services,* which are commonly referred to as CLAS. These standards require all health care institutions that receive federal funds to provide access to 24-hour, no-cost language assistance services for individuals who are unable to speak or understand the English language.

Nurses need to be aware of interpreter resources that should be available in all health care settings. For example, the Language Line Services offer immediate telephone interpretation services for subscribers. In situations where no interpreters are

 Box 2-3 Guidelines for Using Interpreters

Before the Interaction

- Whenever possible, use the services of a professional interpreter. Avoid using visitors or staff from auxiliary services unless permission to do so has been obtained from both the older adult and the interpreter.
- Given that there are more than 140 languages spoken in North America, be certain that the correct language and dialect have been identified before arranging for an interpreter. For example, does the person speak Cantonese or Mandarin Chinese?
- If an interpreter for the primary language is unavailable, determine whether the older adult speaks other languages. For example, many older adults from Vietnam and some African nations are also fluent in French.
- Be aware of age, gender, and socioeconomic class considerations in selecting an interpreter. In general, it is best to use an interpreter who is the same gender and of the same approximate age and socioeconomic class as the older adult.
- Organize your thoughts and plan ahead to ensure that the most important topics are covered.
- Allow sufficient time for the interaction and expect that it will take longer than an interaction with an older adult for whom English is the primary language.

During the Interaction

- Review the importance of confidentiality.
- Talk to the older adult, not the interpreter.
- Talk about only one topic at a time.
- Use short sentences and simple vocabulary.
- Use the active voice. Avoid vague modifiers.
- Avoid professional jargon, idioms, and slang.
- Be aware that many words do not translate into another language. For instance, the English word *depression* has no equivalent in many Asian and other languages.

available, nurses can obtain immediate fee-based telephone interpretation services from Language Line Services by calling 1-800-752-6096. Box 2-3 summarizes guidelines for using interpreters in health care settings with older adults.

CULTURAL PERSPECTIVES ON WELLNESS

As discussed in Chapter 1, nurses have numerous opportunities to promote wellness for older adults, even under the most challenging of circumstances, through holistic nursing interventions to improve physical comfort and psychological and spiritual growth. To achieve this, nurses need to have a good understanding of the meaning of health and wellness to each older adult. Nurses can explore this with older adults by asking questions such as "What does it mean to you to be healthy?" or "How do you achieve wellness in your life?" If appropriate, nurses can explore this topic from the perspective of cultural diversity with a question such as "I'm interested in knowing more about how Chinese people view wellness. Can you tell me your thoughts about this?"

Health care practices and beliefs of individuals are strongly influenced by the **health belief system** (defined

Box 2-4 Cultural Considerations: Major Health Belief Systems

Magico-Religious Paradigm

- Supernatural forces dominate the fate of the world and all those in it depend on the actions of supernatural forces (e.g., God, gods).
- Origins of illness include sorcery, breach of a taboo, intrusion of a disease object, intrusion of a disease-causing spirit, and loss of soul.
- Illness is initiated by a supernatural agent with or without justification, or by a person who practices sorcery or engages the services of sorcerers.
- *Health is* a gift or reward given as a sign of God's blessing and goodwill.
- Health and illness belong first to the community and then to the individual, so there is a strong sense of community.
- The magico-religious perspective is common among Latino, African, Caribbean, African American, and Middle Eastern groups.

Holistic Paradigm

- Forces of nature must be kept in balance or harmony.
- Human life is only one aspect of nature and a part of the general order of the universe.
- The whole person is viewed in the context of the total environment.
- Disease is caused by an imbalance or disharmony between the human, geophysical, and metaphysical forces of the universe.
- Illness is not an intruding agent but is a natural part of life's rhythmic course; health and illness are both natural parts of a continuum.

- Diseases of civilization (e.g., unemployment, discrimination, ghettos, suicide) are just as much illnesses as are biomedical diseases.
- *Health* and *healing reflect* the quality of wholeness associated with healthy functioning and well-being.
- The holistic paradigm is common among Asian, North American, and Indian groups, and was also espoused by Florence Nightingale.

Scientific (Biomedical) Paradigm

- Life is controlled by a series of physical and biochemical processes that can be studied and manipulated by humans.
- Principles of determinism: a cause-and-effect relationship exists for all natural phenomena.
- Principles of mechanism: life processes can be controlled through mechanical, genetic, and other engineered interventions.
- Principles of reductionism: all life can be reduced or divided into smaller parts (e.g., the mind and body are two distinct entities).
- Disease is a breakdown of the human machine as a result of stress, internal damages, or external trauma or invasion.
- *Health is* the absence of disease.
- The scientific perspective is common among most Western cultures, including the United States and Canada.

Source: Andrews, M. M. (2016b). The influence of cultural and health belief systems on health care practices. In M. M. Andrews & J. S. Boyle (Eds.). *Transcultural concepts in nursing care* (pp. 73–88). Philadelphia, PA: Lippincott, Williams & Wilkins.

---

as the health-related attitudes, beliefs, and practices) of one's cultural group. Andrews (2016b) described three major health belief systems that underpin health beliefs and health-related behaviors of individuals, as summarized in Box 2-4. It is important to recognize that many people integrate beliefs from two or all of these paradigms, but some people are firmly entrenched in one health belief system. Nurses need to be aware of the health beliefs that influence their clients, so they can adapt their interventions accordingly. For example, people who adhere to the holistic paradigm described in Box 2-4 may view their condition as an imbalance between "hot" and "cold" energies and request a particular food or herbal remedy for restoring balance.

The influence of religion and spirituality is another cultural aspect pertinent to promoting wellness for older adults. For example, religious affiliation may influence a person's health-related behaviors and is also associated with positive emotions and social support (Spector, 2017). A review of studies about religion and spirituality among three groups of older adults in the United States identified the following findings that are pertinent to promoting wellness (Chatters, Nguyen, & Taylor, 2014):

- African American older adults: Attendance at religious services is associated with improved coping with stressors, greater levels of life satisfaction, higher self-rated health, and lower levels of depression, suicide risk, and obsessive–compulsive behaviors
- Asian American older adults: Religious affiliation is associated with higher levels of life satisfaction and well-being,

as indicated by perceptions of happiness, harmony, acceptance, inner peace, and meaning in life
- Older Mexican Americans: Belief in the efficacy of prayer is associated with greater optimism, more positive perceptions of health, and an increased sense of control

A Student's Perspective

I came from a highly educated, Christian, Caucasian family and this affects how I see the world both consciously and unconsciously. Education is a very important part of my life. My Christian upbringing makes me value honesty, justice, compassion, and forgiveness. I was raised to have an open mind and not judge people until I got to know them. I think that has been the most important idea that I live my life around.

One thing I learned was how I see everyone who was not born in the United States and those who do not speak English as immigrants. I get very frustrated when I don't understand people because of their heavy accent or inability to speak English. Because one of my grandmothers used plenty of home remedies, I was exposed to alternative medicine from an early age. I think it is important to take into consideration other's beliefs and incorporate them as best as you can into their care. I am sure I will continue to discover my true values and beliefs as I grow in nursing. I think it is a good idea to keep reviewing my own cultural beliefs so that I become aware of them and how they affect my practice.

Sarah L.

OVERVIEW OF CULTURAL GROUPS OF OLDER ADULTS IN THE UNITED STATES

To provide culturally competent care, nurses need to learn about the cultural groups in their patient populations. Until recently, the study of aging in the United States has focused almost exclusively on white Americans; however, gerontologists are increasingly addressing interrelationships among race, ethnicity, aging, and health. Studies regarding cultural aspects of aging began with a focus on African Americans during the 1960s and then extended to Hispanic Americans in the 1970s and to other groups in the 1980s. Because little or no census information about various subgroups was available until the early 2000s, researchers are just beginning to address issues related to aging in these population groups. More recently, nonprofit organizations and gerontologists are addressing aging-related concerns of other diverse groups, such as rural, homeless, and LGBT older adults.

Even today, terminology used in reference to subgroups is inconsistent, and definitions of specific groups vary tremendously. For example, Native Hawaiians are categorized with Pacific Islanders in the U.S. Census, but as Native Americans in the Older Americans Act and in other contexts. Categories defined by the U.S. government for the 2010 census are as follows:

- *American Indian* or *Alaska Native:* People who descended from any of the original people of North, South, or Central America, and who maintain their tribal affiliation or community attachment
- *Asian:* People who descended from any of the original people of the Far East, Southeast Asia, or the Indian subcontinent (this includes Cambodia, China, India, Japan, Korea, Malaysia, Pakistan, Philippine Islands, Thailand, and Vietnam)
- *Black* or *African American:* People who descended from any of the black racial groups of Africa (this includes Kenyan, Nigerian, Senegalese)
- *Hispanic* or *Latino:* A person of Cuban, Mexican, Puerto Rican, South or Central American, or other Spanish culture or origin, regardless of race
- *Native Hawaiian* or *Other Pacific Islander:* People who descended from any of the original peoples of Hawaii, Guam, Samoa, or other Pacific islands
- *White:* People who descended from any of the original peoples of Europe, the Middle East, or North Africa (e.g., Arab, Caucasian, German, Irish, Italian, Lebanese, or Moroccan)
- *Some Other Race:* All those who reported entries such as multiracial, mixed, interracial, or a Hispanic or Latino group as race

Although much progress has been made in research related to diverse groups of older adults, many subgroups are combined as one and discussed as a homogeneous group. Thus, it is important to realize that conclusions from studies may not apply to all the subgroups that are categorized as one. For example, considerable health disparities exist among the different Hispanic groups, but the earliest studies focused on Mexican Americans because this is the largest Hispanic group in the United States. Information about the four largest minority groups of older adults is presented in the following sections. The intent of this information is to provide an overview based on current information about the cultural traditions of four population groups in the United States. As already stated, it is imperative to view each person as a unique individual and avoid applying generalization or stereotypes on the basis of a person's race or ethnicity.

African Americans

African Americans are mainly the descendants of as many as 24 million Africans who were forcibly brought to the United States as slaves beginning in the 17th century (Campinha-Bacote, 2013). Slavery, therefore, became the way of life that partially formed the roots of African-American (black) culture in a European-American (white) society. Inherent effects of slavery included racism, poverty, and social and psychological obstacles. The 2010 U.S. Census uses the terms African American interchangeably with "black" and "Negro" with emphasis on the importance of asking African Americans about their preferred term.

In 2010, only 9% of older adults in the United States were African Americans; this figure is expected to increase to 12% by 2060 (Federal Interagency Forum on Aging, 2016). Geographically, African Americans live in all states, with the highest percentages living in Southern states and in large metropolitan areas outside the South. Older adults who identify themselves as black or African American are an extremely heterogeneous group, with a wide range of socioeconomic conditions, including income, educational level, and jobs. Family constellations vary widely and female-headed households are common, as are multigenerational households.

National surveys find that African American older adults have the highest level of religious participation, with common religious affiliations being Baptist, Methodist, Pentecostal, Catholic, and Muslim (Chatters, Nguyen, & Taylor, 2014; Spector, 2017). An important implication for nurses is that Faith Community Nurses (also called Parish Nurses, as described in Chapter 6) and ministers associated with religious organizations have important roles in addressing health care needs of African Americans. African Americans may associate good health with harmony in life and may view illness as a punishment for sin.

All age groups of African Americans experience significant health disparities, but those who are older experience serious cumulative effects. Major consequences of these health disparities include decreased life expectancy and increased levels of disability and poor health. Factors contributing to poor health outcomes among African Americans include discrimination, cultural barriers, and lack of access to health care.

See **ONLINE LEARNING ACTIVITY 2-3: RESOURCES FOR INFORMATION ABOUT OLDER AFRICAN AMERICANS** at http://thepoint.lww.com/Miller8e.

Case Study

Mrs. A. is an 81-year-old African American who lives with her daughter, Mildred, and teenage great-grandson in a two-bedroom apartment in a large metropolitan area of Ohio. Mildred works as a nursing assistant in a nearby nursing home and often works double shifts. Mrs. A. was born in Alabama and lived there until 20 years ago, when her husband died and she moved in with her daughter (who lived alone at the time). Seven years later, Mildred took on responsibility for raising her infant grandson, who is now 13 years old. Mrs. A. has glaucoma, arthritis, and hypertension, and she had a stroke several years ago. She admits to having "a little problem with my memory," but Mildred says "She remembers what she wants to remember." Mrs. A. takes an over-the-counter analgesic as needed for her arthritis and has two prescription medications for hypertension. She also uses prescription eye drops twice daily. Mrs. A. has her blood pressure checked by the parish nurse about once monthly; she sees a doctor and nurse practitioner at a neighborhood clinic for checkups about twice yearly. The parish nurse often tells her that her blood pressure is "a little on the high side" and encourages her to see her doctor, but Mrs. A. has difficulty getting appointments because she depends on Mildred to take her there. Mrs. A. is about 30 lb overweight and she walks very slowly. When she is out of the house, Mildred provides a supportive hand to assist her with steadiness and mobility. Mildred shops for groceries, but Mrs. A. prepares most meals for the family.

THINKING POINTS

- How might Mrs. A.'s living arrangements influence her health and functioning, both positively and negatively?
- What factors are likely to influence the kind of health care Mrs. A. receives?
- If you were the parish nurse, what actions would you take to decrease health risks and promote quality of life for Mrs. A.?
- What additional resources could be used to improve Mrs. A.'s situation?

Hispanics or Latinos

Because the U.S. government counts race and Hispanic origin as two separate categories, the census categorizes people by race and by whether or not they are Hispanic or Latino. Thus, the category of Hispanic includes many heterogeneous groups that immigrated to the United States. In 2010, Hispanics accounted for 7% of the older adult population and by 2060, they will account for 22% of older adults in the United

States (Federal Interagency Forum on Aging, 2016). U.S. distribution of the Hispanic or Latino population in 2010 was as follows (Pew Research Center, 2016):

- Mexican: 64.0%
- Puerto Rican: 9.6%
- Salvadoran: 3.8%
- Dominican: 3.2%
- Guatemalan: 2.4%
- Columbian: 1.9%
- Honduran: 1.5%
- Spaniard: 1.4%
- Ecuadorian: 1.2%
- Peruvian: 1.1%
- Total of other groups with less than 1% each: 9.9%

Although these groups have some characteristics in common, they represent culturally diverse groups that are categorized together for reasons such as census and research.

Hispanics have high regard (*respecto*) for people by virtue of their age, service, or experience, and this carries over to a strong respect for older people. Hispanic groups have a strong sense of family, and they tend to place the needs of the group or family over those of the individual. Hispanics, like African Americans, are more likely than whites to be living with family or extended family and less likely to be living in a nursing home. Older Hispanic Americans, especially those who are Puerto Rican, have higher poverty rates than whites. The educational level of older Hispanics is lower than that of whites or African Americans. Most Hispanics in the United States speak both Spanish and English. Differing immigration patterns of these groups have led to different proportions of elderly, with a high proportion among Cubans and a lower proportion among Mexicans and Puerto Ricans.

Mexicans

The initial wave of Mexican immigrants came during the early 1900s to what was then the southwest territory of the United States because of political turmoil in Mexico and U.S. economic opportunities, such as building railroads. A second wave of immigrants came during the *bracero* period (1940s to 1960s) as experienced farm laborers to work in cotton, sugar beet, and other agricultural fields. The people who came during the *bracero* period currently comprise the population of older Mexican Americans. Recent Mexican immigrants are younger people, including many who are undocumented immigrants. This group will contribute to the significant increase in older Hispanics that is expected to occur over the next decades.

Puerto Ricans

Puerto Ricans first came in the 1830s and began settling in New York City, but they did not come in great numbers until after World War II. In 1917, Puerto Ricans were granted citizenship if they agreed to mandatory military service. By the 1970s, more than 1 million Puerto Ricans had immigrated to more than 20 cities, motivated primarily by economics, employment, social mobility, and family relationships.

Currently, more than 3 million Puerto Ricans live in the United States, with more than half living in the northeastern area. Fluctuating economic conditions in recent years led to a pattern of Puerto Ricans moving back and forth, which is made easier by the fact that they are dual citizens of the United States and Puerto Rico.

Cubans

The Republic of Cuba is a multiracial country with people primarily of Spanish and African descent, but also of Chinese, Haitian, and Eastern European origins. Cubans initially immigrated to the United States in the late 1800s to work in the tobacco industry. A second influx occurred between 1940 and 1950 when Cubans came to help with the war industry. The largest number of Cuban émigrés came to the United States between 1959 and 1979 when many middle- and upper-class citizens fled Cuba for political reasons. This accounts for the higher number of older Cubans in relation to younger Cubans. They are most highly concentrated in Florida but also have significant numbers in New Jersey, New York, Illinois, and California. Because three or four generations of family often live together, many older adults live with other family members.

See ONLINE LEARNING ACTIVITY 2-4: RESOURCES FOR INFORMATION ABOUT OLDER HISPANIC AMERICANS at http://thepoint.lww.com/Miller8e.

Case Study

Both Mr. and Mrs. H. are 64-year-old Mexican Americans who came to an urban area of Texas to live with their son, Jose, and daughter-in-law, Maria, about 10 years ago. Mr. and Mrs. H. provide child care for their four grandchildren. Jose works as a farm laborer, and Maria does domestic work. Mr. and Mrs. H. prefer to speak and read in Spanish, and all family members speak Spanish in the home, but they can speak English well enough to communicate when necessary. Jose and Mr. H. each smoke a couple of packs of cigarettes a day. None of the family members has health insurance, but this is not of concern to Mr. and Mrs. H. because they have relied on folk healers for many years and this has been effective for them. In their *curanderismo* (traditional healing) system, Mrs. H. is the first person consulted and she applies the remedies that have been passed on to her from her mother and grandmother. Her remedies are directed toward restoring balance between hot and cold, and she also encourages prayers and lighting of candles at church. In the rare instances when a family member has not gotten better within a couple of days, Mrs. H. takes him or her to a *yerbero* (herbalist) for herbs and other remedies. Once, when Maria had a more serious "female" problem, Mrs. H. took her to a *curandero* (folk healer), who was able to cure the problem.

You are a community health nurse in the county where Mr. and Mrs. H. reside and you are asked to develop a planning committee for a health fair, which is being held at and cosponsored by the Catholic church attended by many of the community's Mexican Americans. The county health department received a grant from the National Institutes of Health to identify people most at risk for cancer, diabetes, and hypertension as part of the *Healthy People 2020* initiative. At least part of the motivation for receiving this grant was to cut the cost of providing care for people who are not diagnosed until these diseases are advanced. Statistics verify that Hispanics in your county have unusually high rates of diabetes, hypertension, and lung and breast cancer. Statistics also confirm that the cost of treating these conditions is disproportionately high because of complications from untreated and undiagnosed cases. The goal of this health fair, which is part of a larger initiative, is to screen for diabetes and to motivate people to return to future fairs for additional preventive measures. Your target population for this health fair is Hispanic people aged 45 years and older.

THINKING POINTS

- Who would you want to be on your committee?
- What factors will significantly influence participation in this health fair, both positively and negatively? What plans would you suggest for overcoming barriers to participation?
- What health topics would you be sure to address for health promotion?
- How might you incorporate a family perspective in the plans for the health fair?
- What could be done to incorporate folk healers in the planning and implementation of the health fair? What are the benefits and risks in doing this?
- What additional information would you want to have so that you could proceed with planning a successful health fair? How would you go about finding this information?

Asians and Pacific Islanders in the United States

The category of "Asians and Pacific Islanders," like the category of "Hispanics," refers to numerous diverse subgroups of people clustered together for purposes of simplifying data. The 2000 and 2010 census data distinguish between the Asian and the Native Hawaiian and other Pacific Islander populations, but previous census data, and much of the available information about U.S. subgroups, combine many subgroups in the one category labeled as Asian Americans and Pacific Islanders. People in the group labeled as Asian Americans and Pacific Islanders, which makes up 5.4% of the U.S. population, come from nearly 50 countries and ethnic groups and speak more than 100 languages and dialects (Social Security Administration, 2013). Chinese represent the largest Asian group in the United States, followed by Asian Indians,

Filipinos, Vietnamese, Korean, and Japanese (U.S. Census Bureau, 2017). Since 2009, Asians have outnumbered Hispanics as the highest percentage of immigrants arriving in the United States each year (Pew Research Center, 2017).

Despite the great diversity among Asian and Pacific Islander groups, some general characteristics can be identified. Asian and Pacific Islander cultures are very family oriented and place a strong value on care of older family members. Asian older adults are less likely to live alone than the older population in general in the United States. Most American-born Asians speak English, but some immigrants speak only their native language or are bilingual. Immigrant churches and church-sponsored community centers provide support and a sense of belonging for Asian older adults.

In Asian cultures, health is viewed as a state of spiritual and physical harmony, and illness occurs when the yin and yang are out of balance. "Yin" refers to female energy and is associated with wet, cold, and dark; "yang" refers to male energy and is associated with dry, hot, and light. Asian Americans generally enjoy exceptionally good health and longevity, but some subgroups, such as Hmong, Laotian, Vietnamese, and Cambodian, experience significant health and socioeconomic disadvantages (Hummer, Melvin, Sheehan, et al., 2014). Asian Americans as a group have lower mortality rates at all ages, with mortality rates at age 85 years and older being 31% to 37% lower than whites (Hummer, Melvin, Sheehan, et al., 2014).

Chinese

Chinese people first migrated as laborers between 1840 and 1882, after which immigration of Chinese people to America was suspended until 1924, when annual quotas were established. Many of these immigrants came for political or socioeconomic reasons and had little or no education. In 1965, the Quota Act was abolished and many professional and highly educated Chinese came to the United States. Many Chinese live in metropolitan areas; the states with the largest Chinese populations are California, New York, Hawaii, and Texas.

Filipinos

Filipinos came in three waves, beginning in the early 1700s when the "pioneer" group came to New Orleans. This first wave continued through the early 1900s and included agricultural workers in Hawaii and the western states. Beginning in 1934, Filipino immigrants were limited to an annual quota of 50. The second wave of Filipino immigrants occurred between 1946 and 1965 when the annual quota was raised to 100. During this period, many became U.S. citizens by joining the armed services or coming as students, professionals, or war brides. The third wave began after quotas were expanded and includes a large proportion of families and young professionals.

Asian Indians

Asian Indians (also called East Indians) began coming to the United States in the late 1900s as laborers in the lumber, farming, shipping, and railroad industries. This first wave of immigrants continued coming until they were barred from these jobs by Asian Immigration Act of 1917. By the mid-1940s, fewer than 2000 Asian Indians remained in the United States; however, a second wave of highly educated and technically trained Asian Indians began arriving after immigration laws were changed in the mid-1960s.

Vietnamese

Vietnamese people began arriving in the mid-1970s seeking political refuge because of the Vietnam War. Second and third waves of Vietnamese, Cambodians, and Laotians have come as refugees, including many older adults and other extended family members. A fourth wave of immigrants began after the American Homecoming Act of 1987 provided for entry of former South Vietnamese military officers, political detainees, and children of American servicemen and their mothers and close relatives.

Koreans

Koreans began immigrating to the United States in the 1900s, particularly to Hawaii, where they sought plantation work. Between 1950 and 1965, a second major wave of Koreans came, including many war brides of American servicemen. After 1965, many middle-class and college-educated Koreans, including many health care professionals, came.

Japanese

Japanese people began immigrating to America in 1885, and immigration peaked in the early 1900s. In 1924, they were barred from entering the United States, and in 1942, all Japanese people living in the United States were relocated to internment camps. Immigration resumed in the 1950s and increased after 1965 when immigration restrictions were eased. Japanese Americans are the only immigrant group whose members identify themselves according to their generation of birth in the United States. Generation groupings are *issei,* first-generation immigrants; *nisei*, first American-born generation; *sansei*, third generation; and *yonsei, gosei,* and *rokusei* for fourth, fifth, and sixth generations, respectively.

 See ONLINE LEARNING ACTIVITY 2-5: RESOURCES FOR INFORMATION ABOUT OLDER ASIANS AND PACIFIC ISLANDERS IN THE UNITED STATES at http://thepoint.lww.com/Miller8e.

Case Study

Mrs. C. is a 76-year-old Chinese American widow who lives in an apartment in the Chinatown section of San Francisco. She has lived within the same 1-mile radius since her parents brought her to San Francisco from Mainland China when she was 9 years old. All three of her children are married; two live about an hour away, and the other one lives on the East Coast. Although she can speak and read English, Mrs. C. prefers to use her native Chinese dialect, and all of her reading materials are in Chinese. She completed a high school education in Chinatown and married a Chinese immigrant when she was 19 years old. She served as her husband's primary caregiver after he developed lung cancer several years ago until his death last year.

Mrs. C. is enrolled in the On Lok Senior Health Program, a health maintenance organization that provides a wide range of health and social services. She attends a daily meal program and sees the nurse at the center for blood pressure checks every month. She has hypertension, arthritis, and coronary artery disease. Mrs. C. sees a local herbalist every few weeks to obtain the herbal medicines that will keep her yin and yang energies in balance, and she chooses foods according to their yin and yang characteristics. She periodically has acupuncture treatments when her arthritis bothers her. Although Mrs. C. believes she can control her heart problem and high blood pressure with herbs and diet, she takes her two medications as prescribed because the nurse at the On Lok clinic has emphasized that these pills are essential for keeping her energy in balance.

Mrs. C. recently had a stroke and received medical treatment and rehabilitation services. She is being discharged to her apartment with a referral to the On Lok home care services for skilled nursing and speech, physical, and occupational therapies. Discharge orders also include the need to instruct Mrs. C. in a low-sodium diet. In addition to having some aphasia and left-sided paralysis, Mrs. C. has some residual memory impairment from the stroke. Before discharge from the rehabilitation program, she said she would not need any home health aide assistance because she expected that her daughter and daughter-in-law would take turns coming over every day and that they would take care of her. You are the nurse assigned to do the initial assessment and your visit is scheduled for the day after discharge, when the daughter-in-law will be there. Although you have been a visiting nurse for several years, you have recently moved to San Francisco and you began working for On Lok 2 weeks ago.

THINKING POINTS

- What cultural factors might influence Mrs. C.'s acceptance of you, as the skilled care nurse, and of home care services in general?
- What would you do to gain cultural competence to work more effectively with Mrs. C. and other patients in the On Lok health care program?
- What are your specific health care concerns for Mrs. C., and what strategies would you use to develop an effective and acceptable care plan?

American Indians and Alaska Natives

American Indians and Alaska Natives are the only minority groups that are indigenous to the United States, and they comprise 567 federally recognized tribes. According to the U.S. census, 6.6 million people in the United States identify as American Indian and Alaska Native, comprising 2% of the total population (U.S. Census Bureau, 2016). The largest tribal groups of American Indians are (in order of size) Cherokee, Navaho, Choctaw, Mexican American Indian, Chippewa, Sioux, Apache, Blackfeet, Creek, and Iroquois.

Median age for American Indian and Alaska Native population, which is counted as one group, is 6.4 years younger than that of the total United States; only 8% are aged 65 years and older. The states with the largest population of American Indians and Native Alaskans were California, Oklahoma, Texas, Arizona, New York, New Mexico, Washington, North Carolina, Florida, Michigan, Colorado, and Alaska (U.S. Census Bureau, 2016). The typical older American Indian and Alaska Native is poor, has less than a high school education, and is likely to speak an indigenous language rather than English. In recent years, American Indians have been moving from reservations to metropolitan areas; however, they frequently travel back to reservations to maintain cultural and family ties (National Rural Health Association, 2016).

American Indian and Alaska Native groups value older members of the community, particularly with regard to their roles as grandparents and story tellers. Language of the Lakota nation distinguishes between "elderlies" (i.e., those who are frail) and "elders" (i.e., those who are highly esteemed for their service to their community and ability to teach younger generations about traditional Lakota customs) (Rodriguez-Galan, 2014). American Indian and Alaska Native groups hold strong traditions related to spirituality and religious practices, with each tribe having unique expressions. Healing practices common among American Indians include herbalism, spiritual healing, the concept of the healing influence of the connection with the environment, and a strong belief in the connection among body, mind, and spirit (Moss, 2016).

American Indians and Alaska Natives experience disproportionately high rates of all of the following conditions: diabetes, tuberculosis, heart disease, substance abuse, and certain cancers (e.g., liver, cervix, kidney, gallbladder, and colorectal (Weinstein, Geller, Nagussie, et al., 2017). Factors that contribute to poorer health among American Indians and Alaska Natives include geographic isolation, economic conditions, cultural barriers, and mistrust of health care institutions. Access to care is a major barrier, particularly for those who live on reservations.

 See ONLINE LEARNING ACTIVITY 2-6: RESOURCES FOR INFORMATION ABOUT OLDER AMERICAN INDIANS AND ALASKA NATIVES at http://thepoint.lww.com/Miller8e.

Case Study

Mrs. I. is an 82-year-old Navajo who lives with her daughter and son-in-law. In accordance with Navajo traditions, Mrs. I. believes that health is closely linked with being in harmony with the environment, family members, and supernatural forces. She regularly attends native healing ceremonies and protects her family and herself from sickness through songs, stories, rituals, prayers, and sand paintings. Mrs. I.'s mother kept a medicine bundle, called a *jish* containing stones, feathers, arrowheads, and corn pollen and used this for healing and blessings. Mrs. I.'s elder sister now uses the *jish* that was passed on from their mother. Mrs. I. has had diabetes and hypertension for several years, and is about 30 pounds over her ideal weight. She receives medical care at the Indian Health Service, where you are the nurse. During a recent visit, you found Mrs. I.'s blood pressure was 164/98 mm Hg; her random blood sugar level as measured on the glucometer was 196 mg/dL. You know from previous visits that Mrs. I. does not want to take any prescription medications because she thinks they are not in harmony with spiritual forces. When you explain that both her blood sugar and blood pressure are high, she promises you that she will ask her older sister to use the *jish* for healing. You know from your experience with the Indian Health Service that nurses have been successful in persuading Navajos to perform physical exercise if it is viewed in a larger cultural context. For example, when the nurse consulted a tribal leader in developing an exercise program, the American Indians at a community health center were receptive to incorporating mild aerobic exercise into their daily routines in the form of traditional dance movements.

THINKING POINTS

- What cultural factors are likely to influence Mrs. I.'s understanding of diabetes and hypertension?
- How would you use metaphors and cultural knowledge to help Mrs. I. understand her diabetes and hypertension?
- What questions would you ask Mrs. I. to identify teaching strategies and other interventions that might be successful with regard to her diabetes and hypertension?
- What strategies are likely to be successful in implementing dietary and lifestyle interventions for Mrs. I.?
- What steps would you take to improve your cultural competence in working with Mrs. I.?

OLDER ADULTS IN OTHER DIVERSE GROUPS

It is important to recognize that the concept of cultural competence applies even to one's own group because individuals within groups have unique combinations of characteristics. Another consideration is that many culturally based characteristics are subtle, not noticed, or even purposefully hidden (e.g., sexual orientation, religious affiliations). Thus, nurses need to learn about groups of older adults that may be less visible and smaller in numbers but with unique needs. In recent years, gerontologists are identifying the needs of some of these groups, such as those considered rural or homeless. Other groups, such as those who are discriminated against because of sexual orientation or gender identity, are advocating on their own behalf to identify and address their unique needs. Information about some of these groups is discussed in this section and nurses are encouraged to use the resources listed in Online Learning Activity 2–7 to learn more about these and other groups. Again, as with all aspects of cultural diversity, what is known about a group of people does not necessarily apply to individuals within that group.

Older Adults in Rural Areas

The 2010 U.S. Census classifies "rural" as all those areas outside of an urban area, which is an area with a population density of at least 2500 people per square mile with at least 1500 living in noninstitutional settings. Although the percentage of rural population decreased from 21% in 2000 to 19.3% in 2010, the composition of rural America today is predominantly elderly, with 20% of older adults living in rural areas (National Rural Health Association, 2013). The disproportionate increase in rural elderly is due to younger adults moving to urban areas while long-term residents of rural areas are aging in place. Another population trend that occurred between 2000 and 2010 is that minorities accounted for 82.7% of the population increase in rural areas, with significant geographic and minority group variations as indicated by the following (National Rural Health Association, 2013):

- Hispanics are moving from the Southwest into the Southeast and Midwest.
- The large concentrations of African Americans in the Southeast are being joined by an influx of black migrants from other areas.
- Asian Americans are the smallest minority group in rural areas.

Although significant local differences exist among rural areas, researchers have identified some common characteristics and needs. Rural older adults tend to be poorer and less educated and have less access to stores, transportation, social programs, and health care services. Lack of access to grocery stores, known as "food desert" areas, contributes to increased prevalence of obesity and diabetes in these communities (National Rural Health Association, 2013). Health disparities for rural (vs. urban) residents include higher prevalence of chronic conditions (e.g., diabetes, arthritis, cardiovascular disease), poorer self-rated health, increased functional limitations, and higher mortality rates, particularly for cancer and heart disease (Agency for Healthcare Research and Quality, 2013; Miles & Smith, 2014).

Appalachia is a specific, federally defined, rural nonfarming U.S. region established by an act of Congress in 1965. The region spans more than 1500 miles across 13 states: Alabama, Georgia, Kentucky, Maryland, Mississippi,

New York, North Carolina, Ohio, Pennsylvania, South Carolina, Tennessee, Virginia, and West Virginia. Much of the designated area lies in mountainous territory, causing geographic isolation and lack of access to health care. Appalachian people have been characterized as white, of British or Scotch-Irish descent, and predominantly fundamentalist Protestant in religion. Appalachia has a higher poverty rate and a lower level of formal education than the general population. Appalachian families maintain strong bonds, and older family members are honored for their role in transmitting their culture to younger generations. Older family members are likely to live with or very close to their children.

Appalachian people may be reluctant to seek medical care, particularly in a hospital, because they view the hospital as a place to go to die. Similarly, they may be reluctant to use rehabilitative services because they tend to view illness as the will of God and disability as an inevitable consequence of aging. Although access to usual health care services has been improving, access to specialized medical care is limited. Another factor that influences use of health care services is the strong belief in folk medicine.

Homeless Older Adults

The category of "older homeless" typically extends downward to the age of 50 years because homeless people have significant health problems and other characteristics that are typically associated with older chronologic age. During the past 2 decades the average age of homeless single adults has been increasing, largely due to the elevated risk of homelessness among adults who were born between 1954 and 1963 (Brown, Goodman, Guzman, et al., 2016). Because most people between the ages of 50 and 64 years do not qualify for Medicare, Social Security, or subsidized housing, homelessness in this group is due to a combination of poverty and lack of affordable housing. Health disparities among homeless older adults include significantly higher mortality rates, higher levels of disability, higher overall rates of chronic and mental illnesses, and high rates of geriatric syndromes (e.g., falls, frailty, major depression, urinary incontinence, and cognitive and sensory impairment) (Brown, Hemati, Riley, et al., 2016; Kimber, DeWees, & Harris, 2017).

Lesbian, Gay, Bisexual, and Transgender Older Adults

The acronym LGBT is an umbrella term that includes three groups whose sexual orientation is not heterosexual (lesbian, gay, or bisexual) and several groups whose gender identity and/or gender expression differs from the sex they were assigned at birth (e.g., transgender). Although sexual orientation and gender identity are distinct entities, these subgroups share a common bond of being viewed outside the norms of sexual expression and identity and they all experience similar societal stigma, isolation, stereotypes, and prejudices.

Despite the relatively small numbers of LGBT older adults, there is growing recognition of the unique barriers, challenges, and disparities that affect these groups. See Figure 2-3 for examples. These initiatives and reports identify a need for more evidence-based recommendations addressing health-related needs of subgroups that are currently under the umbrella term of LGBT. Research on LGBT older adults has focused disproportionately on whites, lesbians, and gay men, with very limited attention to bisexual, transgender, racial/ethnic minorities, or those who are 85 years and older. Consequently, it is imperative to keep in mind that conclusions about LGBT older adults are based on limited research and do not necessarily apply to individuals or even subgroups within the larger group.

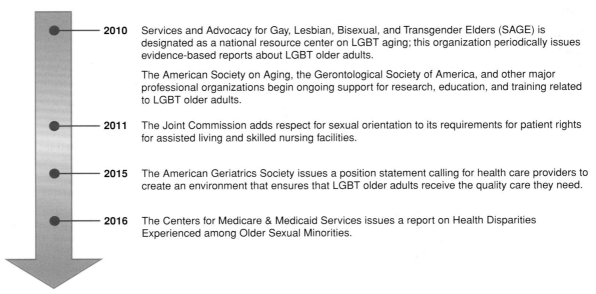

2010 Services and Advocacy for Gay, Lesbian, Bisexual, and Transgender Elders (SAGE) is designated as a national resource center on LGBT aging; this organization periodically issues evidence-based reports about LGBT older adults.

The American Society on Aging, the Gerontological Society of America, and other major professional organizations begin ongoing support for research, education, and training related to LGBT older adults.

2011 The Joint Commission adds respect for sexual orientation to its requirements for patient rights for assisted living and skilled nursing facilities.

2015 The American Geriatrics Society issues a position statement calling for health care providers to create an environment that ensures that LGBT older adults receive the quality care they need.

2016 The Centers for Medicare & Medicaid Services issues a report on Health Disparities Experienced among Older Sexual Minorities.

FIGURE 2-3 Examples of initiatives addressing LGBT older adults.

A common bond among different subgroups of LGBT individuals is their experiences of various levels and types of stigma, but this varies significantly because vastly different sociopolitical forces shape each age group. Cohorts of LGBT older adults older than 70 years entered into young adulthood at a time when homosexuality was considered a crime or a mental illness. This group of older adults has lived through unique experiences including marginalization inside and outside the LGBT community, multidimensional effects of the HIV/AIDS epidemic, and LGBT pride and resilience. Among the subgroups included in LGBT, transgender older adults experience the most stigma, victimization, discrimination, and misunderstandings. Also, Hispanic and African American LGBT older adults experience greater discrimination and lower health-related quality of life than white LGBT older adults (Kim, Jen, & Fredriksen-Goldsen, 2017).

Many LGBT people experience their sexual orientation along a continuum and they do not necessarily live as either heterosexual or gay/lesbian during their entire adult lives. A unique characteristic of LGBT older adults is that more have been in opposite-sex marriages than in same-sex marriages (Fredriksen-Goldsen, Bryan, Jen, et al., 2017). Thus, it is important to recognize that older LGBT individuals vary widely not only in the length of time they have identified themselves as such but also in the ways in which they have addressed their sexual identities.

Some LGBT have biologic, adopted, or step children, grandchildren, or great grandchildren and very close relationships with their families. Other LGBT older adults have no biologic family—or have been rejected by their families—but they have strong bonds with their "family of choice." Studies indicate an important source of strength for most LGBT older adults is support of their friends and peers (Fredrisksen-Goldsen, 2016). Older LGBT vary greatly in their intimate relationships and many have had or continue to have monogamous committed partnerships. In 2015, same-sex marriages became legally recognized in the United States; however, some older LGBT in long-term relationships choose to continue in their unmarried status (sometimes due to financial, legal, or family concerns). An important aspect of providing culturally competent care for LGBT older adults is using gender-neutral terminology in reference to intimate or partner relationships, which is a topic discussed in Chapter 26.

Despite the prominence of health disparities (see Box 2-1) and the effects of other issues that affect LGBT older adults, there is much evidence pointing toward resilience and strengths. On a positive note, many older adults who identify as lesbian, gay, bisexual, or transgender report that their experiences prepare them for aging by helping them overcome adversity. Strengths identified in studies include resiliency, greater inner strength, being more accepting of others, not taking anything for granted, being more resilient, having greater inner strength, having greater self-reliance, having a chosen family, and being more careful about legal and financial matters (Fredriksen-Goldsen, 2017).

 See ONLINE LEARNING ACTIVITY 2-7: RESOURCES FOR INFORMATION ABOUT RURAL, HOMELESS, AND LGBT OLDER AMERICANS at http://thepoint.lww.com/Miller8e.

Chapter Highlights

Cultural Diversity in the United States
- The population of the United States is increasing in diversity to the point that non-Hispanic whites will comprise less than half the population by 2044.
- The older adult population in the United States is increasing in diversity (Figure 2-1).
- Gerontologists are identifying health care needs of many diverse subgroups of older adults by characteristics such as race/ethnicity, socioeconomic factors, rural residency, homelessness, and self-identification as LGBT.

Health Disparities
- Members of racial or ethnic groups experience many health disparities, and these have significant implications for older adults (Box 2-1, Figure 2-2).

Health Literacy
- Health literacy is increasingly addressed as a major determinant of health outcomes and a measure of quality of care.

Cultural Competence
- All nurses are expected to develop cultural competence by assessing their own attitudes (Box 2-2) and learning about culturally diverse groups.
- All health care providers need to be linguistically competent and to use resources to address needs of patients who are not proficient in English (Box 2-3).

Cultural Perspectives on Wellness
- Nurses need to explore what health and wellness mean to individual older adults.
- Definitions of health and wellness are rooted in the three major health belief systems (Box 2-4).

Overview of Cultural Groups of Older Adults in the United States
- Racial and ethnic groups as categorized by the U.S. Census are American Indian and Alaska Native, Asian American, black or African American, Hispanics or Latinos, Native Hawaiian and Pacific Islanders, and multiracial.
- Nurses can develop cultural competence by educating themselves about the cultural traditions of the older adults in their geographic areas.
- Because groups are composed of many subgroups and individuals and there is great diversity within these groups, it is imperative to avoid generalizations.

Older Adults in Other Diverse Groups

- Rural older adults tend to be poorer and less educated and have limited access to stores, transportation, social programs, and health care services.
- The population of older homeless single adults is increasing, with older adults who were born between 1954 and 1963 already being the predominant subgroup.
- Health care professionals need to develop cultural competency related to caring for LGBT older adults.

Critical Thinking Exercises

1. Complete the cultural self-assessment in Box 2-2 and think about how you are similar to and differ from the many cultural groups to which you belong.
2. Reflect on your encounters during the past few weeks with people who differ from you culturally. Make a list of the obvious differences and another list of differences that you may not have recognized but most likely existed (e.g., you most likely interacted with someone who was LGBT). Ask yourself how accepting and nonjudgmental you feel about these people.
3. Identify one culturally diverse group that you are likely to work with in your current geographic area. Contact local agencies and organizations that serve these groups and find out what services they offer; ask about unique health care issues affecting these particular groups.
4. Use Online Learning Activity 2-2 to find information that you might use if you were presenting a health education program to a group of older adults who are of a particular cultural background (e.g., Chinese, American Indian, African American). Think about how the health promotion materials for a specific cultural/ethnic group differ from those that have been developed for whites.
5. Think of the various settings in which you work with older adults and describe what you would do or whom you would call if you needed to communicate with a patient who did not speak English.

 For more information about the topics discussed in this chapter, be sure to check out the interactive Online Learning Activities and other helpful resources at http://thepoint.lww.com/Miller8e.

REFERENCES

Agency for Healthcare Research and Quality. (2013). *2012 National Healthcare Disparities Report.* Rockville, MD: Agency for Healthcare Research and Quality, publication number 13–0003.

American Geriatrics Society. (2016). Achieving high-quality multicultural geriatric care. *Journal of the American Geriatrics Society, 64,* 255–260.

Andrews M. M. (2016a). Culturally competent nursing care. In M. M. Andrews & J. S. Boyle (Eds.). *Transcultural concepts in nursing care* (6th ed., pp. 30–54). Philadelphia, PA: Wolters Kluwer.

Andrews M. M. (2016b). The influence of cultural and health belief systems on health care practices. In M. M. Andrews & J. S. Boyle (Eds.). *Transcultural concepts in nursing care* (6th ed., pp. 102–118). Philadelphia, PA: Wolters Kluwer.

Brown, R., Goodman, L., Guzman, D., et al. (2016). Pathways to homelessness among older homeless adults: Results from the HOPE HOME Study. *PLOS One,* doi: 10.1371/journal.pone.0155065.

Brown, R. T., Hemati, K., Riley, E. D., et al. (2016). Geriatric conditions in a population-based sample of older homeless adults. [Epub] doi: 10.1003/geront/gnw011.

Campinha-Bacote. (2013). People of African American Heritage. In L. D. Purnell (Ed.): *Transcultural health care: A culturally competent approach* (pp. 91–114). Philadelphia, PA: F. A. Davis.

Centers for Medicare and Medicaid. (2017). *Understanding communication and language needs of Medicare beneficiaries.* Available at www.cms.gov

Chatters, L. M., Nguyen, A. W., & Taylor, R. J. (2014). Religion and spirituality among older African Americans. In K. E. Whitfield & T. A. Baker (Eds.). *Handbook of minority aging* (pp. 47–64). New York: Springer Publishing.

Colby, S., & Ortman, J. (2015). Projections of the size and composition of the U. S. population: 2014 to 2060. Available at www.census.gov

Federal Interagency Forum on Aging. (2016). *Older Americans 2016: Key indicators of well-being.* Washington, DC: U.S. Government Printing Office.

Fredriksen-Goldsen, K. I. (2016). The future of LGBT + aging: A blueprint for action in services, policies and research. *Generations, 40,* 6–13.

Fredriksen-Goldsen, K. I. (2017). Dismantling the silence: LGBTQ aging emerging from the margins. *The Gerontologist, 57,* 121–128.

Fredriksen-Goldsen, K. I., Dryan, A., Jen, S., et al. (2017). The unfolding of LGBT lives: Key events associated with health and well-being in later life. *Gerontologist, 57*(Suppl 1), S15–S29.

Giger, J. N. (2017). *Transcultural nursing.* St. Louis, MO: Elsevier.

Go, A. S., Mozaffarian, D., Roger, V. L., et al. (2014). Heart disease and stroke statistics: 2014 update: A report from the American Heart Association. *Circulation, 128,* e1–e267.

Huff, R. M., Kline, M. V., & Peterson, D. V. (2015). *Health promotion in multicultural populations* (3rd ed.). Los Angeles: Sage.

Hummer, R. A., Melvin, J. E., Sheehan, C. M., et al. (2014). Race/ethnicity, mortality, and longevity. In K. E. Whitfield & T. A. Baker (Eds.). *Handbook of minority aging* (pp. 131–152). New York: Springer Publishing.

Institute of Medicine. (2013). Health Literacy: Improving health, health systems, and health policy around the world: Workshop summary. Washington, DC: National Academies Press.

Kim, H. J., Jen, S., & Fredriksen-Goldsen, K. I. (2017). Race/ethnicity and health-related quality of life among LGBT older adults. *The Gerontologist, 57,* S1, S30–S39.

Kimbler, K. J., DeWees, M. A., & Harris, A. N. (2017). Characteristics of the old and homeless: Identifying distinct service needs. *Aging and Mental Health, 21,* 190–198.

Kobayashi, L., Wardle, J., Wolf, M., et al. (2016). Aging and functional health literacy: A systematic review and meta-analysis. *Journals of Gerontology: Psychological Sciences and Social Sciences, 71,* 445–457.

Kopera-Frye, K. (2017). *Health literacy among older adults.* New York: Springer Publishing Company.

MacLeod, S., Musich, S., Gulyas, S., et al. (2017). The impact of inadequate health literacy on patient satisfaction, healthcare utilization, and expenditures among older adults. *Geriatric Nursing.* [Epub] doi: 10.1016/j.gerinurse.2016.12.003.

Matthews, K., Croft, J., Liu, Y., et al. (2017). Health-related behaviors by urban-rural county classification – United States, 2013. Available at www.cdc.gov

Mezuk B., & Gallo J. J. (2013). Depression and medical illness in late life. In H. Lavretsky, M. Sajatovic & C. F. Reynolds, III (Eds.). *Late-life mood disorders* (pp. 270–294). Oxford: Oxford University Press.

Miles, T. P., & Smith, M. L. (2014). Does health care quality contribute to disparities? An examination of aging and minority status issues in America. In K. E. Whitfield & T. A. Baker (Eds.). *Handbook of minority aging* (pp. 237–255). New York: Springer Publishing Company.

Moss, M. P. (2016). *American Indian health and nursing.* New York: Springer Publishing Company.

National Center for Health Statistics. (2016). *Health United States, 2015.* Table 17: Selected causes of death sex, race, and Hispanic origin: United States 2014. Available at cdc.gov/nchs

National Rural Health Association Policy Brief. (2013). *Elder health in rural America.* Available at www.nhra.org

National Rural Health Association Policy Brief. (2016). *American Indian and Alaska Native health.* Available at www.nhra.org

Pew Research Center. (2016). *Hispanic trends: Statistical portrait of Hispanics in the United States.* Available at www.pewresearch.org

Pew Research Center. (2017). *Hispanic trends: Among new arrivals, Asians outnumber Hispanics.* Available at www.pewresearch.org

Purnell, L. D. (2013). *Transcultural health care: A culturally competent approach.* Philadelphia, PA: F. A. Davis.

Rodriguez-Galan, M. B. (2014). The ethnography of ethnic minority families and aging: Familism and beyond. In *Handbook of minority aging* (pp. 435–453). New York: Springer Publishing.

Rooks R. N., & Thorpe R. J. (2014). Understanding age at onset and self-care management to explain racial and ethnic cardiovascular disease disparities in middle- and older-age adults. In K. E. Whitfield & T. A. Baker (Eds.). *Handbook of minority aging* (pp. 471–496). New York: Springer Publishing.

Rose, P. (2017). *Health, disparities, diversity, and inclusion.* Burlington, MA: Jones & Bartlett Learning.

Social Security Administration. (2013). *Asian Americans and Pacific Islanders.* Available at www.ssa.gov/aapi/index.htm

Spector, R. (2017). *Cultural diversity in health and illness.* New York: Pearson.

U.S. Census Bureau. (2016). *American Indian and Alaska Native Heritage Month: November 2016.* Available at www.census.gov.

U.S. Census Bureau. (2017). *Asian-American and Pacific Islander Heritage Month: May* 2017.

Weinstein, J., Geller, A., Negussie, Y., et al. (2017). *Communities in action: Pathways to health equity.* Washington, DC: National Academies Press.

chapter 3

Applying a Nursing Model for Promoting Wellness in Older Adults

LEARNING OBJECTIVES

After reading this chapter, you will be able to:

1. Discuss the concepts that underpin the Functional Consequences Theory in older adults.

2. Define concepts of age-related changes, risk factors, and functional consequences as they relate to nursing care of older adults.

3. Describe the domains of nursing (i.e., person, nursing, health, environment) in the context of the Functional Consequences Theory.

4. Apply the Functional Consequences Theory to the practice of nursing to promote wellness in older adults.

KEY TERMS

age-related changes

environment

functional consequences

Functional Consequences Theory for Promoting Wellness in Older Adults

health

interprofessional collaboration

negative functional consequences

nursing

older adult

person

positive functional consequences

risk factors

wellness

wellness outcomes

As discussed in Chapter 1, myths about aging are insidious and pervasive in society and form the foundation of ageism, which has serious detrimental effects on older adults. Nurses are influenced not only by societal myths and ageist attitudes but also by their experiences with older adults in health care settings, which often reinforce the perception that older adults are frail, confused, depressed, and dependent. These attitudes can lead to a sense of pessimism—or even hopelessness—regarding caring for older adults. Fortunately, knowledge can be an effective antidote to ageism, and the theoretical base of information about aging has expanded exponentially during the past half-century. Research-based information enables health care providers to differentiate between age-related changes that are inevitable and risk factors that can be addressed or even prevented. Chapters in this text provide research-based information about age-related changes and risk factors affecting a particular aspect of functioning, with emphasis on the changes and risks that nurses can address. Nurses can apply this information to promote wellness for older adults by identifying ways of improving functioning and quality of life.

As discussed in Chapter 4, theories about aging and older adults attempt to answer questions about why and how people age, and they provide a base for identifying the risk factors that health care providers can address. However, they do not address *nursing* care of older adults, as does a *nursing theory* that explains relationships among the core concepts of person, nursing, health, and environment. Discipline-specific nursing theories guide nursing care and are essential to promoting wellness for older adults. The Functional Consequences Theory for Promoting Wellness in Older Adults, which is delineated in this chapter and used throughout this text, provides a framework that nurses can use to promote wellness and improve functioning and quality of life for older adults.

A NURSING THEORY FOR WELLNESS-FOCUSED CARE OF OLDER ADULTS

During the 1980s, this author proposed a model for gerontological nursing, which was the organizational framework for the first edition of this book (Miller, 1990). Since its inception, this model has emphasized the significant role of nurses in using health education interventions to promote optimal health, functioning, and quality of life for older adults. In the fifth and sixth editions, some terminology was revised to reflect current emphasis on adding life to years in conjunction with adding years to life. Thus, the model is now called the Functional Consequences Theory for Promoting Wellness in Older Adults. In addition, the updated model reflects and incorporates the evolving understanding of wellness as an integral aspect of health care. Nurses are among the health care professionals who have increasingly emphasized the need to incorporate wellness-oriented goals into their care plans. The Functional Consequences Theory can be used to achieve these goals in all aspects of nursing care for older adults because it addresses essential questions, such as *"What is unique about promoting wellness for older adults?"* and *"How can nurses address the unique wellness needs of older adults?"*

The purpose of nursing theories is to describe, explain, predict, or prescribe nursing care based on scientific evidence. Since the time of Florence Nightingale, nurses have developed theories that address the relationships among the domains of person, nursing, health, and environment. The Functional Consequences Theory is based on a combination of research on aging and health and the author's more than four decades of providing nursing care for older adults. It also draws on theories that emphasize concepts related to wellness, health promotion, and holistic nursing. In this text, up-to-date and evidence-based information about specific aspects of functioning is applied to nursing care of older adults in the framework of the Functional Consequences Theory. Basic premises of the Functional Consequences Theory are as follows:

- Holistic nursing care addresses the body–mind–spirit interconnectedness of each older adult and recognizes that wellness encompasses more than physiologic functioning.
- Although age-related changes are inevitable, many risk factors can be prevented or alleviated.
- Older adults experience positive or negative functional consequences because of a combination of age-related changes and risk factors.
- Interventions can be directed toward alleviating or modifying the negative functional consequences of risk factors.
- Nurses can promote wellness in older adults through health promotion interventions and other nursing actions that address the negative functional consequences.
- Nursing interventions result in positive functional consequences, also called wellness outcomes, which enable older people to function at their highest level despite the presence of age-related changes and risk factors.

This theoretical framework, shown in Figure 3-1, can be illustrated by the following example. Because of age-related visual changes, older adults experience an increased sensitivity to glare and have difficulty seeing clearly when they face bright lights or when lights reflect off shiny surfaces.

For instance, older adults may have difficulty seeing clearly when they are driving toward the sunlight or reading shopping mall maps in glass cases. In addition to this age-related change, older adults are likely to have disease-related conditions, such as cataracts, that further interfere with their visual abilities. In addition, environmental factors, such as bright lights, highly polished floors, and white or glossy paint, can intensify glare. These age-related changes and risk factors can interfere with vision to the extent that older adults stop performing activities or perform them unsafely.

To counteract these functional consequences, the older person or a nurse can initiate any of the following interventions, which are discussed in Chapter 17:

- Wearing sunglasses and using glare-reducing glasses (self-care)
- Addressing environmental conditions by using adequate nonglare lighting (self-care)
- Obtaining periodic evaluations from an ophthalmologist (self-care)
- Teaching about the use of sunglasses and glare-reducing glasses (nursing action)
- Teaching about and facilitating environmental modifications (nursing action)
- Taking actions to avoid glare (e.g., not standing in front of a bright window when talking with an older adult) (nursing action)
- Teaching older adults about the importance of having their eyes evaluated at least annually for treatable conditions (nursing action)

Wellness outcomes resulting from these interventions include improved safety, function, and quality of life.

CONCEPTS UNDERLYING THE FUNCTIONAL CONSEQUENCES THEORY

The Functional Consequences Theory draws from theories that are pertinent to aging, older adults, and holistic nursing. The nursing domain concepts of person, environment, health, and nursing are linked together specifically in relation to older adults. Before discussing these domain concepts, however, the concepts of functional consequences, age-related changes, and risk factors are explained. Box 3-1 summarizes the key concepts in the Functional Consequences Theory for Promoting Wellness in Older Adults.

Functional Consequences

Functional consequences are the observable effects of actions, risk factors, and age-related changes that influence the quality of life or day-to-day activities of older adults. Actions include, but are not limited to, purposeful interventions initiated by either older adults (i.e., self-care) or nurses (i.e., nursing interventions) and other caregivers. Risk factors can originate in the environment or arise from physiologic and psychosocial influences. Functional consequences are

A Nursing Model for Promoting Wellness in Older Adults

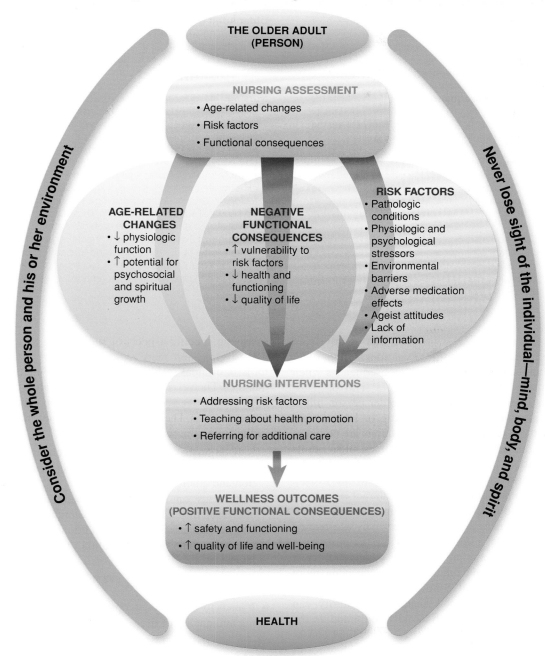

FIGURE 3-1 The Functional Consequences Theory for Promoting Wellness in Older Adults. Age-related changes and risk factors combine to cause negative functional consequences. Nurses holistically assess older adults and initiate interventions to counteract or minimize negative functional consequences. Nursing actions result in wellness outcomes.

negative when they interfere with a person's level of function or quality of life or increase a person's dependency. Conversely, they are positive when they facilitate the highest level of performance and the least amount of dependency.

Negative functional consequences typically occur because of a combination of age-related changes and risk factors, as illustrated in the example of impaired visual performance. They also may be caused by interventions, in which case the interventions become risk factors. For example, constipation resulting from the use of an analgesic medication is an example of a negative functional consequence caused by an intervention. In this case, the medication is both an intervention for pain and a risk factor for impaired bowel function.

Box 3-1 Concepts in the Functional Consequences Theory for Promoting Wellness in Older Adults

Functional Consequences: Observable effects of actions, risk factors, and age-related changes that influence the quality of life or day-to-day activities of older adults. The effects relate to all levels of functioning, including body, mind, and spirit.
- **Negative functional consequences:** Those that interfere with the older adult's functioning or quality of life.
- **Positive functional consequences:** Those that facilitate the highest level of functioning, the least dependency, and the best quality of life. When positive functional consequences are the result of nursing interventions, they are called wellness outcomes.

Age-Related Changes: Inevitable, progressive, and irreversible changes that occur during later adulthood and are independent of extrinsic or pathologic conditions. On the physiologic level, these changes are typically degenerative; however, on psychological and spiritual levels, they include potential for growth.

Risk Factors: Conditions that increase the vulnerability of older adults to negative functional consequences. Common sources of risk factors include diseases, environment, lifestyle, support systems, psychosocial circumstances, adverse medication effects, and attitudes based on lack of knowledge.

Older Adult (Person): A complex and unique individual whose functioning and well-being are influenced by the acquisition of age-related changes and risk factors. When risk factors cause the older adult to be dependent on others for daily needs, their caregivers are considered an integral focus of nursing care.

Nursing: The focus of nursing care is to minimize the negative effects of age-related changes and risk factors and to promote wellness outcomes. Goals are achieved through the nursing process, with particular emphasis on health promotion and other nursing interventions that address the negative functional consequences.

Health: The ability of older adults to function at their highest capacity, despite the presence of age-related changes and risk factors. It is not limited to physiologic function and encompasses psychosocial and spiritual function. Thus, it addresses well-being and quality of life as defined by each older adult.

Environment: External conditions, including caregivers, that influence the body, mind, spirit, and functioning of older adults. Environmental conditions are risk factors when they interfere with function, and they are interventions when they enhance function.

Positive functional consequences can result from automatic actions or purposeful interventions. Often, older adults bring about positive functional consequences when they compensate for age-related changes with or without conscious intent. For example, an older person might increase the amount of light for reading or begin using sunglasses without realizing that these actions are compensating for age-related changes. At other times, older adults initiate interventions in response to a recognized need. In the example cited earlier, improved function would likely result from purposeful interventions, such as cataract surgery or environmental modifications. In a few instances, positive functional consequences are caused directly by age-related changes. For example, a woman may view the postmenopausal inability to become pregnant as a positive effect of aging. Consequently, sexual relationships may become more satisfying in later adulthood. Similarly, positive functional consequences, such as increased wisdom and maturity, can result from psychological growth in older adulthood. In the context of the nursing process, positive functional consequences are called wellness outcomes because they result from purposeful nursing interventions.

The concept of functional consequences draws on concepts and research regarding functional assessment, which focuses on a person's ability to perform activities of daily living that affect survival, overall health, and quality of life, as discussed in Chapter 7. From a research perspective, functional assessment provides a framework for research and a method for planning health services for dependent people. From a clinical perspective, health care practitioners view the multidimensional functional assessment as an important component in the care of older people. Evidence-based tools are widely available for

assessing specific aspects of functioning and activities of daily living, and there is strong support for using these tools in clinical settings. Although the Functional Consequences Theory draws on concepts related to functional assessment, its scope is much broader. The Functional Consequences Theory differs from functional assessment in the following ways:
- It distinguishes between age-related changes that increase a person's vulnerability and risk factors that affect function and quality of life.
- It focuses on functional consequences that can be addressed through nursing interventions.
- It focuses on assessment of conditions that affect functioning, rather than on identification of a person's functional level.
- It leads to interventions that address negative functional consequences.
- It leads to wellness outcomes, such as improved functioning and quality of life.

Many standardized and easy-to-use assessment tools are available for use in clinical settings, and those that are most pertinent to nursing care of older adults are cited in clinically oriented chapters of this text. In addition, all clinically oriented chapters contain comprehensive assessment and intervention boxes that apply evidence-based information to a wellness-oriented approach to nursing care of older adults (see list in the front of this book).

Age-Related Changes and Risk Factors

A unique challenge of caring for older adults is the need to differentiate between age-related changes and risk factors, because the interventions for age-related changes differ from those for risk factors. Age-related changes cannot be reversed or altered, but it is possible to compensate for their effects so that wellness outcomes are achieved. By contrast, risk factors can be modified or eliminated to improve functioning and quality of life for older adults.

In the Functional Consequences Theory, **age-related changes** are the inherent physiologic processes that increase the vulnerability of older people to the detrimental effects of risk factors. From a body–mind–spirit perspective, however, age-related changes are not limited to physiologic aspects but include potential for increased cognitive, emotional, and spiritual development. Thus, nurses holistically focus on the whole person by identifying age-related changes that can be strengthened to improve the older adult's ability to adapt to physiologic decline. For example, nurses can work with older adults to strengthen their coping skills, as discussed in Chapter 12. In addition, nurses have many opportunities to build on the wisdom of older adults, especially their "everyday problem-solving" skills (as discussed in Chapter 11), by teaching about interventions to address risk factors.

The definition of age-related changes in the context of the Functional Consequences Theory draws primarily on research on aging. Biologic theories can help differentiate between age-related and disease-related processes; usually, however, there is some overlap among these processes as discussed in Chapter 4. In addition to biologic theories of aging, other theories about aging and older adulthood can shed light on age-related changes that contribute to the ability of older adults to respond to the challenges of aging. Clinically oriented chapters in this text discuss research on age-related changes pertinent to specific aspects of functioning.

A Student's Perspective

Most older adults live outside nursing homes and are actively involved in maintaining their independence and functional abilities as much as possible. Having worked in an acute care setting for many years, it is very easy for me to assume that all older adults have many underlying chronic diseases and do very little to comply with their medical therapies. It does help to separate what is a part of the aging process from what is part of a chronic condition, since problems resulting from chronic conditions may be receptive to medical and nursing interventions.

Darris C.

Risk factors are the conditions that are likely to occur in older adults and have a significant detrimental effect on their health and functioning. Risk factors commonly arise from environments, acute and chronic conditions, psychosocial conditions, or adverse medication effects. Although many risk factors also occur in younger adults, they are more likely to have serious functional consequences in older adults because of the following characteristics:

- They are cumulative and progressive (e.g., long-term effects of smoking, obesity, inadequate exercise, or poor dietary habits).
- The effects are exacerbated by age-related changes (e.g., effects of arthritis are exacerbated by diminished muscle strength).
- The effects may be mistakenly viewed as age-related changes rather than reversible and treatable conditions (e.g., cognitive changes from adverse medication effects may be attributed to normal aging or dementia).
- They would not have negative functional consequences in a younger person (e.g., glare or background noise would not affect the vision or hearing of someone who is not experiencing age-related sensory changes).

Researchers and health care providers commonly address risk factors in relation to prevention and treatment of medical conditions. For example, evidence-based practice guidelines for pharmacologic or surgical treatments often weigh the probable risks versus benefits. Similarly, researchers focus on identifying risk factors for developing conditions, such as heart disease, so these risks can be addressed through health promotion interventions.

Nurses incorporate the concept of risk factors in many aspects of the nursing process. For example, many nursing diagnoses, interventions, and outcomes address risk control, risk identification, or risk detection. In the context of nursing diagnosis, NANDA-International states that "sometimes a risk diagnosis can be the diagnosis with the highest priority for a patient" (Gallagher-Lepak, 2018, p. 38). A major focus of wellness-focused nursing is to identify risk factors that can be addressed through health promotion interventions. For example, from a health promotion perspective, nurses routinely assess for risks associated with stress, smoking, obesity, poor nutrition, and inadequate physical activity. An aspect that is unique to caring for older adults is the need to identify myths or ageist attitudes that can affect health care. For example, if urinary incontinence is mistakenly attributed to "normal" aging, then the older adult will not receive appropriate evaluation and interventions. Environmental risks are also particularly pertinent to older adults because additional risk factors, such as sensory, mobility, or cognitive impairments, can compromise their safety and functioning. Identification of risk factors is an integral aspect of the Functional Consequences Theory because nurses have numerous opportunities for promoting wellness by identifying and addressing the many modifiable factors that affect functioning and quality of life for older adults.

Person

In the Functional Consequences Theory, the concept of **person** applies specifically to older adults. Because the holistic approach of the theory views each **older adult** as a complex and unique individual whose functioning and well-being are influenced by many internal and external factors, older adults are not defined simply according to chronologic criteria. From this perspective, an older adult is characterized by the acquisition of physiologic and psychosocial characteristics that are associated with increasing maturity. Physiologic characteristics include slowing down of physiologic processes, compromised ability to respond to physiologic stress, and increased vulnerability to pathologic conditions and other risk factors. Psychosocial characteristics include an increased potential for psychosocial strengths, such as wisdom and creativity, and the potential for advanced levels of personal and spiritual growth.

Because aging is a complex and gradual process involving all aspects of body, mind, and spirit, a person does not suddenly become an older adult at a particular chronologic age. Rather, people who live long enough recognize at some point that they have reached a stage of life that society categorizes as older adulthood. When they reach this point, they may or may not identify with social labels, such as elder, senior, or older adult. Although this conceptual approach has the distinct disadvantage of being difficult to measure, it has the advantage of accurately reflecting the realities of older adulthood as one part of the life-course continuum. Because people become more heterogeneous rather than homogeneous as they age, any definition of the older adult must, by its nature, be broad. In the context of the Functional Consequences Theory, an individual is an older adult when he or she manifests several or many functional consequences attributable to age-related changes alone or to age-related changes in combination with risk factors. Stated simply, it is the accumulation of age-related functional consequences that is the core criterion for defining someone as an older adult. Moreover, because aging involves many gradual, interacting, and cumulative processes, each older adult experiences his or her own unique continuum. This concept is applied in the unfolding case examples in chapters of Parts 3 and 4 of this book, with each case illustrating the progression of an individual from young–old to old–old as he or she is affected by functional consequences pertinent to a particular aspect of functioning. These unfolding case examples illustrate roles of nurses in promoting wellness for an older adult as he or she experiences several phases of health and illness during the course of older adulthood.

The older adult is further conceptualized in the context of his or her relationships with others because a person is not an isolated entity but a dynamic being who continually influences and is influenced by the environment and other people. This context is particularly important for older adults, because the more functionally impaired a person is, the more important are support resources and environmental factors. When functional consequences accumulate to the extent that the older adult depends on others for daily needs, nurses broaden their focus to include caregivers during nursing assessments and interventions. In all circumstances, it is important to address the needs of older adults in the context of their relationships because older people have a long history of interpersonal relationships that influence their health behaviors and well-being.

Although no characteristics are universally applicable to all older adults, all are affected by the cumulative effects of aging and all are vulnerable to the effects of risk factors. Thus, it is imperative to be knowledgeable about normal aging so nursing care can address negative functional consequences. The Functional Consequences Theory emphasizes the importance of identifying and respecting the unique characteristics of each older adult that affect his or her functioning and well-being.

Nursing

The conceptualization of **nursing** in the Functional Consequences Theory draws on nursing theories, including those of long-established theorists, as described in Box 3-2. An additional aspect of the Functional Consequences Theory is its emphasis on person-centered care, which focuses on older adults as the center of their own care. The individualized needs of older adults are addressed and there is a sharing of power and responsibility. Nurses involve older adults in decision making because they recognize that older adults are experts in their own health. In addition, the person-centered approach includes families and caregivers as appropriate in all aspects of assessment, planning, and interventions. The approach used throughout this text is consistent with current emphasis on person-centered, family-centered, and culture-centered health care, based on a comprehensive assessment of individual needs and preferences. Content for all clinically oriented chapters is presented in the framework of the nursing process and applied to a particular aspect of functioning. The first figure in most chapters illustrates how nurses can apply the Functional Consequences Theory to their nursing care of older adults in relation to a specific aspect of functioning.

Health and Wellness

The Functional Consequences Theory defines **health** as the ability of older adults to function at their highest capacity,

---

Box 3-2 Nursing Theories That Support the Conceptualization of Nursing in the Functional Consequences Theory

Florence Nightingale: Nurses foster an environment conducive to healing and health promotion.

Virginia Henderson: Nurses provide assistance with daily activities to help patients/clients gain independence as rapidly as possible.

Imogene King: Nurse and client interact to achieve a specific health-related goal.

Jean Watson: Nursing consists of knowledge, thought, values, philosophy, commitment, and action with passion in human care transactions.

Martha Rogers: Nurses promote person–environment interactions for unitary human beings.

Margaret Newman: Nursing is the act of assisting people to use their power to evolve toward higher levels of consciousness.

despite the presence of age-related changes and risk factors. It encompasses psychosocial as well as physiologic function, including well-being and quality of life as defined by each older adult. In this model, health is individually determined, based on the functional capacities that are perceived as important by that person. For example, one person might define the desired level of function as a capacity for intimate relationships, whereas another might define it as being able to perform aerobic exercise for half an hour daily. Definitions of health by major nursing theorists that are consistent with the conceptualization of health in the Functional Consequences Theory are summarized in Box 3-3.

Wellness is a closely related concept that is used throughout this book in reference to the person's highest potential for well-being. A concept analysis of wellness in older adults described it as "a purposeful process of individual growth, integration of experience, and meaningful connection with others, reflecting personally valued goals and strengths, and resulting in being well and living values" (McMahon & Fleury, 2012, p. 48). Similarly, in the context of current emphasis on person-centered care, wellness is conceptualized as "the meaning a person brings to his/her life experience, and yes, that life experience may include living with and managing disease" (Fulton, 2016, p. 136). These concepts are consistent with the Functional Consequences Theory as it is applied to the nursing care of older adults.

Environment

In the Functional Consequences Theory, **environment** is a broad concept that includes all aspects of the setting in which the care is provided; for dependent older adults, the environment also includes their caregivers. Some aspects of

---

Box 3-3 Definitions of Health That Support the Conceptualization of Health in the Functional Consequences Theory

Florence Nightingale: to be well, but to be able to use well every power we have
Imogene King: a dynamic life experience involving continuous adjustment to stressors through optimum use of one's resources to achieve maximum potential for daily living
Callista Roy: a state and process of being and becoming integrated and whole
Jean Watson: unity and harmony within the mind, body, and soul; congruence between the self as perceived and the self as experienced
Margaret Newman: expanding consciousness; evolving pattern of the whole of life
Rosemarie Parse: a way of being in the world; the living of day-to-day ways of being
Madeleine Leininger: a state of well-being that is culturally constituted, defined, valued, and practiced by individuals or groups that enables them to function in their daily lives
Nola Pender: the actualization of inherent and acquired human potential through goal-directed behavior, competent self-care, and satisfying relationships with others

---

Box 3-4 Definitions of Environment From Nursing Theories That Are Pertinent to the Functional Consequences Theory

Florence Nightingale: A healthy environment is essential for healing and includes specific aspects such as noise level, cleanliness, and nutritious food
Madeleine Leininger: The totality of an event, situation, or particular experience that gives meaning to human expressions, interpretations, and social interactions in particular physical, ecologic, sociopolitical, and cultural settings
Imogene King: The background for human interactions, which is both internal and external to the individual
Margaret Newman: All internal and external factors of influences that surround the client or system
Callista Roy: All conditions, circumstances, and influences that surround and affect the development and behavior of humans

---

the conceptualization may seem to be contradictory because the environment can be a source of both negative functional consequences and wellness outcomes. For example, the environment is a risk factor when it interferes with functioning (e.g., glare or poor lighting), but it also can facilitate wellness outcomes when it is used to improve functioning (e.g., grab bars, or bright and nonglare lighting). Box 3-4 summarizes some nursing conceptualizations of the environment that are pertinent to the Functional Consequences Theory.

Since the 1970s, gerontologists have studied the influence of the environment on functioning of older adults. For example, the Person–Environment Fit Theory (discussed in Chapter 4) focuses on the interrelationship between the individual person and his or her environment. This theory has been used in studies of the effects of physical and social environments on many aspects of functioning and quality of life for older adults. Current emphasis is on the need to develop age-friendly environments in communities as well as supportive environments for older adults in long-term care settings (Davis & Weisbeck, 2016; Menec, Newall, & Nowicki, 2016; Rodiek, Nejati, Bardenhagen, et al., 2016). Some of the questions that gerontologists as well as nurses address include the following:

- How does the environment affect the older adult's level of functioning?
- How does the environment affect the older adult's quality of life?
- Is the environment comfortable for the older adult?
- Is the environment a source of risks that interfere with functioning and well-being of the older adults, for example, does it increase the risk for falls?
- How can the environment be adapted to improve functioning for the older adult?

Throughout this text, the Functional Consequences Theory provides a framework for addressing questions such as these as an integral part of the nursing assessment and interventions for specific aspects of functioning.

In addition to focusing on the environment as it affects older adults individually, this text focuses on broader aspects of the older adult's environment, such as social supports, interpersonal relationships, and emotional and spiritual factors. Also, in keeping with current emphasis on the effects of health care environments, this text addresses the practice environments in which nurses care for older adults, including institutional, home, and community settings. This is consistent with the increasing recognition that interprofessional collaboration is an essential component of all health care environments. Nurses have crucial leadership roles in assuring that care for older adults is provided in an environment that is based on interprofessional collaboration. This topic is discussed in more detail in Chapter 6, and throughout this text content related to this topic is designated by the icon or with an IPC bar to the right of the text (as shown here). Online Learning Activity 3-1 provides a link to an article describing environments of care in relation to the nursing theories and the practice of nursing.

See ONLINE LEARNING ACTIVITY 3-1: ARTICLE, A PRACTICE THEORY APPROACH TO UNDERSTANDING THE INTERDEPENDENCY OF NURSING PRACTICE AND THE ENVIRONMENT at http://thepoint.lww.com/Miller8e.

 Interprofessional Collaboration

Characteristics of environments of interprofessional collaboration are: (a) the patient and family are always at the center of care, (b) health care team members communicate effectively, and (c) a shared decision-making approach encourages the full contribution of all involved (Talley, 2016).

APPLYING THE THEORY TO PROMOTE WELLNESS IN OLDER ADULTS

In the context of the Functional Consequences Theory, nurses direct their care toward addressing risk factors and promoting wellness outcomes for older adults. The focus and goals of this type of care vary in different settings. For acute care, the focus is on treatment of pathologic conditions that create serious risks; goals include helping vulnerable older adults recover from illness and maintain or improve their level of functioning. For long-term care, the focus is on addressing multiple risk factors that interfere with functional abilities; goals include improved functioning and quality of life. The Functional Consequences Theory is particularly pertinent in rehabilitation settings, where the focus is on preventing negative functional consequences and promoting wellness outcomes (Gouveia, Jardim, & Martins, 2011). For home and community settings, the focus is on short- and long-term interventions aimed at age-related changes and risk factors; goals include improving or preventing declines in functioning and addressing quality-of-life concerns. In all settings, nurses can incorporate wellness outcomes to address each older

adult's personal aspirations toward well-being of body, mind, and spirit. Examples of these wellness outcomes are delineated in all clinically oriented chapters of this text.

A Student's Perspective

Today I cared for L.C., who has had two previous cerebrovascular accidents, with the second one leading to left-sided hemiplegia. As I was caring for her, I noticed a few things in her room that may have significance for her. First, I noted that she had poles both by her bed and in the bathroom; both were bolted to the ceiling and the floor. These poles made it easier for L.C. to stand on her own with little assistance from anyone else. I feel that these make her more independent and help her use the strong side of her body. L.C. also had a divided box, with different kinds of tea in each section. I feel that this is significant to her because she is able to have the type of tea she likes whenever she wants it. It allows her to make choices each day and provides one of the comforts of "home." A third item was a triangle pillow that she sleeps on rather than a regular one. This is significant because it allows her to breathe better in the night or whenever she is sleeping. Because L.C. has chronic obstructive pulmonary disease, it is hard for her to breathe.

Kelly Z.

Nurses apply the nursing process to assess age-related changes and risk factors, identify nursing diagnoses, plan wellness outcomes, implement nursing interventions to achieve wellness outcomes, and evaluate the effectiveness of their interventions. A major focus of nursing care is on educating older adults and caregivers of dependent older adults about interventions that will eliminate risk factors or minimize their effects. The educational aspects are particularly important when older adults are influenced by myths and misunderstandings about age-related changes. For example, nurses can provide information about the difference between normal aging changes and risk factors to an older person who believes that functional impairments are a necessary consequence of old age and identify ways of minimizing the effects of risk factors and compensating for the effects of age-related changes.

Providing nursing care for older adults can be both challenging and rewarding, despite the common perception that it is futile and discouraging. Although nursing care of older adults is often associated with limited goals, a holistic perspective focuses on the potential of every person to experience wellness by achieving higher levels of psychological or spiritual functioning. Even older adults who have dementia, and other progressive conditions that can profoundly affect functioning and quality of life, may have potential for spiritual growth in ways that are not always observable or measurable. The Functional Consequences Theory helps nurses see older adults as more than an accumulation of age-related physiologic changes and pathologic conditions leading to diminished functioning. Thus, it provides a framework for

TABLE 3-1 Middle Range Theories Applicable to the Care of Older Adults

Middle Range Theory	Application to Care of Older Adults	Theorists and References	Related Chapter(s) in This Text
Health Promotion Model	This model is designed to guide nurses in helping clients achieve improved health, enhanced functional ability, and better quality of life.	First proposed by Nola Pender in 1982 and revised in 1996. McCullagh (2017).	Chapter 5
Self-Efficacy	Self-efficacy (i.e., one's own judgments about one's ability to accomplish a specific task) influences health behaviors such as nutrition, exercise, smoking cessation, bone health, fear of falling, and screening for colon cancer.	Based on Bandura's self-efficacy theory, first proposed in 1977 and revised several times through 1997. Resnick (2017).	Chapters 5, 18, 20, 21, 22
Theory of Generative Quality of Life for the Elderly	Quality of life for older adults is synonymous with connectedness, and a goal of nursing care is to establish patient-centered connections that can result in generativity.	Register and Herman (2010).	Chapters 12 and 13
Chronic Sorrow	Chronic sorrow is viewed as a normal response to the ongoing disparity or void created by significant loss. Family caregivers with chronic sorrow benefit from nursing interventions, such as education about caregiving, taking time to listen, focusing on feelings, and recognizing uniqueness of each individual.	Eakes (2017).	Chapters 15 and 27
Comfort	Comfort is the immediate experience of being strengthened by having needs of relief, ease, and transcendence met in four contexts (physical, psychospiritual, sociocultural, and environmental). Note that comfort involves more than the absence of pain or other physical discomfort.	Kolcaba's Comfort Theory, first developed in 1988. Kolcaba (2017).	Chapter 27
Health-Related Quality of Life	Based on research on health-related quality of life, the patient's perceived satisfaction with health-related quality of life becomes a significant indicator of the success of a nursing intervention.	Sandau, Bredow, and Peterson (2017).	Wellness outcomes in all clinically oriented chapters
Pain: a balance between analgesia and side effects	From a prescriptive nursing perspective, this theory reflects the nursing mission to intervene effectively and holistically to relieve pain and suffering and to prevent their long-term effects.	Good (2017).	Chapter 28

promoting wellness because it addresses the whole-person needs of the older adult and his or her relationships with self, others, and the environment. It reminds nurses to identify strengths and potentials in relation not only to physical aspects of functioning but also to psychological and spiritual well-being. Moreover, it leads to nursing interventions directed toward achieving wellness outcomes, such as improved quality of life for older adults.

ADDITIONAL THEORIES PERTINENT TO THE CARE OF OLDER ADULTS

When the Functional Consequences Theory was initially developed in the late 1980s, it focused primarily on alleviation or prevention of risk factors in healthy older adults. The focus has gradually expanded to include promoting wellness during all stages of health and illness, including end-of-life care. Consistent with this expanded focus, additional theories related to relevant aspects of illness are incorporated in all clinically oriented chapters. These additional theories are rooted not only in nursing but also in other disciplines, as is fitting for addressing complex needs of older adults within the context of interprofessional collaboration. Table 3-1 provides examples of currently evolving middle range nursing theories that are applicable to the content of this text.

See **ONLINE LEARNING ACTIVITY 3-2: RESOURCES FOR ADDITIONAL INFORMATION** at http://thepoint.lww.com/Miller8e.

Chapter Highlights

A Nursing Theory for Wellness-Focused Care of Older Adults (Figure 3-1)

• The Functional Consequences Theory explains the unique relationships among the concepts of person, health, nursing, and environment in the context of promoting wellness for older adults.

Concepts Underlying the Functional Consequences Theory (Boxes 3-1 to 3-4)

- Combinations of age-related changes and risk factors increase the vulnerability of older people to negative functional consequences, which interfere with the person's level of functioning or quality of life.
- Nurses assess the age-related changes, risk factors, and functional consequences, with particular emphasis on identifying the factors that can be addressed through nursing interventions.
- Wellness outcomes enable older adults to function at their highest level despite age-related changes and risk factors.

Applying the Theory to Promote Wellness in Older Adults

- Nurses can incorporate wellness outcomes to address each older adult's personal aspirations for well-being of body, mind, and spirit.
- Nurses educate older adults and caregivers about interventions to minimize risk factors or their effects.
- Providing nursing care for older adults is rewarding when approached from a holistic perspective that sees opportunities for wellness in physical, psychological, and spiritual aspects of function.

Additional Theories Pertinent to Care of Older Adults (Table 3-1)

Critical Thinking Exercises

Bring to your mind a vivid image of an older friend, relative, or patient who is at least 80 years old, and apply the following questions to one obvious functional consequence (e.g., impaired mobility). Develop an opportunity to talk with that person about what you have learned about the Functional Consequences Theory for Promoting Wellness in Older Adults and use Figure 3-1 as a basis for discussion.

1. What age-related changes and risk factors interact to contribute to this functional consequence?
2. What environmental conditions either improve or interfere with the affected aspect of functioning?
3. How can you use your nursing knowledge to improve health and quality of life in relation to that aspect of functioning?

 For more information about the topics discussed in this chapter, be sure to check out the interactive Online Learning Activities and other helpful resources at http://thepoint.lww.com/Miller8e.

REFERENCES

Davis, R., & Weisbeck, C. (2016). Creating a supportive environment using cues for wayfinding in dementia. *Journal of Gerontological Nursing, 42*(3), 36–44.

Eakes, G. (2017). Chronic sorrow. In S. J. Peterson, & T. S. Bredow (Eds.). *Middle range theories: Application to nursing research and practice* (4th ed., pp. 93–105). Philadelphia, PA: Wolters Kluwer.

Fulton, J. S. (2016). Personhood… the place for wellness. *Clinical Nurse Specialist, 30,* 135–136.

Gallagher-Lepak, S. (2018). Nursing diagnosis basics. In T. H. Herdman, & S. Kamitsuru (Eds.). *NANDA International Nursing Diagnoses Definitions and Classification, 2018-2020* (11th ed., pp. 34–44). New York: Thieme Publishers.

Good, M. (2017). Pain: A balance between analgesia and side effects. In S. J. Peterson, & T. S. Bredow (Eds.). *Middle range theories: Application to nursing research and practice* (4th ed., pp. 49–66). Philadelphia, PA: Wolters Kluwer.

Gouveia, B. R., Jardim, H., & Martins, M. M. (2011). Foundation of gerontological rehabilitation nursing: Applicability of the Functional Consequences Theory. *Referencia [Suppl], 1*(4), 475.

Kolcaba, K. (2017). Comfort. In S. J. Peterson, & T. S. Bredow (Eds.). *Middle range theories: Application to nursing research and practice* (4th ed., pp. 196–211). Philadelphia, PA: Wolters Kluwer.

McCullagh, M. (2017). Health promotion. In S. J. Peterson, & T. S. Bredow (Eds.). *Middle range theories: Application to nursing research and practice* (4th ed., pp. 227–238). Philadelphia, PA: Wolters Kluwer.

McMahon, S., & Fleury, J. (2012). Wellness in older adults: A concept analysis. *Nursing Forum, 47*(1), 39–50.

Menec, V. H., Newall, N., & Nowicki, S. (2016). Assessing communities' age-friendliness: How congruent are subjective versus objective assessments? *Journal of Applied Gerontology, 35,* 549–565.

Miller, C. A. (1990). *Nursing care of older adults: Theory and practice.* Glenview, IL: Scott, Foresman/Little, Brown Higher Education.

Register, M. E., & Herman, J. (2010). Quality of life revisited: The concept of connectedness in older adults. *Advances in Nursing Science, 33*(1), 53–63.

Resnick, B. (2017). Self-efficacy. In S. J. Peterson, & T. S. Bredow (Eds.). *Middle range theories: Application to nursing research and practice* (4th ed., pp. 79–92). Philadelphia, PA: Wolters Kluwer.

Rodiek, S., Nejati, A., Bardenhagen, E., et al. (2016). The Seniors' Outdoor Survey: An observational tool for assessing outdoor environments at long-term care settings. *Gerontologist, 56,* 222–233.

Sandau, K. E., Bredow, T. S., & Peterson, S. J. (2017). Health-related quality of life. In S. J. Peterson, & T. S. Bredow (Eds.). *Middle range theories: Application to nursing research and practice* (4th ed., pp. 212–226). Philadelphia, PA: Wolters Kluwer.

Talley, L. B. (2016). Collaborative partnerships: Raising the professional practice of nursing. *Journal of Nursing Administration, 46,* 291–292.

chapter 4

Theoretical Perspectives on Aging Well

LEARNING OBJECTIVES

After reading this chapter, you will be able to:

1. Describe theoretical perspectives on the relationships among aging, disease, health, and quality of life.

2. Discuss pertinent concepts from biologic theories of aging and their relevance to nursing care of older adults.

3. Discuss pertinent concepts from sociocultural theories of aging and their relevance to nursing care of older adults.

4. Discuss pertinent concepts from psychological theories of aging and their relevance to nursing care of older adults.

KEY TERMS

activity theory	life-course theories
age-stratification theory	life expectancy
aging well	life span
caloric restriction theory	paradox of aging
compression of morbidity	person–environment fit
cross-linkage theory	place identity
cumulative advantage/disadvantage theory	program theory
disengagement theory	quadruple jeopardy
double jeopardy	rectangularization of the curve
feminist gerontology	residential normalcy
free radical theory	selective optimization with compensation
gerotranscendence	social competence/breakdown model of aging
healthspan	
immunosenescence theories	

socioemotional selectivity theory	stem cell aging
sociology of knowledge of aging	stress process model
senescence	subculture theory
strength and vulnerability integration theory	wear-and-tear theory

People have always looked for answers to universal questions, such as *How long can we live? Why do we age?* and *How can we prevent the unwanted effects of aging?* Since early times, scientists and philosophers have tried to answer these questions from various perspectives by proposing and testing biologic, sociologic, and psychological theories. As knowledge about unique and variable aspects of aging expanded, it became evident that aging is multidimensional and requires an interprofessional approach. Now, a dominant question is *How can we live both long and well?* and the concept of **aging well** is prominent in studies. The following terms are commonly used in relation to aging well:

- Healthy aging: no illness and preserved functioning in activities of daily living
- Active aging: high physical and cognitive functioning and positive affect and control
- Productive aging: social participation and engagement
- Successful aging: the full concept of aging well
- Effective aging: the capacity to manage life challenges associated with aging
- Optimal aging: high levels of well-being and enjoyment of life

(Fernandez-Ballesteros, Molina, Schettini, et al., 2013; Woods, Rillamas-Sun, Cochrane, et al., 2016)

This chapter describes theoretical perspectives pertinent to aging well and discusses ways in which nurses can apply this information to promote wellness when they care for older adults.

HOW CAN WE LIVE LONG AND WELL?

Questions about how long we can live have traditionally been addressed by measuring life span, life expectancy, and rates of morbidity (i.e., illness) and mortality (i.e., death). Questions about how we can live both long and well—which is the current focus of gerontology—are currently being considered by exploring the relationships among aging, health, and disease. In recent decades, gerontological research has increasingly focused on identifying ways to delay the effects of aging and maintain high levels of functioning and quality of life. Leonard Hayflick, who is well known for the first biologic theory of aging, describes three types of current "seekers" in biologic theory development and their various goals as follows: (1) conservative seekers who simply want to slow the aging process, (2) less cautious believers who wish to stop or reverse it, and (3) a small but vocal majority who seek mortality (Hayflick, 2016). Theories that address these concepts are discussed in the following sections.

Life Span and Life Expectancy

Two measures that gerontologists use to address questions about how long we can live are life span and life expectancy.

Life span, defined as the maximum survival potential for a member of a species, is relatively stable as evident by the barely perceptible extensions that occur over the evolutionary timescale. Studies indicate that the theoretical maximum for the human life span is about 123 to 124 years, with only 1 in 5 million people living beyond 110 years in industrialized nations and far fewer in less developed countries (Andersen, Sebastiani, Dworkis, et al., 2012; Hanayama & Sibuya, 2016). The person verified to be the longest living human, Jeanne Calment, lived for 122 years and 165 days.

Life expectancy is the predictable length of time that one is expected to live from a specific point in time, such as birth or age 65. In contrast to the relatively stable time frame for life span, life expectancy at birth has increased from 47 years in 1900 to a record high of 76.4 years for men and 81.2 for women in 2014 (National Center for Health Statistics, 2016). It is important to recognize that life expectancies vary significantly, not only between developed and developing nations but also by gender and racial characteristics in the United States, as illustrated in Figure 4-1.

Life expectancy has increased not only at birth but also during later adulthood. For example, in 1900 people surviving to the age of 65 could expect to live another 12 years, whereas in 2014 the number of years at this age could expect

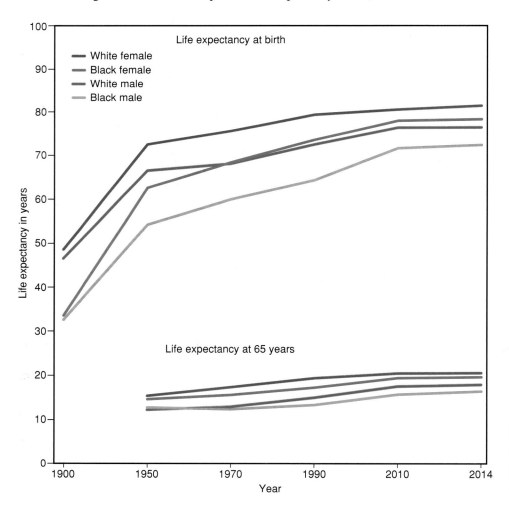

FIGURE 4-1 Life expectancies at birth and age 65, by race and sex: United States, 1900–2014. (From National Center for Health Statistics, Health United States 2016. Hyattsville, MD.)

to live had increased to 19 years (National Center for Health Statistics, 2016). For centenarians in the United States, remaining life expectancy is about 2 years. Gerontologists estimate that between 1994 and 2012, the estimated prevalence of centenarians in developed nations doubled from 1 in 10,000 to 1 in 5000 (Sebastiani & Perls, 2012).

 GLOBAL PERSPECTIVE

The worldwide average life expectancy in 2015 was 68.6 years, representing an increase of 35 years since 1970. In 2015, 24 countries had a life expectancy at birth exceeding 80 years, with the highest life expectancies occurring in Japan, Singapore, and Macau (He, Goodkind, Kowal, 2016).

Rectangularization of the Curve and Compression of Mortality

Mortality rates are graphically represented in a survivorship curve, which illustrates the changes occurring in death rates over different periods of time. The vertical axis designates the percentage of survivors, whereas the horizontal axis represents the age of survivorship. Since the 1980s, the rate of increase in average longevity has continued to rise, but the pace of increase has slowed down. This change in pace has resulted in the squaring of the human survival curve, meaning that life expectancy has not been prolonged as significantly after the age of 75 or 80. This **rectangularization of the curve** is attributed to changes in survival caused by various significant factors occurring at different points in time (see Figure 4-2).

The first major change resulted from improved housing and sanitation, and the second major change is attributable to the advent of immunization programs and other advances

in public health practices. The third major change, which occurred between 1960 and 1980, is attributable to biomedical breakthroughs, such as organ transplants, heart–lung machines, and cancer treatments. Recently, gerontologists have identified a fourth stage—the age of delayed degenerative diseases—characterized by the later onset of death from diseases that cause disability and chronic illness.

James Fries, a physician, first brought attention to this concern in an article on the **compression of morbidity**, in which he argued that the onset of significant illness could be postponed, but that one's life expectancy could not be extended to the same extent. Consequently, disease, disability, and functional decline are "compressed" into a period averaging 3 to 5 years before death. Fries and Crapo emphasized that preventive approaches must be directed toward preserving health by postponing the onset of chronic illnesses (Fries & Crapo, 1981). Results of early studies supported this theory and indicated that cohorts of older adults turning 65 were living longer with less disability, with improvements being attributed to factors such as higher levels of education and interventions that improve function and accessibility. A recent review of studies concluded that disability prevalence among older adults declined during the 1990s, but that trend did not continue into the 2000s (Wolf, 2016). Currently, there is growing concern that this trend toward improved functioning during later life will reverse due to the prevalence of conditions such as diabetes, smoking, obesity, physical inactivity, and poor dietary habits (Bardenheier, Lin, Zhou, et al., 2016; Cao, 2016; Jacob, Yee, Diehr, et al., 2016; Stenholm, Head, Kivimaki, et al., 2016). A recent commentary concluded that "we have yet to experience much compression of morbidity as the age of onset of most health problems has not increased markedly" (Crimmins, 2015).

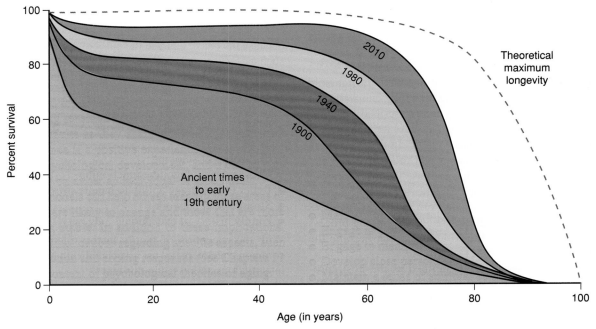

FIGURE 4-2 Illustration of changes in survivorship rates from ancient times to the theoretical maximum longevity.

Healthy Life Expectancy

These concerns have led to a focus on healthy life expectancy, which is measured on a continuum ranging from inability to perform activities of daily living to full independent functioning, as an indicator of quality of life during later adulthood. The term **healthspan** is currently used to describe time spent in good health and functioning, or the "maintenance of functional health with increasing age" (Melov, 2016, p. 2). As described by an interprofessional "think tank" of gerontologists, "The goal of aging science and health care...is not to extend life per se or make everyone live to 110, but rather to provide people with an opportunity to live their lives in a state of good health (healthspan) for as long as possible" (Nikolich-Zugish, Goldman, Cohen, et al., 2016, p. 437). This focus is particularly relevant to health care for older adults because health-promotion measures, such as physical activity, are consistently identified as primary, secondary, and tertiary prevention for chronic disease in older adults (Fried, 2016). Online Learning Activity 4-1 provides a link to a video describing the *Healthspan Imperative*, which is produced by the Alliance for Aging Research.

 See ONLINE LEARNING ACTIVITY 4-1: ADDITIONAL INFORMATION ABOUT THE HEALTHSPAN IMPERATIVE at http://thepoint.lww.com/Miller8e.

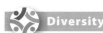 **Diversity Note**

The prevalence of functional impairment varies significantly by race and ethnic groups, with the highest rate for Native Americans, followed by rates (in order of prevalence) for US-born blacks, US-born Hispanics, foreign-born Hispanic women, and US- and foreign-born Asians (compared with whites) (Mehta, Sudharsanan, & Elo, 2014).

Relationships Among Aging, Disease, and Death

Whether age-associated diseases are inevitable or not is an important question related to living both long and well. The noted gerontologist, Leonard Hayflick, described the complex relationship between aging and disease as analogous to the "weak links" in automobiles. According to his analogy, both humans and particular makes and models of cars are characterized by weak links that increase the probability of component failure. For cheap cars, the "mean time to failure" is 4 or 5 years; for Americans born today, it is about 78 years. As Hayflick (2001–2002) stated, "The aging process increases vulnerability to the pathologies that become the leading causes of death" (p. 21).

Theories about **senescence**, defined as the postreproductive period leading to increased probability of death, address questions about the relationships between aging and death. Kohn (1982) proposed a senescence theory based on postmortem studies of 200 people who died at the age of 85 years or older. Kohn compared findings from autopsies with the listed cause of death and found that at least 26% of the subjects had no disease process that would be a cause of death. Kohn concluded that, had the same degree of disease occurred in middle-aged people, the condition would not have been fatal. Thus, he concluded that aging itself was the actual cause of death in a large fraction of the aged population (Kohn, 1982). Kohn further suggested that, when death in older people cannot be ascribed to a disease process that would cause death in middle-aged people, the cause of death should be listed on the death certificate as senescence.

Studies of Older Adults Who Are Healthy and Long-Lived

Studies of long-lived people who are healthy and functional explore the most important question of all: *How can we live a life that is not only long but also functional, productive, and satisfying?* This question is particularly relevant to the growing attention to adding quality, not just quantity, to life. The first study of "extreme longevity" was the Okinawa Centenarian Study, which began in 1975; since then, more than a dozen major longitudinal studies have been ongoing worldwide for a decade or more (Willcox, Willcox, & Poon, 2010). As these studies progressed, they also included "exceptional survivors" or "supercentenarians," defined as the oldest-old population who are 110 years or older. For example, the New England Centenarian Study in the United States currently has the largest sample in the world, with about 107 supercentenarians and about 1600 centenarians as study participants in 2014 (New England Centenarian Study, 2014).

People who survive to 100 years and older are a heterogeneous group with a wide range of health and socioeconomic characteristics. Most centenarians experience good health and relatively good functioning until their mid-90s or later because they have delayed the onset of common pathologies, such as cancer, diabetes, and cardiovascular disease (Ismail, Nussbaum, Sebastiani, et al., 2016). Common characteristics of centenarians include the following:

- Lean or healthy body mass index
- High intake of plant-based foods (e.g., fruits, vegetables, grains)
- No history of smoking
- High levels of cognitive functioning
- Better than average ability to handle stress
- Strong social network
- Family history of exceptional longevity

With the exception of family history factors, all of these common characteristics are associated with health-promotion interventions addressed in this text.

 See ONLINE LEARNING ACTIVITY 4-2: ADDITIONAL INFORMATION ABOUT CENTENARIANS AND SUPERCENTENARIANS at http://thepoint.lww.com/Miller8e.

HOW DO WE EXPLAIN BIOLOGIC AGING?

Biologic theories of aging address questions about the basic aging processes that affect all living organisms. These theories answer questions, such as *How do cells age?* and *What triggers the process of aging?* Biologic aging is the gradual and progressive decline in physiologic functioning that occurs throughout adulthood and ends in death. It is important to recognize that each biologic theory of aging attempts to explain a specific aspect of aging from a particular perspective. As such, each theory provides a narrow lens through which biologic aging can be viewed, but they do not provide a broad vision. Table 4-1 summarizes some of the well-established theories of aging that have been proposed to explain aging from a biologic perspective.

Current Foci of Biologic Aging Theories

Chronic inflammation is a major focus of research on biologic aging, with regard to both normal aging and many age-related pathologic conditions. The concept of cellular senescence (i.e., the failure of cells to divide) is gaining much attention because this biologic process underlying aging leads to chronic inflammation. With aging, senescent cells accumulate in many tissues and contribute to the development of osteoporosis, chronic lung disease, cardiovascular diseases, and neurodegenerative diseases (e.g., Alzheimer's, Parkinson's) (Xu & Kirkland, 2016).

Another emphasis of current studies is stem cell aging. Such research focuses on two basic properties of adult stem cells (also called somatic cells): (1) self-renewal, which is the capacity to produce an offspring cell with similar properties, and (2) multipotency, which is the capacity to generate mature cells to replace their corresponding adult host tissue. With increased age, the loss in stem cell number and activity causes a decline in tissue and organ function (Schultz & Sinclair, 2016). One explanation for this decrease is based on the long-standing free radical theory of aging (described in Table 4-1). Stem cell aging theories underlie current research on rejuvenation strategies and interventions to restore organ function (Sousa-Victor, Neves, & Jasper, 2016).

Conclusions About Biologic Theories

Biologic theories provide insight into the inevitable consequences of normal aging as well as the increased susceptibility of older adults to diseases. In addition, these theories attempt to identify the factors that can predict long as well as healthy lives. Although some of the hundreds of biologic theories of aging that have been proposed during the past several centuries have been disproved, others lay the groundwork for current and future research. As stated in a recent commentary on biologic theories of aging, "Aging research has placed us at the brink of a medical revolution, whereby it might be possible to do what was thought to be impossible: delay human aging." (Kennedy, 2016, p. 107)

TABLE 4-1 Biologic Theories of Aging

Theory	Description
Wear-and-Tear Theory	A human body is like a machine: It functions well for a certain time and broken parts can be fixed or replaced, but eventually it stops working because of accumulated effects of wear and tear. Longevity is affected by the genetic components as well as by the care provided. For humans, the wearing-out process is exacerbated by harmful factors, such as stress, disease, smoking, poor diet, and alcohol abuse
Free Radical Theory	Free radicals are ionized oxygen molecules that are highly unstable because they have an extra electron. They are waste products of metabolism and they can damage cells. Healthy bodies have protective mechanisms that can remove and repair damaged cells; however, these mechanisms become less effective with increased age and cellular damage becomes cumulative
Immunosenescence Theories	Immunosenescence, which is an age-related decline of the immune system, increases the susceptibility of older people to diseases, such as cancer and infections. The immune system may even attack healthy cells, leading to autoimmune conditions, such as rheumatoid arthritis
Cross-Linkage Theory	Biochemical processes create linkages, or connections, among structures that normally are separated. This causes a buildup of collagen-like substances that leads to failure of tissues and organs
Program Theory	The life span of each animal species is predetermined by a genetic program, which allows for a maximum of about 110 years in humans. Abnormal cells, such as cancer cells, are not subject to this predictable program and can proliferate an indefinite number of times
Caloric Restriction Theory	Numerous animal studies have found that reducing caloric intake by 30% to 40% without causing malnutrition results in enhanced ability to protect cells, increased resistance to stress, and overall longer and healthier life expectancy. However, to date, this research has not been applied to humans

Scientists estimate that between 20% and 30% of the variation in human longevity is attributable to genetic factors (Bertozzi, Tosti, & Fontana, 2017; Passarino, De Rango, & Montesanto, 2016). Since the early 2000s, when the Human Genome Project mapped the location of each human gene, gerontologists have had access to a wealth of data that is improving our understanding of genetic factors that influence aging. In particular, gerontologists are applying information from the Human Genome Project to address questions about the relationships among health, diseases, and long life. For example, Bloss, Pawlikowska, and Schork (2011) proposed the following explanations about the relationship between longevity and genetic factors:

1. An individual does not possess disease-predisposing genetic variations, and therefore does not develop life-threatening diseases to the same extent as others.
2. A person lives in a health-enhancing environment and/or engages in healthy behaviors.
3. An individual possesses disease-predisposing genetic variations or lives in an unhealthy environment, but also possesses "protective" genetic variations that mitigate detrimental effects.
4. A person has a combination of these factors.

In conclusion, all biologic theories of aging recognize that aging is a multidimensional process that is directly influenced by many interacting factors. Moreover, because of the great variability among people—which increases with aging—no single theory can explain the complex phenomenon of aging that involves many processes and mechanisms. Although no one theory can explain biologic aging, these theories lead to the following conclusions:

- Biologic aging affects all living organisms.
- Biologic aging is natural, inevitable, irreversible, and progressive with time.
- The course of aging varies from individual to individual.
- The rate of aging for different organs and tissues varies within individuals.
- Biologic aging is an intrinsic process that is independent of external factors but is strongly influenced by nonbiologic factors.
- Biologic aging processes are different from pathologic processes.
- Biologic aging increases one's vulnerability to disease.

Relevance to Nurses

A primary role of nurses is to help older adults identify and address the modifiable factors that can lead to diseases, disability, and death as well as those health-promoting factors that can contribute to a longer and healthier life. Thus, nurses need to understand not only the relationship between aging and disease but also what "causes" healthy aging and longevity. Biologic theories of aging shed light on the differences between age-related changes and the risk factors that affect the health and functioning of older adults. Nurses then can use this knowledge to implement interventions that promote wellness and a higher level of functioning. For example, longitudinal studies have shown that adherence to dietary guidelines, as discussed in Chapter 18, is strongly associated with successful aging and improved healthy life expectancy (Gopinath, Russell, Kifley, et al., 2016).

Biologic theories of aging are applicable to attitudes of health care professionals about aging. If, for example, health care providers hold the perspective of "what do you expect, you're old," reversible disease conditions may go untreated. Similarly, if health care providers view aging as an ultimately fatal disease, their attitude may reflect a hopelessness that affects their care for older patients. Biologic theories of aging can be used to point out that such fatalistic perspectives are outdated. Nurses can base their care on a holistic perspective and use studies of healthy and functional oldest-old people to identify health-promotion interventions that will improve quality of life for older adults. Nurses often are in positions to serve as teachers and advocates for older adults whose care might be based on an outdated or narrow approach that incorrectly equates aging and disease. The Functional Consequences Theory for Promoting Wellness in Older Adults (discussed in Chapter 3) provides a framework for a holistic approach that identifies the risk factors and addresses those that are modifiable in older adults. This text addresses each aspect of functioning from this perspective, with emphasis on those factors that nurses can address through health-promotion interventions.

A Student's Perspective

One thing I feel I did well during my first week of providing patient care was seeing my patient for the person that she is and not just as a set of problems that needed caring for. I can understand how difficult it may be in today's health care settings to stop for a minute and really "see" the patient. When I cared for Mrs. S., I was able to look past the wrinkles and white hair and see the spunky spirit that she really is. It is easy to just categorize someone in your mind as old, senile, or dependent. One very important lesson that I will take with me for the rest of my career is that you cannot categorize someone because everyone is so different. It's amazing what you can discover if you actually take the time to see people for who they truly are. Taking care of a person holistically means taking care of them physically, psychologically, and spiritually as well.

Sarah L.

Biologic theories highlight the need for health-promotion interventions to prevent disease conditions and minimize the negative effects of aging. However, these theories do not address the significant influence of nursing, medical, and psychosocial interventions that can improve a person's functioning and life expectancy. From a broader perspective, aging is more than an unrelenting progression of cellular deterioration. Survival to old age is an accomplishment that denotes strong will and the ability to adapt. As emphasized throughout this text, older adulthood is a dynamic part of the life span continuum and has the potential to be a most rewarding part of the life cycle, during which one experiences personal growth and self-understanding, fulfillment of potential, and the ability to establish clear priorities. These aspects of aging are addressed in the following sections, which describe sociocultural and psychological theories of aging.

Case Study

Imagine that you are 72 years old and your mother and father are 96 and 95 years old, respectively, and they live in an assisted-living apartment. You have a brother who died last year at the age of 70 years and you have a sister who is 69 years old. You have two children, three grandchildren, and two great-grandchildren. Your mother is moderately obese and has osteoarthritis, hypertension, glaucoma, and type 2 diabetes. Functionally, she uses a walker, needs help with getting in and out of the bathtub, and has some trouble reading but can see well enough to watch television and get around familiar environments. Your father has hypertension, osteoarthritis, and a recent diagnosis of prostate cancer. Functionally, he is independent in his basic activities of daily living but is quite hearing impaired. Both of your parents have some memory impairment, but the support services at the facility where they live address their needs for meals, medication administration, and reminders about getting to activities.

THINKING POINTS

- Using the concepts of rectangularization of the curve and compression of morbidity, what would you expect the health, functioning, and life expectancy to be for each of the five generations in your family?
- Pick a biologic theory of aging that you think is applicable for your family and use it to explain to your great-grandchildren why their great-great grandparents are still living.
- Based on information presented, how would you respond to your mother's statement, "I'm 96 years old—what does it matter if I follow a diabetic diet? If the sugar hasn't killed me so far, then eating two donuts this morning isn't going to kill me. It's old age that will take me, not my diet."
- Based on information presented, how would you respond to your father's declaration that "Of course, I have prostate cancer! I'm 95 years old!"
- What perspectives on aging would you want your father's primary care provider to use in addressing your father's prostate cancer?

SOCIOCULTURAL PERSPECTIVES ON AGING

Sociocultural theories of aging attempt to explain the interrelationship between older adults and the societies and environments in which they live. The first sociocultural theories were proposed during the 1960s when gerontology was just beginning to address ideas about age, social structure, the environment, and the life course. Dominant themes of these theories were: (1) aging is a social process, (2) societies are structured according to age-based roles, and (3) new cohorts of people move through the age structure of the population as a group (Settersten, 2016). Historical events and social movements

Box 4-1 Sociocultural Theories of Aging

Early Theories That Focus on the Status of Older People in Society

- **Activity Theory:** Older people remain socially and psychologically fit if they remain actively engaged in life.
- **Disengagement Theory:** Social and psychological withdrawal by the individual is a universal and inevitable part of the aging process.
- **Subculture Theory:** Because older people as a group have their own norms, expectations, beliefs, and habits, they form a unique subculture.
- **Age-stratification Theory:** Each age cohort develops a unique history as it interacts with society and social influences.

Theories That Address the Influence of the Environment

- **Person–Environment Fit** (also called Ecological): Older individuals with functional limitations need to adapt to their environments in order to remain independent.
- **Place Identity** (also called Place Attachment): People form affective, cognitive, behavioral, and social bonds to their environments, thereby transforming "space" into "place" (e.g., "my home" or "my neighborhood").
- **Residential Normalcy:** People who feel comfortable and in control of their environment at home may not feel the need to change anything.

Theories That Evolved Out of Social Movements

- **Feminist Gerontology:** Aging is examined from perspectives of older women and addresses issues such as gender inequalities with regard to diseases, caregiving roles, and economic status.
- **Double Jeopardy:** Black women experience two types of bias—that is, those associated with racism and sexism.
- **Quadruple Jeopardy:** Being black, female, old, and poor exponentially increases the risk of being failed by society and social welfare support.
- **Sociology of Knowledge of Aging:** Maggie Kuhn and Gray Panthers rallied against the common media portrayals of older adults as weak and diminished (i.e., infantilized and dehumanized).

of the 1970s stimulated development of sociologic theories addressing unique needs of older adults related to gender roles, racial and cultural diversity, and economic inequities. Box 4-1 summarizes some of the key theories that paved the way for current theories. More recently, sociocultural theories have expanded to address a wide array of vulnerable populations and the "enormous challenge of individual, societal, and global aging" (Estes & DiCarlo, 2016, p. 102). These sociocultural theories are described in the following sections.

A Student's Perspective

I think that over the past few weeks, I have really been able to see that it doesn't matter if a person is 90 or 50 or 5, they have a story, a family, a life. They have values and friends and things that are important to them. I think that this is what I will take away from this experience the most. I will try to remember in my nursing career that each patient has a story and that I will be a better nurse if I take the time to find out that story and connect with my patients, no matter what age they are.

Erika B.

Social Competence/Breakdown Model of Aging

The Social Competence/Breakdown Model of Aging, which was proposed during the 1970s, is a sociocultural theory of aging that addresses ageism and stereotypes related to problems of aging (Bengston, 2016). According to this model, older adults experience a cycle, or spiral, of social competence or incompetence characterized by the following stages:

1. Vulnerability set in motion because of a health crisis, widowhood, or lowered income.
2. Subsequent crises concerning role losses (e.g., due to social isolation or immobility) that lead to loneliness, depression, and anomie.
3. Dependence on external sources of self-labeling, which reflect stereotypical images of elderly as dependent, incapable, and incompetent.
4. Acceptance of negative labels resulting in behaviors and self-images consistent with dependency.
5. Further reduction of social and psychological competence and corresponding loss of skills involving social and cognitive coping.

This model is particularly pertinent to nursing because the cycle of competence breakdown can be broken through the educational interventions of health care providers (Bengston, 2016).

Sociocultural Theories Addressing Inequalities

Consistent with the current focus of healthy aging, a central focus of recent theorizing is on finding explanations for health inequalities (also called disparities) across the heterogeneous population of older adults (Abramson, 2016; Settersten, 2016). This focus stems in part from the increasing recognition that gains in life expectancy and healthspan vary considerably across nations, as well as across socioeconomic groups within the same nation (Quesnel-Vallee, Willson, & Reiter-Campeau, 2016; Sadana, Blas, Budhwani, et al., 2016). This focus also is based on the studies of health disparities across racial and ethnic groups, and within-group differences associated with education, immigrant status, and economic variables (Angel, Mudrazija, & Benson, 2016). Within this context, gerontologists are exploring questions such as the following:

- What are the sources of health inequalities?
- What variables are associated with stark differences in health and longevity at the population level?
- How do social inequalities affect health status?
- How do we intervene to reduce health inequalities?

The Cumulative Advantage/Disadvantage Theory postulates that trajectories of advantage or disadvantage that begin in earlier life have a persistent and cumulative effect on later status and achievement. For example, educational institutions select and sort students in ways that have lifelong consequences and lead to inequities in later years (O'Rand, 2016). This model is widely used in studies related to health

disparities, wealth accumulation, and gender and race disparities (Crystal, Shea, & Reyes, 2016).

Sociocultural Theories Related to Caregiving

As the roles and stresses of caregiving have become a prominent concern in society, gerontologists have been developing theories to help identify interventions and promote support services for caregivers. The Stress Process Model has been widely used since the 1990s to guide both research and practice related to caregivers' stress. Montgomery, Kwak, and Kosloski (2016) describe key concepts in this model as follows:

- Characteristics of caregiver, such as age, gender, ethnicity, socioeconomic status, employment, relationship with care recipient
- Characteristics of care environment, including availability of support services or resources
- Primary stressors (i.e., challenges or problems that are directly linked to caregiving situation and care recipient's needs), such as type and severity of disease and functional limitations, caregiver's subjective perception of care demands
- Secondary stressors (i.e., those that are produced or affected by primary stressors), such as role strain, and caregiver's personal stresses
- Mediators of stress: level of social support and coping skills of the caregiver
- Outcomes of the stress process on the caregiver's well-being, including physical and mental health
- Proliferation, which is the process whereby stressors in one role or domain of life impact other domains or roles

This model has led to the development of a wide range of psychoeducational interventions that go beyond the approach of simply providing services by addressing caregiver's needs related to coping and self-efficacy (Montgomery, Kwak, & Kosloski, 2016).

Relevance of Sociocultural Theories of Aging to Nurses

Sociocultural theories of aging help nurses view older adults in relation to society and environments. Thus, these perspectives contribute to a better understanding of influences, such as culture, family, education, community, ascribed roles, cohort effects, home and living settings, and personal and political economics. These theories remind health care practitioners that even though older adults within cohorts may share similar characteristics, each person is unique. Some older people achieve their identity in a subculture, others may define successful aging in relation to their activities, and still others may find new roles in society. In addition, these theories emphasize the importance of assessing environmental factors that influence the functioning of an older person. Some of the risk factors discussed throughout this text identify environmental factors that interfere with the health and functioning of older adults. Similarly, many of the nursing interventions discussed in this text identify ways of modifying the environment to improve the functioning of older adults.

Sociocultural perspectives encourage nurses to consider not only the cultural needs of individual older adults but also the role of culture in shaping societal attitudes about aging. Feminist-based theories provide a broad and holistic understanding of the needs of older adults as well as their families and caregivers. Information about diverse aspects of aging, such as cultural or gender differences, is discussed throughout this text, and pertinent information gleaned from studies appears in the Diversity Note. Theories about person–environment interactions are stimulating interest in broadening the environments of institutional settings to include pets and intergenerational activities.

See ONLINE LEARNING ACTIVITY 4-3: ARTICLE ABOUT INDIVIDUALIZED AGING at http://thepoint.lww.com/Miller8e.

Case Study

Imagine that you are 87 years old and have been retired for 10 years. Create an image of yourself at that age, making sure that you incorporate some changes that are likely to occur as you grow older. Describe the people who are an active part of your relationships during a typical month. Describe the activities you would engage in during a typical week for each of the following aspects of your life: leisure activity, physical activity, intellectual stimulation, emotional growth, social interaction, and spiritual nurturing. Are you active in any volunteer organizations? What would your health and functioning be and where would you be living? Based on the image of yourself at 87 years old that you just created, answer the following questions.

THINKING POINTS

- Which of the early theories of aging would you apply to explain the way you expect to be when you are 87?
- What social movements would influence your perception of yourself at that age?
- How would the Cumulative Advantage/Disadvantage Theory apply to your life experiences?

PSYCHOLOGICAL PERSPECTIVES ON AGING

Psychological theories of aging focus on the psychological factors that affect health, longevity, and quality of life. These theories are especially relevant to psychosocial aspects of aging because they address variables such as learning, memory, emotions, intelligence, and motivation. A major focus of current geropsychology research is on the identification of behavioral interventions to remediate age-related declines or to slow the rate of decline and maintain independent function (Schaie, 2016). This approach, which is based on interprofessional collaboration, is particularly pertinent to health promotion for older adults. The following sections review some of the major psychological theories of aging. In addition, relevant psychological theories about cognitive function, stress and coping, and depression are discussed in Chapters 11, 12, and 15, respectively.

Life-Course Theories

Life-course theories have been used for more than half a century to address old age within the context of the life cycle. For example, Maslow's human needs theory is a psychological theory that gerontologists use to address the concepts of motivation and human needs. According to Maslow (1954) theory, the five categories of basic human needs, ordered from lowest to highest, are physiologic needs, safety and security needs, love and belongingness, self-esteem, and self-actualization. The attainment of lower-level needs takes priority over higher-level needs; self-actualization can occur only when lower-level needs are met to some degree. People continually move between the levels but always strive toward higher levels. This theory is particularly applicable to older adults because Maslow describes self-actualized people as fully mature humans who possess such desirable traits as autonomy, creativity, independence, and positive interpersonal relationships.

Erikson's (1963) theory about the eight stages of life has been used widely in relation to older adulthood. Erikson defines the stages of life as trust versus mistrust, autonomy versus shame and doubt, initiative versus guilt, industry versus inferiority, identity versus identity diffusion, intimacy versus self-absorption, generativity versus stagnation, and ego integrity versus despair. Each of these stages presents the person with certain conflicting tendencies that must be balanced before he or she can move successfully from that stage. As in other life-course theories, how one stage is mastered lays the groundwork for successful or unsuccessful mastery of the next stage. In works published between 1950 and 1966, Erikson emphasized the life course from childhood to young adulthood; in later publications, however, he reconsidered the meaning of these stages. In 1982, when he was 80 years old, Erikson described the task of old age as balancing the search for integrity and wholeness with a sense of despair. He believed that the successful accomplishment of this task, achieved primarily through life-review activities, would result in wisdom.

Peck (1968) expanded Erikson's original theory and divided the eighth stage—ego integrity versus despair—into additional stages occurring during middle age and old age. The stages described by Peck as specific to old age are ego differentiation versus work-role preoccupation, body transcendence versus body preoccupation, and ego transcendence versus ego preoccupation.

Some life-course theories concentrate on middle or later adulthood and address tasks of late life such as the following:

- Adjusting to decreasing physical strength and health
- Coping with physical changes of aging
- Adjusting to retirement and reduced income
- Adjusting to the death of a spouse
- Redirecting energy to new roles and activities, such as retirement, widowhood, and grandparenting
- Establishing an explicit association with one's age group
- Adapting to social roles in a flexible way
- Establishing satisfactory physical living arrangements
- Accepting one's own life
- Developing a point of view about death

Psychological Theories of Successful Aging

Consistent with the increasing focus on aging well, recent psychological theories of aging address questions, such as *How is emotional well-being maintained during older adulthood? Does psychological well-being differ in younger and older adults?* and, perhaps most importantly, *How do people define and achieve "successful aging?"* Initial theories of emotion and aging focused on losses and negative emotions; however, more recent longitudinal studies have challenged earlier conclusions. The phrase **paradox of aging** was coined recently to describe the relatively high rates of emotional well-being experienced by older adults despite age-related declines in many physical and cognitive processes (Charles & Hong, 2016). Four psychological theories of aging that help explain this finding are selection, optimization, and compensation; socioemotional selectivity; gerotranscendence; and strength and vulnerability integration.

The theory of **selective optimization with compensation** was proposed to explain successful aging based on a dynamic model of development as a continuous process of specialization and loss. According to this theory, older adults *select* certain goals and tasks while disengaging from other goals; they *optimize* necessary resources to achieve these goals; and they *compensate* by establishing new resources to substitute for lowered or lost abilities and skills. Studies have found that older adults using these compensatory strategies report higher levels of positive emotions and lower levels of loneliness (Charles & Hong, 2016). Morley (2009) describes the following examples of well-known people who illustrate this theory:

- Grandma Moses became a famous painter of miniatures after arthritis limited her ability to make quilts.
- Monet invented modern impressionism when his eyesight was clouded by cataracts.
- Renoir held his paintbrush in his clenched fist after he developed arthritis.
- Maurice Ravel composed his famous *Bolero* after he developed dementia.

This theory is used to explore aspects of successful aging well such as coping with stress, managing careers, and recovering from illness.

The **socioemotional selectivity theory** has been proposed to explain emotional well-being during older adulthood. According to this theory, in contrast to younger adults who view time as unconstrained, older adults recognize that their time is limited, so they focus on emotional goals rather than on knowledge-seeking goals. Studies based on this theory indicate that older adults have smaller social networks, and they report high levels of intimacy, satisfaction, and emotional closeness with their close interpersonal relationships (Charles & Hong, 2016). Another finding from studies based on this theory is that older adults tend to remember and attend to positive emotional information, an effect referred to as "positivity" (Ngo, Sands, & Isaacowitz, 2016).

The **strength and vulnerability integration theory** posits that older adults experience age-related gains as well as losses in emotion-related processes, but overall they maintain a relatively positive level of emotional experience. Strengths of older adults include improved abilities to (1) direct emotional attention away from negative stimuli, (2) appraise situations, and (3) remember experiences more positively. Age-related vulnerabilities are defined as diminished physiologic ability to respond to high levels of stress. Studies based on this theory have found that older adults tend to report fewer stressors and daily hassles than younger adults; however, when they experience stressors, they may experience greater reactivity (Charles & Hong, 2016).

The theory of **gerotranscendence** was proposed in the early 1990s by Tornstam (1994) and has become widely recognized in Sweden and other Scandinavian countries. This theory proposes that human aging is a process of shifting from a rational and materialistic metaperspective to a more cosmic and transcendent vision. This shift includes the following aspects (Tornstam, 1996):

- Decreased self-centeredness
- Less concern with body and material things
- Decreased fear of death
- Discovery of hidden aspects of self
- Increased altruism
- Increased time spent in meditation and solitude
- Decreased interest in superfluous social interaction
- Urge to abandon roles
- Increased understanding of moral ambiguity
- Increased feelings of cosmic union with the universe
- Increased feelings of affinity with past and coming generations
- A redefinition of one's perception of time, space, and objects

Gerotranscendence (i.e., a shift from a materialistic and rational vision to a more cosmic and transcendent one, accompanied by increased life satisfaction) may explain successful aging, or psychological well-being, in older adults with functional limitations (Wong, Low, & Yap, 2016).

A Student's Perspective

My comfort level at the nursing home increases each and every week, and I find myself enjoying my time there more and more. Today there was a children's program in the dining room for all the residents. It was very cute. The kids were great, and most of the residents expressed true appreciation and enjoyment while the kids visited. For instance, my patient Mr. B. was chatting with a young boy and his mother. As the boy got more and more involved in the conversation, Mr. B.'s attitude changed completely; he became so happy and engaged with the young boy. I had seen Mr. B. smile a couple of times before, but not to the extent of how he smiled and laughed with the little one. After the boy left, Mr. B. told me that the boy reminded him of his own grandson, whom he doesn't get to see very much. I think it brought Mr. B. joy and a sense of comfort because he felt like he was with his family. Personally, I was quite touched. Sometimes, everyone gets so caught up in current tasks or problems, when really at the end of the day it comes down to making people smile and helping them to enjoy life to the best of one's abilities.

Caitlin B.

Relevance of Psychological Theories of Aging to Nurses

In caring for older adults, nurses can use psychological theories of aging as a framework for addressing certain issues, such as response to losses and continued emotional development. Maslow's hierarchy of needs framework is useful for conceptualizing the nature of interventions in institutional or home settings. For instance, if older adults are unable to purchase food, they are unlikely to feel secure. Likewise, if older adults feel insecure about being able to meet their shelter needs, they are unlikely to have a sense of trust. Older adults who have already met their lower-level needs, however, can be encouraged to focus on higher-level achievements such as self-actualization.

In addition, psychological theories imply that devoting some time and energy to life review and self-understanding can be beneficial for older adults. Nurses can facilitate this process by asking sensitive questions and by listening attentively to older adults as they share information about their past. Reminiscence is a positive experience that is essential for continued psychological development, and it can be promoted by nurses on either an individual or group basis.

Life-course models can help nurses identify those areas of personality that are likely to change and those that are more likely to remain stable. In addition to these implications, nurses consider implications regarding specific aspects, such as cognitive function and coping responses (see Chapters 11 and 12), in the context of psychological theories of aging.

 See ONLINE LEARNING ACTIVITY 4-4: ADDITIONAL RESOURCES FOR INFORMATION ABOUT THEORIES OF AGING at http://thepoint.lww.com/Miller8e.

Case Study

Imagine, again, that you are 87 years old and add the following information to the description of yourself that you created for the discussion of sociocultural theories. Describe your personality, including, but not limited to, the following characteristics: emotional stability, adjustments to losses, contentedness with life, optimism versus pessimism, engagement in activities versus withdrawal from activities, and feelings of self-efficacy versus feelings of powerlessness. Describe your beliefs about your gender-specific roles (i.e., those aspects of roles that are defined by you being a woman or a man). Based on this image of yourself at 87 years old, answer the following questions:

THINKING POINTS

- Describe what your psychological development would be in the context of a life-course theory and how you would have moved between the levels over the course of your lifetime.
- What aspects of your lifestyle at 87 years old could be explained by the gerotranscendence theory?
- Based on your own experiences, how has your perception of aging changed over time?

A HOLISTIC PERSPECTIVE ON AGING AND WELLNESS

From a holistic perspective—the one that is most pertinent to promoting wellness—it is necessary to consider the body–mind–spirit interconnectedness of each older adult for whom nurses provide care. Thus, questions about how we can live long and well must be answered in the context of the interplay among the many factors that influence health and aging. This requires an integrated perspective on aging, an avoidance of stereotypes, and a commitment to identifying the factors that most directly affect—both negatively and positively—health and quality of life for each unique older adult. Current theories point to the following determinants of living long and well:

- Inherit good genes.
- Avoid oxidative damage (e.g., from tobacco, environmental conditions).
- Protect from oxidative damage with antioxidants from natural sources (e.g., fruits and vegetables).
- Maintain optimal weight.
- Engage in physical exercise.
- Engage in meaningful social interactions.
- Develop close personal relationships.
- Maintain a sense of spiritual connectedness.
- Reject ageist stereotypes.

The Functional Consequences Theory for Promoting Wellness in Older Adults that was presented in Chapter 3 provides a nursing framework for addressing the factors that affect the health and functioning of older adults. Although it is beyond the scope of any nursing text to address all aspects of body–mind–spirit interconnectedness, nurses can use the functional consequences perspective, in conjunction with information from theories discussed in this chapter, to help older adults answer their own questions about aging. When older adults express resignation in the "What-do-you-expect-you're-old?" outlook, nurses can rephrase that viewpoint and ask "So, what *do* you expect because you are older?" or "What *will* you expect when you are older?" Nurses can challenge ageist stereotypes and approach the question from a holistic perspective that acknowledges the interconnectedness among one's body, mind, and spirit. From this point of view, nurses can emphasize that even though some degenerative changes affect one's body with increasing age, one's mind and spirit can continue to thrive and even improve.

Because self-responsibility is an essential component of wellness, nurses can ask older adults to identify for themselves those factors that most significantly influence their health and functioning and can focus care on those aspects that are within the scope of nursing. Nurses also need to avoid communicating ageist stereotypes, which requires that we examine our own attitudes about aging and make sure that our nursing care of older adults is based on accurate, theory-based information. Nurses can check their attitudes about their own aging and periodically ask, *What do I expect (or wish) for my own wellness when I am older tomorrow?… a week from now?… a month from now?… a year?… 10 years?… 20 years?* Even more important, ask, *What am I doing today that will affect how well I am aging tomorrow?… 10 years from now?* If we acknowledge that no matter what else is happening, we are aging biologically, we are likely to pay careful attention to health-related behaviors that affect how well we age. Likewise, if we approach our care of older adults holistically, we will be able to identify interventions that promote wellness of body, mind, and spirit.

Chapter Highlights

How Can We Live Long and Well? (Figures 4-1 and 4-2)

- Theories of aging attempt to explain from various professional perspectives how and why we age.
- The rectangularization of the curve illustrates the changes in survivorship and life expectancy that have been occurring in developed countries.
- The compression of morbidity describes the phenomenon of postponing disability until the last years before death.
- Major current emphasis is on identifying ways to promote a healthy life expectancy, or healthspan.
- Studies of people who are healthy and long-lived provide insights into characteristics of healthy aging.
- From a holistic perspective, the most important question is *How can we live a life that is both long and healthy?* Nurses address this question by promoting wellness and facilitating an optimal level of functioning for older adults.

How Do We Explain Biologic Aging? (Table 4-1)

- Biologic theories of aging address questions about inevitable consequences of normal aging.
- Examples of biologic theories of aging are wear and tear, free radical, immunosenescence, cross-linkage, program, and caloric restriction.
- Two foci of current biologic aging theories are cellular senescence and stem cell aging.
- Nurses can apply information about biologic theories of aging to teach older adults about health-promotion interventions.

Sociocultural Perspectives on Aging

- Sociocultural theories of aging attempt to explain how a society influences its old people and how old people influence their society.
- Early theories (e.g., activity, disengagement, activity, subculture, and age stratification) focus on the status of older people in society.
- Theories that address the influence of the environment include person–environment fit, place identify, and residential normalcy.
- Theories that evolved out of social movements include feminist gerontology, double or quadruple jeopardy, and sociology of knowledge of aging.
- Currently evolving sociocultural theories include the social competence/breakdown model of aging, cumulative advantage/disadvantage theory, and the stress process model related to caregiving.
- Nurses can apply information from sociocultural theories to holistically address the multidimensional needs of older adults.

Psychological Perspectives on Aging

- Life-course theories (e.g., Maslow, Erikson, and Peck) address old age within the context of the life cycle.
- Gerontologists are especially interested in theories to explain successful aging, such as selective optimization with compensation; socioemotional selectivity; strength and vulnerability integration; and gerotranscendence.
- Psychological theories of aging help nurses address the psychosocial needs of older adults.

A Holistic Perspective on Aging and Wellness

- Nurses can use theories of aging developed by other disciplines in conjunction with the Functional Consequences Theory (see Chapter 3) to develop and implement a holistic approach to promoting wellness in older adults.

Critical Thinking Exercises

You are assessing an 87-year-old woman who is being admitted to the hospital with heart failure for the third time in the past 2 years. She does not have any cognitive impairment and she lives alone in her own home. When you ask her why she came to the hospital, she states, "I'm 87 years old, you know. Isn't that a good enough reason to be sick? Don't you think you'll be in the hospital when you're my age?"

1. How do you respond to her?
2. What additional assessment information would you want?
3. What health teaching would you think about incorporating into your care plan?

 For more information about topics discussed in this chapter, be sure to check out the interactive Online Learning Activities and other helpful resources at http://thepoint.lww.com/Miller8e.

REFERENCES

Abramson, C. M. (2016). Unequal aging: Lessons from inequality's end game. *Public Policy & Aging Report, 26*, 68–72.

Andersen, S. L., Sebastiani, P., Dworkis, D. A., et al. (2012). Health span approximates life span among many supercentenarians: Compression of morbidity at the approximate limit of life span. *Journals of Gerontology: Biological Sciences and Medical Sciences, 67*(4), 395–405.

Angel, J. L., Mudrazija, S., & Benson, R. (2016). Racial and ethnic inequalities in health. In L. K. George & K. F. Ferraro (Eds.). *Handbook of aging and the social sciences* (8th ed., pp. 123–142). Oxford: Academic Press.

Bardenheier, B. H., Lin, J., Zhou, X., et al. (2016). Compression of disability between two birth cohorts of US adults with diabetes, 1992–2012: A prospective longitudinal analysis. *Lancet Diabetes and Endocrinology, 4*, 686–694.

Bengston, V. L. (2016). How theories of aging became social: Emergence of the Sociology of Aging. In V. L. Bengston & R. A. Settersten (Eds.), *Handbook of theories of aging* (3rd ed., pp. 67–86). New York: Springer Publishing Company.

Bertozzi, B., Tosti, V., & Fontana, L. (2017). Beyond calories: An integrated approach to promote health, longevity, and well-being. *Gerontology, 63*, 13–19.

Bloss, C. S., Pawlikowska, L., & Schork, N. J. (2011). Contemporary human genetic strategies in aging research. *Ageing Research Review, 10*(2), 191–200.

Cao, B. (2016). Future healthy life expectancy among older adults in the US: A forecast based on cohort smoking and obesity history. *BioMed Central, CAO Population Health Metrics, 14*, 23.

Charles, S. T., & Hong, J. (2016). Theories of emotional well-being and aging. In V. L. Bengston & R. A. Settersten (Eds.), *Handbook of theories of aging* (3rd ed., pp. 193–212). New York: Springer Publishing Company.

Crimmins, E. M. (2015). Lifespan and healthspan: Past, present, and promise. *Gerontologist, 55*, 901–911.

Crystal, S., Shea, D. G., & Reyes, A. M. (2016). Cumulative advantage, cumulative disadvantage, and evolving patterns of late-life disability. *Gerontologist,* doi: 10.1093/geront/gnw056 [Epub ahead of print].

Erikson, E. H. (1963). *Childhood and society* (2nd ed.). New York: W.W. Norton & Company.

Estes, C. L., & DiCarlo, N. R. (2016). Social movements and social knowledge: Gerontological theory in research, policy, and practice. In V. L. Bengston & R. A. Settersten (Eds.), *Handbook of theories of aging* (3rd ed., pp. 87–106). New York: Springer Publishing Company.

Fernandez-Ballesteros, R., Molina, M. A., Schettini, R., et al., (2013). The semantic network of aging well. *Annual Review of Gerontology and Geriatrics, 33*, 79–107.

Fried, L. P. (2016). Investing in health to create a third demographic dividend. *Gerontologist, 56*, S167–S177.

Fries, J. F., & Crapo, L. M. (1981). Vitality and aging: Implications of the rectangularization of the curve. San Francisco, CA: W. H. Freeman & Company.

Gopinath, B., Russell, J., Kifley, A., et al. (2016). Adherence to dietary guidelines and successful aging over 10 years. *Journals of Gerontology: Biological Sciences and Medical Sciences, 71*, 349–355.

Hanayama, N., & Sibuya, M. (2016). Estimating the upper limit of lifetime probability distribution, based on data of Japanese centenarians. *Journals of Gerontology: Biological Sciences and Medical Sciences, 71*, 1014–1021.

Hayflick, L. (2001–2002). Anti-aging medicine hype, hope, and reality. *Generations, 20*, 20–26.

Hayflick, L. (2016). Unlike aging, longevity is sexually determined. In V. L. Bengston & R. A. Settersten (Eds.), *Handbook of theories of aging* (3rd ed., pp. 31–52). New York: Springer Publishing Company.

He, W., Goodkind, D., Kowal, P., U.S. Census Bureau. (2016). *An aging world 2015.* Washington, D.C.: U.S. Government Publishing Office.

Ismail, K., Nussbaum, L., Sebastiani, P., et al. (2016). Compression of morbidity is observed across cohorts with exceptional longevity. *Journal of the American Geriatrics Society, 64*, 1583–1591.

Jacob, M. E., Yee, L. M., Diehr, P. H., et al. (2016). Can a healthy lifestyle compress the disabled period in older adults? *Journal of the American Geriatrics Society, 64*, 1952–1961.

Kennedy, B. K. (2016). Advances in biological theories of aging. In V. L. Bengston & R. A. Settersten (Eds.), *Handbook of theories of aging* (3rd ed., pp. 107–111). New York: Springer Publishing Company.

Kohn, R. R. (1982). Cause of death in very old people. *Journal of the American Medical Association, 247*, 2793–2797.

Lawton, M. P. (1982). Competence, environmental press, and the adaptation of older people. In P. G. Windley & T. O. Byerts (Eds.), *Aging and the environment: Theoretical approaches* (pp. 33–59). New York: Springer.

Maslow, A. H. (1954). Motivation and personality. New York: Harper & Row.

Mehta, N. K., Sudharsanan, N., & Elo, I. T. (2014). Race/ethnicity and disability among older Americans. In K. E. Whitfield & T. A. Baker (Eds.), *Handbook of minority aging* (pp. 131–161). New York: Springer.

Melov, S. (2016). Geroscience approaches to increase healthspan and slow aging. *F1000 Faculty Rev, 5*, 785. doi: 10.112688/f1000research.7583.1.

Montgomery, R., Kwak, J., & Kosloski, K. D. (2016). In V. L. Bengston & R. A. Settersten (Eds.), *Handbook of theories of aging* (3rd ed., pp. 443–462). New York: Springer Publishing Company.

Morley, J. E. (2009). Successful aging or aging successfully. *Journal of the American Medical Directors Association, 10*(2), 85–86.

National Center for Health Statistics. (2016). *Health, United States, 2015.* Washington D.C.: U.S. Government Printing Office.

New England Centenarian Study. (2014). *Why study centenarians? An overview.* Available at www.bumc.bu.edu/centenarian/overview.

Ngo, N., Sands, M., & Isaacowitz, D. M. (2016). Emotion-cognition links in aging: Theories and evidence. In V. L. Bengston & R. A. Settersten (Eds.), *Handbook of theories of aging* (3rd ed., pp. 213–234). New York: Springer Publishing Company.

Nikolich-Zugish, J., Goldman, D. P., Cohen, P. R., et al. (2016). Preparing for an aging world: Engaging biogerontologists, geriatricians, and the society. *Journals of Gerontology: Biological Sciences and Medical Sciences, 71*, 435–444.

O'Rand, A. (2016). Long, broad, and deep: Theoretical approaches in aging and inequality. In V. L. Bengston & R. A. Settersten (Eds.), *Handbook of theories of aging* (3rd ed., pp. 365–379). New York: Springer Publishing Company.

Passarino, G., De Rango, F., & Montesanto, A. (2016). Human longevity: Genetics or lifestyle? It takes two to tango. *Immunity & Aging, 13*,12.

Peck, R. C. (1968). Psychological developments in the second half of life. In B. L. Neugarten (Ed.), *Middle age and aging* (pp. 88–92). Chicago, IL: University of Chicago Press.

Quesnel-Vallee, A., Willson, A., & Reiter-Campeau, S. (2016). Health inequalities among older adults in developed countries: Reconciling theories and policy approaches. In L. K. George & K. F. Ferraro (Eds.), *Handbook of aging and the social sciences* (8th ed., pp. 483–502). Oxford: Academic Press.

Sadana, R., Blas, E., Budhwani, S., et al. (2016). Healthy ageing: Raising awareness of inequalities, determinants, and what could be done to improve health equity. *Gerontologist, 56,* S178–S194.

Schaie, K. W. (2016). The psychology of aging. In V. L. Bengston & R. A. Settersten (Eds.), *Handbook of theories of aging* (3rd ed., pp. 53–66). New York: Springer Publishing Company.

Schultz, M. B., & Sinclair, D. A. (2016). When stem cells grow old: phenotypes and mechanisms of stem cell aging. *The Company of Biologists Ltd/Development, 143,* 3–14.

Sebastiani, P., & Perls, T. (2012). The genetics of extreme longevity: Lessons from the New England Centenarian Study. *Frontiers in Genetics, 3,* Article ID 277. doi:10.3389/fgene.2012.00277.

Settersten, R. A. (2016). Advances in social science theories of aging. In V. L. Bengston & R. A. Settersten (Eds.), *Handbook of theories of aging* (3rd ed., pp. 301–304). New York: Springer Publishing Company.

Sousa-Victor, P., Neves, J., & Jasper, H. (2016). Theories of stem cell aging. In V. L. Bengston & R. A. Settersten (Eds.), *Handbook of theories of aging* (3rd ed., pp. 153–172). New York: Springer Publishing Company.

Stenholm S., Head, J., Kivimaki, M., et al. (2016). Smoking, physical inactivity and obesity as predictors of health and disease-free life expectancy between the ages of 50 and 75: A multicohort study. *International Journal of Epidemiology,* 1–11. doi: 10.1093/ije/dyw126.

Tornstam, L. (1994). Gerotranscendence: A theoretical and empirical exploration. In L. E. Thomas & S. A. Eisenhandler (Eds.), *Aging and the religious dimension.* Westport, CT: Greenwood.

Tornstam, L. (1996). Gerotranscendence: A theory about maturing into old age. *Journal of Aging & Identity, 1,* 37–50.

Willcox, D. C., Willcox, B. J., & Poon, L. W. (2010). Centenarian studies: Important contributors to our understanding of the aging process and longevity. *Current Gerontology and Geriatrics Research,* Article ID 484529. doi:10.1155/2010/484529.

Wolf, D. (2016). Late-life disability trends and trajectories. In L. K. George & K. F. Ferraro (Eds.), *Handbook of aging and the social sciences* (8th ed., pp. 77–99). Oxford: Academic Press.

Wong, G., Low, J. A., & Yap, P. (2016). Active ageing to gerotranscendence. *Annals of the Academy of Medicine, 45*(2), 41–43.

Woods, N. F., Rillamas-Sun, E., Cochrane, B. B., et al. (2016). Aging well: Observations for the Women's Health Initiative Study. *Journals of Gerontology: Biological Sciences and Medical Sciences, 71,* S3–S12.

Xu, M., & Kirkland, J. L. (2016). Inflammation and aging. In V. L. Bengston & R. A. Settersten (Eds.), *Handbook of theories of aging* (3rd ed., pp. 137–152). New York: Springer Publishing Company.

Nursing Considerations for Older Adults

**Unfolding Patient Stories:
Sherman "Red" Yoder · Part 2**

Sherman "Red" Yoder, age 80, lives alone on his farm, which is managed by his son, Jon, who lives nearby. Red drives 20 miles into town at least once a week to visit with friends. The home health nurse has come to evaluate his diabetes management and an open foot wound. Red's daughter-in-law, Judy, has expressed concern about his driving ability. How does the nurse initiate the discussion with Red to assess his ability to drive safely? What age-related changes and conditions can increase the risk for unsafe driving? What interventions should the nurse consider if driving risks are identified?

Care for Red and other patients in a realistic virtual environment: **vSim** *for Nursing* (thepoint. lww.com/vSimGerontology). Practice documenting these patients' care in DocuCare (thepoint.lww.com/ DocuCareEHR).

**Unfolding Patient Stories: Julia Morales
and Lucy Grey · Part 2**

Recall from Part 1 Julia Morales, who is receiving chemotherapy and radiation for lung cancer. She has decided to stop treatment. Lucy, her partner for more than 25 years, is supportive of her choice and wants to care for Julia in their home. Julia's son, Neil, is urging her to try one more round of chemotherapy. How can the nurse assist them with care decisions? Why is it important for the nurse to discuss advance directives and the appointment of a health care proxy with Julia and her family? How can the nurse establish and support Julia's values and preferences for care? What other health care practitioners could the nurse call on to provide an interprofessional approach in this situation?

Care for Julia, Lucy, and other patients in a realistic virtual environment: **vSim** *for Nursing* (thepoint. lww.com/vSimGerontology). Practice documenting these patients' care in DocuCare (thepoint.lww.com/ DocuCareEHR).

chapter 5

Gerontological Nursing and Health Promotion

What emerges from the information in Part 1 is an image of older adults as a diverse group of individuals from varied sociocultural backgrounds who are more heterogeneous than homogeneous. Clearly, even among same-age cohorts, as people age, they become less and less like others of the same age. Indeed, the most universal characteristic of increasing age is increasing individuality and diversity. Because the provision of health care and other services to this population is complex, several branches of science have evolved to address the unique issues related to aging and older adults. In recent years, there has been increasing attention to the importance of all nurses becoming competent in addressing the unique health care needs of older adults and applying evidence-based guidelines to nursing practice. There also has been increasing attention to the importance of health promotion interventions and the roles of nurses in promoting wellness.

GERONTOLOGY AND GERIATRICS

Gerontology, which is the study of aging and older adults, was first recognized as a specialty in the mid-1940s with the establishment of the Gerontological Society of America and the publication of the first issue of the *Journals of Gerontology*. Since its beginning, gerontology has addressed problems through a multidisciplinary perspective. Gerontology continues to be multidisciplinary and is a specialized area within various disciplines, such as nursing, psychology, social work, and certain allied health professions. Although the initial focus of gerontology was primarily on *problems of aging and older adults*, the focus has shifted to an emphasis on *healthy and successful aging*.

In addition to focusing on healthy aging, gerontologists are addressing the increasing diversity among older people and the increasing complexity of providing health care for older adults. Consequently, the health care specialties of geriatric medicine and gerontological nursing have emerged. **Geriatrics** (also called geriatric medicine) is a subspecialty of internal medicine or family practice that focuses on the medical problems of older people. The American Geriatrics Society was established in 1942 and published the first issue of its professional journal, *Geriatrics*, in 1946. In 1953, the society changed the name of its journal to the *Journal of the American Geriatrics Society* and broadened its focus to address multidimensional issues that affect the overall health and functioning of older adults. In recent decades, geriatric practitioners shifted their focus from curing to caring. This does not mean, however, that decisions about interventions are based primarily on chronologic age. Rather, decisions about interventions are based on a holistic assessment of the individual, with emphasis on quality-of-life issues, interventions to maintain optimal functioning, and health promotion as a means of delaying the onset of disability.

GERONTOLOGICAL NURSING AS A SPECIALTY AND A RESPONSIBILITY

Although nurses first recognized the importance of addressing the unique needs of older adults in the early 1900s, geriatric nursing was not considered a specialty until the 1960s. By the mid-1970s, the American Nurses Association (ANA) was advocating the use of the term *gerontological nursing*, instead of *geriatric nursing*, to more accurately reflect the broader scope of nursing care rather than a focus on disease conditions. For more than a half century, the ANA has shown strong support of gerontological nursing as a specialty, which includes the recent revision of the *Gerontological Nursing Scope and Standards of Practice* (ANA, 2010). This document describes the responsibilities for gerontological nurses, who are the health care professionals consistently responsible for the 24-hour care of older adults in all clinical settings. **Gerontological nursing** includes the following responsibilities:

- Use of evidence-based information to address the unique physiologic, psychosocial, developmental, economic, cultural, and spiritual needs related to the process of aging and care of older adults
- Collaboration with older adults and their significant others to promote autonomy, wellness, comfort, optimal functioning, and quality of life from healthy aging to end of life
- Leadership in interprofessional teams in a holistic and person-centered approach

(ANA, 2010).

The American Nurses Credentialing Center is another nursing organization that recognizes gerontological nursing as a specialization by offering certification as a gerontological nurse, a clinical specialist in gerontological nursing, or a gerontological nurse practitioner. In addition, the American Association of Colleges of Nursing (AACN) has worked collaboratively with other organizations for several decades to develop, update, and promulgate recommended competencies for baccalaureate and advanced practice nursing programs. Since 2010, this organization has published the following competencies that are pertinent to gerontological nursing: Baccalaureate Competencies for Nursing Care of Older Adults, Adult-Gerontology Primary Care Nurse Practitioner Competencies, Adult-Gerontology Acute Care Nurse Practitioner Competencies, and Adult-Gerontology Clinical Nurse Specialist Competencies.

Medicare began paying for services of nurse practitioners in 2003, and opportunities for advance practice nurses in geriatric care setting have been expanding since then. An advanced practice gerontological nurse holds a degree higher than a baccalaureate and demonstrates clinical expertise in caring for older adults at all levels of wellness and illness. Roles of advanced practice nurses include teacher, researcher, consultant, administrator, expert clinician, independent practitioner, care/case manager, individual/group counselor, and multidisciplinary team member/leader. The expansion of opportunities for advanced practice nurses that began during the early 2000s was accompanied by wide variability of licensure requirements among the states. In 2008, the Advanced Practice Registered Nurse Consensus Group and the National Council of State Boards of Nursing APRN Advisory Committee addressed these concerns and recommended the merger of adult and gerontological nursing as one area of advanced practice nursing. Based on these recommendations, graduate schools of nursing began offering Adult-Gerontology Advanced Practice Nursing programs in 2015. These programs prepare advanced practice nurses to provide comprehensive care to the entire adult population, including healthy and frail older adults.

Competencies for Older Adult Care

In conjunction with the growth of gerontological nursing as a specialty, there has been increasing recognition that *all nurses who work with adults* need to be competent in addressing the unique health issues of *older adults*. This recognition has evolved from a combination of demographic changes discussed in Chapter 1 and the increasing concerns about quality of care for older adults. A major theme of the 2008 Institute of Medicine report on *Retooling for an Aging America: Building the Health Care Workforce* was that much more needs to be done to ensure that all professionals are competent to care for older adults (Institute of Medicine, 2008). The *Recommended Baccalaureate Competencies for the Nursing Care of Older Adults*, published in 2010 by the AACN, describes 19 competencies that are essential for all nurses who provide care for older adults. Some competencies that are included in this document are as follows:

- Incorporate professional attitudes, values, and expectations about aging in the provision of person-centered care for older adults and their families.
- Assess the living environment as it influences functional, physical, cognitive, psychological, and social needs of older adults.
- Recognize and respect the variations of care, the increased complexity, and the increased use of health care resources inherent in care of older adults.
- Facilitate ethical, noncoercive decision making by older adults, families, and caregivers.
- Facilitate safe and effective transitions across levels of care.
- Implement and monitor strategies to prevent risk and promote quality and safety.

Links to the full document discussing application of the 19 gerocompetency statements to essential competencies for baccalaureate nursing are provided in Learning Activity 5-1.

Initiatives and Resources for Improving Gerontological Nursing Competencies

In 2010, the Institute of Medicine published a landmark report on *The Future of Nursing: Leading Change, Advancing Health* (Institute of Medicine, 2010). One outgrowth of this report was the establishment of the Campaign for Action, a national initiative of AARP, the AARP Foundation, and the Robert Wood Johnson Foundation for the purpose of guiding implementation of the Future of Nursing report. In October 2013, John Rowe, MD, who served on the Future of Nursing committee, accepted a leadership award from the AACN and spoke about the opportunities and challenges facing nursing that are being addressed by the Campaign for Action. Dr. Rowe's first point in his acceptance speech was in relation to the aging of the population and the role of nurses in caring for older adults:

> As you all are aware, previously unimagined numbers of individuals are living to be very old in America and our health care system, including nursing, is ill prepared to cope with the increasing demand for sophisticated geriatric care. We need more, better, and better prepared providers of geriatric care and new models of care designed to address common geriatric syndromes. Nursing will be called upon to provide much of the needed care.

Additional points emphasized by Dr. Rowe that are especially relevant to nursing care for older adults are (1) the need for more content in nursing education on geriatrics, gerontology, prevention, and palliative care; (2) the rapid development of new models of care and care coordination; (3) the importance of interdisciplinary teams; and (4) the critical role of nurses in improving quality of care and reducing costs (e.g., by reducing hospital readmission rates by 25%) (Rowe, 2013). In 2016, Dr. Rowe and other prominent professionals, including nurse leaders, stated that "geriatric competence of all health care providers may be the number one problem we face in delivering needed care for older persons" (Rowe, Berkman, Fried, et al., 2016, p. 4).

The Campaign for Action is an example of current programs that are working toward the goal of assuring that all nurses are competent in caring for older adults in all adult health care settings. Since the early 1990s, the John A. Hartford Foundation has been forming partnerships with schools of nursing and professional nursing organizations to develop and update evidence-based resources related to improving care for older adults. Of particular importance to practicing nurses and nursing students, the Hartford Institute for Geriatric Nursing supports the development of evidence-based assessment tools and information related to nursing interventions for older adults. Resources include tools and related material for general assessment, for older adults with dementia, and for specialized care, such as pain, caregiving, and risks for cardiovascular disease. Periodically, assessment tools are updated and new ones are added, including resources developed in conjunction with specialty nursing organizations. All resources are readily accessible through the ConsultGeriRN section of Hartford Institute for Geriatric Nursing, which can be accessed through the link in Online Learning Activity 5-1.

Valuable resources for learning about nursing care of older adults also are available through the Center for Geriatric Clinical Simulation at the University of North Carolina, which has developed simulations of nursing case studies with federal funding from the Health Services and Resources Administration. These 26 peer-reviewed simulations address nursing care for older adults who experience a sudden change in health status, an exacerbation of a chronic condition, or a sentinel event such as a fall. Pertinent clinical simulations are cited in Online Learning Activities in many chapters of this text. Figure 5-1 provides a timeline of significant events related to nursing care of older adults as a specialization for some and a responsibility for all nurses in adult care settings.

 See ONLINE LEARNING ACTIVITY 5-1: LINKS TO RECOMMENDED BACCALAUREATE COMPETENCIES AND ADDITIONAL RESOURCES FOR IMPROVING COMPETENCY IN PROVIDING NURSING CARE FOR OLDER ADULTS at http://thepoint.lww.com/Miller8e.

HEALTH, WELLNESS, AND HEALTH PROMOTION

Nurses often use the terms *health* and *wellness* interchangeably because of the shifting paradigm from the traditional health–illness continuum to a whole-person model and person-centered care. This paradigm shift is evident in holistic nursing definitions of health and wellness. For example, a holistic nursing definition of health is "an individually defined state or process in which the individual (nurse, client, family, group, or community) experiences a sense of well-being, harmony, and unity such that subjective experiences about health, health beliefs, and values are honored; a process of becoming an expanded consciousness" (Mariano, 2016, p. 54). Similarly, a holistic nursing definition of wellness is "integrated, congruent functioning aimed toward reaching one's highest potential" (Mariano, 2016, p. 55). In this text, *health* is defined as the ability of older adults to function at their highest capacity despite the presence of age-related changes and risk factors, whereas *wellness* is an outcome (also called a positive functional consequence) for older adults whose well-being and quality of life is improved through nursing interventions. The growing emphasis on wellness recognizes the importance of health promotion and broadens the focus on self-responsibility.

HEALTH PROMOTION FOR OLDER ADULTS

Health promotion refers to programs or interventions that focus on behavior changes directed toward improved

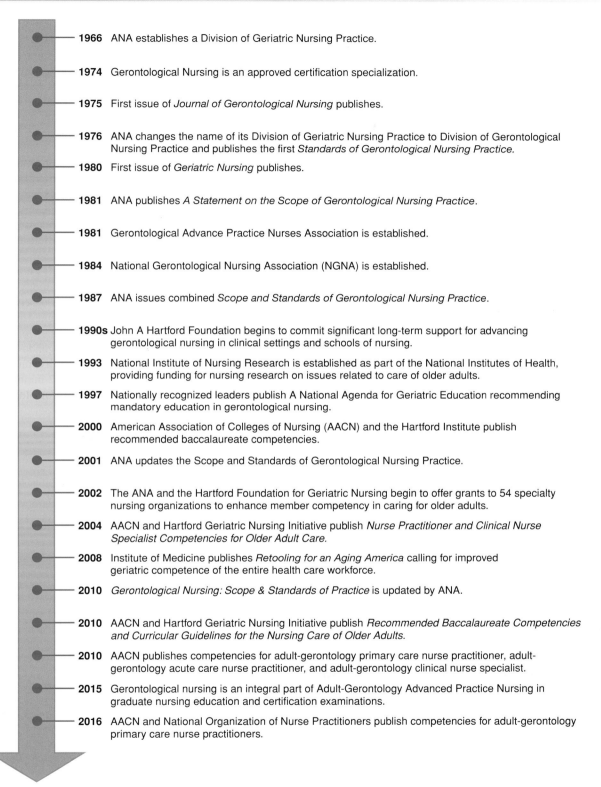

1966 ANA establishes a Division of Geriatric Nursing Practice.

1974 Gerontological Nursing is an approved certification specialization.

1975 First issue of *Journal of Gerontological Nursing* publishes.

1976 ANA changes the name of its Division of Geriatric Nursing Practice to Division of Gerontological Nursing Practice and publishes the first *Standards of Gerontological Nursing Practice.*

1980 First issue of *Geriatric Nursing* publishes.

1981 ANA publishes *A Statement on the Scope of Gerontological Nursing Practice.*

1981 Gerontological Advance Practice Nurses Association is established.

1984 National Gerontological Nursing Association (NGNA) is established.

1987 ANA issues combined *Scope and Standards of Gerontological Nursing Practice.*

1990s John A Hartford Foundation begins to commit significant long-term support for advancing gerontological nursing in clinical settings and schools of nursing.

1993 National Institute of Nursing Research is established as part of the National Institutes of Health, providing funding for nursing research on issues related to care of older adults.

1997 Nationally recognized leaders publish A National Agenda for Geriatric Education recommending mandatory education in gerontological nursing.

2000 American Association of Colleges of Nursing (AACN) and the Hartford Institute publish recommended baccalaureate competencies.

2001 ANA updates the Scope and Standards of Gerontological Nursing Practice.

2002 The ANA and the Hartford Foundation for Geriatric Nursing begin to offer grants to 54 specialty nursing organizations to enhance member competency in caring for older adults.

2004 AACN and Hartford Geriatric Nursing Initiative publish *Nurse Practitioner and Clinical Nurse Specialist Competencies for Older Adult Care.*

2008 Institute of Medicine publishes *Retooling for an Aging America* calling for improved geriatric competence of the entire health care workforce.

2010 *Gerontological Nursing: Scope & Standards of Practice* is updated by ANA.

2010 AACN and Hartford Geriatric Nursing Initiative publish *Recommended Baccalaureate Competencies and Curricular Guidelines for the Nursing Care of Older Adults.*

2010 AACN publishes competencies for adult-gerontology primary care nurse practitioner, adult-gerontology acute care nurse practitioner, and adult-gerontology clinical nurse specialist.

2015 Gerontological nursing is an integral part of Adult-Gerontology Advanced Practice Nursing in graduate nursing education and certification examinations.

2016 AACN and National Organization of Nurse Practitioners publish competencies for adult-gerontology primary care nurse practitioners.

FIGURE 5-1 Significant events in the growth of gerontological nursing.

health and well-being of individuals, groups, communities, and nations in relation to their environments. Traditionally, health promotion programs emphasized disease prevention (i.e., risk reduction) and health maintenance (i.e., sustaining a neutral state of health), but more recently, health promotion also emphasizes personal responsibility for health and self-care actions to achieve high-level wellness. Based on this broader approach, promoting wellness for older adults inherently involves helping older adults incorporate health-enhancing behaviors into their daily lives. The scope of health promotion interventions for older adults includes all the following aspects:

- Regularly engaging in several types of physical exercise
- Assuring optimal nutritional intake and avoiding foods associated with risk for disease
- Engaging in recommended screening and preventive services, such as blood pressure checks and immunizations
- Using stress-reduction methods, such as meditation and relaxation
- Fostering healthy relationships with others
- Engaging in self-wellness actions (e.g., getting adequate rest and sleep, taking time for enjoyable activities alone or with others)
- Attending to spiritual growth
- Engaging in holistic wellness practices (e.g., yoga, tai chi)

In addition, engaging older adults in developing advance care planning is a topic that is receiving attention as an aspect of health behavior change using the Stages of Change model (Ernecoff, Keane, & Albert, 2016; Fried, Redding, Robbins, et al. 2016).

Because of the importance of reducing health care costs and improving quality of care, health promotion programs increasingly focus on evidence-based interventions to prevent, detect, and manage conditions that are leading causes of death and disability. Major organizations such as the American Heart Association, the American Cancer Association, and the American Diabetes Association publish evidence-based information related to primary and secondary prevention. Another focus of health promotion for older adults is on effective self-management, of chronic conditions that occur more commonly among older adults and affect independent functioning and quality of life, as discussed in the section on Roles of Nurses in Promoting Self-Management of Chronic Conditions.

In addition to having an impact on cost of care, health promotion can have a positive effect on quality of life. A commonly cited goal of gerontological health care is to *add life to years, not just more years to life*, which is synonymous with improved quality of life. The concept of **health-related quality of life** was proposed by the National Center for Chronic Disease and Health Promotion (at the Centers for Disease Control and Prevention) in 1993 and has been used as a measure of Medicare health outcomes since 2003. Health-related quality of life is measured by a standard set of questions, called "Healthy Days Measures," addressing one's perception of physical and mental health and functioning. Currently, there is increasing attention to improved health-related quality of life as an outcome of health promotion interventions related to specific conditions.

Even though health promotion interventions are cost-effective ways of preventing disease and disability and improving functioning and quality of life for older adults,

older adults as a group receive fewer prevention and screening services than other populations. This is due to misperceptions, such as (1) older adults are less responsive to health promotion interventions and (2) preventive services are less effective after the onset of chronic illness. In reality, health promotion is essential for older adults precisely because they have more chronic conditions, have complex health care needs, and use considerably more health care services than younger adults. In addition, longitudinal studies show that even after the age of 75 or 80 years, health-promoting interventions for older adults are effective for improving functioning and quality of life and increasing life expectancy (Behm, Eklund, Wilhelmson, et al., 2016; Duplaga, Grysztar, Rodzinka, & Kopec, 2016). Another current concern is that significant health disparities exist among older adults related to use of clinical preventive services, as illustrated in Figure 5-2.

The *Healthy People* initiative is a well-known program that began in the 1990s and continues today as a major source of recommendations for evidence-based health promotion interventions. The program—designed as a road map for improving the health of all people in the United States—outlines a comprehensive, nationwide agenda for promoting health and preventing illness, disability, and premature death. *Healthy People 2020* identifies 12 major objectives specifically related to promoting health for older adults, as summarized in Box 5-1.

 GLOBAL PERSPECTIVE

Since 2001, the World Health Organization has encouraged the development of health promotion initiatives focused on needs of older adults.

A Student's Perspective

On our first day at the facility, we interviewed Teri, the registered nurse who oversees all the clinical care. She has been a nurse for about 15 years and she was very animated and passionate about her job. Throughout her years as a nurse, she has worked in settings such as hospitals, the ICU, a dermatologist's office, and now in long-term care. She did not think she'd be working in gerontological nursing, but she is very happy and fulfilled.

Teri talked about some of the different ways the staff promotes wellness for residents including things such as life-enriching activities that include health and fitness programs, special outings, and cultural events to enhance a resident's mind, body, and spirit. Another way they promote wellness that really caught my attention is the fact that the staff of nurses and other employees work hard to keep residents in their current living situation. For example, they will do whatever is necessary to keep clients in the independent living apartment before moving them to assisted living. They strive to help the residents keep their independence as long as possible and I really enjoyed that aspect of their care.

Molly D.

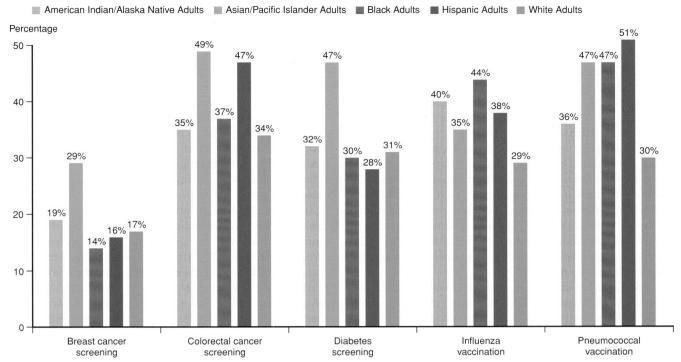

■ American Indian/Alaska Native Adults   ■ Asian/Pacific Islander Adults   ■ Black Adults   ■ Hispanic Adults   ■ White Adults

FIGURE 5-2 Percentage of adults who need clinical preventive services by race and ethnicity. (Adapted from Centers for Disease Control and Prevention, Administration on Aging, Agency for Healthcare Research and Quality, and Centers for Medicare and Medicaid Services. *Enhancing Use of Clinical Preventive Services Among Older Adults*. Washington, DC: AARP. 2011. Available at www.cdc.gov/aging)

 ## TYPES OF HEALTH PROMOTION INTERVENTIONS

Interventions to promote physical and psychosocial well-being include screening programs, risk-reduction interventions, environmental modifications, and health education. This section reviews these types of programs in relation to promoting wellness for older adults. All clinically oriented chapters of this text emphasize health promotion because this is a central focus of the Functional Consequences Model for Promoting Wellness. Thus, nursing interventions are directed toward improved health, functioning, and quality of life for older adults, with emphasis on teaching older adults and their caregivers about health-promoting activities.

Screening Programs

Screening programs are an essential component of disease prevention because they may detect serious and progressive conditions as early as possible. The National Guideline

---

Box 5-1   Objectives of *Healthy People 2020* Pertinent to Nursing Care of Older Adults

Objectives Related to Health Promotion Activities

Increase the proportion of older adults who:
● Use Medicare preventive services benefit
● Engage in light, moderate, or vigorous leisure-time activities
● Are up-to-date on core clinical preventive services (e.g., colorectal cancer screening)
● Report confidence in managing their chronic conditions
● Have moderate to severe functional limitations
● Participate in diabetes self-management programs

Objectives Related to Resources for Older Adults

● Reduce the proportion of community-living older adults with disabilities who have an unmet need for long-term care services and supports
● Reduce the proportion of unpaid caregivers who report an unmet need for caregiver support services

Objectives Related to Care of Older Adults

● Reduce the rate of pressure ulcer–related hospitalizations
● Reduce the rate of emergency department visits due to falls

Objectives Related to Elder Abuse

● Improve data collection and dissemination of information from States, the District of Columbia, and Native American Tribes related to characteristics of victims, perpetrators, and case of elder abuse, neglect, and exploitation

Objectives Related to the Health Care Workforce

● Increase the proportion of registered nurses with geriatric certification

Healthy People 2020, available at www.healthypeople.gov.

Clearinghouse, the U.S. Preventive Services Task Force, and many professional organizations publish numerous evidence-based recommendations for screening related to conditions such as glaucoma, diabetes, hypertension, hyperlipidemia, osteoporosis, cognitive impairment, and many types of cancer. Most recently, screening guidelines have been developed for lung cancer and obstructive sleep apnea (Jonas, Amick, Feltner, et al., 2017; van der Aalst, ten Haaf, & de Koning, 2016).

Screening programs focus on conditions that can be accurately detected and effectively treated before they progress to a serious or fatal stage. Cost-effectiveness of a screening test is determined according to criteria such as its ability to detect a condition or risk factor at an early stage and without excessive false-positive or false-negative results. Another requirement for recommending a screening test is that early intervention must be superior to waiting until signs or symptoms of disease are present.

Guidelines for starting and stopping certain screening procedures are based on chronological age or life expectancy. It is imperative to consider chronologic age as only one criterion for decisions about screening for, or treatment of, diseases. Most importantly, decisions need to be based on an assessment of the individual's risk factors and current and anticipated status with regard to health, functioning, and quality of life. Also, primary care practitioners and older adults should engage in shared decision making about benefits and harms of screening tests (Braithwaite, Demb, & Henderson, 2016).

Risk-Reduction Interventions

Risk-reduction interventions, which are based on an assessment of the risk for developing a particular condition, are directed toward reducing the chance of developing that condition. Some risk-reduction interventions (e.g., immunizations) apply to all older adults, and other interventions vary according to specific risk factors and the health level of an older person. Risk-assessment tools have been developed for various conditions pertinent to older adults, such as falls, anxiety, depression, heart disease, pressure ulcers, and elder abuse and neglect, as discussed in this textbook. These tools often include a rating scale to identify people who are most likely to develop a particular condition so that health care professionals can plan and implement preventive interventions for them. These tools also serve to identify risk factors that can be addressed through preventive interventions.

Even without formal assessment tools, however, health care professionals can usually identify risk factors that can be addressed to prevent disease or disability. Typically, priority is given to reducing the risk factors that are most dominant or likely to have the most serious negative consequences. For example, health promotion interventions for a relatively healthy older adult with a history of hypertension and hypercholesterolemia and family history of heart attacks would address risk factors for heart disease. Health promotion interventions for a frail older adult who is in a skilled care unit and who is recovering from a fractured hip would focus on risk for falls.

For all older adults, risk-reduction interventions include lifestyle factors, such as weight management, optimal nutrition, adequate physical activity, sufficient sleep, avoidance of secondhand smoke, and appropriate stress-relieving techniques. Smoking cessation is a risk-reduction activity for all people who smoke. Health promotion activities to reduce risk may also include the use of dietary supplements (e.g., vitamins, minerals), and complementary and alternative therapies (e.g., yoga).

Immunizations (also called vaccinations) are an effective but often overlooked risk-reduction intervention for older adults that nurses can routinely incorporate in their care (Hale & Marshall, 2016). In addition to the immunizations for influenza, pneumonia, and tetanus that have been routinely recommended for decades, since 2006, a herpes zoster immunization has been recommended for people aged 60 years and older. Figure 5-3 illustrates an easy-to-read educational handout that nurses can use to teach older adults about immunizations.

Environmental Modifications

Environmental modifications are health promotion activities when they reduce risks or improve a person's level of functioning. The Functional Consequences Model for Promoting Wellness addresses environmental modifications as health promotion interventions in relation to many aspects of functioning in clinically oriented chapters of this text. For example, environmental modifications can be effective health promotion interventions when their implementation reduces fall risks (Chapter 22), improves hearing and vision (Chapters 16 and 17), and prevents urinary incontinence (Chapter 19).

Health Education

Health education is an essential component of health promotion because it focuses on teaching people to engage in self-care activities that are preventive and wellness enhancing. Health education interventions address specific conditions as well as overall health and functioning. For example, engaging in regular exercise is a major focus of health education because lack of physical activity is well recognized as a risk factor that contributes to numerous unhealthy conditions. Additional topics of health education that are important for all adults are nutrition, dental care, and avoidance of smoking and secondhand smoke (see Chapters 18 and 21). Clinically oriented chapters of this text contain intervention boxes with guidelines for teaching older adults and their caregivers about specific aspects of health and functioning (refer to list at the end of the table of contents in the front of this book). It is imperative to incorporate cultural considerations in health education and to address health literacy as discussed

Attention Older Adults!
Vaccines are not just for kids!

Many people think that only young children need to get vaccinated. However, THOUSANDS OF OLDER ADULTS die or have serious complications each year from vaccine-preventable diseases.

What vaccines do *I* need?

The Centers for Disease Control and Prevention (CDC) recommends that older adults get the following vaccines:

 Shingles vaccine

One shot reduces the risk of shingles and long-term pain after shingles in adults 60 years old and older.

- Shingles causes a painful, blistering rash.

- One in five people with shingles will develop severe, long-term pain after the rash heals.

- Shingles is more common and more serious in older adults.

 Pneumococcal vaccine

One shot reduces the risk of pneumococcal disease.

- Pneumococcal disease can cause serious infections: pneumonia, bacteremia, and meningitis.

- Pneumococcal disease is one of the most common causes of vaccine-preventable death in the United States and is particularly dangerous for older adults.

 Influenza (flu) vaccine

Get the flu vaccine every year to avoid getting the flu and spreading it to loved ones.

- Every year in the United States, an average of 24,000 people die from the flu. Most of these deaths are among adults 65 years old and older.

 Tetanus, diphtheria, pertussis (Tdap) vaccine

One shot of Tdap vaccine reduces the risk of getting potentially deadly infections and the risk of spreading some of these infections to others.

- Parents and grandparents can be ill with pertussis (whooping cough) for months and can pass the infection to babies who are too young to be vaccinated.

- Tetanus is a severe and painful infection, with most deaths from tetanus occurring in older adults.

National Center for Immunization & Respiratory Diseases
Immunization Services Division

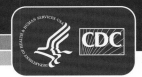

CS226523C   10/2011

FIGURE 5-3 Example of an educational handout to teach older adults about immunizations. (Adapted from National Center for Immunization and Respiratory Diseases, Immunization Services Division. Available at http://www.cdc.gov/vaccines/pubs/downloads/f_imz_oldadults_pr.pdf.)

Box 5-2 Guidelines for Prevention and Health Promotion Interventions for Older Adults

Screening for Healthy Older Adults

- Blood pressure checks: at least annually, more frequently if risk factors are present (e.g., diabetes, African-American race)
- Serum cholesterol: every 5 years, more frequently for people with risk factors, such as personal or family history of cardiovascular disease
- Screening for colorectal cancer as recommended by primary care practitioner
- Visual acuity and glaucoma screening: annually
- Breast examination: self-examination: monthly, annually by primary care practitioner

For Women
- Pap smear and pelvic examination: annually until three consecutive negative examinations, then every 2 to 3 years until 65 years of age
- Mammogram, age 50 to 74 years: every 1 to 2 years

For Men
- Digital rectal examination annually

Screening for Older Adults With Risk Factors

- Blood glucose level
- Thyroid function
- Heart function (electrocardiography)
- Bone density
- Mental status assessment
- Screening for dementia, depression, substance abuse
- Urinary incontinence assessment

- Functional assessment
- Screening for potentially inappropriate medications
- Skin cancer assessment
- Fall risk assessment
- Pressure ulcer assessment
- Elder abuse or neglect assessment
- HIV screening
- Lung cancer screening
- Abdominal aortic aneurysm

For Men
- Prostate-specific antigen blood test

Health Promotion Counseling for Older Adults (Unless Contraindicated)

- Exercise: at least 30 minutes of moderate-intensity physical activity daily
- Nutrition: adequate intake of all vitamins and minerals, especially calcium and antioxidants
- Dental care and prophylaxis: every 6 months
- Protective measures: seat belts, sunscreens, smoke detectors, fall risk prevention

Health Promotion Counseling for Older Adults If Applicable

- Smoking cessation
- Substance abuse cessation
- Weight loss
- Dietary supplements

---

in Chapter 6. Nurses can use Box 5-2 as a guide to teaching older adults about the most widely agreed-on guidelines for health promotion interventions.

RESOURCES FOR HEALTH PROMOTION

Many national nonprofit and governmental organizations provide publications and web-based information related to prevention of specific conditions, such as cancer and cardiovascular disease. National organizations also provide valuable information related to self-management of chronic conditions (e.g., arthritis and diabetes) that can be used for health promotion. In addition, links to pertinent resources are provided in the Online Learning Activities in this textbook. Nurses can access resources related to the national programs for health promotion for older adults listed in Box 5-3 through the links in Online Learning Activity 5-2.

 See ONLINE LEARNING ACTIVITY 5-2: RESOURCES FOR HEALTH PROMOTION MATERIALS AND GUIDELINES at http://thepoint.lww.com/Miller8e.

PROMOTION OF PHYSICAL ACTIVITY AS A NURSING INTERVENTION FOR WELLNESS

Articles about the need for increased physical activity are ubiquitous in lay and professional literature, and physical

activity has emerged as the most widely heralded health promotion intervention today. In recent years, there is increasing emphasis on the premise that moderate-intensity physical

Box 5-3 National Programs for Health Promotion for Older Adults

Medicare Preventive Health Services

- Initial preventive physical examination, within the first 12 months after enrollment
- Annual wellness visits
- Screening and preventive services as detailed in Box 5-2

Centers for Disease Control and Prevention, Healthy Aging Program

- Healthy Brain Initiative: A National Public Health Road Map to Maintaining Cognitive Health (2013–2018)
- Enhancing Use of Clinical Preventive Services Among Older Adults: Closing the Gap
- Opportunity Knocks for Preventive Heath
- Advance Care Planning
- Depression
- Emergency Preparedness
- Oral Health
- Shingles Immunization
- Smoking Cessation

National Center for Health and the Aging

- 2013 Monograph: Evidence-Based Programs and Resources for Changing Behavior in Older Adults activity can improve overall health and quality of life and lower the risk for disease. Numerous studies identify all the following health benefits of physical activity for older adults (e.g., Bouaziz, Vogel, Schmitt, et al., 2017; Layne, Hsu, Blair, et al., 2017; Liberman, Forti, Beyer, & Bautmans, 2017; Stubbs, Koyanagi, Hallgren, et al., 2017):

- Weight control
- Decreased risk of cardiovascular disease, diabetes, metabolic syndrome, and some cancers
- Strengthening of bones and muscles
- Reduced risk for falls
- Improved mental health and mood, including alleviation of depression
- Improved functioning in daily activities
- Increased longevity

Despite the wealth of well-established evidence about the beneficial effects of physical activity for older adults, less than one-third of older people in the United States engage in it regularly. Nurses take many roles in promoting physical activity for older adults—in particular, teaching older adults about the health benefits of physical activity. Nurses also assess for and address other factors that positively or negatively influence an older adult to participate in regular physical activity. Nurses can use Figure 5-4 to teach older adults about recommended exercises.

MODELS OF BEHAVIOR CHANGE FOR HEALTH PROMOTION

Health promotion interventions for preventing disease often require a change from detrimental health-related behaviors to those that enhance wellness. Even after people adopt new behaviors, they need to maintain these healthier behaviors and not revert to unhealthy ones. The more ingrained and rewarding or pleasurable the behaviors that must be changed, the more difficult it is to refrain from these activities. Some unhealthy behaviors, such as cigarette smoking, have a strong addictive component that increases the difficulty of behavior change. Similarly, the more comfortable a person is with the absence of healthy behaviors, such as physical activity, the more difficult it will be to develop healthier behaviors.

Initiation and maintenance of healthy behaviors involve both motivation and action steps. The role of gerontological health care professionals in health promotion interventions is to lead and support the older person in replacing unhealthy behaviors with health-promoting behaviors. The **Stages of Change model** (also called the Transtheoretical model) has been widely used by health care professionals to explain stages of behavior change. During the last three decades, the Stages of Change model has been used successfully in programs for stress management, sun exposure, smoking cessation, medication compliance, alcohol and drug cessation, diet and weight control, and screening for cancers. As the name implies, the Stages of Change model describes five specific stages through which a person progresses in accomplishing behavior changes (Table 5-1).

In the first stage, *precontemplation*, the person is unaware of the problem, is in denial of the need for change, or is resistant to change. At this stage, the person has no intention of changing his or her behaviors within the next 6 months. Appropriate health promotion interventions for a person in this stage include providing information about the problem behavior and providing unconditional encouragement for thinking about behavior change. When working with an older adult in this stage, gerontological nurses can offer information, discuss their own beliefs, and help the person identify the personal benefits of the health-promoting behaviors. The nurse also can acknowledge the person's perspective and point out the negative consequences of current behaviors.

The second stage, *contemplation*, is characterized by an intention to change in the foreseeable future, based on some acknowledgment of the negative consequences of current behaviors and positive consequences of different behaviors. The person is likely to ask questions and to seek information about the short- and long-term risks and benefits of various behaviors. He or she is likely to be ambivalent about giving up a rewarding activity or taking on an activity that is viewed as difficult or less enjoyable. During this stage, the gerontological nurse can help the person see that the benefits outweigh the disadvantages, even though the person may not experience the benefits immediately. Appropriate health promotion interventions for this stage include providing additional information about the risks and benefits and exploring with the person how he or she can begin establishing personal goals for a healthier lifestyle. Interventions also include increasing the person's sense of self-efficacy by helping the person to see himself or herself practicing these new behaviors. When working with an older adult in this stage, it is helpful to express confidence in the person's ability to develop health-promoting behaviors.

Stage three, the *preparation* stage, is characterized by some ambivalence about the unhealthy behavior but a stronger inclination to change to healthier behaviors. The person acknowledges the need for change, expresses serious intent to adopt the healthier behaviors within the next month, and begins to identify strategies for implementing them. During this stage, people usually benefit from support from family and friends, and they are likely to state their intentions and seek help from others in accomplishing their goals. Gerontological nurses can support and provide positive reinforcement for the person's intent to change; they also can point out the progress that the person already has made in developing an action plan. An important role for nurses is to assist with developing a plan and identifying the person's goals and small-step strategies to achieve them. Although discussing the barriers to changing behaviors might be necessary, it is important to focus on the benefits of the new behavior. Planning strategies for dealing with anticipated difficulties in implementing the plan is also helpful.

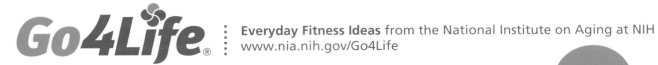

Go4Life®   Everyday Fitness Ideas from the National Institute on Aging at NIH
www.nia.nih.gov/Go4Life

ENDURANCE
STRENGTH
FLEXIBILITY
BALANCE

Include All 4 Types of Exercise

**Exercise generally falls into four main types:
endurance, strength, balance, and flexibility.**

Some activities fit into more than one type of exercise; for example, some endurance activities help build strength, and some flexibility exercises also improve balance. Be creative and choose exercises from each of the four types to see the benefits!

Endurance. Activities that increase your heart rate and breathing for an extended period of time, such as walking, jogging, swimming, dancing, yard work, climbing stairs.
BENEFITS: Everyday activities, like gardening or shopping, become easier to do.
HOW MUCH & HOW OFTEN: Build up to at least 30 minutes of moderate-intensity endurance activity on most or all days of the week.

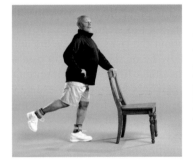

Strength. Activities that increase your muscle strength, such as using resistance bands or small weights (even cans of food) to strengthen groups of muscles.
BENEFITS: Improve ability to do everyday and enjoyable activities and remain independent.
HOW MUCH & HOW OFTEN: Aim for a 30-minute session two or more days a week and include all major muscle groups.

Balance. Activities that improve your balance, such as tai chi, standing on one foot, heel-to-toe walking.
BENEFITS: Help prevent falls and improve safety when performing activities such as standing on tiptoe to reach for objects on high shelves.
HOW MUCH & HOW OFTEN: Do these often, anywhere and anytime; be sure to use a wall or sturdy object for support as needed for safety.

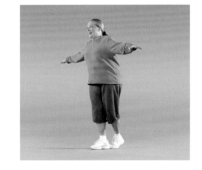

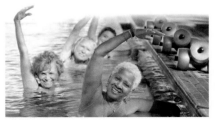

Flexibility. Activities that stretch groups of muscles, or shoulder and upper arm stretches.
BENEFITS: Give you more freedom of movement for daily activities, such as getting dressed.
HOW MUCH & HOW OFTEN: Stretch a group of muscles as far as possible without pain, hold the position for 10 to 30 seconds, relax, breathe, then repeat three to five times.

FIGURE 5-4 Example of an educational handout about recommended types of exercise for older adults. (Adapted from Everyday Fitness Ideas from the National Institute on Aging at NIH. Available at www.nia.nih.gov/Go4Life)

TABLE 5-1 Applying the Stages of Change Model to Mrs. H.

Stage	Nurse	Mrs. H.
I: Precontemplation		
Assessment	"I know you're concerned about preventing heart disease because you've talked with me about your high blood pressure and you pay attention to avoiding high-fat foods. How do you think you rate on a scale of 1 to 10, with 1 being the lowest level and 10 being the best, in level of physical activity for preventing heart disease?"	"I would rate myself about 10. I take the dog out for a 5-minute walk every morning. My friend says we don't need more than 10 minutes of walking a day after we're 70 years old."
Intervention	"Did you know that there is extremely good evidence that 30 minutes of physical activity every day—even if it's not done all at once—is a good measure for protecting against heart disease? Would you be willing to read this pamphlet from the American Heart Association and let me know what you think when I see you again next week?"	"I've seen that before, but I'll try to read it this week if I have a chance."
II: Contemplation		
Assessment	"Now that you've had a chance to read that brochure, what's your understanding of the role of physical activity in preventing heart problems?"	"I think the Heart Association is on an exercise kick—they must think we all want to participate in marathons! Maybe they have a point about walking more than 15 minutes a day, but don't they realize that those of us who are in our 70s have a lot of problems walking? Most of us have arthritis. I think that brochure was written for people in their 20s, but on the other hand, maybe they do know what they're talking about."
Intervention	"From what I know, the Heart Association focuses on help-ing people prevent heart disease through healthy habits. They strongly urge everyone to do physical exercise for 30 minutes every day to keep the heart healthy. Many studies of people of all ages support this recommen-dation. You already walk 5 minutes with your dog every day, so you've gotten a good start on daily exercise. I bet your dog would love to go just a little farther each day and you would be quite capable of increasing your walk by just a little bit."	"Well, the dog is getting pretty fat, and it would probably do her good to get out for another walk in the evening. But it's hard enough for me to get out once a day with the weather as cold as it is right now. With my arthritis, I think I should wait a couple of months until the weather is warmer."
III: Preparation		
Assessment	"Since we met a couple of months ago, what are your cur-rent thoughts about increasing your walking?"	"I've been doing a lot of thinking about what we discussed, and now that spring is finally here, I think it's time to increase my walking time by a little bit each day. I just hope my arthritis doesn't get worse if I walk more."
Intervention	"So, have you thought of a plan that might work for you? Can you identify people who might be helpful in sup-porting your efforts?"	"Well, to begin with, I thought I could walk for 10 minutes every morning instead of 5—my dog sure would like that. I could increase that by 5 minutes every few weeks until I get up to 30 minutes a day. I've told my daughter that I'm trying to do more walking, and she said she might come over and walk with me and the dog on Saturdays. I do worry about my arthritis, though."
IV: Action		
Assessment	"It's so good to hear that you've been increasing your walking time for 3 months now. Congratulations on getting up to 30 minutes a day. How are you feeling about that?"	"My dog sure likes it, but I'm not sure that it's doing any good for me. I guess it feels good to pay attention to my health, but I haven't noticed that I'm feeling any better physically—at least not yet. My daughter came with me for the first few weeks and that was a good chance to see her, but she hasn't been coming for the last 3 weeks."
Intervention	"You deserve a lot of credit for accomplishing your goal—do you give yourself any rewards? It sounds as though you're disappointed that your daughter stopped walking with you—is there anyone else who might walk with you?"	"I guess I do deserve some credit—I did buy myself a new pair of walking shoes last week. A neighbor lady has talked to me about my walking and she said she'd like to get out there and join me, but I didn't encourage that because I thought my daughter would be coming with me. Maybe I'll invite her along—she could use the exercise, too."

(continued)

TABLE 5-1 Applying the Stages of Change Model to Mrs. H. (*Continued*)

Stage	Nurse	Mrs. H.
V: Maintenance		
Assessment	"Congratulations on walking for 30 minutes every day for 7 months—that's quite an accomplishment and a nice gift for yourself and your health. You also deserve credit for getting your neighbor to join you at least a couple of days a week. Are you concerned about any temptations to cut down on your walking routine?"	"Thanks for the encouragement—my neighbor says she appreciates me inviting her along, and I enjoy the chance to keep up on neighborhood happenings by chatting with her when we walk. I am a little concerned about keeping up with the walking during the winter. I don't even take the dog out when it snows."
Intervention	"Have you thought about walking in the mall when the weather is bad? I'm not sure if you can take the dog along, but the mall opens every day an hour before the stores open so that walkers can come. I understand there's quite a group that walks there in the mornings."	"That sounds like a good idea—my neighbor mentioned that we might go there in bad weather. I think I'll try that out—maybe if I went to the mall, I could get my daughter to meet me there on Saturdays."

Action, the fourth stage, occurs when the person has already made the behavior change, but the changes have been practiced for less than 6 months. At this stage, people usually do not fully experience the benefits of the new behavior and are vulnerable to resuming prior unhealthy behaviors or giving up the new healthy behaviors. At the same time, they are likely to have high levels of self-efficacy and to feel good about the progress they have made. Health promotion interventions during this stage are directed toward reinforcing the progress that has been made as well as toward identifying any barriers to continuing the healthy behaviors. Gerontological nurses can help the older adult identify motivators, establish a reward system, and plan strategies for overcoming the identified obstacles. They also can ask about support from friends and family and help the person identify ways of extending their support system if necessary.

Stage five, *maintenance*, occurs when the person has continued the healthy behaviors for 6 months or longer. By this time, the person is experiencing positive effects of the healthier behavior and the risk of relapse is less. During this stage, levels of self-efficacy are usually high and the person is motivated to maintain the healthier lifestyle. Because the person has less need for external support, the role of the gerontological nurse diminishes. Health promotion interventions during this stage include reinforcement of progress and positive feedback about the healthier behaviors. In addition, the nurse can ask about any difficulties in maintaining the progress and help the person identify strategies to overcome any difficulties.

Models of behavior change that have been developed more recently are based on a positive approach and build on the person's strengths. Motivational interviewing is an example of a positive model in which the health care professional assumes the role of a "change coach" and works in partnership with the person. This model emphasizes all the following:

- Personal autonomy and self-responsibility
- Capacity rather than incapacity
- Actions to facilitate change, rather than reasons for avoiding change

- Communication techniques of affirmation, summarizing, reflective listening, open-ended questions, and avoid argumentation or direct persuasion
- Discussion about the person's awareness of the problem, main concerns, intention to change, and confidence about changing
- Exploration of goals and the costs and benefits of changing versus not changing
- Communicating empathy, caring, and a genuine interest in the person's perspective

Although the full use of motivational interviewing requires extensive training, nurses can apply a brief form to health promotion interventions (Howard & Williams, 2016; McCarthy, Dickson, Katz, & Chyun, 2016). Online Learning Activity 5-3 provides a link to an article describing the application of brief motivational interviewing to effectively improve the health behaviors of a challenging patient with heart failure.

 See ONLINE LEARNING ACTIVITY 5-3: ARTICLE DESCRIBING APPLICATION OF MOTIVATIONAL INTERVIEWING TO NURSING CARE OF A PATIENT WITH HEART FAILURE at http://thepoint.lww.com/Miller8e.

Appreciative inquiry is another positive model that has recently been applied to promoting behavior change in health care settings. This model replaces deficit thinking with possibility thinking and uses a set of questions to appreciate and value the best of what is, to envision a future of what might be, and to dialogue about and create what will be. The process is divided into four steps designated as discover, dream, design, and delivery. Moore and Charvat (2007) propose that nurses use the appreciative inquiry approach to explore the person's experiences of what works or has worked to promote health, as in the following questions for each of the four steps:

- Discover: Describe a time when you had an exceptionally healthy lifestyle and consider the following questions: What did you appreciate about the experience? How did

Box 5-4 Communication Techniques for Encouraging Behavior Change

Self-efficacy: increasing the older adult's confidence in accomplishing the desired behavior
- "You deserve a lot of credit for losing those first 5 pounds. Sometimes those are the hardest ones to lose, so you can be confident that you can keep making progress pound by pound."
- "Think about a time when you were successful in the face of a challenge, even though you weren't confident."
- "Describe a personal characteristic that helps you accomplish your goals."

Values clarification: helping older adults identify values in order to reconcile differences between expectations and behaviors
- "People often have mixed feelings about changing behaviors. For example, you know that being overweight increases the risks to your health, but at the same time, you enjoy eating. Let's talk about the ways in which your health is important to you."
- "It sounds like you have a conflict between believing that getting more exercise is good for your health and believing that you have time for this. Let's talk about how you can use your time to support your health."

Consciousness raising: increasing the older adult's awareness about risks that are identified objectively (e.g., elevated blood pressure or abnormal laboratory values for lipids) but are not associated with immediate symptoms
- "Your blood pressure has been around 156/90 for several weeks lately. Are you aware that the ideal range is below 120/80?"
- "Your weight has been increasing during the last 3 years and it is at the point that you are at an increased risk for diabetes, especially because you also have high blood pressure."

Restructuring: using positive thinking to focus on ways of overcoming barriers
- "I know it's hard to get outside in the winter, so let's try to identify some ways of getting more exercise indoors during your usual

activities. For instance, are there times that you could walk in shopping malls or even around your house?"
- "You've identified several barriers to achieving your goal. Can you pick the one that is the easiest to tackle and we'll see if we can find some ways to overcome that. I know that one of your strengths is facing your challenges, so let's look at one of those challenges and come up with a strategy that might work for you."

Focusing on benefits (also called reinforcing rewards): immediately and frequently reinforcing benefits, which are classified as tangible, social, or self-generated
- "Describe how you felt the last time you were at your ideal body weight."
- "Can you identify a healthy reward for engaging in physical activity, for example, by treating yourself to fresh fruit after you come back from the park?"
- "Let's talk about the benefits of quitting smoking. For example, within a day of quitting you've already decreased your risk for heart attack Can you think of another benefit?"

Strengthening social support: involving family and friends in healthy behaviors
- "That's an excellent idea to walk with your friend for a half-hour right after you both come back from the lunch program at the senior center."
- "When your grandchildren visit, would it be feasible to take them to the park or a playground?"

Adapted from C. A. Miller. (2013). *Fast facts for health promotion in nursing: Promoting wellness in a nutshell*. Used with permission from Springer Publishing Company.

---

you make this happen? What people or situational factors supported this positive experience?
- Dream: Imagine that you are so physically active that you feel very fit and healthy and consider the following questions: What would you feel like on a daily basis? What would you be doing? How would you look? What would you be doing for exercise? How do you think it would help your heart?
- Design: What could you do now to be more in charge of your own health and care? Who would you go to for help?
- Delivery: What are we going to do to start this process?

Through this interaction, the nurse and client engage in a cooperative search for strengths, passions, and life-giving forces, so the patient is open to new possibilities.

Nurses can apply principles from these models as they work with older adults to promote healthy behaviors related to nutrition, physical activity, weight management, and other lifestyle factors that increase the risk for disease and affect the person's health and functioning. Although most nurses are not professional health coaches, all nurses can incorporate communication techniques for encouraging behavior change such as the following: self-efficacy, values clarification, consciousness raising, restructuring, focusing on

benefits, and strengthening social support. Box 5-4 briefly describes these interventions and provides examples of communication techniques that can be used to help older adults increase healthy behaviors or decrease those that endanger their health.

Case Study

Mrs. H. is 72 years old and visits the local senior center three times weekly for meals and social activities. Once a month she comes to see you to have her blood pressure checked. You have recently studied the Stages of Change model and are interested in applying it to your clinical work in the senior wellness program. Mrs. H. takes medication for high blood pressure and has expressed concern about heart disease. When you discuss risk factors for heart disease with Mrs. H., she says that she would like to incorporate more physical activity into her daily life, as long as it doesn't worsen her arthritis. She agrees to begin meeting with you regularly to develop a plan. Table 5-1 shows how you might apply the Stages of Change model to your work with Mrs. H.

THINKING POINTS

Precontemplation Stage

- From a health promotion perspective, how would you assess Mrs. H.'s understanding of the role of exercise in preventing heart disease? What misconceptions would you want to address?
- What are the goals of your teaching interventions at this stage?

Contemplation Stage

- How would you assess Mrs. H.'s perception of the advantages and disadvantages of increased levels of exercise?
- What are the goals of your teaching interventions at this stage?
- What additional teaching points would you incorporate in your health promotion interventions at this time?

Preparation Stage

- What additional assessment questions would you ask Mrs. H.?
- What are the goals of your teaching interventions at this stage?
- What additional teaching points would you incorporate, particularly with regard to Mrs. H.'s concerns about her arthritis?

Action Stage

- What concerns would you have about Mrs. H. during this stage, and what additional questions would you ask?
- What additional teaching points would you make?

Maintenance Stage

- What additional assessment questions would you ask Mrs. H.?
- What additional teaching points would you make?

TECHNOLOGY TO PROMOTE WELLNESS IN OLDER ADULTS

The pervasive influence of technology is evident in every aspect of health care, ranging from ways in which clinicians deliver, document, and track health care to implementation of high-tech interventions for diagnosis and treatment of pathologic conditions. More recently, health care providers are increasingly using technology-based apps and interactive programs to improve access to health care. For example, patients can connect with their health care providers through smartphone or laptop apps for assessment and management of chronic and nonlife-threatening acute conditions without visiting a medical facility. In addition, there is much current interest in developing technology-based products to improve functioning and quality of life for people living with functional limitations and chronic conditions. There also is growing awareness of the important ways in which technology contributes to health promotion, particularly regarding self-management of chronic conditions. For example, technology is successfully used to achieve improved diabetes self-management in older adults through all of the following interventions: education, videoconferencing, case management, remote monitoring and screening, interactive feedback and coaching (Walker, Kopp, Binford, & Bowers, 2017). Based on their review of studies, Walker and colleagues concluded that "the use of technology to remotely educate, coach, and monitor "has been shown to decrease cognitive decline, mortality, admissions, and healthcare costs, and may increase knowledge and improve adherence and self-efficacy" (p. 209).

Nurses necessarily need to learn and maintain skills related to the use of technology in clinical practice; however, nurses also need to keep up-to-date on technological developments that can be used to promote wellness in older adults. This is challenging, in part because of misperceptions that older adults are not interested in or capable of using technological devices and programs. Although older adults are the age group least likely to use the internet, the percentage of people age 65 and older who do use it doubled between 2006 and 2016 from 32% to 64% (Pew Research Center, 2017a). Similarly, the percentage of older adults using smartphones has increased to 42% in 2016 (Pew Research Center, 2017b). Moreover, adults now entering older adulthood (often called the "Baby Boomers") are increasingly incorporating personal technology into every part of their lives.

Another aspect of the challenge is obtaining accurate information about technological advances that are currently available and being used to promote wellness in older adults. To address this challenge in the context of the wellness focus of this textbook, a new feature of this edition is the inclusion of "Technology to Promote Wellness in Older Adults" boxes, designated with the ☀ icon. These boxes inform nurses about practical ways in which technology can be used to promote wellness for older adults and ways in which technology presents new opportunities to promote wellness for older adults. Content in the next subsections presents background information about ways in which technology has emerged as an important focus of care for older adults. It also discusses roles of nurses related to the use of technology to promote wellness.

Overview of Gerontechnology

The term **gerontechnology** was coined in 1988 to describe the multidisciplinary field that aims to develop technology to meet the needs of older adults and their caregivers (Graafmans, 2017). In 1991, an interprofessional collaboration of scientists, engineers, and service providers from Europe, Japan, and the United States held the first International Conference on Gerontechnology in the Netherlands. The overriding goal of the conference was to improve the quality of life for older adults and people with disabilities by focusing on three goals derived from public health: (1) delay of age-associated changes in health and daily functioning (primary prevention); (2) compensation for common functional declines (secondary prevention), and (3) improved care for individuals with disabilities (tertiary prevention) (Graafmans, 2017).

Gerontechnology has been rapidly evolving as a major interest at many levels as in the following examples:

- The National Institutes of Nursing Research has funded initiatives led by schools of nursing to test sensors embedded in homes or senior living facilities to prevent falls. Study results are published in peer-reviewed nursing journals.
- Universities are establishing interdisciplinary Centers for Gerontechnology (or Centers for Technology and Aging), with many involving schools of nursing (e.g., Pace University in New York involving professors from the Lienhard School of Nursing).
- For-profit businesses recognize the increasing need for devices and applications that are usable by, and useful to, the rapidly growing population of older adults, their caregivers, and their social network.
- In 2016, the National Institutes of Health launched a 4-year, $7 million initiative, the Collaborative Aging-in-Place Research Using Technology (CART), to develop and test technology-based devices.

Technology for Health Promotion

Telehealth (also called telemedicine or telecare), which involves the use of electronic devices and communication technologies to provide health services to individuals who cannot easily access them, is the most well established type of technology that has been used to connect health care providers with other providers and with patients. Two commonly used telehealth methods are (1) video-conferencing using mobile or laptop devices and (2) telemonitoring, which involves the use of portable devices that are developed for collecting and transmitting assessment information.

Potential benefits of telehealth for older adults include the following (Gray, 2017):

- Increased access to health care services for people who live in rural areas and remote communities and for those who have mobility or transportation limitations
- Improved follow-up and monitoring in home care settings
- Greater autonomy for older adults and their caregivers in accessing health care
- Reduced rate of admission to hospital and long-term care
- Reduced cost of health care

An example of telehealth for health promotion is the delivery of the Gerofit exercise program via video to rural veterans in Virginia who have limited access to in-person wellness

---

Box 5-5 Considerations Related to Technology and Older Adults

Examples of Telehealth Applications for Care of Older Adults

- Video conferencing for assessment and management of acute conditions, such as stroke
- Video conferencing for determination of the need for further evaluation.
- Telemonitoring for chronic conditions including all of the following: falls, hypertension, diabetes, heart failure, chronic obstructive pulmonary disease
- Specialist consultation via video conference for comprehensive geriatric assessment
- Video-conference consultation by dermatologist for skin problems in long-term care residents
- Video-conference consultation by mental health professionals for assessment and monitoring

Examples of Technologies for Improving Health, Function, Safety, and Quality of Life

- Environmental control systems to automate lights, appliances, temperature, communication devices
- Wearable technologies (e.g., reminder watch, activity monitors, dietary monitoring)
- Cognitive training programs
- Assistive robots that perform functions such as fetching objects and that facilitate the performance of daily activities (housekeeping, meal preparation, medication management, financial management)
- Companion robots for cognitive and emotional stimulation

---

programs. Box 5-5 delineates examples of telehealth applications for the care of older adults.

Technology to Promote Wellness in the Daily Lives of Older Adults

Assistive devices have been available for decades to compensate for functional limitations related to hearing, vision, mobility, and other aspects of daily living, as discussed in many chapters of this text. In recent years, technology is increasingly being incorporated in these devices to extend their functionality. For example, emergency alert systems, which have been widely used in homes to call for help after a person falls, now include features such as wearability and wireless communication.

An evolving trend related to telehealth technology among older adults is the increasing use of apps that provide support and feedback for a healthy lifestyle (Kampmeijer, Pavlova, Tambor, et al., 2016). These apps, referred to as mHealth, are used in conjunction with smartphones or other wearable mobile or wireless devices to monitor and provide feedback about health behaviors. For example, wearable devices such as the popular Fitbit device can be combined with telephone counseling to improve physical activity in older adults (Lyons, Swartz, Lewis, et al., 2017). Box 5-5 provides examples of technologies for improving health, function, safety, and quality of life.

Roles of Nurses Related to Technology and Aging

Nurses and other health care professionals have key roles in developing and implementing care plans that may include recommendations about the use of technology. In clinical settings, these roles involve all of the following (1) identification of the need; (2) general and/or specialist assessment; (3) prescription, acquisition, training, and/or education; and (4) follow-up and/or ongoing monitoring (Mihalidis, Wang, & Boger, 2017). Nurses also have essential roles as members of interdisciplinary teams developing person-centered mobile apps to improve functioning in older adults—for example, for those with mild cognitive impairment (Hill, 2017).

Even though some of the featured technological devices are not widely available or easily affordable, it is imperative to be aware of technology-based interventions that are becoming increasingly available to improve function and quality of life for older adults and their caregivers. By being aware of the possibilities, nurses can encourage older adults and their caregivers to explore resources that are available, including participation in clinical trials that involve the use of technology-based interventions.

Chapter Highlights

Gerontology and Geriatrics

- Gerontology and geriatrics are areas of professional specialization that have evolved since the mid-1940s to address the unique needs of older adults.
- The original focus of these specialties was on problems associated with aging, but the current focus is on quality-of-life issues and promoting optimal health and functioning.

Gerontological Nursing as a Specialty and a Responsibility

- Gerontological nursing was first recognized as a specialty during the 1960s; major strides have been made in advancing this specialization through professional nursing organizations and philanthropic foundations (Figure 5-1).
- There is increasing recognition that all nurses in adult health care settings need to be competent in addressing the complex and unique health care needs of older adults.
- The current perspective of health care providers and policy-makers recognizes the dual need for specialized gerontological nurses and for all nurses in adult clinical settings to develop skills in caring for older adults.
- Many evidence-based resources are available for nurses and nursing students to develop competency in care of older adults.

Health, Wellness, and Health Promotion

- Health is the ability of older adults to function at their highest capacity despite the presence of age-related changes and risk factors.

- Wellness is an outcome for older adults whose well-being and quality of life is improved through nursing interventions.

Health Promotion for Older Adults

- Nurses have important roles in health promotion interventions, which are essential for preventing chronic conditions, reducing mortality, and improving quality of life for older adults.
- *Healthy People 2020* identifies 12 major objectives specifically related to promoting health for older adults (Box 5-1).

Types of Health Promotion Interventions for Older Adults (Box 5-2, Figure 5-3)

- Screening programs focus on conditions that can be accurately detected and effectively treated before they progress to a serious or fatal stage.
- Risk-reduction interventions focus on primary or secondary prevention of chronic conditions.
- Environmental modifications reduce risk or improve a person's level of functioning.
- Health education focuses on teaching older adults to engage in self-care activities to promote health.

Resources for Health Promotion

- Many national nonprofit and governmental organizations provide publications and web-based information for health promotion related to specific conditions (Box 5-3).

Promotion of Physical Activity as a Nursing Intervention for Wellness

- Nurses have important roles in teaching older adults about the benefits of physical activity and promoting exercise (Figure 5-4).

Models of Behavior Change for Health Promotion

- The Stages of Change model has been used to address disease prevention and health promotion interventions that require a change in health-related behaviors (Table 5-1).
- Motivational interviewing and appreciative inquiry are models of behavior change based on positive feedback.
- Nurses can incorporate communication techniques to address all the following: self-efficacy, values clarification, consciousness raising, restructuring, focusing on benefits, and strengthening social support (Box 5-4).

Technology to Promote Wellness in Older Adults (Box 5-5)

- Technology is increasingly important in providing health care for older adults.
- Gerontechnology describes the growing multidisciplinary field that aims to develop technology to meet the needs of older adults and their caregivers.

- Telehealth involves the use of electronic devices and communication technologies to increase access to care.
- Technology-based devices are available to improve safety, functioning, and quality of life for older adults.
- Nurses have key roles in developing and implementing care plans that may include recommendations about the use of technology.

Critical Thinking Exercises

1. Describe the development of gerontological nursing from the 1960s to the present.

2. You are asked to give a presentation to beginning nursing students to recruit them for an elective class called "Nursing for Wellness in Older Adults." What topics would you expect to be covered in this course and what points would you make to encourage them to enlist in this course?

3. You are discussing with your fellow students the choices you will be making about a practice area after graduation. You tell them that you are planning to specialize in gerontological nursing, and they challenge your decision with statements such as "You'll be bored to death taking care of old folks. Why don't you specialize in something exciting like trauma care? Besides, there's not much to do about the conditions of older folks, and what's the challenge in taking care of people who aren't going to get better?" How do you respond to these statements?

4. Identify one health-related behavior that you would like to change in your life (e.g., smoking cessation, increased level of exercise, decreased dietary fat intake) and develop a care plan for your behavior change using the Stages of Change of Health Promotion (as in the case study).

5. Identify a clinical situation or a personal experience with someone whose functioning or quality of life is limited due to illness. Then explore internet resources to find technology-based interventions that the person could use to improve his or her wellness.

 For more information about the topics discussed in this chapter, be sure to check out the interactive Online Learning Activities and other helpful resources at http://thepoint.lww.com/Miller8e.

REFERENCES

American Nurses Association. (2010). *Gerontological nursing: Scope and standards practice*. Silver Spring, MD: Author.

Behm, L., Eklund, K., Wilhelmson, K., et al. (2016). Health promotion can postpone frailty: Results from the RCT elderly persons in the risk zone. *Public Health Nursing, 33*, 303–315.

Bouaziz, W., Vogel, T., Schmitt, E., et al. (2017). Health benefits of aerobic training programs in adults aged 70 and over: A systematic review. *Archives of Gerontology and Geriatrics, 69*, 110–127.

Braithwaite, D., Demb, J., & Henderson, L. (2016). Optimal breast screening strategies for older women: Current perspectives. *Clinical Interventions in Aging, 11*, 111–125.

Duplaga, M., Grysztar, M., Rodzinka, M., & Kopec, A. (2016). Scoping review of health promotion and disease prevention interventions

addressed to elderly people. *BioMed Central Health Services Research, 16*(Suppl 5). Doi: 10.1186/s12913-016-1521-4.

Ernecoff, N., Keane, C., & Albert, S. (2016). Health behavior change in advance care planning: An agent-based model. *BioMed Central Public Health, 16*. Doi: 10.1186/s12889-016-2872-9.

Fried, T., Redding, C., Robbins, M., et al. (2016). Development of personalized health messages to promote engagement in advance care planning. *Journal of the American Geriatrics Society, 64*, 359–364.

Graafmans, J. (2017). The history and incubation of gerontechnology. In S. Kwon (Ed.), *Gerontechnology: Research, practice, and principles in the field of technology and aging* (pp. 3–11). New York: Springer Publishing Company.

Gray. L. C. (2017). Telemedicine applications in geriatrics. In H. M., Fillit, K. Rockwood, & John Young (Eds.), *Brocklehurst's textbook of geriatric medicine and gerontology* (8th ed., pp. 1082–1086). Philadelphia, PA: Elsevier.

Hale, D., & Marshall, K. (2016). The benefits of immunizations for older adults. *Home Healthcare Now, 34*, 458–459.

Hill, N. (2017). Person-centered technology for older adults. *Journal of Gerontological Nursing, 43*(4), 3–4.

Howard, L., & Williams, B. (2016). A focused ethnography of baccalaureate nursing students who are using motivational interviewing. *Journal of Nursing Scholarship, 48*, 472–481.

Institute of Medicine. (2008). *Retooling for an aging America: Building the health care workforce*. Washington, DC: National Academies Press.

Institute of Medicine. (2010). *The future of nursing: Leading change, advancing health*. Washington, DC: National Academies Press.

Jonas, D. E., Amick, H. R., Feltner, C., et al. (2017). Screening for obstructive sleep apnea in adults: Evidence report and systematic review of US Preventive Services Task Force. *Journal of the American Medical Association, 317*, 415–433.

Kampmeijer, R., Pavlova, M., Tambor, M., et al. (2016). The use of e-health and m-health tools in health promotion and primary prevention among older adults: A systematic literature review. *BioMed Central Health Services Research, 16*(Suppl 5), 290.

Layne, A. S., Hsu, F. C., Blair, S. N., et al. (2017). Predictors of change in physical function in older adults in response to long-term, structured physical activity: The LIFE Study. *Archives of Physical Medicine and Rehabilitation, 98*, 11–24.

Liberman, K., Forti, L. N., Beyer, I., & Bautmans, I. (2017). The effects of exercise on muscle strength, body composition, physical functioning and the inflammatory profile of older adults: A systematic review. *Current Opinion in Clinical Nutrition and Metabolic Care, 20*, 30–53.

Lyons, E. J., Swartz, M. C., Lewis, Z. H., et al. (2017). Feasibility and acceptability of wearable technology physical activity intervention with telephone counseling for mid-aged and older adults: A randomized controlled pilot trial. *Journal of Medical Internet Research Mhealth Uhealth, 5*, e28. Doi: 10.2196/mhealth.6967.

Mariano, C. (2016). Holistic nursing: Scope and standards of practice. In B. M. Dossey & L. Keegan (Eds.), *Holistic nursing: A handbook for practice* (7th ed., pp. 53–76). Boston, MA: Jones and Bartlett Publishers.

McCarthy, M., Dickson, V., Katz, S., & Chyun, D. (2016). An exercise counseling intervention in minority adults with heart failure. *International Journal of Nursing Studies*. Doi: 10.1002/rnj.265.

Mihalidis, A., Wang, R., & Boger, J. (2017). Gerontechnology. In H. M. Fillit, K. Rockwood, & J. Young (Eds.), *Brocklehurst's textbook of geriatric medicine and gerontology* (8th ed., pp. 1087–1094). Philadelphia, PA: Elsevier.

Moore, S. M., & Charvat, J. (2007). Promoting health behavior change using appreciative inquiry: Moving from deficit models to affirmation models of care. *Family & Community Health Nursing, 30*(15 Suppl 1), S64–S74.

Pew Research Center. (2017a). Internet/broadband fact sheet. *Pew Research Center Internet, Science & Technology*. Available at www.pewinternet.org/fact-sheet.

Pew Research Center. (2017b). Mobile fact sheet. *Pew Research Center Internet, Science & Technology*. Available at www.pewinternet.org/fact-sheet.

Rowe, J. (2013). Dr. John Rowe receives John P. McGovern Lectureship Award from AACN. Available at http://campaignforaction.org/news/dr-john-rowe-receives-john-p-mcgovern-lecturship-award.

Rowe, J., Berkman, L., Fried, L., et al. (2016). *Preparing for better health and health care for an aging population. Perspectives: Expert voices in health & health care*. Washington, DC: National Academy of Medicine.

Stubbs, B., Koyanagi, A., Hallgren, M., et al. (2017). Physical activity and anxiety: A perspective from the World Health Survey. *Journal of Affective Disorders, 208*, 545–552.

Van der Aalst, C. M., ten Haaf, K., & de Koning, H. J. (2016). Lung cancer screening: Latest developments and unanswered questions. *Lancet Respiratory Medicine, 4*, 749–761.

Walker, C., Kopp, M., Binford, R., & bowers, C. (2017). Home telehealth interventions for older adults with diabetes. *Home Healthcare Now, 35*, 202–210.

chapter 6

Health Care for Older Adults in Various Settings

LEARNING OBJECTIVES

After reading this chapter, you will be able to:

1. Describe commonly available types of community-based services for older adults.

2. Describe the types of home-based services and explain how people obtain these services.

3. Explain the difference between skilled nursing home care and long-term nursing home care.

4. Discuss issues related to quality of care in nursing homes and efforts of the nursing home culture change movement to address these issues.

5. Discuss ways in which concerns about quality of care for hospitalized older adults are being addressed.

6. Describe ways in which nurses are involved with interprofessional collaboration when caring for older adults.

7. Discuss the ways in which nurses address concerns about quality and safety of care through Quality and Safety in Nursing (QSEN) competencies and transitional care interventions.

8. Describe caregiver burden, caregiver wellness, and ways in which nurses address needs of caregivers.

9. Describe sources of payment for health care services for older adults.

KEY TERMS

acute care for elders (ACE)

adult day centers

caregiver wellness

Centers for Medicare and Medicaid Services (CMS)

culture change

faith community nursing

geriatric care manager

geriatric resource nurse (GRN)

interprofessional collaboration

long-term care insurance

Medicare

Medigap insurance

nonmedical home care

nursing home

Older Americans Act (OAA)

person-centered care

Program of All-Inclusive Care for the Elderly (PACE)

Quality and Safety Education for Nurses (QSEN)

respite care

skilled home care

transitional care

Although nurses have always cared for older adults, only since the late 1960s have programs been developed to address the unique health care needs of older adults. This chapter presents information about the wide array of services that address the needs of older adults, starting with those that are community based and proceeding to those that are institutional based. However, even this distinction is not always clear because older adults typically receive care in several places, and some services, such as skilled care and hospice, are provided in both community and institutional settings. Because health care providers and policy-makers are currently focusing on major concerns related to both quality and coordination of care, this chapter discusses the roles of nurses in addressing these issues.

The establishment of **Medicare** in 1965 (discussed later in this chapter) stimulated major changes in the delivery of health care services to older adults, primarily in terms of increased access to care for older adults. In recent years, increasing concerns about costs and quality of care have led to the current emphasis on the "triple aim" of improving care, improving health, and reducing costs. The **Centers for Medicare and Medicaid Services (CMS)**, the 2010 Affordable Care Act, and national organizations are addressing these concerns, resulting in another wave of major changes in delivery of health care services to older adults. It is important to recognize that all programs and institutions that receive

Medicare and Medicaid funds—which includes virtually all health care facilities and programs—are directly affected by policies of the CMS. Even when services are not covered by insurance, if the providing agency receives public funds, the services must comply with CMS regulations. Thus, any references to CMS in this chapter apply to virtually all health care services for older adults.

COMMUNITY-BASED SERVICES FOR OLDER ADULTS

Public and private agencies have provided many types of community support resources for older adults for decades, and the range of these services has been broadening in recent decades (see Figure 6-1). For example, home-delivered meals programs have been available in most metropolitan areas for decades, and in recent years, groceries and prepared meals have become available for delivery within 24 hours through Internet sites or toll-free phone numbers. Although community-based services are widely available, older adults and their caregivers often are not aware of the great variety of services available to meet the health needs of older adults in their own homes. Even when they are aware of such services, they may not know the eligibility criteria for publicly funded services to which they are entitled. Also, if community-based services are not culturally relevant, older adults or their families may not use them, even when they are aware of their existence.

Because the use of these resources may improve the health, functioning, and quality of life of older adults, nurses need to address any lack of information about these services. In addition, it is important to address other barriers, such as resistance by caregivers. Nurses have important roles in encouraging the use of services by teaching about the positive effects of services on both the older adult and family caregivers (Macleod, Tatangelo, McCabe, & You, 2017)). Box 6-1 summarizes community-based services and resources that are widely available to address the needs of older adults. These services are particularly important for older adults living in their own homes or other independent settings, which includes 93% of all adults aged 65 years and over (see Figure 6-2). Online Learning Activity 6-1 provides links to additional information about these types of programs.

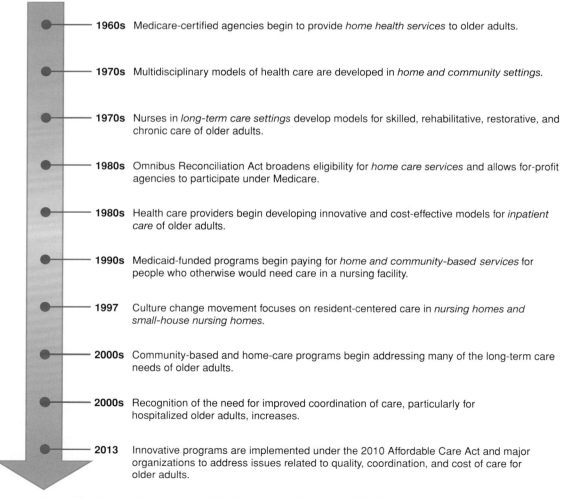

1960s Medicare-certified agencies begin to provide *home health services* to older adults.

1970s Multidisciplinary models of health care are developed in *home and community settings.*

1970s Nurses in *long-term care settings* develop models for skilled, rehabilitative, restorative, and chronic care of older adults.

1980s Omnibus Reconciliation Act broadens eligibility for *home care services* and allows for-profit agencies to participate under Medicare.

1980s Health care providers begin developing innovative and cost-effective models for *inpatient care* of older adults.

1990s Medicaid-funded programs begin paying for *home and community-based services* for people who otherwise would need care in a nursing facility.

1997 Culture change movement focuses on resident-centered care in *nursing homes and small-house nursing homes.*

2000s Community-based and home-care programs begin addressing many of the long-term care needs of older adults.

2000s Recognition of the need for improved coordination of care, particularly for hospitalized older adults, increases.

2013 Innovative programs are implemented under the 2010 Affordable Care Act and major organizations to address issues related to quality, coordination, and cost of care for older adults.

FIGURE 6-1 Significant events that have spurred the development of various models of care for older adults.

Box 6-1 Community Resources for Older Adults

National Eldercare Locator: Provides free information about many types of resources in any part of the United States according to the zip code

Senior Information and Referral Service: Local programs, sometimes called an "Infoline," that provide information about agencies to address specific needs

Area Agency on Aging: Governmental agencies that provide a wide range of services, including referrals, case management, and nonmedical home care workers

Senior Centers: Community-based centers providing services for older adults, such as meals, limited transportation, and social and educational programs

Home-Delivered Meals: Programs that provide home delivery of hot meals to homebound people, sponsored by local senior centers, churches, or hospitals

Companions and Friendly Visitors: Programs that offer services such as socially oriented home visits, assistance with errands, or accompaniment to appointments

Telephone Reassurance: Service providers make scheduled telephone calls to older people to provide support and reminders

Personal Emergency Response Systems: An emergency response system that involves the use of a "call button" (e.g., necklace or bracelet) to initiate a phone call to designated people when assistance is needed (e.g., if the person falls)

Energy Assistance Programs: State and local programs that offer financial assistance for utility bills for people with low incomes

Home Weatherization and Home Repair Service: Contractors paid by government agencies to provide home repairs and maintenance (e.g., insulation, window caulking, and installation) for people with low incomes

 See **ONLINE LEARNING ACTIVITY 6-1: ADDITIONAL INFORMATION ABOUT COMMUNITY-BASED SERVICES FOR OLDER ADULTS** at http://thepoint.lww.com/Miller8e.

Health Promotion Programs

Because of the growing emphasis on health and wellness, many community-based programs for older adults incorporate health promotion activities. Senior centers and other places where older adults gather often offer periodic health screenings and health education activities. Among the health promotion activities offered by these programs are blood pressure checks; safe driving courses; smoking cessation classes; health screening (e.g., cancer, vision, hearing); flu shots and other immunizations; medication assessment, management, and education; and various types of exercise, such as walking, aerobics, aquatics, or tai chi. Health education topics include nutrition, stress management, general health care, and seasonal health issues such as hypothermia, heat-related illness, and colds and flu.

Organized group activities, such as senior wellness programs, frequently take place in, or are sponsored by, community-based senior centers that are available in almost every community. Hospitals and other health care institutions are becoming more involved in providing a broad range of health promotion programs and are employing nurses to address the needs of older adults in the community. Senior centers and health care agencies often cosponsor programs to address specific health issues, such as diabetes, glaucoma, cholesterol levels, or blood pressure. For example, senior health fairs provide the opportunity for follow-up and referral of identified medical issues. Thus, these programs can provide a valuable health promotion service for older adults and at the same time increase the potential patient base for health care providers.

With the current emphasis on improving quality and outcomes and reducing costs, health care providers are developing innovative models of care that involve robust roles for nurses. A review of current models of community care identified the

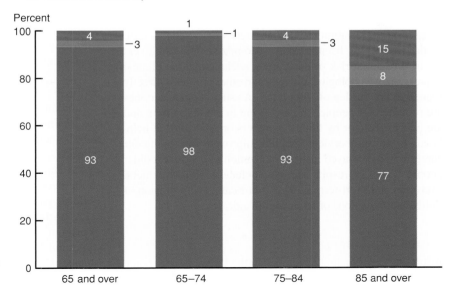

FIGURE 6-2 Percentage of Medicare enrollees age 65 years and over residing in selected residential settings, by age group, 2013. (Adapted from Federal Interagency Forum on Aging-Related Statistics, *Older Americans 2016: Key Indicators of Well-Being*.)

following roles for nurses: team leadership, initial contact, care management/coordination, education, health coaching, and consultation (Mullins, Skemp, & Maas, 2016). Health promotion programs such as these that address the needs of older adults are likely to continue developing as essential components of innovative and comprehensive models of care.

Faith Community Nursing

Faith community nursing (also called parish nursing) has been recognized by the American Nurses Association (ANA) as a specialty practice since 1998. The ANA *Faith Community Nursing: Scope and Standards of Practice*, which was first published in 2005, describes faith community nursing as "a specialized practice of professional nursing that focuses on the intentional care of the spirit as well as on the promotion of wholistic health and prevention or minimization of illness within the context of a faith community" (American Nurses Association, 2012, p. 6). In 2014, the ANA's American Nurses Credentialing Center began offering a portfolio-based certification for Faith Community Nursing. Although the majority of faith community nurses focus on Christian models, some are based in other religious and cultural traditions, such as Hindi, Latino, and Muslim (Harris & Longcoy, 2016).

Faith community nurses provide spiritual care in conjunction with various types of health services, such as education, referrals, screenings, coaching, counseling, and advocacy. For example, a 3-month blood pressure self-monitoring and coaching intervention offered by faith community nurses was effective in promoting lifestyle changes to improve blood pressure (Cooper & Zimmerman, 2017). In addition, the spiritual support provided by faith community nurses is an essential component of health promotion that contributes to improved outcomes for older adults and caregivers (Judge and Hall, 2016).

Respite Services

Respite care refers to any service whose primary goal is to relieve caregivers periodically from the stress of their usual caregiving responsibilities. Gerontologists first used this term in the late 1970s because they recognized that caregivers are at substantial risk of developing social isolation, clinical depression, psychological distress, and other problems directly related to the burden of caregiving. As such, respite services are provided for people who are living in a home setting and are being cared for by family members or other unpaid help. Goals of respite services include improved well-being for caregivers and delayed institutionalization of dependent older people. Types of respite services include adult day centers, overnight and short-term nursing home care, and provision of in-home companions or home health aides.

Adult Day Centers

Adult day centers, first developed in the 1970s, have become a major community-based resource for the care of dependent older adults. These centers provide structured social and recreational activities for functionally impaired older people in a group setting. In addition to group social activities, adult day centers provide meals and any of the following services: transportation, medication management, assistance with personal care, and other health-related services and therapies. Adult day centers generally provide supervised care on weekdays for 8 hours a day, with approximately 5 hours of formal programming during that time and 3 hours of social interaction and other unstructured activities. Less commonly, services are available for longer hours and on weekends and holidays.

Participants in adult day centers usually are impaired to the point that they need supervision or assistance in several functional areas. Most participants are cognitively impaired, but depression and physical disabilities are common conditions among adult day center participants. Participants typically live with a family member, but some live independently or in group settings. The goals of these programs are to maintain or improve the functional abilities of impaired older people; to provide relief for caregivers of dependent older adults; and to improve the quality of life for impaired older adults and their caregivers. Studies have found the following benefits of adult day centers: decreased stress and fewer behavioral problems in people with dementia, and decreased stress, burden, and depression for family caregivers of people with dementia (Klein, Kim, Almeida, et al., 2016; Vandepitte, Van Den Noortgate, et al., 2016; Williams, Tappen, Wiese, et al., 2016). In many situations, the use of adult day centers delays or prevents a move to an institutional setting (Kelly, Puurveen, & Gill, 2016).

Geriatric Care Managers

Identification and coordination of appropriate services have become increasingly more important as the range of programs expands. Decisions related to the selection of care providers are complex because they are based on many variables, including, but not limited to, factors such as cost, availability, and acceptability. Older adults and their families may not be prepared to take on the tasks associated with identifying, arranging, and coordinating appropriate services. Two societal trends that have affected the ability and availability of families to manage care for older adults are the entry of more women into the paid workforce and the common occurrence of adult children moving away from their hometowns to other parts of the country or even to other countries. These factors, along with the significant increase in the number of people aged 85 years and older, have led to the need for independent community-based professional geriatric care management services.

A **geriatric care manager** serves as the primary care coordinator who is responsible for implementing immediate and long-term plans as the needs of the older adult change. Care management services involve comprehensive assessment, care planning, implementation, monitoring, and reassessment. Care managers typically work not only with older adults but also with other professionals, family members, caregivers, and support resources. When family members provide care or coordinate services, care managers often provide counseling and education to address the needs of caregivers, who may or may not be older adults themselves. Nurses are in an ideal position to assume the role of a geriatric care manager because they can comprehensively assess the needs for immediate and long-term care services and then plan, coordinate, and oversee the services.

Geriatric care managers work either as independent contractors or through nonprofit and for-profit groups and organizations. Although the terms care manager and case manager are sometimes used interchangeably, these roles differ in that case management services are usually part of a broader institution-based program. Hospitals and health insurance companies use case managers to make sure that patients receive the most appropriate and cost-effective services.

HOME-BASED SERVICES

Older people and other dependent populations have always received much of their health care at home, and visiting nurse services have existed in the United States since the 1800s. However, the delivery of home care services dramatically changed after 1965 when Medicare began funding these services. By the late 1970s, thousands of home care agencies had been established, and their number escalated exponentially during the next two decades. Although Medicare home health care services were established as a short-term supplement to acute care services for people who needed skilled care, consumers came to view these services as an extension of long-term care for people with chronic illnesses. During the 1980s, two major factors affected the provision of home care services: (1) many restrictions on Medicare-covered home care services were lifted and (2) the Medicare prospective payment system resulted in shorter hospital stays and more referrals for home care services. By the 1990s, home care had become the fastest growing component of the Medicare program, and costs had increased so drastically that Congress included cost-containment measures in the Balanced Budget Act of 1997. Because of this legislation and other federal mandates, the pendulum swung back and it became increasingly more difficult for people to receive skilled home care services. Consequently, fewer Medicare beneficiaries received care, beneficiaries received fewer visits, and home care agencies received lower payments.

At the same time that the federal government was cutting funds for home care, state governments were addressing the high cost of care in nursing homes—which placed a heavy financial burden on state Medicaid programs—by providing more funds for home- and community-based services. Thus, motivated both by cost containment and by consumer preference, state long-term care policy began shifting to community-based services. Although many state-funded programs are limited to people who would be eligible for Medicaid if they were in a nursing home, many affordable services have become widely available through public, private, and nonprofit agencies.

Because of the changing trends in home care since the mid-1960s, two types of home care services—skilled home care and nonmedical home care—have evolved to address different needs. **Skilled home care** services address the needs of people who are recovering from an illness or injury and have potential for returning to their previous level of functioning. In contrast, **nonmedical home care** services address the needs of people with chronic or declining conditions who do not qualify for skilled care.

Skilled Home Care

Home care services provided under Medicare and other health insurance programs have always been limited to skilled home care and restricted to people who meet all of the following criteria:

- The person must be homebound (i.e., leaving the home requires considerable and taxing effort).
- The services must be ordered by a primary care provider.
- There must be a need for skilled nursing or rehabilitative services.
- The person must require intermittent, but not full-time, care.

For people who meet these criteria, Medicare covers the following types of home care services: skilled nursing, physical therapy, occupational therapy, nutrition counseling, speech–language therapy, medical social work, home health aide, and medical supplies and equipment. In addition to nursing assessment and interventions, skilled nursing services can include case management, medication management, infusion therapy, intravenous antibiotics, and psychiatric nursing care. Examples of home health aide services that can be provided under the directions of a licensed nurse or therapist include assistance with bathing, linen changes, range-of-motion exercises, and assistance with transfers and ambulation. People often qualify for skilled home care after a hospitalization or a stay in a skilled nursing or rehabilitation setting for an acute episode, or they may qualify when they experience a change in their condition but have not needed care in a hospital or nursing home.

Because skilled home care services are meant to be short term, a major focus is on teaching the older person and caregivers about self-care activities. Typical skilled care recipients are (1) people who are homebound but able to manage most of their daily care at some level of independence and (2) people who, although homebound and dependent in many functional areas, receive help from families, friends, or paid caregivers to supplement the skilled care services. If people reach a level of independence such that they are no longer homebound, they cannot continue receiving skilled care services under Medicare. Likewise, people no longer qualify for skilled care after they achieve self-care goals. Many people receiving skilled care, however, still need some level of home care services after they no longer qualify for Medicare-funded skilled care and services are discontinued.

Nonmedical Home Care

A wide spectrum of nonmedical home care services are available for the large majority of older adults who need home-based services but do not meet the criteria for skilled home care. At one end of the spectrum is nonskilled care provided by companions, homemakers, and home health aides. The most common services are meal preparation, light housekeeping, assistance with personal care, accompaniment to medical appointments, and grocery shopping and other errands. These services are often supplemented by community-based services such as transportation and home-delivered meals, as described in Box 6-1. Frequency of service ranges from a couple of hours monthly to 24 hours daily. A licensed nurse may assess the client and supervise the services, and a registered nurse usually assists with medication management, if needed.

Sources of Home Care Services

Home care services are available through formal sources (e.g., agencies) or informal sources (e.g., independent caregivers). People who self-pay for home care can obtain services from agencies or from informal sources, but when home care services are covered by insurance or public funds, they traditionally have been provided by agencies under contractual arrangements. This is changing, however, and some states now allow care recipients to choose and direct independent providers (including family members) who are paid under Medicaid.

Agencies usually provide initial assessments, arrange for services, assign workers, provide ongoing supervision, and collect payment for services. They are responsible for hiring, training, directing, scheduling, and firing workers. Some agencies provide a wide range of services, including licensed nurses and care managers. Other agencies provide only a limited type of nonmedical service, such as companions or light housekeeping. Some so-called agencies, however, are little more than a registry or referral service. When services are obtained from informal sources rather than from agencies, the care recipient or a surrogate decision maker is responsible for performing the organizational tasks that agencies normally perform (e.g., hiring, firing, and supervising the caregiver). In this case, a geriatric care management service (discussed later in this chapter) can be helpful for arranging services and overseeing the care. A common way of finding independent caregivers and other home care resources is through a word-of-mouth network, in which names are obtained from friends, families, churches, or local offices on aging.

Roles for Nurses in Home Care

Nurses who provide skilled home care services typically assume a primary coordinating role working with a multidisciplinary team that can include all or any of the following: primary care providers, psychiatrists, social workers, rehabilitation therapists, and home health aides. Nursing responsibilities are usually long term and involve all the following skills: assessments, care planning, hands-on care, health education, coordination of care, and referrals for additional services. In most home settings, nurses direct their interventions as much toward the caregivers of dependent older people as toward the older people themselves. In this role, they also provide teaching and role modeling about interventions to provide adequate care for the older adult. In addition, they address needs of the caregiver related to information about resources and ways to reduce caregiver stress.

 Technology to Promote Wellness in Older Adults

A challenge for nurses working in home care agencies is to keep up-to-date with technologic advances that increasingly are an integral part of health care services, as discussed in Chapter 5. For example, videoconferencing and telemonitoring are used in home settings to improve access to resources for ongoing assessment and diagnosis from specialized professionals. Today, home care nurses commonly use telehealth as a tool for improving health outcomes in people with chronic conditions such as diabetes, heart failure, and chronic obstructive pulmonary disease. Nurses have increasingly important roles in teaching patients and families about the effectiveness and advantages that can be provided through technology in home care settings (Wessel, 2017).

NURSING HOME SETTINGS

The term **nursing home**, or *nursing facility*, refers to a residential institutional setting for people who need assistance with several activities of daily living (ADLs). Nursing homes are licensed by a state or federal agency and must be certified as a Medicare or Medicaid facility if they receive funds from these programs. Nursing homes are required to have continuous on-site supervision by a registered nurse or a licensed practical nurse. In addition to medical care and nursing services, nursing homes must provide dental, podiatry, medical specialty consultation services, and rehabilitation therapies (e.g., physical and occupational therapies). There is some overlap between health care services provided in acute care and nursing home settings, but the care recipients are called *residents* rather than *patients* because these are residential facilities. Nursing home care can be categorized as skilled care, which is usually short term, or long term, which has traditionally been called intermediate care.

To qualify *for skilled care in a nursing home*, people must meet the following Medicare criteria:

- Have an inpatient hospitalization of at least 3 consecutive days within the previous 30 days for a medical condition that is associated with the need for skilled care
- Have a physician referral for services that must be provided by licensed professionals, such as nurses or therapists

● Require daily skilled care that can be provided appropriately in a Medicare-certified skilled nursing facility

For people who meet the criteria for skilled care in a nursing facility, Medicare and other insurance programs will cover all or part of the care for up to 100 days of care, *but only as long as the person continues to require the skilled level of services.* Typical diagnoses associated with skilled care in a nursing home are stroke, fractured hip, heart failure, and rehabilitation after acute illnesses (e.g., pneumonia, myocardial infarction). The expectation is that the person will be able to progress to a higher level of functioning and show some recovery from the acute episode. If his or her condition declines, for example, with dementia, the person may continue to require a significant level of care without meeting the relatively narrow criteria for skilled care. In these situations, the person usually begins paying for needed care unless family members can provide it.

Long-term care in a nursing home refers to services provided for chronically ill people who need significant assistance with daily activities. In contrast to admissions for skilled nursing care that usually occur following a hospitalization, admissions for long-term care in a nursing home typically occur after a period of gradual decline in functioning because of a chronic condition, such as dementia. Also in contrast to skilled nursing home care, insurance programs rarely cover long-term care in a nursing home. Most nursing homes provide a combination of skilled care services for short-term residents and intermediate care services for long-term residents.

In recent decades, changes in health care services for older adults have significantly influenced both long-term and short-term nursing home care. On any given day, about 5% of older adults are residing in a nursing facility; however, almost half of people older than 65 years are likely to spend some time in a nursing home. These statistics reflect the following major trends in health care for older adults in the United States:

● Shorter lengths of hospital stays and subsequent increased use of skilled care in a nursing home
● Increased availability of community-based programs that address needs for long-term care
● Higher percentages of nursing home residents returning to community settings
● Increased use of skilled home care services

One result of these trends is that the percentage of long-term residents who are more dependent on assistance with ADLs has gradually increased in recent years, because people who are less dependent now receive care in other settings, such as assisted living facilities.

During the 1990s, nursing homes began developing dementia special care units; however, at that time, the care in these units was similar to that in other nursing home units. During the early 2000s, the Alzheimer's Association and regulatory agencies demanded more accountability for programs that were advertised as dementia special care units. The increasing popularity of assisted living and other residential care facilities during this same time stimulated the development of dementia special care units within residential care communities. In 2014, 22% of residential care communities had a designated dementia special care unit, and 58% offered disease-specific programs for Alzheimer's disease (Lendon, Rome, & Sengupta, 2017).

Quality of Care in Nursing Homes

During the past two decades, health care consumers, providers, and organizations have increasingly focused on concerns about quality of care and quality of life for people who need long-term care. This focus stems in part from consumer pressure that began during the 1970s through the National Citizens Coalition for Nursing Home Reform and, in part, from the Nursing Home Reform Act of 1987 (discussed in Chapter 9). At the same time, many types of community-based residential care facilities, such as assisted living facilities and residential dementia special care units, were developing. Because of influences such as these, a new era in nursing home care has evolved.

The term **culture change** has been used since 1997 to describe a major movement toward implementing fundamental reforms in the way that nursing homes provide care. A major goal of culture change is to transform the philosophy and practice in nursing homes from an overemphasis on safety, uniformity, and medical care to a consumer-directed focus on health promotion, quality of life, and individualized care. The Pioneer Network, the Eden Alternative, and the Green House Project are models of long-term care that are based on the culture change movement, as described in Box 6-2.

The culture change movement has been gaining momentum, not only in the private sector but also in the public sector. For example, the CMS publishes a self-study tool, called the Artifacts of Culture Change Tool, to help nursing homes assess their progress toward improved quality of care. In addition, the CMS helped launch a voluntary public–private coalition in 2006, called Advancing Excellence in America's Nursing Homes, to address quality of care concerns. In 2014, the CMS began requiring all nursing homes to implement a Quality Assurance Performance Improvement program to assess the quality of care provided to residents and to improve outcomes. In addition, consumers have access to information about quality of care in every nursing home that received Medicare or Medicaid funds through the CMS Five-Star Rating System, which was expanded in 2016 to include additional quality measures.

Person-centered care (also called person-directed care or resident-centered care), defined as care that emphasizes personal choices and quality of life, is a core component of the culture change movement. Person-centered care focuses on promoting a sense of dignity and honoring individual preferences (Bangerter, Van Haitsman, Heid, & Abbott, 2016). Key components of person-centered care for residents

---

Box 6-2 Long-Term Care Settings Based on the Culture Change Movement

Pioneer Network

- Formed in 1997, is the umbrella organization of the culture change movement
- Focuses on 13 core values related to individualized and holistic care; optimal use of all aspects of the physical, organizational, and psychosocial/spiritual environment; and ongoing growth and continuous quality improvement
- Is expanding its scope to promote person-directed care in all settings that provide services for older adults, including home and community-based services

Eden Alternative

- Was developed in the mid-1990s by William Thomas, MD, with the intent of creating small group neighborhoods of residents
- Is a comprehensive program to transform the organizational culture as well as the physical, spiritual, psychosocial, and interpersonal environments of a facility

- Incorporates pets, plants, and children into the environment to create a homelike setting and improve the residents' quality of life
- Also incorporates strategies to engage and empower staff in bringing about environmental change

Green House Project

- Was developed in 2003 as a small-house nursing home by William Thomas, MD, the founder of the Eden Alternative
- Typically houses 7 to 12 residents in a home that blends in with neighboring houses
- In small-house nursing homes provides a full range of licensed and certified nursing home services in a normal household setting to older people with high levels of disability, including those associated with dementia
- Emphasizes relationships and meaning-making in interventions for dementia-related behavioral disturbances

---

include having choices about sleep and wake times, being heard by organizational leaders, and having consistent staff assignments (Harrisom & Frampton, 2017).

Delivery of person-centered care involves an interprofessional approach to not only developing, but also consistently implementing, a care plan based on a comprehensive assessment of the needs and preferences of the individual who is receiving care (i.e., the resident). In addition to strong nursing input, the care plan integrates assessments and interventions from team members such as social workers, rehabilitation therapists, primary care practitioners, mental health practitioners, dental care providers, and spiritual care providers. Nurses can use a simple question like "What do I need to know about you as a person to give you the best care possible?" as a starting point for developing a person-centered plan (Pan, Chochinov, Thompson, & Clement, 2016).

A Student's Perspective

This week in the nursing home, I found it was important to listen to Mrs. R. while allowing her to make her limitations known to me. I asked if she needed help, and didn't just provide it. I paid close attention to her body language and nonverbal communication. After finding her fast asleep sitting up during breakfast, I woke her and allowed her to tell me what was next. She determined that going to the bathroom and then getting washed would be best. After she was ready, I helped her down to the beauty salon to get her hair done, which is something she does every Friday afternoon. It can be easy to fall into the patient care aspect of a nursing home where you expect them to be on a schedule; however, you have to treat it as their home and allow them to pick and choose their activities and rest periods.

Jillian B.

Roles for Nurses in Nursing Home Settings

Nurses have always assumed strong leadership roles in nursing homes and other long-term care settings, and opportunities for role expansion are associated with the increasing complexity of care. Also, because of the focus on improved quality of care in nursing home settings, nurses have many opportunities to implement innovative changes in delivery of care. Roles for registered nurses in long-term care settings include team leader, nursing supervisor, wellness nurse, director of nursing, and assistant director of nursing. Nurses also have very strong roles in teaching nursing assistants about the best care for nursing home residents. Medicare and Medicaid began to pay for nurse practitioner services in nursing homes during the 1990s and the 2010 Affordable Care Act encourages the use of advanced practice nurses for improved quality of care. In addition to direct care of residents, advanced practice nurses may provide staff education, assist with program development, act as consultants in planning and implementing care, establish support groups for clients and families, and act as advocates for clients and their families.

Models of care based on the culture change movement present many challenges, as well as opportunities, for nurses because culture change involves philosophical and organizational changes that affect all staff. The Pioneer Network has collaborated with gerontological nursing leaders to develop 10 competencies deemed most relevant and critical for nurses implementing culture change models of care, as described in Box 6-3.

Online Learning Activity 6-2 provides links to additional information related to improving the quality of care and quality of life for nursing homes residents.

 See ONLINE LEARNING ACTIVITY 6-2: ADDITIONAL INFORMATION RELATED TO IMPROVING QUALITY OF CARE AND QUALITY OF LIFE FOR NURSING HOME RESIDENTS at http://thepoint.lww.com/Miller8e.

Box 6-3 Roles for Nurses in Implementing Nursing Home Culture Change

- Modeling, teaching, and using effective communication skills, including active listening, giving meaningful feedback, and addressing emotional behaviors
- Implementing and modeling person-directed care practices
- Identifying and addressing barriers to person-directed care
- Maintaining consistency of caregivers for residents
- Solving complex problems related to resident choice and risk
- Involving residents, families, and all team members in problem solving, decision making, and planning
- Viewing the care setting as the resident's home and works to create attributes of home

Adapted from Nurse Competencies for Nursing Home Culture Change. Available at www.PioneerNetwork.net.

HOSPITAL SETTINGS

Hospital settings (also called acute care settings) are an important part of the continuum of care because of the complexity of care associated with illnesses in older adults (as discussed in detail in Chapter 27). The increasing awareness of unique needs of hospitalized older adults is leading to the development of programs to address these needs. This section presents information about specialized programs and resources that currently are available. Because issues related to quality of care are multifaceted, they need to be addressed in policies and practices by the institution and by each professional group within the institution. This section discusses current efforts to address concerns about quality of care in hospitals, with attention on roles of nurses.

Acute Care Units for Elders

Since the early 1980s, hospitals in the United States have been establishing comprehensive geriatric assessment units, called **acute care for elders (ACE)** units, based on the underlying premise that older adults have complex and unique needs that can be addressed by a specially trained multidisciplinary team to prevent functional decline during hospitalization. Key elements of ACE units are patient-centered care, interprofessional team management, frequent medical review, early discharge planning, a specially adapted physical environment, and assessment and interventions for common geriatric syndromes (e.g., mobility, fall risk, self-care, skin integrity, continence, confusion, depression, anxiety). In addition to gerontological nurses, the health care teams in ACE units typically include a geriatrician, pharmacist, social worker, various rehabilitation therapists (e.g., speech, physical, or occupational therapists), mental health professionals (e.g., psychologists or psychiatrists), and supportive therapies such as music or activity. If a dedicated ACE unit is not feasible, nurses in all acute care settings should focus on (1) patient-centered care, including individualized preventive care interventions based on comprehensive assessments;

(2) daily review of medications, treatments, and planned procedures; and (3) referrals for rehabilitation therapists and geriatric specialists.

Resources for Improving Care of Hospitalized Older Adults

In 1992, the Hartford Foundation funded a major initiative called the Nurses Improving Care for Healthsystem Elders (NICHE). The NICHE program is ongoing and was active in 500 hospitals nationwide in 2014. A unique characteristic of NICHE is its focus on developing a positive nurse practice environment by involving nurses at all levels in decisions regarding care of older adults (Capezuti, Parks, Boltz, et al., 2016). An integral component of NICHE is the **geriatric resource nurse (GRN)**, who serves as a consultant and role model for other nurses. These nurses are skilled at identifying and addressing specific geriatric syndromes, such as falls and confusion, and implementing interventions that discourage using restrictive devices and promote patient mobility. Evaluation of the GRN model has identified reductions in costs and improvements in all the following areas: nursing knowledge, quality of care, implementation of geriatric protocols, and clinical outcomes related to conditions such as delirium (Capezuti, Parks, Boltz, et al., 2016).

In 2011, NICHE and the Joint Commission published standards of care and information about resources to address the needs of hospitalized older adults. Box 6-4 delineates some of these standards that nurses can implement, even if NICHE or other specialized geriatric resources are not readily available. Online Learning Activity 6-3 provides access to an article with a case study illustrating the application of NICHE recommendations to care of a critically ill older adult.

See ONLINE LEARNING ACTIVITY 6-3: ARTICLE AND EVIDENCE-BASED INFORMATION ABOUT ADDRESSING NEEDS OF HOSPITALIZED OLDER ADULTS at http://thepoint.lww.com/Miller8e.

INTERPROFESSIONAL COLLABORATION

Interprofessional collaboration is an essential common element in all models of care that address needs of older adults. As discussed throughout this chapter, roles of nurses vary significantly according to the health needs of older adults and the resources available. For example, interprofessional collaboration for relatively healthy older adults may involve a broad range of staff in community-based organizations, but for older adults with functional impairments and complex medical conditions it would involve highly specialized professionals. In all settings, nurses are responsible for seeking resources and initiating contact when care of older adults can be improved through interprofessional collaboration. Box 6-5 lists examples of professionals with whom

---

Box 6-4 Examples of Standards of Care for Hospitalized Older Adults Established by the Joint Commission and Nurses Improving Care for Healthsystem Elders (NICHE)

Nursing and Human Resources

- The GRN model is implemented and evaluated.
- Specialized needs of hospitalized older adults are discussed in staff orientation, interdisciplinary continuing education, and competency-based training for nursing staff.
- NICHE coordinator and managers evaluate the learning needs of the staff related to care of hospitalized older adults.

Provision of Care

- The care, treatment, and services provided to hospitalized older adults is interdisciplinary.
- The interdisciplinary team utilizes evidence-based assessment practices and individualized interventions to prevent and manage pain, falls-related injuries, and other geriatric syndromes.
- The unique needs of older adult patients are integrated within palliative care and end-of-life services.
- The learning needs of hospitalized older adults and their families are addressed.

- Policies and practices support alternatives to physical restraints.
- Transitional care needs of older adults and their families are addressed through comprehensive assessment, planning, and interventions.

Medication Management

- Administration and prescription of medications for older adults is consistent with evidence-based practice (e.g., using American Geriatrics Society Beers' Criteria).

Environments of Care

- Physical environment reflects aging-sensitive principles to provide for basic safety: nonglare flooring, adequate lights, grab bars, adjustable height beds, and appropriate use of alarms.
- All practitioners are familiar with their roles and responsibilities relative to the environment of care.

Source: Nurses Improving Care for Healthsystem Elders. (2011). A Crosswalk: Joint Commission Standards & NICHE Resources. Available at www.nicheprogram.org.

---

nurses are likely to initiate collaboration in various settings. Please note that (1) this list is not all-inclusive, but it provides examples of resources that might be available, and (2) the availability of the professionals is highly dependent on resources within the institution or community.

Although community-based workers are not necessarily defined as professionals, they are included in the context of interprofessional collaboration because nurses have essential roles in working with a diverse and flexible team, particularly for chronic disease management in community settings (Bookey-Bassett, Markle-Reid, Mckey, & Akhtar-Danesh, 2017). In addition, community-based workers are important resources for promoting wellness in older adults who live in home or community settings, and nurses in hospitals and long-term care facilities have important roles in initiating or suggesting referrals as components of discharge plans.

Care of older adults with complex needs inherently involves numerous opportunities for interprofessional collaboration; however, these opportunities also exist when caring for relatively healthy older adults in community-based settings. Throughout this textbook, information about interprofessional collaboration is highlighted with 👥 or ▬▬ to draw attention to roles of nurses when interacting with other professionals in caring for older adults in any setting. This emphasis is consistent with the recent National League of Nursing recommendation that content related to interprofessional collaboration be incorporated in the nursing curriculum (National League for Nursing, 2016). In addition to the text that is highlighted in this visual way, it is important to consider the less obvious content that addresses roles of nurses in working with caregivers and other support people. These support

---

Box 6-5 Examples of Nurse-Initiated Interprofessional Collaboration in Different Settings

Community-Based Settings

- Primary care practitioners (often per phone, text, or e-mail)
- Nurses and other professionals in home care agencies
- Social workers in community agencies
- Staff in aging network services
- Staff in culturally specific organizations
- Staff in faith-based organizations
- Adult protective services in at-risk situations (see Chapter 10)

Rehabilitation and Long-Term Care Facilities

- Primary care practitioners
- Physical therapists
- Occupational therapists
- Speech language therapists
- Registered dieticians and dietary staff

- Social workers
- Mental health specialists
- Recreational and activities staff
- Dental care providers
- Podiatrists

Acute Care Settings

- Geriatric nurse specialists
- Geriatricians
- Social workers
- Rehabilitation therapists
- Registered dieticians
- Geriatric consultants (e.g., for neurology, psychiatry, oncology)
- Geropsychologists and other specialized mental health professionals

people may not be considered professionals per se, but they are essential team members for care of older adults.

CONCERNS ABOUT QUALITY AND SAFETY OF CARE

All sectors of health care and the larger society have identified quality and safety issues as a high priority that is being addressed by professional disciplines including nursing. Although these concerns are not specific to older adults, they disproportionately affect nursing care of older adults. Because concerns about quality of care in hospitals have escalated in recent years, the CMS supported initiatives to improve care and decrease the cost of care, particularly for older adults. For example, the CMS denies payment for certain hospital-acquired conditions that are deemed to be preventable, including catheter-associated urinary tract infections, fall-related injuries, and pressure ulcer stages III and IV. All these conditions disproportionately affect frail older adults and are discussed in Chapters 19, 22, and 23 of this text. Another major focus is on reducing unnecessary hospitalizations, with emphasis on readmissions within 30 days of discharge and hospitalizations of nursing home residents. This issue is addressed in the section on transitional care.

Quality and Safety in Nursing: QSEN

Concerns about quality of health care for older adults need to be addressed at an institutional level, with essential input from all involved professionals. One way in which nurses are addressing this issue is through the rapidly growing network of nurses working toward widespread implementation of a framework called **Quality and Safety Education for Nurses (QSEN)**. The QSEN project evolved from a series of grants from the Robert Wood Johnson Foundation in response to the Institute of Medicine's report, published in 2000, called *To Err is Human*. This was the first of a series of reports that addressed aspects of the "quality chasm" that existed in the US health care systems. Initiatives such as QSEN are congruent with national priorities related to health care such as the following:

- Making care safer
- Ensuring person- and family-centered care
- Promoting effective communication and coordination of care
- Promoting the most effective strategies for preventing and treating leading causes of mortality, starting with cardio-vascular disease
- Promoting wide use of best practices that support healthy living
- Making quality care more affordable

Nurses have developed QSEN competencies with the goal of improving the delivery of health care services in all of the following areas: patient-centered care, teamwork and collaboration, evidence-based practice, quality improvement, safety, and informatics. Competencies for each of the six areas are identified for knowledge (K), skills (S), and attitudes (A), or KSA. Some of the competencies apply more directly to the work environment, but all competencies affect direct care of patients in some way. In this textbook, QSEN competencies that are most directly related to care of older adults are applied to case study examples in the clinically oriented chapters. Table 6-1 summarizes these QSEN competencies—which are patient-centered care, teamwork and collaboration, and evidence-based practice—and their

TABLE 6-1 Selected Quality and Safety in Nursing (QSEN) Competencies and Related Knowledge, Skills, and Attitudes

QSEN Competency	Knowledge/Skill/Attitude
Patient-centered care	(K) Integrate understanding of multiple dimensions of patient-centered care
	(K) Describe how diverse backgrounds function as a source of values
	(K) Describe strategies to empower patients in all aspects of the health care process
	(K) Examine common barriers to active involvement in patients
	(K) Discuss principles of effective communication
	(K) Examine nursing roles in ensuring coordination, integration, and continuity of care
	(S) Elicit patient values, preferences, and expressed needs
	(S) Provide patient-centered care with sensitivity and respect for diversity of the human experience
	(S) Assess own level of communication skill in encounters with patients and families
	(S) Communicate care provided and needed at each transition in care
	(A) Value seeing health care situations "through patients' eyes"
Teamwork and collaboration	(K) Describe scopes of practice and role of health care team members
	(K) Recognize contributions of other individuals and groups in helping patient achieve health goals
	(K) Describe impact of own communication style on others
	(S) Integrate the contributions of others who play a role in helping patient achieve health goals
Evidence-based practice	(K) Describe how the strength and relevance of available evidence influence the choice of intervention
	(S) Base individualized care plan on patient values, clinical expertise, and evidence
	(S) Read original research and evidence reports related to clinical practice
	(A) Value evidence-based practice as integral to determining the best clinical practice

associated KSA. Although other QSEN competencies are equally important in clinical practice, the application of QSEN to case study examples in this textbook focuses on the ones that nurses can most directly incorporate in their care of older adult patients.

Transitional Care

A foremost concern related to cost, safety, and quality care is the lack of coordination during transitions in care, which refers to the numerous transfers of older adults during the course of an illness. Problems with transitions in care occur during transfers from one setting to another, whether those are institutions, homes, or community settings. Older adults with complex medical problems or combinations of chronic and acute problems (e.g., dementia and heart failure) are particularly vulnerable to experiencing problems as they transfer between care settings, including different departments within the same institution. Major organizations such as the CMS, the Institute of Medicine, and the Joint Commission (JCAHO) consider this a high priority, because poor coordination of care across health care settings is associated with many serious outcomes, such as high rates of readmission to hospitals within 30 days of discharge.

In 2003, the American Geriatrics Society defined **transitional care** as "a set of actions designed to ensure the coordination and continuity of health care as patients transfer between different locations or different levels of care within the same location" (American Geriatrics Society, 2003, p. 556). Effective transitional care interventions result in the following positive outcomes related to quality, safety, and cost of care: reduced all-cause readmissions, decreased mortality and reduced hospitalizations for heart failure (Coffey, Mulcahy, Savage, et al., 2017; Le Berre, Maimon, Sourial, et al., 2017).

The 2010 Affordable Care Act includes incentives for better care coordination and improved outcomes for hospitalized patients as a goal for reducing Medicare costs. For example, in October 2012, the CMS began reducing Medicare payments to hospitals if their readmission rate for certain conditions (e.g., pneumonia and heart failure) is higher than expected. Also, starting in 2018, similar penalties are being extended to skilled nursing facilities as a measure to prevent re-hospitalizations. This goal is noteworthy because almost one-fifth of Medicare beneficiaries are readmitted within 1 month of their discharge, and one-fifth are readmitted within the first 3 months, with many of these readmissions being considered preventable (Schuller, Kash, & Gamm, 2017).

Although problems with transitions of care need to be addressed at the institutional level, all professionals within the setting share responsibility for aspects of transitions. Numerous models have been developed to address the contributing factors, and nurses have assumed primary roles in developing and implementing interventions. The first step is to identify those older adults who are at high risk for poor outcomes related to poor transitions in care. Nurses have developed an easy-to-use and evidence-based screening tool called the Transitional Care Model (TCM): Hospital Discharge Screening Criteria for High Risk Older Adults to identify older adults who are at risk for poorly managed transitions. Nurses are encouraged to use this tool, which is available through Online Learning Activity 6-4, to identify older adults who need special attention for transitional care interventions (Lim, Foust, & Van Cleave, 2016).

After identifying patients at risk for poor outcomes, a transitional care intervention needs to be implemented through interprofessional collaboration. Successful transitional care programs are based on the following components:

- Patient engagement
- Caregiver engagement
- Management of medications
- Patient education
- Caregiver education
- Care continuity
- Accountability
- Patients' and caregivers' well-being

(Naylor, Shaid, Carpenter, et al., 2017).
Box 6-6 describes characteristics of effective transitional care interventions, and Online Learning Activity 6-4 provides links to resources for additional information about transitional care. In the Spotlight on Transitional Care sections in Chapters 27, 28, and 29, unfolding case examples illustrate application of transitional care interventions.

 See ONLINE LEARNING ACTIVITY 6-4: ARTICLE AND ADDITIONAL INFORMATION ABOUT TRANSITIONAL CARE INTERVENTIONS at http://thepoint.lww.com/Miller8e.

ADDRESSING NEEDS OF CAREGIVERS

The term **caregiver burden** is commonly used to describe the emotional, physical, social, financial, and spiritual negative functional consequences experienced by family members when caring for dependent older adults. Specific functional consequences associated with caregiver burden include depression; disturbed sleep; social isolation; family discord; career interruptions; financial difficulties; lack of time for self; poor physical health; psychological/emotional/mental strain; and feelings of anger, guilt, grief, anxiety, hopelessness, and helplessness. The following factors are associated with increased risk for experiencing caregiver burden: lower socioeconomic status, residing with the care recipient, self-reported depression, social isolation, financial stress, and lack of choice in assuming the caregiving role (Musich, Wang, Kraemer, et al., 2017).

Although most studies have focused on the burdens of caregiving, caregivers typically experience a combination of negative and positive feelings associated with both the burdens and inconveniences of caregiving and the satisfaction of

---

Box 6-6 Characteristics of an Effective Transitional Care Intervention

Overall Considerations

- Begins at preadmission or admission and continues until discharge or postdischarge
- Is interdisciplinary and incorporates information from all health care professionals
- Delineates method of documenting and communicating pertinent information among all those involved with care and follow-up across settings

Assessment of Patient and Caregiver

- Assesses strengths and needs of patient and family, including all of the following: cultural considerations, motivational factors, health literacy, educational levels, socioeconomic background, level of knowledge about condition
- Assesses knowledge and understanding of all health conditions
- Identifies barriers to care (e.g., knowledge deficit, caregiver burden issues)
- Identifies risks for progression of disease, readmission, poor follow-up, lack of coordination, and other potential issues
- Identifies need for medical equipment, skilled care, and other supports postdischarge
- Identifies resources that can be used for follow-up

Patient and Caregiver Education

- Is based on assessment as outlined in previous section
- Begins early and is ongoing as needs change based on reassessments

- Focuses on all the following topics: recognition and management of signs and symptoms of the patient's conditions and complications, nutritional considerations, medication management, information about how and when to seek health care
- Incorporates teach-back techniques and individualized and person-centered methods to promote understanding of content
- Incorporates culturally and linguistically appropriate educational resources, such as printed materials, Web site resources, and audiovisual materials
- Includes written information about follow-up appointments

Medication Reconciliation (described in Chapter 8)

- Is performed on admission and at all points of transfer across settings and within settings
- Addresses patient and caregiver understanding of medications
- Includes documentation of prescription and nonprescription medications being used regularly or periodically
- Includes information about accessibility to medications postdischarge

Follow-Up Interactions

Follow up with patient and caregiver via telephone, home visits, telehealth, or other technology-based methods for the following purposes:
- To answer questions
- To provide education and support
- To provide advice about symptom management
- To facilitate recognition of complications
- To address concerns about self-care and recovery

---

helping others. Positive outcomes related to the experience of caregiving include feelings of satisfaction, personal gratification, experiences of social approval, increased patience and tolerance, increased personal relationship, and finding meaning in the caregiver role (Cheng, Mak, Lau, et al., 2016).

For older adults who have dementia or other conditions that cause progressive declines in functioning, the role of caregiver usually evolves gradually and can last for years. Even in situations in which older adults do not have progressively declining conditions, families of older adults frequently deal with intermittent and cumulative conditions that require intense medical care or rehabilitative services. It is not uncommon for families of older adults to take on roles of care managers and find themselves negotiating health care services for at least one and sometimes several parents, grandparents, aunts, uncles, and other relatives or friends.

Nurses have important roles in promoting **caregiver wellness**. For example, because increased feelings of self-efficacy are associated with improved caregiver well-being, simple communication techniques, such as providing positive feedback when teaching caregivers, can be interventions for caregiver wellness. Nurses address teaching needs of older adults' families, partners, and significant others as an essential nursing responsibility related to continuity of care for patients in all health care settings. Consistent with this responsibility, nurses follow standards of care and document the teaching they provide regarding caregiving instructions, but they do not necessarily address the broader needs

of caregivers because of barriers, such as time constraints and perception of this as a nonessential aspect of care. However, when nurses care for dependent older adults, it is important to recognize that even the basic needs of the older adult cannot be met without a strong support system. Thus, nurses need to identify outcomes and interventions to prevent caregiver burnout and enhance the ability of families and other caregivers to provide the necessary care, as discussed in Chapter 27. As with all aspects of caring for older adults, there is great individual variation among families, caregivers, and care recipients, so there are many varied interventions to address caregiver issues. Many of the chapters in Parts 3 and 4 of this textbook highlight nurses' roles in promoting caregiver wellness.

PAYING FOR HEALTH CARE SERVICES FOR OLDER ADULTS

Sources of payment for health care services are self-pay, private insurance, and government-supported programs such as Medicare, Medicaid, and the Veterans Administration. The 2010 Affordable Care Act stimulated changes in health insurance and health care services that are comparable to the unprecedented changes stimulated by the enactment of Medicare and Medicaid legislation 1965. Because these developments are ongoing and many of the newer programs are available only in certain geographic location, it is difficult to keep up-to-date on all the options available to older adults today. Despite the complexity and limitations of programs, however, nurses need to know enough about common types of programs so they can understand and address some of the barriers to, and challenges of, implementing nursing care plans and discharge plans. For example, knowing the Medicare criteria for skilled home care services, which has not changed in decades, enables the nurse to make referrals for this type of nursing care when appropriate. This section presents information about the programs that most directly influence health care services for older adults, including those that play a major role in the ability of older adults to live in home settings.

Out-of-Pocket Expenses

Despite the major contribution of health insurance programs in paying for health care services, out-of-pocket health care expenses have been increasing steadily in recent decades and that burden falls disproportionately on poor people. Older adults with lower incomes and those aged 85 years and older experience disproportionately higher increases in out-of-pocket expenses, as illustrated in Figure 6-3. Except for the limited coverage for skilled nursing home care, Medicare does not cover costs of care in nursing homes or in assisted living facilities. Because assisted living facilities are residential places, however, Medicare will pay for skilled home care services and hospice care for people who meet the criteria for these services. A national survey found that the median rate for a private room was $3628 per month in assisted living facilities and $7698 per month in nursing homes in 2016 (Genworth Financial, 2016).

Medicare

As a federal health insurance program for people who are eligible for Social Security benefits, Medicare covers primarily hospital and physician services, with very limited coverage for some skilled care services in homes and nursing homes (as reviewed previously in this chapter). The original Medicare plan is divided into Part A, funded through payroll taxes, and Part B, financed through monthly premiums paid by beneficiaries and by general revenues. Medicare, therefore, is part of the national budget and is subject to the same political processes that affect other budget items. Thus, the program has changed many times in response to concerns about cost and quality of care and pressure from consumers and health care providers. Box 6-7 summarizes information about the Medicare-covered services as they have evolved since 1965.

Medicare-Supported Comprehensive Models

Medicare-supported comprehensive models of care address long-term care needs of older adults by providing care across several community-based health care settings. The On Lok Senior Services program, which began in 1971 as a senior day health center in the Chinatown area of San Francisco, is the first program of comprehensive care that received CMS support. On Lok—Cantonese for "peaceful happy abode"—continues in a greatly expanded form as a successful model of community-based, comprehensive, and cost-effective care for older adults. The success of On Lok prompted the development of a similar program, called **Program of All-Inclusive Care for the Elderly (PACE)**, in the late 1980s. This program has gradually expanded, and in 1997, the federal government designated PACE models as permanent Medicare and Medicaid providers. This publicly funded model is consistently identified as "one of the oldest and most successful nursing home alternative models that provides comprehensive community-based team care that is family- and person-centered" (Cortes & Sullivan-Marx, 2016). The 2010 Affordable Care Act provides incentives

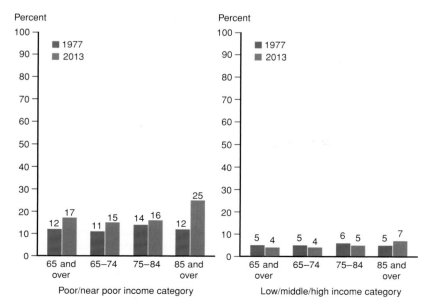

FIGURE 6-3 Out-of-pocket expenditures as a percentage of household income, among people aged 65 years and over, by age group and income category, 1977 and 2013. (Adapted from Federal Interagency Forum on Aging-Related Statistics, *Older Americans 2016: Key Indicators of Well-Being.*)

Box 6-7 Medicare-Covered Services as They Have Evolved Since 1965

Original Medicare Part A, Also Called Hospital Insurance

- Available since 1965 without charge
- Helps pay for medical care for people 65 years and older and people under 65 years with certain conditions
- Covers acute care in hospitals, skilled care in a licensed facility, home health care, and hospice care
- Requires beneficiaries to be responsible for a copay amount for most services, which can be covered by other insurance

Original Medicare Part B, Also Called Supplemental Insurance

- Available since 1965 in conjunction with Medicare Part A
- Requires beneficiaries to pay a monthly premium and copay amount
- Helps pay for outpatient care (e.g., physicians and advance practice nurses, diagnostic tests); some ambulance services; and some durable medical equipment

Medicare Advantage Plans (Also Called Medicare Part C)

- Allows beneficiaries to enroll in one of the following types of private insurance plans, such as a health maintenance organization or a preferred provider organization
- Covers all benefits covered under Medicare Parts A and B, plus some additional services, such as preventive care and prescription medications

Medicare Part D

- Available since 2006, provides limited coverage for prescription medications for Medicare beneficiaries

- Requires a monthly premium and cost-sharing amounts
- Applies limits to the annual amount covered and excludes some drugs
- Approved drug plans vary in coverage for specific drugs and beneficiaries are expected to compare available plans to determine which one best meets their needs

Medicare Changes Associated with the 2010 Affordable Care Act

- Expansion of preventive care services covered with no out-of-pocket expense, including wellness visits and recommended screenings and immunizations (listed in Box 5-2)
- Additional coverage for prescription drugs
- Creation of the Center for Medicare & Medicaid Innovation to implement models of care that address safety, effectiveness, timeliness, efficiency, and inequities
- Increased funding for nurse-managed health centers

Innovative Models of Care Evolving from the 2010 Affordable Care Act

- Expansion of Program of All-Inclusive Care of the Elderly (PACE)
- Partnerships for Patients
- Accountable Care Organizations
- Patient-Centered Medical Home
- Independence at Home

---

for expansion of PACE, with further support from the 2015 Program of All-Inclusive Care for the Elderly Innovation Act.

Distinguishing features of the PACE model are (1) the provision of comprehensive and community-based long-term care services to nursing-home-eligible clients, (2) an emphasis on preventive services, (3) integrated service delivery through adult day health centers, (4) case management through multidisciplinary teams, and (5) full funding on a capitation basis (similar to health maintenance organizations). Core components of PACE programs are nutrition, transportation, home care, acute care, respite care, primary care, social services, restorative therapies, prescription drugs, long-term care, adult day care, medical specialty care, durable medical equipment, and multidisciplinary case management.

Medigap Insurance

The many limitations of the original Medicare program have led to the development of **Medigap insurance** policies, which are supplemental policies that attempt to fill the gap between the services covered by original Medicare and those that are paid for out of pocket. All supplemental policies, which are regulated by federal and state laws, cover the premiums and copayments for services covered by Medicare Parts A and B, but additional benefits vary according to each

policy. The National Association of Insurance Commissioners has developed 10 standard plans that insurance companies must follow in the provision of Medigap policies. Plan A contains basic benefits, such as coverage for coinsurance payments and additional payments for hospital days. Other plans (B through J) cover Part A deductible and additional services, such as prescription medications, preventive medical care, skilled nursing coinsurance, and medical care in foreign countries. It is important to know that Medigap policies were designed as supplements to original Medicare Parts A and B, and they are not applicable to Medicare Advantage plans or the newer models that are being developed under the 2010 Affordable Care Act. Because health insurance choices have become increasingly complex, nurses can encourage older adults and their caregivers to seek information from organizations that are not directly involved with selling insurance policies, such as local senior centers.

Medicaid

Medicaid legislation was enacted at the same time as Medicare to provide health insurance for poor people. Medicaid is a federal/state partnership that has evolved to become the nation's largest health insurer. To qualify for Medicaid, people must meet medical and financial criteria, which are established by both state and federal regulations. States limit liquid assets to no more than about $2000, and the value of the home is generally exempt up to a maximum amount. Medicaid rules include strict policies to prevent the transfer of assets from one family member to another for 5 years before applying for Medicaid; however, the income and assets of a spouse are usually exempt from these restrictions. Older adults typically "spend down" their liquid assets and they meet Medicaid eligibility when the cost of required care exceeds their ability to pay.

Although states have some discretion about what services are covered by Medicaid, the federal government mandates that certain medical services, including skilled home care and all levels of nursing home care, are covered for all eligible adults. Initially, Medicaid paid primarily for care in institutional rather than community-based settings; however, in the early 1990s, the focus shifted toward paying for community-based services for people who otherwise would need nursing home care. Medicaid funds often are available for home care services for people who otherwise would need nursing home care, but the cost of home care must be lower than the cost of care in an institutional setting. Availability of and criteria for receiving the Medicaid-supported community-based services vary widely from state to state and accurate information about these programs is available through local Area Agencies on Aging.

Older Americans Act

The **Older Americans Act (OAA)** was enacted in 1965 to support programs to help older adults remain independent in their own homes and communities. The OAA funds all the following types of programs to varying degrees: group and home-delivered meals; assistance with chores, personal care, and light housekeeping; transportation; adult day care; respite care; and family caregiver supports. In 2006, the OAA Reauthorization Act included major provisions for improving coordination and delivery of long-term services and supports. This reauthorization act also funded an initiative called the Administration on Aging's Choice for Independence to provide information and support for consumers with regard to long-term care services. OAA-funded programs vary significantly among the states and localities and they are administered through local senior centers. Nurses have important roles in facilitating referrals and suggesting that older adults and their families explore these resources by their local senior center.

Long-Term Care Insurance

Long-term care insurance policies are designed to cover some long-term care expenses that are not covered by health insurance programs. When long-term care insurance policies were first promoted in the late 1980s, they were unregulated and many of the policies contained large loopholes and significant barriers to receiving benefits. In recent years, many states enacted laws mandating standards suggested by the National Association of Insurance Commissioners.

Suggested requirements for long-term care insurance policies include inflation protection and caps on rates. A good long-term care policy will provide payment for a range of options, including home care services, assisted-living facilities, and nursing home care. In addition, policies should be open enough that they include services that may be developed in the future but are not available at the time the policy is initiated. For example, the first long-term care policies that were developed were limited to nursing home care because few other options were available at that time. A major drawback of this type of insurance for older people is that the premiums are based on the age of the person when he or she initially signs up for the policy. For most older adults, therefore, the cost of the policy will outweigh the benefits.

Chapter Highlights

Community-Based Services for Older Adults

- Public and private agencies have provided many types of services for older adults, with the range of services continually broadening (Figure 6-1, Box 6-1).
- Health promotion programs provide organized screening and health education services in community settings, such as senior centers
- Faith community nursing is a holistic approach to addressing the physical, emotional, and spiritual needs of members of church-based congregations.
- Respite care refers to any service whose primary goal is to relieve caregivers periodically from the stress of their usual caregiver responsibilities.
- Adult day centers provide structured activities for functionally impaired older people in a group setting.
- Geriatric care management services involve comprehensive assessment, care planning, implementation, monitoring, and reassessment to address immediate and long-term needs of older adults.

Home-Based Services

- Skilled home care services, including nursing, therapies, and home health aides, provide skilled care for homebound older adults who meet criteria established by the CMS.
- A wide spectrum of services ranging from housekeeping and companionship to full-time hands-on nursing care is available under the auspices of nonmedical home care.
- Sources of home care services are formal sources, such as agencies, or informal sources, including independent caregivers and family and friends.
- Nurses working in home care agencies have many responsibilities, including using telehealth technology as an integral part of assessment and nursing care.

Nursing Home Settings

- Nursing homes are residential institutional settings for people who need assistance with several daily activities.
- Skilled care in a nursing home addresses short-term needs of people who need nursing care and/or rehabilitation

therapies for people who have had an acute illness and are expected to progress to a higher level of functioning.
- Long-term care in a nursing home refers to services provided for chronically ill people who need significant assistance with daily activities.
- The nursing home culture change movement was initiated in 1997 with the goal of transforming the philosophy and practice in nursing homes to emphasize resident-centered care (Box 6-2).
- Nurses have many roles in addressing issues related to quality of care in nursing homes (Box 6-3).

Hospital Settings
- Specialized ACE units address the complex needs of hospitalized older adults though multidisciplinary assessments and interventions.
- The NICHE program offers many resources for implementing standards of care for hospitalized older adults (Box 6-4).

Interprofessional Collaboration
- Interprofessional collaboration is an essential common element in all models of care that address needs of older adults.
- Box 6-5 lists examples of professionals with whom nurses are likely to collaborate in various settings.

Concerns About Quality and Safety of Care
- Quality and Safety in Nursing (QSEN) competencies have been developed to help nurses address national priorities related to improving quality of health care services (Table 6-1).
- Older adults are at risk for serious negative functional consequences associated with poor coordination of care during transitions from one setting to another.
- Transitional care is a set of actions implemented to improve coordination of care, as described in Box 6-6.
- Application of transitional care interventions is illustrated in the unfolding case example in Chapters 27 to 29.

Addressing Needs of Caregivers
- The term caregiver burden describes the emotional, physical, social, financial, and spiritual negative functional consequences experienced by family members who provide extensive care for dependent older adults.
- Nurses have important roles in promoting caregiver wellness, as discussed in Chapter 27 and highlighted in many chapters in Parts 3 and 4 of this textbook.

Paying for Health Care Services for Older Adults
- Sources of payment for health care services are self-pay (also called out-of-pocket), public funds for people who qualify, and insurance policies for people who have them (Figure 6-3).

- Medicare is the health insurance program that covers hospital and medical care and some skilled care services for people who are eligible for Social Security (Box 6-7).
- PACE is a widely supported model of comprehensive care that addresses long-term care needs of older adults in community-based settings.
- Medigap insurance policies are available from many sources to supplement original Medicare policies.
- Medicaid is a federal/state partnership that was established in 1965 to provide medical care for poor people, but it has become the primary source of payment for nonskilled long-term care for older adults.
- The OAA funds services to help older adults remain independent in their own homes; in recent years, it has expanded to include programs that support caregivers and provide services for people who are at high risk for nursing home placement but are not eligible for Medicaid.
- Long-term care insurance policies are available to cover the cost of some long-term care services, but the costs outweigh the potential benefits for most older adults.

Critical Thinking Exercises

1. Mrs. S. is 84 years old. She was recently diagnosed with dementia. She is able to care for herself as long as someone reminds her to eat her meals and take her medications. Two months ago, she began living with her daughter who works full time and is involved with several church-related activities. Three days a week, Mrs. S.'s daughter takes her to an adult day center at 8:30 and picks her up at 4:30. Twice weekly, Mrs. S. receives home-delivered meals. Find local resources for the types of services delineated in Box 6-1 and obtain information about four or five additional services that Mrs. S.'s daughter may need to use.

2. Mrs. F. is a resident in the skilled care section of the nursing home where you work. She had been living alone in her own home before being admitted to the hospital with a fractured hip 4 weeks ago. She has regained much of her independence and walks with a walker and one-person assist. She expects to ambulate independently using a walker within 2 weeks, at which time she expects to return to her own home. She asks you what kind of services would be available in her home. What additional information would you want to know before you answered her questions? What information would you give to her? What suggestions would you make?

3. Your great aunt, who is 84 years old, is being admitted to a nursing home for long-term care. Her diagnoses include dementia, arthritis, and heart failure. Her daughter (who is your aunt) asks your advice about what to look for when she is selecting a nursing home. Use the resources in Online Learning Activity 6-2 to explore information about culture change and quality of care in nursing homes.

For more information about topics discussed in this chapter, be sure to check out the interactive Online Learning Activities and other helpful resources at http://thepoint.lww.com/Miller8e.

REFERENCES

American Geriatrics Society. (2003). Improving quality of transitional care for persons with complex care needs. American Geriatrics Society position statement. *Journal of the American Geriatrics Society*, *51*(4), 556–557.

American Nurses Association. (2012). *Faith community nursing: Scope and standards of practice*. Silver Spring, MD: Author.

Bangerter, L. R., Van Haitsma, K., Heid, A. R., and Abbott, K. (2016). "Make me feel at ease and at home": Differential care preferences of nursing home residents. *Gerontologist*, *56*, 702–713.

Bookey-Bassett, S., Markle-Reid, M., Mckey, C. A., & Akhtar-Danesh, N. (2017). Understanding interprofessional collaboration in the context of chronic disease management for older adults living in communities: A concept analysis. *Journal of Advanced Nursing*, *73*, 71–84.

Capezuti, E., Parks, A. J., Boltz, M., et al. (2016). Acute care models. In M. Boltz, E. Capezuti, T. Fulmer, & D. Zwicker (Eds.), *Evidence-based practice protocols for best practice* (5th ed., pp. 621–631). New York: Springer.

Cheng, S. T., Mak, E. P., Lau, R. W., et al. (2016). Voices of Alzheimer caregivers on positive aspects of caregiving. *Gerontologist*, *56*, 451–460.

Coffey, A., Mulcahy, H., Savage, E., et al. (2017). Transitional care interventions: Relevance for nursing in the community. *Public Health Nursing*. Doi: 10.1111/phn.12324. [Epub ahead of print]

Cooper, J., & Zimmerman, W. (2017). The effect of a faith community nurse network and public health collaboration on hypertension prevention and control. *Public Health Nursing*. Doi: 10.1111/phn.12325. [Epub ahead of print]

Cortes, T., & Sullivan-Marx, E. (2016). A case exemplar for national policy leadership: Expanding Program of All-inclusive Care for the Elderly (PACE). *Journal of Gerontological Nursing*, *42*(3), 9–14.

Genworth Financial. (2016). *Genworth 2016 cost of care*. Available at http://www.genworthfinancial.com.

Harris, M., & Longcoy, R. (2016). Collaborative efforts in the community: Faith community nurses as partners in healing. *Home Healthcare Now*, *34*, 146–150.

Harrison, J., & Framptom, S. (2017). Residnet-centered care in 10 U.S. nursing homes: Residents' perspectives. *Journal of Nursing Scholarship*, *49*, 6–14.

Judge, D., & Hall, M. (2016). Spirituality and health education in a faith community. *Home Healthcare Now*, *34*, 532.

Kelly, R., Puurveen, G., & gill, R. (2016). The effect of adult day services on delay to institutional placement. *Journal of Applied Gerontology*, *35*, 814–835.

Klein, L. C., Kim, K., Almeida, D., et al. (2016). Anticipating an easier day: Effects of adult day services on daily cortisol and stress. *Gerontologist*, *56*, 303–312.

Le Berre, M., Maimon, G., Sourial, N., et al. (2017). Impact of transitional care services for chronically ill older patients: A systematic evidence review. *Journal of the American Geriatrics Society*. Doi: 10.1111/jgs.14828. [Epub ahead of print]

Lim, F., Foust, J., & Van Cleave, J. (2016). Transitional care. In M. Boltz, E. Capezuti, T. Fulmer, & D. Zwicker (Eds.), *Evidence-based practice protocols for best practice* (5th ed., pp. 633–650). New York: Springer.

Lendon, J. P., Rome, V., & Sengupta, M. (2017). *Maps of selected characteristics of residential care communities and residents in the United States. Data from the National Study of Long-Term Care Providers, 2013–2014*. Washington, DC: National Center for Health Statistics.

Macleod, A., Tatangelo, G., McCabe, M., & You, E. (2017). "There isn't an easy way of finding the help that's available." Barriers and facilitators of service use among dementia family caregivers: A qualitative study. *International Psychogeriatrics*, *29*, 765–776.

Mullins, L., Skemp, L., & Maas, M. (2016). Community models of care: A scoping review. *Journal of Gerontological Nursing*, *42*(12), 12–20.

Musich, S., Wang, S., Kraemer, S., et al. (2017). Caregivers for older adults: Prevalence, characteristics, and health care utilization and expenditures. *Geriatric Nursing*, *38*, 9–16.

National League for Nursing. (2016). NLN releases: A vision for interprofessional collaboration in education and practice. Available at www.neponline.net. Doi: 10.1097/01.NEP.0000476111/94472.a6.

Naylor, M. D., Shaid, E. C., Carpenter, D., et al. (2017). Components of comprehensive and effective transitional care. *Journal of the American Geriatrics Society*, *65*(6), 1119–1125.

Nurses Improving Care for Healthsystem Elders. (2011). A crosswalk: Joint commission standards & NICHE resources. Available at www.nicheprogram.org.

Pan, J., Chochinov, H., Thompson, G., & McClement, S. (2016). The TIME questionnaire: A tool for eliciting personhood and enhancing dignity in nursing homes. *Geriatric Nursing*, *37*, 273–277.

Vandepitte, S., Van Den Noortgate, N., Putman, K., et al. (2016). Effectiveness of respite care in supporting informal caregivers of persons with dementia: A systematic review. *International Journal of Geriatric Psychiatry*, *31*, 1277–1288.

Schuller, K., Kash, B., & Gamm, L. (2017). Enhanced transitions of care: Centralizing discharge phone calls improves ability to reach patients and reduces hospital readmissions. *Journal for Healthcare Quality*, *39*(2), e10–e21.

Wessel, K. (2017). How an aging population is transforming nursing. *Home Healthcare Now*, *35*, 221–223.

Williams, C., Tappen, R., Wiese, L., et al. (2016). Stress in persons with dementia: Benefits of a memory center day program. *Archives of Psychiatric Nursing*, *30*, 531–538.

chapter 7

Assessment of Health and Functioning

LEARNING OBJECTIVES

After reading this chapter, you will be able to:

1. Discuss factors that contribute to the complexity of assessing older adults.

2. Use assessment tools to assess specific aspects of functioning, including activities of daily living and instrumental activities of daily living.

3. Discuss the importance of a function-focused approach to promote optimal level of functioning, particularly for hospitalized older adults.

4. Describe how the older adult's environment, use of adaptive and assistive devices, and cognitive abilities can affect functioning.

5. Discuss the relevance of comprehensive geriatric assessments and the Minimum Data Set in relation to care of older adults.

6. Assess safety of older adults in their home setting.

7. Discuss nursing roles related to concerns about safe driving by older adults.

KEY TERMS

activities of daily living (ADLs)

complexity of assessing health in older adults

comprehensive geriatric assessment

everyday competence

functional assessment

function-focused care

instrumental activities of daily living (IADLs)

Minimum Data Set (MDS)

nursing assessment tools

safe driving

Assessment of health and functioning of older adults is an essential and complex component of nursing care. This chapter discusses approaches to and tools for assessing the older adult's health and functioning. It also discusses currently evolving information about function-focused care. In addition, because health and functioning significantly affect the ability to drive a motor vehicle—which is a major safety concern with implications for society and individual older adults—this chapter discusses how nurses can assess and address risk factors that interfere with safe driving by older adults.

ASSESSING HEALTH OF OLDER ADULTS

A major challenge of caring for older adults is the complexity of assessing their health, especially from a comprehensive and holistic nursing perspective. Many factors contribute to the **complexity of assessing health in older adults**:

- Older adults commonly have one or more chronic conditions, in addition to any acute health conditions for which they are being assessed. These conditions often interact, causing older adults' health to fluctuate unpredictably.

- Manifestations of illness, even acute illness, tend to be obscure and less predictable in older adults than in younger adults. For example, in older adults, a common manifestation of illness or an adverse medication effect is a change in behavior or mental status.

- For any one manifestation of illness in an older adult, there are usually several possible explanations. For example, changes in function can be caused by a combination of several conditions, such as acute illness, psychosocial factors, environmental conditions, age-related changes, a new chronic illness, an existing chronic illness, or an adverse effect of medication(s) or other treatments.

- Treatments are often directed toward the symptoms while the source of a problem is unidentified and unresolved. This treatment approach can mask the underlying problem even further and cause additional complications (e.g., when adverse medication effects are not recognized as such and are treated with additional medications).

- Cognitive impairments can make it difficult for older adults to accurately report or describe a physiologic problem and reliable sources of information may be scarce or inaccessible.
- In many cases, by the time illness in an older adult is detected and addressed, the underlying physiologic disturbance is in an advanced stage, and additional complications have developed.
- Myths and misunderstandings can lead health care providers, family members, or older adults to falsely attribute treatable conditions to aging.

Because of these factors, a detective-like approach is needed for assessing older adults. This approach requires nurses to assess all aspects of the person's body, mind, and spirit to look for clues—which are usually many and complicated and range from subtle to obvious—to underlying causes of changes in health or functioning.

The Functional Consequences Model for Promoting Wellness in Older Adults (described in Chapter 3) is applied to specific aspects of functioning throughout this text. Clinically oriented chapters of this text include detailed guides to assessment of specific aspects of functioning along with guides to nursing interventions directed toward improved functioning and quality of life (refer to the list of assessment and intervention boxes in the front matter of this book). Clinically oriented chapters of this text also include information about normal age-related variations that nurses need to consider when assessing specific aspects of health and functioning. In addition, Table 7-1 can be used as a guide to age-related variations in laboratory values that are pertinent to overall nursing assessment of older adults. Chapter 27 provides information about unique and atypical manifestations of illness in older adults and additional information about promoting wellness for older adults during illness.

NURSING ASSESSMENT TOOLS

Since the late 1980s, the Hartford Institute for Geriatric Nursing has been in the forefront of developing, promulgating, and updating evidence-based and easy-to-use **nursing assessment tools** for use in various settings. These assessment guides, called *Try This: Best Practices in Nursing Care to Older Adults,* and cost-free web-based articles and videos demonstrating the application of these tools can be accessed through the online learning activities in clinically oriented chapters of this text. These tools do not replace a comprehensive assessment but are useful for identifying specific areas to address in the care plan. Also, it is important to consider that the purpose of some assessment tools is to screen for indicators of certain conditions, such as depression or dementia, and in these situations, they are a stepping stone to further assessment.

TABLE 7-1 Age-Related Variations in Laboratory Values	
Laboratory Values That Are NOT Affected by Normal Aging	
• Hematocrit and hemoglobin • Electrolytes (sodium, potassium, chloride, bicarbonate) • Calcium • Phosphorus	• Liver function tests • Blood urea nitrogen • Thyroid tests • White blood cell count • Platelet count

Laboratory Values That Often Are Abnormal in Older Adults	**Clinical Considerations**
Sedimentation rate	Elevations between 10 and 20 mm may be within normal for older adults
Glucose	Glucose may be elevated during acute illness and return to normal when the physiologic stress resolves
Albumin	Average values decline slightly with increased age, especially during acute illness, but significant decreases indicate undernutrition
Alkaline phosphatase	May be mildly elevated with normal aging, but significant elevations may occur with serious illness (e.g., liver or Paget disease)
Serum iron, iron-binding capacity, ferritin	Decreased values may usually indicate undernutrition and/or gastrointestinal blood loss
Urinalysis	Hematuria requires further evaluation; slight pyuria or bacteriuria is common and does not necessarily require treatment

Source: Adapted from Kane, R. L., Ouslander, J. G., Abrass, I. B., et al. (2013). *Essentials of clinical geriatrics* (7th ed.). New York: McGraw-Hill Education.

The Fulmer SPICES tool has been widely used since 1991 to identify the following common syndromes that require nursing interventions: **S**leep disorders, **P**roblems with eating or feeding, **I**ncontinence, **C**onfusion, **E**vidence of falls, and **S**kin breakdown. Standardized instruments also are used for assessing safe mobility as a particularly important aspect of functional assessment. For example, the "Get Up and Go" test, as described in Chapter 22, is widely used to assess mobility. Online Learning Activity 7-1 provides additional information about the SPICES and other assessment tools.

 See ONLINE LEARNING ACTIVITY 7-1: ADDITIONAL INFORMATION ABOUT ASSESSMENT TOOLS AND FUNCTION-FOCUSED CARE at http://thepoint.lww.com/Miller8e.

Wellness Opportunity

When assessing older adults, nurses try to identify the conditions that affect not only the health status and level of functioning but also the quality of life.

FUNCTIONAL ASSESSMENT AND FUNCTION-FOCUSED CARE

A **functional assessment** is an integral component of nursing care because an essential part of promoting wellness for older adults is identifying areas where function can be improved. The concept of functional assessment originated during the 1920s, when workers' compensation programs needed to determine a cash value to impairments that affected loss of function in jobs. Initially, there were no standards for this and the determination was based solely on a physician's opinion. When rehabilitation services were developed after World War II, tools were needed to measure changes in functional abilities. Functional assessment tools measure **activities of daily living (ADLs)**, which are the tasks associated with meeting one's basic needs, and **instrumental activities of daily living (IADLs)**, which are the more complex tasks that are essential in community-living situations.

In recent years, health care practitioners have increasingly recognized the value of functional assessment, particularly with regard to chronic conditions and care of older adults. In contrast to a medical diagnosis approach, a functional assessment approach focuses on improved functioning in daily life, regardless of diagnosis. In clinical settings, there is increasing emphasis on using functional assessments as a core component of **function-focused care**, which includes measures to prevent functional decline and maintain or improve an older adult's level of functioning. Figure 7-1 lists major trends related to functional assessment and function-focused care in gerontological health care settings today.

Functional Assessment

Assessment of ADLs is important in determining the level of assistance needed on a daily basis for the following activities: bathing, dressing, mouth care, hair care, dietary intake, transfer mobility, ambulation, bed mobility, and bladder and bowel elimination. When assessing ADLs, it is important to determine whether limitations are attributable, at least in part, to cognitive impairments, rather than primarily to physical limitations. For example, the ability to dress independently can be limited by difficulties with processing information, as is common in people with dementia. Also, it is important to assess any relationship between cognitive impairment and difficulty with maintaining bowel and bladder control because this information is pertinent to planning effective interventions.

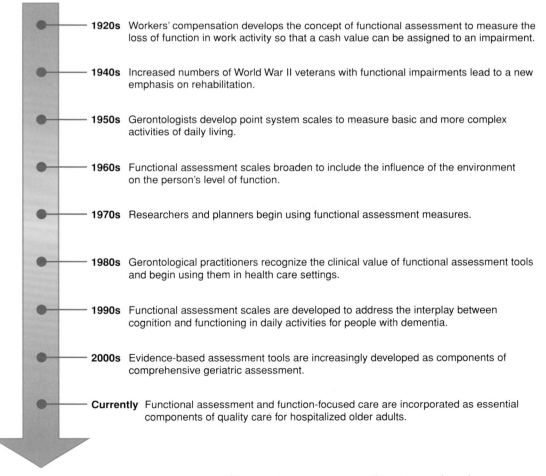

1920s Workers' compensation develops the concept of functional assessment to measure the loss of function in work activity so that a cash value can be assigned to an impairment.

1940s Increased numbers of World War II veterans with functional impairments lead to a new emphasis on rehabilitation.

1950s Gerontologists develop point system scales to measure basic and more complex activities of daily living.

1960s Functional assessment scales broaden to include the influence of the environment on the person's level of function.

1970s Researchers and planners begin using functional assessment measures.

1980s Gerontological practitioners recognize the clinical value of functional assessment tools and begin using them in health care settings.

1990s Functional assessment scales are developed to address the interplay between cognition and functioning in daily activities for people with dementia.

2000s Evidence-based assessment tools are increasingly developed as components of comprehensive geriatric assessment.

Currently Functional assessment and function-focused care are incorporated as essential components of quality care for hospitalized older adults.

FIGURE 7-1 Significant trends related to the use of functional assessment approaches in gerontological health care settings today.

IADLs are shopping, laundry, transportation, housekeeping, meal preparation, money management, medication management, and use of telephone. Although these IADLs are less important for residents or patients in institutional settings, an assessment is essential for discharge planning. When older adults cannot perform IADLs and have no caregiver to help with the task, community resources, such as home-delivered meals, are available to meet these needs.

 Interprofessional Collaboration

Nurses obtain information for the functional assessment from multiple sources, with much current emphasis on the importance of interprofessional assessment, communication, and care planning. When older adults are able to accurately describe their level of function before admission, information is obtained by interviewing the patient/resident soon after admission. If older adults are not able to provide this information, it should be obtained from a family member or other person who is knowledgeable about the person's level of function before admission. In all direct-care situations, nurses have numerous opportunities to observe the person's current level of function in performing ADLs and identify conditions that affect independent functioning. In addition to observing the person's level of functioning, nurses use assessment questions to obtain subjective information. Rather than asking open-ended questions such as "Do you have any difficulty with …?" it is better to ask for specific details about how tasks are accomplished, such as "Describe how you get your grocery shopping done." Also, consider the relevance of IADLs in relation to the person's support system and living arrangements. For example, a person who lives with other people might never have to participate in grocery shopping, whereas a person who lives alone may need to be able to use a telephone or emergency response system to beckon help when needed.

Function-Focused Care

Function-focused care is an approach to care that focuses both on evaluating a person's underlying capability with regard to functional and physical activity and on implementing interventions to optimize and maintain functional abilities and increase physical activities (Resnick, Galik, & Boltz, 2013). The philosophy of function-focused care addresses direct care issues as well as broader considerations, such as environmental factors, education and training of staff, and institutional policies that affect care. Studies find that this approach is effective in improving outcomes for older adults with acute and chronic conditions, including trauma and dementia (Boltz, Chippendale, Resnick, et al., 2015; Resnick, Wells, Galik, et al., 2016). Evidence-based practice guidelines for geriatric nursing have incorporated this approach in relation to assessment of physical function and preventing functional decline in acute care settings, as summarized in Box 7-1 (Boltz, Resnick, & Galik, 2016; Kresevic, 2016). This attention is warranted because studies have found that 35% to 45% of hospitalized older adults report a hospital-acquired functional decline at discharge, and this rate increased to 50% for those aged >85

(Palese, Gonella, Moreale, et al., 2016). The article available through Online Learning Activity 7-2 describes application of the function-focused care to orthopedic trauma patients. Although initial attention has focused on function-focused care in acute care settings, there is increasing attention to function-focused care in other settings, such as assisted-living facilities (Resnick, Galik, Vigne, et al., 2016).

 See ONLINE LEARNING ACTIVITY 7-2: ARTICLE ABOUT FUNCTION-FOCUSED CARE at http://thepoint.lww.com/Miller8e.

A Student's Perspective

During my first week with Mr. M., I was able to sit with him while he was having breakfast, and I used this time to consider his strengths and weaknesses. While studying his interactions with others, I observed that he had difficulty being understood. He struggled to articulate his various wants and needs. This seemed to lead to Mr. M. being more isolated than would otherwise be the case. One of his strengths was his ability to feed himself. Initially, I had hoped to read his chart more before meeting him. However, this interaction allowed me a more accurate assessment of his abilities than what would have been recorded in his chart.

After breakfast, we returned to his room to do oral care and to shave. After this, I helped transfer Mr. M. to his bed and he asked for a drink, which I gave him and he started choking. I was terrified, but fortunately my senior student was with me and together we managed the situation and he was okay. I learned from this experience to assess the person's entire environment before addressing patient needs and desires. Mr. M. choked because I gave him a cup of water that was not thickened.

Kimberly S.

Wellness Opportunity

Nurses identify factors that affect the older adult's quality of life by asking a question, such as "Are there enjoyable activities that you used to do but are no longer able to do because of health problems?"

Functional Assessment in People Who Are Cognitively Impaired

Because cognitive status and psychosocial functioning can significantly affect one's level of functioning, it is particularly challenging to assess function in older adults who have any cognitive or psychosocial limitations (e.g., dementia, delirium, depression). Some functional assessment scales have been developed specifically to address the interplay between cognition and abilities to perform ADLs. The Cleveland Scale for Activities of Daily Living (CSADL) (see Figure 7-2) is an example of a reliable and valid tool for assessing the ADLs in people with cognitive impairment.

Box 7-1 Evidence-Based Practice: Functional Assessment and Function-Focused Care

Background: Physical Functional Assessment

- Functional status describes the capacity and performance of ADLs and IADLs.
- Functional status of an individual, which is a sensitive indicator of health or illness in older adults, is an essential component of nursing assessment.
- Some types of functional decline can be prevented or ameliorated through prompt and aggressive nursing interventions, such as the ones described in function-focused care.

Background: Function-Focused Care

- Functional decline is a common complication in hospitalized older adults.
- Patient risk factors for functional decline during hospitalization that have been identified in studies include the following: pain, depression, nutritional problems, cognitive impairment, fear of falling, adverse medication effects, and prehospitalization functional loss, the presence of two or more comorbidities, taking five or more medications, having had a hospitalization or emergency department visit within the past 12 months.
- Risks within the care environment that are associated with low mobility include curtailing mobility and using restraints and tethering devices.
- Outcomes of poor physical function include increased likelihood of being discharged to a nursing home setting, increased rehabilitation costs, and decreased functional recovery.
- Outcomes of immobility associated with functional decline include infections, pressure ulcers, falls, ongoing decline in function, and recurrent hospital admissions.
- Outcomes of bed rest include loss of muscle strength and lean muscle mass, decreased aerobic capacity, diminished pulmonary ventilation, altered sensory awareness, and reduced appetite and thirst.

Assessment Related to Functional Status and Function-Focused Care

- Comprehensive functional assessment of older adults includes all the following components: independence in performing ADLs, IADLs, and social activities; assistance needed to accomplish these tasks; cognitive level; sensory ability; pain level; and capacity to ambulate.
- Function should be assessed over time, including baseline, on admission, and daily.

- Assessment of baseline function provides a benchmark when developing discharge goals.

Interprofessional Collaboration

- Interprofessional communication regarding functional status, changes, and expected trajectory should be part of all care settings and should include the patient and family whenever possible.
- The interprofessional team approach should address risk factors that affect goal achievement (e.g., cognitive status, nutritional status, pain, fear of falling, fatigue, medications, adverse medication effects).

Nursing Interventions to Maximize Functional Status and Prevent Decline

- Maintain the individual's daily routine as much as possible (e.g., encourage ambulation, allow flexible visitation, include pets).
- Educate older adults, family, and caregivers about the value of independent functioning and the consequences of functional decline.
- Explore alternatives to physical restraints.
- Assess and treat for pain.
- Facilitate referrals for rehabilitation therapies (e.g., physical therapy, occupational therapy).

Nursing Interventions to Help Older Adults Cope With Functional Decline

- Help older adults and family members establish realistic goals with interprofessional consultation.
- When decline cannot be prevented, provide caregiver education and support and consider consultation for palliative care consultation.
- Educate patient and family about safety concerns, including falls, injuries, and common complications.
- Provide sufficient protein and caloric intake to prevent further decline.
- Consider referrals for community-based services, such as home care, rehabilitation services, senior centers, and Meals on Wheels.

Source: Boltz M., Resnick, B., & Galik, E. (2016). Preventing functional decline in the acute care setting. In M. Boltz, E. Capezuti, T. Fulmer, et al. (Eds.), *Evidence-based geriatric nursing protocols for best practice* (5th ed., pp. 197–209). New York: Springer Publishing Co.; Kresevic, D. (2016). Assessment of physical function. (2016). In M. Boltz, E. Capezuti, T. Fulmer, et al. (Eds.), *Evidence-based practice protocols for best practice* (5th ed., pp. 89–102). New York: Springer Publishing Co.

Wellness Opportunity

When assessing the impact of cognitive abilities on functioning, nurses can try to identify simple interventions, such as putting labels on drawers that can improve the person's self-esteem by promoting independence.

Assessing the Use or Potential Use of Adaptive and Assistive Devices

The actual or potential use of items, such as mobility aids (e.g., canes, walkers, wheelchairs) and adaptive equipment (e.g., grab bars), should be assessed as factors that can significantly affect safety, functioning, and quality of life for older adults. Physical, occupational, and rehabilitation therapists are skilled in assessing for the use of these aids, but nurses need to be familiar with the array of adaptive and assistive devices so that they

can make recommendations or facilitate referrals for further evaluation. Online Learning Activity 7-3 provides information about many helpful and innovative devices that can be used to improve functioning and independence in daily activities. Additional assistive devices are illustrated and discussed in many chapters of this book (see Chapters 16, 17, 18, and 22).

Nurses also can identify problems related to the use of assistive devices and request further evaluation by a qualified therapist. For example, nurses can assess comfort and function of wheelchairs because improper fit leads to specific problems, such as the ones delineated in Table 7-2. Another nursing responsibility is making sure that wheelchairs are used appropriately for responsible patient care rather than for staff convenience, as is sometimes the case in long-term care facilities.

(*text continue on page 107*)

CLEVELAND SCALE FOR ACTIVITIES OF DAILY LIVING (CSADL)

Name or ID of Subject _____   Date _ _/_ _/_ _   Rater _____
                                                                 m m d d y y

Name of Informant _____

Relation of Informant to Subject *(Circle one.)*   Contact with Subject   Interview Type

1 Spouse   4 Friend or other family   1 2 days/week   1 Visit
2 Child   5 Professional: _____   2 3–4 days/week   2 Telephone
3 Sibling   6 Other: _____   3 5 or more days/week

To administer this scale, the rater must be thoroughly familiar with the Manual, which includes the full instructions. Place rating in blank after each item number. Several items have specific rating instructions. In particular, some require special questioning if the subject is rated as dependent (rating of 1, 2, or 3).

Rating	*Meaning of Rating*
0	**Never Dependent.** [S] does this effectively, quite independently, without any direction or help.
1	**Sometimes Dependent.** [S] usually does this independently, but sometimes or in some situations [S] needs direction or help.
2	**Usually Dependent.** [S] usually requires some direction or help, but sometimes or in some situations [S] does it independently.
3	**Always Dependent.** [S] always requires direction or help. [S] never does it independently.
9	Cannot rate because of insufficient information

Bathing

1. _____   Initiates bath or shower with appropriate frequency and at appropriate times

2. _____   Prepares bath/shower (draws water of proper temperature, ensures soap and towel are present, etc.)

3. _____   Gets in and out of tub or shower

4. _____   Cleans self

Toileting

5. _____   Able to physically control timing of urination

6. _____   Able to physically control timing of bowel movements

7. _____   Recognizes need to eliminate

8. _____   After toileting, cleans and re-clothes self appropriately

Personal Hygiene and Appearance

9. _____   Initiates personal grooming with appropriate frequency and at appropriate times

10. _____   Washes hands and face

11. _____   Brushes teeth

12. _____   Combs hair, shaves (as appropriate)

FIGURE 7-2 The Cleveland Scale for Activities of Daily Living (CSADL). This functional assessment form was specifically designed for use with people with Alzheimer disease. (Used with permission from the University Memory and Aging Center, Case Western Reserve University, Cleveland, OH. © 1994.)

Dressing

13. _____   Initiates dressing at appropriate time

14. _____   Selects clothes

15. _____   Puts on garments, footwear, etc.

16. _____   Fastens clothing (buttons, shoelaces, zippers, etc.)

Eating

17. _____   Initiates eating at appropriate times of day and with appropriate frequency

18. _____   Carries out physical acts of eating (including using utensils)

19. _____   Eats with acceptable manners, e.g., with appropriate speed, does not speak with food in mouth, etc.

20. _____   Prepares own meals (includes cooking on stove). *This item requires special questioning.*

Mobility

21. _____   Initiates actively moving about the environment, as opposed to sitting, not attempting to get about, etc.

22. _____   Actively moves about environment (with or without assisting device)

22a.   Does subject have physical limitations of mobility? *(Circle one of following codes.)*

    0   No physical limitations of mobility

    1   Yes, there are physical limitations of mobility. *(Circle all that apply.)*

Needs assistance of other persons to walk	Trouble getting in or out of bed	Other Mobility Problems
Needs cane	Trouble getting in or out of chair	*(describe):*
Needs walker	Trouble getting on or off toilet	
Needs wheelchair	Trouble climbing or descending stairs	

Medications

23. _____   Takes medications as scheduled and in correct dosages. *If subject has taken no medications during prior year, rate item as 9. This item requires questioning.*

Shopping

24. _____   Does necessary grocery shopping, buying appropriate items and quantities. *This item requires special questioning.*

25. _____   Does necessary clothes shopping, buying appropriate items and quantities. *This item requires special questioning.*

Travel

26. _____   Finds way about in familiar surroundings

27. _____   Orients to unfamiliar surroundings without undue difficulty

28. _____   Travels beyond walking distance (i.e., driving own vehicle or using public transportation)

29. _____   Drives motor vehicle. *This item requires special questioning.*

FIGURE 7-2 *(Continued)*

Hobbies, personal interests, employment

30. _____   Initiates activities of personal interest (e.g., card playing, woodworking, others). *This item requires special questioning.*

31. _____   Carries out such activities. *This item requires special questioning.*

32. _____   Does subject work for pay? *If subject does not work because of having reached an age appropriate to retirement from his or her occupation, rate 9. This item requires special questioning.*

Housework/home maintenance (as appropriate to individual situation)

33. _____   Initiates work around house as needed. *This item requires special questioning.*

34. _____   Carries out work effectively, e.g., cleanly, neatly, accurately, efficiently. *This item requires special questioning.*

Types of work done *(Don't score, just circle)*

Dish washing	Vacuuming	Mowing lawn
Sweeping	Scrubbing floors	Gardening
Personal laundry	Small home repairs	Minor car care
Other types of work *(Describe)*:		

Telephone

35. _____   Looks up numbers

36. _____   Dials numbers

37. _____   Answers phone

38. _____   Takes messages

Money Management

39. _____   Pays for purchases (selecting appropriate amount and determining correct change). *This item requires special questioning.*

40. _____   Manages financial responsibilities beyond paying for immediate purchases (e.g., paying monthly bills, managing checking or savings account, etc.). *This item requires special questioning.*

Communication Skills

41. _____   Spontaneously expresses thoughts and needs to others

42. _____   Responds accurately to spoken instructions and conversation

43. _____   Reads and understands single words and short phrases (signs, lists, etc.)

44. _____   Reads and understands complex material (books, newspapers, etc.)

45. _____   Writes short phrases (lists, brief messages)

46. _____   Writes complex material (letters, diary, etc.)

FIGURE 7-2 *(Continued)*

Social Behavior

47. _____   Behaves in a socially appropriate manner. Socially inappropriate behaviors encompass a **wide** range of behavior, including but not limited to such things as making rude remarks, belching, touching private parts, showing little regard for personal privacy, etc. For this item, dependency refers to the extent to which other people must direct or manage the subject to ensure that he or she behaves in a socially appropriate fashion.

Other Problems — Are there any situations in which patient does not behave in an independent and responsible fashion that have not been covered by these questions? *(Circle one of following codes.)*

48.   0   No other dependent behaviors

           1   Yes, there are other dependent behaviors.   *(Please provide details below.)*

QUALITY OF INTERVIEW (Rater's Judgment)

Interview appeared valid   0

Some questions about interview, but it is probably acceptable   1

Information from interview is of doubtful validity   2

Rater should record the basis for judging the interview of questionable or doubtful validity.

Comments:

FIGURE 7-2 *(Continued)*

See **ONLINE LEARNING ACTIVITY 7-3: RESOURCES FOR INFORMATION ABOUT HELPFUL AND INNOVATIVE DEVICES TO IMPROVE FUNCTIONING AND INDEPENDENCE** at http://thepoint.lww.com/Miller8e.

COMPREHENSIVE GERIATRIC ASSESSMENTS

As gerontologists and health care providers began addressing the complexity of care for older adults, they recognized the need for assessment models that were more comprehensive than those that focused on particular aspects of health or functioning. A **comprehensive geriatric assessment** includes medical, psychosocial, cognitive, and functional components and involves input from several professionals. Comprehensive geriatric assessments are particularly important for older adults who are cognitively impaired or frail, as discussed in Chapters 14 and 27, respectively. They also are essential in situations where the older adult's decision-making capacity is questionable, as discussed in the chapters on legal and ethical considerations and elder abuse (Chapters 9 and 10, respectively). In acute care and community settings these assessments are performed by an interprofessional team of clinicians who have additional expertise in geriatrics and gerontology. In addition to assessing the older adult, the health care team involves family members and caregivers in the

TABLE 7-2 Negative Effects of Improper Wheelchair Fit

Seating Problem	Result on Body	Potential Effect
Wheelchair too high	Feet do not touch the floor Unable to self-propel Pelvis moves forward	Edema and decreased circulation in legs Decreased activity Poor sitting posture
Poor back support	Compression of trunk, chest, abdomen Sliding out of chair Increased pelvic tilt	Skin breakdown on back and sacrum Impaired gastrointestinal and respiratory function
Wheelchair too heavy	Difficulty moving chair	Decreased activity
Wheelchair too wide	Pelvic shifting laterally Forward leaning Difficulty using hand rims	Shear stress on skin Poor posture, circulation Decreased mobility
Seat not firm enough ("sling" effect)	Scoliosis Sliding out of chair	Poor posture, circulation Shear stress on skin
Footrest too high	Poor femoral support Unequal pressure distribution Increased ischial tuberosity	Poor posture Skin breakdown

Source: Rader, J., Jones, D., & Miller, L. (2000). The importance of individualized wheelchair seating for frail older adults. *Journal of Gerontological Nursing, 26*(11), 24–32.

assessment process and in implementing recommendations. Assessment information is usually presented to the older adult and family members as part of a problem-solving approach so a plan of ongoing care can be developed.

The Omnibus Budget Reconciliation Act of 1987 mandated that all Medicaid- and Medicare-funded nursing homes use a standardized form, called **Minimum Data Set (MDS)**, to comprehensively assess each resident's functional, medical, mental, and psychosocial status. The form and overall process has been revised several times, with increasing emphasis on broader aspects of function and on the resident's quality of life. The Centers for Medicare & Medicaid Services issues guidelines that address all aspects of implementation including updated standardized forms. Beginning in 2015, the assessment process involves the MDS, the Resident Assessment Instrument (RAI), and the Care Area Assessments. The value of the MDS has been internationally recognized, and the MDS forms have been translated, validated, and implemented in many countries, including Canada, Australia, and Asian and European countries. Box 7-2 summarizes components of the MDS form, with examples of items related to each topic and Figure 7-3 shows the section on Functional Status, with details related to assessment of ADLs.

> **Wellness Opportunity**
>
> Keep in mind that formal assessment tools fulfill requirements for documentation, but their primary purpose is to improve care and quality of life for older adults.

ASSESSMENT OF SAFETY IN HOME SETTINGS

In addition to assessing the older adult's health and functioning, nurses need to be aware of environmental factors that influence the person's safety, functioning, and quality of life. Researchers and practitioners increasingly are addressing the interrelationship between people and their environments, and this is particularly pertinent to care of older adults. In the late 1990s, the term **everyday competence** was used to describe the effects of cultural, physical, cognitive, emotional, social, and contextual factors on a person's daily functioning. This is particularly important to consider when assessing older adults because these factors can appreciably hinder or improve functional abilities. For example, environmental factors that significantly affect hearing, vision, and mobility are discussed in Chapters 16, 17, and 22, respectively.

Home assessments provide an excellent base for assessing the relationship between older adults and their environments. These assessments are essential not only for identifying fall risks (as discussed in Chapter 22) but also for identifying environmental conditions that positively or negatively affect safety, functioning, and quality of life. For example, proper lighting is essential for performing enjoyable activities, such as reading, playing cards, and engaging in hobbies. Similarly, the ability to regulate the temperature is important not only as a safety consideration for preventing hypothermia and hyperthermia but also for comfort. Nurses can use Box 7-3 as a guide to assessing home environments for safety and optimal functioning.

> **Wellness Opportunity**
>
> In addition to assessing conditions that affect functioning, nurses pay attention to environmental factors that affect quality of life.

DRIVING SAFETY

Nurses are among the health care professionals responsible for addressing complex decisions about driving,

Box 7-2   Minimum Data Set Categories and Examples of Assessment Items

Hearing, Speech, and Vision

- Ability to hear, use of hearing aid
- Speech clarity, abilities to make self understood and to understand others
- Ability to see in adequate light, use of corrective lenses

Cognitive Patterns

- Repetition and recall of three words
- Orientation to year, month, day
- Short- and long-term memory
- Ability to make decisions about tasks of daily life
- Signs and symptoms of delirium

Mood (Interview or Self-Assessment)

- Symptoms of depression during the past 2 weeks
- Evidence of depression

Behavior

- Hallucinations or delusions
- Physical or verbal behavioral symptoms directed toward others
- Rejection of care
- Wandering
- Changes in behavior

Preferences for Customary Routine, Activities, and Community Setting

- Preferred routine for daily activities (e.g., personal care, communication, social and religious activities)
- Potential for returning to the community

Functional Status (see Figure 7-3)

Bladder and Bowel

- Ability to maintain urinary and bowel continence
- Toileting program for urinary elimination (e.g., scheduled toileting, prompted voiding, bladder training) or bowel continence
- Bowel patterns

Active Disease Diagnosis (i.e., Currently Listed Diagnoses)

- Cancer
- Conditions related to any of the following systems: thermoregulation, circulatory, gastrointestinal, genitourinary, musculoskeletal, pulmonary, neurologic, or metabolic
- Nutritional conditions
- Infection
- Psychiatric or mood disorder

Health Conditions

- Pain management and assessment
- Cough or shortness of breath (dyspnea)

- Chest pain or angina
- Current tobacco use
- Prognosis related to chronic disease that may result in shortened life expectancy
- Falls assessment and history

Swallowing/Nutrition Status

- Swallowing disorder
- Height and weight
- History of weight loss of 5% or more during the last month or 10% or more in the last 6 months
- Nutritional approaches (e.g., feeding tube, mechanically altered diet, therapeutic diet)

Oral/Dental Status

- Condition of teeth and gums
- Absence of teeth
- Mouth or facial pain

Skin Conditions

- Presence of pressure ulcers in the last 5 days
- Pressure ulcer stages
- Healed pressure ulcers
- Other skin problems (e.g., venous or arterial ulcers, surgical wounds, burns, open lesions)
- Skin treatments (e.g., pressure-reducing devices, repositioning program, dressings, nutrition or hydration interventions to manage skin problems)

Medications

- Injections
- Use of any of the following medications during the last 5 days: antipsychotic, antianxiety, antidepressant, hypnotic, anticoagulant

Special Treatments and Procedures

- Cancer treatments
- Respiratory treatments
- Dialysis
- Hospice care
- Vaccination status (influenza, pneumococcal)
- Therapies (e.g., speech-language, occupations, physical, respiratory, psychological, recreational)
- Nursing rehabilitation and restorative care
- Physician examination and orders during the past 5 days

Restraints

- Any method that the person cannot remove easily, which restricts freedom of movement or normal access to one's body

Source: Recommended MDS 3.0, available at www.cms.gov

---

not only as a personal safety issue for older adults, but also as an ethical issue to protect individuals and society. **Safe driving** is receiving much attention as a multifaceted issue involving personal safety, safety of others, and quality-of-life considerations. Decisions about driving safety are complex because of considerations such as the following:

- Older adult drivers are more likely to incur higher rates of at-fault crashes.
- Older adult drivers have a higher fatality rate per mile driven than any other age group older than 25.
- Older adult drivers have a disproportionately higher rate of poor outcomes in accidents, due in part to chest and head injuries.

Resident _____　Identifier _____　Date _____

Section G	Functional Status

G0110. Activities of Daily Living (ADL) Assistance
Refer to the ADL flow chart in the RAI manual to facilitate accurate coding

Instructions for Rule of 3
■ When an activity occurs three times at any one given level, code that level.
■ When an activity occurs three times at multiple levels, code the most dependent, exceptions are total dependence (4), activity must require full assist every time, and activity did not occur (8), activity must not have occurred at all. Example, three times extensive assistance (3) and three times limited assistance (2), code extensive assistance (3).
■ When an activity occurs at various levels, but not three times at any given level, apply the following:
　○ When there is a combination of full staff performance, and extensive assistance, code extensive assistance.
　○ When there is a combination of full staff performance, weight bearing assistance and/or non-weight bearing assistance code limited assistance (2).
If none of the above are met, code supervision.

1. ADL Self-Performance
Code for **resident's performance** over all shifts - not including setup. If the ADL activity occurred 3 or more times at various levels of assistance, code the most dependent - except for total dependence, which requires full staff performance every time

Coding:
Activity Occurred 3 or More Times
0. **Independent** - no help or staff oversight at any time
1. **Supervision** - oversight, encouragement or cueing
2. **Limited assistance** - resident highly involved in activity; staff provide guided maneuvering of limbs or other non-weight-bearing assistance
3. **Extensive assistance** - resident involved in activity, staff provide weight-bearing support
4. **Total dependence** - full staff performance every time during entire 7-day period
Activity Occurred 2 or Fewer Times
7. **Activity occurred only once or twice** - activity did occur but only once or twice
8. **Activity did not occur** - activity did not occur or family and/or non-facility staff provided care 100% of the time for that activity over the entire 7-day period

2. ADL Support Provided
Code for **most support provided** over all shifts; code regardless of resident's self-performance classification

Coding:
0. **No** setup or physical help from staff
1. **Setup** help only
2. **One** person physical assist
3. **Two+** persons physical assist
8. ADL activity itself **did not occur** or family and/or non-facility staff provided care 100% of the time for that activity over the entire 7-day period

	1. Self-Performance	2. Support
	↓ Enter Codes in Boxes ↓	
A. Bed mobility - how resident moves to and from lying position, turns side to side, and positions body while in bed or alternate sleep furniture	☐	☐
B. Transfer - how resident moves between surfaces including to or from: bed, chair, wheelchair, standing position (**excludes** to/from bath/toilet)	☐	☐
C. Walk in room - how resident walks between locations in his/her room	☐	☐
D. Walk in corridor - how resident walks in corridor on unit	☐	☐
E. Locomotion on unit - how resident moves between locations in his/her room and adjacent corridor on same floor. If in wheelchair, self-sufficiency once in chair	☐	☐
F. Locomotion off unit - how resident moves to and returns from off-unit locations (e.g., areas set aside for dining, activities or treatments). **If facility has only one floor**, how resident moves to and from distant areas on the floor. If in wheelchair, self-sufficiency once in chair	☐	☐
G. Dressing - how resident puts on, fastens and takes off all items of clothing, including donning/removing a prosthesis or TED hose. Dressing includes putting on and changing pajamas and housedresses	☐	☐
H. Eating - how resident eats and drinks, regardless of skill. Do not include eating/drinking during medication pass. Includes intake of nourishment by other means (e.g., tube feeding, total parenteral nutrition, IV fluids administered for nutrition or hydration)	☐	☐
I. Toilet use - how resident uses the toilet room, commode, bedpan, or urinal; transfers on/off toilet; cleanses self after elimination; changes pad; manages ostomy or catheter; and adjusts clothes. Do not include emptying of bedpan, urinal, bedside commode, catheter bag or ostomy bag	☐	☐
J. Personal hygiene - how resident maintains personal hygiene, including combing hair, brushing teeth, shaving, applying makeup, washing/drying face and hands (**excludes** baths and showers)	☐	☐

FIGURE 7-3 Functional Status section of MDS 3.0 Version 1.13.2. Effective 10/01/2015 available at www.cms.gov

Resident _____   Identifier _____   Date _____

Section G	**Functional Status**

G0120. Bathing

How resident takes full-body bath/shower, sponge bath, and transfers in/out of tub/shower (**excludes** washing of back and hair). Code for **most dependent** in self-performance and support

Enter Code | **A. Self-performance**
0. **Independent** - no help provided
1. **Supervision** - oversight help only
2. **Physical help limited to transfer only**
3. **Physical help in part of bathing activity**
4. **Total dependence**
8. **Activity itself did not occur** or family and/or non-facility staff provided care 100% of the time for that activity over the entire 7-day period

Enter Code | **B. Support provided**
(Bathing support codes are as defined in item **G0110 column 2, ADL Support Provided**, above)

G0300. Balance During Transitions and Walking

After observing the resident, **code the following walking and transition items for most dependent**

Coding:
0. **Steady at all times**
1. **Not steady, but able to stabilize without staff assistance**
2. **Not steady, only able to stabilize with staff assistance**
8. **Activity did not occur**

↓ **Enter Codes in Boxes**

- **A. Moving from seated to standing position**
- **B. Walking** (with assistive device if used)
- **C. Turning around** and facing the opposite direction while walking
- **D. Moving on and off toilet**
- **E. Surface-to-surface transfer** (transfer between bed and chair or wheelchair)

G0400. Functional Limitation in Range of Motion

Code for limitation that interfered with daily functions or placed resident at risk of injury

Coding:
0. **No impairment**
1. **Impairment on one side**
2. **Impairment on both sides**

↓ **Enter Codes in Boxes**

- **A. Upper extremity** (shoulder, elbow, wrist, hand)
- **B. Lower extremity** (hip, knee, ankle, foot)

G0600. Mobility Devices

↓ **Check all that were normally used**

- ☐ **A. Cane/crutch**
- ☐ **B. Walker**
- ☐ **C. Wheelchair** (manual or electric)
- ☐ **D. Limb prosthesis**
- ☐ **Z. None of the above** were used

FIGURE 7-3 (*Continued*)

- Driving cessation is associated with all the following serious negative health consequences: increased depressive symptoms, social isolation, and difficulty with IADL.

(Chihuri, Mielenz, DiMaggio, et al., 2016; Choi & DiNitto, 2016; Douroudgar, Chuang, Perry, et al., 2017; Edwards, Lister, Lin, et al., 2016)

Thus, a current focus is on how best to support older adults who need to stop driving and at the same time promote continued participation within the community (American Geriatrics Society & Pomidor, 2016; Liddle, Gustafsson, Mitchell, et al., 2016). Psychosocial implications related to driving cessation are discussed in Chapter 12, and in this chapter, safe driving is discussed as an IADL.

Risks for Unsafe Driving

Age-related changes in vision, musculoskeletal function, and central and autonomic nervous systems can affect driving abilities even in healthy older adults. In addition, older adults typically have other conditions that increase the risk for unsafe driving, such as medical conditions, cognitive impairment, functional limitations, medication use, and alcohol consumption. For example, visual impairments due

Box 7-3 Guidelines for Assessing the Safety of the Environment

Illumination and Color Contrast

- Is the lighting adequate but not glare producing?
- Are the light switches easy to reach and manipulate?
- Can lights be turned on before entering rooms?
- Are night lights used in appropriate places?
- Is color contrast adequate between objects, such as a chair and the floor?

Hazards

- Are there highly polished floors, throw rugs, or other hazardous floor coverings?
- If area rugs are used, do they have a nonslip backing, and are the edges tacked to the floor?
- Are there cords, clutter, or other obstacles in pathways?
- Is there a pet that is likely to be running underfoot?

Furniture

- Are chairs the right height and depth for the person?
- Do the chairs have armrests? Are tables stable and of the appropriate height?
- Is small furniture placed well away from pathways?

Stairways

- Is lighting adequate?
- Are there light switches at the top and bottom of the stairs?
- Are there securely fastened handrails on both sides of the stairway?
- Are all the steps even?
- Are the treads nonskid?
- Should colored tape be used to mark the edges of the steps, particularly the top and bottom steps?

Bathroom

- Are grab bars placed appropriately for the tub and toilet?
- Does the tub have skid-proof strips or a rubber mat in the bottom?
- Has the person considered using a tub or shower seat?
- Is the height of the toilet seat appropriate?
- Has the person considered using an elevated toilet seat?
- Does the color of the toilet seat contrast with surrounding colors?
- Is toilet paper within easy reach?

Bedroom

- Is the height of the bed appropriate?
- Is the mattress firm at the edges to provide enough support for sitting?
- If the bed has wheels, are they locked securely?
- Would full or partial side rails be a help or a hazard?
- When side rails are in the down position, are they completely out of the way?
- Is the pathway between the bedroom and bathroom clear of objects and adequately illuminated, particularly at night?

- Would a bedside commode be useful, especially at night?
- Is there a light near the bed, and does the person have sufficient physical and cognitive ability to turn it on before getting out of bed?
- Is furniture positioned to allow safe use of assistive devices for ambulation?
- Is a telephone situated near the bed?

Kitchen

- Are storage areas used to the best advantage (e.g., are objects that are frequently used in the most accessible places)?
- Are appliance cords kept out of the way?
- Are nonslip mats used in front of the sink?
- Does the person know how to use the oven, stove, or microwave safely?

Assistive Devices

- Is a call light available, and does the person know how to use it?
- What assistive devices are used?
- Would the person benefit from any assistive devices that are not being used?
- Are assistive devices being used safely and properly, or do they present additional hazards?

Temperature

- Is the temperature of the room(s) comfortable?
- Can the person read the markings on the thermostat and adjust it appropriately?
- During cold months, is the room temperature high enough to prevent hypothermia?
- During hot weather, is the room temperature cool enough to prevent hyperthermia?

Overall Safety

- How does the person obtain objects from hard-to-reach places?
- How does the person change overhead light bulbs?
- Are doorways wide enough to accommodate assistive devices?
- Do door thresholds create hazardous conditions?
- Are telephones accessible, especially for emergency calls? Would it be helpful to use a cordless portable phone?
- Would it be helpful to have some emergency call system available?
- Does the person wear sturdy shoes with nonskid soles?
- Does the person keep a list of emergency numbers by the phone?
- Does the person have an emergency exit plan in the event of fire?
- Are smoke alarms present and operational?
- Is there a carbon monoxide detector in an appropriate place (if the house has gas appliances, wood-burning stoves, or another object that produces carbon monoxide)?

---

to cataracts or glaucoma have specifically been identified as risks for unsafe driving (Agramunt, Meuleners, Fraser, et al., 2016; Wood, Black, Mallon, et al., 2016).

Nursing Assessment of Driving

Questions about the older person's perception of or concerns about his or her driving can be used to open the discussion of this important—and often sensitive—topic. Nurses can open

the discussion by indicating that questions about driving are routinely incorporated into an assessment so that any identified safety concerns can be addressed proactively. The following questions can be used for this part of the assessment:

- Do you have any concerns about your ability to drive safely?
- Have you adjusted your driving patterns to avoid certain situations, such as driving at night, on highways, or at intersections involving left-hand turns?

- Has anyone expressed or discussed concerns about your driving? For example, friends, family members, or health care professionals?
- Have you gotten lost while driving in places that are usually familiar?
- Have you been in any accidents during the past couple of years? (If yes, ask about circumstances.)
- Have you had any citations related to unsafe driving or driving under the influence?

When appropriate, nurses can use these same kinds of question to elicit assessment information from family members who are likely to have observations and concerns.

If answers to any of these questions raise concerns about driving safety, a more comprehensive assessment is warranted, as discussed in the next section. In addition, if the older person has any condition that is associated with risks for driving (e.g., dementia, functional impairment, significant vision impairment), arrangements should be made for appropriate assessments, which usually are performed by specialized rehabilitation specialists. In all situations, interventions should be directed toward improving the safety of the older adult and others within the context of maintaining quality of life for the older adult. When risks are identified it is important to assess the older adult's insight into the effect of these risks on safe driving. Whereas some older adults appropriately self-regulate their driving in relation to their limitations, others have little insight or continue to drive despite their awareness of risks.

Wellness Opportunity

Nurses can promote personal responsibility by encouraging older adults to use self-assessment tools, which are available through the resources listed in Online Learning Activity 7-4.

Interprofessional Team Approach Related to Older Adult Drivers

In 2016, the American Geriatrics Society (AGS) and the National Highway Traffic Safety Administration (NHTSA) called upon all health care professionals to use a collaborative team approach to not only address serious safety-related concerns about older adult drivers but also to "be supportive in the face of what may be a devastating loss of independence, and to use available resources and professionals who can assist with transportation to allow older adults to maintain independence" (American Geriatrics Society & Pomidor, 2016, p. 6). Recent articles in nursing journals have echoed the call for nurses to address this complex issue as a public health nursing opportunity (Wiese & Wolff, 2016) and as an essential gerontological nursing responsibility (Counsell, 2016; Resnick, 2016). These articles encourage nurses to become familiar with the AGS/NHTSA

Clinician's Guide to Assessing and Counseling Older Drivers report, which is listed as a resource in Online Learning Activity 7-4 Box 7-4 highlights key points of that report that are most pertinent to nursing assessment and interventions related to older adult drivers.

Box 7-4 Clinician's Guide to Addressing Concerns Related to Older Drivers

Clinical Team Members

- All clinical team members can help identify and counsel older adults who may be at risk for unsafe driving.
- All clinical team members have opportunities for screening and assessment or referral to another team member or specialist for further evaluation.

Roles of Nurses

- Nurses contribute to the assessment by monitoring vital signs and by evaluating functional abilities, disease risk factors, medication adherence and adverse effects, and personal health behaviors such as alcohol use, and health literacy.
- Information from nursing assessments can be used to facilitate changes in the care plan.
- Home health nurses and direct care assistants have unique opportunities to closely observe, counsel, and support older adults at home in their daily activities.
- Nurses may also serve as case managers, health counselors, resources for older adults and caregivers, and liaisons with other clinical team members to address health-related concerns.
- Nurses identify risks through a comprehensive geriatric assessment that includes the following components:
  - Full visual examination
  - Cognitive tests, including skills related to attention, executive function, and visuoperceptual processing
  - Motor performance, including gait, balance, postural control, and speed of walking
  - Medication review
  - Self-report questions
  - Questions for family members and caregivers

Clinical Interventions

- Identify, correct, or stabilize any functional deficits that may impair driving performance.
- Optimize management of all medical conditions.
- Refer to a driver rehabilitation specialist.
- Provide information about resources for transportation.

Functions of Driver Rehabilitation Specialists

- Evaluate sensory, cognitive, and motor function abilities that affect driving skills.
- Provide assessment and/or training in the vehicle and on the road.
- Recommend rehabilitation when restoration of abilities is possible.
- Recommend modifications (e.g., hand controls, left foot accelerator) to compensate for physical impairment.
- Recommend strategies to improve driving safety, such as route modifications.
- Suggest restrictions to support ongoing driving, such as limited routes.

Adapted from American Geriatrics Society & Pomidor A. (Ed.). (2016). *Clinician's guide to assessing and counseling older drivers.* 3rd ed. (Report No. DOT HS 812 228). Washington, DC: National Highway Traffic Safety Administration.

Nursing Interventions Related to Safe Driving

Addressing risk factors that affect driving abilities is an important health promotion activity that should be integrated into usual care for older adults, preferably before significant safety concerns arise. Some risks for unsafe driving can be minimized through interventions that address contributing factors, such as vision impairments, hearing impairments, and medication-related issues (discussed in Chapters 17, 16, and 8, respectively). When pathologic conditions affect neuromuscular functioning, nurses may suggest a referral for physical or occupational therapy to improve particular aspects of functioning that affect driving. For example, an older person with arthritis or Parkinson disease may benefit from working with a therapist who has additional training for driving rehabilitation. Even if the therapist does not have special training, the older adult can focus on the goal of improved safety and functioning for driving skills as part of the therapy program. For all older adults who want to maintain driving independence and safety, nurses have essential roles in teaching about the benefits of physical activity on overall health and driving ability in particular (Miller, Taylor-Piliae, & Insel, 2016).

Referrals for Driving Evaluation and Recommendations

Families are likely to seek guidance from nurses and other health care professionals to address their safety concerns about driving abilities of older adults. For example, nurses in home care settings often need to guide family and caregivers on how to open the conversation about "giving up the keys" (Pastor, Jones, & Arms, 2017). One way of addressing caregivers' concerns about driving safety is to provide information about resources that families can use to approach this issue. Driving evaluation programs, which usually are administered by occupational therapy departments, provide recommendations related to driving and appropriate follow-up for those who can benefit from education and rehabilitation. When suggesting this referral, it is important to emphasize that the purpose is not to take away the person's driving privileges but rather to identify interventions to improve safety for the older driver and others.

Recommendations of driving evaluation programs fall within a wide range and may include modifying vehicles to compensate for physical limitations, participating in driving rehabilitation therapy, or refraining from or restricting driving. Examples of adaptive equipment include pedal extenders, distance sensors, left foot accelerators, steering wheel adaptations, touch pads to operate auxiliary controls, and spot mirrors to compensate for visual and range-of-motion deficit. Examples of recommendations related to driving restrictions are no highways, short distances or familiar areas only, daytime or fair weather driving only, and requiring the presence of a navigator. Driving rehabilitation, specialists also may counsel older adults about considerations related to the purchase of a new vehicle—for example, safety features that are best matched to the needs of the purchaser.

Driver education programs are another type of resource that helps older adults recognize driving issues and improve safety. These programs are available through organizations such as AARP (Mature Driving Program) and the American Automobile Association (Safe Driving for Mature Operators). Use Online Learning Activity 7-4 to find information about resources related to education, evaluation, and rehabilitation related to driving.

In addition to suggesting programs that directly address safe driving, nurses can suggest referrals to programs that provide transportation for older adults. For example, senior centers are available in every area of the country under the Area Agency on Aging and they generally provide transportation services and information about local resources.

See **ONLINE LEARNING ACTIVITY 7-4: RESOURCES RELATED TO EDUCATION, EVALUATION, AND REHABILITATION RELATED TO DRIVING** at **http://thepoint.lww.com/Miller8e.**

Chapter Highlights

Health Assessment of Older Adults

- Assessment of health and functioning in older adults is challenging because of many factors that contribute to the complexity of assessing older adults (e.g., presence of multiple interacting conditions, unique manifestations of illness, treatments that mask the underlying problem, and myths and misunderstandings about aging.
- Consider age-related variations in some laboratory values when assessing older adults (Table 7-1).

Nursing Assessment Tools

- Easy-to-use and evidence-based nursing assessment tools and related resources are available through online learning activities in clinically oriented chapters of this text.

Functional Assessment and Function-Focused Care

- Approaches to functional assessment have evolved since the 1920s, with current emphasis on function-focused care and comprehensive geriatric assessments (Figure 7-1).
- Functional assessment tools provide a structure for assessing the person's ability to perform ADLs and IADLs.
- Function-focused care focuses both on evaluating a person's underlying capability with regard to functional status and physical activity and on implementing interventions to optimize and maintain functional abilities and increase physical activities (Box 7-1).
- The CSADL can be used for older adults who are cognitively impaired (Figure 7-2).
- Assessing the use of adaptive equipment and assistive devices is important for identifying factors that affect safety, comfort, and functioning.

Comprehensive Geriatric Assessments

- Comprehensive geriatric assessments, such as the MDS for Resident Assessment and Care Screening, are used to provide information about all aspects of functioning (Box 7-2 and Figure 7-3).

Assessment of Safety in Home Settings

- Assessment of the home environment is important for identifying factors that affect safety, comfort, functioning, and quality of life (Box 7-3).

Driving Safety

- Nurses have essential roles in addressing issues related to older adult drivers through an interprofessional team approach (Box 7-4).
- Common risk factors include conditions that affect vision, cognition, motor responses, and reaction time.
- Nurses incorporate questions about driving to identify the need for a more comprehensive assessment.

- Risks for unsafe driving can be minimized through interventions that address contributing factors (e.g., vision and hearing impairments, medication-related issues).
- Nurses have important roles in facilitating referrals for further evaluation or for programs related to driving safety, education, and rehabilitation.

Critical Thinking Exercises

1. Review the factors that contribute to the complexity of assessing health of older adults and apply these to an older adult in a clinical setting or someone you know personally.
2. Using Online Learning Activity 7-1, select a nursing assessment tool that would be easy to use in clinical settings, and apply the information to an older adult for whom you have cared.
3. Read the evidence-based information in Box 7-1 and identify ways in which this information is applicable to older adults in hospitals or nursing homes.
4. Identify an older adult (in a clinical setting or someone you know personally) who has some functional impairment as well as some cognitive impairment and perform a functional assessment on him or her, using Figure 7-2.
5. Identify an older adult (in a clinical setting or someone you know personally) who has risk factors that affect his or her driving safety; then explore one or more of the resources listed in Online Learning Activity 7-4 to find information applicable to addressing concerns about safe driving for this person.

 For more information about topics discussed in this chapter, be sure to check out the interactive Online Learning Activities and other helpful resources at http://thepoint.lww.com/Miller8e.

REFERENCES

Agramut, S., Meuleners, L. B., Fraser, M. L. et al. (2016). Bilateral cataract, crash risk, driving performance, and self-regulation practices among older drivers. *Journal of Cataracts and Refractory Surgery, 42*, 788–794.

American Geriatrics Society & Pomidor, A. (Ed.). (2016). *Clinician's guide to assessing and counseling older drivers,* 3rd ed. (Report No. DOT HS 812 228). Washington, DC: National Highway Traffic Safety Administration.

Boltz, M., Chippendale, T., Resnick, B., et al. (2015). Testing family-centered, function-focused care in hospitalized persons with dementia. *Neurodegenerative Disease Management, 5,* 203–215.

Boltz, M., Resnick, B., & Galik, E. (2016). Preventing functional decline in the acute care setting. In M. Boltz, E. Capezuti, T. Fulmer, et al. (Eds.), *Evidence-based practice protocols for best practice* (5th ed., pp. 197–209). New York: Springer Publishing Co.

Boot, W. B., & Scialfa, C. T. (2017). The aging road user and technology to promote safe mobility for life. In Kwon, S. (Ed.), *Gerontechnology: Research, practice, and principles in the field of technology and aging* (pp. 207–222). New York: Springer Publishing Company

Chihuri, S., Mielenz, T. J., DiMaggio, C. J., et al. (2016). Driving cessation and health outcomes in older adults. *Journal of the American Geriatrics Society, 64*, 332–341.

Choi, N. G., & DiNitto, D. M. (2016). Depressive symptoms among older adults who do not drive: Association with mobility resources and perceived transportation barriers. *The Gerontologist, 56,* 432–443.

Counsell, S. R. (2016). Driving expert eldercare forward–on and off the road. *Journal of Gerontological Nursing, 42,* 47–48.

Doroudgar, S., Chuang, H. M., Perry, P. J., et al. (2017). Driving performance comparing older versus younger drivers. *Traffic and Injury Reports, 18,* 41–46.

Edwards, J. D., Lister, J. J., Lin, F. R., et al. (2016). Association of hearing impairment and subsequent driving mobility in older adults. *The Gerontologist,* doi: 10.1093/geront/gnw009 [Epub ahead of print, February 25, 2016].

Kresevic, D. (2016). Assessment of physical function. In M. Boltz, E. Capezuti, T. Fulmer, et al. (Eds.), *Evidence-based practice protocols for best practice* (5th ed., pp. 89–102). New York: Springer Publishing Co.

Liddle, J., Gustafsson, L., Mitchell, G., et al. (2016). A difficult journey: Reflections on driving and driving cessation from a team of clinical researchers. *The Gerontologist,* doi: 10.1093/geront/gnw079 [Epub ahead of print, April 21, 2016].

Miller, S. M., Taylor-Piliae, R. E., & Insel, K. C. (2016). The association of physical activity, cognitive. processes and automobile driving ability in older adults: A review of the literature. *Geriatric Nursing, 37,* 313–320.

Palese, A., Gonella, S., Moreale, R., et al. (2016). Hospital-acquired functional decline in older patients cared for in acute medical wards and predictors: Findings from a multicenter longitudinal study. *Geriatric Nursing, 37,* 192–199.

Pastor, D. K., Jones, A., & Arms, T. (2017). Where the rubber hits the road: What home healthcare professionals need to know about driving safety for persons with dementia. *Home Healthcare Now, 35,* 26–32.

Resnick, B. (2016). Optimizing driving safety: It is a team sport. *Geriatric Nursing, 37,* 257–259.

Resnick, B., Galik, E., & Boltz, M. (2013). Function focused care approaches: Literature review of progress and future possibilities. *Journal of the American Medical Directors Association, 14,* 313–318.

Resnick, B., Galik, E., Vigne, E., et al. (2016). Dissemination and implementation of function-focused care for assisted living. *Health Education Behavior, 43,* 296–304.

Resnick, B., Wells, C., Galik, E., et al. (2016). Feasibility and efficacy of function-focused care for orthopedic trauma patients. *Journal of Trauma Nursing, 23,* 144–155.

Wiese, L. K., & Wolff, L. (2016). Supporting safety in the older adult driver: A public health nursing opportunity. *Public Health Nursing, 33*(5), 460–471.

Wood, J. M., Black, A. A., Mallon, K., et al. (2016). Glaucoma and driving: On-road driving characteristics. *PLoS One, 11*(7), e0158318.

Medications and Other Bioactive Substances

Although the topic of medications and older adults is not a distinct category of function in the same sense as physiologic and psychosocial aspects of function (e.g., vision and cognition), it can be addressed from a similar perspective. This chapter presents information in the context of the functional consequences theory for promoting wellness to address issues related to medications and older adults, with particular attention to the role of nurses.

OVERVIEW OF BIOACTIVE SUBSTANCES

In addition to discussing prescription and over-the-counter (OTC) medications in relation to older adults, this chapter addresses other bioactive substances that are used for therapeutic purposes (e.g., herbs and homeopathic remedies). Bioactive substances that can affect medication action also are addressed in the section on Medication Interactions. Nurses need to be aware of the special considerations related to commonly used types of bioactive substances so that they can promote safe and effective use for older adults.

Considerations Regarding Medications

Effects of medications in the body are usually considered in relation to **pharmacokinetics** (i.e., how the drug is absorbed, distributed, metabolized, and excreted) and **pharmacodynamics** (i.e., how the body is affected by the drug at the cellular level and in relation to the target organ). Absorption refers to the passage of a medication from its site of introduction, usually the gastrointestinal tract, into the general circulation. Absorption of oral medications can be affected by diminished gastric acid, increased gastric pH, delayed

Promoting Safe and Effective Medication Use in Older Adults

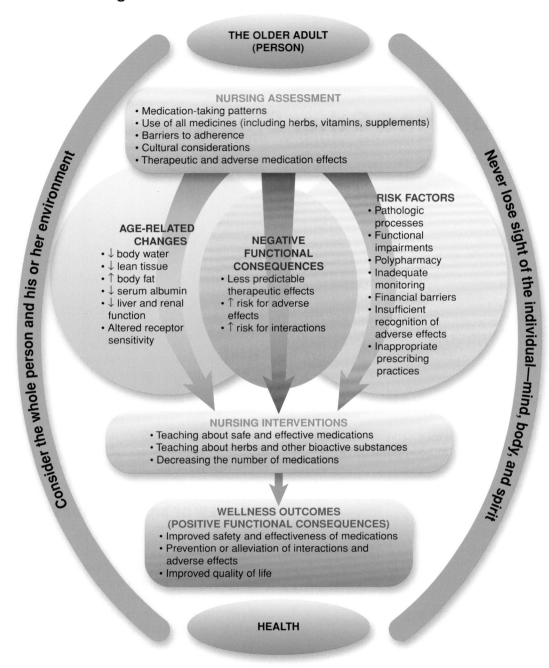

gastric emptying, and the presence of other substances (e.g., food, nutrients, other medications, medication additives). Because most oral medications are absorbed by passive diffusion across the small intestine—a process that is not pH dependent—they are not usually affected by any alterations in gastric acidity. The unique chemical properties of each medication determine the degree to which it is susceptible to any gastrointestinal changes, regardless of age. For example, pH-sensitive medications, such as penicillin and ferrous sulfate, are more likely to be affected by altered gastric acid levels or by prolonged exposure to these acids because of delayed emptying.

Two measures of the efficiency of metabolism and elimination of a drug are elimination half-time and clearance rate. **Elimination half-time** (also called serum half-life) is the time required to decrease the drug concentration by one-half of its original value. It takes five half-times to reach steady-state concentrations after a drug is initiated or to completely eliminate a drug from the body after a drug is discontinued. The **clearance rate** measures the volume of blood from which the drug is eliminated per unit of time. An increase in serum half-time or a decrease in clearance rate may result in accumulation of the drug. The results are that the therapeutic effect is likely to be altered, and the risk of adverse effects is likely to be increased.

Considerations Regarding Herbs and Homeopathy

Herbs are the most commonly used complementary health approach by adults in midlife and older in the United States (Johnson, Jou, Rhee, et al., 2016). In recent years, concerns have been raised about the increasing use of herbs, particularly with regard to potential herb–drug interactions. Concerns also are related to the fact that patients do not discuss their use of herbs with their health care practitioners unless they are asked (Jou & Johnson, 2016). These concerns have important nursing implications because nurses are responsible for assessing and teaching about safety, effectiveness, and potential interactions of herbal products (Schaffer, Curry, & Yoon, 2016). In addition, health care practitioners need to be prepared to address questions that their patients may ask about alternative practices, as discussed in the section on Teaching About Medications and Herbs.

Herbs

Herbs were perhaps the original OTC products, used by people who found these medicinal remedies in their natural environments. **Herbs** (also called botanicals or phytotherapies) are plant-based products that are used for medicinal properties. Action of herbs can be similar to that of commonly used plant-derived medications (see Table 8-1 for examples). Because herbal products and medications are affected by the same pharmacokinetic and pharmacodynamic factors, herbal products can affect circulating levels of drugs by interacting in the liver, kidney, and intestine and at target sites. Also, even when taken alone, herbs can be affected by the same age-related changes and risk factors that affect medications in older adults.

It is important to recognize that herbs are categorized by the U.S. Food and Drug Administration (FDA) as dietary supplements, so there is no requirement that they be tested for safety or efficacy. In addition, although manufacturers are required to list the active ingredients, labels do not necessarily include accurate information about inactive ingredients, potential harmful effects, quantity of active ingredients, or suitability of form for human use. Despite the lack of strict requirements, however, some safeguards are in place to protect consumers from false claims. In the United States, the FDA is responsible for addressing false claims on product labels and the Federal Trade Commission monitors advertising claims in the media.

Safeguards also are in place to address concerns about safety of herbal products and other dietary supplements. The United States Pharmacopoeia (USP) established the Dietary Supplement Verification Program in 2001 to assure

TABLE 8-1 Drugs and Herbs With Similar Bioactivity

Drug	Herb
Aspirin	Birch bark
	Willow bark
	Wintergreen
	Meadowsweet
Anticoagulants	Garlic
	Ginger
	Ginkgo
	Ginseng
	St. John's wort
Caffeine	Guarana
	Kola nut
Ephedrine	Ephedra
Estrogen	Black cohosh
	Fennel
	Red clover
	Stinging nettle
Lithium	Thyme
	Purslane
Monoamine oxidase inhibitors	Ginseng
	St. John's wort
	Yohimbe
Nicotine	Lobelia
Calcium channel blockers	Angelica

consumers that they are buying a quality product that has been held to rigorous standards. This voluntary program ensures that all ingredients of a dietary supplement meet standards for quality in both the product and the manufacturing process. Products that meet these rigorous standards display a USP Verified Mark (illustrated in Figure 8-1) on the label. Additional safeguards are provided through the Dietary Supplement and Nonprescription Drug Consumer Protection Act, which was signed into law in December 2006. This legislation requires manufacturers of dietary supplements and nonprescription medications to maintain records of adverse events and report serious ones to the FDA.

Although most dietary supplements are safe if they have been obtained from reliable sources, the risk for adverse effects increases for people with certain conditions, such as

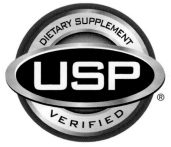

FIGURE 8-1 The United States Pharmacopoeia (USP) mark affixed to approved dietary supplements is an assurance of quality.

heart disease, liver disorders, and any condition requiring anticoagulation therapy. Also, surgical care can be complicated by effects of certain herbs, such as those that affect coagulation or electrolyte balance or prolong the effects of anesthetics. Thus, surgeons generally recommend that all herbs and supplements be discontinued at least 2 weeks prior to surgery. Some of the more serious effects of herbs (listed in Table 8-2) include altered liver function, electrolyte imbalance, elevated blood pressure, diminished blood clotting mechanisms, and alterations of the heart rate and rhythm. A review of literature found that overdoses and allergic reactions were the most common adverse effects of herbs for patients presenting to emergency departments (Jatau, Aung, Kamauzaman, et al., 2016). Less serious adverse effects include nausea, vomiting, and other gastrointestinal

symptoms from oral preparations, especially if they are taken with medications that have similar adverse effects. Another concern is that herbs and other dietary supplements have the potential for interactions with other drugs, as discussed in the section on Medications and Herbs.

Homeopathic Remedies

Three concepts are crucial to understanding homeopathy, as it was proposed two centuries ago by the German physician Samuel Hahnemann. First, according to the law of similars, or "like cures like," homeopathy stimulates the body's self-healing abilities through the use of a small amount of a substance similar to that which caused the illness. For example, quinine can produce symptoms of malaria in a healthy person, and it can cure malaria when administered in minute doses. Second, based on the concept that potency of a substance increases the more it is diluted, homeopathic remedies are diluted repeatedly and shaken vigorously each time. Third, based on the concept that treatment must be individualized to match each episode of illness, homeopathic practitioners focus on treating the person, not the disease. Homeopathy is widely used in India, Russia, Mexico, and European countries, and it is gaining acceptance in the United States as a safe alternative to conventional medicine.

Although most homeopathic remedies are now available for self-treatment, a few are available only through health care practitioners. Unlike herbs, homeopathic remedies are regulated by the FDA as OTC products. Remedies come in a variety of single-substance or combination forms, including powders, wafers, small tablets, and alcohol-based liquids. Because OTC homeopathic products are too weak to cause adverse effects, there is little concern about the safety of these products.

AGE-RELATED CHANGES THAT AFFECT MEDICATIONS IN OLDER ADULTS

Age-related changes that affect medications in older adults are discussed in relation to those that affect therapeutic effects and those that affect the skills involved with taking them. The factors that have the most significant impact on the effectiveness of medications in older adults are not age-related changes, but risk factors, and are considered in the section on Risk Factors That Affect Medications in Older Adults.

Changes That Affect the Action of Medications in the Body

An age-related decline in glomerular filtration rate, which begins in early adulthood and progresses at an annual rate of 1% to 2%, can decrease renal clearance and increase serum levels of medications. This is especially problematic for medications that are highly water soluble and those that have a narrow therapeutic range (see Box 8-1 for examples).

TABLE 8-2 Potential Adverse Effects of Some Herbs	
Herb	**Potential Effect**
Black cohosh	Bradycardia, hypotension, joint pains
Bloodroot	Bradycardia, arrhythmia, dizziness, impaired vision, intense thirst
Boneset	Liver toxicity, mental changes, respiratory problems
Coltsfoot	Fever, liver toxicity
Dandelion	Interactions with diuretics, increased concentration of lithium or potassium
Ephedra	Anxiety, dizziness, insomnia, tachycardia, hypertension
Feverfew	Interference with blood clotting mechanisms
Garlic	Hypotension, inhibition of blood clotting, potentiation of antidiabetic drugs
Ginseng	Anxiety, insomnia, hypertension, tachycardia, asthma attacks, postmenopausal bleeding
Ginseng	Anxiety, insomnia, hypertension, tachycardia, asthma attacks, postmenopausal bleeding
Ginkgo	Increased anticoagulation
Goldenseal	Vasoconstriction
Guar gum	Hypoglycemia
Hawthorn	Hypotension
Hops, skullcap, valerian	Drowsiness, potentiation of antianxiety or sedative medications
Kava	Damage to the eyes, skin, liver, and spinal cord from long-term use
Licorice	Hypokalemia, hypernatremia
Lobelia	Hearing and vision problems
Motherwort	Increased anticoagulation
Nettle	Hypokalemia
Senna	Potentiation of digoxin
Yohimbe	Anxiety, tachycardia, hypertension, mental changes

Box 8-1 Effects of Age-Related Changes on Medication Effectiveness

Medications With Decreased Clearance Caused by Renal Changes

Amantadine
Atenolol
Ceftriaxone
Cephalexin
Chlorpropamide
Cimetidine
Ciprofloxacin
Colchicine
Digoxin
Enalapril
Furosemide
Gentamicin
Glyburide
Hydrochlorothiazide
Levofloxacin
Lisinopril
Metformin
Penicillins
Ranitidine

Medications With Decreased Clearance Caused by Hepatic Changes

Acetaminophen
Amitriptyline
Barbiturates
Benzodiazepines
Codeine
Labetalol
Lidocaine
Meperidine
Morphine
Phenytoin
Propranolol
Quinidine
Salicylates
Theophylline
Warfarin

Medications With Increased Concentrations Caused by Changes in Body Composition

Cimetidine
Digoxin

Ethanol (alcohol)
Gentamicin
Morphine
Propranolol
Quinine
Warfarin

Medications With Decreased Concentrations Caused by Changes in Body Composition

Phenobarbital
Prazosin
Thiopental
Tolbutamide

Medications With Increased Potency Caused by Increased Receptor Sensitivity

Angiotensin-converting
  enzyme inhibitors
Diazepam
Digoxin
Diltiazem
Enalapril
Felodipine
Levodopa
Lithium
Midazolam
Morphine
Temazepam
Verapamil
Warfarin

Medications Whose Signs of Toxicity May Be Delayed Because of Decreased Receptor Sensitivity

Beta-blockers
Bumetanide
Dopamine
Furosemide
Isoproterenol
Propranolol
Tolbutamide

medications, herbs, nutrients, and nicotine. The cytochrome P-450 system is particularly important with regard to certain medications because competition at the enzyme sites can cause adverse effects and interactions, as discussed in the section on Medication Interactions. In particular, many psychotropic medications and herbs that are used for mental health issues are metabolized through the cytochrome P-450 system, causing adverse effects and interactions (Tang, Tang, & Leonard, 2017). Box 8-1 lists examples of medications that are affected by age-related hepatic changes.

Age-related changes in body composition (i.e., decreased body water and lean tissue and increased body fat) can affect substances according to their degree of fat or water solubility. Consequently, medications that are distributed primarily in body water or lean body mass may reach higher serum concentrations in older adults and their effects may be more intense. Similarly, the serum concentration of highly fat-soluble substances can increase, so the immediate therapeutic effects are diminished, but the overall effects are prolonged or erratic.

Protein-binding capacity of a medication (i.e., the extent to which their molecules are bound to serum albumin and other proteins) is an important determinant of both therapeutic and adverse effects. Low serum albumin levels, which are common in older adults, lead to an increased amount of the active portion of protein-bound substances. In addition, when two or more protein-bound substances compete for the same binding sites, adverse effects are more likely to occur. Medications that are likely to have adverse effects when they are taken together or when serum albumin levels are low include aspirin, digoxin, furosemide, nonsteroidal anti-inflammatory drugs (NSAIDs), hypoglycemics, phenytoin, sertraline, and sulfonamides.

In addition to changes that affect pharmacokinetics, age-related changes in receptor sensitivity can influence pharmacodynamics and cause older adults to be more or less sensitive to particular substances (see Box 8-1 for examples). For instance, an increased sensitivity of the older brain to centrally acting psychotropic medications may potentiate both the therapeutic and adverse effects of these drugs. This is particularly true for anticholinergic medications, as discussed in the section on Inappropriate Prescribing Practices. Age-related change in homeostatic mechanisms, such as thermoregulation, fluid regulation, and baroreceptor control over blood pressure, can also affect pharmacodynamics. For example, inefficient fluid regulation may alter the action of medications, such as lithium, that are particularly sensitive to fluid and electrolyte balance.

Changes That Affect Medication-Taking Behaviors

For any adult, all the following factors affect the appropriate use of medications:

• Motivation
• Knowledge about the purpose of the substance

Hepatic blood flow declines progressively, beginning around the age of 40 years, and this age-related change can increase serum levels of substances that are metabolized more extensively by the liver. In addition, factors such as diet, caffeine, smoking, alcohol, genetic variations, and pathologic conditions can affect liver metabolism of substances. In recent years, there has been increasing attention to the role of enzyme systems in the liver that are responsible for the metabolism of orally administered bioactive substances, including

- Cultural and psychosocial influences
- Ability to obtain correct amounts (influenced by factors such as cost and accessibility)
- Ability to distinguish the correct container
- Ability to read and comprehend directions
- Ability to hear and remember verbal instructions
- Knowledge about correct timing for consumption
- Ability to follow the correct dosage regimen
- Physical ability to remove the substance from the container and administer it
- Ability to swallow oral preparations
- Additional skills related to coordination, manual dexterity, and visual acuity for substances that are administered nasally, transdermally, subcutaneously, or by other routes.

Even for healthy older adults, age-related changes and functional impairments often interfere with these skills. For example, hearing or vision changes can interfere with the ability to understand instructions and read directions and labels on bottles. Any limitations in fine motor movement of the hands may interfere with the ability to remove lids from containers, especially when the lids are tamper resistant. Although age-related change can influence skills related to taking medications, risk factors that commonly occur in older adults exert a stronger influence.

 ## RISK FACTORS THAT AFFECT MEDICATIONS IN OLDER ADULTS

Risk factors that influence medications in older adults can arise from the person's own attitudes, level of knowledge, and socioeconomic circumstances or can be attributed to outside sources (e.g., health care providers). The consumption of more than one bioactive substance greatly increases the potential for adverse and altered therapeutic effects. Because older adults typically take several or many medications, they are more likely to experience interactions and adverse effects. Additional risks arise from myths and misunderstandings that affect the medication consumption patterns of older adults. Finally, certain factors unrelated to age, such as weight, sex, and smoking habits, combine with age-related changes and risk factors to increase further the risk of adverse and altered effects.

> ### Wellness Opportunity
>
> Nurses provide holistic care when they explore the wide range of factors that affect medications and medication-taking behaviors, with emphasis on identifying those that are most amenable to health promotion interventions.

Pathologic Processes and Functional Impairments

Because the purpose of any medication is to relieve or control symptoms, one can assume that people who take medications have at least one underlying pathologic process.

The increased prevalence of chronic conditions in older adults adds complexity to prescribing the safest and most appropriate medication regimen. For example, pain management for the many older adults who have both arthritis and hypertension is complicated by the common occurrence of increased blood pressure as an adverse effect of NSAIDs.

Medication–disease interactions manifest themselves in any of the following ways:

- Pathologic processes can exacerbate age-related changes that would otherwise have little or no impact on the medication. For example, malnutrition further decreases serum albumin, thereby increasing both the therapeutic and adverse effects of highly protein-bound medications.
- Pathologic processes can alter therapeutic and adverse effects of substances. For instance, heart failure decreases both the metabolism and the excretion of most medications.
- Medications can cause serious adverse effects for people with pathologic conditions. For example, anticholinergics may cause urinary retention in men with prostatic hyperplasia.

Pathologic conditions not only influence the action of substances in the body but also contribute to nonadherence, especially in combination with functional limitations. For example, dementia can significantly affect the older adult's ability to understand directions, remember instructions, and self-manage medication regimens. Dysphagia is an example of a physical limitation that can interfere with the ability to take substances orally.

Behaviors Based on Myths and Misunderstandings

Myths and misunderstandings influence attitudes held by older adults, as well as their caregivers, about the use of medications. An attitude that can be potentially harmful for older adults is that medications provide a "quick fix" for problems that commonly occur during later adulthood. For example, messages promoting medications for overactive bladder can reinforce false beliefs about urinary incontinence and lead to inappropriate use of medications without proper evaluation (as discussed in Chapter 19). Although adults of any age can be influenced by these attitudes, older adults are more likely than their younger counterparts to experience adverse effects and drug interactions.

Another potentially harmful belief is that OTC remedies are always safe, even in extra-strength doses. Although OTC preparations may be relatively safe for healthy younger adults, they can cause problems for older adults, particularly when combined with other substances. For example, OTC preparations for colds and insomnia typically contain anticholinergic ingredients that are strongly associated with delirium and other serious adverse effects in older adults. In these situations, the addition of a seemingly harmless OTC product to an already complex regimen of prescription medications can be the factor that tips the scale of safety and causes a serious effect, such as delirium. NSAIDs are another category of OTC drugs that commonly have serious adverse effects in older adults, either alone or with other substances (e.g., anticoagulants, prednisone). Acetaminophen, also a commonly used OTC product, can have serious adverse effects, including liver failure and death, when used in high doses.

Attitudes and expectations about medications as quick-fix remedies can influence the prescribing patterns of primary care practitioners. For example, a nonpharmacologic remedy may be safer than, and just as effective as, a prescription medication, but these remedies usually demand more of the practitioner's time and some degree of patient motivation. Sleep and anxiety complaints are examples of conditions that respond to evidence-based nonpharmacologic treatments, but these conditions are often addressed by prescription medications because of the attitudes of the patient or primary care practitioner.

Wellness Opportunity

By taking time to identify an older adult's beliefs about illness and treatments (including pharmacologic and nonpharmacologic approaches), nurses pave the way for teaching about the safest and most effective interventions.

Communication Barriers

Another factor that may contribute to an increased use of prescriptions by older adults is their reluctance to challenge or question the primary care practitioner, whom they perceive as "all-knowing." Although the image of the infallible physician is subsiding, older adults are still inclined to accept advice from prescribing practitioners without question. Additional communication barriers include lack of confidence in one's communication skills and fear of appearing ignorant. Hearing and vision impairments also may interfere with patient-directed discussions of a treatment plan. An attitude of impatience on the part of the health care practitioner also may thwart discussion. In addition, language barriers on the part of either the older adult or the health care practitioner can interfere with a discussion of health issues and lead to misunderstandings.

Polypharmacy and Inadequate Monitoring of Medications

The term **polypharmacy** initially meant numbers of medications taken (e.g., five or more), but more recently, it typically refers to the appropriateness of medications—for example, the use of more medications than are clinically indicated, or the use of unnecessary or harmful prescriptions (Levy, 2017). Polypharmacy occurs because of many factors, including any of the following: patient self-medication, inappropriate overtreatment, uncoordinated transitions in care, lack of coordination among prescribers, excessive application of clinical guidelines, and inappropriate treatment of adverse

drug events with medications (Stefanacci & Khan, 2017). Polypharmacy is common in older adults, particularly those in long-term care facilities. Although multiple medications may be necessary for older adults with several pathologic conditions, polypharmacy can lead to drug interactions and adverse medication effects.

As the number and sources of medications increase, the need for monitoring becomes more important, from the time of the initial prescription until the termination of treatment. The following risk factors can interfere with medication monitoring in older adults:

- Patient's use of multiple health care providers, who usually do not communicate with each other about the patient's care
- Health care practitioners' lack of information about medications obtained from a variety of sources (i.e., prescription medications offered by friends and relatives, or nonprescription products, such as herbs, nutritional supplements, and OTC products)
- Health care practitioners' lack of information about a patient's nonadherence to a treatment regimen
- A patient's fear of disclosing information about folk remedies or medications obtained from sources other than the prescribing health care practitioner
- A patient's reluctance to disclose information about self-directed changes in the medication regimen
- An assumption by the patient or health care practitioner that once most medications are started, they should be continued indefinitely
- An assumption by the patient or health care practitioner that once an appropriate medication dosage is established, it will not need to be changed
- An assumption by the patient or health care practitioner that a lack of adverse effects early in the course of treatment indicates that adverse effects will never occur
- Changes in the patient's weight, especially weight loss, which may affect pharmacokinetic processes
- Changes in the patient's daily habits (e.g., smoking, activity level, or nutrient and fluid intake), which may affect pharmacokinetic processes
- Changes in the patient's mental–emotional status, which may affect medication consumption patterns
- Changes in the patient's health status, which may affect medication actions, increasing the potential for adverse effects

Medication Nonadherence

Medication nonadherence refers to medication-taking patterns that differ from the prescribed pattern, including missed doses, failure to fill prescriptions, or medications taken too frequently or at inappropriate times. Medication nonadherence occurs in about half of adults of all ages taking prescription medications for chronic conditions; however, because older adults typically take medications for more than one condition, they experience worse health outcomes when nonadherence occurs (Marcum, Hanlon, & Murray, 2017). Medication nonadherence is associated with multiple interacting factors including all of the following that are consistently identified in studies: frequent doses, high number of medications, cognitive impairment, social isolation, asymptomatic disease, low health literacy, long treatment duration, poor communication between the patient and provider, and misunderstandings about the medication or disease (Hudani & Rojas-Fernandez, 2016; Jin, Kim, & Rhie, 2016; Lo, Chau, Woo, et al., 2016). Additional barriers to medication adherence include difficulty opening or reading prescription bottles, feeling worse when taking the medication, and difficulty paying for the medications (Campbell, Zhan, Tu, et al., 2016).

Financial Concerns Related to Prescription Drugs

Prescription drug benefits are available for older adults through the Medicare Modernization Act of 2003, which created **Medicare Part D**, and the Patient Protection and Affordable Care Act (ACA) of 2010. Medicare Part D plans are offered by private insurance companies and they vary according to the specific drugs that are covered and the amount covered varies according to the specific drugs that are prescribed. Enrollees who do not qualify for the low-income supplement have a gap in coverage after a certain point is reached and then the coverage resumes when the enrollee reaches an out-of-pocket expenditure threshold. The Patient Protection and Affordable Care Act of 2010 provides for gradually closing this gap—known as the "donut hole"—by 2020. Under these Medicare plans, the average annual Medicare spending for prescriptions will increase from $2203 per beneficiary in 2015 to $3861 in 2025 (Kaiser Family Foundation, 2016). Parallel to this trend toward increasing costs for Medicare, older adults will be paying higher out-of-pocket costs for prescriptions, with higher increases in their costs if Medicare benefits are reduced through governmental actions.

Despite the benefits of health insurance, 35% of older adults with prescription coverage reported financial hardship from medication purchases in 2015 (Olson, Schommer, Mott, et al., 2016). Older adults with certain conditions, such as cancer or rheumatoid arthritis, pay significantly higher costs for necessary medications. For example, Medicare beneficiaries who did not receive low-income subsidies and required ongoing cancer treatment paid between $4000 and $10,000 out of pocket for oral chemotherapy drugs in 2014 (Dusetzina & Keating, 2016).

Insufficient Recognition of Adverse Medication Effects

Another problem specific to older adults is that adverse effects are likely to be misinterpreted or not recognized as such because of their similarity to age-related changes or commonly occurring pathologic conditions. When an older adult experiences an adverse medication reaction, two or

three potential causes other than the medication usually can be identified, with medications being a common cause. Although adverse effects are not unique to older adults, they occur more commonly with increasing age and are more likely to be attributed erroneously to pathologic conditions or age-related changes and circumstances. Current guidelines emphasize that adverse medications should be considered as a potential cause of nonspecific symptoms in older adults, including falls, fatigue, cognitive decline, or constipation (Lavan & Gallagher, 2016). Table 8-3 summarizes adverse medication effects that are likely to remain unrecognized in older adults because of their similarity to age-related changes.

The term **prescribing cascade** has been applied to the following commonly occurring scenario: an adverse drug reaction is misinterpreted as a new medical condition, a drug is prescribed for this condition, another adverse drug effect occurs, the patient is again treated for the perceived additional medical condition, and the sequence perpetuates new adverse events. For example, proton pump inhibitors (e.g., omeprazole), which have been widely used for ongoing treatment of gastrointestinal symptoms, are often prescribed inappropriately in nursing home residents to counteract adverse effects of medications. In turn, the long-term use of a proton pump inhibitor can cause additional adverse effects, such as diarrhea, iron or vitamin B12 deficiency, and increased risk for fractures or pneumonia (Rababa, Al-Ghassani, Kovach, et al., 2016).

> ### Wellness Opportunity
>
> Nurses promote self-responsibility by addressing factors that interfere with adherence and, at the same time, supporting independence.

INAPPROPRIATE PRESCRIBING PRACTICES

Despite the fact that older adults are the primary consumers of prescription and OTC medications, research on the influence of age-related changes on the therapeutic and adverse effects of medications was virtually nonexistent before the 1980s, and the few cross-sectional studies that were done identified age differences rather than age-related changes. A series of initiatives implemented by governmental and health care organizations that began during the 1980s has led to the development of evidence-based practices that are widely used today (see Figure 8-2).

The phrase **potentially inappropriate medications** refers to medications that pose more risks than benefits for older adults, particularly when safer alternatives exist. A recent review of studies identified benzodiazepines, NSAIDs, antihistamines, and antipsychotics as the most commonly identified drugs reported as potentially inappropriate for older adults (Lucchetti & Lucchetti, 2017). Potentially inappropriate medications are associated with increased risk for serious

TABLE 8-3 Some Adverse Medication Effects That May Remain Unrecognized in Older Adults

Manifestation of Effect	Medication Type	Specific Examples
Cognitive impairment	Antidepressants; antipsychotics; antianxiety agents; anticholinergics; hypoglycemics; OTC cold, cough, and sleeping preparations	Perphenazine, amitriptyline, chlorpromazine, diazepam, chlordiazepoxide, benztropine, trihexyphenidyl, cimetidine, digoxin, barbiturates, tolazamide, tolbutamide, chlorpheniramine, diphenhydramine
Depression	Antihypertensives, antiarthritics, antianxiety agents, antipsychotics	Reserpine, clonidine, propranolol, indomethacin, haloperidol, barbiturates
Urinary incontinence	Diuretics, anticholinergics	Furosemide, doxepin, thioridazine, lorazepam
Constipation	Narcotics, antacids, antipsychotics, antidepressants	Codeine, chlorpromazine, calcium carbonate, aluminum hydroxide, amoxapine
Vision impairment	Digitalis, antiarthritics, phenothiazines	Digoxin, indomethacin, ibuprofen, chlorpromazine
Hearing impairment	Mycin antibiotics, salicylates, loop diuretics	Gentamicin, aspirin, furosemide, bumetanide
Postural hypotension	Antihypertensives, diuretics, antipsychotics, antidepressants	Guanethidine, furosemide, propranolol, chlorpromazine, imipramine, clonidine
Hypothermia	Antipsychotics, alcohol, salicylates	Haloperidol, aspirin, alcohol, fluphenazine
Sexual dysfunction	Antihypertensives, antipsychotics, antidepressants, alcohol, antihypertensives	Timolol, clonidine, thiazides, haloperidol, amitriptyline, alcohol, cimetidine, propranolol, methyldopa
Mobility problems	Sedatives, antianxiety agents, antipsychotics, ototoxic medications	Chloral hydrate, diazepam, furosemide, gentamicin
Dry mouth	Anticholinergics, corticosteroids, bronchodilators, antihypertensives	Chlorpromazine, haloperidol, prednisone, furosemide, sertraline, theophylline
Anorexia	Digitalis, bronchodilators, antihistamines	Digoxin, theophylline, diphenhydramine
Drowsiness	Antidepressants, antipsychotics, OTC cold preparations, alcohol, barbiturates	Amitriptyline, haloperidol, chlorpheniramine, secobarbital
Edema	Antiarthritics, corticosteroids, antihypertensives	Ibuprofen, indomethacin, prednisone, reserpine, methyldopa
Tremors	Antipsychotics	Haloperidol, chlorpromazine, thioridazine

adverse effects, including higher mortality rates in older adults (do Nascimento, Mambrini, Lima-Costa, et al., 2017; Heider, Matschinger, Meid, et al., 2017; Muhlack, Hoppe, Weberpals, et al., 2017).

The **Beers Criteria** (complete title is Beers Criteria for Potentially Inappropriate Medication Use in Older Adults) list is a widely used evidence-based tool that identifies medications that should trigger careful evaluation when used for older adults (Mion and Sandhu, 2016). As delineated in Figure 8-2, this tool has been used since 1991 and has been updated several times, with the most recent revision in 2015. In the United States, the Beers Criteria are considered a "gold standard" for evidence-based decisions about prescribing medications for older adults (Simonson, 2016a). Online Learning Activity 8-1 provides links to the Beers Criteria and additional information about the use of this tool.

 See ONLINE LEARNING ACTIVITY 8-1: LINKS TO ADDITIONAL INFORMATION ABOUT BEERS CRITERIA at http://thepoint.lww.com/Miller8e.

Developed more recently, the **STOPP/START criteria** is a two-part evidence-based screening tool that is used

for improving prescribing practices and facilitating decisions about medications that should be stopped or started (Blanco-Reina, Garcia-Merino, Ocana-Riola, et al., 2016; Khodyakov, Ochoa, Olivieri-Mui, et al., 2017; Lonnbro & Wallerstedt, 2017). The STOPP (Screening Tool of Older Persons' Prescriptions) part identifies potentially inappropriate medications, and the START (Screening Tool to Alert doctors to Right Treatment) part identifies medications that are not being used but are recommended for improved management of specific conditions. In 2016, the STOPP/START tool was updated, and a STOPPFrail tool was developed to identify medications that are potentially inappropriate for frail older adults with limited life expectancy (Lavan, Gallagher, Parsons, et al., 2017).

The Harford Institute for Geriatric Nursing recommends that the Beers Criteria be used in conjunction with other criteria such as the STOPP/START to best guide health care practitioners through the medication decision-making process (Greenberg, 2016). It is important to recognize that despite the ongoing development and revisions of tools to improve medication decision making, older adults continue to experience high rates of adverse effects, drug interactions, and serious functional consequences due

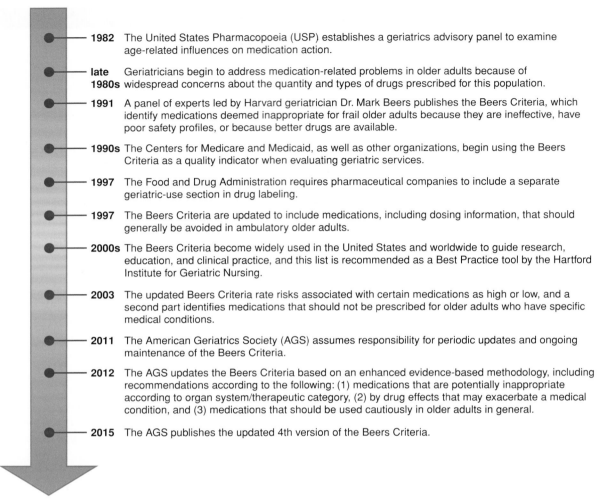

1982   The United States Pharmacopoeia (USP) establishes a geriatrics advisory panel to examine age-related influences on medication action.

late 1980s   Geriatricians begin to address medication-related problems in older adults because of widespread concerns about the quantity and types of drugs prescribed for this population.

1991   A panel of experts led by Harvard geriatrician Dr. Mark Beers publishes the Beers Criteria, which identify medications deemed inappropriate for frail older adults because they are ineffective, have poor safety profiles, or because better drugs are available.

1990s   The Centers for Medicare and Medicaid, as well as other organizations, begin using the Beers Criteria as a quality indicator when evaluating geriatric services.

1997   The Food and Drug Administration requires pharmaceutical companies to include a separate geriatric-use section in drug labeling.

1997   The Beers Criteria are updated to include medications, including dosing information, that should generally be avoided in ambulatory older adults.

2000s   The Beers Criteria become widely used in the United States and worldwide to guide research, education, and clinical practice, and this list is recommended as a Best Practice tool by the Hartford Institute for Geriatric Nursing.

2003   The updated Beers Criteria rate risks associated with certain medications as high or low, and a second part identifies medications that should not be prescribed for older adults who have specific medical conditions.

2011   The American Geriatrics Society (AGS) assumes responsibility for periodic updates and ongoing maintenance of the Beers Criteria.

2012   The AGS updates the Beers Criteria based on an enhanced evidence-based methodology, including recommendations according to the following: (1) medications that are potentially inappropriate according to organ system/therapeutic category, (2) by drug effects that may exacerbate a medical condition, and (3) medications that should be used cautiously in older adults in general.

2015   The AGS publishes the updated 4th version of the Beers Criteria.

FIGURE 8-2 Timeline of significant initiatives to improve prescribing practices for older adults.

to inappropriate prescribing practices. Nurses have essential roles in working with other health care practitioners, including pharmacists and all prescribers, to raise questions about medications that may be inappropriately prescribed. This process requires an interprofessional approach that addresses the individualized needs of each older person.

Wellness Opportunity

Nurses have many opportunities to prevent adverse medication effects by raising questions about the use of medications that are potentially inappropriate.

MEDICATION INTERACTIONS

Medications can interact with any other biologically active substance, including other medications, herbs, nutrients, alcohol, caffeine, and nicotine. These interactions occur not only with prescription medications but also with commonly used OTC products, including antacids, analgesics, and remedies for coughs, colds, and sleep problems. Interactions result in altered therapeutic effects and an increased potential for adverse effects.

Another concern is that some adverse effects and medication–medication interactions are identified only after a medication has been on the market for several years. Because older adults are most likely to have the highest risk for adverse effects and interactions, it is important to recognize that recently approved medication should be used cautiously in older adults because of the lack of information about adverse effects and unpredictable interactions.

Medication–Medication Interactions

The risk of adverse effects from interactions between two or more medications increases exponentially according to the number of medications being consumed. Because older adults often take two or more medications concurrently, they are at increased risk for medication–medication interactions. Medication–medication interactions are typically

TABLE 8-4 Types and Examples of Medication–Medication Interactions

Type of Interaction	Interaction Example	Effect
Binding effect (e.g., an oral drug diminishes the absorption of another drug in the stomach)	Magnesium- or aluminum-containing antacids may bind with tetracycline in the stomach	Decreased effects of tetracycline
Metabolism interference effect (e.g., one drug interferes with hepatic metabolism of another drug)	Ciprofloxacin and anticonvulsants inhibit metabolism of warfarin	Increased effects of warfarin
Metabolism-enhancing effect (e.g., one drug activates the drug-metabolizing enzymes in the liver)	Phenobarbital increases metabolism of warfarin	Decreased effects of warfarin
Elimination interference effect (e.g., one drug interferes with the renal elimination of another drug)	Furosemide can interfere with elimination of salicylates	Increased effects of salicylates
Elimination enhancement effect (e.g., renal reabsorption is blocked because of altered urinary pH)	Sodium bicarbonate can enhance excretion of lithium, tetracyclines, and salicylates	Decreased effects of lithium, tetracycline, or salicylate
Competitive or displacement effect (e.g., two drugs compete at receptor sites)	Diphenhydramine may interfere with effect of cholinergic agents (e.g., tacrine and donepezil)	Decreased effects of tacrine or donepezil
Potentiating effect (e.g., two drugs produce greater effects when taken together even though they have different actions)	Acetaminophen taken with codeine has a greater analgesic effect than either medication taken alone	Increased analgesic effect
Additive effect (e.g., two drugs produce greater effect because they have similar action)	Verapamil or diltiazem may have additive effect when taken with a beta-blocker	Increased effect on blood pressure

caused by competitive action at binding sites, but they can be caused by any mechanism that influences the absorption, distribution, metabolism, or elimination of any of the medications. Effects of medication–medication interactions include increased or decreased serum levels of either one or both of the medications, with subsequent altered therapeutic effects and increased risk of adverse or toxic effects. Medication–medication interactions can cause serious functional consequences and are a major cause of unnecessary hospital admissions (Dalleur, Beeler, Schnipper, et al., 2017).

Although it is impossible to know details about all potential medication–medication interactions, nurses can be aware of specific mechanisms that are most commonly associated with these interactions in older adults, as listed in Table 8-4, which also lists examples of each type. It is important to be aware of serious interactions that occur more frequently with certain medications. For example, warfarin (Coumadin) requires close monitoring because serum levels are easily altered by interactions with other medications, foods, and herbs.

Medications and Herbs

Many medication–herb interactions have been identified in recent years because of the increased use of herbs and increased attention to interactions. Although the more widely recognized medication–herb interactions are sometimes listed in pharmacology references, the FDA does not require that information about these interactions be made public because these products are classified as dietary supplements. Significant medication–herb interactions can occur when herbs are taken with medications that have a narrow therapeutic window or potential life-threatening toxicity (such as warfarin, anticancer drugs, and immunosuppressants) (Mouly, Lloret-Linares, Sellier, et al., 2017). For example,

studies consistently find that certain herbs, including ginkgo, St. John's wort, and ginseng, can interact with warfarin to increase the risk for bleeding due to a combination of anticoagulation activity of the herbs and the narrow therapeutic range for warfarin (Hirsch, Viecili, deAlmeida, et al., 2017; Leite, Martins, & Castilho, 2016).

Medications and Nutrients

In the context of medication–nutrient interactions, the term nutrient includes foods, beverages, enteral formulas, and dietary supplements. Older adults are likely to experience medication–nutrient interactions because of a combination of age-related changes and other risk factors. For example, changes in the gastrointestinal tract can delay or diminish the absorption of medications. Another widely recognized example is the effect of grapefruit juice on increasing the bioavailability of certain drugs, such as statins, triazolam, buspirone, calcium channel blockers, and phosphodiesterase type-5 inhibitors (Nicoteri, 2016). Table 8-5 lists examples of nutrient–medication interactions.

Medications and Alcohol

Alcohol interacts with medications in the same way as other central nervous system depressants, but health care practitioners do not always inquire about a patient's use of alcohol, and even when people are asked, they might not accurately acknowledge the amount of alcohol used. Alcohol is consumed not only in beverages but also in OTC preparations, such as vitamin and mineral tonics, and liquid cough and cold preparations. When taken with medications, alcohol can alter the therapeutic action of medications and increase the potential for adverse effects. Older adults may be more susceptible to

TABLE 8-5 Medication–Nutrient Interactions

Effect on Medication	Example of Interaction Effect
Delayed absorption rate, no effect on amount absorbed	Ingestion of food may delay absorption of cimetidine, digoxin, and ibuprofen
Reduced rate and amount of absorption	Calcium decreases absorption of tetracycline. A high-protein or high-fiber meal decreases absorption of levodopa. Grapefruit juice can decrease absorption of antifungals and antihistamines
Reduced absorption because of nonnutrient components	Caffeinated tea and fiber intake interfere with iron absorption
Increased absorption	High-fat foods increase serum levels of griseofulvin
Decreased therapeutic effect	Vitamin K decreases the effectiveness of warfarin. Charcoal broiling of foods diminishes the effectiveness of aminophylline or theophylline
Increased rate of metabolism	A high-protein diet increases the metabolism of theophylline
Increased concentrations and bioavailability	Potential effect of grapefruit juice and amiodarone, atorvastatin, buspirone, calcium channel blockers, carbamazepine, diazepam, lovastatin, simvastatin, and triazolam

medication–alcohol interactions because age-related changes in receptor sensitivity and body composition lead to higher blood-alcohol levels. Table 8-6 lists some of the medication–alcohol interactions that can occur in older adults.

Medications and Nicotine

Medication–nicotine interactions can be associated with tobacco smoking, smokeless tobacco, and the many

TABLE 8-6 Medication–Alcohol Interactions

Type of Interaction	Example of Interaction Effect
Altered metabolism of benzodiazepines when combined with alcohol	Increased psychomotor impairment and adverse effects
Altered metabolism of barbiturates and meprobamate when combined with alcohol	Central nervous system depression
Altered metabolism of alcohol when combined with chlorpromazine	Increased serum levels of alcohol and acetaldehyde; increased psychomotor impairment
Enhanced vasodilation as a result of a combination of alcohol and nitrates	Severe hypotension and headache, enhanced absorption of nitroglycerin
Altered metabolism of oral hypoglycemics in the liver	Potentiation of oral hypoglycemics by alcohol

TABLE 8-7 Medication–Nicotine Interactions

Effect of Nicotine	Example of Interaction Effect
Altered metabolism	Decreased efficacy of analgesics, lorazepam, theophylline, aminophylline, beta-blockers, and calcium channel blockers
Vasoconstriction	Increased peripheral ischemic effect of beta-blockers
Central nervous system stimulation	Decreased drowsiness from benzodiazepines and phenothiazines
Stimulation of antidiuretic hormone secretion	Fluid retention, decreased effectiveness of diuretics
Activation of neuroendocrine pathways	Interacts with insulin, aggravates insulin resistance, interferes with alpha-blockers
Increase in platelet activity	Decreased anticoagulant effectiveness (heparin, warfarin); increased risk of thrombosis with estrogen use
Increased gastric acid secretion	Decreased or negated effects of H_2 antagonists (cimetidine, famotidine, nizatidine, ranitidine)

nicotine-based products (e.g., gum, patches, e-cigarettes) that are increasingly being used as substitutes for smoking or alternatives to traditional cigarettes. Because nicotine can interfere with the therapeutic action of medications, smokers may require higher doses of a medication and it may be necessary to adjust doses when smoking patterns change either voluntarily or involuntarily (e.g., during a hospitalization). Also when nicotine products, such as patches, are initiated or discontinued, doses may need to be adjusted. Table 8-7 lists some common medication–nicotine interactions.

FUNCTIONAL CONSEQUENCES ASSOCIATED WITH MEDICATIONS IN OLDER ADULTS

Age-related changes can alter therapeutic effects of medications and increase the potential for adverse effects even in healthy older adults, as discussed in this section. As already discussed in the section on Risk Factors That Affect Medications in Older Adults, when adverse effects are not recognized in older adults, this leads to additional serious consequences. This section discusses additional functional consequences that are more uniquely associated with medications in older adults and have implications for nurses.

Altered Therapeutic Effects

Age-related changes alone can alter the therapeutic action of some substances; however, most of the altered therapeutic effects that occur in older adults are caused by risk factors, such as polypharmacy. Consequently, the therapeutic effectiveness of substances is less predictable, even in healthy older adults. The main implication is that medications need to be monitored more closely in older adults, especially initially and when there is any change in the person's medical status or treatment regimen. Thus, the commonly accepted principle for geriatric drug prescribing is "start low and go slow."

Increased Potential for Adverse Effects

Adverse drug events (also called adverse drug reactions or adverse medication effects) are the unintended and undesired outcomes of a medication that occur in doses normally used in humans. Consequences of adverse drug events include a decline in function, an increased risk for falls and fractures, an increased number of visits for health care services, admission to a hospital or prolongation of a hospital stay, and death. There is much agreement that adverse medication events occur commonly, have serious consequences, and frequently are avoidable. Older age and increased number of medications are the two conditions most strongly and consistently associated with adverse drug events (Mihajlovic, Gauthier, & MacDonald, 2016). Box 8-2 lists some of the factors that can increase the risk for adverse drug events.

In recent years, there has been increasing attention to adverse drug events as a preventable cause of hospitalizations for older adults, with studies indicating that up to 30% of hospital admissions of older adults are caused by an adverse drug event (Zwicker & Fulmer, 2016). Medications most frequently cited as causes of emergency hospitalizations are anticoagulants, antibiotics, diabetes agents, and NSAIDs (Oscanoa, Lizaraso, & Carvajal, 2017; Shehab, Lovegrove, Geller, et al., 2016). Polypharmacy, older age, and drug–drug interactions are commonly identified as risk factors (Kanagaratnam, Drame, Novella, et al., 2017; Pedros, Formiga, Corbella, et al., 2016).

Several aspects of adverse medication effects are particularly important for the care of older adults. As discussed in the section on Risk Factors That Affect Medications in Older Adults, adverse effects may not be recognized as such because they are similar to the manifestations of pathologic conditions or they are mistakenly attributed to aging. Three concerns of particular importance are anticholinergic adverse effects, changes in mental status, and tardive dyskinesia.

Anticholinergic Adverse Effects

In recent years, geriatricians have increasingly recognized that older adults are particularly susceptible to the anticholinergic adverse effects from medications, including some medications that are not widely recognized as having anticholinergic effects in the body. Many OTC agents commonly used for coughs, colds, and sleep problems contain anticholinergic ingredients. Anticholinergic adverse effects also can occur from systemic absorption of commonly used topical medications or ophthalmic agents (e.g., mydriatics and cycloplegics). Common types of medications with anticholinergic properties include antidepressants, first-generation antihistamines, antipsychotics, cardiovascular agents, gastrointestinal agents, and urinary antispasmodics (see Box 8-3 for examples).

Studies in the United States and other countries have consistently identified anticholinergic agents as a causative factor for significant functional and cognitive decline in older adults (Boccardi, Baroni, Paolacci, et al., 2017; Collamati, Martone, Poscia, et al., 2016; Pfistemeister, Tumena, Gaismann, et al., 2017). Anticholinergic drugs are commonly

---

Box 8-2 Factors That Increase the Risk for Adverse Medication Effects

- Increased numbers of medications
- Frailty
- Malnourishment or dehydration
- Multiple illnesses
- An illness that interferes with cardiac, renal, or hepatic function
- Cognitive impairment
- History of medication allergies or adverse effects
- Fever, which can alter the action of certain medications
- Recent change in health or functional status
- Medications in any of the following categories: anticoagulant/ antiplatelet, antidiabetics, NSAIDs, central nervous system drugs

---

Box 8-3 Examples of Medications With Anticholinergic Effects

High Anticholinergic Effects

Amitriptyline
Atropine
Benztropine
Chlorpheniramine[a]
Clozapine
Darifenacin
Desipramine
Dicyclomine
Diphenhydramine[a]
Doxepin
Flavoxate
Hydroxyzine
Hyoscyamine
Imipramine
Meclizine
Methocarbamol
Nortriptyline
Olazapine
Oxybutynin
Paroxetine
Promethazine
Quetiapine
Tolterodine

Medium Anticholinergic Effects

Amantadine
Belladonna

Carbamazepine
Loxapine
Meperidine

Low Anticholinergic Effects

Alprazolam
Atenolol
Bupropion
Captopril
Cetirizine[a]
Chlorthalidone
Cimetidine
Codeine
Digoxin
Diazepam
Dipyridamole
Fentanyl
Furosemide
Haloperidol
Hydrocortisone
Loratadine[a]
Isosorbide
Loperamide
Nifedipine
Ranitidine
Risperidone
Theophylline
Venlafaxine
Warfarin

[a]Medication that is available over-the-counter (OTC).

identified as a risk factor for delirium (Bishara, Harwood, Sauer, et al., 2016; Swami, Cohen, Kairalla, et al., 2016). Specific adverse effects commonly associated with anticholinergic medications include falls, constipation, somnolence, urinary retention, dry mouth, and dry eyes. Adverse effects are directly associated with the cumulative effects of all the medications a person takes that contain anticholinergic ingredients, a condition referred to as anticholinergic burden (also called anticholinergic drug load) (Simonson, 2016b; Wouters, van der Meer, & Taxis, 2017). Another concern related to anticholinergic agents is that their pharmacologic action can counteract the effects of cholinesterase inhibitors, which are prescribed as a primary treatment for dementia. The Beers Criteria and evidence-based guidelines emphasize the importance of avoiding medications with anticholinergic effects because they are inappropriate for use in older adults and safer alternatives are usually available (American Geriatrics Society, 2012).

Altered Mental Status

Although medications can cause mental changes in anyone, older adults are at increased risk for medication-related altered mental status. In addition, when older adults experience changes in their mental status, these changes are likely to be attributed to dementia or another pathologic condition, rather than being recognized as adverse medication effects. Nurses need to be alert to the possibility that even a simple OTC product, such as diphenhydramine, is a common cause of mental changes in older adults.

Delirium is an acute confusional state that can be precipitated by any medication or by medication interactions (refer to Chapter 14 for further discussion of delirium). Older adults are particularly susceptible to medication-induced delirium because of altered neurochemical activity in the brain. Moreover, some pathologic conditions (e.g., dementia, dehydration, malnutrition, head injury, or central nervous system infection) can increase the risk for medication-induced delirium. Even at nontoxic serum levels, or at doses considered normal, medications can cause mental changes in older adults. It is important to keep in mind that medication-induced mental changes may not subside immediately after the offending medication is discontinued. In some cases, it may take several weeks or even months after the medication is decreased or discontinued for mental function to return to the premedication level. Medications that are likely to cause mental changes in older adults, as well as the mechanisms underlying these adverse actions, are discussed in Chapter 11.

Antipsychotics in People With Dementia

The use of psychotropic drugs in long-term care facilities has been a particular focus of concern since 1987, when the Nursing Home Reform Act mandated that the Health Care Financing Administration address this issue. The strong association between serious adverse effects and the first-generation antipsychotics (e.g., haloperidol and phenothiazines) led to the development of atypical (also called second-generation) antipsychotics (e.g., aripiprazole, olanzapine, quetiapine, risperidone, and ziprasidone). During the past two decades, studies have focused on both the therapeutic effectiveness and the risk of adverse effects related to the use of atypical antipsychotics. Recent reviews have concluded that although atypical antipsychotics may be relatively safer than first-generation antipsychotics, they are limited in their effectiveness for management of behavioral symptoms of dementia. Moreover, they are associated with serious adverse effects, including increased risk for all of the following: falls, fractures, strokes, arrhythmias, acute myocardial infarction, hospitalization, and death (Cioltan, Alshehri, Howe, et al., 2017; Farlow & Shamliyan, 2017; Forlenze, Loureiro, Pais, et al., 2017; Johnell, Jonasdottir Bergman, Fastbom, et al., 2017). Because of major concerns about adverse effects, there is increasing emphasis on non-pharmacologic management of neuropsychiatric symptoms in people with dementia, as discussed in Chapter 14. In 2012, the Centers for Medicare & Medicaid launched the National Partnership to Improve Dementia Care and Reduce Unnecessary Antipsychotic Drug Use in Nursing Homes to address these concerns. Online Learning Activity 8-2 provides links for additional information about this ongoing program.

 See Online Learning Activity 8-2: ADDITIONAL INFORMATION ABOUT THE NATIONAL PARTNERSHIP TO IMPROVE DEMENTIA CARE AND REDUCE UNNECESSARY ANTIPSYCHOTIC DRUG USE IN NURSING HOMES at http://thepoint.lww.com/Miller8e.

Tardive Dyskinesia and Drug-Induced Parkinsonism

Tardive dyskinesia and drug-induced parkinsonism are two adverse effects that may be overlooked as potentially reversible conditions if the adverse effect is recognized as such and the causative medication is discontinued. Nurses have key roles in observing for indicators for these conditions and facilitating referrals for further evaluation before the conditions progress.

Tardive dyskinesia refers to a constellation of rhythmic and involuntary movements of the trunk, extremities, jaw, lips, mouth, or tongue. The earliest signs are usually fine, wormlike movements of the tongue. Other early signs include chewing, grimacing, lip smacking, jaw clenching, eye blinking, and side-to-side jaw movements. Manifestations can begin as early as 3 to 6 months after initiation of antipsychotic medications, and they usually persist even after the causative agent is discontinued. Tardive dyskinesia is a common adverse effect of first-generation antipsychotics (e.g., haloperidol, phenothiazines); however, it also can occur with second-generation antipsychotics (e.g., amoxapine, olanzapine, queitiapine) (Carbon, Hsieh, Kane, et al., 2017; O'Brien, 2016; Rakesh, Muzyk, Szabo, et al., 2017).

Advanced age correlates with both an earlier onset and increased severity of tardive dyskinesia. Moreover, when combined with age-related changes and risk factors, tardive dyskinesia can seriously impair the older adult's ability to perform activities of daily living.

Drug-induced parkinsonism is the occurrence of Parkinson-like manifestations as an adverse medication effect. Manifestations can be reversed if the offending drug is stopped, but many times the condition is misdiagnosed as Parkinson disease and treated inappropriately with an anti-Parkinson medication. First-generation antipsychotics (e.g., haloperidol, chlorpromazine) are the most commonly identified causative drugs, with second-generation antipsychotics (e.g., risperidone, olanzapine) and calcium channel blockers also being associated with increased risk for drug-induced parkinsonism (Munhoz, Bertucci Filho, & Teive, 2017; Shuaib, Rajput, Robinson, et al., 2016). Despite its common occurrence, this condition is often not diagnosed correctly and is treated inappropriately with medications rather than with the more effective approach of discontinuing the causative drug.

NURSING ASSESSMENT OF MEDICATION USE AND EFFECTS

Nurses assess medication regimens and medication-taking behaviors of older adults to accomplish the following:

- Determine the effectiveness of the medication regimen
- Identify any factors that interfere with the correct regimen
- Ascertain risks for adverse effects or altered therapeutic actions (with particular attention to older adults at increased risk)
- Detect adverse medication effects
- Identify teaching needs with regard to medications

During a medication assessment, nurses should clarify the prescribed medication regimen and identify actual medication-taking behaviors so that they can assess for adherence to the treatment regimen.

Communication Techniques for Obtaining Accurate Information

Some of the many barriers to obtaining accurate information about medications and medication-taking behaviors include time limitations, complex medication regimens, and lack of a trusting relationship. Because medication assessments can be time-consuming, and because the older adult may not think of all the information during the first interview or may initially be reluctant to reveal accurate information, it may be necessary to conduct the medication assessment over the course of two or more visits. Many older adults have learned not to ask questions about their health care because they are unsure of what to ask or they falsely believe that they are not entitled to medical information. Reluctance to openly discuss medications may be caused by fear of being judged, especially if the prescribed regimen is not being followed exactly,

or if the person uses folk remedies, alternative therapies, or OTC medications. When people do not follow the medication regimen exactly as prescribed, they are likely to recite the orders rather than describe their actual medication-taking behaviors. Another factor that contributes to this reluctance is anxiety about discussing the underlying reason for not following the regimen. For example, older adults who cannot afford medications may be embarrassed to discuss their limited finances.

Nurses can address the barriers by asking open-ended questions in a matter-of-fact way and conveying a nonjudgmental attitude during the medication interview. Keep in mind the importance of eliciting information about the use of herbs, folk remedies, OTC preparations, and complementary and alternative care practices. For example, "What do you do to help you sleep?" is more open ended than "Do you take any medications for sleep?" because the latter may be interpreted only in relation to prescription medications.

Another interview technique is to use leading questions related to potential risk factors that interfere with the older person's ability to adhere to the prescribed regimen. For example, if the cost of medications is a problem, ask a question such as "I know that some of these prescribed medications can be quite expensive; do you have any problems with getting them?" Similarly, asking a question such as "I know you don't drive, do you have someone who helps you get them from the pharmacy?" may elicit information about transportation barriers.

Nurses should ask additional questions about the person's ability to take his or her medications as prescribed based on specific observations. For example, if the older adult has limited hand strength, an appropriate assessment question would be "Do you have any difficulty getting the caps off your medication bottles?" Another technique for eliciting information is to ask about the person's method of organizing medications. For example, people taking medications often have a method of organizing their regimen by using divided medication boxes or written charts or schedules. They usually are willing to show this organizational system to the nurse and, in fact, may be proud to discuss their method with the nurse during the medication assessment.

Wellness Opportunity

Nurses can build on their trusting relationship with older adults to encourage open discussion of factors that interfere with adherence to medication regimens.

Scope of a Medication Assessment

Medication assessments include information about all of the following:

- Prescription and OTC medications, used orally and by all other routes (e.g., nasal, aural, topical, optical, injectable, dermal methods)
- Medications that are used only sporadically, or as needed

- Vitamins, minerals, and dietary supplements (including dosages and frequency)
- Alcohol and caffeine
- Tobacco smoking and use of nicotine products (including information about recent changes)
- Folk remedies and complementary and alternative modalities, including all herbal products and homeopathic remedies

Information about doses of vitamins and minerals is important because megavitamins can be harmful, and even low doses can cause interactions or produce adverse effects (e.g., iron or calcium carbonate can be constipating). Information about the brand names of OTC medications can help identify additives that may be causing problems or increasing the risk of altered medication action (e.g., analgesics with caffeine, antacids with lactose, or bronchodilators with sulfites). Information about folk remedies and complementary and alternative health care practices can help identify health beliefs that affect adherence and other aspects of medication-taking behaviors.

Nurses also need to assess the person's understanding of the purpose of medications. As with other parts of the medication assessment, it is essential to phrase questions in as open-ended and nonjudgmental a manner as possible. Asking "What do you take this pill for?" with a tone of curiosity will likely elicit more information than asking questions such as, "What do you take for your heart?" or "Why do you take furosemide?"

Obtaining information about allergies and adverse reactions is essential because anyone with a history of medication-related problems will need to be closely monitored, especially if the medications being administered are similar to those that caused the reaction. Sometimes people state that they are allergic to a medication, but when they are asked about the symptoms, they describe an adverse effect, rather than an allergic reaction. Therefore, rather than simply documenting that the person is allergic to a certain medication, nurses should document the specific reaction that occurred. Nurses can use Box 8-4 as a guide to assessing medication regimens and medication-taking behaviors.

It is also important to obtain and document information about the person's perception of and preferences for various forms of medications because this information can influence prescribing decisions, especially when there are several options that may be equally effective. Similarly, nurses should identify any cultural factors that might influence medication-taking behaviors. For example, according to some Asian traditions, illness is perceived as an imbalance of hot and cold forces, and remedies are selected according to their ability to restore

---

 Box 8-4 Guidelines for Medication Assessment

Information About the Therapeutic Agents

- Prescription pills, liquids, injections, eye drops, ear drops, nasal sprays, transdermal methods, and topical preparations
- OTC preparations that are used regularly or occasionally
- Vitamins, minerals, and nutritional supplements
- Pattern of alcohol, caffeine, or tobacco use
- Herbs and herbal preparations
- Homeopathic remedies
- Home folk remedies
- Sources of health care, including complementary and alternative practitioners

Interview Questions to Assess Medication-Taking Behaviors

- How would you describe your usual daily routine for taking medications and remedies, beginning when you get up in the morning?
- Is there anything else you do or use to treat illness or to maintain your health, such as using herbs, ointments, home remedies, or nutritional supplements?
- Are you taking anyone else's medications?
- What do you do when you miss a dose of medication?
- What do you take for constipation? What do you do to help you sleep (or to alleviate any other identified problem)?
- How do you get your prescriptions filled? (Where do you get your remedies?)
- Do you have any difficulty taking your pills?
- What method do you use to keep track of your medications and remedies?
- Is there anything you do to help you remember to take your medicines or remedies at the appropriate time?

Interview Questions to Assess the Person's Understanding of the Purpose of Medications and Other Remedies

- What is this medication (or herb, etc.) for?
- For medications (or remedies) that are used as needed (PRN): How do you decide when to take this pill (or remedy)?
- What did your health care practitioner tell you about this medication (or herb, etc.)?
- What problems were you having when the health care practitioner prescribed this medication (or suggested that you use this remedy)?

Interview Questions to Elicit Additional Information

- Are there any medications or remedies you were taking at one time but are no longer taking?
- Have you ever had an allergic reaction, or any other bad reaction, to a medication or remedy? (If yes, describe what happened.)
- Where do you store your medications and remedies?

Questions and Observations Based on Reading of Prescription Labels

- Who is the prescribing health care practitioner?
- If there is more than one health care practitioner, does each practitioner know all the medications that are being used?
- Are any medications the same or similar and prescribed by different health care practitioners?
- If the dates on various prescriptions are different, were the later medications supposed to be added to the medication regimen, or were they intended to replace previously prescribed medications?
- Are the date of the last refill and the number of pills in the bottle consistent with the prescribed regimen?

Box 8-5 Cultural Considerations: Culturally Competent Medication Assessment and Interventions

Overview

- Teaching about medications should be done in the context of culturally based beliefs about health, illness, and remedies.
- Medications that are not readily available or that are available by prescription only in the United States may be available OTC in other countries, such as Mexico, Canada, and Latin America.
- Older Hispanic people may view wine and other forms of alcohol as a food staple, not as a social drug, because they may be used as a healthy alternative to potentially contaminated water in their home country.
- People of Vietnamese and other cultural groups may view injections as being more effective than pills, and pills as being more effective than drops.
- People of Asian, Latino, and Middle Eastern heritage believe that it is important to take medicine with certain foods or beverages (e.g., tea or warm water rather than cold water) to provide the necessary balance.
  - Some Chinese and other Asian people may have the following preferences:
  - Balms and ointments rather than pills for local pain
  - Teas and soups rather than antacids for indigestion
  - Herbs rather than prescription drugs

Biocultural Variations in the Metabolism of Medications

Biocultural variations may affect the metabolism of medications in the following groups:

African Americans

- Increased risk for adverse effects from psychotropics (e.g., lithium toxicity, delirium from tricyclic antidepressants, agranulocytosis from clozapine)
- Increased risk for angioedema due to angiotensin-converting enzyme (ACE) inhibitors
- Diminished therapeutic response to propranolol and ACE inhibitors
- Respond best to diuretics, calcium antagonists, and alpha-blockers for hypertension

- Increased incidence of adverse effects, such as depression, with thiazides
- Decreased therapeutic response to analgesics and increased risk of adverse gastrointestinal effects, especially with acetaminophen
- Diminished eye dilatation in response to mydriatic drug

Arab Americans

- Require lower dose of antiarrhythmics, antihypertensives, neuroleptics, and psychotropics
- May need a higher dose of opioids for adequate analgesic effects

Asian/Pacific Islanders

- Sensitivity to propranolol and other beta-blockers, manifest by decreased blood levels accompanied by seemingly more profound response
- Respond best to calcium antagonists for hypertension
- Require lower doses of antidepressants and neuroleptics (e.g., benzodiazepines, haloperidol)
- Increased gastrointestinal adverse effects associated with analgesics
- Decreased therapeutic effects of opiates
- May require dose adjustment for fat-soluble vitamins and other drugs
- Increased sensitivity to alcohol

Filipino

- Increased sensitivity to central nervous system depressants (e.g., haloperidol)

Hispanics

- Require lower doses of antidepressants and experience more adverse effects

Source: Andrews, M. M. (2016). Cultural competence in the health history and physical examination. In M. M. Andrews & J. S. Boyle (Eds.), *Transcultural concepts in nursing care* (6th ed.). Philadelphia, PA: Lippincott Williams & Wilkins; Purnell, L. D. (2013). *Transcultural health care: A culturally competent approach* (4th ed.). Philadelphia, PA: F. A. Davis Company.

balance. Box 8-5 lists some cultural factors that are pertinent to a medication assessment.

Another aspect of a comprehensive medication assessment is the identification of biocultural variations that can affect the metabolism of medications. These variations can have important implications related to doses of medications and assessment of both therapeutic and adverse effects. Nurses can use the information in Box 8-5 to be aware of ways in which some groups may respond differently to certain medications. Keep in mind that these are only examples of biocultural variations that have been identified in some studies. As with all aspects of cultural variations, it is imperative to be aware of possible influence of biologically based differences while at the same time avoiding generalizations. It also is imperative to consider that altered response or nonresponse to medications may be due to ethnic or genetic differences rather than because of nonadherence (Woods, Mentes, Cadogan, & Phillips, 2017).

Another component of a comprehensive medication assessment is obtaining information about various sources of health care. This information is particularly important when someone receives care from more than one health care practitioner, as is often the case. Nurses can ask nonjudgmentally about whether the person receives care from non-Western health care practitioners, such as herbalists, spiritual healers, naturopathic practitioners, or Ayurvedic doctors. Box 8-6 summarizes some culturally specific sources of health care and treatment modalities that older adults might use.

Wellness Opportunity

Nurses promote personal responsibility for health by encouraging discussion of various sources of care.

Observing Patterns of Medication Use

In addition to using good communication techniques, nurses obtain essential assessment information by reviewing the person's array of medications. When nurses conduct the medication assessment in the home setting, they can ask to

Box 8-6   Cultural Considerations: Culturally Specific Health Care Sources and Practices

Cultural Group	Sources of Care[a]	Health Practices[a]
African Americans	Home remedies, faith, and root healers (herbalists)	Folk remedies (e.g., teas, herbs); magic or voodoo (especially in rural areas)
Amish	Folk healers (braucher orbrauch-doktor)	Physical manipulation, massage, herbs, teas, reflexology
Chinese	Herbalists, acupuncturists	Herbs, food, beverages, and other remedies to balance yin and yang
Filipino	Folk healers (hilot)	Prayer, exorcism, hot/cold balance
Hindu	Traditional healers (nattuvaidhyars)	Ayurvedic medicine (herbs and roots)
Japanese	Herbalists	Herbs, prayer at temple, church, or small shrines at home
Mexicans	Folk healer (curandero) or spiritualist (espirituista)	Herbs, teas, soups, rituals, physical modalities (massage, manipulation), prayer, candles
Puerto Ricans	Healers (espiritistas and santeros)	Tea, herbs, folk remedies, liquid astringent
Russians	Folk remedies	Herbal teas, sweet liquor, physical modalities (oils, ointments, enemas, mud baths)
Vietnamese	Asian physicians, folk healers, spiritual healers, magicians (sorcerers)	Herbs, acupuncture, cup suctioning, skin pinching

[a]In the United States, Western practitioners and medicine often are used with these sources of care and health practices.
Source: Purnell, L. D. (2013). *Transcultural health care: A culturally competent approach* (4th ed.). Philadelphia, PA: F. A. Davis Company.

see all the medications that the older person uses. In settings other than the home, the nurse can ask the older adult ahead of time to bring in all of his or her medications. In community settings, nurses might sponsor a "brown bag" medication review session. Program participants are asked to bring all their medications to an educational session, during which the nurse provides group education and individual assessment and counseling regarding the medications. Because older people often are very comfortable discussing medications with their peers, this method is both nonthreatening and quite effective.

Direct observation of medication containers provides useful information about adherence, dates of original prescription and refills, duplication of similar medications, and pharmaceutical treatments for pathologic conditions. For example, if three types of antihypertensive medications have been prescribed at different times, inquire whether the second or third medication was supposed to replace or supplement the original medication. Also assess whether the bottles contain the original medications, and ask additional questions when the contents are not consistent with expectations. For example, if the label indicates that the original prescription was for 30 pills, but it has not been refilled for 1 year, the nurse might inquire about the reason. Patients may explain that they cannot afford the prescription or they cannot manipulate the childproof lid. Another purpose for examining medication containers is to discover information about sources of care and duplication of medications. It is not unusual to find that patients are getting prescriptions from more than one health care practitioner, with the same or similar medications from different sources or under more than one name (e.g., generic and brand names).

Linking the Medication Assessment to the Overall Assessment

The nurse uses information from the medication interview with the overall health assessment in several ways. First, information about past and present medication patterns can provide clues to identified problems or complaints. For example, if the person complains of morning lethargy or experiences mental changes, the nurse can inquire about the use of medications with anticholinergic properties, including OTC products (e.g., diphenhydramine). Information about changes in health-related behaviors can also shed light on current problems, such as the recurrence of symptoms that once were controlled by medications. For example, if an insulin-dependent diabetic stopped smoking, it is important to consider whether the dose of insulin needs to be decreased. Another way that the medication history is pertinent to overall health assessment is that latent adverse medication effects may explain current symptoms. For example, a common residual adverse effect is the onset of diarrhea after a course of antibiotics.

Second, an assessment of aspects of function that affect medication-taking behaviors helps answer the question "Can the person or caregivers safely and effectively administer medications?" The environment also should be assessed in relation to conditions that affect the person's ability to take medications, such as the availability of a refrigerator if necessary for medication storage. The overall assessment also might provide information about financial limitations, mobility, or transportation problems that interfere with obtaining medications.

Third, if the home environment can be observed as part of the overall assessment, important clues to health problems and medication-taking behaviors may be disclosed. For example, observing that nitroglycerin is stored on a sunny window sill may explain why the medication is not effective in relieving angina. An assessment of the home environment may lead to additional pertinent information. For example, when the nurse observes OTC preparations and folk remedies in the home, she or he has the opportunity to ask about the use of these items.

Finally, the overall health assessment serves as the basis for identifying many factors that can increase the risk for nonadherence, altered therapeutic effects, and adverse medication effects. For example, the nursing assessment of the older adult's cognitive abilities and abilities to perform daily activities provides valuable information about factors that can significantly influence medication-taking behaviors. Similarly, the nursing assessment of depression and other psychosocial aspects of functioning can provide important information about motivational and behavioral factors that can influence medication-taking behaviors.

Identifying Adverse Medication Effects

The first, and sometimes most difficult, step in alleviating adverse medication effects is to recognize their existence. Because many adverse effects are subtle and superimposed on one or more symptoms of illness, they may be attributed to pathologic conditions rather than to the treatment of the condition. Nurses often are the first to recognize adverse medication effects because they generally spend more time with patients than do primary care practitioners. Nurses also are more attentive to long-term monitoring of changes in day-to-day function, in contrast to the medical practitioner's focus on acute illness. Particularly in long-term care and home settings, the nurse is the health professional most likely to notice subtle changes in function that may be attributable to adverse medication effects.

Health care practitioners may hesitate to discuss adverse medication effects with patients for several reasons: (1) they may be uncertain about the potential adverse effects of a prescribed drug, especially when newer medications are prescribed; (2) they may be concerned that the power of suggesting possible adverse effects will become a self-fulfilling prophecy; or (3) they may fear that the patient will choose not to take the medication. The nurse can serve as an "interpreter" between the prescribing practitioner and the patient by emphasizing the medication's benefits as well as pointing out the problems that are most likely to arise. The nurse also can provide health education about ways to avoid adverse effects. For example, if a medication is likely to cause stomach irritation, taking the medication after meals or with milk may prevent this effect. Nurses do not automatically initiate a discussion of all the potential adverse effects of a medication, but when a change in health status is potentially related to adverse medication effects, nurses can raise that possibility.

Changes in mental status are a potentially devastating adverse medication effect that is often overlooked as such, especially when superimposed on existing dementia. Medication-induced mental status changes (e.g., confusion, lethargy, depression, or agitation) can be sudden and obvious, or subtle and gradual. For example, delirium or hallucinations usually are obvious, but they may be attributed mistakenly to pathologic processes rather than to medication effects. Thus, whenever an older person experiences an alteration in mental status, medication intake must be assessed carefully. Besides considering all prescription drugs, alcohol and OTC medications (especially those with anticholinergic properties) must be considered as potential contributing factors. When medications are a potential cause of altered mental status, consideration must be given to discontinuing or lowering the dose of the medication. Assessment also addresses the possibility that the altered mental state interferes with proper dosing (e.g., when memory impairment contributes to overdosing or underdosing). Another aspect of assessing the relationship between mental changes and medications is to recognize that it may take days or even months after discontinuation of the medication before mental status returns to baseline. The resolution time depends on the particular medication involved, the length of time it was consumed, and the person's general health status.

NURSING DIAGNOSIS

When the nursing assessment identifies factors that interfere with safe and accurate medication self-administration (e.g., cognitive or functional impairments affecting medication-taking ability), an applicable nursing diagnosis is Ineffective Health Management. This diagnosis is defined as a "pattern of regulating and integrating into daily living a therapeutic regimen for the treatment of illness and its sequelae that is unsatisfactory for meeting specific health goals" (Herdman & Kamitsuru, 2018, p. 157). Related factors that might be identified include complex medication regimens, inadequate social support, adverse effects of medication(s), lack of money or transportation, and lack of understanding of instructions.

If the nursing assessment identifies adverse effects of medications, particularly those that affect one's safety or quality of life, the nurse might address these through a nursing diagnosis that is specific to the adverse effect. Examples of these diagnoses include Confusion, Constipation, Urinary Incontinence, Imbalanced Nutrition, Impaired Memory, and Risk for Falls.

Wellness Opportunity

Nurses can use the wellness nursing diagnosis of Readiness for Enhanced Self-Health Management when caring for older adults who are interested in addressing potential adverse effects.

PLANNING FOR WELLNESS OUTCOMES

The following Nursing Outcomes Classification terminology can be used in care plans to identify wellness outcomes that are pertinent to medications and older adults: Adherence Behavior, Health Promoting Behavior, Knowledge: Medication, Medication Response, Risk Detection, and Self-Care: Non-Parenteral Medication, and Self-Management: Chronic Disease.

Wellness Opportunity

Participation in health care decisions is an outcome that is applicable when nurses empower older adults to make responsible decisions about the use of OTC products, such as herbs and medications.

NURSING INTERVENTIONS TO PROMOTE SAFE AND EFFECTIVE MEDICATION MANAGEMENT

Promoting safe and effective medication-taking patterns in older adults is multidimensional and depends on coordinated efforts from several health care providers, including nurses, pharmacists, and prescribing practitioners. Nurses have essential roles in teaching older adults about medications, identifying interventions to support adherence to the therapeutic regimen, and preventing and identifying adverse effects. The following sections describe practical interventions that nurses can use to promote adherence, prevent adverse effects, and encourage safe and effective medication-taking behaviors in older adults. Box 8-7 summarizes a protocol for reducing adverse drug events developed by Zwicker and Fulmer (2016), and Learning Activity 8-3 provides additional information related to this protocol.

 See ONLINE LEARNING ACTIVITY 8-3: PROTOCOL FOR REDUCING ADVERSE DRUG EVENTS at http://thepoint.lww.com/Miller8e.

Medication Reconciliation

Medication reconciliation is the process of identifying a patient's medication errors–such as omissions, duplications, dosing errors, or drug interactions—during transitions in care. This intervention has been mandatory in hospital settings since January 2006 and is now widely recommended in all health care settings and during any transition, even within the same setting. A process for medication reconciliation is warranted because medication errors represent the most common patient safety error in hospital settings, with

---

 Box 8-7 Evidence-Based Practice: Reducing Adverse Drug Events

Statement of the Problem

- Adverse drug events are undesirable medical occurrences that develop during treatment with a pharmaceutical product.
- Adverse drug events may occur because of a medication error or under the following circumstances: during normal use of medications, poor adherence, self-medication, inappropriate use, inappropriate or suboptimum prescribing.
- Up to 30% of older adult hospital admissions are secondary to an adverse drug event, with more than half of these being preventable.
- Reasons for medication-related adverse effects: age-related physiologic changes that alter pharmacokinetics and pharmacodynamics, polypharmacy, incorrect doses of medications, inappropriate prescribing practices (e.g., use of medications to treat symptoms that are not disease specific), adverse drug reactions and interactions, nonadherence, and medication errors

Recommendations for Nursing Assessment

- Consider age-related changes in pharmacokinetics and pharmacodynamics: absorption, distribution, metabolism, clearance.
- A comprehensive medication assessment includes all of the following: currently prescribed drugs, including doses, routes, frequency, and duration; OTC and herbal remedies; drugs taken recently but not currently; and focused questions about nicotine, alcohol, folk remedies, and all nonprescription products.
- Assess all of the following in relation to medications: renal and liver function, ability to self-administer medications, potential inappropriate medications, and drug–drug or drug–disease interactions.
- Examples of assessment tools include Beers Criteria, STOPP criteria, START criteria, brown bag method, computer software programs.
- Identify medications associated with high risk for adverse drug reactions.

- Identify patient characteristics associated with potential adverse medication effects, such as dementia, polypharmacy, renal insufficiency, multiple chronic conditions.
- Identify potential interactions with other prescriptions and with all nonprescription products.

Nursing Interventions for Reducing Adverse Drug Events During and After Hospitalization

- Consider any new symptoms as a possible adverse medication effect.
- Empower patients by providing information and involving them in decisions.
- Collaborate with interdisciplinary team for the following interventions: discontinuing unnecessary drugs, using safer drugs, optimizing the regimen, avoiding the prescribing cascade, avoiding inappropriate medications, and using nonpharmacologic approaches for symptoms.
- Follow the prescribing principle of "start low and go slow."

Nursing Interventions for Reducing Adverse Drug Events at Discharge

- Use medication reconciliation during all transitions in care, even within the same setting.
- Assess patient's abilities and limitations with regard to self-administration of medications.
- Address adherence issues that are likely to occur.
- Provide patient and caregiver education about safe and effective medication management.

Source: Zwicker, D. E., & Fulmer, T. (2016). Reducing adverse drug events. In E. Capezuti, D. Zwicker, M. Mezey, & T. Fulmer (Eds.), *Evidence-based geriatric nursing protocols for best practice* (4th ed., pp. 311–341). New York: Springer Publishing Co.

more than 40% of these errors being caused by inadequate reconciliation during transitions (Volpi, Giannelli, Toccafondi, et al., 2017). In long-term care settings, common medication discrepancies are incorrect indication (e.g., allopurinol for heart failure), no monitoring parameters, omission of medication name on admission to facility, incorrect dose, and incorrect frequency (Tong, Oh, Thomas, et al., 2017).

Medication reconciliation involves the following steps: (1) verification by collecting an accurate list; (2) clarification of questions about drugs, dosages, frequency, and other pertinent information; and (3) reconciliation of any discrepancies or concerns by communicating with prescribing practitioners. This process requires interprofessional collaboration involving nursing, pharmacy, primary care practitioners, and the staff responsible for transmitting chart information.

Important nursing interventions for a successful medication reconciliation have been described by Pincus (2013) as follows:

- Determine who administers medications.
- View all the medications.
- Be aware of medications that are commonly implicated in discrepancies (e.g., as-needed medications, medications used prophylactically during hospitalization).
- Address ability to get prescriptions filled.
- Address issues that affect adherence (e.g., administration difficulties).
- Allow the patient to ask questions.

Flanagan and Beizer (2016) describe the application of the Beers Criteria to guide the medication reconciliation process in home care settings. This article is available at the link provided in Online Learning Activity 8-4.

GLOBAL PERSPECTIVE

The Joint Commission International and the World Health Organization recognize medication reconciliation as an essential component of patient safety and quality of health care services.

See ONLINE LEARNING ACTIVITY 8-4: ARTICLE ABOUT MEDICATION RECONCILIATION USING THE 2015 BEERS CRITERIA AND LINKS TO RESOURCES FOR ADDITIONAL INFORMATION ABOUT MEDICATION RECONCILIATION at http://thepoint.lww.com/Miller8e.

Teaching About Medications and Herbs

Medications are safest and most therapeutic when they are taken as prescribed and when the regimen is periodically reevaluated for maximum effectiveness and minimal risk of adverse reactions. An effective way to initiate health education about medications is to have the person write a list of all medications and OTC agents taken and to include a history of medication allergies and adverse effects. Emphasize that this information should be available to health care

practitioners during all interactions because it is essential that all practitioners keep track of the person's medications. This list is especially important when more than one health care practitioner is involved. Nurses should explain that a medication list facilitates communication and reminds the health care practitioner periodically to reevaluate the medication regimen.

It is imperative to discuss each medication on the list and provide appropriate information based on assessment of the person's knowledge and understanding. Morrow and Conner-Garcia (2013) have summarized the following recommendations for communicating with older adults about medications:

- Use concrete, active, and direct language with emphasis on how the medication helps the person.
- Use patient education materials that are concrete, matched to patient needs, and reinforced with graphics.
- Explore patient concerns by empathic listening.
- Verify patient understanding by "teachback" techniques, such as asking older adults to state information in their own words or having them demonstrate how they organize their medications.

Because older adults may be reluctant to question their health care practitioners, nurses can suggest pertinent questions for discussion with prescribing practitioners. In addition, nurses can teach older adults and their caregivers about obtaining medication-related information from knowledgeable sources, such as pharmacists. People need to understand that prescribing practitioners are skilled in diagnosing illnesses and deciding the most appropriate interventions, and that pharmacists are the health care practitioners who are most knowledgeable about the specific actions and interactions of medications. Nurses can use Box 8-8 to teach older adults about which medication questions are best answered by prescribing practitioners and which are best addressed by pharmacists. In addition, nurses can suggest ways of communicating effectively with pharmacists and other health care practitioners. For example, nurses can help older adults develop a list of questions about specific medications that they can discuss with pharmacists or health care practitioners.

Wellness Opportunity

Nurses find opportunities to empower older adults by teaching them effective ways of communicating with health care providers so that they can knowledgeably observe for therapeutic and adverse medication effects.

As discussed in the Nursing Assessment section, nurses need to ask about the use of herbs and other bioactive substances so that they can observe for and teach about interactions and adverse effects, when appropriate. Although information about the use of complementary and alternative therapies needs to be an integral part of the assessment, nurses cannot know all the details about these products.

Box 8-8 Tips for Safe and Effective Medication Use

Nurses are in a key position to teach patients ways to ensure safe and effective ways to take their medications. Some tips for patients follow:

Carry an up-to-date list of all your medications, including herbs and OTC preparations, and show the list to your health care practitioner(s).

When your health care practitioner suggests a medication, ask if there is any way to take care of the problem without medication.

Ask your health care practitioner the following questions about each new, regularly scheduled medication:
- What is the reason for taking the medication?
- How will I know if it's doing what it's meant to do?
- How soon can I expect to feel the beneficial effects?
- What will happen if I don't take it?
- How often am I supposed to take it?
- How long should I continue taking it?
- What should I do if I miss a dose?
- When will you want to see me again, and what will you want me to tell you so that you can determine whether the medication is effective?

Ask your health care practitioner the following questions at follow-up visits:
- Do I still need to take this medication?
- Can the dosage be reduced?

Ask your health care practitioner the following questions about each medication that is prescribed on an "as-needed" (PRN) basis:
- What is the reason for taking the medication, and how should I determine whether I need the medication?
- How often can I take it? Is there a range of frequency?
- What is the maximum dose I can take within 24 hours?
- What should I do if the medication does not relieve the symptoms (e.g., if chest pain continues after taking several nitroglycerin tablets)?

Ask your pharmacist the following questions:
- What are the generic and brand names for this medication?
- Is it likely to interact with the other medications I'm taking?
- Is it likely to interact with herbs, cigarettes, alcohol, or any nutrient?
- What is the best time of day to take it?
- Does it matter if I take it before or after meals?
- Are there any side effects I should watch for?
- Is there anything I can do to minimize the risk of side effects (e.g., taking the medication with milk or meals to reduce stomach irritation)?
- Is there anything I should avoid while I'm taking this medication (e.g., milk, certain foods, driving)?
- Are there any special instructions for storing this medication?

At a minimum, however, they need to know how to teach about these remedies, just as they teach about pharmacologic and medical interventions. Nurses can use Box 8-9 as a tool to teach their patients about general precautions for the use of herbs and homeopathic remedies, such as being aware of potential interactions and adverse effects and making sure that all health care practitioners are aware of all OTC products that are used.

Another important nursing role—and a way of promoting personal responsibility—is teaching patients and caregivers about reliable sources of information on which they can base decisions. The National Institutes of Health established the

National Center for Complementary and Integrative Health to fund research and provide evidence-based information about herbs and other nonprescription remedies commonly used for managing disease and promoting health. This and other resources for reliable information are described in Online Learning Activity 8-5.

See ONLINE LEARNING ACTIVITY 8-5: RESOURCES FOR HEALTH EDUCATION MATERIALS FOR TEACHING OLDER ADULTS ABOUT MEDICATIONS AND HERBS at http://thepoint.lww.com/Miller8e.

Box 8-9 Tips on the Use of Herbs

- Before treating any symptom with a nonprescription product, make sure you are not overlooking a condition that requires medical attention.
- Discuss the use of any nonprescription product with your primary health care provider(s).
- Be cautious about substituting herbs or any OTC product for prescribed medications.
- Seek information from objective sources and check any warnings on the label or package.
- Keep in mind that dietary supplements are not fully regulated by the FDA.
- Look for a recognized mark of quality verification on the label before purchasing herbs or other dietary supplements.
- Observe for beneficial and harmful effects (it may take several months before these are noticed).
- Report any possible side effects to your primary health care provider for evaluation.

- Herbs can interact with all of the following: other herbs, food, beverages, nutrients, prescription medications, and OTC medications.
- Some herbs are contraindicated in people with the following conditions: stroke, glaucoma, diabetes, hypertension, heart disease, thyroid disorder, and any bleeding disorder or condition requiring anticoagulation.
- Common side effects of herbs include stomach problems, skin rashes, or allergic reactions.
- Herbs that are used for anxiety or insomnia should not be taken before driving a car.
- Be skeptical about exaggerated claims; if it sounds too good to be true, it probably is!

Source: Adapted from information at the U.S. Food and Drug Administration (www.fda.gov).

Addressing Factors That Affect Adherence

When older adults have trouble adhering to their medication regimen, nurses can work with them and their caregivers to identify ways to improve adherence. For example, unit-dose medication systems, which have been widely used in institutional settings, are becoming more available for use in home settings, and may be helpful in improving medication adherence, especially when medication regimens are complex. A variety of simple pill organizers (i.e., containers with separate compartments designated for each day of the week and with one or more compartments for each day) are widely available in stores. In addition, more sophisticated devices to enhance independence and improve adherence are available and may be particularly helpful for people with cognitive or functional impairments. For example, human voice recordings, telephone–computer services, and beeping watches or key chains can be used to remind the person to take medications at designated times. Medication-dispensing systems, which can be filled monthly and programmed to dispense medications at specific times, also are available. Nurses can encourage older adults and their caregivers to investigate different types of devices and systems that can be used to improve medication adherence.

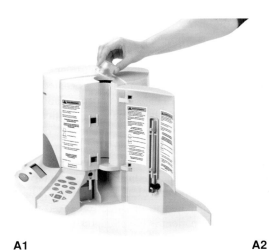

A1

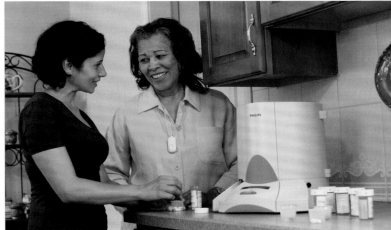

A2

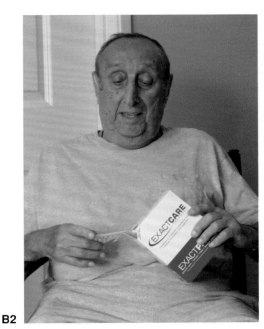

B2

JOE SAMPLE 1/1
Take April 16, 2009 @09:00 AM

Colace 100MG Qty 1
red oval capsule n 512

Glucophage 500MG Qty 1
white round tablet BMS 6060

Motrin 600MG Qty 1
white oblong tablet 600

Norvasc 5MG Qty 1
white octagonal tab NOR

Prilosec 20MG Qty 1
purple oblong capsule 742

B1

FIGURE 8-3 Examples of devices and systems designed to improve medication adherence and independence. (**A**) An automatic pill dispenser with a tamper-proof locking system and an audible alarm, with 28 compartments that can be programmed for taking medications up to four times a day. (**B**) An individualized dosing system for prescription and nonprescription medications, for use in homes and institutions, with each tear-apart compartment printed with patient name, date and time of administration, medication name and dose, and pill description. ((A) used with permission from Philips Healthcare.com and (B) used with permission from ExactCarepharmacy.com.)

Technology to Promote Wellness in Older Adults

Nurses can encourage older adults and their caregivers to explore the many options for automated medication management systems to support independence and adherence. Examples of these systems can be found online, as follows:

- MedCenter Systems, www.medcentersystems.com
- Medminder pill dispensers, www.medminder.com
- MedReady, www.medreadyinc.net
- MedActionPlan, www.mymedschedule.com
- Reminder Rosie, www.reminder-rosie.com

Wellness Opportunity

Nurses promote wellness when they challenge ageist attitudes and identify adverse effects falsely attributed to aging or pathologic conditions.

Even with the increased availability of prescription drug benefits through Medicare, older adults and people with chronic conditions are burdened by the high cost of prescription medications. Thus, nurses often need to address financial barriers that affect adherence to medication regimens because even a person who has an adequate income may decide that a medication is not worth the high cost, especially on an ongoing basis. Nurses can encourage older adults to be candid with their health care practitioners and ask about the availability of less costly but equally safe and effective medications. One way of addressing high costs is to use **generic medications**, which are regulated by the FDA and required to be bioequivalent (i.e., identical) to their brand name counterparts in dosage form, safety, purity, strength, quality, intended use, performance characteristics, and route of administration.

Additional ways of decreasing the cost of medications include obtaining free samples of medications from prescribing practitioners and enrolling in **prescription assistance programs**, which provide medications at little or no cost to consumers. Until recently, it was difficult to obtain information about these programs; however, in April 2005, the Partnership for Prescription Assistance was established to increase awareness and improve access. This partnership provides a single point of access to about 500 organizations, including pharmaceutical companies, that provide free or low-cost medications to people who earn less than 200% of the federal poverty level.

Decreasing the Number of Medications

Because the chance of adverse medication effects increases in proportion to the number of medications consumed, a key intervention is to decrease the number of medications to as few as possible. **Deprescribing** is an interprofessional process of identifying and discontinuing medications that are prescribed inappropriately (i.e., because actual or potential harms outweigh the benefits). Nurses accomplish this by coordinating the efforts of the prescriber(s) to discontinue duplicate medications or medications that are no longer appropriate and by educating the older person about the judicious use of medications that are not medically necessary. In home and community settings, nurses can teach older adults to review their medications with their health care practitioners at every visit. An important role for nurses in this process is to discuss goals of care with older adults and to provide support to older adults and their family caregivers regarding medication decision making (Brandt, 2016).

When older adults are admitted to the hospital, they often are under the care of primary care practitioners who were not the ones who prescribed the medications taken before the admission. Nurses usually obtain the medication history, and the prescribing practitioner may automatically order the medications that are listed on the admission assessment. Because the hospital admission is an ideal time to re-evaluate the safety, efficacy, and necessity of medications, nurses should ask older adults or their caregivers about the purpose and potential adverse effects of each medication. This assessment, which should be done with the medication reconciliation process, may provide important clues to medications or interactions that contributed to or directly caused the problem for which the patient is hospitalized.

When medications are prescribed for behavioral reasons rather than for a medical condition, nurses can teach older adults and their caregivers about these medications and about nonpharmacologic alternatives. For example, caregivers of people with dementia may use medications to address behaviors that might respond equally well to nonpharmacologic interventions that do not have any risk of adverse effects. Once these medications are prescribed, they are likely to be used over long periods without re-evaluation. Nurses need to recognize that the efficacy may diminish (e.g., with hypnotics), the underlying reason may resolve or change (e.g., with situational anxiety), and adverse effects may develop gradually and not be recognized (e.g., with anticholinergic agents). Thus, it is imperative to review periodically all medications and to consider whether nonpharmacologic approaches could be used to address the symptoms or behaviors. Behavioral problems are one example of the types of symptoms that can be managed medically but might be managed just as well, and with fewer risks, through nonpharmacologic interventions. Other types of problems that can often be managed without pharmacologic agents are those related to sleep, comfort, anxiety, and chronic illnesses.

In community settings, it is important to make sure that older adults and caregivers understand the appropriate use of medications that are prescribed as needed (i.e., prn). For example, a caregiver of someone with dementia may be instructed to give a behavior-modifying medication when the person becomes agitated. Although the episodes of agitation may be precipitated by environmental factors (e.g., noise or overstimulation), the caregiver might not realize that nonpharmacologic interventions could be equally effective and carry no risk of adverse effects. In contrast to this situation, a caregiver may withhold medications that could improve the quality of life for the older person and for himself or herself because of misunderstandings or lack of information about the appropriate use of medications. Nurses can teach caregivers about nonpharmacologic interventions, as well as the appropriate use of medications for behavior management, particularly for people with dementia (discussed in Chapter 14).

Wellness Opportunity

Nurses promote wellness by talking with older adults and their caregivers when appropriate about choosing interventions, such as relaxation techniques, that can improve health and quality of life, rather than using medications.

EVALUATING EFFECTIVENESS OF NURSING INTERVENTIONS

Nurses evaluate interventions related to medication management according to the degree to which the older adult follows a safe and effective medication regimen. This process involves an evaluation of medication-taking behaviors as well as an evaluation of the therapeutic effects of the medication. Another evaluation criterion is the extent to which negative functional consequences, such as interactions and adverse effects, are prevented, alleviated, or controlled. In home settings, nurses can evaluate the effectiveness of their interventions by observing the medication-taking patterns of the older adult. In any setting, nurses can evaluate the knowledge of safe and effective use of prescription and OTC medications. Another measure of effectiveness is the degree to which barriers to adherence are eliminated or addressed.

Case Study

Mrs. M., who is 76 years old, is being discharged to her home after a stay in a nursing home for rehabilitation after a stroke. Residual problems from the stroke include left-sided weakness and visual–perceptual difficulties. In addition to the stroke, Mrs. M.'s diagnoses include glaucoma, depression, and heart failure. Her medications include the following: multivitamin, one tablet daily; furosemide (Lasix), 20 mg, two tablets daily; aspirin (Ecotrin), 81 mg daily; clopidogrel (Plavix), 75 mg daily; diltiazem (Cardizem), 60 mg, three times daily; metoprolol (Lopressor), 50 mg twice daily; simvastatain (Zocor), 40 mg at bedtime; sertraline (Zoloft), 50 mg at bedtime; and timolol ophthalmic (Timoptic), 0.25% twice daily. The nursing home regimen for administering the medications is as follows:

7:30 AM:	Cardizem 60 mg
	Furosemide 20 mg, 2 tablets
	Ecotrin 81 mg
	Timoptic, 0.25% in each eye
9:00 AM:	Lopressor 50 mg
1:00 PM:	Multivitamin, 1 tablet
	Cardizem 60 mg
3:30 PM:	Furosemide 20 mg, 2 tablets
7:30 PM:	Timoptic, 0.25% in each eye
	Cardizem 60 mg
	Plavix 75 mg
9:00 PM:	Lopressor 50 mg
	Zoloft 50 mg
	Zocor 40 mg daily

NURSING ASSESSMENT

Your assessment reveals that, before her hospitalization and nursing home stay, Mrs. M. administered her medications independently, but the only medications she took were the eye drops, furosemide (20 mg once daily), and digoxin, which she is no longer taking. The functional assessment indicates that Mrs. M. has weakness and limited use of her left arm and hand, causing difficulty performing tasks that require fine motor movements. She has full use of her right upper extremity, and she is right-hand dominant. She ambulates independently, but slowly, with a walker. A mental status assessment reveals that Mrs. M. is alert, oriented, and has no memory deficits; however, her abstract thinking and time perception have been impaired by the stroke. She has some expressive aphasia, but she seems to understand instructions, especially if ideas are reinforced with concrete examples and demonstrations.

(continued)

NURSING ASSESSMENT *(Continued)*

Mrs. M. expresses motivation to take her medications, but she admits to being overwhelmed by the complexity of the regimen, stating that at the nursing home, they administered her medications at six different times. She is also concerned about self-administering her eye drops because she used to use her left hand to hold her eyelids open. With regard to furosemide, she says she does not like taking it twice a day because it makes her go to the bathroom too much. While at the nursing home, she has not had any trouble with incontinence, but she worries about what she'll do at home because there is no bathroom on the first floor. She asks whether she can take the entire dose of furosemide at night so that she will only have to get up during the night to go to the bathroom, which is located near the bedroom.

In response to your questions about medication management routines before her stroke, Mrs. M. reports using a compartmentalized medication container and taking her two medications and the eye drops after breakfast, around 9:30 am. She would administer the second dose of eye drops around 9:30 pm, before getting ready for bed. She had no difficulty remembering the medications because she kept the pill container and one bottle of eye drops near the toaster, and she kept a second bottle of eye drops on her nightstand. Now, however, she expresses concern about the number of times she must take medications if the regimen remains the same as in the nursing home, and she thinks she will need six pill containers but is not sure where she should put all of them. Mrs. M. also tells you that she is worried about paying for so many medications because when she signed up for Medicare Part D, she was taking only two generic medications and eye drops. Now that she is on so many new pills—and she knows that some are very expensive—she needs to have her prescription drug plan reviewed and perhaps changed.

Mrs. M. lives with her husband, who is physically healthy but has early-stage Alzheimer's disease. Their daughter lives nearby and visits two or three times weekly to assist with grocery shopping, laundry, and household chores. She also provides transportation to stores and appointments.

NURSING DIAGNOSIS

You decide on a nursing diagnosis of Ineffective Health Management because Mrs. M. expresses a desire to take her medications, but several factors deter adherence to the current regimen. Related factors include functional impairments, complex medication regimens, negative side effects of furosemide, and concern about the cost of medications.

NURSING CARE PLAN FOR MRS. M.

Expected Outcome	Nursing Interventions	Nursing Evaluation
Mrs. M.'s medication routine will be simplified	• Work with the pharmacist and the prescribing practitioner to simplify the medication regimen • Discuss with Mrs. M.'s prescribing practitioner the problem of the complexity of the regimen and the cost of medications. Ask Mrs. M.'s prescribing practitioner if she can take Cardizem CD, 180 mg daily, rather than Cardizem, 60 mg three times a day (This will be less expensive and will eliminate two doses of medication daily.) • Ask the pharmacist about combining medications to allow twice-daily administration • Assist Mrs. M. in establishing a routine for self-administering medications that will fit in with her usual activities • At least 3 days before discharge from the nursing home, arrange for Mrs. M. to assume responsibility for her own medication management, using pill containers that she herself fills	• Mrs. M. will be able to follow a twice-daily medication dosing schedule
Mrs. M.'s concerns about furosemide will be addressed	• Explain the importance of taking furosemide, as ordered, to control heart failure effectively • Suggest that Mrs. M. obtain a portable commode for use downstairs during the day	• Mrs. M. will take furosemide as directed and will not experience difficulty with urinary incontinence

NURSING CARE PLAN FOR MRS. M. (Continued)

Expected Outcome	Nursing Interventions	Nursing Evaluation
Mrs. M.'s concerns about the cost of medications will be addressed	• Encourage Mrs. M. to talk with her primary care practitioner about her concerns over the cost of the prescribed medications • Suggest that Mrs. M. talk with her usual pharmacist about her current prescription drug plan and ask if there might be a better plan for her	• Mrs. M. will be able to afford her prescribed medications
A system for self-administering eye drops will be identified	• Ask an occupational therapist to evaluate Mrs. M.'s ability to self-administer her eye drops and to identify any assistive devices that may increase her independence and reliability in performing this task • Have Mrs. M. practice self-administering her eye drops before she is discharged from the nursing home, with staff providing whatever assistance is necessary • Talk with Mrs. M. about the possibility of her husband assisting with the eye drop procedure if she is unable to do this independently • Ask Mrs. M.'s ophthalmologist whether the eye drop regimen can be simplified to once-daily dosing by prescribing an extended-action eye drop formula	• Mrs. M. will self-administer her eye drops or will receive the assistance she needs for eye drop administration from her husband

THINKING POINTS

- What are the factors that influence Mrs. M.'s ability to manage her medications independently?
- What additional assessment information would be helpful in establishing a plan for Mrs. M. to manage her medications independently?
- What health education would you provide to address Mrs. M.'s concerns about the cost of her medications?
- What steps would you take to ensure that expected outcomes are achieved after Mrs. M. is back in her own home?

Chapter Highlights

Overview of Bioactive Substances

- Pharmacokinetics, pharmacodynamics, and elimination half-time of medications
- Herbs and homeopathic remedies
- Herbs and medications with similar bioactivity (Table 8-1)
- Potential adverse effects of herbs (Table 8-2)

Age-Related Changes That Affect Medications in Older Adults

- Age-related changes that affect medications in the body (Box 8-1)
- Changes that affect medication-taking behaviors

Risk Factors That Affect Medications in Older Adults

- Pathologic processes and functional impairments
- Behaviors based on myths and misunderstandings (e.g., attitudes about and expectations for medications)
- Communication barriers between older adults and prescribing practitioners
- Polypharmacy and inadequate monitoring

- Medication nonadherence
- Financial concerns related to prescription drugs
- Insufficient recognition of adverse effects (Table 8-3)

Inappropriate Prescribing Practices (Figure 8-2)

- Beers Criteria
- STOPP/START criteria

Medication Interactions

- Medication–medication interactions (Table 8-4)
- Medication–herb interactions
- Medications and nutrients (Table 8-5)
- Medications and alcohol (Table 8-6)
- Medications and nicotine (Table 8-7)

Functional Consequences Associated With Medications in Older Adults

- Altered therapeutic effects
- Increased potential for adverse drug events (Box 8-2)
- Anticholinergic adverse effects (Box 8-3)
- Increased potential for altered mental status
- Antipsychotics in people with dementia
- Tardive dyskinesia and drug-induced parkinsonism

Nursing Assessment of Medication Use and Effects

- Communication techniques for obtaining accurate information
- Scope of a medication assessment (all bioactive substances, older adult's understanding of regimen, preferences) (Box 8-4)
- Cultural considerations (factors that influence medication-taking behaviors, culturally specific health care sources and practices) (Boxes 8-5 and 8-6)
- Patterns of medication use
- Medication assessment as it relates to the overall assessment
- Identifying adverse medication effects

Nursing Diagnoses

- Ineffective Self-Health Management
- Adverse effects: Confusion, Risk for Falls, Instrumental Self-Care Deficit
- Readiness for Enhanced Self-Health Management

Planning for Wellness Outcomes

- Knowledge: Medication
- Self-care: Non-Parenteral Medication

Nursing Interventions to Promote Safe and Effective Medication Management

- Implementing evidence-based interventions (Box 8-7)
- Medication reconciliation
- Teaching about medications and herbs (Boxes 8-8 and 8-9 patient teaching tools)
- Addressing factors that affect adherence (Figure 8-3)
- Decreasing the number of medications

Critical Thinking Exercises

1. You are asked to give a half-hour presentation titled "Medications and Aging" to a local senior citizens group. Describe the following:
   - What points would you cover about age-related changes in terms that would be easily understood by older adults?
   - How would you address the risk factors that affect medication action and medication-taking behaviors?
   - What tips would you give about taking medications?
   - What educational materials would you use?
   - How would you promote group participation in the discussion?
2. Carefully read the interview questions in Box 8-4 and decide which questions you would use and how you would phrase the questions in your own words for each of the following situations:
   - You are doing an admission interview for a 78-year-old man who lives alone and has been admitted to the hospital for the third time in 18 months for heart failure.

- You are working in a senior wellness program in an urban setting with a large number of older adults who were born in Mexico. You are preparing for 15-minute interviews with older adults who have agreed to participate in an educational session to which they must bring all their pills in a bag and ask the nurse about them.
3. Carefully read the information in Boxes 8-8 and 8-9 and describe what information you would be likely to use in each of the following situations.
   - Discharge planning for the 78-year-old man described in Exercise 2, bullet 1.
   - Health education for people described in the senior wellness program in Exercise 2, bullet 2.

 For more information about topics discussed in this chapter, be sure to check out the interactive Online Learning Activities and other helpful resources at http://thepoint.lww.com/Miller8e.

REFERENCES

American Geriatrics Society 2012 Beers Criteria Update Expert Panel. (2012). American Geriatrics Society updated Beers Criteria for potentially inappropriate medication use in older adults. *Journal of the American Geriatrics Society, 60*(4), 616–631.

Bishara, D., Harwood, D., Sauer, J., et al. (2016). Anticholinergic effect on cognition of drugs commonly used in older people. *International Journal of Geriatric Psychiatry, 32*(6), 650–656.

Blanco-Reina, E., Garcia-Merino, M. R., Ocana-Riola, R., et al. (2016). Assessing potentially inappropriate prescribing in community-dwelling older patients using the updated version of STOPP-START criteria: A comparison of profiles and prevalences with respect to the original version. *PLOS One, 11*(12), e0167586.

Boccardi, V., Baroni, M., Paolacci, L., et al. (2017). Anticholinergic burden and functional status in older people with cognitive impairment: Results from the Regal Project. *Journal of Nutrition Health and Aging, 21*, 389–396.

Brandt, N. (2016). Optimizing medication use through deprescribing. *Journal of Gerontological Nursing, 42*, 10–14.

Campbell, N. L., Zhan, J., Tu, W., et al. (2016). Self-reported medication adherence barriers among ambulatory older adults with mild cognitive impairment. *Pharmacotherapy, 35*, 196–202.

Carbon, M., Hsieh, C. H., Kane, J. M., et al. (2017). Tardive dyskinesia prevalence in the period of second-generation antipsychotic use: A meta-analysis. *Journal of Clinical Psychiatry, 78*(3), e264–e278.

Cioltan, H., Alshehri, S., Howe, S., et al. (2017). Variation in use of antipsychotic medications in nursing homes in the United States: A systematic review. *BioMed Central Geriatrics, 17*, 32.

Collamati, A., Martone, A. M., Poscia, A., et al. (2016). Anticholinergic drugs and negative outcomes in the older population: From biological plausibility to clinical evidence. *Aging and Clinical Experimental Research, 28*, 25–35.

Dalleur, O., Beeler, P., Schnipper, J., et al. (2017). 30-day potentially avoidable readmissions due to adverse drug events. Doi: 10.1097/PTS.0000000000000346. [Epub ahead of print].

do Nascimento, M. M., Mambrini, J. V., Lima-Costa, M. F., et al. (2017). Potentially inappropriate medications: Predictor for mortality in a cohort of community-dwelling older adults. *73*(5), 615–621.

Dusetzina, S., & Keating, N. (2016). Minding the gap: Why closing the doughnut hole is insufficient for increasing Medicare Beneficiary access to oral chemotherapy. *Journal of Clinical Oncology, 34*, 375–380.

Farlow, M. R., & Shamliyan, T. A. (2017). Benefits and harms of atypical antipsychotics for agitation in adults with dementia. *European Neuropsychopharmacology*, 27, 217–231.

Flanagan, N., & Blazer, J. (2016). Medication reconciliation and education for older adults: Using the 2015 AGS Beers criteria as a guide. *Home Healthcare Now*, 34, 542–549.

Forlenza, O., Loureiro, J. C., Pais, M. V., et al. (2017). Recent advances in the management of neuropsychiatric symptoms of dementia. *Current Opinion in Psychiatry*, 30, 151–158.

Greenberg, S. (2016). The 2015 American Geriatrics Society Updated Beers Criteria for Potentially Inappropriate Medication Use in Older Adults. Available at http://consultgerirn.org.

Heider, D., Matschinger, H., Meid, A. D., et al. (2017). Health service use, costs, and adverse events associated with potentially inappropriate medication in old age in Germany: Retrospective matched cohort study. *Drugs and Aging*, 34, 289–301.

Herdman, T., & Kamitsuru, S (Eds.). (2018). NANDA International Nursing Diagnoses Definitions and Classification, 2018–2020 (11th ed., pp. 34–44). New York: Thieme Publishers.

Hirsch, G. E., Viecili, P. R., de Almeida, A. S., et al. (2017). Natural products with antiplatelet action. *Current Pharmaceutical Design*, 23. Doi: 10.2174/1381612823666161123151611

Hudani, Z. K., & Rojas-Fernandez, C. H. (2016). A scoping review on medication adherence in older patients with cognitive impairment or dementia. *Research in Social and Administrative Pharmacology*, 12, 815–823.

Jatau, A., Aung, M., Kamauzaman, T., et al. (2016). Use and toxicity of complementary and alternative medicine among patients visiting emergency department: Systematic review. *Journal of Intercultural Ethnopharmacology*, 5, 191–197.

Jin, H., Kim, Y., & Rhie, S. J. (2016). Factors affecting medication adherence in elderly people. *Patient Preference and Adherence*, 10, 2117–2125.

Johnell, K., Jonasdottir Bergman, G., Fastbom, J., et al. (2017). Psychotropic drugs and the risk of fall injuries, hospitalizations and mortality among older adults. *International Journal of Geriatric psychiatry*, 32, 414–420.

Johnson, P. J., Jou, J., Rhee, T. G., et al. (2016). Complementary health approaches for health and wellness in midlife and older US adults. *Maturitas*, 89, 36–42.

Jou, J., & Johnson, P. J. (2016). Nondisclosure of complementary and alternative medicine use to primary care physicians: Findings from the 2012 National Health Interview Survey. *JAMA Internal Medicine*, 174, 545–546.

Kaiser Family Foundation. (2016). 10 essential facts about Medicare and prescription drug spending. Available at www.kff.org.

Kanagaratnam, L., Drame, M., Novella, J. L., et al. (2017). Risk factors for adverse drug reactions in older subjects hospitalized in a dedicated dementia unit. *American Journal of Geriatric Psychiatry*, 25, 290–296.

Khodyakov, D., Ochoa, A., Olivieri-Mui, B. L., et al. (2017). Screening tool of older person's prescriptions/screening tools to alert doctors to right treatment medication criteria modified for U. S. nursing homes. *Journal of the American Geriatrics Society*, 65, 586–591.

Lavan, A., & Gallagher, P. (2016). Predicting risk of adverse drug reactions in older adults. *Therapeutic Advances in Drug Safety*, 7, 11–22.

Lavan, A., Gallagher, P., Parsons, C., et al. (2017). STOPPFrail (screening tool of older persons prescriptions in frail adults with limited life expectancy): Consensus validation. *Age and Ageing*. [Epub]. Doi: 10.1093/ageing/afx005.

Leite, P. M., Martins, M. A., & Castilho, R. O. (2016). Review on mechanisms and interactions in concomitant use of herbs and warfarin therapy. *Biomedical Pharmacotherapeutics*, 83, 14–21.

Levy, H. B. (2017). Polypharmacy reduction strategies: Tips on incorporating American Geriatrics Society Beers and Screening Tool of Older Peoples Prescription criteria. *Clinical Geriatric Medicine*, 33, 177–187.

Lo, S. H., Chau, J. P., Woo, J., et al. (2016). Adherence to antihypertensive medication in older adults with hypertension. *Journal of Cardiovascular Nursing*, 31, 296–303.

Lonnbro, J., & Wallerstedt, S. M. (2017). Clinical relevance of the STOPP/START criteria in hip fracture patients. *European Journal of Clinical Pharmacology*, 73, 499–505.

Lucchetti, G., & Lucchetti, A. L. (2017). Inappropriate prescribing in older persons: A systematic review of medications available in different criteria. *Archives of Gerontology and Geriatrics*, 68, 55–61.

Marcum, Z., Hanlon, J., & Murray, M. (2017). Improving medication adherence and health outcomes in older adults: An evidence-based review of randomized controlled trials. *Drugs and Aging*, 34, 191–201.

Mihajlovic, S., Gauthier, J., & McDonald, E. (2016). Patient characteristics associated with adverse drug events in hospital: An overview of reviews. *Canadian Journal of Hospital Pharmacology*, 69, 294–300.

Mion, L. C., & Sandhu, S. (2016). Adverse drug events in older hospitalized adults: Implications for nursing practice. *Geriatric Nursing*, 37, 153–155.

Morrow, D. G., & Conner-Garcia, T. (2013). Improving comprehension of medication information. *Journal of Gerontological Nursing*, 39(4), 22–29.

Mouly, S., Lloret-Linares, C., Sellier, P. O., et al. (2017). Is the clinical relevance of drug-food and drug-herb interactions limited to grapefruit juice and Saint John's Wort? *Pharmacology Research*, 118, 82–92.

Muhlack, D. C., Hoppe, L. K., Weberpals, J., et al. (2017). The association of potentially inappropriate medication at older age with cardiovascular and overall mortality: A systematic review and meta-analysis of cohort studies. *Journal of the American Medical Directors Association*, 18(3):211–220.

Munhoz, R. P., Bertucci Filho, D., & Teive, H. A. (2017). Not all drug-induced parkinsonism are the same: The effect of drug class on motor phenotype. *Neurological Sciences*, 38, 319–324.

Nicoteri, J. A. (2016). Food-drug interactions: Putting evidence into practice. *The Nurse Practitioner*, 41(2), 1–7.

O'Brien, A. (2016). Comparing the risk of tardive dyskinesia in older adults with first-generation and second-generation antipsychotics: A systematic review and meta-analysis. *International Journal of Geriatric Psychiatry*, 31, 683–693.

Olson, A. W., Schommer, J. C., Mott, J. C., et al. (2016). Financial hardship from purchasing medications for senior citizens before and after the Medicare Modernization Act of 2003 and the Patient Protection and Affordable Care Act of 2010: Findings from 1998, 2001, and 2015. *Journal of Managed Care and Specialty Pharmacy*, 22, 1150–1158.

Oscanoa, T. J., Lizaraso, F., & Carvajal, A. (2017). Hospital admissions due to adverse drug reactions in the elderly: A meta-analysis. *European Journal of Clinical Pharmacology*, 73(6), 759–770.

Pedros, C., Formiga, F., Corbella, X., et al. (2016). Adverse drug reactions leading to urgent hospital admission in an elderly population: Prevalence and main features. *European Journal of Clinical Pharmacology*, 72, 219–226.

Pincus, K. (2013). Transitional care management services. *Journal of Gerontological Nursing*, 39(10), 10–15.

Pfistermeister, B., Tumena, T., Gaismann, K. G., et al. (2017). Anticholinergic burden and cognitive function in a large German cohort of hospitalized geriatric patients. *PLOS One*, 12, e0171353.

Rababa, M., Al-Ghassani, A. A., Kovach, C., et al. (2016). Proton pump inhibitors and the prescribing cascade. *Journal of Gerontological Nursing*, 42(4), 23–31.

Rakash, G., Muzyk, A., Szabo, S. T., et al. (2017). Tardive dyskinesia: 21st century may bring new treatments to a forgotten disorder. *Annals of Clinical Psychiatry*, 29, e9–e20.

Schaffer, S., Curry, K., & Yoon, S-J. (2016). Herbal supplements for health promotion and disease prevention. *The Nurse Practitioner*, 41(10), 39–45.

Shehab, N., Lovegrove, M. C., Geller, A., et al. (2016). U. S. Emergency department visits for outpatient drug events, 2013–2014. *Journal of the American Medical Association*, 316, 2115–2125.

Shuaib, U., Rajput, A., Robinson, C., et al. (2016). Neuroleptic-induced parkinsonism: Clinicopathological study. *Movement Disorders, 31,* 360–367.

Simonson, W. (2016a). The 2015 updated Beers Criteria: The evolution continues. *Geriatric Nursing, 37,* 61–62.

Simonson, W. (2016b). Anticholinergic properties of medications. *Geriatric Nursing, 37,* 302–303.

Stefanacci, R. G., & Khan, T. (2017). Can managed care manage polypharmacy? *Clinics in Geriatric Medicine, 33,* 241–255.

Swami, S., Cohen, R. A., Kairalla, J. A., et al. (2016). Anticholinergic drug use and risk to cognitive performance in older adults with questionable cognitive impairment: A cross-sectional analysis. *Drugs & Aging, 33,* 809–818.

Tang, S., W., Tang, W., & Leonard, B. (2017). Patients on psychotropic medications and herbal supplement combinations: Clinical considerations. *International Clinical Psychopharmacoloty, 32,* 63–69.

Tong, M., Oh, Y., Thomas, J., et al. (2017). Nursing home medication reconciliation. *Journal of Gerontological Nursing, 43*(4), 9–14.

Volpi, E., Giannelli, A., Toccafondi, G., et al. (2017). Medication reconciliation during hospitalization and in hospital-home interface: An observations retrospective study. *Journal of Patient Safety.* [Epub] Doi: 10.1097/PTS.0000000000000360.

Woods, D., Mentes, J., Cadogan, M., et al. (2017). Aging, genetic variations, and ethnopharmacology: Building cultural competence through awareness of drug responses in ethnic minority elders. *Journal of Transcultural Nursing, 28,* 56–62.

Wouters, J., van der Meer, H., & Taxis, K. (2017). Quantification of anticholinergic and sedative drug load with the Drug Burden Index: A review of outcomes and methodological quality of studies. *European Journal of Clinical Pharmacology, 73,* 257–266.

Zwicker, D., & Fulmer, T. (2016). Reducing adverse drug events. In M. Boltz, E. Capezuti, T. Fulmer, & D. Zwicker (Eds.), *Evidence-based practice protocols for best practice* (5th ed., pp. 311–341). New York: Springer Publishing Co.

chapter **9**

Legal and Ethical Concerns

LEARNING OBJECTIVES

After reading this chapter, you will be able to:

1. Define the following terms: autonomy, competency, and decision-making capacity.

2. Describe the following advance directives: living wills, medical directives, and durable power of attorney for health care.

3. Discuss ethical issues that nurses commonly address when caring for older adults.

4. Describe cultural considerations that affect autonomy, decision making, and advance directives.

5. Describe nursing responsibilities regarding advance care planning and decisions about care.

KEY TERMS

advance care planning	incompetent
advance directives	living wills
allow a natural death (AND)	Nursing Home Residents' Bill of Rights
artificial nutrition and hydration (ANH)	Omnibus Budget Reconciliation Act (OBRA) of 1987
autonomy	Patient Self-Determination Act (PSDA)
competency	
decision-making capacity	
do not resuscitate (DNR) order	physical restraint
	Physician Orders for Life-Sustaining Treatment (POLST)
durable power of attorney for health care	
guardianship	values clarification
health care proxy	

Since the early 1980s, various legislative efforts have addressed the rights of older adults beginning with issues pertaining to vulnerable elders. Later in the 1980s, legislative efforts focused on issues related to end-of-life decisions, the rights of patients and nursing home residents, and the quality of care provided under Medicaid and Medicare programs. Currently, autonomy and shared decision making are emphasized, particularly regarding medical interventions. Many of these legislative and policy initiatives involve ethical issues for gerontological health care practitioners. For example, nurses commonly address questions about the extent to which an older person is able to be involved with decisions about his or her health care. Although legislation provides guidelines, laws do not resolve ethical dilemmas that arise when no advance directive is provided or when conflicts exist about how an advance directive should be interpreted or implemented. The next sections review some of the pertinent legal and ethical issues that are relevant to nursing care of older adults. Additional legal and ethical considerations regarding vulnerable or abused elders are addressed in Chapter 10.

AUTONOMY AND RIGHTS

Autonomy is the personal freedom to direct one's own life as long as it does not infringe on the rights of others. An autonomous person is capable of rational thought and is able to recognize the need for problem solving. In addition, an autonomous person is capable of identifying the problem, searching for alternatives, and selecting a solution that allows his or her continued personal freedom. People may be denied the right to autonomy if the outcome of their decisions or their lack of decision-making ability jeopardizes their safety, or the rights, safety, or property of others. Loss of autonomy and, therefore, loss of independence, is a very real fear among older adults. Moreover, for older adults with dementia and other conditions that affect decision-making abilities, loss of autonomy is a challenge that is frequently addressed by families and health care professionals throughout the course of the condition, which can last for many years.

Because autonomy is highly valued in many European and North American cultures and there is no easy way to evaluate decision-making abilities, which can fluctuate from day to day, questions often arise about medical interventions and health care decisions. Thus, nurses need to be familiar with legal and ethical guidelines related to competency and decision-making capacity. Nurses are responsible for assisting older adults and their families, often as impartial mediators, when issues concerning personal autonomy arise. However, if the safety of the older person is threatened because of risky behaviors arising from impaired decision-making abilities, nurses must refer older people to the appropriate community agencies (e.g., adult protective services) for further evaluation, as discussed in Chapter 10.

Competency

Competency is a *legal term* that refers to the ability to fulfill one's role and handle one's affairs in a responsible manner. All adults are presumed to be competent, and state laws designate the age of competency—usually 18 years—for participating in legally binding decisions. Because competent people are guaranteed all the rights granted by the U.S. constitution and state laws, all adults who have not been declared **incompetent** by a judge have the legal right to make their own decisions about medical treatment and health care. However, in reality, families and health care providers often raise questions about an older person's ability to make reasonable decisions, particularly when the person is cognitively impaired.

When questions are raised about a person's ability to participate in health care decisions, a legally appointed surrogate decision maker, if one has been designated, assumes decision-making responsibility (see the discussion of health care proxy in the section on Advance Directives). In the absence of a surrogate decision maker or when conflicts exist among the people involved with making and implementing decisions, a petition can be filed with a probate court to determine whether the person is competent. Often, these petitions are filed because a health care provider (usually a physician) is concerned that appropriate decisions be made for a person who is not making safe and reasonable medical decisions independently. Usually a family member files the petition, but if no qualified family member is available, or if family members are in conflict about the petition, an attorney or other person may file. If the court determines that the person is incompetent (i.e., incapable of making decisions on his or her own behalf), the judge assigns either a partial or a full **guardianship** (also called a conservatorship).

With a partial guardianship, the incompetent person continues to make limited decisions; with a full guardianship, the person loses all of his or her rights to make decisions. Although additional court action can revoke or reverse a guardianship after it has been granted, the guardianship typically remains in place until the incompetent person dies. Usually, guardianship is initiated only as a last resort when no other legal intervention is appropriate because it is a drastic measure that takes away rights and entails court proceedings and ongoing court monitoring. Most often the need for guardianship can be avoided if a person makes his or her wishes known in a comprehensive and legally binding manner, including the appointment of a surrogate decision maker, before any questions arise about his or her mental capacities. In the absence of these documents, however, or when conflict arises about the ability of designated people to honor the person's wishes, legal and ethical issues are generally addressed through probate court proceedings, such as guardianship.

Decision-Making Capacity

Decision-making capacity is a measure of a person's ability to make an informed and logical decision about a particular aspect of his or her health care. It is a *clinical term* that describes the person's ability to understand, make, and be responsible for the consequences of health care decisions. In contrast to competency—which is determined by a court of law—decision-making capacity is determined by health care practitioners and it relates to a single decision rather than a global determination of one's ability to manage one's own affairs. Decision-making capacity requires that the person be able to do all of the following:

- Understand and process information that is relevant to the decisions about diagnosis, prognosis, and treatment options
- Weigh the relative risks, benefits, and outcomes of decisions in relation to one's own situation
- Apply personal values to the situation
- Arrive at a decision that is consistent over time
- Communicate the decision to others

Nurses need to recognize the influence of differing religious and culturally based beliefs when assessing the rationality of the person's conclusions and decision-making capacity. For example, a belief in miracles may be culturally appropriate for some clients/patients but seem to be delusional to a Western-trained care provider. It is important to consider that treatment preferences are not always based on logical reasons and may be strongly influenced by religious or cultural beliefs.

An additional consideration pertinent to older adults is that determination of decision-making capacity should not be based on chronologic age or a particular diagnosis. This is especially important with regard to older adults who have dementia because they may retain the ability to make safe and sufficient decisions during early stages; however, this ability gradually diminishes as the dementia progresses. During mild-to-moderate stages of dementia, assessment of decision-making ability is based on the person's ability to describe the importance or implications of the choice on his or her future health (Post & Boltz, 2016b). As dementia progresses from early to later stages, everyday decision-making processes transitions from shared decision making by the person with dementia and family caregivers, to surrogate decision making, which is done by family caregivers based on their knowledge of the person's wishes (Fetherstonbaugh, McAuliffe, Bauer, et al., 2017).

Rather than basing conclusions on a person's age or diagnosis, health care professionals focus on a specific situation and evaluate the person's ability to understand the issues involved, to weigh the pros and cons of choices, and to communicate about them. For example, a person with dementia may be able to decide about the appointment of a surrogate decision maker but may not be able to participate in a complex decision about medical treatment options for cancer. In this situation, it might be reasonable for the person to designate a family member to make the treatment decision.

It is important to recognize that rather than being an "all or nothing" process, decision making typically involves considerations related to both the individual and his or her family and others whose opinions the person values. More often than not, decision making is a complex process in which information is shared between patients and clinicians and among family and others who are affected by the outcomes. Another consideration is that rather than being based primarily on logic and deliberation, decisions are strongly influenced by needs, values, habits, emotions, and cultural factors (discussed in the section on Cultural Aspects of Legal and Ethical Issues).

Nurses have dual roles in helping surrogate decision makers involve the older adult as much as possible and at the same time supporting shared or surrogate decision makers in assuming responsibility for decisions. This role is especially complex when decisions involve conflicting needs and values of the older adult and the caregivers. For example, spouses and families of people with dementia may experience conflict related to the value of caring for the person at home—a decision that involves sacrifices for the caregiver as well as benefits for the care recipient—and the decision to have care provided in an assisted living or nursing facility. Additional responsibilities of nurses include documenting the person's specific abilities and limitations in the care plan and ensuring that decision-making abilities are periodically reevaluated.

It is also important to recognize that decision-making capacity can fluctuate from day to day and hour to hour and may be significantly influenced by factors that can be addressed, such as delirium, depression, polypharmacy, and sleep deprivation. Thus, an important role of nurses is to promote optimal decision-making capacity by identifying and addressing the factors that influence cognitive functioning. For example, even such a relatively simple measure as ensuring that a hearing-impaired person uses his or her hearing aid may improve communication and thereby have a positive effect on decision-making abilities. Similarly, if a person with dementia has better cognitive abilities in the morning

or when rested, then efforts can be made to discuss health care decisions during this time, rather than when the person is more confused.

The phrases *decisional autonomy* and *executional autonomy* are sometimes used in relation to decision-making capacity. Decisional autonomy refers to the ability and freedom to make decisions without external influence, whereas executional autonomy (also called executive autonomy) refers to the ability to implement the decisions. These concepts call attention to the complexity of assessing decision-making capacity and the importance of evaluating a person's ability not only to make reasonable decisions but also to carry out all of the actions necessary for implementing them. This point is particularly important in relation to people with impaired executive control functions, which are the cognitive skills involved in successfully planning and carrying out goal-oriented behavior, such as self-care tasks. Conditions that are likely to cause impaired executive control functions include stroke, dementia, major depression, Parkinson's disease, traumatic brain injury, and any conditions affecting frontal lobe functioning. These situations are particularly difficult to evaluate because the person may retain the capacity to understand and make decisions (decisional autonomy) but may not have the capacity to carry them out (executive autonomy). Chapter 13 discusses guidelines for nursing assessment of executive control functions, and this topic is addressed in Online Learning Activity 9-1.

 See ONLINE LEARNING ACTIVITY 9-1: EVIDENCE-BASED INFORMATION RELATED TO HEALTH CARE DECISION MAKING at http://thepoint.lww.com/Miller8e.

ADVANCE DIRECTIVES

Advance directives (also called advance medical directives) are legally binding documents that allow competent people to document what medical care they would or would not want to receive if they were not capable of making decisions and communicating their wishes. Advance directives also enable a person to appoint a **health care proxy** (also called a proxy decision maker), who is responsible for communicating the person's wishes if he or she becomes incompetent or unable to communicate them.

The **Patient Self-Determination Act (PSDA)**, which became effective on December 1, 1991, provides the legal mandate for advance directives. This legislation protects health care consumers by requiring that providers do all of the following:

- Inform patients of their right to refuse treatments and make health care decisions.
- Provide written information about their state's provisions for implementing advance directives.
- Ask each person whether an advance directive has been completed.

- Include documentation of patients' advance directives in their medical records.
- Provide education for the staff and the community on advance directives.

The PSDA applies to all hospices, hospitals, home health agencies, extended care facilities, and health maintenance organizations that receive federal funds. Because of this legislation, nurses in all settings routinely inquire about advance directives and facilitate communication about patients' wishes.

Advance directive documents must be drawn up when the person is capable of understanding their intent, and they become effective only when the person lacks the capacity to make a particular health-related decision. Thus, it is imperative to address advance directives before the onset of any condition, such as dementia, that can affect functioning and cognitive abilities. When the diagnosis of dementia has already been made, it is imperative that decision-making capacity be evaluated and documented as early in the process as possible and specifically in relation to the task of executing advance directive documents. This often requires a comprehensive assessment by an interdisciplinary team including a mental health professional such as a geropsychologist or geropsychiatrist. An important nursing responsibility is to facilitate referrals for comprehensive assessments, particularly when conflicts among family members or decision makers exist or are probable in the future. Keep in mind that it may be prudent to periodically reassess decision-making abilities as the older adult's condition changes.

Although federal and state laws do not *require* that people have advance directive documents, these laws encourage discussions about health care decisions and *suggest* that people have advance directives. State laws vary regarding details (e.g., scope, type of document, conditions for application of advance directives, and requirements for updates) of advance directives, and not all states honor out-of-state advance directives. This policy is particularly problematic for older adults who travel between or reside in more than one state. Up-to-date information about state laws related to advance directives can be found by using Online Learning Activity 9-2. Common types of advance directives are discussed in the following sections.

 See ONLINE LEARNING ACTIVITY 9-2: RESOURCES FOR INFORMATION ABOUT STATE LAWS RELATED TO ADVANCE DIRECTIVES at http://thepoint.lww.com/Miller8e.

Durable Power of Attorney for Health Care

A **durable power of attorney for health care** is an advance directive that takes effect whenever someone cannot, for any reason, provide informed consent for health care treatment decisions. Because it enables a surrogate health care decision maker, also called a health care proxy (as previously discussed), to represent the person during any time of incapacity, it is often considered the most important advance directive. Like other powers of attorney, the durable power of attorney for health care must be initiated when the person is competent, and it takes effect only when the person is incapacitated. When used with other advance directives, this document provides written guidelines stating the person's wishes on issues, such as termination of life support measures. It is imperative that the health care proxy has a copy of all advance directives and periodically discusses the person's wishes about medical treatments and end-of-life issues. Because language in advance directive documents can sometimes be vague, nurses should encourage older adults to discuss their wishes with their primary care provider, other health care workers, and their designated surrogate before a crisis develops.

Do Not Resuscitate Orders

A **do not resuscitate (DNR) order** is a very specific type of advance directive that compels health care providers to refrain from cardiopulmonary resuscitation if the person is no longer breathing and has no heartbeat. Sometimes, families, as well as health care professionals, mistakenly associate DNR orders with directives to withhold other medical treatments. For example, questions may arise about not sending someone to a hospital or not requesting certain diagnostic or treatment procedures simply because a DNR order is in place. Other times, DNR orders are overlooked, particularly in emergencies or when the health care power of attorney is not immediately available. Nurses have important roles in discussing this document with the patient and the health care proxy so that additional and appropriate advance medical directives, or variations of DNR orders, are in place to cover the circumstances that are most likely to arise. It is also imperative to teach older adults, all care providers, and health care powers of attorney to have copies of DNR orders readily accessible.

In 2000, the Reverend Chuck Meyers proposed that the designation of **allow a natural death (AND)** be used instead of DNR, with the intent to replace negative terms (i.e., "do not") with a positive statement. Patients, families, and health care professionals have indicated that they prefer this term over DNR terminology and advocacy groups are working toward legislative changes to include this designation (Fairlie, 2017; Levin & Coyle, 2015). Although the designation of AND is not recognized in state laws, many states and health care institutions allow—and even encourage—variations of the DNR order, such as Comfort Care DNR (also called DNR Comfort Care, CC/DNR, or Comfort Care-Only DNR). These legal interventions direct health care professionals (including emergency care workers and first responders) to provide designated comfort care measures but not resuscitative therapies (e.g., cardioversion, chest compression, artificial airway, resuscitative drugs, drugs to correct heart rhythm) if the person is in full respiratory or cardiac arrest or if the person is near this condition. Comfort care measures defined in these documents include oxygen therapy, positioning, airway suctioning, pain medication, control of bleeding, and emotional support of patient and family. State procedures for implementing these documents usually require that they be signed by a primary care practitioner and encourage people to make sure these directives are readily available whenever they may be needed. Some states have also implemented identification procedures with the use of officially recognized bracelets, wallet cards, or other items.

Living Wills

Living wills are a type of advance directive whose purpose is to guide decisions about care that is provided or withheld under certain circumstances, usually at the end of life or when the person is considered terminally ill. Living wills evolved as a component of the first right-to-die statute, which was enacted in 1976 in California. People must be competent to initiate a living will and they can revoke or change it at any time as long as they remain competent. It is imperative that living wills, and all advance directives, reflect the person's values and goals. A major goal of living wills is to affirm the right of a person to receive or refuse treatment; a limitation is that they do not cover all foreseeable options.

Living wills are not the same as DNR orders because these documents address preferences for a broad range of medical treatments that the person wishes to have or not have in certain circumstances. For example, these advance directives can provide instructions about specific interventions, such as antibiotics, food and nutrition, and admission to the hospital. These documents afford reassurance to people who fear that treatments or pain control and comfort measures will not be provided when they are sick and cannot express their own wishes. Although advance directives cannot guarantee that a medical intervention will be provided regardless of the circumstances, they provide legal assurance that the person's preferences will be considered. Because of the inability to predict medical treatments that might become available, and because of the changing health condition of the person executing the document, medical directives should be reviewed and updated periodically.

An important consideration is that living wills typically apply only to situations in which the person is considered terminally ill, whereas other advance directives may apply to a broader range of circumstances, such as irreversible brain damage or temporary incapacity. Another limitation is that definitions of terminal illness are not always clear, and there may be disagreement about whether the person is terminally ill. In general, someone is considered to be terminally ill when a physician determines that his or her predictable life expectancy is 6 months or less. Some laws or policies require that two physicians document that the person is terminally ill.

Most states and the District of Columbia recognize the validity of living wills, but the scope and details of living wills differ from state to state. For example, some states require that living wills specifically address certain procedures, such as the withholding or withdrawal of artificial sustenance. Advocacy groups and health care professionals are encouraging all adults to draw up living wills and to take steps to ensure that all their health care providers have copies of these documents.

Medical Orders for Life-Sustaining Treatment

The **Physician Orders for Life-Sustaining Treatment (POLST)** is an evolving development, which has been available for general use since 1995 after it was tested in Oregon for 4 years. In 2017, only three states were not implementing or endorsing a POLST program, and many states offered the documents in other languages. Several states use the term Medical Orders for Life-Sustaining Treatment (MOLST) or Medical Orders for Scope of Treatment (MOST), with the same intent as POLST. These medical directives are effective for ensuring that patient preferences are known and honored in all settings and situations, including emergencies and long-term care.

POLST directives do not replace advance directives, and they differ from advance directives in the following ways:

- They are designed specifically for seriously ill or frail patients who are likely to die or lose decision-making capacity during the next year
- They are signed by the patient or his or her legally recognized decision maker and a health care professional (i.e., physician, nurse practitioner, or physician assistant)
- Because they are a legally valid physician's order, they serve as a medical order for providing or withholding treatment
- Health care professionals are legally obligated to follow the instructions in any health care setting

POLST documents usually are printed on brightly colored forms and are transferred across settings.

Although there is increasing use of POLST documents, concerns have been raised about whether the documents accurately reflect current preferences of patients, particularly when their conditions change (Hickman, Hammes, Torke, et al., 2017; Rahman, Bressette, & Enguidanos, 2017). Similarly, concerns have been raised about the possibility that documents will not be reviewed and updated as the patient's condition changes, causing the patient to receive care that is more or less aggressive than the patient prefers (Kendra, Rubin, & Halpern, 2016).

Five Wishes

Advocacy groups encourage all adults to establish advance directives and to make their wishes known to their families and health care providers regarding health care decisions, particularly end-of-life care issues. For example, the organization Aging with Dignity promotes the use of the *Five Wishes* document for use as an advance directive. The *Five Wishes* document addresses the following:

- Who you want to make care decisions for you when you cannot make them.

- What kind of medical treatment you want or do not want.
- The level of comfort you want.
- How you want people to treat you.
- What you want your loved ones to know.

This document was introduced in 1997 with support from the Robert Wood Johnson Foundation and is now widely accepted in the United States and is available in Braille and 28 languages. It is used in all 50 states and in countries around the world. The document meets the legal requirements for advance directives in 42 states, and in other states it can be attached to the state-issued forms (Aging with Dignity, 2017).

ADVANCE CARE PLANNING

Advance care planning is defined as "a process that supports adults at any age or stage of health in understanding and sharing their personal values, life goals, and preferences regarding future medical care" (Sudore, Lum, You, et al., 2017, p. 821). The primary goal of advance care planning is to ensure that medical care is consistent with an individual's values, goals, and preferences. Initially, the focus was on the individual signing documents related to specific medical procedures, such as cardiopulmonary resuscitation. More recently, the process has evolved to address all of the following components (Bravo, Trottier, Arcand, et al., 2016):

- Identification of trusted relatives or friends to make decisions on their behalf if the person becomes incapacitated
- Clarification of the person's preferences and goals of care before a serious health event occurs
- Communication of these wishes to designated proxies
- Discussion of the person's values, for example, related to autonomy
- Documentation of legal documents and conversations related to patient's wishes in medical records

Current emphasis is on the importance of communication about advance care planning, which is usually initiated by the person's primary care practitioner. Because the process is ongoing, it requires collaborative participation of nurses and other interprofessional team members (Nediat-Hajem, Carrion, Gonzalez, et al., 2017). A crucial role for nurses is communicating with and teaching older adults about advance directives and dispelling myths and misperceptions about these documents (Splendore & Grant, 2017). The American Nurses Association Code of Ethics for Nurses states that "nurses should promote advance care planning conversations and must be knowledgeable about the advantages and disadvantages of various advance directive documents" (American Nurses Association, 2015, p. 3).

Advance care planning is an ongoing process that includes teaching, listening, and incorporates discussions about personal values and goals of care. Prince-Paul and DiFranco (2017) proposed that advance care planning conversations be considered an essential aspect of health promotion activities.

Nurses can open the conversation by helping older adults discuss their personal values and preferences, what quality of life means for them, the importance of preserving life, and the effects of the patient's illness and death on others (Ko, Lee, & Hong, 2016; Post & Boltz, 2016a). Nurses also can teach older adults to discuss their wishes with all health care providers and with family and surrogate decision makers.

When care is provided over long periods, documents and preferences need to be reviewed periodically and updated as appropriate, and at all times, current documents need to be included in patient charts. In addition, nurses encourage people to provide copies of advance directives to their family members, designated surrogate, and anyone likely to be involved with decisions about their medical care. If written advance directives have not been completed, it is important to initiate a discussion of relevant medical care and end-of-life treatment preferences and document any statements made that express a patient's wishes. Nurses can use information in Box 9-1 as an assessment guide for discussing advance directives and goals of care when decisions are complex. Box 9-2 can be used to teach caregivers about advance care planning.

💡 Technology to Promote Wellness in Older Adults

Most recently, technologic advances are helping people engage in advance care planning as a self-learning and ongoing process through interactive "e-planning" websites. Making Your Wishes Known is an example of a comprehensive website that provides educational materials and thought-provoking questions to help participants understand complex issues related to medical care and develop advance planning documents that communicate their preferences about care to health care providers. Studies indicate that interactive e-planning programs are effective for generating an advance directive that reliably reflects the person's values and goals (Markahm, Levi, Green, et al., 2015; Sudore, Boscardin, Feuz, et al., 2017). Online Learning Activity 9-3 provides detailed information about this and other e-planning tools that nurses can use to discuss advance care documents with older adults and their caregivers (as discussed in the section on Nursing Interventions).

See ONLINE LEARNING ACTIVITY 9-3: ADDITIONAL INFORMATION ABOUT ADVANCE DIRECTIVES AND ADVANCE CARE PLANNING at http://thepoint.lww.com/Miller8e.

LEGAL ISSUES SPECIFIC TO LONG-TERM CARE SETTINGS

As the regulator of Medicare and Medicaid programs, Congress is responsible for ensuring that dollars expended for health care are well spent. In response to public concern about the quality of care in nursing homes during the 1960s, Congress mandated an Institute of Medicine study entitled *Improving the Quality of Care in Nursing Homes*, which

Box 9-1 Examples of Assessment Questions Related to Health Care Decisions

Questions to Assess the Person's Understanding of Decisions About Treatments

- What is your understanding of your current health condition?
- What do you understand about your treatment choices?
- What do you think you would gain from the proposed intervention?
- What would be the risks involved with the intervention?
- What questions do you have about your condition or the treatment choices?
- Would you like more information from anyone about your choices?

Questions About the Person's Supports

- Whom do you usually rely on to help make important decisions?
- Is there anything I can do to help support you during this time?
- What are the areas of concern for your family?

Questions About the Person's Values Related to Comfort

- What are the things and people who bring you enjoyment or pleasure?
- What is most important to you in terms of everyday comfort (e.g., music, privacy, physical comfort, social interactions)?
- Are there circumstances that would make you feel that life is unbearable

Questions About the Person's Values Related to Autonomy

- How much do you want your family or others to be involved with decisions about your care?

- Is there anyone you do not want involved with decisions about your care?
- How important is it to maintain your ability to be independent?
- If you need help with activities of daily living, whom would you turn to for help, and how would you feel about that?

Questions About the Person's Connections With Others

- What relationships are most important to you during this time?
- What role does religion or spirituality have in your life?
- Has your current health situation affected your relationships with others?
- Do you have concerns about the effects of your health on your relationships with others?
- Is there anything I can do to support your relationships with others during this time?

Questions for Families When the Person Cannot Make Independent Decisions

- What discussions have you had with _____ about health care decisions?
- What do you understand about the choices _____ would make if he or she were able to do so?
- What was important to _____ in terms of independence and quality of life?

was published in 1986. Recommendations of the study included the increased use of registered nurses, the use of standardized resident assessments, and the implementation of training and certification for nurse's aides. Subsequently, the Nursing Home Reform Act was included as part of the **Omnibus Budget Reconciliation Act (OBRA) of 1987**. This legislation has had far-reaching consequences, including increased emphasis on residents' rights and quality of life and major initiatives to improve quality of care (as discussed in Chapter 6). The provisions of OBRA that apply to nursing homes were developed through joint efforts of the health care professionals, the Health Care Financing Administration, the National Citizens Coalition for Nursing Home Reform, AARP, and representatives from the long-term care industry.

OBRA states that each resident in a long-term care facility is to be at his or her highest practicable level of physical, mental, and psychosocial well-being and that the long-term care facility is to accomplish this goal in an atmosphere that emphasizes residents' rights. To assist facilities in accomplishing this task, OBRA mandates that all Medicaid- and Medicare-funded facilities use a standardized form, known as the Minimum Data Set (MDS) for Resident Assessment and Care Planning, as described and discussed in Chapter 7. OBRA requires that within 14 days of admission, and at least annually thereafter, nursing facility staff perform a comprehensive, interdisciplinary assessment of every resident. Also, a care plan must be developed from that assessment,

with the goal of continually evaluating the resident's highest functional level and preventing any deterioration unless it is assessed and clearly documented as unavoidable. A primary responsibility of nurses is to ensure that the comprehensive assessment is performed at appropriate times. In addition, the nurse must ensure that the assessment tool is used as a basis for planning care that addresses the changing needs of the resident.

In addition to addressing the development and documentation of care plans in nursing homes, OBRA strengthened the government oversight of nursing homes and addressed the many issues related to quality of care, which had been a focus of consumer advocacy groups since the 1970s. Improvements in nursing home care that have been attributed to the enactment of OBRA include decreased use of indwelling catheters, decreased prevalence of dehydration and pressure ulcers, increased presence of geriatricians and nurse practitioners, and reduced use of physical restraints and psychotropic drugs.

The **Nursing Home Residents' Bill of Rights** is a component of OBRA that has had far-reaching consequences for nursing home staff and residents. Under this provision, federal law requires that all residents of long-term care facilities are informed of their rights and that all long-term care facilities must have a mechanism in place for addressing complaints if residents think that their rights have been compromised. Moreover, facilities must post the Residents' Bill of Rights and the resources for investigating complaints in a

Box 9-2   Caregiver Wellness: Information About Health Care Decisions

Advance Care Planning

Advance care planning is an ongoing process that involves learning about types of decisions related to health care, discussing these decisions with family members and health care providers, and making your wishes known in legal documents called advance directives.

Actions to Take if You are a Family Caregiver

- Recognize that it is imperative to engage in advance care planning before any questions arise about the person's ability to express his or her wishes related to health care decisions.
- Explore the resources listed below to obtain information and engage in interactive educational activities related to advance care planning.
- Initiate discussions about advance directives.
- Facilitate the process of preparing appropriate documents and make sure that a health care power of attorney is designated.

What are Advance Directives?

- *Advance directives* are legal documents that direct decisions about medical care that is provided or withheld.
- Common types of advance directives include living will, do-not-resuscitate orders, and durable health care power of attorney.
- The *health care power of attorney* (also called *proxy decision maker*) is extremely important because this gives authority for all health care decisions to a trusted surrogate; it is used only when someone is not able to express one's own wishes.
- A *living will*, *do-not-resuscitate order,* and other advance directive documents provide guidelines on which the durable power of attorney for health care can base decisions about treatments.
- Examples of medical care that are addressed in advance directives are cardiopulmonary resuscitation, ventilator use, artificial nutrition and hydration, and comfort care.

How are Advance Directives Prepared?

- Advance directives must be prepared when the person is competent to make decisions.

- It is best to prepare advance directives before the actual need arises.
- Because requirements for advance directives are determined by each state, legally recognized documents must be obtained from each person's state of residence.
- Appropriate forms and information about preparation of advance directives are readily available from the websites listed in the next section and from any health care institution.
- Although advance directives do not need to be notarized or drawn up by an attorney, if conflicts among family members are likely to arise, it may be advisable to seek legal advice.

What to do After Preparing Advance Directives

- Make sure that copies of all advance directives are readily available for health care providers and all those who will be involved with decision making (i.e., health care power of attorney).
- Periodically review the advance directives and update them when there are major changes in health status.
- Initially and periodically discuss the documents with anyone who will be involved with health care decisions.

Resources for Information About Health Care Decisions and Advance Care Planning

- AARP, www.aarp.org
- American Bar Association Commission on Law and Aging, www.americanbar.org
- Caring Connection, www.caringinfo.org
- Coalition to Transform Advanced Care, http://advancedcarecoalition.org
- Compassion and Support at the End of Life, www.compassionandsupport.org/index.php
- Family Caregiver Alliance, http://caregiver.org
- Health in Aging, www.healthinaging.org
- Helpguide, www.helpguide.org/elder/advance_directive_end_of_life_care.htm
- U.S. Living Will Registry, http://uslivingwill.com/

---

prominent place. According to this law, "the resident has a right to a dignified existence, self-determination, and communication with and access to persons and services inside and outside the facility" (Code of Federal Regulations, Title 42, Section 483.10). Box 9-3 lists some of the rights explicitly defined by this bill. The National Long-Term Care Ombudsman program was established under the Older American Act with the mandate to advocate for rights of residents of nursing homes, assisted living facilities, and board and care homes. The program also investigates complaints and provides information about quality of care in long-term care facilities. Local offices on aging in every part of the United States provide assistance with accessing these services.

ETHICAL ISSUES COMMONLY ADDRESSED IN GERONTOLOGICAL NURSING

Although ethical questions are often associated with major issues as already discussed, many daily care issues related to patients' values, preferences, and quality of life involve ethical dilemmas. These issues are omnipresent in health care settings, and they range from seemingly inconsequential concerns like being able to choose the time that meals are served to decisions about how to provide nutrition and hydration to people who are at risk for aspiration. As with all ethical questions, answers are more often in the "gray area" rather than being "black and white." This section first provides an overview of a nursing approach to addressing these issues and then discusses issues commonly encountered when caring for older adults.

Holistic Nursing Ethics

Principles underlying holistic nursing ethics, which emphasize the caring process when curing is not possible, are particularly appropriate in relation to gerontological nursing. Questions such as the following can guide nurses in holistic decision making about ethical issues (Burkhardt, 2016):

- Am I wise and courageous enough to perceive and respect others' differences and honor them as I honor my own beliefs?

Box 9-3 Some Rights of Nursing Home Residents

The Right to be Fully Informed

- The right to daily communication in their language
- The right to assistance if they have a sensory impairment
- The right to be notified in advance of any plans to change their room or roommate
- The right to be fully informed of all services available and the charge for each service

The Right to Participate in Their Own Care

- The right to receive adequate and appropriate care
- The right to participate in planning their treatment, care, and discharge
- The right to refuse medications, treatments, and physical and chemical restraints
- The right to review their own record

The Right to Make Independent Choices

- The right to make personal choices, such as what to wear and how to spend their time
- The right to reasonable accommodation of their needs and preferences
- The right to participate in activities, both inside and outside the nursing home
- The right to organize and participate in a resident council

The Right to Privacy and Confidentiality

- The right to private and unrestricted communication with any person
- The right to privacy in treatment and in personal care activities

- The right to confidentiality regarding their medical, personal, or financial affairs

The Right to Dignity, Respect, and Freedom

- The right to be treated with the fullest measure of consideration, respect, and dignity
- The right to be free from mental and physical abuse
- The right to self-determination

The Right to Security of Possessions

- The right to manage their own financial affairs
- The right to be free from charge for services covered by Medicaid or Medicare

Rights During Transfers and Discharges

- The right to remain in the facility unless a transfer or discharge is necessary, appropriate, or required
- The right to receive a 30-day notice of transfer or discharge

The Right to Complain

- The right to present grievances without fear of reprisal
- The right to prompt efforts by the nursing home to resolve grievances

The Right to Visits

- The right to immediate access by their relatives
- The right to reasonable visits by organizations or individuals providing health, social, legal, or other services

Adapted from the U.S. Code of Federal Regulations, Title 42, Section 483.10.

- What does the patient want?
- Does the patient understand his or her choices?
- Is the patient being coerced?
- What does quality of life mean for this patient?
- How are others responding to the patient's perceptions of quality of life?
- Does having the technology always mean it should be used?

Although answers to these questions may not be evident, a process of values clarification can be used to guide nurses in ethical decision making. **Values clarification** is an ongoing process in which an individual becomes increasingly aware of what is important and just—and why (Burkhardt, 2016). Burkhardt (2016) suggests the following ways in which nurses can facilitate this process for patients: (1) listen carefully and reflect back so the patient clarifies what is personally important and (2) list several health behaviors or values, such as health, happiness, independence, and good relationships, and ask patients to rank them or identify how they incorporate them into their lives.

Decisions About the Use of Restraints

Since the late 1990s, governmental and health care organizations have addressed the use of physical restraints as a major ethical issue that is relevant to older adults in acute and long-term care settings. A **physical restraint** is defined as "any action or procedure that prevents a person's free body movement to a position of choice and/or normal access to his or her body by the use of any method, attached or adjacent to a person's body that he or she cannot control or remove easily" (Bleijlevens, Wagner, Capezuti, et al., 2016). Examples of physical restraints are belts, hand mitts, soft wrist or leg restraints, certain types of chairs, and full side rails in certain circumstances. In recent years, the use of physical restraints is an indicator of quality of care in institutional settings, and health care organizations are initiating major initiatives to limit or eliminate the use of any restrictive devices that infringe upon patient rights.

Although restraints have been used for decades presumably to protect patients from harm, studies find that these measures are associated with serious harm including increased risks for fractures, delirium, soft tissue injury, and even death (Bradas, Sandhu, & Mion, 2016; Lach, Leach, & Butcher, 2016). Increasingly, physical restraints are viewed as an ethical issue related to preservation of autonomy and dignity versus patient safety and protection. Reducing the use of restraints for older adults requires a nurse-driven and multicomponent intervention that includes institutional policy change, staff education, legal support, and practical support (e.g., availability of alternative interventions) (Kong, Choi, & Evans, 2017; Lach, Leach, & Butcher, 2016). Alternatives to physical restraints are addressed in Chapter 14 on delirium and Chapter 22 on fall prevention.

See ONLINE LEARNING ACTIVITY 9-4: EVIDENCE-BASED INFORMATION AND CASE STUDY ABOUT PHYSICAL RESTRAINTS at http://thepoint.lww.com/Miller8e.

Issues Related to Artificial Nutrition and Hydration

Nurses frequently address ethical issues about artificial nutrition and hydration when they care for older adults who have poor nutritional intake or limited ability to chew and swallow. **Artificial nutrition and hydration (ANH)** refers to methods of bypassing the upper gastrointestinal tract to deliver nutritional substances. A percutaneous endoscopic gastrostomy (PEG) tube (sometimes referred to as a "feeding tube" or "tube feeding") is a surgically inserted tube that is used to deliver nutrients directly to the stomach. In addition to PEG tubes, methods of ANH include jejunostomy tubes, nasogastric tubes, hypodermoclysis through the subcutaneous tissue, and total parenteral nutrition delivered through a central or peripheral vein.

In recent years, ANH has become widely used as a life-sustaining treatment that is considered for patients who cannot meet their nutritional needs by mouth or for people with conditions that gradually affect their ability to chew and swallow safely. Because PEG tubes are considered in a variety of circumstances, many studies have addressed safety, efficacy, and outcome issues associated with this commonly used intervention. In particular, concerns have been raised about the use of PEG tubes as an intervention for people who have advanced dementia.

Discussions about ANH are often initiated because the person is losing weight or requires considerable and time-consuming assistance with feeding. Another reason these issues arise is because families and caregivers may have unrealistically optimistic expectations about benefits of a feeding tube. Also, families sometimes receive well-intentioned but not evidence-based information about potential benefits of ANH. In all these situations, nurses are responsible for providing up-to-date and evidence-based information about the advantages and disadvantages of ANH. Fortunately, a strong foundation of evidence-based information is now available in position statements of major organizations including the American Nurses Association (2011), the Hospice and Palliative Nurses Association (2011), and the American Geriatrics Society (2014). Current scientific evidence on which these position statements are based concludes that ANH in advanced dementia is not beneficial (i.e., it does not prolong life or prevent suffering) and treatment burdens outweigh any potential benefits (Ayman, Khoury, Cohen, et al., 2017). The concept of "comfort feeding only" (i.e., patients should be fed only as long as it is comfortable for them to eat) is the recommended approach to address nutritional needs during late-stage dementia (Smith & Ferguson, 2017). Information in Box 9-4 can be used as an evidence-based guide to decisions about ANH and alternative methods of meeting nutritional needs.

Even with the broad base of currently available information, however, decisions related to ANH are complex and emotional for families, caregivers, and professionals. Conflicts often arise between the previously expressed wishes of the person with advanced dementia and the wishes of the family who are involved with decisions. In many situations, the person with dementia has expressed the desire to forego ANH; however, the surrogate decision makers express a desire to allow the insertion of a PEG tube (Somers, Grey, & Satkoske, 2016). One way of addressing the complexity of this issue is to encourage families to use a "decision aid," such as the interactive tool on Making Your Wishes Known (described in Online Learning Activity 9-3).

An important nursing responsibility is to involve other team members in decisions and care plans related to meeting nutritional needs of people who have difficulty with oral intake. Speech-language therapists are a major resource for evaluating and advising about the safest and most effective way of providing nutrients by mouth. Registered dietitians are another resource because they make recommendations on providing, withdrawing, or withholding nutrition for individual situations and they also serve as active members of institutional ethics committees.

See ONLINE LEARNING ACTIVITY 9-5: ADDITIONAL INFORMATION RELATED TO DECISIONS ABOUT MEETING NUTRITIONAL NEEDS OF OLDER ADULTS at http://thepoint.lww.com/Miller8e.

Issues Specific to Long-Term Care Settings

The increasing attention to quality of care in long-term care settings in recent years has led to more emphasis on autonomy, individual rights, and quality of life for residents (as discussed in Chapter 6). Ethical issues are often associated with this approach because it is not always easy to balance needs of individual residents with those of others and the institution itself. Ethical issues are also associated with questions about safety versus freedom. For example, conflicts arise when a resident with a history of falls desires to walk freely around the facility, but staff members want to limit that person's activity. Additional examples of ethical decisions that nurses in long-term care settings commonly address are as follows:

- Using restrictive measures to address potential risks to safety (as already discussed)
- Restricting cigarette smoking
- Allowing residents to refuse therapies, social activities, and food or fluid
- Providing more care assistance than necessary because it is more time-efficient for the staff

Box 9-4 Evidence-Based Practice: Key Points About Artificial Nutrition and Hydration (ANH)

Evidence-Based Recommendations Related to the Use of ANH

- The preponderance of evidence *does not support* the effectiveness of ANH in people with advanced dementia or other serious progressive conditions.
- ANH can be beneficial for patients with a potentially reversible condition or with mechanical blockage of the upper gastrointestinal tract.
- Numerous studies have shown that tube feeding in patients with serious progressive conditions does not prolong life and in fact is associated with increased risk of mortality, medical complications (including increased risk for infections), fluid overload, and skin excoriation around the tube.
- ANH does *not* protect against aspiration, and in some patient populations may increase the risk of aspiration and its complications.
- Contrary to common beliefs, ANH is associated with an increased risk of developing new pressure ulcers and slower rate of healing for existing pressure ulcers.
- Patient outcomes, such as weight gain, increased caloric intake, or improved laboratory values, are not adequate reasons for ANH in the absence of improved overall well-being.
- Patients with advanced illness often experience a loss of interest in eating and drinking and some may experience dysphagia; at some point most patients with advanced illness will refuse food.
- Families and caregivers fear that undernourished patients experience hunger and other troublesome symptoms; however, studies show that most actively dying patients do not experience hunger even if they have poor intake.
- Terminally ill patients may experience thirst or dry mouth, but these symptoms are associated with factors other than fluid intake, so ANH is unlikely to alleviate that.

Issues Related to Decisions About ANH

- ANH is a medical therapy that can be declined or accepted by the patient's surrogate decision maker in accordance with advance directives or other indicators of the patient's wishes.

- Decisions to initiate, withhold, or withdraw ANH are made by the patient and family with accurate and nonjudgmental input from the health care team.
- ANH is incorporated into the patient's plan only when medically appropriate and consistent with the patient's beliefs.
- Health care providers are responsible for promoting choices, endorsing shared and informed decision making, and honoring patient preferences.
- Perspectives of the patient, family, and surrogate decision makers should be assessed with cultural sensitivity by an interdisciplinary team.

Evidence-Based Recommendations Related to Care

- Nurses and all members of the health care team are responsible for understanding and implementing a care plan that is consistent with the previously expressed wishes of the patient.
- Primary responsibilities of nurses include teaching about evidence-based information related to ANH, supporting surrogate decision makers, promoting the use of advance directives, and facilitating early discussions about goals of care and treatment choices.
- Usual care of people with advanced dementia should include efforts to enhance oral feeding by altering the environment and creating patient-centered approaches to feeding.
- Food and water offered to patients by mouth is the usual means of providing nutrition and hydration to patients.
- Good oral care, ice chips, and moistening the mouth are interventions that are likely to relieve thirst.

Source: American Geriatrics Society. (2014). American Geriatrics Society feeding tubes in advanced dementia position statement. *Journal of the American Geriatrics Society, 62,* 1590–1593; American Nurses Association. (2011). Position statement on forgoing nutrition and hydration. Available at www.ana.org; Hospice and Palliative Nurses Association. (2011). *HPNA position statement: Artificial nutrition and hydration in advanced illness.* Available at www.hpna.org

---

- Scheduling resident care practices for the convenience of the staff rather than according to individual preferences
- Accommodating residents who wish to express sexual interests and activities

Long-term care settings address these ethical issues by establishing policies and procedures that are based on best practices. An important nursing responsibility is to involve residents and their surrogate decision makers in developing a plan that is safe, individualized, respectful of the person's preferences, and appropriate for addressing everyday ethical issues.

CULTURAL ASPECTS OF ETHICAL ISSUES

Religious teachings and other cultural factors have a strong influence on ethical issues, particularly with regard to advance directives and decisions about ANH and end-of-life care. Because cultural factors influence health care providers as well as their patients/clients, examining one's own biases and assuring culturally competent care (as discussed in Chapter 2) is especially important when addressing ethical

issues. A major issue is that legal requirements related to advance directives are strongly biased toward Anglocentric cultures, with emphasis on individual autonomy. This is in stark contrast to cultural groups, such as Chinese Americans and Latin Americans, that value family-centered decision making or other approaches to health care decisions (Rising, 2017). For example, some families may believe that it is a sign of respect to protect an elder from the burdens of receiving information about his or her health status, or from making decisions about medical interventions and long-term care plans. This attitude may be in conflict with that of health care professionals who believe that all competent adults are entitled to information about their own health. Thus, nurses need to identify and accept individual and family decision-making preferences when they discuss advance directives and other aspects of health care decisions.

Another major area of concern in the United States is the need to accommodate people who do not speak English. Language barriers can significantly increase the difficulty of understanding advance directives and participating in complex decisions about treatment and other aspects of care. Even when advance directives are available in the person's primary language, it is difficult to communicate the intent of these documents when there are conflicting cultural views on decisions about health care choices. Interventions to address language barriers are discussed in Chapter 2. Nurses also can use the *Five Wishes* document, which is available in more than 27 languages, as a base for discussing advance directives.

The importance of applying principles of cultural competency to all legal and ethical aspects of nursing care cannot be overemphasized, nor is this a simple process. Box 9-5 describes characteristics of some cultural groups that potentially influence legal and ethical issues related to care of older adults in the United States. This information is not intended to promote stereotypes, rather it is meant as a brief guide to culturally based beliefs that should be considered when developing care plans. In all situations, it is imperative to use excellent communication skills to nonjudgmentally assess and discuss issues related to health care decisions (see Chapter 2 for a guide to culturally sensitive communication).

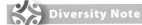 **Diversity Note**

African Americans, Asian Americans, and other minority populations are less likely than White Americans to engage in advance care planning, nor do they view advance directives as relevant (Post & Boltz, 2016a; Sun, Bui, Tsoh, et al., 2017).

 Box 9-5 Cultural Considerations: Legal and Ethical Aspects of Care

Cultural Factors That Influence Ethical Decision Making

- The intent of advance directives is based on Western values of individual autonomy, but many cultures believe that the fate of human beings is beyond their control.
- Values of filial piety and respect for authority of one's elders—rather than the model of individual autonomy—guide decisions about care in traditional Asian cultures.
- In collectivist cultures (e.g., the Xhosa tribe in South Africa), tribal elders make decisions about care of their members, based on distribution of human and material resources.
- Traditional Chinese and many other cultures rely on family members and their physicians to make decisions, rather than expecting to receive information and being involved in decision making.
- Ethnoreligious groups, including Jews, Muslims, and Hindus, are likely to base end-of-life decisions on their beliefs on the sanctity of life.
- Religious beliefs may take precedence over scientific reasoning (e.g., opposition of blood transfusions as a life-saving measure by members of Jehovah's Witnesses).
- Some groups may prefer their own religious and spiritually based healing practices to those of scientific medicine (e.g., Christian scientists).

Cultural Considerations Related to Ethical and Legal Issues in Specific Groups

- *African Americans:* It is important to include women and extended family members in decision making and dissemination of health information.
- *Amish:* Grandparents and other extended family are involved with health care decisions, which are based on consideration of the type of health problem, accessibility of health care services, and perceived cost of the care.
- *Appalachian:* Individuals may abdicate self-responsibility for decision making and prefer that physicians take charge of their care completely.
- *Arab:* Older males assume decision-making roles; most patients expect physicians to select treatments.
- *Chinese:* Each family has a recognized male head who has great authority and assumes all major responsibilities.
- *Cuban:* Traditional patriarchal family structure is the most important social unit and the primary spokesperson needs to be involved in decision making.
- *European American:* There is great variation among families, but high value is generally placed on egalitarian relationships and decision making; advance directives allow patients to specify their wishes and designate a decision maker.
- *Filipino:* Because planning for one's death is taboo, many are adverse to discussing advance directives or living wills.
- *German:* Extended family should be included in decision making.
- *Greek:* Older people hold positions of respect; extended nuclear family members should be included in decision making.
- *Haitian:* The family council, composed of influential family members, is an important unit for decision making.
- *Hindu:* The patriarchal joint family, based on the principle of superiority of men over women, is the primary authority for decisions.
- *Hmong:* Traditional decision making requires that the male head of the family or clan make decisions for family members; individuals do not have the right to make their own decisions about health care.
- *Iranian:* The father and/or older male siblings have authority to make decisions for family.
- *Irish:* Families make end-of-life decisions and these are usually influenced by all the following: their definition of extraordinary means, financial considerations, quality of life, and effects on the family.
- *Italian:* Traditional families recognize the father's absolute authority and they accept his decisions as law.
- *Japanese:* Discussion of serious illness and death is taboo, so it is difficult to obtain information.
- *Jewish:* Rabbis may be included in making decisions about health care (e.g., organ donation or transplant).
- *Korean:* Older adults are frequently consulted on important family matters as a sign of respect for their experience.
- *Mexican:* Families are not necessarily patriarchal, but men are expected to be the spokesperson for the family, so it is important to ask who makes which decisions.
- *Puerto Rican:* Adults, especially women, may prefer to consult with close family members before making health care decisions.
- *Russian:* It is important to ask clients whom they want to include in medical decisions because extended family is very important.
- *Somali:* Discussing advance directives and end-of-life care is taboo because faithful Muslims believe that Allah will determine how long a person will live; thus, these issues should be addressed indirectly.
- *Turkish:* Traditional families are patriarchal but less traditional ones are more egalitarian, so it is important to identify the family spokesperson and accept decision-making patterns without judgment.
- *Vietnamese:* Women often make family health care decisions.

Source: Purnell, L. D. (2013). *Transcultural health care: A culturally competent approach* (4th ed.). Philadelphia, PA: F. A. Davis Co.

A Student's Perspective

In working with "G.," an 82-year-old Chinese woman, I have learned a lot about her background. She and her three brothers, two sisters, and parents were all born in China. Her parents moved the children to Jakarta, a city in Indonesia, which was a Dutch colony at the time, to get a better education. Chinese culture emphasizes respect for elders, especially the father, who is head of the family. G. giggles and comments, "When father said 'eat that,' we ate it, whether we liked it or not." As an adult, she worked for a time in the front lobby of the U.S. embassy as a translator. Her position led her on many journeys throughout the world, working in Russia, Germany, France, and eventually to the United States. G. didn't marry until she was 70, when she married an American. She now lives in a quiet neighborhood with her husband.

A difficulty in learning more about G. and her culture regarding health care has been her acceptance of her disease process. Her cultural background taught her to view authority figures, such as physicians, with incredible esteem. Until I learned more about her culture, I wasn't always certain she understood what was being said because she would sit with her head down and only nod, or simply say, "yes." I now realize those behaviors are her way of showing respect to an authority figure. She seldom looks you in the eye, another form of showing respect. She is also hesitant to ask questions so as not to appear disrespectful. G. looks to her husband many times to make decisions for her.

Deborah L.

ROLES OF NURSES REGARDING LEGAL AND ETHICAL ISSUES

Nurses have important roles with regard to implementing advance directives and facilitating decisions about care. Although these issues are often addressed within the context of a multidisciplinary team and always with the primary care practitioner, nurses have unique and important responsibilities. Responsibilities related to facilitating decisions about care and promoting caregiver wellness are discussed in this section. Chapter 29 discusses roles of nurses related to legal and ethical considerations about care at the end of life.

Facilitating Decisions About Care

Nurses play key roles not only in implementing advance directives but also in working with family members and other caregivers who are involved with making decisions related to care and treatment issues. Advance directives designate surrogate decision makers, but the surrogates do not always have a good understanding of the person's wishes, and this can be a barrier to appropriate implementation. Nurses facilitate these discussions by providing accurate information on rights and statutes, addressing questions about care options, listening to the needs and concerns of all involved, attending to concerns about treatment options and end-of-life care, and acting as liaisons with primary care providers when necessary.

As discussed previously, decisions about care are particularly complicated when working with older adults who have cognitive impairments. Evidence-based guidelines for nurses summarize the following nursing care strategies for health care decision making (Post & Boltz, 2016b):

1. Communicate with patient, family, and surrogate decision makers to enhance their understanding of treatment options.
2. Be sensitive to racial, ethnic, religious, and cultural influences with regard to care decisions, disclosure of information, and end-of-life planning.
3. Be aware of available resources for conflict resolution.
4. Observe, document, and report the patient's ability to state preferences, follow directions, make simple choices, and communicate consistent care wishes.
5. Observe and document fluctuations in patient's mental status and factors that affect it.
6. Assess the patient's understanding specifically in relation to a particular decision (e.g., ask what the patient understands about the risks and benefits of the intervention).
7. Use appropriate decision aids.
8. Help the patient express what he or she understands about the clinical situation and the potential outcomes.
9. Help the patient identify who should participate in discussions and decisions.

Another important role of nurses is to involve other professionals and support resources when complex decisions must be made or when the decision makers seek additional help. In some settings, an interdisciplinary team—composed of a social worker, a religious leader, therapists, nurses, and a primary care provider—may provide information and support to proxy decision makers. Decision-making assistance from professionals may relieve families and proxy decision makers of some of the guilt they could experience when making and implementing decisions, particularly difficult end-of-life decisions. Hospitals and long-term care facilities that are accredited by the Joint Commission (formerly the Joint Commission on Accreditation of Healthcare Organizations [JCAHO]) are required to have ethics committees that provide a formal mechanism for addressing medical ethical dilemmas within their institutions.

Nurses in intensive care units often address issues related to surrogate decision making for patients who are unable to communicate their wishes about medical interventions. These situations require interprofessional collaboration with major roles for nurses, for example, through nurse-led family meetings that include the following nursing actions:

- Prior to the meeting: ask the family to bring documents related to advance care planning to the meeting; instruct the family to prepare any questions or concerns; arrange for privacy
- During the meeting: assess the family's understanding of the patient's condition; review the patient's condition, focusing on the big picture; assess family member's understanding

---

Box 9-6 Model for Facilitating Decisions About the Care of People With Dementia

Step I: Assess the Decision-Making Situation

- What is the decision-making ability of the person with dementia?
- What are the typical decision-making patterns in the family?
- Who influences the decision making, either directly or indirectly?
- How do family relationships help or hinder the decision-making process?
- Are there patterns of passive nondecisions as well as active decisions?
- What is each person's perception of the situation?
- How objective are the perceptions of the various decision makers?
- What does each person in the decision-making process have to gain or lose based on various decisions?

Step II: Obtain Consensus About Problems and Needs

- Have each person involved with the care describe the problems and needs from their perspective.
- Provide additional assessment information about the needs of the person with dementia.
- Address the needs of the caregivers as well as the needs of the person with dementia.
- Summarize the identified needs of the older adult and the caregivers.

Step III: Discuss Potential Resources

- Ask caregivers to suggest potential solutions and resources.
- Identify resources for the caregivers' needs as well as for those of the person with dementia.
- Supplement the family's knowledge about resources and potential solutions.
- Discuss the positive and negative consequences of each option for the person with dementia and for the caregivers.

- As the family members discuss solutions, assess their attitudes about using various services and spending family resources to purchase services.
- Provide information about the long-range benefits that the caregivers might not perceive.
- Summarize important points on paper or a blackboard for all participants to review.

Step IV: Agree on a Plan of Action

- Obtain agreement about the most appropriate actions to take.
- Emphasize the fact that any plan of action will be given a trial period and should not be viewed as a permanent decision.
- Suggest a time frame and criteria for evaluating the plan of action.
- Identify one or two people who will evaluate the plan and make appropriate changes.

Step V: Involve the Person With Dementia

- Discuss the ability of the person with dementia to understand the decision.
- Identify the most realistic level of involvement for the person with dementia.
- Identify the best approach to take in involving the person with dementia.
- Identify the roles of caregivers and professionals in assisting the person with dementia to understand the decision.

Step VI: Summarize the Plan and Clarify Roles

- Review and summarize the plan of action.
- Have the caregivers state their roles in very specific terms.
- Clarify the role of the nurse and other professionals.
- Assure caregivers that you will be available for further discussion and problem solving, or provide the name of someone who can assume this role.

---

of what was discussed; answer questions; explain medical terms; help family understand what to expect; discuss patient's values, goals, wishes, and care preferences

- After the meeting: document summary of meeting; communicate with other health care team members; arrange follow-up with other health care team members; conduct on-going assessment of family and patient

(Wu, Ren, Zinsmeister, et al., 2016).

Nurses also take a strong role in supporting and facilitating decisions about care during chronic conditions and end-of-life care. In particular, nurses provide information about the best types of services (e.g., hospice programs, palliative care) or place of care (e.g., hospital admission for nursing home residents when medical problems arise). Box 9-6 summarizes a nursing model for facilitating decisions about long-term care for people with dementia.

Promoting Caregiver Wellness

As discussed previously, decisions about medical treatments are usually stressful and complex, not only for the older adult but also for families and caregivers. Stress is magnified when caregivers are responsible for decisions—including decisions that shorten life expectancy—with little

or no input from the older adult. For example, when an older person is cognitively impaired and the surrogate decision makers have not previously discussed the care alternatives, the caregiver's stress is compounded by feelings of guilt and uncertainty. Similarly, stress is magnified when family decision makers (e.g., siblings, spouses, in-laws) have differing perspectives or hold conflicting values about treatments. In all situations, nurses are the health care professionals who assume key support roles for caregivers, including teaching and advocacy. In addition to applying information in this chapter (e.g., online learning activities, communication strategies in Box 9-1), Box 9-2 can be used to teach caregivers about health care decision making; it includes a list of helpful resources that caregivers can be encouraged to explore for additional information.

Chapter Highlights

Autonomy and Rights

- Autonomy is the personal freedom to direct one's own life as long as it does not infringe on the rights of others.
- Adults are presumed to be competent and have the right to make health-related decisions unless they have been declared incompetent by a judge.

- Decision-making capacity describes one's ability to understand and process information, weigh alternatives, apply personal values, arrive at a decision, and communicate that decision to others.
- If an adult's decision-making capacity is questionable or compromised, his or her rights can be protected through legal documents, such as advance directives.

Advance Directives

- Advance directives (e.g., durable power of attorney for health care, DNR orders, living wills) are legal documents that make a person's wishes about medical treatments known to care providers and surrogate decision makers.
- Legal requirements for advance directives are specified in state laws.
- Advance directives must be drawn up when a person is competent and they need to be available when questions arise about the person's wishes.
- Nurses have essential roles in teaching older adults and their caregivers about advance directives and respecting each person's values related to health care decisions.

Advance Care Planning

- Advance care planning is an ongoing process designed to ensure that medical care is consistent with an individual's values, goals, and preferences.
- Nurses have crucial roles in talking with older adults about advance care planning (Box 9-1).
- Nurses can teach caregivers about advance care planning (Box 9-2).

Legal Issues Specific to Long-Term Care Settings

- Federal legislation enacted in the 1980s requires nursing homes to meet certain standards of care, to perform and document assessments, and to implement interdisciplinary care plans that comprehensively address residents' needs.
- The Nursing Home Bill of Rights states that residents are entitled to dignity, self-determination, and the opportunity to communicate (Box 9-3).

Ethical Issues Commonly Addressed in Gerontological Nursing

- Values clarification is a process that can be applied when addressing ethical issues in everyday care of older adults.
- Decisions about use of restraints are complex and must be based on evidence-based guidelines.
- ANH is a life-sustaining intervention that involves complex ethical issues (Box 9-4).

Cultural Aspects of Legal and Ethical Issues

- Language barriers and cultural influences are important to consider when discussing advance directives.
- Nurses should identify culturally influenced patterns of decision making when discussing advance directives and end-of-life care with patients and their families (Box 9-5).

Roles of Nurses Regarding Legal and Ethical Issues

- Nurses facilitate decision making about advance directives by providing information about advance directives and care options to older adults and to proxy decision makers. Nurses facilitate decisions about care of people with dementia by using the model in Box 9-6.

Critical Thinking Exercises

1. You have been assigned to work with Mrs. M., an 85-year-old, white, widowed woman who is in the hospital with heart failure. Her son and daughter tell you that they would like to arrange for her to be discharged to a nursing home because they don't think she takes her medications correctly, and they are tired of her being admitted to the hospital every couple of months "to get her straightened out." The son and daughter live in another state and visit only when their mother is in the hospital. Mrs. M. has told you that she thinks her son and daughter would like to have her "put away in one of those homes" but she is adamantly opposed to leaving her home. She also has told you that they think she is "senile" and that she should stop driving her car, but she thinks she is quite capable of living alone, driving her car, and taking care of herself. Your observations are that she needs a lot of direction to take medications and participate in self-care activities, and she seems to be somewhat confused later in the day. What steps would you take to address her competency and decision-making abilities?

2. A 78-year-old Mexican American woman is being admitted to the hospital with hemiplegia after a stroke. There are no advance directives on her chart. What information would you want to know before you approached her about a living will and durable power of attorney for health care? How would you explain these documents to her?

3. Mr. S. is 78 years old and has been admitted for hip surgery after a fall-related fracture. He has had dementia for 5 years and his family provides care for him in his home. His son is his durable power of attorney for health care, but he will not make any decisions unless his three sisters agree to them. Mr. S. does not have any other advance directives and the family says he never talked much about what medical care services he would want. He always told his family that they could make whatever decisions are best for him. The physician has asked the family to consider placement of a PEG tube because Mr. S.'s food and fluid intake are inadequate to meet his needs and one pressure area is beginning to develop on his buttocks. Mr. S.'s son and one daughter think that their father would have wanted to have every intervention possible in such a situation, and they think the PEG tube will improve his comfort and prevent the pressure ulcer. The other two daughters adamantly state that their father would never agree to such an invasive procedure and they are not sure it will make him any more comfortable. They also

worry about complications from having the tube. You are a member of the multidisciplinary team that is meeting with the family to help them come to a decision about a PEG tube. What points would you want to make during this family conference?

 For more information about the topics discussed in this chapter, be sure to check out the interactive Online Learning Activities and other helpful resources at http://thepoint.lww.com/Miller8e.

REFERENCES

Aging with Dignity. (2017). *Five wishes in my state.* Available at http://agingwithdignity.org

American Geriatrics Society. (2014). American Geriatrics Society feeding tubes in advanced dementia position statement. *Journal of the American Geriatrics Society, 62,* 1590–1593.

American Nurses Association. (2011). *Position statement on forgoing nutrition and hydration.* Available at www.ana.org

American Nurses Association. (2015). *Code of ethics for nurses with interpretive statements.* Silver Spring, MD: American Nurses Association.

Ayman, R. A., Khoury, T., Cohen, J., et al. (2017). PEG insertion in patients with dementia does not improve nutritional status and has worse outcomes as compared with PEG insertion for other indications. *Journal of Clinical Gastroenterology, 51,* 417–420.

Bleijlevens, M. H., Wagner, L. M., Capezuti, E., et al. (2016). Physical restraints: Consensus of a research definition using a modified Delphi technique. *Journal of the American Geriatrics Society, 64,* 2307–2310.

Bradas, C. M., Sandhu, S. K., & Mion, L. C. (2016). Physical restraints and side rails in acute and critical care settings. In M. Boltz, E. Capezuti, T. Fulmer, & D. Zwicker (Eds.). *Evidence-based practice protocols for best practice* (5th ed., pp. 381–394). New York: Springer Publishing Co.

Bravo, G., Trottier, L., Ancand, M., et al. (2016). Promoting advance care planning among community-based older adults: A randomized controlled trial. *Patient Education and Counseling, 99,* 1785–1795.

Burkhardt, M. A. (2016). Holistic ethics. In B. M. Dossey & L. Keegan (Eds.). *Holistic nursing: A handbook for practice* (7th ed., pp. 121–134). Boston, MA: Jones & Bartlett Publishers.

Fairlie, D. E. (2017). Specific words and experience matter to surrogates when making end of life decisions. *Health Communications.* doi: 10.1080/10410236.2017.1283560.

Fetherstonbaugh, D., McAuliffe, L., Bauer, M., et al. (2017). Decision-making on behalf of people living with dementia: How do surrogate decision-makers decide? *Journal of Medical Ethics, 43,* 35–40.

Hickman, S. E., Hammes, B. J., Torke, A. M., et al. (2017). The quality of physician orders for life-sustaining treatment decisions: A pilot study. *Journal of Palliative Medicine, 20,* 255–262.

Hospice and Palliative Nurses Association. (2011). *HPNA position statement: Artificial nutrition and hydration in advanced illness.* Available at www.hpna.org

Kendra, A., Rubin, E., & Halpern, S. (2016). The problem with physician orders for life-sustaining treatment. *Journal of the American Medical Association, 315,* 259–260.

Ko, E., Lee, J., & Hong, Y. (2016). Willingness to complete advance directives among low-income older adults living in the USA. *Health and Social Care in the Community, 24,* 708–716.

Kong, E. H., Choi, H., & Evans, L. K. (2017). Staff perceptions of barriers to physical restraint-reduction in long-term care: A meta-analysis. *Journal of Clinical Nursing, 26,* 49–60.

Lach, H., Leach, K., & Butcher, H. (2016). Evidence-based practice guideline: Changing the practice of physical restraint use in acute care. *Journal of Gerontological Nursing, 42*(2), 17–25.

Levin, T. T., & Coyle, N. (2015). A communication training perspective on AND versus DNR directives. *Palliative and Supportive Care, 13,* 385–387.

Markham, S. A., Levi, B. H., Green, M. J., et al. (2015). Use of a computer program for advance care planning with African American participants. *Journal of the National Medical Association, 107,* 26–32.

Nedjat-Haiem, F. R., Carrion, I. V., Gonzalez, K., et al. (2017). Exploring health care providers' views about initiating end-of-life care communication. *American Journal of Hospice and Palliative Care, 34,* 308–317.

Post, L. F., & Boltz, M. (2016a). Advance care planning. In M. Boltz, E. Capezuti, T. Fulmer, & D. Zwicker (Eds.). *Evidence-based practice protocols for best practice* (5th ed., pp. 691–709). New York: Springer Publishing Co.

Post, L. F., & Boltz, M. (2016b). Health care decision making. In M. Boltz, E. Capezuti, T. Fulmer, & D. Zwicker (Eds.). *Evidence-based practice protocols for best practice* (5th ed., pp. 43–56). New York: Springer Publishing Co.

Prince-Paul, M., & DiFranco, E. (2017). Upstreaming and normalizing advance care planning conversations – A public health approach. *Behavioral Sciences,* doi: 10.3390/bs7020018.

Rahman, A. N., Bressette, M., & Enguidanos, S. (2017). Quality of physician orders for life-sustaining treatment forms completed in nursing homes. *Journal of Palliative Medicine, 20,* 538–541.

Rising, M. (2017). Truth telling as an element of culturally competent care at the end of life. *Journal of Transcultural Nursing, 28,* 48–55.

Smith, L., & Ferguson, R. (2017). Artificial nutrition and hydration in people with late-stage dementia. *Home Healthcare Now, 35,* 321–325.

Somers, E., Grey, C., & Satkowske, V. (2016). Withholding versus withdrawing treatment: Artificial nutrition and hydration as a model. *Current Opinion in Supportive and Palliative Care, 10,* 208–213.

Splendore, E., & Grant, C. (2017). A nurse practitioner-led community workshop: Increasing adult participation in advance care planning. *Journal of the American Association of Nurse Practitioners,* [Epub] doi: 10.1002/2327–6924.

Sudore, R. L., Boscardin, J., Feuz, M. A., et al. (2017). Effect of PREPARE website vs an easy-to-read advance directive on advance care planning documentation and engagement among veterans: A randomized clinical trial. *Journal of the American Medical Association Internal Medicine,* [Epub] doi: 10.1001/jajainternmed.2017.1607.

Sudore, R. L., Lum, H. D., You, J. J., et al. (2017). Defining advance care planning for adults: A consensus definition from a multidisciplinary Delphi panel. *Journal of Pain and Symptom Management, 53,* 821–832.

Sun, A., Bui, Q., Tsoh, J. Y., et al. (2017). Efficacy of a church-based, culturally tailored program to promote completion of advance directives among Asian Americans. *Journal of Immigrant and Minority Health, 19,* 381–391.

Wu, H., Ren, D., Zinsmeister, G., et al. (2016). Implementation of a nurse-led family meeting in a neuroscience intensive care unit. *Dimensions of Critical Care Nursing, 35*(5), 268–276.

chapter 10

Elder Abuse and Neglect

Elder abuse and neglect is one of the most complex and serious functional consequences that affects vulnerable older adults—and one of the most challenging aspects of gerontological nursing. Situations of elder abuse and neglect require an interdisciplinary approach, with nurses assuming essential roles in preventing, detecting, reporting, assessing, and intervening in situations that are actually or potentially abusive. This chapter presents the topic with emphasis on the key roles of nurses in addressing this complex issue.

OVERVIEW OF ELDER ABUSE AND NEGLECT

Certain members of any population are vulnerable to abuse and neglect by virtue of being physically or psychosocially impaired or subjugated. In industrialized societies today, vulnerable groups are protected and cared for through legislative mandates and social programs. In the United States and many other countries, for example, children and people with developmental disabilities have been protected for many decades. In recent decades, additional groups have been recognized as needing protection: victims of domestic violence and abused or neglected older people. Although abuse or neglect of older adults is not new, in recent years elder abuse has received increased recognition and attention as a social problem, crime, and major health care concern.

Definitions and Forms of Elder Abuse

Definitions of elder abuse have changed over time in response to shifts in political climate, public sentiment, available funding, and increased knowledge and professional interest. The terms *elder abuse* and *elder mistreatment* are often used interchangeably and without clear distinctions. Currently, there is a significant lack of consensus on the meaning of elder abuse among experts and an even greater gap in concept understanding between experts and the general public (Volmert & Lindland, 2016). The Administration on Aging defines elder abuse as "any knowing, intention, or negligent act that causes harm or a serious risk of harm to a vulnerable older adult." Box 10-1 identifies seven types of elder abuse as they are defined by the Administration on Aging.

Definitions proposed by professionals and scholars may differ from the ways in which older adults themselves perceive and define elder abuse. Studies have found that older adults view elder abuse on both a personal and societal level and associate it with ageism, family breakdown, power and control imbalances, and the marginalized social position of older adults (Killick, Taylor, Begley, et al., 2015; Mysyuk, Westendorp, & Lindenberg, 2016). In addition, older adults often define elder abuse in terms of violation of their rights.

For example, issues identified as abusive by older adults but rarely addressed by professionals or researchers include lack of privacy, unnecessary loss of independence, being treated like a child, lack of control over their own affairs, and being forced to do things against their will.

Although these definitions provide an overview of types of elder abuse, they do not describe the complexity of elder abuse as it occurs in different settings and under unique circumstances. Each elder abuse situation involves an older adult who is the victim and a perpetrator who is responsible for the action or inaction leading to neglect or abuse. In situations of self-neglect, the older adult is viewed as both the perpetrator and the victim. Anetzberger (2012) proposed an elder abuse taxonomy that recognizes variations among elder abuse forms, settings, and victim/perpetrator relations. Figure 10-1, which is based on Anetzberger's taxonomy, identifies variables according to setting, perpetrator, and type of abuse. Regardless of the variables, and whether the motivation is unintentional or intentional, the outcomes for older adults can involve physical, psychological, social, financial, and sexual harm, as discussed in the section on Functional Consequences Associated With Elder Abuse.

Recognition of Elder Abuse in the United States and the World

Issues related to vulnerable older adults were initially brought to public and professional attention during the 1960s when the federal government and major organizations recognized the need to protect the increasing numbers of older adults who lived alone in community settings and needed assistance to provide for their own care or protection. Although public and professional attention to elder abuse has evolved slowly, efforts have been increasing exponentially during the past decade, as illustrated in Figure 10-2. In addition to the public and professional attention as described in Figure 10-2, philanthropic and nonprofit organizations have increasingly provided support for concerns related to elder abuse. For example, the first Judith D. Tamkin International Symposium on Elder Abuse took place in 2016 and is committed to ongoing support for research to identify evidence-based interventions for preventing and addressing elder abuse. Currently, there is much emphasis on addressing the multidimensional nature of elder abuse from all the following perspectives: public health, social services, family violence, crime, gender, civil rights, and human rights (Jackson, 2016).

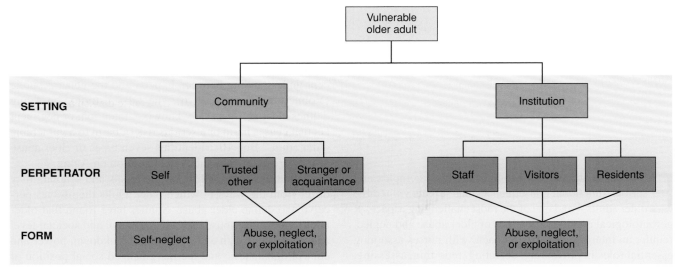

FIGURE 10-1 Variables for elder abuse according to setting, perpetrator, and type of abuse. (Adapted with permission from Anetzberger, G. J. (2012). An update on the nature and scope of elder abuse. *Generations*, *36*(3), 12–30.)

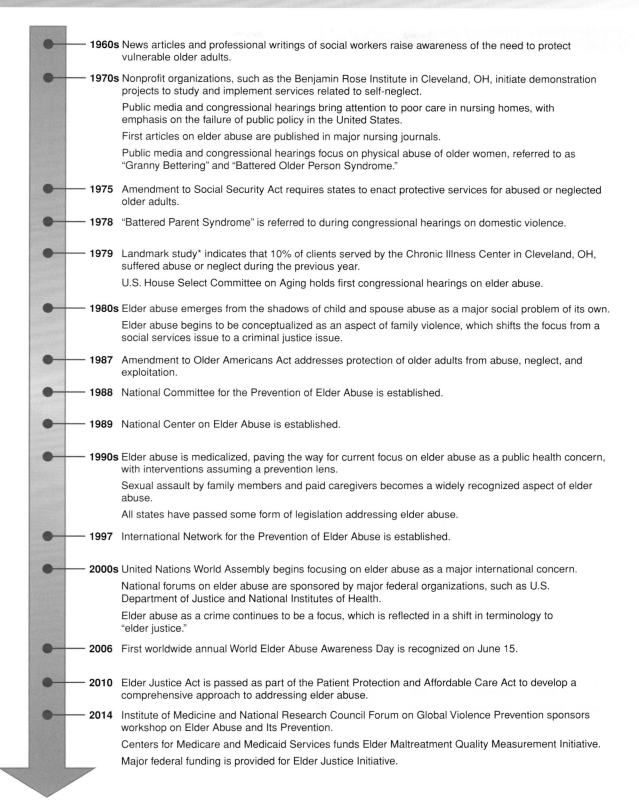

1960s News articles and professional writings of social workers raise awareness of the need to protect vulnerable older adults.

1970s Nonprofit organizations, such as the Benjamin Rose Institute in Cleveland, OH, initiate demonstration projects to study and implement services related to self-neglect.

Public media and congressional hearings bring attention to poor care in nursing homes, with emphasis on the failure of public policy in the United States.

First articles on elder abuse are published in major nursing journals.

Public media and congressional hearings focus on physical abuse of older women, referred to as "Granny Bettering" and "Battered Older Person Syndrome."

1975 Amendment to Social Security Act requires states to enact protective services for abused or neglected older adults.

1978 "Battered Parent Syndrome" is referred to during congressional hearings on domestic violence.

1979 Landmark study* indicates that 10% of clients served by the Chronic Illness Center in Cleveland, OH, suffered abuse or neglect during the previous year.

U.S. House Select Committee on Aging holds first congressional hearings on elder abuse.

1980s Elder abuse emerges from the shadows of child and spouse abuse as a major social problem of its own.

Elder abuse begins to be conceptualized as an aspect of family violence, which shifts the focus from a social services issue to a criminal justice issue.

1987 Amendment to Older Americans Act addresses protection of older adults from abuse, neglect, and exploitation.

1988 National Committee for the Prevention of Elder Abuse is established.

1989 National Center on Elder Abuse is established.

1990s Elder abuse is medicalized, paving the way for current focus on elder abuse as a public health concern, with interventions assuming a prevention lens.

Sexual assault by family members and paid caregivers becomes a widely recognized aspect of elder abuse.

All states have passed some form of legislation addressing elder abuse.

1997 International Network for the Prevention of Elder Abuse is established.

2000s United Nations World Assembly begins focusing on elder abuse as a major international concern.

National forums on elder abuse are sponsored by major federal organizations, such as U.S. Department of Justice and National Institutes of Health.

Elder abuse as a crime continues to be a focus, which is reflected in a shift in terminology to "elder justice."

2006 First worldwide annual World Elder Abuse Awareness Day is recognized on June 15.

2010 Elder Justice Act is passed as part of the Patient Protection and Affordable Care Act to develop a comprehensive approach to addressing elder abuse.

2014 Institute of Medicine and National Research Council Forum on Global Violence Prevention sponsors workshop on Elder Abuse and Its Prevention.

Centers for Medicare and Medicaid Services funds Elder Maltreatment Quality Measurement Initiative.

Major federal funding is provided for Elder Justice Initiative.

FIGURE 10-2 Timeline of significant trends related to elder abuse. (*The landmark study referred to in this figure is Lau, E., & Kosberg, J. (1979). Abuse of the elderly by informal care providers. *Aging*, 299–300, 10–15.)

Prevalence

Elder abuse is neither a rare nor an isolated phenomenon, with all indicators suggesting that mistreatment of vulnerable older adults is widespread and occurs among all subgroups. In the United States, a population-based survey of 5777 community-dwelling, cognitively intact adults aged 60 years and older found that 1 in 10 reported neglect or emotional, physical, or sexual abuse during the previous years, with many experiencing multiple forms (Acierno, Hernandez-Tejeda, Muzzy, et al., 2010). Prevalence of elder abuse in people with dementia varies according to type of abuse, with a review of 28 studies identifying the following rates:

- Psychological abuse: 27.9% to 62.3%
- Physical abuse: 3.5% to 23.1%
- Neglect by caregivers: 20.2%
- Financial exploitation: 15%
- Self-neglect: 13.6% to 18.8%

(Dong, Chen, & Simon, 2014).

It is important to note that prevalence rates for elder abuse are based on known cases and do not reflect the majority of cases, which go undetected and unreported. Elder abuse scholars have discussed this tip-of-the-iceberg theme for decades, and it was substantiated by a report called *Under the Radar: New York Elder Abuse Prevalence Study*. This landmark report found that for every known case of elder abuse that was known to authorities, 23.5 cases were unknown, with financial exploitation having the highest percentage of unreported cases (Lifespan of Greater Rochester, Inc., Weill Cornell Medical Center of Cornell University, & New York City Department of Aging, 2011). Thus, even the most up-to-date data on elder abuse prevalence does not accurately reflect the actual occurrence. Also, because definitions and types vary, there is little consistency among the studies.

SPECIFIC TYPES OF ELDER ABUSE MOST RELEVANT TO NURSING

Because of the wide-ranging scope of elder abuse, as is illustrated in Figure 10-1, it is impossible to address all forms and settings in this chapter. Thus, content focuses primarily on information that is pertinent to nursing care of older adults in home, community, and institutional settings who are in actually or potentially abusive situations. This section discusses self-neglect and neglect by caregivers as forms that are commonly addressed by nurses in clinical settings. Other types of elder abuse discussed in this chapter are elder abuse in nursing homes (under the heading Elder Abuse in Nursing Homes) and indicators of physical abuse as an aspect of assessment.

Self-Neglect

Self-neglect differs from other types of neglect in that the only perpetrator is the older person himself or herself. In cases of self-neglect, the older person fails to meet essential needs to the point that his or her health and safety is threatened. Although self-neglect is not specifically identified as a form of abuse in all state laws, it is the type most frequently encountered and addressed by adult protective services agencies. It also is commonly addressed by nurses in home care settings and is recognized by geriatric health care practitioners as a complex clinical issue. An ethical issue that is central in many—if not most—cases of self-neglect is determination of the person's capacity to refuse services that may be unwanted, as discussed in Chapter 9.

Self-neglect develops gradually and is often associated with lack of resources, such as food, money, and housing; other times adequate resources are available, but the older adult may refuse services. Self-neglect occurs within the context of interactions among several risk factors in the older adult and his or her social and physical environments. Typically, older adults who become self-neglecting experience a combination of the following risks: (1) physical disability or medical conditions, (2) cognitive impairments or mental illness, and (3) inadequate social supports. Also, prior traumatic personal experiences, such as physical or sexual abuse or exposure to violence, are associated with increased prevalence of self-neglect in older adults who have no cognitive impairment (Lien, Rosen, Bloeman, et al., 2016).

In 2008, Self-Neglect was designated as a NANDA nursing diagnosis because of its relevance to nursing care of older adults. The current NANDA definition of Self-Neglect is "A constellation of culturally framed behaviors involving one or more self-care activities in which there is a failure to maintain a socially accepted standard of health and well-being" (Herdman & Kamitsuru, 2018, p. 248). Defining characteristics of Self-Neglect are inadequate personal hygiene, inadequate environmental hygiene, and nonadherence to health activities.

Self-neglect as a unique form of elder abuse is most pertinent to nursing care across all clinical settings because all the following interventions are within the scope of usual nursing care:

- Facilitation of referrals for comprehensive and interdisciplinary assessment
- Interventions to address functional limitations (e.g., making suggestions about assistive devices, facilitating referrals for rehabilitation therapists)

- Interventions to improve management of chronic conditions (e.g., medication management strategies, education about self-care)
- Assessment and interventions related to risks for falls and other safety concerns
- Facilitation of appropriate and acceptable support services (e.g., home-delivered meals, personal care assistance)

Interventions for self-neglect typically involve interprofessional collaboration, and nurses can take the lead in identifying the needs, contributing assessment and intervention skills from a nursing perspective, and working with other professionals to address the complex needs of self-neglecting older adults.

See ONLINE LEARNING ACTIVITY 10-1: CASE EXAMPLES AND JOURNAL ARTICLE DESCRIBING ELDER ABUSE AND SELF-NEGLECT at http://thepoint.lww.com/Miller8e

Neglect by a Trusted Other

A trusted other is defined as a spouse/partner, friend, relative, neighbor, paid caregiver, family caregiver, or anyone on whom the older adult relies for support or assistance. Neglect by trusted others can be intentional, unintentional, or both, depending on factors such as motivation, knowledge, and skill level of the responsible person. Also, neglect may evolve gradually as the health and functional levels of the caregiver or the dependent older adult change. For example, caregivers may initially be well intentioned and provide good care, but become overwhelmed or lack the skills as the needs of the care recipient increase. Other times, caregivers may experience functional or cognitive impairments and not only become incapable of providing care to others but also be in a position of needing care for themselves.

Neglect by a caregiver is particularly pertinent to nursing care of older adults for all the following reasons:

- These situations often involve a combination of acute and chronic risk factors that can be addressed by health care professionals.
- Nurses are in key positions to identify risks for actual or potential domestic elder abuse.
- Nurses have key roles in working with family caregivers who are actual or potential perpetrators of elder abuse.
- Nursing interventions such as caregiver education or referrals to appropriate resources may be effective in preventing or resolving some situations of domestic elder abuse.

CULTURAL CONSIDERATIONS

Cultural factors strongly influence how elder abuse is defined and perceived as well as broader aspects of elder abuse, as in the following examples:

- African Americans may consider more situations as abusive than do other ethnic groups (National Center on Elder Abuse, 2016).
- The cultural value of *la familia* (i.e., the emphasis on the family as a cohesive unit) for Latinos is associated with unwillingness to report abuse (National Center on Elder Abuse, 2014).
- Behaviors that seem abrupt, rude, or demanding toward elderly family members may be considered abusive in the context of Chinese values regarding respect for older adults (Dong, 2015).
- American Indians may view substance abuse and "culture loss" (i.e., the breakdown of traditional valuing of the wisdom of native elders) as underlying factors leading to elder mistreatment (Jervis, Sconzert-Hall, & the Shielding American Indian Elders Project Team, 2017).
- Sixty-five percent of lesbian, gay, bisexual, and transgender (LGBT) elders report victimization due to sexual orientation, and those who seek help from abuse may be further marginalized or even experience retaliation for complaining (National Center on Elder Abuse, 2013; Rawles, 2016).

As discussed in Chapter 2, it is imperative to avoid generalizations related to any topic; however, this is especially important with regard to cultural dimensions of elder abuse because of limitations in the current base of knowledge. A few studies related to elder abuse in culturally diverse groups in the United States were published in the 1980s, but this topic did not gain national attention until the late 1990s. In 2011, the National Center on Elder Abuse began publishing research briefs and tips on elder abuse specific to minority groups, such as African Americans, Asian Pacific islanders, Latino, and LGBT elders. Other governmental and nonprofit agencies are addressing cultural aspects of abuse in specific groups, such as American Indians, as described in Online Learning Activity 10-2.

See ONLINE LEARNING ACTIVITY 10-2: CULTURAL CONSIDERATIONS RELATED TO ELDER ABUSE at http://thepoint.lww.com/Miller8e

Several themes recur in literature about elder abuse in specific groups, particularly related to obligations to provide care and financial support for older family members. For example, a theme common across many cultural groups is that having an elderly parent cared for in a nursing home is considered abusive because of cultural beliefs in filial piety and family-based elder care (Lee, Kaplan, and Perez-Stable, 2014). Another common theme is that many cultural groups hold a strong sense of family self-reliance and tradition of resolving conflicts within the family. This cultural value promotes feelings of shame and a need to maintain secrecy about mistreatment by family members. Themes related to disrespect for elders also are common and are often manifest in culturally specific ways. For example, Asian older adults report experiences of "silent treatment" as a form of mistreatment by families.

Perhaps the most important consideration is that information about cultural influences reflects general characteristics of particular groups, but this information cannot accurately describe characteristics of individuals within a group. In addition, each individual and situation is influenced by a combination of cultural factors from many sources, as described in Box 10-2. As with all information in this chapter, it is imperative to avoid stereotypes and seek the perspectives of individual older adults who may be at risk for, or victims of, elder abuse, as well as that of caregivers who are at risk for becoming perpetrators of elder abuse.

 ## CAUSES OF, AND RISK FACTORS FOR, ELDER ABUSE AND NEGLECT

During the late 1970s, theories about the etiology of elder abuse focused on caregiver stress as an underlying causative factor. At that time, elder abuse was considered primarily physical abuse of vulnerable elders by their caregivers. As the scope of elder abuse gradually broadened, researchers recognized that causation is multifaceted and varies significantly according to variables such as type of abuse,

characteristics of the older adult and the perpetrators, relationship factors, and the larger societal environment in which elder abuse occurs. Current theories do not discount the effects of stress associated with the demands of caregiving, but they emphasize the need to address interacting conditions within the broader situation. These interacting conditions include all of the following: cognitive impairment, physical function and psychological distress of the older adult; caregiver burden, psychological characteristics and mental health status of the perpetrator; poor social relationships; less supportive environments; and previous exposure to traumatic events (Dong & Wang, 2016). Box 10-3 summarizes risk factors for elder abuse that have most often been identified in research. Although it is beyond the scope of this chapter to discuss larger societal factors, information in Chapter 1 related to ageism and attitudes toward aging is pertinent to elder abuse.

Because causes of elder abuse are multifaceted, a logical approach in clinical settings is to identify those risk factors that can be addressed by health care professionals, as discussed in the section on Nursing Assessment of Abused or Neglected Older Adults. Risk factors that tend to be common across elder abuse situations are vulnerability of the

---

 Box 10-2 Cultural Considerations: Assessing Elder Abuse and Neglect

Expectations Related to Interpersonal Relationships

- What conduct is considered abusive in the family, by the community, and in the country of the person's origin?
- How do culturally based views of gender roles influence the perception of spousal and interfamilial relationships between men and women?
- How do personal, familial, and societal experiences influence one's perceptions of violence in general and in interpersonal relationships specifically?

Perceptions of Autonomy and Independence Versus Safety and Dependency

- Does ageism or other factors influence perceptions of an older adult's right to choose to live in situations involving risks to safety?
- Do family members differ in their perceptions of the older adult's right to make decisions about his or her care?

Expectations About Family Caregiving

- Who within the family is expected to care for frail and dependent older members, and what happens if they fail to do so?
- Is it acceptable to employ paid caregivers?
- Do family members differ in their perceptions of caregiving responsibilities, especially across generations?
- How might cultural perspectives influence the roles of family related to expectations for caregiving?
- Are older grandparents expected to care for grandchildren and great-grandchildren?

Decisions About Family Resources

- How might cultural perspectives influence family expectations related to financial support across generations?
- Who makes decisions about how family resources are expended?

- Who, within the family, is expected to provide financial support for older members?
- Does the family consider it appropriate to use the older member's resources for the benefit of other family members?

Attitudes About Using Nonfamily Resources

- How do religious beliefs, past experiences, and attitudes affect decisions about accepting services from outsiders?
- What are the acceptable sources of help from outsiders (e.g., extended family, religious leaders, respected members of the community, healers within the community)?

Considerations Related to Immigrant Older Adults or Those With Communication Barriers

- When did the older and younger generations of the family come to the United States (e.g., together or at different times, which generation came first)?
- What were the circumstances of immigration for the different members of the family?
- Were there sponsorship agreements between the older and younger family members, and if so, what were the expectations related to financial or caregiving support?
- What is the legal status of the older adults and other members of the family?
- Do communication barriers influence the care that is provided or limit the caregiving resources?

Considerations Related to Nursing Assessment of Physical Abuse

- How does skin color affect assessment of bruises, pressure sores, and other skin changes?

Adapted with permission from Miller, C. A. (2017). *Elder abuse and nursing: What nurses need to know and can do about it.* New York: Springer Publishing Company.

Box 10-3 Risk Factors for Elder Abuse

Risk Factors Associated With any Type
Older Adult Factors
- Physical dependence
- Dementia
- Problem behaviors

Perpetrator Factors
- Mental illness (e.g., history of psychiatric hospitalization)
- Substance abuse
- Hostility in general or directed toward victim
- Financial or housing dependence

Risk Factors in the Relationship Between the Older Adult and Perpetrator
- Shared living arrangements
- Social isolation
- Lack of social supports

Risks Factors According to Forms of Abuse
Emotional Abuse
- Lack of social support
- Physical dependence
- Prior traumatic experiences

Physical Abuse
- Substance abuse (perpetrator)
- Mental illness (perpetrator)

- Unemployment (perpetrator)
- Social isolation
- Lack of social support for the older adult

Neglect
- Low income
- Poor health
- Inadequate social support

Financial
- Physical disability
- Female sex
- African-American race

Sexual
- Low social support
- Prior traumatic events

Self-Neglect
- Physical disability
- Medical conditions
- Cognitive impairment
- Mental illness
- Inadequate social supports

older person, invisibility of the problem, and psychosocial and caregiver risk factors.

Vulnerability of the Older Adult

As indicated in Box 10-3, vulnerability in many forms is a common characteristic for older adults who are victims of any form of abuse. This characteristic is associated with a combination of social, personal, situational, and environmental factors. For example, older adults may have significant psychosocial limitations resulting from conditions such as dementia, depression, and other mental disorders. These conditions can increase their vulnerability to self-neglect or abuse or exploitation by others; they also can affect the ability to seek help from others. In situations of domestic elder abuse, vulnerability often is associated with dependency, which can be bidirectional. For example, an older adult may be dependent on the perpetrator for care, and the perpetrator may be dependent on the older person for financial support, and both may depend on each other for mutual support. Another factor that leads to vulnerability is the absence of close relatives or other support people who are able and willing to provide adequate and appropriate assistance. For example, a study found that living a perpetrator only was the living arrangement associated with higher severity of neglect and physical and emotional abuse (Burnes, Pillemer, & Lachs, 2016).

Social Isolation and Lack of Social Support

Social isolation and lack of social support are closely related risk factors that are consistently identified as conditions that underlie many elder abuse situations. Both factors can apply to either or both the older adult who becomes a victim and the family caregivers who become perpetrators. Although lack of social support goes hand in hand with social isolation, it also has a broader societal-level aspect in that needed social supports may not be available for older adults or caregivers. In some situations, social support is available but barriers exist to the use of these services, as discussed in Chapter 13. For example, a common scenario associated with self-neglect is that older people who live alone may be afraid of acknowledging impairments because they fear that they will be required to receive services or move to a long-term care facility. This fear may lead to social isolation, the overlooking of treatable or reversible causes of impairment, or a progressive but unnecessary decline in function.

Social isolation can arise from the older adult, the perpetrator, or social circumstances, as in the following examples:

- An older adult self-isolates as a means of maintaining privacy, autonomy, and control over her life
- An older adult self-isolates to avoid the imposition of unwanted services
- An older adult with dementia self-isolates because of embarrassment, impaired decision-making abilities, or impaired ability to initiate actions and solve problems
- An older adult who is depressed self-isolates to avoid unwanted social interactions, even with family
- A family caregiver who engages in abusive behaviors purposely isolates the older adult to avoid detection
- A family caregiver uses social isolation as a component of psychological abuse

- Social isolation is inherent in the geographic environment—for example, in rural areas
- The older adult is socially isolated because of communication barriers, such as hearing impairment or lack of English language skills
- The older adult is socially isolated because of cultural barriers, such as being an immigrant
- The older adult is socially isolated because of stigma or discrimination—for example, based on religious affiliation or sexual orientation

---

Wellness Opportunity

By sensitively communicating care and concern, nurses encourage vulnerable older adults to talk about conditions that can be addressed to prevent abuse or neglect.

Dementia, Depression, and Mental Illness

Dementia is frequently identified as a risk factor for elder abuse, with studies reporting prevalence rates between 25% and 55%, and higher rates associated with minority groups and people with a history of intimate partner violence (Tronetti, 2014). Impaired judgment, lack of insight, inability to make safe decisions, and loss of contact with reality are dementia-related impairments that can lead to abuse and self-neglect. Moreover, when the older adult denies the cognitive impairment or refuses help or evaluation, the risk for elder abuse increases as the dementia progresses. Following are examples of ways in which dementia increases the vulnerability of older adults to abuse:

- During early stages, an older adult may have difficulty managing his or her financial affairs, even though he or she functions well in all or many other aspects of daily living.
- Cognitive impairments interfere with the ability of an older adult to perceive and self-report elder abuse.
- The credibility of an older adult with cognitive impairment or a diagnosis of dementia may be questioned when elder abuse is suspected or reported.
- Dementia-related behaviors such as anxiety, aggression, agitation, and neuropsychiatric manifestations increase the risk for abuse.
- Dementia causes functional dependency, which increases the risk for all types of abuse.

Depression is another condition that is associated with elder abuse, both as a risk factor for self-neglect and a consequence of all types of abuse (Hansen, Flores, Coverdale, et al., 2016; Roepke-Buehler, Simon, & Dong, 2015). Characteristics of depression that contribute to its role in self-neglect include social isolation, a negative outlook, and lack of interest in self-care. Long-term mental illness also may predispose an older adult to abuse or neglect, especially in combination with other factors, such as dementia or the loss of a significant social support.

Caregiver Factors

Caregiving itself does not cause elder abuse; however, it can lead to abuse when those assuming the caregiving role are additionally challenged because of life stresses, pathologic characteristics, personality characteristics, insufficient resources, or lack of understanding of the older adult's condition. Characteristics of caregivers who become abusive include the following: depression; alcohol or substance abuse; diagnosis of mental illness; inadequate coping skills; financial pressures; high levels of general hostility or anger; and history of social, mental, and/or legal problems. It is not unusual to have a mutually neglectful or abusive situation—for example, when an older married couple has several of the psychosocial risk factors just identified and is also socially isolated.

ELDER ABUSE IN NURSING HOMES

Although most elder abuse occurs in community settings, it also happens in long-term residential care settings, including nursing homes, assisted living facilities, and board and care homes (defined in Chapter 6). Despite the fact that nursing homes are held to clearly defined standards of care established by the Centers for Medicare and Medicaid Services, as of 2016 elder abuse was not specifically addressed in these federal regulations. Data about deficiencies that cause harm to residents indicate that in 2014, more than one in five facilities received a deficiency for actual harm or jeopardy (Harrington, Carrillo, & Garfield, 2015).

Risk Factors Related to Elder Abuse in Nursing Homes

Although research is just beginning to unravel elder abuse risk factors in nursing homes, many factors stem from administrative problems within the institution, such as lack of abuse prevention policies, insufficient staff screening, and staff shortages and turnover. A risk factor most pertinent to nursing staff is inadequate education and training with regard to interventions for dementia-related behaviors (see Chapter 14 for discussion of this issue). For example, staff may view their own abusive actions as justifiable responses in retaliation to aggressive behaviors of residents. Dementia and dependency on others for care are the characteristics of residents that are associated with increased risk for elder abuse. The risk is heightened when the resident's dementia-related behaviors are viewed as difficult or disturbing (e.g., aggressive or combative behaviors).

Forms of Elder Abuse in Nursing Homes

All forms of elder abuse can occur in a long-term care setting, arising from any of the following sources: administrators, direct care workers, families, friends, visitors, and other residents. Examples of elder abuse abound, from stealing personal belongings to name-calling to slapping to rape, with recent attention focused on invasive videos and photos of residents posted by staff on social media (Centers for Medicare & Medicaid Services, 2016). This section focuses on the two forms that are most directly within the jurisdiction of nurses, whether as direct care providers or as supervisors of nursing assistants: abuse by direct care staff and resident-to-resident mistreatment.

Elder Abuse by Direct Care Staff

Physical mistreatment and inadequate care (i.e., neglect) are two types of elder abuse commonly associated with direct care staff in long-term care facilities. Staff actions or omissions, which may be intentional or unintentional, are considered abusive when they harm the resident. Acts of omission, such as not answering call lights in a timely manner, or acts of commission, such as verbal abuse, may or may not cause immediate physical harm, but they can cause immediate and long-term emotional harm. Residents may perceive some actions that are unintentional on the part of direct care staff as abusive or neglectful. For example, staff may talk to residents using a disrespectful, impatient, or infantilizing tone of voice or choice of words. Similarly, residents commonly complain that they feel rushed and are not allowed to perform self-care tasks, whereas direct care staff feel they are doing the best they can within the limits of their time. Acts of omission that are considered negligent include lack of ambulation, oral care, or other essential care activities. Acts of commission that are considered abusive include unnecessary or unwanted touching, especially around breasts or genitalia, and invasive procedures, such as rectal examinations, that are unnecessary for patient care.

Misuse of psychotropic medications is an important care issue related to elder abuse in long-term care facilities that is directly within the scope of licensed nurses. The federal government has been addressing this issue in nursing homes since the 1980s, and some progress has been made; however, in 2014, 26% of nursing home citations were related to the inappropriate and unnecessary use of psychotropic medications (Harrington, Carrillo, & Garfield, 2015). Elder abuse also occurs when nursing staff deny access to medication or inappropriately delay the administration of medications (Castle, Ferguson-Rome, & Teresi, 2015). Use of physical restraints is another nursing care issue that is viewed as a form of elder abuse. Nursing issues related to use of physical restraints and psychotropic medications for dementia-related behaviors are addressed in Chapters 9 and 14, respectively.

Resident-to-Resident Mistreatment

Resident-to-resident mistreatment (also called resident-to-resident abuse, violence, or aggression) is considered a unique type of elder abuse that occurs in all types of long-term care settings. Resident-to-resident aggression is defined as "negative, aggressive and intrusive verbal, physical, sexual, and material interactions between long-term care residents that in a community setting would likely be unwelcome and potentially cause physical or psychological distress or harm to the recipient" (McDonald, Hitzig, Pillemer, et al., 2015). This definition encompasses a broad range of experiences ranging from the imposition of unwanted assistance to serious physical injury, sexual abuse, or even death.

A study of 2011 residents in 10 nursing homes in the state of New York found a 1-month prevalence rate of 20.2% for resident-to-resident mistreatment, with verbal abuse most common and sexual abuse least common. Factors associated with higher rates of mistreatment included severe levels of cognitive impairment, residence in a dementia unit, and higher caseloads for nursing assistants (Lachs, Teresi, Ramirez, et al., 2016). A 2010 survey of 6846 assisted living residents in the United States found that 9.5% had exhibited verbal abuse, 7.6% had engaged in physical abuse, and 2.0% had engaged in sexual abuse toward other residents during the previous month, with dementia and mental illness being the most significant risk factors (Gimm, Chowdhury, & Castle, 2016). Interventions to address resident-to-resident mistreatment are discussed in the section on Nursing Interventions to Address Elder Abuse.

Recently, the experience of "bullying" has been addressed as a concern related to resident-to-resident aggression. This concept is typically associated with an imbalance of power, which can be very subtle among residents of long-term care facilities. For instance, a resident who is limited in one aspect of functioning (e.g., memory loss) may talk loudly in a demeaning manner about someone with another type of disability (e.g., mobility impairment). Another example occurs in group dining room settings, when a resident refuses to sit with certain other residents. Although the rights of individual residents need to be respected, staff also need to take action when this type of resident-to-resident interaction is detrimental to one of the residents. Also, health care providers need to take action to prevent these behaviors from escalating to the level of abuse (D'Angelo, 2016).

Resources for Addressing Elder Abuse in Long-Term Care Settings

Major concerns about quality of care in nursing homes that began during the 1960s led to the establishment of the Nursing Home Ombudsman program in 1972. This program has gradually expanded—as reflected in changing the name to the Long-Term Care Ombudsman program in 1981—and has become a major resource for addressing issues related to care in all nursing homes and residential care facilities. A major mandate of all Long-Term Care Ombudsman programs is to "identify, investigate, and resolve complaints that (1) are made by or on behalf of residents; and (2) relate to actions, inactions, or decisions, that may adversely affect the health, safety, welfare and rights of residents" (Federal Register, 2015, p. 7761). Although state reporting laws vary, the local adult protective services agency and the Nursing Home Ombudsman program investigate reports of abuse. If a report

Unfolding Case Study

Part 1: Mrs. B. at 82 Years of Age

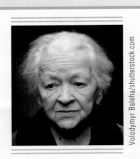

Mrs. B. is an 82-year-old divorced and widowed mother of four. She lives in a senior citizens' apartment located in the downtown area of a large city. The building is regularly serviced by subsidized transportation to grocery stores and shopping malls and has a nutrition center on the ground floor. Mrs. B.'s eldest son died in an accident 12 years ago. Her daughter lives 65 miles away but visits once a week to do the grocery shopping and other errands. Two sons live within 4 miles of their mother's apartment. Mrs. B. lived in the home of one son and his wife until they argued 1 year ago. The other son lives alone in a small apartment and visits his mother two or three times weekly and frequently takes her to lunch or dinner. Mrs. B. has been hospitalized for major depression eight times since her eldest son's death. She also has been diagnosed as having hypertension, rheumatoid arthritis, and type 2 diabetes.

Mrs. B. was referred to a home health agency for follow-up after her last hospital stay because her medication regimen, which she had followed for 6 years, had been changed while she was in the hospital. At the time of discharge, Mrs. B. was given a 30-day supply of medications set out in daily-dose medication containers for her. She was to take glyburide, 2.5 mg once a day; propranolol, 40 mg twice a day; paroxetine, 25 mg once a day; folic acid, 1 mg once a day; and methotrexate, four 2.5 mg tablets each Wednesday. Scheduled medication times were 8 AM and 8 PM. The home health nurse was to instruct Mrs. B. in her medication regimen, including what medications she was to take, how she was to take them, what each medication was expected to do, and possible side effects. The nurse was also to assess Mrs. B.'s ability to follow instructions and her adherence to the medication regimen.

Because Mrs. B.'s vision was impaired from diabetes, she had difficulty managing her complex medication regimen. The visiting nurse arranged for unit-dose packaging for Mrs. B.'s prescriptions and visited twice a day for 2 days to observe Mrs. B.'s ability to take her medications accurately. On the third morning, which was Monday, the nurse telephoned Mrs. B. at 8:15 AM and asked Mrs. B. if she had any problems taking her pills. Mrs. B. happily reported that she had taken all the pills, including the four methotrexate tablets, without any difficulty. The nurse then scheduled Mrs. B. to be seen three times a week for ongoing assessment for several weeks.

THINKING POINTS

- What are the factors that contribute to the risk of Mrs. B. becoming abused or neglected?
- What are the factors that protect Mrs. B. from becoming abused or neglected?

- As the visiting nurse, what concerns would you have about Mrs. B. when you discharge her from home care, and how would you address these concerns?

is substantiated, further investigation is carried out by the state agency responsible for licensure and certification and also by the state professional licensing authority when the abuse is committed by a professional.

 See ONLINE LEARNING ACTIVITY 10-3: RESOURCES FOR INFORMATION ABOUT ELDER ABUSE IN LONG-TERM CARE FACILITIES at http://thepoint.lww.com/Miller8e

 ## FUNCTIONAL CONSEQUENCES ASSOCIATED WITH ELDER ABUSE

Older people who have several risk factors are likely to become victims of elder abuse, as illustrated by the following case examples:

1. A middle-aged alcoholic man hit his aged father during an argument. In turn, both were beaten by their sons/grandsons, who wanted money for drugs.
2. An elderly woman never left home because she feared her memory lapses would prevent her from finding the way back. When she did venture out, she fell on the porch, and the local office on aging was called. Outreach workers found she had no food in the house and was malnourished.
3. An unemployed couple kept their impaired grandparents confined to the house, refusing them visitors, abandoning them for days without adequate food, and denying them help for fear of losing access to their Social Security checks.
4. A son visited his mother in the nursing home and sexually assaulted her when staff members were not present.

5. A depressed elderly woman refused to take a needed medication with the result that her legs became so swollen that she could not leave her chair.

6. A woman in her 80s—who was weak, incontinent, and hypertensive—was abandoned in an emergency department with a note reading "Totally dependent! Handle with care."

Older adults who become victims of elder abuse experience serious functional consequences, both immediate and long term. Studies have identified all the following personal consequences for older adults who become victims of abuse:

- Overall health and functioning: pain, injury, increased morbidity, functional impairment, increased dependency
- Psychological/emotional effects: fear, anxiety, depression; decreased self-esteem; feelings of shame, guilt, powerless, self-blame
- Social effects: isolation, depression, stigma
- Increased risk for being admitted to a long-term care setting
- Shorter life expectancy

(Dong & Wang, 2016; Wong & Waite, 2017).

Shorter life expectancy, or premature mortality, has gained attention as the most serious functional consequence of elder abuse, with increasing recognition that elder abuse can be life limiting as well as life threatening. For example, a study of mortality rates across five categories of substantiated elder abuse found that victims of caregiver neglect and financial exploitation had the shortest 5-year survival rates (Burnett, Jackson, Sinha, et al., 2016).

In addition to identifying personal consequences for victims of elder abuse, legislators, gerontologists, and social service providers have discussed consequences of elder abuse from a societal perspective. In particular, there is increasing attention to the cost of elder abuse due to greater utilization of health care services.

Case Study

When Mr. P.'s wife died, Mr. P., a frail man, sought care in the home of a neighbor who offered both board and care in exchange for his monthly Social Security check. In reality, the neighbor provided neither, but locked Mr. P. in the basement and gave him little food. If Mr. P. complained about the treatment or refused to sign over the income or property, the caregiver hit or kicked him. After 4 years, the situation was discovered and reported to the county protective services agency. Mr. P. later sat in the social worker's office and sadly commented, "So this is what it's like to be a protective case."

THINKING POINTS

- What type(s) of abuse does this case represent?
- What are some of the psychosocial consequences that Mr. P. is likely to have experienced in the past 4 years?
- What are some factors that contribute to this situation going on for 4 years?

NURSING ASSESSMENT OF ABUSED OR NEGLECTED OLDER ADULTS

Elder abuse is not so much *assessed* as it is *detected,* so nurses often must assume the role of detective putting together clues. Because elder abuse by its very nature is a hidden problem, assessment begins with a suspicion about its existence. Information may be purposefully withheld, and it is rarely volunteered, except in situations in which the older person or caregiver is desperate for help. Clues to elder abuse might first be noted when an older person is seen in an emergency department or admitted to a hospital. Often, a home visit is an essential component of the assessment process, and gaining admission to the home usually is the first assessment challenge. Many times, the situation deteriorates so gradually that it is hard to determine the onset of abuse. In questionable situations, people who suspect that elder abuse is occurring may ignore the clues in hopes that the situation will resolve by itself.

See ONLINE LEARNING ACTIVITY 10-4: EVIDENCE-BASED INFORMATION AND ASSESSMENT TOOL FOR ELDER MISTREATMENT at http://thepoint.lww.com/Miller8e

Wellness Opportunity

Nurses pay particular attention to the older adult's relationships with others so that they can detect clues to elder abuse.

Unique Aspects of Elder Abuse Assessment

Assessment of elder abuse differs from usual nursing assessment in several respects. First, situations of elder abuse often involve elements of fear, secrecy, and resistance on the part of the older person or perpetrators (who may also be the primary caregivers). When indicators of abuse are identified by health care professionals in a clinical setting, this may be a prime opportunity for the older adult to confide about a situation that he or she has been afraid to reveal. Thus, nurses need to recognize their important roles in identifying clues and asking probing—and at the same time nonjudgmental—questions so actual or potential situations of elder abuse can be addressed.

Second, a major purpose of the assessment is to determine whether the safety of the older adult is jeopardized and whether legal interventions are appropriate or necessary for protection of the older adult. If the older adult is assessed as being at risk to self or others, the assessment must address the person's decision-making ability and his or her right to refuse services if he or she so chooses. This assessment often involves consideration of legal interventions, as discussed in the section on Legal Interventions and Ethical Issues. Because the determination of safety is based on professional assessment information, the role of the nurse is especially important. In home settings in particular, the nursing assessment may be a major factor with regard to interventions, including legal actions.

Third, in contrast to most health care situations, the nurse may be viewed as a threat rather than a help, particularly in community-based situations involving the perpetrator who also is a caregiver or family member. Thus, it may be difficult to gain access or to obtain adequate assessment information. When this is the case, it is important to minimize the perceived threat even before the initial contact. This can be achieved by identifying someone who acknowledges that a problem exists and is willing to facilitate the assessment process. Any of the following people can be helpful in gaining access and acceptance:

- Neighbors or friends
- Relatives (especially family members who do not live in the problematic home setting)
- Staff from senior centers, offices on aging, or health care or community agencies
- Physicians or any other health professionals
- Church-based people (e.g., clergy, parish nurses)

Finally, the nurse's personal safety is an assessment consideration in many elder abuse situations, especially when home visits involve contact with a known or suspected perpetrator. In any situation that places a nurse at risk, it is essential to ensure that appropriate protections and precautions are in place. For example, nurses can arrange their visits in conjunction with protective services worker visits or, if warranted, law enforcement officers. Some communities have law enforcement officers who are specially trained to deal with elder abuse situations. In addition, it is imperative that nurses are vigilant about potential risks and attentive to an escape route.

Wellness Opportunity

When making home visits, nurses pay particular attention to self-wellness by protecting themselves from risks.

Assessment of Risks to Health and Safety

A major focus of nursing assessment in elder abuse situations is the identification of risks to health and safety of the older adult and others because the consequences can be life threatening if the safety issues are not addressed. In emergency departments, this assessment may influence decisions about admission and treatment. In acute care and long-term care settings, this assessment may be an important factor in discharge plans. In home settings, this assessment may be essential for determining whether the older adult can remain in his or her environment. In all settings, assessment of safety in the context of elder abuse is both essential and wide ranging. It is essential because the choice and immediacy of interventions are influenced by both the degree of risk and the decision-making

capacity of the older adult. It is wide ranging because safety issues related to elder abuse are integral to all the following aspects:

- Self-neglect for older adults who live alone
- Neglect for older adults whose care is inadequate
- Protection from abuse or neglect perpetrated by others
- Protection of other people and properties due to risky behaviors of the older adult
- Protection of one's personal assets in situations of exploitation

As with other aspects of elder abuse, assessment of safety must be multidimensional and based on information from several professionals. Nurses can use Box 10-4 as a guide to assessment of indicators of elder abuse that are within the scope of nursing. The following sections provide information about nursing assessment of health-related indicators most relevant to elder abuse situations. In addition, assessment information from other chapters is applicable to elder abuse assessment (e.g., Assessment of Safety in Home Settings in Chapter 7, Assessing the Risks for Suicide in Chapter 15, Identifying Risks for Falls and Injuries in Chapter 22, and Risk Identification Under Pressure Injury in Chapter 23). In situations in which the caregiver is the abuser, it is imperative to assess the degree to which the caregiver presents a threat to the life of the dependent older person.

Physical Assessment

Any of the following conditions can be key indicators of abuse or self-neglect: burns, bruises, fractures, leg ulcers, pressure ulcers, dependent edema, poor wound healing, and fall-related injuries. More than one of these indicators at the same time, or over a short period of time, should raise high levels of suspicion about neglect or abuse. A challenging aspect of physical assessment indicators is that these conditions are not unique to elder abuse situations, so nursing assessment needs to consider patterns of injuries and collect information about broader circumstances. A guiding principle for assessment is to consider whether the observed injuries match the explanation given by the older adult or the caregiver.

Bruises and Injuries

Assessment of bruises and injuries is particularly relevant to elder abuse because it is imperative to identify whether the cause was accidental (i.e., unintentional), inflicted by others (i.e., intentional), or self-inflicted (least commonly). For example, the following characteristics would suggest that the injuries were intentionally inflicted by others:

- Similar bruises on both upper arms that would result from being grabbed or shaken harshly
- Bruises that reflect the shape of objects, such as a belt or hairbrush
- Burns from cigarettes
- Puncture wounds
- Bite marks

Box 10-4   Guide to Nursing Assessment of Signs of Elder Abuse

Health-Related Indicators of Elder Abuse

- Untreated or poorly managed medical conditions
- Untreated wounds or infections
- Untreated injuries
- Suspicious bruises or injuries
- Dementia without appropriate support resources
- Inability to meet, or have met by others, basic needs (e.g., nutrition, hydration, personal hygiene, urinary and bowel elimination)
- Inability to manage therapeutic regimens
- Inappropriate use of drugs or alcohol, either self- or caregiver induced
- Suicidal ideation or actions

Threats to Safety of the Older Adult

- Inability to recognize an unsafe situation
- Inability to call for help
- Inability of the older adult to escape from abusive situation
- Frequent falls, especially if explanations do not match patterns of injuries or if the person lives alone and cannot call for help
- Episodes of getting lost or wandering in unsafe neighborhoods or in very cold weather without proper clothing
- Living in environmental conditions associated with undue risk for disease, physical harm, hypothermia, hyperthermia, or becoming a victim of crime
- Access to toxic substances or dangerous tools or cutlery in the household without the ability to recognize the dangers

Risks to the Safety of Others due to Behaviors of the Older Adult

- Unsafe driving of vehicles
- Unsafe use of appliances (e.g., gas stoves)
- Unsafe smoking (e.g., falling asleep with lighted cigarette)
- Access to weapons without the ability to make safe and appropriate decisions about their use

Considerations Related to the Older Adult With Dementia

- Is the person receiving appropriate medical evaluation and management?
- Are additional risk factors for elder abuse present?
- How does dementia affect the person's decision-making capacity and safe functioning?
- Do other people use the diagnosis of dementia to impose decisions or control assets?
- How are dementia-associated behaviors addressed?

Considerations Related to the Older Adult's Decision-Making Capacity

- Has the person had a comprehensive evaluation done by qualified professionals?
- Does impaired decision making create risks for elder abuse?
- Does the older adult's decision-making capacity affect the provision of services?

If evidence of fall-related injuries is present, consider the following: (1) whether the person was shoved or otherwise caused to fall by someone else, (2) whether the fall may be associated with alcohol or substance abuse, or (3) whether the person fell because of balance and mobility problems due to overmedication by the caregiver.

Evidence-based information is emerging to help health care professionals identify bruises and injuries that are red flags for abusive situations. For example, a landmark study has identified the most common places for accidental bruises in older adults and for bruises in older adults who were identified as victims of elder abuse, as illustrated in Figure 10-3 (Wiglesworth, Austin, Corona, et al., 2009). More recent studies of intentionally caused injuries in older adults presenting to emergency departments identified the following characteristics associated with possible abuse:

- Intentional injuries occurred most commonly on the head, neck, upper trunk, and upper extremities.
- Maxillofacial injuries were the most common suspicious presentation.
- Intentional injuries involved contusions, abrasions, lacerations, or punctures.
- The most common suspicious circumstance was the occurrence of the injury more than 1 day prior to the presentation in the emergency department.
- Intentionally injured older adults were much more likely to be struck by or against an object.

- Fractures of the back, head, and face raised suspicions about abuse.

(Gironda, Nguyen, & Mosqueda, 2016; Rosen, Bloemen, LoFaso, et al., 2016; Yonashiro-Cho, Gassoumis, & Wilber, 2015).

Pressure Ulcers and Other Skin Indicators

Although pressure ulcers can develop even with good care, they also can be a key indicator of neglect. Important considerations with regard to pressure ulcers are: (1) whether medical care is being provided and treatment has been initiated, (2) whether the treatment is effective, (3) whether caregivers understand how to manage pressure ulcers, and (4) whether caregivers implement interventions to prevent pressure ulcers when the older adult has risk factors (e.g., poor nutrition, limited mobility, exposure of skin to moisture). Skin also should be assessed for indicators of poor hygiene or infections. Body areas that are most commonly neglected are feet, groin and genital area, and any intertriginous areas (e.g., breast or abdominal folds). Refer to Chapter 23 for information about pressure ulcers.

Infections

Infections are common in older adults and usually are not associated with elder abuse; however, it is important to consider that they also can be caused by abusive or neglectful

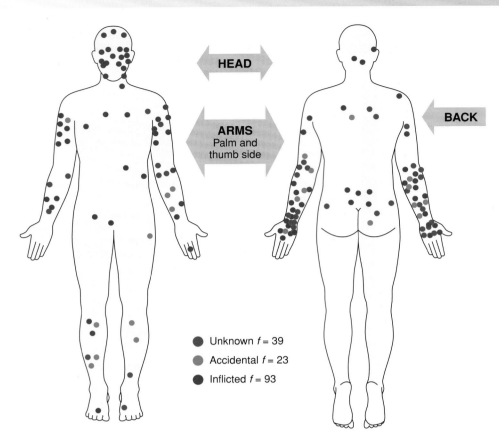

FIGURE 10-3 Bruising in older adults as reported by abused elders. (Adapted from NCEA Research to Practice Translation. Bruising in Older Adults. Available at https://ncea.acl.gov/resources/docs/Research-Translation-bruising-NCEA-2014.pdf; based on data from Wiglesworth, A., Austin, R., Conona, M., et al. (2009). *Journal of the American Geriatrics Society, 57*(7), 1191–1196.)

conditions. The following examples of infections may be indicators of elder abuse:

- Infected wounds, leg ulcers, and pressure ulcers may be due to neglect or self-neglect.
- Recurrent urinary tract infections may be due to sexual abuse or poorly managed incontinence.
- Aspiration pneumonia can be caused by inappropriate feeding methods used by caregivers.
- Sexually transmitted infections can be an indicator of sexual abuse.

As with all aspects of assessment of older adults in abusive situations, these conditions need to be considered within the broader context.

Nutrition and Hydration

Nutrition and hydration are important in determining not only the existence of physical neglect but also the seriousness and urgency of the situation. In community settings, nutrition and hydration status are often key factors in determining the need for immediate interventions. Nursing assessment of nutrition and hydration status is discussed in Chapter 18 (see the section on Using Physical Assessment and Laboratory Information, Table 18-1, and Box 18-5).

When indicators of malnutrition or dehydration are identified, the next step is to determine whether the hydration or nutritional status can be improved adequately without removing the person from the setting. The role of the nurse can be especially important in assessing not only the nutrition

and hydration status but also the measures required to alleviate these risks immediately. Sometimes, the provision of water and food is the most important intervention in neglect situations. In addition, this intervention is inexpensive and readily available, and can be quite effective in establishing a relationship with a hungry or thirsty person.

Activities of Daily Living and Functional Assessment

A major focus of assessment in elder abuse situations is to determine the older adult's ability to safely meet his or her daily needs. Personal dress, hygiene, and grooming are among the most visible and commonly appraised aspects of daily function; however, it is important to consider whether these aspects affect safety. In most situations, the priority is to address basic human needs related to adequate nutrition, hydration, and the ability to obtain help in an emergency. In addition, it is imperative to assess functional abilities in relation to safety and self-care considerations. For example, if the 75-year-old wife of an alcoholic man can easily escape when he becomes violent, and she chooses to remain in the situation, she would not necessarily be considered a protective case. In contrast, if the woman who is the target of violence when her husband is inebriated is cognitively impaired, physically frail, or unable to move quickly, the situation could be defined as elder abuse. Specific functional abilities also need to be assessed in relation to risks for elder abuse. For instance, it is imperative to address bowel and bladder

TABLE 10-1 Risks to Safety Associated With Functional Limitations

Functional Limitation	Risks to Safety
Any mental or physical impairment, especially combined with social isolation and lack of a support system	Nutrition and hydration
Mobility limitations or seriously impaired vision, especially combined with poor judgment	Falls
Cognitive impairments in ambulatory people	Wandering, getting lost
Immobility, poor nutrition, incontinence	Pressure sores
Cognitive impairment, especially poor judgment	Inability to get help
Poor judgment, especially when living in an unsafe neighborhood	Basic safety and security

elimination for people who are confined to bed or a chair and lack the appropriate assistance. Table 10-1 summarizes some of the specific functional and environmental conditions that present risks to basic needs.

Wellness Opportunity

Nurses promote self-determination for older adults by respecting their rights to make decisions about their care, as long as their actions do not jeopardize safety for themselves or others.

Administration of Medications

For certain medical conditions, it is essential to assess the older adult's ability to follow medical regimens and the consequences of not following prescribed regimens. Failure to do so can constitute abuse or neglect; for example, consequences can be quite serious when a person with heart failure does not take medications correctly and lives alone or relies on a caregiver whose competence is questionable. When a medication regimen is complex, it is important to determine if it can be simplified to improve adherence and support the person's ability to remain in an independent setting. A thorough nursing assessment can lead to interventions to achieve adequate adherence, as discussed in Chapter 8.

Another assessment consideration is that elder abuse may involve caregivers withholding therapeutic medications or interfering with medical care. For example, caregivers may decide not to purchase prescriptions or provide nursing care, medical equipment, or comfort items because they do not want to spend the money, even though this care is recommended or even prescribed. If the older adult has not freely chosen to forego treatments, medications, or assistance, this may constitute neglect. If the caregiver is likely to inherit the money that is being saved, this may represent financial exploitation as well.

A third major consideration related to the administration of medications is the inappropriate use of psychoactive medications, either by the older adult or imposed by caregivers. For example, caregivers may administer excessive and unnecessary amounts of psychoactive medications solely to control behaviors of the older adult for the caregiver's benefit. Similarly, caregivers—particularly those who abuse alcohol—may administer alcohol to older adults who prefer not to drink. Nurses are likely to observe any of the following indicators of overmedication in an elder: ataxia, confusion, slurred speech, excessive sleeping, problems with balance or mobility, or neurologic adverse effects.

Psychosocial Function

Information in Chapters 13 (Psychosocial Assessment), 14 (Delirium and Dementia), and 15 (Depression) is pertinent to assessing psychosocial function in relation to elder abuse. In addition to assessing psychosocial function from a nursing perspective, nurses collaborate with mental health professionals, such as geropsychiatrists, geropsychologists, and social workers. The possibility of substance abuse by the older adult also should be considered in all situations of suspected abuse or self-neglect, especially if the older adult is depressed, grieving, socially isolated, or has a history of substance abuse. In addition, an important aspect of psychosocial function for abuse situations is assessment of the elder's capacity for reasonable judgments about self-care. Thus, the crucial element of psychosocial assessment for elder abuse cases is a determination of *risk* (i.e., danger to the person) rather than a determination of whether other people would judge the decision as *good* or *appropriate*. There are no federal guidelines for determining the mental capacity of abused or neglected older adults, and the legal criteria differ from state to state. The ethical and legal considerations related to elder abuse are discussed later in this chapter and more extensively in Chapter 9.

Caregivers and Support Resources

Support resources include those people, such as caregivers and friends, who influence a person's physical and psychosocial function. Some or all of the support people may directly cause the abusive situation or may actively or passively contribute to it. Therefore, nurses assess the support resources in terms of both helpful and detrimental effects. In addition, support resources not currently being used are identified as potential sources of help. Nurses base their assessment on their own observations and, whenever possible, they collaborate with social workers for a more comprehensive assessment.

When the caregivers who perpetrate the abuse are also the support resources, nurses assess the potential for working with them to alleviate the negative consequences. Although it is not always easy to work with abusive caregivers, it may be even more difficult to eliminate their influence over an older adult. For example, it is not unusual to address situations in which an alcoholic son or daughter lives with a parent and provides emotional support while at the same time neglecting the parent's needs and financially exploiting the situation. During the assessment, therefore, nurses identify any strengths of the caregiver and any willingness to change the situation voluntarily. If the caregiver is extremely stressed, then respite, along with individual or group support and counseling, may be effective interventions. In mutually abusive situations in which the designated caregiver, often a spouse, also is abused or neglected, the nurse tries to identify any outside sources of support that have not been tapped. For example, in a mutually abusive situation involving a socially isolated married couple, the nurse might identify a relative, friend, or paid caregiver who is willing to provide appropriate assistance.

Because a caregiver's lack of knowledge can be an underlying factor in elder abuse, nurses assess the caregiver's understanding of the elder's needs. For example, caregivers may use adult briefs for the control of incontinence, but they may not understand the potential for skin breakdown or the effect on the person's self-esteem. Another example is the administration of excessive amounts of psychoactive medications because caregivers do not understand the importance of avoiding adverse effects by using nonmedication interventions. In situations such as these, nursing assessment of the caregiver's knowledge is especially important because educational interventions, role modeling, or the provision of additional services may alleviate the abuse.

In situations of self-neglect, there usually are very few support services to assess, and the major nursing task is to identify potential sources of help and the barriers that interfere with the use of these resources. The assessment of barriers to the use of resources is discussed in Chapter 13 and is summarized in Box 13-11. It is especially important to identify these barriers because simple interventions, such as provision of information or assistance with transportation, may be effective in eliminating them. Cultural influences also must be assessed in relation to the use of support resources, as discussed in Chapter 2.

Cultural Aspects of Assessment

Definitions and perceptions of elder abuse and neglect are influenced to a great extent by cultural norms. For example, Asian Indians may consider not visiting an older family member to be a form of psychological neglect, but Anglo Americans may consider it a way of respecting privacy and autonomy. Cultural factors also have a strong influence on caregiver roles and responsibilities. Most families have culturally influenced expectations about which family members should provide care to dependent older adults and about whether it is acceptable to enlist the aid of paid caregivers. In some families, there may be conflicts about these expectations, particularly between older and younger generations. Sometimes, these conflicts may need to be identified and addressed before elder abuse or neglect can be resolved.

Nurses identify cultural factors that influence the care that is provided—or not provided—to older adults. When assessing family caregiver relationships, it is important to be sensitive to cultural variations in perspectives on family caregiving and respect differences, while also addressing abusive situations. In addition, cultural assessment information on the following topics should be considered: Communication and Psychosocial Assessment (see Chapter 13), Nutrition (see Chapter 18), Dementia (see Chapter 14), and Depression (see Chapter 15).

Environmental Influences

For community-living older adults, it is essential to assess the home environment and the elder's level of functioning in that environment as a crucial aspect of identifying risks for, or the actual occurrence of, elder abuse. The primary purposes of this part of the nursing assessment are to identify conditions that create risks and to determine which of these factors can be alleviated through interventions. In addition, nurses often need to obtain information from caregivers. Home care workers provide valuable information, and they provide a different perspective than family members. In some circumstances, it may be appropriate to involve occupational or physical therapists in the home assessment. When a difference of opinion exists, or when it is difficult to determine the safety of the situation, it may be helpful to have a team conference that includes all of the people who function in assessment or caregiving capacities and who have some degree of objectivity. In cases of suspected elder abuse, the assessment team often includes input from many informal sources of help, such as family and neighbors, as well as formal sources of help, such as nurses, home care workers, and social workers.

With regard to the immediate living conditions, assess whether minimal standards of safety and cleanliness are being maintained. When home environments are extremely cluttered, it is important to assess both the meaning and the consequences of the clutter. For example, a massive and long-developing collection of clutter from hoarding may be indicative of an underlying disorder and may or may not be a risk to safety that requires immediate attention. Because consequences of hoarding range from socially unacceptable appearances to serious risks to health and safety, it is important to assess the person's ability to safely maneuver in the environment during daily activities as well as during emergency situations, such as a fire. When nurses and other workers are initially exposed to massive amounts of clutter, their first inclination may be to think of a way to eliminate some of it. If this reaction is communicated to the resident of the cluttered home, however, it may become impossible to establish an accepting relationship, and the older adult may reject any further interventions. Thus, it is imperative to convey a nonjudgmental attitude, while at the same time addressing the risks that require immediate action.

Another assessment aspect for community-dwelling older adults is to identify risks to safety in the neighborhood environment. This is especially important when the older person lives in an area of high crime or extreme isolation and is vulnerable by virtue of impaired judgment, physical frailty, or a combination of physical and psychosocial impairments. For example, people who are only moderately forgetful may be safe in an apartment or a suburban neighborhood where neighbors watch out for them. In a high-crime neighborhood, however, forgetting to lock the doors or to take other precautions may place the person at increased risk for physical harm, financial exploitation, or other serious abuses. Likewise, in a rural environment, social isolation may increase the risks for vulnerable older adults.

Finally, seasonal conditions can influence the degree of risk for self-neglect in people who are cognitively impaired and live in climates characterized by extreme heat or cold. For example, people who do not pay utility bills may not be in any danger as long as the weather is mild, but when the temperature turns cold, they would be at risk for hypothermia. Similarly, older adults may lack cognitive capacity to sense that temperatures are not appropriate or to operate thermostats properly. The same is true for people who occasionally wander outside without dressing appropriately. As long as the neighborhood is safe and the weather is mild, they may be relatively safe; however, they may be at increased risk during the cold months or very hot months, especially if they do not wear proper clothing. In situations of neglect, caregivers may fail to assure that the temperatures in living areas are appropriate for the older adult. For example, caregivers may not want to spend money for providing adequate heating or cooling or for repairing or replacing equipment that is not functional. Nursing assessment of risk factors for hypothermia or heat-related illness is discussed in Chapter 25.

Case Study

Mrs. K. is 80 years old and had resided in a nursing facility for 1 year until she recently was discharged at her request but "against medical advice" with no prescriptions for her medications or medical referral for home care. She has complex health conditions, including osteoarthritis, coronary artery disease, heart failure, chronic obstructive pulmonary disease, depression, and insulin-dependent diabetes. Although alert and oriented, Mrs. K. has major deficits in her ability to perform daily living tasks. She also depends on a walker for ambulation and has a history of falling, including a fall that resulted in a hip fracture and her admission to a nursing facility.

Mrs. K.'s support system is limited. Her son lives in another state but functions as power of attorney and provides some telephone reassurance. Her daughter is estranged from Mrs. K., and at their last meeting was verbally abusive to her. Mrs. K.'s older brother visits a few times weekly to help with meal preparation, grocery shopping, transportation, and medication pickups; however, his own health problems prevent him from providing more help.

Shortly after returning home, Mrs. K.'s precarious health status rapidly deteriorated. She became severely short of breath, requiring continuous oxygen. She began to hallucinate in the evening, believing that she alone had the responsibility of feeding all of the children in the neighborhood. As her fears increased, so too did the calls to her brother. Eventually, she made several calls every night, overwhelming and exhausting him.

THINKING POINTS

- What form(s) of elder abuse is (are) represented?
- What are signs or indicators of abuse that you as a nurse would be able to identify?
- What factors contribute to Mrs. K.'s current risks?
- How will you proceed in conducting a nursing assessment of Mrs. K.?
- What barriers might you encounter in conducting the assessment? How will you overcome them?

NURSING DIAGNOSIS

Because elder abuse and neglect is so broad and complex, various nursing diagnoses are applicable, depending on the situation. A nursing diagnosis that would apply to many elder abuse situations where family members are caregivers is Compromised Family Coping, defined as "a usually supportive primary person (family member, significant other, or close friend) provides insufficient, ineffective, or compromised support, comfort, assistance, or encouragement that may be needed by the client to manage or master adaptive tasks related to his or her health challenge" (Herdman & Kamitsuru, 2018, p. 331). In more serious cases of elder abuse, the nursing diagnosis of Disabled Family Coping might be applicable. This is defined as "behavior of primary person (family member, significant other, or close friend) that disables his or her capacities and the client's capacities to effectively address tasks essential to either person's adaptation to the health challenge" (Herdman & Kamitsuru, 2018, p. 333).

If stress is a contributing factor related to family caregiving, the nursing diagnosis of Caregiver Role Strain, or Risk for Caregiver Role Strain, might be applicable. Related caregiver factors include ineffective coping patterns, functional or cognitive impairments, and insufficient resources (e.g., respite, financial assets, assistance with care). Related factors involving the dependent older adult include increased dependence and the presence of difficult or unsafe behaviors (e.g., paranoia, wandering, incontinence).

The nursing diagnosis of Risk for Injury is applicable when older adults are in self-neglecting situations, especially if the person lives alone and is functionally and cognitively impaired. The nursing diagnosis of Decisional Conflict might apply to abused or neglected older adults who live in an environment that places them at risk for harm because they are unable to make decisions about alternative environments. Related factors include fear, lack of information about alternatives, and impaired decision-making ability.

> ### Wellness Opportunity
>
> Nurses address body–mind–spirit interrelatedness by identifying nursing diagnoses that address fear and other psychosocial consequences of abuse or neglect.

PLANNING FOR WELLNESS OUTCOMES

Nurses direct care for abused or neglected older adults toward addressing the complex needs of the elder as well as those of the family caregivers. Some Nursing Outcomes Classification terminology that is likely to pertain to the abused older adult includes Abuse Cessation, Abuse Protection, Abuse Recovery (Emotional, Financial, Physical, Sexual), Neglect Cessation, Neglect Recovery, Self-Care Status, and Social Support. Outcomes related to abusive caregivers or family members include Abusive Behavior Self-Restraint, Caregiver Emotional Health, Caregiver–Patient Relationship, Caregiver Stressors, Caregiver Well-Being, Family Coping, Family Social Climate, Knowledge: Health Resources, Role Performance, and Stress Level.

> ### Wellness Opportunity
>
> Quality of Life is a wellness outcome that is applicable to older adults and their caregivers when conditions contributing to abuse or neglect are alleviated.

 ## NURSING INTERVENTIONS TO ADDRESS ELDER ABUSE AND NEGLECT

From a health care perspective, abused elders can be described as the intensive care patients of the community because they require the highest level of skill from a variety of professionals. Unlike intensive care patients in hospitals, however, not all the team members are specialized health care professionals, and many are community-based workers and people who provide informal support. Nurses often assume the role of coordinator or team leader in implementing interventions that address the older adults, the caregivers, and the environment for these inherently complex and challenging situations.

Because of the extensive scope of elder abuse, there are numerous Nursing Interventions Classification terms that could be applicable to both the abused or neglected elder and the caregiver. Some that would be appropriate in most situations are Abuse Protection Support: Elder, Crisis Intervention, Referral, and Risk Identification for the Elder; and Caregiver Support, Coping Enhancement, Referral, Role Enhancement, and Teaching for Caregivers.

Elder abuse interventions often involve legal actions when decision-making abilities of the older adult are impaired or when reliable and competent caregivers are not available to ask in the best interest of the elder. Thus, many cases of elder abuse involve legal and ethical questions about the competency of the elder and the caregivers. Nurses often have a key role in advocating for the older adult and may feel unprepared or uncomfortable either making or participating in decisions that affect the rights of others. Similarly, nurses may feel torn between the right of the person to refuse treatment and the obligation to report abuse and neglect situations, as discussed later in this chapter.

Interventions for elder abuse are implemented in community settings, over a long period of time, by a team of formal and informal care providers. Nurses working in home and community settings have the most direct opportunities for both the prevention of and interventions for elder abuse. In institutional settings commonly used nursing interventions include education and support of caregivers and facilitation of referrals to appropriate community agencies. Because the opportunities for intervention in institutional settings differ significantly from those in community settings, each of these areas is discussed separately in the following sections. In all settings, nursing interventions that address caregiver issues, such as the ones delineated in Box 10-5, may prevent or alleviate situations of elder abuse.

> ### Wellness Opportunity
>
> When vulnerable older adults are in an acute or long-term care setting, nurses address psychosocial needs of family caregivers by providing support and education; these are effective tools for preventing elder abuse.

Interventions in Acute Care Settings

Nurses in health care settings have opportunities to intervene in and prevent elder abuse when they interact with caregivers, who often seek advice from nurses about ways of providing care. For example, nurses can encourage caregivers to use a period of institutionalization to reevaluate the demands of the situation and to consider resources for support and assistance. Family may express ambivalence about managing the older adult's care at home, or they may be unsure or unrealistic about their own ability to provide appropriate care or to cope with the stress of the situation. In some cases, caregivers may be seeking approval for not providing care at home. In these situations, nurses can facilitate communication among all the decision makers, including the primary care provider, the older adult (as appropriate), and the various family members who are responsible for care. Sometimes, it is appropriate to suggest individual counseling or support groups or make referrals for social

Box 10-5 Nursing Interventions to Address Caregiver Issues

Examples of Abusive or Neglectful Actions That can be Addressed by Nurses

- Use of adult briefs for managing urinary incontinence without understanding the importance of changing them frequently to prevent skin breakdown
- Lack of knowledge about preventing pressure ulcers
- Restriction of fluid intake in an effort to reduce urinary incontinence
- Administration of excessive amounts of psychoactive medications
- Nonadherence to medication regimen
- Use of physical restraints

Nursing Interventions to Address Caregiver Stress

- Use communication techniques to elicit feelings and expectations about caregiving responsibilities.
- Communicate empathy for caregiver role and emphasize importance of self-care.
- Validate the feelings of the caregiver but also discuss inappropriate expression of feelings (e.g., physical abuse of older adult due to anger or impatience).
- Address unhealthy methods that the caregiver may be using to cope with the situation (e.g., substance abuse, overeating, social isolation).
- Encourage healthy methods of coping with the stress of the caregiving situation (e.g., support groups, body–mind interventions).
- Suggest professional resources for management of mental health issues such as anxiety, depression, or substance abuse.
- Explore the role of religion and religiously oriented resources to reduce stress.
- Address barriers to the use of resources.

Box 10-6 Services Generally Available in Health Care Settings

Resources for Overall Assessment of Actual or Potential Elder Abuse Situations

- Adult and gerontological advanced practice nurses
- Geriatric resource nurses
- Geriatric assessment programs
- Geriatric behavioral health programs

Consultations and Evaluations About Decision-Making Capacity

- Geriatric assessment programs
- Geropsychiatrists
- Geropsychologists
- Ethics committees

Rehabilitation Therapists for Assessment and Recommendations Related to Safety and Self-Care

- Physical therapists: assessment of and recommendations about functioning and safety, particularly regarding mobility, balance, and prevention of falls
- Occupational therapists: assessment of and recommendations related to safety, self-care, and cognitive abilities
- Speech therapists: assessment of and recommendations related to communication, cognitive abilities, swallowing problems, and feeding and eating techniques to prevent aspiration

Social Services

- Assessment of family dynamics and issues related to caregiving
- Assessment and recommendations about long-term care or community-based services
- Assistance with identifying resources for care, including those that are culturally appropriate

Adapted with permission from Miller, C. A. (2017). *Elder abuse and nursing: What nurses need to know and can do about it.* New York: Springer Publishing Company.

services, particularly when caregivers are very stressed about care-related decisions.

When elder abuse is rooted in the caregiver's lack of information, nurses can teach about appropriate caregiving measures and serve as a role model for best care practices. When caregivers need additional health education or support services, a referral to a home care agency for follow-up can be initiated. An important nursing role is to identify needs for postdischarge skilled nursing care or rehabilitation therapies that would be covered by health insurance. When questions arise about the adequacy of a discharge plan, a referral for community-based services or a protective services agency for further assessment and ongoing services should be initiated.

When elder abuse is identified in acute care settings, specialized geriatric resources may be available to provide direct care or consultation to the nursing staff. In addition, rehabilitation therapists are often overlooked as professional resources for addressing many issues related to elder abuse. Nurses providing care in medical, surgical, or intensive care units can consider requesting a consultation for services that are generally available within health care settings, as delineated in Box 10-6.

Interventions in Long-Term Care Settings

Nurses in long-term care facilities usually have a combination of administrative or supervisory responsibilities and direct care activities. Although nursing assistants bear much of the responsibility for interventions related to resident-to-resident mistreatment, licensed nurses are responsible for staff education and role modeling. For example, nurses have important roles in educating nursing assistants about management of dementia-related behaviors as a proactive approach to preventing resident-to-resident mistreatment (Rose, Lachs, Teresi, et al., 2016). In these roles, nurses can address elder abuse in all the following ways:

- Use appropriate interventions to address dementia-associated behaviors and avoid using psychotropic medications
- Support restraint-free care
- Assure that direct care staff are respectful in verbal and nonverbal interactions with residents

- Assure that care plans address needs of residents while at the same time allowing and encouraging self-care within the abilities and wishes of each resident
- Advocate for appropriate staffing levels
- Advocate for staff training, particularly with regard to effective management of behavioral manifestations of dementia

Box 10-7 summarizes strategies for managing resident-to-resident mistreatment based on the evidence-based model called the SEARCH approach (i.e., Support, Evaluate, Act, Report, Care Plan, and Help Avoid). Information about management of dementia-related behaviors, as discussed in Chapter 14, also is pertinent to elder abuse in long-term care facilities.

Interventions in Community Settings

In home settings, professional advice about managing difficult behaviors of people with dementia is an important intervention for preventing elder abuse.

Box 10-7 Strategies for Managing Resident-to-Resident Abuse

Support
- Attend to injuries
- Listen to all residents involved
- Validate residents' fears and frustrations

Evaluate
- Identify needed actions
- Evaluate all residents involved, including those who witnessed the event

Act
- Attend to the needs of all residents involved
- Separate the residents
- Acknowledge grievances and concerns of all residents

Report
- Report to nursing supervisor and all appropriate authorities or agencies
- Contact families if appropriate
- Document the event in residents' charts

Care Plan
- Update care plans for all residents involved
- Talk with care team to identify ways of intervening and avoiding episodes
- Assess and document residents' preferences for privacy and routines
- Obtain appropriate medical and psychiatric evaluations

Help Avoid
- Avoid overcrowding of residents
- Recognize and address risk factors
- Separate residents known to have negative interactions

Source: Ellis, J., Teresi, J. A., Ramirez, M., et al. (2014). Managing resident to resident elder mistreatment (R-REM) in nursing homes: the SEARCH approach. *Journal of Continuing Education in Nursing, 45*(3), 112–123.

Nurses in community settings have many opportunities for teaching caregivers about adequate care through role modeling and verbal and written instruction. For example, nurses may suggest innovative ways of meeting the nutritional requirements of an elderly person who does not eat (use Online Learning Activities 18-3 and 18-6 to explore information about this topic).

When elder abuse is rooted in caregiver stress, nurses can suggest services and help find ways of providing care so that the caregiver can use these resources for self-care. The following are examples of services aimed at reducing caregiver stress or dealing with caregiver problems:

- Alzheimer's Association for support and education groups
- Individual counseling to learn coping skills
- Alcoholics Anonymous for caregivers with alcoholism
- Al-Anon for situations involving substance abuse
- In-home or day care for respite
- Veterans Administration for veterans and their caregivers

Home health aides and paid companions are the formal service providers who are most likely to care for abused elders in home settings, but they often are ill prepared to recognize or address elder abuse. Nurses who provide home-based services, therefore, have a tremendous responsibility to help home care workers identify and intervene in situations that are actually or potentially abusive. For example, nurses can teach home care workers about risks for elder abuse, and they can address concerns about questionable conditions. If nurses cannot openly discuss the situation during home visits, they may have to arrange for a phone conversation with the home care worker. In situations in which the older adult requires a significant degree of physical care or supervision, the services of home care workers may be effective for addressing situations of actual or potential elder abuse. Often, however, the retention of a home care worker in challenging situations depends largely on the degree of support and guidance provided by a professional nurse.

Nurses in other community settings, such as clinics or senior centers, have opportunities to intervene in elder abuse. For example, faith community nurses (also called parish nurses) may be the only contact for older adults who neglect themselves or care for a dependent spouse and are not aware of the many resources to address their needs. Nurses can prevent or alleviate elder abuse by facilitating referrals for appropriate community-based resources, such as adult day care or group or home-delivered meals. Even if nurses are not familiar with specific community services, they can discuss the advantages of various types of services and encourage older adults to call their local office on aging. At a minimum, nurses need to be familiar with the phone number for the area agency on aging that serves as an information center about local resources in every geographic area of the United States. Information about local agencies on aging also is available by calling the Eldercare Locator at (800) 677–1116 or www.eldercare.gov.

Nurses also can initiate or suggest referrals for services for specific groups of people. Older adults and caregivers who identify with a particular group may perceive resources related to their religious denomination or cultural group as more acceptable. The National Center on Elder Abuse provides culturally specific resources, including consumer educational materials in many languages. The Veterans Administration provides many home and community-based services, and these programs are available for veterans of any age and their caregivers. A wide range of services also is available through faith-based organizations, such as Jewish or Catholic Family Services and the Interfaith Partnership Against Domestic Violence and Elder Abuse. Additional information about community-based programs is provided in Online Learning Activity 10-5.

See ONLINE LEARNING ACTIVITY 10-5: RESOURCES FOR INFORMATION ABOUT ELDER ABUSE AND INTERDISCIPLINARY EFFORTS at http://thepoint.lww.com/Miller8e

Wellness Opportunity

Nurses help caregivers maintain self-wellness by identifying ways of alleviating stress associated with the demands of caregiving.

Multidisciplinary Teams

Nurses serve as essential members of **multidisciplinary teams** (also called interdisciplinary teams) that are responsible for initial and ongoing assessment and implementation of plans to address complex elder abuse situations. Multidisciplinary teams are regarded as a hallmark for effective elder abuse response, with national efforts currently underway to expand and strengthen the multidisciplinary teams throughout the country (Breckman, Callahan, & Solomon, 2015). Interdisciplinary teams for elder abuse generally include professionals who offer the perspectives of law, nursing, medicine, psychiatry, social work, and rehabilitation therapy, with additional disciplines included when required. When legal interventions are being considered, the interdisciplinary team conducts a comprehensive assessment, including all aspects of the person's functioning and decision-making capacity, the involvement of the family and significant others in meeting basic needs, and the ability of the older person to participate in developing a safe and realistic plan of action.

Interdisciplinary teams provide a holistic perspective, which is essential for thoroughly assessing the problem and determining appropriate solutions. In addition, team members collaborate in handling complex and difficult cases, and they can establish effective approaches to elder abuse prevention and treatment (Anetzberger, In Press). In recent years, specialized teams have evolved to address particular elder abuse forms or situations, such as older adult hoarding and elder abuse forensics (Navarro, Wysong, DeLiema, et al., 2016).

If nurses do not have access to the resources of an interdisciplinary team, they need to be creative in finding other professionals with whom they can work. For example, when working with homebound elders, nurses may need to identify resources for an initial and ongoing medical evaluation and care. In many areas of the country, primary care providers are resuming the practice of making home visits. In addition, with the growing demand for home health services, an increased number of diagnostic tests are performed in the home (e.g., radiography, blood tests, and electrocardiography). In many situations, these diagnostic tests are essential for determining whether involuntary care measures are justified. For instance, if the older adult refuses to go out of the home, blood tests or radiography done in the home may provide the evidence needed to determine whether a hospitalization is warranted.

Referrals

An important nursing role is to initiate and facilitate referrals for services that improve functioning for the older adult and decrease the burden of caregiving responsibilities. For instance, speech, physical, and occupational therapies may be useful in improving the older person's ability to communicate, ambulate, and perform ADLs. Referrals for skilled home care services usually are made at the time of discharge from an institution; however, the older adult or family may have refused the services at that time. Older adults who are not admitted to health care facilities may not know they qualify for skilled home care services, and a nurse making a home visit may be the first health professional to suggest these resources. Although older adults or their families may not know about or may have refused such services, nurses need to assess their willingness to accept help as conditions change.

Nurses also assess whether recent changes in the elder qualify the person for skilled home care services. For example, a change in medications might qualify a person for skilled nursing care, and a fall might qualify a person for skilled physical therapy. Staff in home care agencies usually are happy to discuss skilled care services with anyone who calls for information. Nurses also can advise about the possibility of having services covered by health insurance, and they can obtain orders from the primary care provider for those services that are covered under Medicare or other health insurance programs.

Another important role for nurses is suggesting types of medical equipment, disposable supplies, and assistive devices to improve function and safety for the elder and ease caregiver burden. For example, caregivers may respond positively to suggestions from the nurse about obtaining and using grab bars for preventing falls in the bathroom. Some durable medical equipment is covered by health insurance, and medical supply companies usually are quite helpful in advising people about specific equipment.

Services for Prevention and Treatment

Abused elders and their caregivers or abusers typically need a wide range of interventions, which can be categorized according to basic function:

- Core, or essential, integrative services
- Emergency services, during crises or just before or after abuse or neglect occurs
- Support services for managing the problem and improving the situation
- Rehabilitative services to address problems of either the victim or the perpetrator
- Preventive services, including programs directed toward changing society in ways that diminish the likelihood of mistreatment or self-neglect

Figure 10-4 identifies some of the specific types of services, arranged by function, that may be needed in elder abuse situations. Nurses are the health care professionals who are most accepted and qualified for implementing or arranging for many of the services for both the caregivers and abused or neglected older person(s).

Elder abuse scholars emphasize that evidence is lacking with regard to the effectiveness of interventions

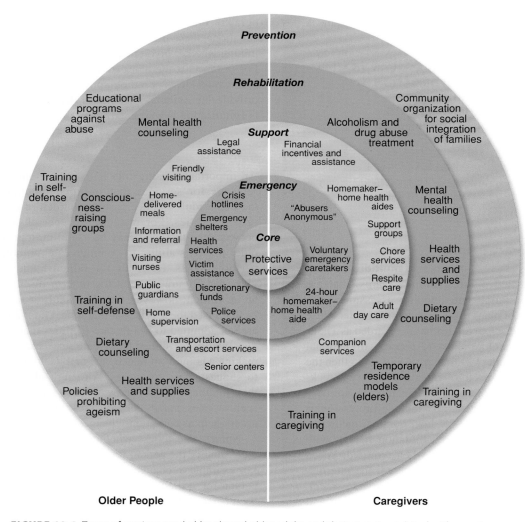

FIGURE 10-4 Types of services needed by abused older adults and their caregivers. (Used with permission from Anetzberger, G. J. (2010). Report of the elder abuse project: Recommendations for addressing the problem of elder abuse in Cuyahoga County. Cleveland, OH: Federation for Community Planning. Originally published in 1982.)

to prevent or treat elder abuse (Pillemer, 2016). Using multiple case studies or program descriptions, five interventions were recently identified as international elder abuse "promising practices": caregiver interventions (e.g., respite care and support groups); money management programs; helplines; emergency shelters; and multidisciplinary teams (Pillemer, Burnes, Riffin, et al., 2016). This is precisely the intent of the Abuse Intervention Model (AIM), currently being tested by the Keck School of Medicine at the University of Southern California to prevent elder abuse against adults with dementia (Mosqueda, Burnright, Gironda, et al., 2016). A university-community partnership, AIM attempts to address elder abuse risk factors using a toolkit of established interventions, such as individual counseling for caregiver depression and in-home care agency for ADL dependency on the part of the adult with dementia.

Case Study

Mr. and Mrs. G. have been married for over 50 years and have six children, four of whom live in their area. Because of Mrs. G.'s memory loss in recent years, Mr. G. has allowed home care workers into the house to assist with ADLs and provide care at night because she does not sleep much. The workers report that Mr. G. yells at his wife when she forgets things. On more than one occasion, they witnessed him attempting to force-feed her when she failed to eat an entire meal. When the couple is in their bedroom, workers have reported hearing screams, crying, and slapping sounds coming from behind the closed door. In the morning, Mrs. G. had bruises on her body and bumps on her head. When asked, Mr. G. denied hitting his wife. Mrs. G. cried when questioned, never providing an explanation for her injuries.

Mr. G. is reluctant to consider additional services, such as adult day care, fearing that the couple's savings will evaporate. He had Mrs. G. change doctors several times in recent years because "they don't do anything to really help her." The children who live nearby have said that they do not want to get involved in their parents' situation. They describe years of their father physically and verbally abusing their mother and fear what might happen if any action is taken now.

THINKING POINTS

- What interventions might be helpful in addressing the elder abuse evident in this situation?
- What is the role of the home care nurse in introducing and implementing these interventions?
- What barriers might be encountered in acceptance of the interventions?
- As the home care nurse in this situation, how will you help to overcome these barriers?

Financial exploitation is an aspect of elder abuse that can be prevented through relatively simple and widely available measures to protect assets. For example, nurses can suggest that a trusted family member establishes a joint account with the older adult and keep track of all transactions. Out-of-town families can oversee financial transactions through online banking.

LEGAL INTERVENTIONS AND ETHICAL ISSUES

Many elder abuse situations require consideration of voluntary or involuntary legal interventions. Whenever feasible, problems should be remedied without the use of involuntary legal intervention. Because voluntary legal interventions require the consent of the older person, they cannot be initiated if the person is not mentally competent. Competent adults can revoke voluntary legal interventions at any time. Money management, power of attorney, and various types of bank accounts, such as joint or direct deposit, are all interventions of this nature. Other legal interventions that are pertinent to older adults are discussed in Chapter 9.

Some legal interventions, such as guardianship or civil commitment, are either voluntary or involuntary but are most commonly used on an involuntary basis when the older person's safety or property is in jeopardy. Because these legal interventions involve a much more extensive loss of personal freedom than voluntary ones, they should be used with extreme caution. A key consideration in the choice of legal interventions is determining the capacity of the person to make decisions, as discussed in Chapters 9 and 13. Some measures, such as guardianship, may be easier to initiate than to discontinue. Others, such as civil commitment, may be accompanied by long-term stigma, even when the intervention is terminated.

Involuntary legal interventions are used when mental impairments, such as limited insight, judgment, memory, or cognition, affect the ability of older people to function safely and meet their basic human needs. In general, involuntary legal intervention is indicated when assessment reveals all of the following conditions:

- Decisions must be made about the older person's health, living arrangements, money, or property.
- The older person is not capable of making reasonable decisions.
- There is a risk to the older person's health, safety, money, or property.
- The risk would be reduced or eliminated if someone else were empowered to make and implement decisions.

Legal interventions that address the abuser include domestic violence law and the criminal code. Adult protective services law is particularly limited when considerable property needs protection, the mistreatment is significant and repeated, the older person's mental impairment is substantial and permanent, or the goal is to prevent mistreatment rather than to treat it. Under these conditions, other legal interventions should be considered with, or as alternatives to, adult protective services.

Wellness Opportunity

Nurses support autonomy for older adults by identifying the least invasive legal interventions, while also ensuring the least amount of endangerment.

Adult Protective Services Laws

Philosophically, **adult protective services laws** (also called elder abuse statutes or elder abuse reporting laws) provide protection for the person who is abused, for the person offering assistance, and for society from possible dangers posed by the person. Adult protective services laws differ among states, but all are directed toward the following purposes:

- Facilitating the identification and referral of abuse or neglect
- Conveying public and centralized authority for addressing protective matters
- Establishing a system of protective services to prevent, correct, or discontinue abuse or neglect
- Permitting, under certain circumstances, involuntary access to the suspected victim of abuse for the purpose of investigation and service delivery

Usually, local departments of social services receive reports of abuse, but in some states, departments of aging or prosecutors' offices receive them.

The scope of reports includes neglect; exploitation; and physical, sexual, and psychological abuse; in several states, laws include abandonment and cruel punishment. In all states but New York, reporting suspected abuse is mandatory for health, social service, and safety professionals and paraprofessionals. State laws typically protect the confidentiality of reports and the identity of the people involved in making them. The usual penalty for failure to report is a charge of misdemeanor, with or without financial penalty. In some states, however, failure to report can result in imprisonment, civil liability for damages, or notification of the state licensing board.

The public authority responsible for elder abuse law implementation must investigate promptly; sometimes, the law mandates a specific response time, often within 24 to 72 hours. Investigation generally includes a home visit with the alleged victim and consultation with people knowledgeable about the situation. Interventions

for at-risk older people can include health care, support services, protective placement, emergency care, or financial management. Most laws emphasize due process, self-determination, least restrictive interventions, and voluntary acceptance of services by mentally capacitated adults. Although protective services workers have the primary responsibility for implementing elder abuse laws, nurses have essential roles in reporting and collaborating, assessing, consulting, testifying in court, and providing care. Nursing responsibilities associated with each of these roles are discussed in the subsequent sections.

Reporting and Collaborating

Nurses are among the health care workers most commonly identified as mandatory reporters in adult abuse and protective services laws. This is appropriate because the usual duties assumed by nurses place them in a key position for witnessing the consequences of abuse and neglect. In addition, a primary role of nurses is to foster collaboration between health care professionals as abuse reporters and adult protective services or law enforcement officials as abuse investigators or service providers.

Mandatory reporting laws do not require reporters to *know* whether abuse or neglect has occurred, but merely to report it if they *suspect* its occurrence. The responsibility for problem verification rests with the public agency charged with law implementation, not with the reporter or referral source. Suspecting elder abuse means detecting signs of violence, such as bruises, welts, or fractures. It also means recognizing conditions associated with neglect or deprivation, such as frostbite, malnutrition, dehydration, oversedation, mental changes, or uncontrolled medical conditions.

Because most reporting laws provide immunity for mandatory reporters, nurses who act in good faith and without malicious intent can report suspected cases without fear of liability. Some laws offer immunity in the workplace; in these cases, nurses cannot be fired, transferred, or demoted for making a report. In all states, responsibility for making the report rests with the individual nurse, so nurses cannot delegate reporting to anyone else. The nurse alone has the responsibility for reporting, and for the consequences—both legal and moral—of failing to do so. Even though individual nurses are responsible for reporting, most agencies and hospitals have established protocols to clarify roles and enhance the credibility of the report. Excellent examples of elder abuse detection protocols are available, and they should be considered for use by nurses in all health care settings involving multiple professions and levels of authority. Box 10-8 illustrates a typical protocol for hospital- or agency-based nurses.

Box 10-8 Sample Protocol for Nurses With Regard to Elder Abuse

Assessment

- Use usual assessment forms and observe for clues to elder abuse
- If there is reason for suspicion, use a formal elder abuse assessment tool
- Observe and interview caregivers and caregiver–older adult interactions
- Analyze data that raise a suspicion of abuse, neglect, or exploitation
- Consider whether objective findings fit the explanation

Consulting the Abuse Detection Team as Appropriate

- Report pertinent findings to the team leader and the primary care provider as soon as possible
- Summarize findings from the assessment guide on progress notes
- Determine the need to report abuse or neglect to authorities
- Document additional facts, and whether a report was made, in the progress notes
- Document discussions with the older adult and caregivers

Follow-Up Actions

- Summarize action steps taken and recommended by team
- Implement any security measures to protect the older adult
- Implement appropriate interventions

Assessing

Protective services workers often call upon nurses to assess their older adults, especially when there is concern about endangerment or questions about the effects of neglect or abuse. Nurses commonly are involved with assessments of older adults who are newly referred or experiencing a change in health status. Nurses are the preferred health care worker for such assessments because of their holistic approach, their availability through nursing agencies, their willingness to make home visits, and the relative ease with which older people usually accept nurses.

Because assessment was discussed earlier in this chapter, only one aspect requires further examination here. Formal elder abuse assessment instruments are used to collect and organize all pertinent information; summarize observations; and provide a base for planning referrals, services, or legal actions. These tools assess and document all of the following:

- Background data (e.g., older adult's name and address)
- Signs of mistreatment or self-neglect according to type (e.g., bruises or welts in cases of suspected physical abuse)
- Severity of signs (e.g., an immediate life threat)

- Indicators of mistreatment intentionality (e.g., a caregiver who will not allow the nurse to be alone with the older adult)
- Symptoms of acute or chronic illness or impairment (e.g., incontinence)
- Functional incapacity (e.g., an inability to dress or toilet without assistance)
- Aggravating social conditions (e.g., an older adult who lives alone and is socially isolated)
- Source of information (e.g., agency referral)
- Recommended action (e.g., referral of the case to home health care service providers)

Consulting

In addition to providing direct assessment, nurses often provide consultation when questions arise regarding the health status of older adults. Typical questions relate to medications, continence, nutrition and hydration, and disease signs. Often, consultation services are part of networks among service providers in a given community; sometimes, they are formally organized through clinical consultation teams that are integral parts of protective services coalitions. Another role for nurses is in staff education for protective services workers on topics such as health assessment, recognition of endangerment, and disease prevention and detection.

Testifying in Court

Although very few cases of elder abuse involve court actions, adult protective services workers may need legal assistance to gain access, deliver services, or obtain a comprehensive assessment. In these situations, the older person usually is mentally impaired and unable to make decisions that would alleviate or eliminate the neglect or abuse. Legal intervention may also be appropriate when older adults in life-endangering circumstances refuse help. Before legal interventions are permitted, the protective services worker must present evidence to a judge or referee about all of the following:

- Abuse or neglect
- Need for protective services
- Inability to gain voluntary cooperation
- No other way to alleviate the problems

Most of the evidence is provided by physicians, mental health providers, and protective services workers; however, nurses are sometimes asked to testify or submit reports about their assessments or services.

Testimony involves two types of evidence: direct observation and expert opinion. Nurses are likely to be called upon to provide in-person testimony about their direct observations because they can provide a professional assessment of the health status or function of the older person. In addition, nursing documentation about assessments and care plans may be used as evidence in court proceedings. Thus, nurses need to carefully, accurately, and objectively document all pertinent information with the understanding that their documentation may be used in legal proceedings.

Providing Care

As discussed in the nursing interventions section of this chapter, nurses provide essential care and treatment for abused and neglected older people. They help correct conditions caused by mistreatment and self-neglect, and they prevent their recurrence through activities such as treating injuries, monitoring medication, educating caregivers, obtaining assistive devices, and facilitating service referrals. In this role, as in others, nurses work cooperatively with other professionals and with paraprofessionals and use their knowledge and expertise to help the victims of elder abuse.

Ethical Issues

Ethical issues related to abused and neglected elders are similar to ethical issues in medicine and other fields. Rather than having clear answers and absolute rights and wrongs, there are usually differing perspectives and different implications, depending on what course of action is taken. Ethical issues in adult protective services are influenced by the fact that all adults in American society have rights—including freedom from intrusion, the right to fair treatment, freedom from unnecessary restraint, and the right to self-determination—but these rights can be taken away through the use of legal measures. Professionals often face a dilemma when they need to initiate legal measures that take away the rights of other adults. For example, unless an older adult has been judged to be incompetent by a court of law, he or she has the right to be protected from intrusion. In adult protective services situations, however, this right can be threatened when services are deemed to be necessary and the older person does not willingly agree to assistance.

Another dilemma involves the characteristics of protective situations that sometimes make respecting personal rights so difficult. The following are examples of situations that present ethical dilemmas in relation to respecting personal rights:

- In situations that are urgent or dangerous, it is hard to walk away, even when the older person asks to be left alone.
- Public pressure to do something, no matter what, places pressure on care providers who are trying to resolve the situation while respecting the rights of the older person.
- Contradictory societal values may pit individual rights against other values, such as paternalism and protectionism.

- Because nursing is directed toward helping others, it is difficult to deal with vulnerable elders who do not accept help, especially when the lack of help has detrimental consequences.
- It may be necessary to make a serious decision based on little information because the older adult may be cognitively impaired, the situation may require immediate actions, or pertinent information may be withheld by the older person or the caregivers.
- The questionable mental status of many abused or neglected elders places decision-making responsibility in the hands of other people. Involuntary legal interventions may unnecessarily deprive the person of certain rights, but inaction can mean that basic human needs are not being met adequately, or at all.
- The intrusive nature of legal interventions, including mandatory reporting, can deprive people of their fundamental rights.

Nurses can apply the hierarchy of principles summarized in Box 10-9 to address ethical dilemmas about particular situations. These principles of adult protective services

---

Box 10-9 Hierarchy of Principles of Adult Protective Services

I. **Freedom Over Safety.** The older adult has a right to choose to live at risk of harm, providing he or she is capable of making that choice, harms no one, and commits no crime.

II. **Self-Determination.** The older adult has a right to personal choices and decisions until such time that he or she delegates, or the court grants, the responsibility to someone else.

III. **Participation in Decision-Making.** The older adult has a right to receive information to make informed choices and to participate in all decisions affecting his or her circumstances to the extent that he or she is able.

IV. **Least Restrictive Alternative.** The older adult has a right to service alternatives that maximize choice and minimize lifestyle disruption.

V. **Primacy of the Adult.** The practitioner's primary responsibility is to serve the older adult, not anyone else (e.g., community members concerned about appearances or a family member concerned about finances).

VI. **Confidentiality.** The older adult has a right to privacy and confidentiality.

VII. **Benefit of Doubt.** If there is evidence that the older adult is making a reasoned choice, the practitioner has a responsibility to ensure that the benefit of doubt is in his or her favor.

VIII. **Do no Harm.** The practitioner has a responsibility to take no action that places the older adult at greater risk of harm.

IX. **Avoidance of Blame.** The practitioner has a responsibility to understand the origins of any mistreatment and to commit no action that would antagonize the perpetrator and so reduce the chances of terminating the mistreatment.

X. **Maintenance of the Family.** If the perpetrator is a family member, the practitioner has a responsibility to deal with the mistreatment as a family problem and to try to find appropriate services to resolve the problem.

TABLE 10-2 Ethical Questions and Suggested Solutions Regarding Abused Elders

Ethical Question/Implications	Suggested Solution
When do I report elder abuse? (If I report too soon, I may needlessly invade someone's privacy. If I wait, the situation may worsen)	Report elder abuse when you believe that, without intervention, the situation will deteriorate or endanger the elder
What if my report places the elder in more danger, or labels someone inaccurately? What if it causes the elder to shy away from me and my agency?	Report elder abuse if you believe that the protective services system can reduce the risk better than the current interventions
How do I decide if the elder or the caregiver receives priority? (If my priority is the elder, I may alienate his or her family members, who serve as the primary sources of care. If my priority is the family, then the care plan may be contrary to the elder's wishes and may not adequately respect his or her rights)	With certain exceptions, the elder should receive priority. These exceptions are limited to circumstances in which the elder has been judged to be incompetent by a court of law or is endangering others by his or her behavior
Is it more important to maintain standards of confidentiality than to comply with a reporting law?	State law takes precedence over professional standards
Does the right of an elder to refuse services extend to total self-neglect and intentional suicide? How can I know that endangered elders clearly understand the consequences of their self-neglect? How can I accept abandoning the situation?	Ethical dilemmas such as these often can be resolved through the use of a hierarchy of values or principles, such as those summarized in Box 10-8
Can emergency services be thrust upon an elder who would have refused them under ordinary circumstances? If the elder's life is endangered, then is it not my primary responsibility to use my nursing skills in life-saving ways, no matter what the elder chooses? Even if the elder might have refused services in the past, does that mean he or she absolutely would refuse them now?	If the elder is incapable of deciding whether to accept or reject emergency services, then these services should be provided, subject to the constraints of the protective services law. This offers the elder essential protection, but recognizes his or her right to refuse ongoing services when the emergency has subsided and he or she is capable of making decisions on his or her own behalf

are arranged from the most to the least important considerations with regard to interventions for abused or neglected elders.

Adult protective services are fraught with ethical dilemmas. Some of these dilemmas are related to the five basic roles—reporter, investigator, service provider, administrator, and planner—assumed by professionals. Each role has a particular sphere of responsibility in addressing elder abuse and neglect. The reporter detects the situation and describes it to someone authorized by law to deal with it. The investigator is the legal agent who assesses the situation and determines the need for protective services. The service provider offers interventions for correcting or discontinuing mistreatment or self-neglect. The administrator manages a protective services program. Finally, the planner develops policies and programs, as well as community education initiatives, aimed at preventing or treating the problem.

Professional workers in each of these roles face different ethical issues. Issues of the reporter role include questions about making a report and the consequences of doing so. The role of the investigator involves confronting questions about privacy, openness, and confidentiality. The service provider deals with issues about the rights of the elder, the rights of the caregivers, and the degree of risk for the elder. Program planners and administrators face dilemmas about service priorities and funding, staff, and other critical resources. Nurses most often deal with ethical issues in their roles as reporters,

investigators, and service providers. Table 10-2 identifies some of the ethical problems, as well as related solutions, that nurses may encounter in their roles in adult protective services.

See ONLINE LEARNING ACTIVITY 10-6: RESOURCES FOR INFORMATION ABOUT ADULT PROTECTIVE SERVICES AND LAWS RELATED TO ELDER ABUSE at http://thepoint.lww.com/Miller8e

EVALUATING EFFECTIVENESS OF NURSING INTERVENTIONS

Nursing care of abused or neglected older adults is evaluated by the extent to which nursing goals are achieved. If a nursing goal is to alleviate the contributing factor of unnecessary dependence, the care is evaluated by whether the older adult is functioning at a higher level of independence. If a nursing goal is to address caregiver stress, the nursing care might be evaluated by the caregiver accepting help with the care, attending caregiver support groups, and expressing less stress about his or her caregiving responsibilities. When the nursing goal is to protect an incompetent older adult from harm, nursing care might be evaluated by the extent to which the least restrictive legal interventions are implemented. In such cases, nursing care is evaluated in terms of protecting the older adult from harm while also protecting his or her rights.

Unfolding Case Study

Part 2: Mrs. B. at 82 Years of Age

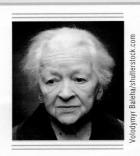

Volodymyr Baleha/shutterstock.com

Recall that Mrs. B. is 82 years old and lives in a senior citizens' apartment. After 2 months of receiving skilled nursing visits, Mrs. B. was discharged from the home care agency because she was successfully managing her medications and other aspects of functioning adequately. Several months after she was discharged, the nurse in the wellness clinic at the senior citizens apartment noted a change in her mannerisms, accompanied by slurred speech and an unbalanced gait. Mrs. B. had bruises on her arms, knees, and forehead, but insisted that she had not fallen. After further investigation, the nurse found that her blood pressure was 210/104 mm Hg and that her blood glucose level was 410 mg/dL on the glucometer that the nurse kept in the clinic. A pill count revealed that Mrs. B. had not taken her medications for 2½ days. After a consultation with her primary care provider, Mrs. B. was admitted to the hospital. Tests revealed that she had suffered a stroke, resulting in left-sided weakness and short-term memory loss.

Mrs. B. left the hospital against medical advice and returned to her apartment, initially refusing visits from the home health nurse. She insisted that her children come and administer her medications and prepare her meals because she was unable to do this for herself. Mrs. B. reasoned that she had cared for her children when they were young, so they should come when she needed them. The children tried to assist Mrs. B. for 4 days but were unable to meet both her demands and those of their jobs and families. Mrs. B. reluctantly agreed to a visit from the home health nurse who had visited her before. She expected that she would see the nurse once and that the nurse would "make my children do right."

Mrs. B.'s children were present for the initial assessment. Mrs. B. was unable to stand or transfer to the commode without help. She could not use her chart and color-coded boxes to take her pills. Mrs. B. flatly refused to consider admission to a nursing facility to receive therapy to regain her strength, and she would not consider living with her daughter or either son. The family told the nurse that they were exhausted and on the "verge of a breakdown" and could not continue to provide the care that Mrs. B. needed. The nurse explained to Mrs. B. that it was not safe for her to remain in her apartment without assistance. She suggested that she hire an aide until other arrangements could be made, because her children were not obligated to lose their jobs or jeopardize their family relationships to care for her. Mrs. B. accused her children of being greedy and caring only about themselves. She said that children have a duty to care for their parents and that she wasn't going to "have strangers doing the things that decent children should be doing." She directed her concluding remarks at the nurse, stating, "What's more, I don't need you to come back either, because all you want to do is side with my children."

THINKING POINTS

- What strategies would you use to establish a relationship with Mrs. B.?
- What additional assessment information would you want to obtain, and how would you obtain it?
- What would your next steps be in working with Mrs. B.?
- How would you work with the family?
- What other resources would you involve in planning and providing care for Mrs. B.?
- What criteria would you use for making a referral for adult protective services?

Chapter Highlights

Overview of Elder Abuse and Neglect

- Definitions and forms (Box 10-1, Figure 10-1)
- Recognition of elder abuse in the United States and the world (Figure 10-2)
- Prevalence

Specific Types of Elder Abuse Most Relevant to Nursing

- Self-neglect
- Neglect by a trusted other

Cultural Considerations

- Cultural considerations affect numerous aspects of elder abuse (Box 10-2).

Causes of, and Risk Factors for, Elder Abuse and Neglect (Box 10-3)

- Vulnerability of the older adult
- Social isolation and lack of social support
- Dementia, depression, and mental illness
- Caregiver factors

Elder Abuse in Nursing Homes

- Risk factors related to elder abuse in nursing homes
- Elder abuse by direct care staff
- Resident-to-resident mistreatment
- Resources for addressing elder abuse in long-term care settings

Functional Consequences Associated With Elder Abuse

- Examples of older adults who become victims of elder abuse in its many forms and guises
- Effects of elder abuse on older adults

Nursing Assessment of Abused Older Adults (Figure 10-3, Box 10-4)

- Unique aspects of elder abuse assessment
- Risks to health and safety
- Physical assessment: bruises and injuries, pressure ulcers and other skin indicators, infections, nutrition and hydration
- Psychosocial function
- Administration of medications
- Environmental influences
- Caregivers and support resources
- Cultural aspects of assessment

Nursing Diagnosis

- Compromised (or Disabled) Family Coping
- Caregiver Role Strain (or Risk for)
- Risk for Injury
- Decisional Conflict

Planning for Wellness Outcomes

- Quality of life
- Abuse cessation, protection, recovery
- Neglect cessation
- Caregiver stressors, emotional health
- Family coping
- Social support

Nursing Interventions to Address Elder Abuse and Neglect

- Interventions to address caregiver issues (Box 10-5)
- Interventions in acute care settings (Box 10-6)
- Interventions in long-term care settings (Box 10-7)
- Multidisciplinary teams and community-based interventions
- Referrals for services for prevention and treatment (Figure 10-4)

Legal Interventions and Ethical Issues (Box 10-8)

- Voluntary and involuntary types of legal interventions
- Roles of nurses in adult protective services: reporting and collaborating, assessing, consulting, testifying in court, providing care
- Ethical issues: principles of adult protective services (Box 10-9)
- Ethical questions and suggested solutions (Table 10-2)

Evaluating Effectiveness of Nursing Interventions

- Higher level of functioning of older adult
- Alleviation of caregiver stress
- Use of least restrictive legal interventions
- Protection of the older adult

Critical Thinking Exercises

1. Identify factors in each of the following categories that currently contribute to elder abuse and neglect in the United States:
   - Demographic statistics
   - Changes in families
   - Health care systems
   - Health status and other characteristics of older adults
   - Social awareness
2. What is different about the nursing assessment of abused or neglected elders compared with the nursing assessment of other older adults?
3. What do you believe about family caregiving responsibilities? How would you deal with a family whose values about caregiving differ significantly from yours?
4. What are your beliefs about the degree of risk a frail elder should be allowed to take?
5. Under what circumstances should an elder be denied the right to remain in his or her own home?

 For more information about the topics discussed in this chapter, be sure to check out the interactive Online Learning Activities and other helpful resources at http://thepoint.lww.com/Miller8e

REFERENCES

Acierno, R., Hernandez, M., Amstadter, A., et al. (2010). Prevalence and correlates of emotional, physical, sexual, and financial abuse and potential neglect in the United States: The National Elder Mistreatment Study. *American Journal of Public Health, 100*(2), 292–297.

Anetzberger, G. J. (2012). An update on the nature and scope of elder abuse. *Generations, 36*(3), 12–30.

Anetzberger, G. J. (In Press). Elder abuse multidisciplinary teams. In X. Dong (Ed.): *Elder abuse: Research, practice, and policy.* New York: Springer Publishing Company.

Breckman, R., Callahan, J., & Soloman, J. (2015). *Elder abuse multidisciplinary teams: Planning for the future.* New York: NYC Elder Abuse Center, Brookdale Center for Healthy Aging, and The Harry and Jeanette Weil Elder Abuse Prevention Center.

Burnes, D., Pillemer, K., & Lachs, M. (2016). Elder abuse severity: A critical but understudied dimension of victimization for clinicians and researchers. *The Gerontologist*, doi: 10.1093/geront/gnv688 [Epub]

Burnett, J., Jackson, S., Sinha, A., et al. (2016). Five-year all-cause mortality rates across five categories of substantiated elder abuse occurring in the community. *Journal of Elder Abuse & Neglect, 28*, 59–75.

Castle, N., Ferguson-Rome, J. C., & Teresi, J. A. (2015). Elder abuse in residential long-term care: An update to the 2003 National Research Council report. *Journal of Applied Gerontology, 34*, 407–443

Centers for Medicare & Medicaid Services. (2016). Memorandum on protecting resident privacy and prohibiting mental abuse related to photographs and audio/video recordings by nursing home staff. Available at www.cms.gov

D'Angelo, G. M. (2016). Does anyone remember Tommy? *Geriatric Nursing, 37*, 244–246.

Dong, X. (2015). Elder abuse: Systematic review and implications for practice. *Journal of the American Geriatrics Society, 63*(6), 1214–1238.

Dong, X., Chen, R., & Simon, M. A. (2014). Elder abuse and dementia: A review of the research and health policy. *Health Affairs, 33*(4), 1–8.

Dong, X., & Wang, B. (2016). Rosalie Wolf Memorial Award lectures: Past, present, and future of elder abuse. *Journal of Elder Abuse & Neglect*, [Epub] doi: 10.1080/08946566.2016.1237318.

Federal Register. (2015). *Rules and regulations. Part 1327—Allotments for vulnerable elder rights protections activities.* Washington, DC: U.S. Department of Health and Human Services.

Gimm, G., Chowdhury, S., & Castle, N. (2016). Resident aggression and abuse in assisted living. *Journal of Applied Gerontology*, [Epub] doi: 10.1177/0733464816661947.

Gironda, M., Nguyen, A., & Mosqueda, L. (2016). Is this broken bone because of abuse? Characteristics and comorbid diagnoses in older adults with fractures. *Journal of the American Geriatrics Society, 64*, 1651–1655.

Hansen, M., Flores, D., Coverdale, J., et al. (2016). Correlates of depression in self-neglecting older adults: A cross-sectional study examining the role of alcohol abuse and pain in increasing vulnerability. *Journal of Elder Abuse, 28*, 41–56.

Harrington, C., Carillo, H., & Garfield, R. (2015). *Nursing facilities, staffing, residents and facility deficiencies, 2009 through 2014.* The Kaiser Commission on Medicaid and the uninsured. Available at kdf.org

Herdman, T., & Kamitsuru, S. (Eds.). (2018). *NANDA International Nursing Diagnoses Definitions and Classification, 2018–2020* (11th ed., pp. 34–44). New York: Thieme Publishers.

Jackson, S. L. (2016). The shifting conceptualization of elder abuse in the United States: From social services, to criminal justice, and beyond. *International Psychogeriatrics, 28*, 1–8.

Jervis, L. L., Sconzert-Hall, W., & The Shielding American Indian Elders Project Team. (2017). The conceptualization of mistreatment by older American Indians. *Journal of Elder Abuse & Neglect, 29*, 43–58.

Killick, C., Taylor, B. J., Begley, E., et al. (2015). Older people's conceptualization of abuse: A systematic review. *Journal of Elder Abuse & Neglect, 27*(2), 100–120.

Lachs, M. S., Teresi, J. A., Ramirez, M., et al. (2016). The prevalence of resident-to-resident elder mistreatment in nursing homes. *Annuals of Internal Medicine*. Advance online publication. doi: 10.7326/M15–1209.

Lee, Y.-S., Kaplan, C., & Perez-Stable, E. J. (2014). Elder mistreatment among Chinese and Korean immigrants; The roles of sociocultural contexts on perceptions and help-seeking behaviors. *Journal of Elder Abuse & Neglect, 26*, 244–269.

Lien, C., Rosen, T., Bloemen, E. M., et al. (2016). Narratives of self-neglect: Patterns of traumatic personal experiences and maladaptive behaviors in cognitively intact older adults. *Journal of the American Geriatrics Society, 64*(11), e195–e200.

Lifespan of Greater Rochester, Inc., Weill Cornell Medical Center of Cornell University, & New York City Department of Aging. (2011). *Under the Radar: New York Elder Abuse Prevalence Study.* New York: Author.

McDonald, L., Hitzig, S. L., Pillemer, K. A., et al. (2015). Developing a research agenda on resident-to-resident aggression: Recommendations from a consensus conference. *Journal of Elder Abuse & Neglect, 27*(2), 146–167.

Mosqueda, L., Burnright, K., Gironda, M. W., et al. (2016). The Abuse Intervention Model: A pragmatic approach to intervention for elder mistreatment. *Journal of the American Geriatrics Society, 64*, 1879–1883.

Mysyuk, Y., Westendorp, R., & Kindenberg, J. (2016). Perspectives on the etiology of violence in later life. *Journal of Interpersonal Violence, 31*, 3039–3062.

National Center on Elder Abuse. (2013). *Research brief, mistreatment of lesbian, gay, bisexual, and transgender (LBGT) elders.*

National Center on Elder Abuse. (2014). *Research to practice: Mistreatment of Latino elders.* Washington, DC: Administration for Community Living.

National Center on Elder Abuse. (2016). *Research to practice: Mistreatment of African American elders.* Washington, DC: Administration for Community Living.

Navarro, A. E., Wysong, J., DeLiema, M., et al. (2016). Inside the black box: The case review process of an elder abuse forensic center. *The Gerontologist, 56*(4), 772–781.

Pillemer, K. (2016). Addressing barriers: Overview. In L. Mosqueda (Chair). *Closing the research gaps—Moving the field forward.* Los Angeles, CA: University of Southern California Judith D. Tamkin International Symposium on Elder Abuse.

Pillemer, K., Burnes, D., Riffin, C., et al. (2016). Elder abuse: Global situation, risk factors, and prevention strategies. *The Gerontologist, 56*(S2), S194–S205.

Rawles, T. (2016). Elderly lesbian woman abused by retirement home residents for being gay, staff "ignores" pleas. San Diego Gay and Lesbian News. Available at http://sdgln.com/news/2016/08/02/elderly-lesbian-woman-abused-retirement-home-residents-being-gay-staff-ignores-pleas

Roepke-Buehler, S., Simon, M., & Dong, X. (2015). Association between depressive symptoms, multiple dimensions of depression, and elder abuse: A cross-sectional, population-based analysis of older adults in urban Chicago. *Journal of Aging & Health, 27*, 1003–1025.

Rosen, T., Bloemen, E., LoFaso, V., et al. (2016). Emergency department presentation of injuries in older adults independently known to be victims of elder abuse. *Journal of Emergency Medicine, 50*, 518–526.

Rosen, T., Lachs, M. S., Teresi, J., et al. (2016). Staff-reported strategies for prevention and management of resident-to-resident elder mistreatment in long-term care facilities. *Journal of Elder Abuse & Neglect, 28*, 1–13.

Tronetti, P. (2014). Evaluating abuse in the patient with dementia. *Clinics in Geriatric Medicine, 30*, 825–838.

United Nations Human Rights Council. (2016). *Report of the Independent Expert on the enjoyment of all human rights by older persons.* New York: United Nations General Assembly.

Volmert, A., & Lindland, E. (2016). *"You can only pray that somebody would step in": Mapping the gaps between expert and public understanding of elder abuse in America.* Washington, DC: FrameWorks Institute.

Wiglesworth, A., Austin, R., Corona, M., et al. (2009). Bruising as a marker of physical elder abuse. *Journal of the American Geriatrics Society, 57*(7), 1191–1196.

Wong, J., & Waite, L. (2017). Elder mistreatment predicts later physical and psychological health: Results from a national longitudinal study. *Journal of Elder Abuse & Neglect, 29*, 15–42.

Yonashiro-Cho, J., Gassoumis, Z., & Wilber, K. (2015). *Characteristics of intentional injuries among older adults presenting to hospital emergency departments 2001–2010.* Orlando, FL; Presentation at Gerontological Society of America Scientific Meeting.

p a r t **3**

Promoting Wellness in Psychosocial Function

Unfolding Patient Stories: Sherman "Red" Yoder · Part 2

Recall from Part 2 **Sherman "Red" Yoder**, who has lived alone on his farm for 10 years since his wife died and drives 20 miles into town weekly to visit with friends. Red's son and daughter-in-law live nearby and manage the farm. He has a diabetic foot wound, which makes it difficult for him to walk and drive. What effect can life events of older adulthood have on his psychosocial function? What nursing interventions by the home health nurse can promote psychosocial wellness for Red? What technology resources can contribute to his quality of life and psychosocial well-being?

Care for Red and other patients in a realistic virtual environment: **vSim** *for Nursing* (thepoint.lww.com/vSim Gerontology). Practice documenting these patients' care in DocuCare (thepoint.lww.com/DocuCareEHR).

Unfolding Patient Stories: Millie Larsen · Part 2

Recall from Part 1 **Millie Larsen**, an 84-year-old who lives alone. While visiting her at home recently, Millie's daughter, Dina, notices she is acting strangely and not making sense. Millie is admitted to the hospital with the diagnosis of a urinary tract infection and dehydration. The daughter tells the nurse, "I'm worried that my mom may have dementia because she is more forgetful and appears confused." How would the nurse explain to the daughter the difference between the clinical manifestations of delirium and dementia? How would the nurse address the daughter's concern? How would the nurse facilitate an interprofessional approach to addressing Millie's symptoms?

Care for Millie and other patients in a realistic virtual environment: **vSim** *for Nursing* (thepoint.lww.com/vSim Gerontology). Practice documenting these patients' care in DocuCare (thepoint.lww.com/DocuCareEHR).

chapter 11

Cognitive Wellness

LEARNING OBJECTIVES

After reading this chapter, you will be able to:

1. Describe age-related changes that affect cognitive abilities.

2. List risk factors that influence cognitive function in older adults.

3. Discuss the functional consequences associated with cognition in older adults.

4. Identify nursing interventions to help older adults maintain or improve cognitive abilities.

KEY TERMS

automatic and effortful processing theory

cognitive reserve

contextual theories

continuum of processing

crystallized intelligence

empowerment theories

fluid intelligence

levels of processing theories

lifespan theories

memory

mild cognitive impairment (MCI)

neuroplasticity

scaffolding theory of aging and cognition

speed of processing theories

Three-Dimensional Wisdom Model

evidence-based information that has emerged in recent decades. Ongoing major national and international initiatives are focusing on finding causes of, and cures for, conditions that affect cognition, including Alzheimer's disease and other dementias. Although many questions remain unanswered, we are moving toward a better understanding of—and a more positive outlook on—maintaining optimal cognitive function during older adulthood. An exciting and significant evidence-based finding from recent studies is that cognitive abilities can improve throughout older adulthood through health promotion interventions. This chapter presents current information about the multidimensional aspects of cognitive aging, with emphasis on how nurses can apply this information to promoting cognitive wellness for older adults.

A Student's Perspective

The residents at Heritage continue to amaze me with their stories. There is so much one can learn just by listening, and the residents just want to share their stories and have our company more than anything—at least that is the impression I continually receive from them. They are all friendly, open people who are no different than the rest of us, but they have gained a large amount of knowledge over the years that many of us who are students probably have not acquired yet.

Megan S.

WHAT IS KNOWN ABOUT COGNITION AND AGING

During the past 50 years, developments in theories about aging and cognition have led to significant improvements in our understanding of "how and why certain components of cognitive function are or are not affected by aging" (Anderson & Craik, 2017, p. 1). Early studies concluded that a global decline in cognitive abilities was a normal and expected part of aging. However, as knowledge about cognitive aging has

Cognition encompasses many processes, including those involved with thinking, learning, and remembering. Myths, such as the one perpetuated by adages such as "you can't teach an old dog new tricks," are pervasive, long-standing, and detrimental to older adults. Fortunately, many myths and misunderstandings can be dispelled by evolved, all of the following conclusions have become clear: (a) there is a great deal of individual variability in cognitive abilities, (b) multiple interacting factors influence cognitive aging, and (c) each older adult experiences a mixture of decline, preservation, and improvement in cognitive abilities (Kensinger & Gutchess, 2017; Salthouse, 2017). Based on the knowledge that the brain maintains the ability to change in positive ways throughout life, gerontologists currently are focusing on identifying interventions that prevent cognitive decline or improve cognitive abilities. A major report on public health dimensions of cognitive aging focused on the interplay between cognitive abilities and factors such as health, education, life experiences, socioeconomic influences, and psychosocial conditions (National Academies of Sciences, 2015). In this context, cognitive aging can be addressed through interventions directed toward risk and protective factors.

Age-Related Changes in the Central Nervous System

Knowledge about brain aging is gleaned from many sources, including clinical, neuropsychological, neuropathologic, neurochemical, and neuroimaging investigations. Initial studies of brain aging relied on autopsy findings, but the evolving use of neuroimaging techniques (e.g., functional magnetic resonance imaging, magnetoencephalography) has significantly broadened the knowledge base. Brain imaging studies show diminished brain volume and loss of brain cells in some regions. Studies also show that these changes are associated with declines in some aspects of cognitive function, even in the absence of pathologic changes. In contrast to studies showing these losses, recent studies indicate that the brain and neural circuits maintain the ability to change and develop throughout the adult life span, which is a process called **neuroplasticity** (also called *neural plasticity*). There is much current interest in identifying conditions that support neuroplasticity, such as lifestyle interventions (as discussed later in this chapter).

The closely related concept of **cognitive reserve** refers to the capacity to continue to function at an adequate cognitive level despite age-related or pathologic processes that affect the neural structures. This theory posits that a higher baseline of cognitive functioning, for example, through education or intellectual pursuits, protects an older adult from cognitive decline under challenging conditions, such as medical illness (Cheng, 2016; Edelstein, Pergolizzi, & Alici, 2017). Moreover, the cognitive reserve model suggests that cognitive abilities can be improved through participation in creative and intellectually stimulating activities, such as art, storytelling, reading, writing, group discussions, and playing musical instruments.

Gerontologists emphasize that because the brain and nervous system continue to develop during adulthood, structural changes in the brain do not necessarily determine cognitive abilities. Researchers have proposed the **scaffolding theory of aging and cognition** as a way of explaining the adaptive response of the brain to the declining neural structures and function. According to this theory, scaffolding is a normal process that involves the development and use of complementary and alternative neural circuits to achieve a cognitive goal. This process serves to buffer the negative effects of age-related and pathologic cognitive aging (Smith, 2016). Moreover, this model proposes that formal interventions and training can enhance cognitive reserve and have a positive effect on neuroplasticity (Willis & Belleville, 2016)

Fluid and Crystallized Intelligence

Cattell and Horn's theory of fluid and crystallized intelligence, first proposed in the late 1960s, is one of the first theories that attempted to explain age-related changes in some cognitive abilities. Fluid intelligence depends primarily on central nervous system functioning and a person's inherent abilities, such as memory and pattern recognition. **Fluid intelligence** is associated with the cognitive skills of integration, inductive reasoning, abstract thinking, and flexible and adaptive thinking. This cognitive characteristic enables people to solve problems and to identify and draw conclusions about complex relationships. **Crystallized intelligence** refers to cognitive skills, such as vocabulary, information, and verbal comprehension, that people acquire through culture, education, informal learning, and other life experiences. This cognitive characteristic is strongly associated with wisdom, judgment, and life experiences.

According to this theory, fluid and crystallized intelligence develop concurrently during infancy and childhood and are indistinguishable as the central nervous system is maturing. Age-related changes in neural structures cause a decline in fluid intelligence, which is primarily related to decreased speed of processing (Scheiber, Chen, Kaufman, et al.,2017). Crystallized intelligence continues to develop during adulthood because of accumulated experiences and learning. Crystallized intelligence does not decline with age, and it may even increase because of experiences that improve wisdom.

Memory

Memory is the cognitive ability that is often conceptualized as a computer-like information processing system in which information is first perceived, then stored, and finally retrieved when needed or wanted. *Short-term memory* has a short duration and a very small capacity, and it serves as a holding tank for events of the immediate past few seconds. Information in the short-term memory can be either recalled for a brief time or transmitted to long-term storage. *Long-term memory* is essential for storage and retrieval of information. Many theories have been proposed to explain the declines in memory functions that are associated with both normal aging (i.e., those that affect all older adults, regardless of pathologic conditions) and pathologic aging processes (e.g., mild cognitive impairment [MCI], dementia).

Since the 1960s, the focus of theory development has shifted from a narrow focus on single mechanisms to multifactorial models that address the vast complexity of the aging brain (Park & Festini, 2017). The following are examples of theoretic models about memory that have been proposed:

- **Speed of processing models**: Age-related declines in speed of processing accounted for diminished memory skills in older adults.
- Levels of processing models: Memory skills depend on levels of processing, ranging from shallow to deep levels; the deeper the level at which information is stored, the longer the memory will last. This framework suggests that poor memory function in older adults is associated with faulty processing mechanisms.
- **Contextual theories**: Memory skills develop in the context of many variables, including all of the following: health, motivation, expectations, experiences, education, personality, task demands, learning habits, sociocultural background, and style of processing information. These theories suggest that memory and other cognitive skills of older adults are as good as or better than those of younger adults under some conditions.
- **Automatic and effortful processing theory**: Memory tasks are conceptualized on a continuum from automatic processing (i.e., tasks that do not require attention or awareness and do not improve with practice) at one end to effortful processing (i.e., tasks that demand high levels of attention and cognitive energy) at the other end. With

practice, effortful tasks require less attention and become more automatic. Older adults maintain skills related to automatic processing (e.g., walking, tying shoes, writing letters) but decline in tasks that require effortful processes (e.g., mental imagery, verbal fluency, and selective attention).

A recent review of theories related to memory and aging concluded that there is a great deal of individual variation among older adults, with some being able to maintain relatively high levels of performance and others performing as well as or even better than young adults (Lustig & Lin, 2016).

 See ONLINE LEARNING ACTIVITY 11-1: INSIDE THE BRAINS OF OLDER ADULTS at http://thepoint.lww.com/Miller8e.

Wellness Opportunity

Nurses can influence attitudes by conveying positive beliefs about the ability of older adults to improve memory skills.

Theories About Adult Cognitive Development

Theories about cognitive development often overlap with psychological theories of successful aging, which are discussed in Chapter 4, and theories related to stress, coping, and resilience, which are discussed in Chapter 12. Additional theories pertinent to adult cognitive development include lifespan theories and empowerment theories, as described in Box 11-1.

Box 11-1 Theories About Cognitive Development in Older Adults

Lifespan Theories

Lifespan theories focus on psychological gains and losses that occur during various life stages. The Schaie and Willis Stage Theory of Cognition identifies the following stages:

- *Achieving stage* (early adulthood): Adults apply acquired knowledge to demands and commitments, such as career and family; they use their intellectual abilities to establish their independence and develop goal-oriented behaviors.
- *Responsible stage* (late 30s to early 60s): Adults integrate long-range goals and attend to the needs of their family and society.
- *Executive stage* (a variation of the responsible stage): Applies to people who have high levels of social responsibilities.
- *Reintegration stage* (later adulthood): Older adults apply acquired knowledge to current interests and values, and they direct efforts toward assuring that their resources meet their anticipated needs.
- *Reorganizational stage* (later adulthood): Older adults engage in activities to maximize quality of life, often with the additional objective of not becoming a burden for the next generation.
- *Legacy-creating stage* (advanced old age): Older adults engage in processes such as life review or memoir-writing, and assuring that legal affairs are in order.

(Schaie, 2016).

Empowerment Theories

Empowerment theories focus on promoting self-determination, choice, and control. These models address the following concepts:

- Empowerment is a process of moving from a state of powerlessness and passivity to one of control (both perceived and actual) over one's life.

- The empowered individual sees oneself as capable of change, able to use his or her knowledge and skills to solve problems and meet goals, and to work in partnership with professionals.
- Empowerment potential exists not only in terms of an individual's resources and abilities, but also in terms of external conditions, which must change in response to the needs of the individual.
- There is a fundamental difference between inability to act because of a lack of choices and a lack of ability to act.

(Hooyman, Mahoney, & Sciegaj, 2016).

Three-Dimensional Wisdom Model

The **Three-Dimensional Wisdom Model** integrates the following theoretical dimensions:

- Cognitive wisdom, which entails the following components: a desire to know the truth; a deep and thorough understanding of life; and knowledge and acceptance of human nature, of the inherent limits of knowledge, and of life's unpredictability and uncertainty.
- Reflective wisdom, which is characterized by the following abilities: to perceive phenomena and events from multiple perspectives, to overcome subjectivity and projections, and to accept reality as it is.
- Compassionate wisdom, which is characterized by the following: a more thorough understanding of life and the human condition combined with a reduction in self-centeredness, which generates sympathetic and compassionate love for others and the motivation to foster others' well-being.

(Ardelt & Oh, 2016).

A topic of current interest is wisdom, which is viewed as a multidimensional characteristic consisting of cognitive, reflective, and benevolent components that are mutually interdependent and benefit the person and others (Bengston, 2016). Wisdom is a cognitive dimension that is strongly associated with subjective well-being in older adults, particularly during times of great challenge (Ardelt & Edwards, 2016). Box 11-1 describes key components of the Three-Dimensional Wisdom Model.

> ### Wellness Opportunity
>
> Nurses acknowledge the wisdom of older adults by asking questions such as "Do you have some words of wisdom to share about that valuable experience?"

FACTORS THAT AFFECT COGNITIVE WELLNESS

As more information about brain aging and cognition has emerged, researchers have been able to identify conditions that affect cognitive function in older adults—both as risk factors and as protective factors. A major focus is on identifying conditions that can be addressed through health promotion interventions. This chapter focuses on factors that affect overall cognitive wellness, with an emphasis on those that can be addressed through nursing interventions. Chapter 14 provides extensive information about risk factors associated with serious cognitive impairment due to dementia, including the many pathological conditions that affect cognitive function.

Sociocultural Influences

Numerous personal, social, and attitudinal factors affect cognitive abilities in people of any age, and researchers have tried to identify those that most significantly affect older adults. Quality and length of formal education has been identified in hundreds of publications as the variable most strongly associated with better cognitive performance and more cognitive reserve in older adults (Leggett, Clarke, Zivin, et al., 2017). Other factors that affect cognitive function include occupation, social relations, socioeconomic status, and leisure and intellectual activities (Binder, Bezzola, Haueter, et al., 2017; Bourassa, Memel, Woolverton, et al., 2017; Oltmanns, Godde, Winneke, et al., 2017). Another important consideration is that commonly used assessment methods are based on cognitive standards developed for English-speaking white Americans. Thus, it is imperative to consider the influence of culture, occupation, literacy, education, and life experiences that affect cognitive aging (National Academies of Sciences, 2015).

Ageism and diminished expectations of older adults in modern societies can negatively affect cognitive function (Robertson, King-Kallimanis, & Kenny, 2016). Studies indicate that older adults internalize stereotypes about memory decline as an inevitable outcome of aging and that these perceptions worsen their performance on tests of memory and other cognitive skills (Mesiner & Levy, 2016; Mogle, Munoz, Hill, et al., 2017; Stephan, Sutin, Caudroit, et al., 2016).

> ### Wellness Opportunity
>
> Be aware of opportunities to dispel negative stereotypes about cognitive aging when talking with older adults.

Nutrition

Much current research focuses on nutrition as a modifiable condition that affects cognitive wellness. Although low levels of certain nutrients are associated with poor cognitive function, dietary approaches to preventing cognitive decline emphasize the importance of overall dietary patterns rather than the use of dietary supplements (Dominguez & Barbagallo, 2017). Systematic reviews consistently identify Mediterranean-style dietary patterns as most effective for preventing cognitive decline (Canavelli, Lucchini, Quarta, et al., 2016; Knight, Bryan, & Murphy, 2016; Vauzour, Camprubi-Robles, Miquel-Kergoat, et al., 2016). See Chapter 18 for details about this dietary pattern.

Physical Activity

Along with dietary patterns, physical activity is being addressed as a modifiable lifestyle behavior that affects cognitive function in beneficial or detrimental ways (Jackson, Pialoux, Corbet, et al., 2016). Studies consistently find a positive association between increased physical activity and both reduced brain atrophy and improved cognitive function (Gallaway, Miyake, Buchowski, et al., 2017; Jonasson, Nyberg, Kramer, et al., 2017).

Vision and Hearing Impairments

Vision and hearing impairments can affect cognitive because they interfere with one's ability to receive information. Recent studies are identifying a link between neurological pathways involved with age-related hearing loss and cognitive impairment (Mudar & Husain, 2016; Zheng, Fan, Liao, et al., 2017). Studies also are finding that the effects on cognitive abilities are magnified when both senses of vision and hearing are impaired (Humes & Young, 2016). Because sensory input significantly influences learning and other cognitive processes, nurses need to ensure optimal visual and hearing conditions when communicating with older adults (as discussed in Chapters 16 and 17).

Medication Effects

Prescription and over-the-counter medications can interfere with memory and other cognitive functions in a variety of ways, as delineated in the examples in Table 11-1.

TABLE 11-1 Mechanisms of Action for Mental Changes Caused by Adverse Medication Effects

Mechanism of Action	Examples
Anticholinergic effects	Atropine, scopolamine, antihistamines, antipsychotics, antidepressants, antispasmodics, anti-parkinsonian agents
Decreased cerebral blood flow	Antihypertensives, antipsychotics
Depression of respiratory center	Central nervous system depressants
Fluid and electrolyte alterations	Diuretics, alcohol, laxatives
Altered thermoregulation	Alcohol, psychotropics, narcotics
Acidosis	Diuretics, alcohol, nicotinic acid
Hypoglycemia	Hypoglycemics, alcohol, propranolol
Hormonal disturbances	Thyroid extract, corticosteroids

Anticholinergic ingredients, which are contained in numerous prescription and over-the-counter medications, are a common cause of changes in mental status in older adults. Because many medications have anticholinergic effects, in recent years, researchers and clinicians have paid particular attention to the cumulative effects of these medications on neurotransmitters that directly affect cognitive function. Chapter 8 provides detailed information about adverse effects of anticholinergics and other types of medications that can be addressed through nursing interventions.

 Wellness Opportunity

From a holistic perspective, nurses help older adults identify risk factors, such as nutrition and over-the-counter medications, that can be addressed through self-care actions.

FUNCTIONAL CONSEQUENCES AFFECTING COGNITION

Healthy older adults will not experience any significant cognitive impairment that interferes with daily life, but they will notice minor deficits in some aspects of cognitive function and improvements in other aspects. These changes can be summarized as follows:

- Age-related declines in some cognitive skills begin around the age of 40; however, not all adults experience these changes.
- There is a great deal of individual variation in cognitive changes.
- The earliest cognitive changes are due to decreased perceptual speed.
- Cognitive functions that depend on experience and accumulated knowledge do not decline in healthy older adults, and may even improve.

- Age-related cognitive changes occur gradually, any major or rapid changes are due to pathologic processes.
- Intellectually stimulating activities and higher levels of education are associated with the development of cognitive reserve.
- Pathologic processes, such as those related to inflammatory processes and cardiovascular diseases, are associated with greater degrees of cognitive impairment.
- Health promotion interventions to protect and even improve cognitive abilities during older adulthood include activities that involve social engagement and cognitive stimulation, and all actions that promote good overall health (e.g., optimal nutrition, physical activity, stress management, not smoking, healthy weight).

Box 11-2 summarizes some of the research-based conclusions about cognitive aging that are most relevant for identifying and implementing health education interventions for older adults.

 See ONLINE LEARNING ACTIVITY 11–2: RESOURCES FOR INFORMATION ABOUT HEALTHY BRAIN AGING at http://thepoint.lww.com/Miller8e.

Wellness Opportunity

Nurses promote wellness by encouraging older adults to identify ways in which their cognitive abilities have improved (e.g., wisdom based on experiences).

 Box 11-2 Functional Consequences Affecting Cognition in Older Adults

Cognitive Abilities in Healthy Older Adults

- Skills that stay the same or improve: wisdom, creativity, common sense, coordination of facts and ideas, and breadth of knowledge and experience.
- Skills that decline slightly and gradually: abstraction, calculation, word fluency, verbal comprehension, spatial orientation, inductive reasoning, and episodic memory.
- Word finding may be more difficult (i.e., "tip-of-the-tongue" experiences), but total vocabulary increases.
- Factors that can cause cognitive impairment: anxiety, depression, diminished sensory input, poor health, negative beliefs, ageist attitudes, pathologic processes (e.g., dementia).
- Factors that improve cognitive function: good nutrition, physical exercise, mental stimulation, challenging leisure activities, strong social networks, and activities that provide a sense of control and mastery.

Learning Abilities

- Older adults are as capable of learning new things as younger people, but the speed with which they process information is slower.
- Older adults are more cautious in their responses and make more errors of omission.
- Potential barriers to learning in older adults include distractions, sensory deficits, lack of relevance, teacher–learner age differences, and values that are incongruent with new knowledge.

PATHOLOGIC CONDITION AFFECTING COGNITION: MILD COGNITIVE IMPAIRMENT

The concept of mild cognitive impairment (MCI) has evolved over the past several decades to describe a state of cognitive function that is between normal aging and dementia. During the early 1960s, symptoms that are now categorized as MCI were referred to as *benign senescent forgetfulness*. During the 1980s and 1990s, labels of *age-associated memory impairment*, *mild neurocognitive decline*, or *cognitive impairment no dementia* were commonly applied to this constellation of symptoms. During the early 2000s, MCI was viewed as a precursor to Alzheimer's disease, but it is now considered a distinct syndrome with symptoms that can remain stable, resolve, or progress. It is now known that MCI increases the risk for developing dementia, but it does not necessarily progress to dementia (Malek-Ahmadi, 2016). Studies indicate that between 5% and 17% of older adults with MCI progress to dementia every year (Cheng, Chen, & Chiu, 2017; Petersen, 2016). A longitudinal study with a mean follow-up of 7.9 years found that 46.8% of the participants initially diagnosed with MCI died with a diagnosis of dementia, 39.2% died with a diagnosis of MCI, and 3.9% died with normal cognitive function (Abner, Kryscio, Schmitt, et al., 2017).

Two subtypes of MCI are amnesic MCI, which involves memory loss, and nonamnesic MCI, which is the less common type. Because MCI has only recently been defined as a distinct syndrome, diagnostic criteria are imprecise and current guidelines emphasize the need for a combination of clinical judgment, functional assessment, and neuropsychological testing (Healey, 2012). Diagnosis of MCI depends on identifying declines in one or more cognitive domains (e.g., memory, attention, visuospatial abilities, and executive functioning) without concurrent major effects on global cognition or daily functioning. Table 11-2 lists cognitive changes associated with normal aging and MCI. In addition to cognitive characteristics, behavioral symptoms, such as anxiety, depression, and aggressiveness, have been identified in 13% of people with MCI, as compared with 39% of

those with Alzheimer's disease and 3% of controls (Van Der Mussele, Le Bastard, Vermeiren, et al., 2013). Because of recent changes in the Medicare program, primary care practitioners can provide cognitive screening and make referrals for more comprehensive neuropsychological testing. Nurses can encourage older adults with noticeable cognitive deficits to obtain an appropriate evaluation, with emphasis on the importance of implementing interventions at a stage when progression to dementia could be delayed.

NURSING ASSESSMENT OF COGNITIVE FUNCTION

Formal assessment of intellectual performance involves neuropsychological testing, but nurses can assess cognitive skills by using evidence-based tools. In addition, it is important to assess for risk factors that are likely to interfere with cognitive function. Because nursing assessment of cognition is an integral part of the psychosocial assessment, it is addressed comprehensively in Chapter 13 (Psychosocial Assessment) rather than in this chapter. Nursing assessment of impaired cognitive function is addressed in Chapter 14 (Delirium and Dementia).

NURSING DIAGNOSIS

Healthy older adults experience some changes in cognitive function, but, in the absence of pathologic conditions and other risk factors, these changes do not significantly affect their overall functioning. The nursing diagnosis of Readiness for Enhanced Knowledge is appropriate for addressing normal cognitive aging, because the focus is on health promotion interventions to maintain optimal cognitive functioning. Impaired Memory may be appropriate for older adults with the amnesic type of MCI or memory limitations that affect daily functioning. Nursing diagnoses related to cognitive impairment associated with dementia, confusional states, and other serious cognitive impairments are discussed in Chapter 14.

TABLE 11-2 Distinguishing Characteristics of Normal Cognitive Aging and Mild Cognitive Impairment

Characteristic	Normal Cognitive Aging	Mild Cognitive Impairment (MCI)	Mild Dementia
Short-term memory changes	Preserved	Impaired in amnesic MCI, preserved in nonamnesic MCI	Noticeably impaired
Awareness of memory loss	Recognizes and remembers details about memory limitations	Little or no recognition and memory of details about limitations	Limited or absent awareness
Mental status assessment	No significant changes from baseline	Mild or no significant impairment	Measurable declines from baseline
Social skills	No significant changes	Usually unchanged from normal	Impaired
Activities of daily living	Preserved	Preserved	Impaired
Instrumental activities of daily living	No significant changes from baseline	Limited changes, apparent in complex tasks (e.g., managing finances, and using appliances)	Impaired

Source: Patel, B. B., & Holland, N. W. (2012). Mild cognitive impairment: Hope for stability, plan for progression. *Cleveland Clinic Journal of Medicine, 79*(12), 857–864.

Wellness Opportunity

Recognize the detrimental influence of myths and negative attitudes about cognitive aging and address these by using the nursing diagnosis of Readiness for Enhanced Knowledge.

PLANNING FOR WELLNESS OUTCOMES

A wellness-oriented outcome criterion related to cognitive function is that older adults take responsibility for addressing risk factors and compensating for age-related cognitive changes. The following are examples of outcomes that address risk factors: improved sensory function, control of cardiovascular diseases, smoking cessation, healthy lifestyle practices, and social and intellectual engagement. Nurses can use the following Nursing Outcomes Classification (NOC) terminology related to cognitive wellness: Cognition, Concentration, Exercise Participation, Information Processing, Knowledge: Health Promotion, Stress Level, Leisure Participation, Hearing Compensation Behavior, and Vision Compensation Behavior.

A Student's Perspective

At the beginning of the 5 weeks at Friendship Village, I didn't know what to expect. I assumed we would just be taking vital signs and making small talk with a few of the clients. I didn't realize I would learn so much by just listening to the life story of someone who is 96 years old. I realized that many of these individuals have had quite the amazing life and have a lot of wisdom and knowledge to pass down.

Needless to say, my expectations changed dramatically! They went from just getting the 5 weeks over with, to me not wanting to leave after the 5 weeks. Many of the residents were still "with it" and could remember a lot about their childhood and past experiences. This is the information that I did my best to take in. How did they get to live to be 96 years old and be able to look back on their life and be proud of their accomplishments. That's the life I want to live!!

Kim V.

Wellness Opportunity

Address the detrimental influence of myths and negative attitudes about cognitive aging and address these by using the NOC of Health Beliefs in relation to the nursing diagnosis of Readiness for Enhanced Knowledge.

NURSING INTERVENTIONS TO PROMOTE COGNITIVE WELLNESS

Many of the health promotion interventions discussed throughout this text provide specific examples of these types of activities. For example, interventions related to nutrition, physical activity, and cardiovascular wellness are particularly relevant to promoting optimal cognitive function. Also, because vision and hearing impairments can interfere with cognitive abilities, any interventions directed toward improving sensory function (discussed in Chapters 16 and 17) may also be effective in improving cognitive function.

The following Nursing Interventions Classification terminology identifies interventions related to cognitive wellness: Cognitive Stimulation, Communication Enhancement: Hearing Deficit, Communication Enhancement: Visual Deficit, Exercise Promotion, Health Education, Learning Facilitation, Learning Readiness Enhancement, Meditation Facilitation, Progressive Muscle Relaxation, Role Enhancement, Self-Awareness Enhancement, Self-Responsibility Enhancement, and Risk Identification.

Wellness Opportunity

Nurses promote personal responsibility for wellness by helping older adults identify ways of incorporating "brain fitness" activities into their daily lives.

Health Education About Cognitive Wellness

Teaching older adults about techniques to maintain or improve cognitive skills is within the realm of nursing responsibilities, in the same way as is teaching about maintaining and improving physical function. Box 11-3, which can be used as a patient teaching tool, summarizes evidence-based information about self-care actions to improve or maintain cognitive wellness. The box also includes tips for improving memory as an important aspect of cognitive function in everyday activities.

Nurses have an important role in addressing beliefs about cognition and aging because these can significantly influence one's ability to learn. Thus, health education needs to include all of the following aspects:

- Correcting myths and misinformation
- Providing accurate information about age-related changes
- Communicating positive expectations
- Identifying goals for self-learning
- Providing information about techniques to enhance cognitive abilities
- Identifying the techniques that are most effective for the individual

 GLOBAL PERSPECTIVE

The Global Council on Brain Health is a global initiative supported by AARP in the United States and Age UK with the goal of teaching older adults about brain health as they age. Resources are available at www.GlobalCouncilOnBrainHealth.org.

 See ONLINE LEARNING ACTIVITY 11-3: ARTICLE ABOUT A NURSE-LED PROGRAM FOR MEMORY TRAINING PLUS YOGA FOR OLDER ADULTS at http://thepoint.lww.com/Miller8e.

Box 11-3 Self-Care Activities for Promoting Cognitive Wellness

Actions for Overall Cognitive Wellness

- Eat foods high in antioxidants (e.g., fruits and vegetable) and omega-3 fatty acids (e.g., fatty fish); limit salt, cholesterol, and saturated fat.
- Maintain a healthy weight.
- Engage in regular physical activity, including aerobic activity, strengthening exercises, and flexibility and balance exercises.
- Engage in new learning experiences that are appealing and challenging.
- Practice body–mind activities, such as tai chi and mindfulness-based meditation.
- Participate in leisure activities, such as dancing, playing board games, playing a musical instrument, doing crossword puzzles, and reading.
- Choose activities in which there is a sense of control and mastery, such as playing computer games or learning a new skill.
- Maintain strong and frequent social relationships with family and friends

Techniques for Improving Memory Skills

- Minimize distractions.
- Pay close attention to the details of what is going on around you.
- Write things down (e.g., use lists, calendars, and notebooks).

- Use auditory cues (e.g., timers and alarm clocks) combined with written cues.
- Assign specific places for specific items and keep the items in their proper place (e.g., keep keys on a hook near the door).
- Use visual images (e.g., create a picture in your mind when you want to remember something).
- Make associations between names and mental images (e.g., Carol and Christmas carol).
- Use self-instruction (e.g., say things aloud to yourself).
- Devise systems to organize routine tasks, such as taking medications.
- Divide information into small parts that can be remembered easily.
- Use rhyming cues (e.g., "In 1492, Columbus sailed the ocean blue.").
- Use first-letter cues and make associations (e.g., to remember to buy soup, tea, oranges, rice, and eggs, remember the word STORE).
- Make word associations (e.g., to remember the letters of your license plate, make a word, such as camel, out of the letters CML).
- Make up a story to connect things you want to remember (e.g., if you have to go to the cleaners and the post office, create a story about mailing a pair of pants).

Wellness Opportunity

Nurses holistically address learning needs of older adults by encouraging participation in group programs, which have the additional benefit of offering social support.

Improving Concentration and Attention

When one's ability to attend to the environment and concentrate on visual and auditory cues is limited, the ability to learn and remember is also impaired. Thus, techniques, such as relaxation, imagery, and meditation, which enhance attention and concentration, may also improve memory and learning. Likewise, any method that reduces environmental distractions may also improve one's cognitive abilities. Mindfulness (also called *mindfulness meditation*), which is the practice of focused awareness of the environment and one's reactions to it, is a self-care practice that can improve attention and other cognitive skills. Many self-help books describe techniques for meditation, mindfulness, and relaxation as ways of maintaining or improving cognitive function and opening the mind to new learning. Nurses can teach the relaxation technique outlined in Chapter 24 to older adults for a variety of uses, including the enhancement of mental skills.

Encouraging Participation in Mentally Stimulating Activities

Because there is much evidence that participation in mentally stimulating activities is effective for promoting cognitive wellness, nurses can encourage older adults to participate in adult learning activities. In some settings, nurses can address health-related concerns of older adults through group health education programs, which have the additional benefit of providing social support. A process for implementing a nurse-led health education group is described in Chapter 12.

 Technology to Promote Wellness in Older Adults

Nurses can also promote the use of technology-based interventions for mental stimulation and practical benefits, such as increased communication with others and the acquisition of information that is relevant to their health and daily functioning, as indicated by the following studies:

- Cognitive training interventions, such as computer-based brain exercises, are effective in improving cognitive abilities in older adults (Shah, Weinborn, Verdile, et al., 2017).
- Increased "digital literacy" (i.e., the use of internet, online cognitive stimulation games, word processing) is beneficial for preventing cognitive decline in healthy older adults (Klimova, 2016).
- Focus groups of older adults with MCI had positive attitudes about assistive robots for cognitive stimulation and object-finding systems (Wu, Cristancho-Lacroix, Fassert, et al., 2016).

Another nursing intervention is to encourage older adults to participate in lifelong learning programs in local communities. Some universities and colleges (particularly community colleges) offer reduced-rate or no-fee courses for students 60 years and older. Some programs also offer associate degrees, certification programs, or a general equivalency diploma. The Institutes for Learning in Retirement is a community-based organization for retirement-age learners that develops and implements educational programs in affiliation with a college or university. These sessions typically involve homework and usually are held for a few hours weekly for several months. Less formal education programs often are available through local senior centers and adult education programs affiliated with local school districts. Older adults can contact local colleges and information to find courses that are offered under this program.

See ONLINE LEARNING ACTIVITY 11-4: RESOURCES FOR HEALTH INFORMATION ABOUT BRAIN AGING at http://thepoint.lww.com/Miller8e.

Wellness Opportunity

Nurses promote personal responsibility by helping older adults identify activities that address their unique learning needs based on their life experiences and current interests.

Adapting Health Education Materials

Much of the research on cognitive aging has centered on factors that affect learning in older adulthood. Because many nursing interventions include patient teaching or health education, information about cognitive aging can be used to adapt educational methods and materials to older adults as summarized in Box 11-4. The suggestions presented in this text for communicating with older adults and compensating for hearing and vision deficit (see Chapters 13, 16, and 17) can be applied to health education.

Adaptations of health education materials may also be necessary to ensure they are culturally appropriate. For instance, many federal government sites provide health education materials that are available in Spanish and other languages. Because there is growing emphasis on addressing the needs of culturally diverse populations, it is important to check Internet resources periodically and explore the availability of teaching materials for specific groups. In addition, local community centers and senior centers often provide culturally specific health education materials related to culturally diverse populations in their service area. For example, organizations and state governments have developed advance directive forms and teaching tools that address learning needs of specific cultural groups, as discussed in Chapter 9. Chapter 2 of this text further addresses the topic of culturally sensitive health education.

Box 11-4 Guidelines for Health Education for Older Adults

Environmental Conditions That Promote Learning

- Establish a warm, friendly environment.
- Eliminate distractions (e.g., noise and excessive visual stimulation).
- Provide good lighting and eliminate sources of glare as much as possible.
- Make sure older adults are using hearing aids and eyeglasses as appropriate.
- Use amplifying devices, such as microphones.

Teaching Strategies That Promote Learning

- Emphasize application of knowledge and experience, rather than the acquisition of irrelevant information.
- Use praise and positive feedback.
- Present one idea or small amounts of information at one time.
- Allow enough time for processing information.
- Use concrete rather than abstract teaching materials in all forms (verbal, written, audiovisual).
- Make sure that the information is personally relevant.
- Relate the information to the person's past experiences.
- As much as possible, adapt presentation to individualized rates of procession.
- Arrange for follow-up to reinforce teaching points.

Teaching Aids That Enhance Learning

- Use audio and visual aids that are relevant to older adults.
- Ensure that examples illustrate healthy aging and do not reinforce myths or stereotypes.
- Provide advance organizers, such as outlines and summaries.
- Explain how to use organizing aids.

EVALUATING EFFECTIVENESS OF NURSING INTERVENTIONS

Effectiveness of nursing interventions is evaluated by the degree to which older adults who have mild memory impairments are able to use their cognitive abilities to meet their daily needs. For example, older adults who forget to keep appointments might learn to use a calendar or other organizational aids to remember the appointments. In these situations, the effectiveness of interventions is measured by how well these persons remember to keep appointments. Effectiveness of nursing interventions also can be measured subjectively, based on the degree to which older adults express positive perceptions of their cognitive abilities and satisfaction with interventions, including self-care actions.

Case Study

Mrs. C. is 71 years old and lives alone in her own home. She attends a local senior wellness clinic for blood pressure checks, health screenings (e.g., cholesterol levels), and her annual flu shot. During her monthly visit for a blood pressure check, she confides that she is embarrassed about missing a doctor's appointment last week. She says she has been noticing increased difficulties with memory, and one of her friends has told her that she probably has Alzheimer's disease. She asks if there is a place where she can get a test for Alzheimer's disease.

Case Study (Continued)

NURSING ASSESSMENT

Your nursing assessment indicates that Mrs. C. has missed a couple of health care appointments during the past year. She said she missed a dental appointment 6 months ago when she was very worried about her daughter, who was undergoing diagnostic tests for a lump in her breast. Last week, when she missed her doctor's appointment, she had been busy shopping for presents for her grandson's wedding. When you ask about additional problems with memory, Mrs. C. admits that she has more difficulty remembering people's names than she used to have. You do not identify any risk factors that might affect Mrs. C.'s cognitive abilities (e.g., depression, medication effects, poor nutrition). Mrs. C. has never used calendars, and she says she remembers her doctor's appointments by keeping the appointment cards in her desk drawer along with her bills and her checkbook. She says that she checks her appointment cards every month, but she had not noticed the cards for the two appointments she missed.

NURSING DIAGNOSIS

You use the nursing diagnosis of Health-Seeking Behaviors because Mrs. C. is interested in learning about memory training skills to assist her in remembering appointments. Mrs. C. has a poor understanding of age-related cognitive changes, and she indicates that she is interested in learning about ways to improve her memory.

NURSING CARE PLAN FOR MRS. C.

Expected Outcome	Nursing Interventions	Nursing Evaluation
Mrs. C. will express an interest in improving her memory skills	• Use information in Box 11-2 to teach Mrs. C. about age-related changes that affect cognitive abilities • Discuss the characteristics of normal cognitive aging, mild cognitive impairment, and dementia • Emphasize that memory skills can be developed through memory training techniques	• Mrs. C. will agree to participate in a discussion of memory training skills
Mrs. C. will use memory training techniques to improve her functional level	• Give Mrs. C. a copy of Box 11-3 and review the information • Assist Mrs. C. in identifying one or two strategies for remembering appointments (e.g., begin using a calendar) • Assist Mrs. C. in identifying one or two strategies for remembering the names of people she meets (e.g., using visual images)	• Mrs. C. will report success in using a method for remembering appointments • Mrs. C. will report success in using a method for remembering names of people
Mrs. C. will be aware of resources for assessment if memory does not improve	• Provide information about local geriatric assessment program for cognitive assessment	• Mrs. C. will follow up, as needed, with obtaining a comprehensive assessment of cognitive function

THINKING POINTS

- What factors are likely to be contributing to Mrs. C.'s forgetting about her appointments?
- What is the most effective way of using information in Boxes 11-2 and 11-3 to facilitate learning for Mrs. C.?
- What additional interventions would you suggest for Mrs. C.?

(continued)

Case Study (Continued)

QSEN APPLICATION

QSEN Competency	Knowledge/Skill/Attitude	Application to Mrs. C.
Patient-centered care	(K) Integrate understanding of multiple dimensions of patient-centered care	Empower Mrs. C. to improve her memory skills by teaching her about normal cognitive aging and interventions to improve memory
	(K) Describe strategies to empower patients in all aspects of the health care process	Use good communication skills to express understanding of Mrs. C.'s concerns and at the same time dispel any myths about cognitive aging
	(S) Assess own level of communication skill in encounters with patients and families	
	(A) Value seeing health care situations "through patients' eyes"	
Teamwork and collaboration	(S) Integrate the contributions of others who play a role in helping the patient achieve health goals	Provide information about obtaining a comprehensive geriatric assessment for cognitive function
Evidence-based practice	(S) Base individualized care plan on patient values, clinical expertise, and evidence	Use evidence-based information summarized in Table 11-2 to teach Mrs. C. about characteristics of normal cognitive aging, mild cognitive impairment, and dementia
	(S) Read original research and evidence reports related to clinical practice	

Chapter Highlights

What is Known About Cognition and Aging

- Age-related changes that affect cognition include degenerative changes of the brain and, on the positive side, the effects of cognitive reserve and neuroplasticity
- Fluid intelligence (inductive reasoning, abstract thinking) declines, but crystallized intelligence (wisdom and judgment) improves
- Some, but not all, memory functions decline in healthy older adults
- Life span theories, empowerment theories, and the Three-Dimensional Wisdom Model focus on cognitive development during older adulthood (Box 11-1)

Factors That Affect Cognitive Wellness

- Sociocultural influences include ageism, education, cultural factors, and socioeconomic status
- Nutrition and physical activity are lifestyle factors that affect cognitive wellness
- Medication effects, especially from anticholinergic ingredients, can adversely affect cognitive function (Table 11-1)

Functional Consequences Affecting Cognitive Function (Box 11-2)

- Cognitive skills that decline with age: perceptual speed, numerical ability, episodic memory, verbal ability, inductive reasoning, executive functions

- Cognitive skills that improve with age: word lexicon, general knowledge
- Rapid or significant declines are due to pathologic processes (e.g., strokes, dementia)

Pathologic Condition Affecting Cognition: Mild Cognitive Impairment

- MCI is a heterogeneous syndrome characterized by cognitive function that is impaired beyond "normal aging" but does not meet the criteria for mild dementia (Table 11-2)
- Symptoms of MCI may improve, remain stable, or progress to Alzheimer's disease

Nursing Assessment of Cognitive Function

Refer to Chapter 13

Nursing Diagnosis

- Readiness for Enhanced Knowledge
- Health-Seeking Behaviors

Planning for Wellness Outcomes

- Cognition
- Concentration
- Health Beliefs
- Health-Seeking Behavior
- Information Processing
- Knowledge: Health Promotion
- Leisure Participation

Nursing Interventions to Promote Cognitive Wellness

- Evidence-based strategies for cognitive health include the following: nutrition, mental exercise, physical exercise, challenging leisure activities, strong social networks, activities that foster a sense of control and mastery
- Nurses can teach about interventions to promote cognitive wellness, including techniques to improve memory function (Box 11-3)
- Body-mind interventions can be used to improve concentration and attention
- Nurses can encourage the older adult to participate in mentally stimulating activities (computers, classes) and lifelong learning programs
- Health education materials can be adapted for older adults (Box 11-4)

Evaluating Effectiveness of Nursing Interventions

- Expresses satisfaction with improved cognitive abilities
- Able to use cognitive skills in daily activities

Critical Thinking Exercises

1. Identify the factors in your own life that interfere with cognitive function.
2. What memory aids do you use in your life? Are they effective? Would you like to develop additional memory aids?
3. You are working in a senior center and have suggested that the center sponsor a series of classes on the memory problems of older adults. This suggestion is based on your observation that many of the older adults have asked you questions about memory problems, and some are concerned about Alzheimer's disease. Address each of the following issues:
   - The center director is a firm believer in the adage, "You can't teach an old dog new tricks." How would you convince the director that the classes you wish to offer are worthwhile?
   - How would you structure the sessions (number and length of sessions, number of participants, etc.)?
   - Describe the content you would cover and the approach you would use for each topic. Include information about normal cognitive aging, risk factors for impaired cognitive function, techniques for improving memory, and other aspects of cognition.
   - What audiovisual aids, including written materials, would you use?
   - How would you adapt your teaching method and materials for the group?
   - How would you evaluate the sessions?

 For more information about the topics discussed in this chapter, be sure to check out the interactive Online Learning Activities and other helpful resources at http://thepoint.lww.com/Miller8e.

REFERENCES

Abner, E. L., Kryscio, R. J., Schmitt, F. A., et al. (2017). Outcomes after diagnosis of mild cognitive impairment in a large autopsy series. *Annals of Neurology*. [Epub] 2017 Feb 22. Doi: 10.1002/ana.24903.

Anderson, N., & Craik, F. (2017). 50 years of cognitive aging theory. *Journals of Gerontology: Psychological Sciences, 72*, 1–6.

Ardelt, M., & Edwards, C. (2016). Wisdom at the end of life: An analysis of mediating and moderating relations between wisdom and subjective well-being. *Journals of Gerontology: Psychological Sciences, 71*, 502–513.

Ardelt, M. & Oh, H. (2016). Theories of wisdom and aging. In V. L. Bengston & R. A. Stettersten (Eds.), *Handbook of theories of aging* (3rd ed., pp. 599–619). New York: Springer Publishing Company.

Bengston, V. L. (2016). Advances in transdisciplinary perspectives on theories of aging. In V. L. Bengston & R. A. Stettersten (Eds.), *Handbook of theories of aging* (3rd ed., pp. 531–537). New York: Springer Publishing Company.

Binder, J., Bezzola, L., Haueter, A., et al. (2017). Expertise-related functional brain network efficiency in health older adults. *BioMed Central Neurology, 18*, 2.

Bourassa, K. J., Memel, M., Woolverton, C., & Sbarra, D. A. (2017). Social participation predicts cognitive functioning in aging adults over time: Comparisons with physical health, depression, and physical activity. *Aging and Mental Health, 21*, 133–146.

Canavelli, M., Lucchini, F., Quarta, F., et al. (2016). Nutrition and dementia: Evidence for preventive approaches? *Nutrients, 8*, 144.

Cheng, S-T. (2016). Cognitive reserve and the prevention of dementia: The role of physical and cognitive activities. *Current Psychiatry Reports, 18*, 85. Doi: 10.1007/s11920-016-0721-2.

Cheng, Y.-W., Chen, T.-F., & Chiu, M.-J. (2017). From mild cognitive impairment to subjective cognitive decline: Conceptual and methodological evolution. *Neuropsychiatric Disease and Treatment, 13*, 491–498.

Dominguez, L. J., & Barbagallo, M. (2017). The relevance of nutrition for the concept of cognitive frailty. *Current Opinion in Clinical Nutrition and Metabolic Care, 20*, 61–68.

Edelstein, A., Pergolizzi, D., & Alici, Y. (2017). Cancer-related cognitive impairment in older adults. *Current Opinion in Supportive and Palliative Care, 11*, 60–69.

Gallaway, P., Miyake, H., Buchowski, M., et al. (2017). Physical activity: A viable way to reduce the risks of mild cognitive impairment, Alzheimer's Disease, and vascular dementia in older adults. *Brain Sciences, 7*, 22.

Healey, W. E. (2012). Mild cognitive impairment and aging. *Topics in Geriatric Rehabilitation, 28*(3), 157–162.

Hooyman, N., Mahoney, K., & Sciegaj, M. (2016). Theories that guide consumer-directed/person-centered initiatives in policy and practice. In V. L. Bengston & R. A. Stettersten (Eds.), *Handbook of theories of aging* (3rd ed., pp. 3-427-442). New York: Springer Publishing Company.

Humes, L. E., & Young, L A. (2016). Sensory-cognitive interactions in older adults. *Ear & Haring, 37*(Suppl 1), 52S–61S.

Jackson, P. A., Pialoux, V., Corbett, D. et al. (2016). Promoting brain health through exercise and diet in older adults: A physiological perspective. *Journal of Physiology, 594*, 4485–4498.

Johasson, L S., Nyberg, L., Kramer, A. F., et al. (2017). Aerobic exercise intervention, cognitive performance, and brain structure: Results from the Physical Influences on Brain in Aging (PHIBRA) study. *Frontiers in Aging Neuroscience, 18*(8), 336.

Kensinger, A., & Gutchess, A. (2017). Cognitive aging in a social and affective context: Advances over the past 50 years. *Journals of Gerontology: Psychological Sciences, 72*, 61–70.

Klimova, B. (2016). Use of the internet as a prevention tool against cognitive decline in normal aging. *Clinical Interventions in Aging, 11*, 1231–1237.

Knight, A., Bryan, J., & Murphy, K. (2016). Is the Mediterranean diet a feasible approach to preserving cognitive function and reducing risk of dementia for older adults in Western countries? New insights and future directions. *Ageing Research Review, 25,* 85–101.

Leggett, A., Clarke, P., Zivin, K., et al. (2017). Recent improvements in cognitive functioning among older U.S. adults: How much does increasing education attainment explain? *Journals of Gerontology: Psychological Sciences, 72.* [Epub] Doi. 10.1093/geronb/gbw210.

Lustig, C., & Lin, Z. (2016). Memory: Behavior and neural basis. In K. Warner Schaie & S. L. Willis (Eds.), *Handbook of the psychology of aging* (8th ed., pp. 147–163). Boston, MA: Elsevier Academic Press.

Malek-Ahmadi, M. (2016). Reversion from milder cognitive impairment to normal cognition: A meta-analysis. *Alzheimer's Disease and Associated Disorders, 30,* 324–330.

Mesiner, B., & Levy, B. (2016). Age stereotypes' influence on health: Stereotype embodiment theory. In V. L. Bengston & R. A. Stettersten (Eds.), *Handbook of theories of aging* (3rd ed., pp. 259–275). New York: Springer Publishing Company.

Mogle, J., Munoz, E., Gill, N. et al. (2017). Daily memory lapses in adults: Characterization and influence on affect. *Journals of Gerontology: Psychological Sciences, 72.* [Epub] Doi: 10.1093/geronb/gbx012.

Mudar, R., & Hussain, F. (2016). Neural alteration in acquired age-related hearing loss. *Frontiers in Psychology, 7.* Doi. 10.3389/fpsyg.2016.00828.

National Academies of Sciences. (2015). *Cognitive aging: Progress in understanding and opportunities for action.* Washington, DC: The National Academies Press.

Oltmanns, J., Godde, B., Winneke, A., et al. (2017). Don't lose your brain at work – the role of recurrent novelty at work in cognitive and brain aging. *Frontiers in Psychology, 8.* Doi: 10.3389.fpsyg.g.2017.00117.

Park, D. & Festini, S. (2017). Theories of memory and aging: A look at the past and a glimpse of the future. *Journals of Gerontology: Psychological Sciences, 72,* 82–90.

Petersen, R. (2016). Mild cognitive impairment. *Continuum, 22,* 408–414.

Robertson, D. A., King-Kallimanis, B. L., & Kenny, R. A. (2016). Negative perceptions of aging predict longitudinal decline in cognitive function. *Psychology and Aging, 31,* 71–81.

Salthouse, T. (2017). Contributions of the individual differences approach to cognitive aging. *Journals of Gerontology: Psychological Sciences, 72,* 7–15.

Schaie, K. W. (2016). Theoretical perspectives for the psychology of aging in a lifespan context. In K. Warner Schaie & S. L. Willis (Eds.), *Handbook of the psychology of aging* (8th ed., pp. 3–14). Boston, MA: Elsevier Academic Press.

Scheiber, C., Chen, H., Kaufman, A. S., & Weiss, L. G. (2017). How much does WAIS-IV perceptual reasoning decline across the 20 to 90-year lifespan when processing speed is controlled? *Applied Neuropsychology: Adult, 24,* 116–131.

Shah, T. M., Weinborn, M., Verdile, G., et al. (2017). Enhancing cognitive functioning in healthy older adults: A systematic review of the clinical significance of commercially available computerized cognitive training in preventing cognitive decline. *Neuropsychology Review.* [Epub] Doi: 10.1007/s11065-016-9338-9.

Smith, J. (2016). Advances in psychological theories of aging. In V. L. Bengston & R. A. Stettersten (Eds.), *Handbook of theories of aging* (3rd ed., pp. 189–191). New York: Springer Publishing Company.

Stephan, Y., Sutin, A., Caudroit, J., & Terracciano, A. (2016). Subjective age and changes in memory in older adults. *Journals of Gerontology: Psychological Sciences, 71,* 675–683.

Van Der Mussele, Le Bastard, N., Vermeiren, Y., et al. (2013). Behavioral symptoms in mild cognitive impairment as compared with Alzheimer's disease and healthy older adults. *International Journal of Geriatric Psychiatry, 28*(3), 265–275.

Vauzour, D., Camprubi-Robles, M., Miquel-Kergoat, S., et al. (2016). Nutrition for the ageing brain: Towards evidence for an optimal diet. *Ageing Research Review.* Doi: 10.1016/j.arr.2016.09.010.

Willis, S. L., & Belleville, S. (2016). Cognitive training in later adulthood. In K. Warner Schaie & S. L. Willis. *Handbook of the psychology of aging* (8th ed., pp. 219–243). Boston, MA: Elsevier Academic Press.

Wu, Y-H., Cristancho-Lacroix, V., Fassert, C., et al. (2016). The attitudes and perceptions of older adults with mild cognitive impairment toward an assistive robot. *Journal of Applied Gerontology, 35,* 3–17.

Zheng, Y., Fan, S., Liao, W., et al. (2017). Hearing impairment and risk of Alzheimer's disease: A meta-analysis of prospective cohort studies. *Neurological Sciences, 38,* 233–239.

chapter 12

Psychosocial Wellness

<table>
<tr><td colspan="2">

LEARNING OBJECTIVES

</td></tr>
<tr><td colspan="2">

After reading this chapter, you will be able to:

1. Identify the life events that commonly occur during older adulthood.

2. Discuss theories related to stress and coping as they apply to older adults.

3. Identify the risk factors and cultural factors that influence psychosocial function in older adults.

4. Describe the functional consequences associated with psychosocial function in older adults.

5. Identify nursing interventions that promote psychosocial wellness in older adults.

6. Describe how to teach a "healthy aging class" for a small group of older adults.

</td></tr>
</table>

<table>
<tr><td colspan="2">

KEY TERMS

</td></tr>
<tr><td>

culture-bound syndromes

elderspeak

infantilization

life events

life review

loneliness

</td><td>

religion

reminiscence

resilience

self-esteem

spirituality

stress

stressors

</td></tr>
</table>

Although the physiologic changes and chronic illnesses associated with older adulthood may affect a person's functional abilities, the psychosocial changes are often the most challenging and demanding in terms of coping energy. Of course, many psychosocial challenges are strongly associated with compromised health and

functioning, but some are attributable to changes in roles, relationships, and living environments. Because many of the psychosocial changes are inevitable and somewhat predictable, older adults can prepare for and respond to psychosocial challenges by developing and using effective coping strategies. Nurses promote psychosocial wellness by supporting effective coping mechanisms and assisting in the development of new coping strategies.

 LIFE EVENTS: AGE-RELATED CHANGES AFFECTING PSYCHOSOCIAL FUNCTION

Life events are the major changes that occur at various times during the life cycle and significantly affect daily life. Certain events are commonly associated with different periods in one's life. For example, younger adults are likely to experience the following life events: establishing a career, moving away from the nuclear family, committing to a partner, creating a home, and beginning a family. The major life events of younger adulthood are familiar to us through either personal experiences or the shared experiences of friends. People usually view these events as positive gains and choose them purposefully. By contrast, life events of older adulthood might be unknown, unexpected, inevitable, and, in fact, unwanted or even feared. Thus, older adults may experience a greater loss of control or fear of losing control over their lives. In addition, life events during older adulthood are likely to involve losses of significant others and objects that have been part of life for many decades. Moreover, they tend to occur close together, with less time available to adjust to each event. Some life events evolve into chronic stresses. Dealing with ageist attitudes and behaviors of others is a life event that is specific to older adults.

Life events that are most likely to occur during older adulthood include ageism, retirement, relocation, chronic illness and functional impairments, decisions about driving a vehicle, widowhood, and death of friends and family. Figure 12-1 illustrates some of the major life events that

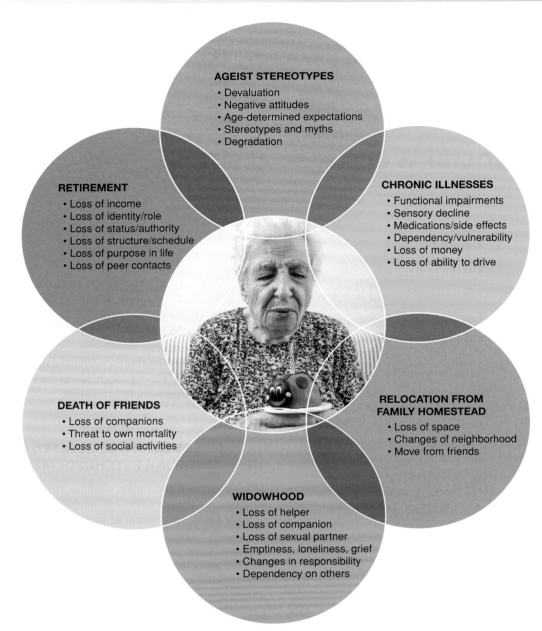

FIGURE 12-1 Psychosocial challenges of older adulthood.

are likely to occur in older adulthood, as well as the related consequences. Although most of the consequences are negative, some consequences can be positive. For example, because of these life events, older adults may focus on achieving integrity and meaning in life, and they may develop a greater acceptance of things that cannot be controlled. The illustration attempts to show the interrelatedness among the life events of older adulthood.

Wellness Opportunity

Nurses promote wellness by asking older adults to talk about the meaning of life events that they have experienced.

Ageist Attitudes

A life adjustment that is unique to older adulthood is defending against negative ageist stereotypes and attitudes, which are pervasive in Western societies. Although stereotypes of older adults can be both positive (e.g., wise, respected, accomplished) and negative (e.g., slow, confused, incompetent), the negative ones far outweigh the positive ones in Western societies. Although these characterizations may be discounted as harmless, studies consistently find that negative stereotypes of aging can have subtle but serious detrimental effects on the health and functioning of older adults. For example, negative age stereotypes, including self-stereotyping, can have a detrimental effect on cognitive skills and performance during mental status assessments (Hagood & Gruenewald, 2016; Marquet, Missotten, & Adam, 2016; Mazerolle, Regner, Barber, et al., 2016). Negative age stereotypes also are associated with poor recovery from illness and decreased physical well-being (Hicks & Siedlecki, 2016; Nelson, 2016). Equally important, positive age stereotypes are associated with better cognitive performance and improved ability to respond to stress (Bellingtier & Neupert, 2016; Bock & Akpinar, 2016; Weiss, 2016). Findings from studies such as these underscore the importance of nursing interventions focused on promoting positive views of aging and empowering older adults to recognize and build on their strengths.

Retirement

Although retirement from employment has traditionally been viewed as a milestone that marks the passage into older adulthood, there is a growing trend toward a gradual transition from full-time to part-time employment before full retirement. For example, older adults are likely to move into self-employment, change their occupation, or become consultants as they phase into full retirement. This change is associated with societal influences such as the outlawing of mandatory retirement for most workers, the gradual increase in the age for older adults to qualify for full Social Security benefits, and financial incentives that favor continued work later in life (Cahill, Giandren, & Quinn, 2016).

Societal attitudes can influence one's adjustment to retirement, particularly in societies with a strong work ethic. In these societies, working people have a higher status than unemployed people and, among working people, status is based on the kind of job one holds and the salary one earns. Therefore, when people retire, they inevitably cope with a change in social status, and the psychosocial challenge may be the greatest for people whose **self-esteem** (the feelings one has about one's self) and self-concept are based on job status. The following factors commonly influence the decision to retire: health, financial assets, job conditions, pension availability, family circumstances (e.g., caregiving responsibilities), opportunities for continued employment, and continued ability to perform job responsibilities. For married couples, both the worker and the spouse, or partner, must adjust to retirement. Sometimes the adjustment is more difficult for the partner who has not been employed.

Positive and negative outcomes of retirement vary significantly among older adults and are influenced by many factors, such as health, family and friendship relationships, and social and economic resources. A major determinant of the degree to which retirement is experienced as negative or positive is whether it is forced or voluntary. Research indicates that people who retire involuntarily or for health-related reasons are more likely to experience decreased psychological well-being; whereas, those who retire voluntarily and engage in volunteer work, bridge employment, and leisure activities have improved psychological well-being (Wang & Shi, 2016).

Relocation

Another common psychosocial adjustment for older adults is the decision to move from the family home because of factors, such as loss of spouse, lack of available assistive services, lack of a kinship network or caregiver, chronic conditions and declining functional abilities, and cognitive impairment or psychiatric illness. Increased dependence on others because of health problems is a common reason for older adults to move to a facility where they can receive support services. Additional reasons for moving to another geographic location include being closer to younger family members, preferring a warmer climate, or desiring a lower cost of living.

In addition to family and personal factors, neighborhood conditions are a major factor that affect the ability of older adults to remain in their own homes (Aneshensel, Harig, & Wight, 2016). For example, older people in urban areas may find they are unsafe or socially isolated because the neighborhood around them has changed gradually and they are no longer surrounded by people with whom they can easily relate. In rural areas, geographic distance and lack of support services can have serious consequences for older adults who are functionally impaired, especially if they have few social supports. Problems also arise for older homeowners who find it more difficult to physically and financially maintain their home and pay for utilities.

Relocation to a residential or skilled care facility is a significant life event for some older adults, and these decisions have serious emotional and economic consequences. Although options for long-term care settings have expanded significantly since the 1990s (discussed in Chapter 6), these decisions are complex and psychologically challenging. When older adults experience an abrupt or major change in health status, it is important to view these decisions as short term rather than permanent. Nurses are in key positions to address these decisions holistically by ensuring that psychosocial issues are considered along with medical concerns. Also, nurses can ensure that older adults are involved as much as possible in decisions and that these decisions are periodically reviewed as the older adult's needs change.

Wellness Opportunity

Nurses promote psychosocial wellness by encouraging older adults to express their feelings about decisions related to long-term care plans and by helping them identify effective ways of coping, even when they are not happy about the decision.

Chronic Illness and Functional Impairments

Another major life adjustment for many older adults is coping with chronic illnesses and functional limitations, particularly limitations that curtail their independence. Although most older adults experience one or more chronic conditions that affect their daily functioning, 80% of people aged 65 to 74 years and 68% of those aged 85 years and older rated their health as good to excellent (Federal Interagency Forum on Aging-Related Statistics, 2016). Most functional limitations necessitate only minor adjustments in daily living, but some, such as considerable cognitive, mobility, or visual impairments, are associated with consequences such as:

- Increased dependence on others
- Threats to self-esteem and altered self-concept
- Changes in lifestyle
- Unpredictability about one's ability to do what one wants
- Expenditures for assistance, medications, and medical care
- Frequent trips to health care providers
- Adverse medication effects, which sometimes cause further functional impairments
- Increased vulnerability to personal crimes and fear of crime

Decisions About Driving a Vehicle

Decisions about driving a vehicle are often one of the most emotionally charged issues that older adults, their families, and health care professionals face. In the United States, access to an automobile and the possession of a valid driver's license not only provide transportation but also serve as significant indicators of autonomy. In fact, for many older adults, the ability to drive is synonymous with independence, and the possession of a driver's license, even one that goes unused, is a symbol of one's ability to shield oneself from dependence on others. Cessation of driving is considered a normal transition of older adulthood; however, for many older adults, driving cessation is associated with serious negative consequences including depression, decreased social engagement, and loss of autonomy. In addition to increasing age, conditions associated with driving cessation are functional limitations, cognitive impairment, major illness, and significant vision impairment.

The loss of an independent means of transportation affects every aspect of an older person's life, from the acquisition of food and medicine to opportunities for social interaction. Because of this far-reaching impact, families and older persons may avoid dealing with driving-related issues. Family members may be reluctant to suggest that an older relative give up driving for a number of reasons. For example, family members may not want to assume an authority role, or they may lack acceptable alternatives for transportation. It is not surprising, then, that older adults and their families may avoid or resist the decision to stop driving. Neither is it surprising that when older adults give up or significantly curtail their driving, they face a difficult psychosocial challenge that may be viewed as a major life event. Implications for nursing assessment and interventions related to safe driving are discussed in Chapter 7 as an aspect of functional assessment.

Widowhood

The example of widowhood as a life event of older adulthood illustrates all of the characteristics discussed earlier. For most older couples, widowhood is inevitable, and the chances are greater that women become widowed more than men. When widowhood occurs, additional consequences follow. Common additional consequences include the following:

- Loss of companionship and intimacy
- Loss of one's sexual partner
- Feelings of grief, loneliness, and emptiness
- Increased responsibilities
- Increased dependence on others
- Loss of income and less efficient financial management
- Changes in relationships with children, married friends, and other family members.

When a marriage or partnership has lasted for many decades, as is common in people who are in their 70s and 80s, the impact of the loss can be tremendous, and the feelings of grief, loneliness, and emptiness may be overwhelming.

Psychological consequences of widowhood vary widely and are significantly influenced by factors such as the quality and emotional meaning of social relationships that continue (Barry & Byers, 2016). Longitudinal studies on widowhood among older couples identified the following trajectories that occur (described in order of most common to lease common):

- Rebound trajectory: The bereaved person rebounds within a few weeks—not because the death did no matter but because the person had good coping skills when faced with adversity.
- Recovery trajectory: The bereaved person experiences significant difficulty adjusting for 18 to 24 months, followed by an ability to re-engage in relationships with others and the wider external world.
- Enduring trajectory: The bereaved person manifests symptoms of complicated grief.

(Falk, 2016.)

Another characteristic of widowhood in older adulthood is that the chance of remarriage diminishes with advancing age. This is especially true for women because there are disproportionately fewer older men than older women due to greater longevity of women. Other reasons that older adults do not remarry include family issues, financial factors (e.g., decreased Social Security benefits), and preference for their newly independent lifestyle. Even when widows or widowers do remarry, they need to adjust to entirely different roles with a new partner. If the married couple had clearly divided roles, as is common in the cohort of people who are currently older than 75 years, loss of the partner means an adjustment in important day-to-day tasks that traditionally have been gender-typed (Perrig-Chiello, Spahni, Hopfliner, et al., 2016). For example, older couples often divide tasks so that only one of the two manages money, drives the vehicle, cleans the house, shops for groceries, and does household repairs and maintenance. When the person responsible for a task no longer performs the role, the other person may be unable, unwilling, or unprepared to assume this role.

Death of Friends and Family

Like other life events of older adulthood, the loss of friends and family becomes inevitable with increasing age. Many people who are in their 90s have outlived most, if not all, of their friends and many of their relatives. Indeed, people who are in their 90s may not even know anyone who is older than they are. Moreover, as people are confronted with the death of others who are younger than or similar to them in age, they become increasingly aware of their own mortality. Older people may read obituaries and death notices in the newspaper as a daily activity. Although families may view this activity as a morbid preoccupation, it may, in fact, be an effective way for older people to learn what is happening to their friends or acquaintances. For older adults, this experience of facing the finitude of life can be a positive perspective that is a source of wisdom (Baars, 2016).

THEORIES ABOUT STRESS AND COPING IN OLDER ADULTS

Theories about stress and coping attempt to answer questions such as *How do life events affect older adults? Do coping patterns change in older adulthood?* and *How do stress and coping patterns affect health and functioning?* In keeping with the perspective of this text, these theories are discussed in relation to positive or negative functional consequences on psychosocial function. Additional psychological theories pertinent to older adults are discussed in Chapter 4.

Theories About Stress

Hans Selye, who proposed the first major theory about stress in the mid-1950s, defined **stress** as the sum of all the effects of factors that act on the body (Selye, 1956). According to Selye's theory, **stressors** include normal activities and disease states; and all factors, whether pleasant or unpleasant, are equally important. Moreover, people respond to stressors in three stages: alarm, resistance, and exhaustion. Limitations of this theory include the broad conceptualization of stress, the lack of distinction between pleasant and unpleasant stressors, and the failure to address the meaning of events for the person.

Holmes and Rahe (1967) proposed that stress causes physical and psychological harm in proportion to the intensity of the impact on and duration of a disruption in one's usual life pattern. They developed the Social Readjustment Rating Scale as a tool for measuring the duration and intensity of 43 commonly experienced life events, with relative weights assigned to each according to the usual amount of adaptive effort required by each event. This rating scale has been criticized because it suggests that life events consistently have a negative impact for all people. Since the 1970s, researchers have developed stress scales that account for the meaning of life events for the individual or that measure effects of life events of particular age groups.

In addition to addressing the impact of major life events (e.g., acute stress), studies examine the impact of chronic stressors, such as those associated with health, finances, work, family, relationships, caregiving, and neighborhood. Daily hassles (i.e., relatively minor events arising from day-to-day living) are another source of stress that can negatively affect cognitive function and psychological well-being. Examples of hassles are misplacing or losing things and not having resources to meet demands (e.g., food, money, medications). When chronic stressors and daily hassles occur together—as is often the case—the negative effects are magnified, leading to declines in physical and cognitive functioning in older adults.

Theories About Coping

Initial theories about age-related differences in coping addressed the following types of internal mechanisms that people use to deal with stressful situations: seeking information; reframing the situation; maintaining a hopeful outlook; using stress-reduction techniques; channeling energy into physical activity; creating fantasies about various outcomes; finding reassurance and emotional support; identifying limited and realistic goals; identifying a positive purpose for the event; getting involved in other activities, such as work and family; and expressing oneself creatively, for example, through music, art, or writing. These coping styles are categorized as problem focused (i.e., directed toward altering the source of stress) or emotion focused (i.e., directed toward regulating one's response). Older adults are more likely to use coping mechanisms that involve management of thoughts and feelings, whereas younger adults are likely to take direct approaches to modify the events or challenging situations in their lives.

Theories about coping and aging also focus on both the meaning of the event to the individual and the coping resources available to him or her. Studies consistently identify strong social supports, especially religious supports and higher-quality relationships with families and friends as a way of facilitating coping in older adults (Morrow-Howell & Greenfield, 2016; Uchino, Ong, Queen, et al., 2016). Social resources include instrumental support (e.g., meals, transportation, personal care), informational support (e.g., information about resources and services), and emotional support (e.g., communication that provides comfort, companionship, and other evidence that the person is loved, valued, esteemed, and cared for).

Current theories of coping and aging focus on how older adults adapt to stressful situations and draw on past experiences to develop new coping skills. For example, many older adults can cope better with major stress because they have learned that they can overcome difficult life events, adapt to adversity, and return to prior levels of psychological functioning (Brown & Frahm, 2016). Recent studies about coping and aging conclude that older adults use more adaptive strategies and are better at emotion regulation as compared with younger adults. In addition, they are more likely to use positive reappraisal and less likely to express hostility or use the following coping mechanisms: rumination, wishful thinking, emotional numbing, or escape/avoidant strategies (Aldwin & Igarashi, 2016). Studies also indicate that older adults who are aging successfully cope with functional decline by establishing new goals and planning strategies to compensate for limitations (Carpentieri, Elliott, Brett, et al., 2017).

Relevance for Nurses

Nurses can use theories about stress and coping to identify interventions that help older adults maintain optimal functioning and quality of life when faced with the many challenges of aging. A nursing study identified strategies used by older adults with chronic comorbid conditions to enable them to remain at home safely (see Figure 12-2). Themes related to coping with functional limitations were (1) getting around at home and (2) expanding life beyond self and home (Westra, Paitich, Ekstrom, et al., 2013). Many sources of stress, such as decreasing eyesight and hearing, can be addressed through nursing interventions to improve functional abilities, as discussed in all chapters of Part 4 in this text. Other significant stresses, such as losses of, or changes in, relationships, can be addressed through the psychosocial interventions discussed in the section on nursing interventions in this chapter.

FACTORS THAT INFLUENCE PSYCHOSOCIAL FUNCTION IN OLDER ADULTS

Psychosocial function is influenced by numerous factors, including personality, experiences, physical and emotional health, and socioeconomic and environmental conditions. Because many of the factors are beyond the usual scope of nursing, this section focuses on two aspects that are particularly pertinent to usual nursing care of older adults: religion and spirituality and cultural considerations. Additional information about these topics is addressed in Chapter 13 (section on Assessing Religion and Spirituality) and Chapter 2 (Addressing Diversity of Older Adults).

Religion and Spirituality

Religion and spirituality are widely recognized as major coping resources that have a positive effect on many aspects of

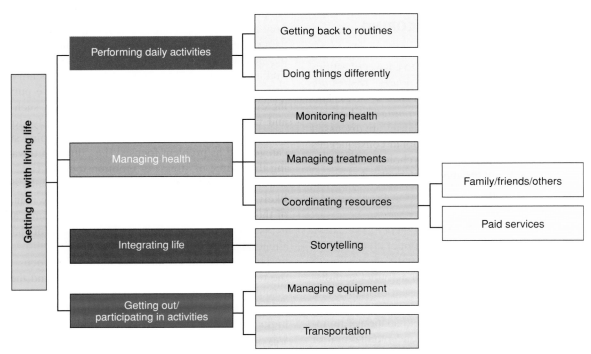

FIGURE 12-2 Strategies used by older adults to get on with living life. (Adapted with permission from Westra, B. L., Paitich, N., Ekstrom, D., et al. (2013). Getting on with living life: Experiences of older adults after home care. *Home Healthcare Nurse, 31*(9), 493–501.)

psychosocial function for older adults. Religion and spirituality are closely related but distinct concepts. **Religion** and religiosity, which have a strong social component, refer to an organized system of beliefs and behaviors that are shared by a group of people who are associated with a defined faith community. Examples of religious practices are rituals, prayers, meditation, worship services, attendance at church, and adherence to certain dietary practices and style of clothing.

Religious practices nurture spiritual development; however, spirituality is broader and less structured and does not necessarily include membership in a formal religious group. Gerontologists consistently find that religion becomes more important with age and that attendance at religious services is associated with many beneficial outcomes including better health and longer life expectancy (Krause & Hayward, 2016).

Florence Nightingale viewed **spirituality** as intrinsic to human nature and emphasized that it was an individual's deepest and the most potent resource for healing. Definitions of spirituality generally include the following concepts: healing; wholeness; social justice; personal growth; interpersonal relationships; a sense of meaning and purpose to life; a transcendent relationship with a higher being; an association with reverence, mystery, and inspiration; connectedness with nature, other people, and the universe; and feelings of and behaviors arising from love, faith, hope, trust, and forgiveness. Current nursing references (e.g., Burkhardt & Nagai-Jacobson, 2016; Westra, 2017) describe the following components of spirituality:

- Connectedness to self: joy, love, surrender, serenity, self-forgiveness, and meaning and purpose in life
- Connectedness with others: service, compassion, loving sexuality, forgiveness of others, shared genuine presence, meaningful interactions with significant others, and reciprocal giving and receiving
- Connectedness with power greater than self: awe, prayer, ritual, reverence, meditation, reconciliation, and mystical experiences
- Engagement in creative activities: art, music, nature, poetry, writing, singing, and spiritual literature

Religion and spirituality are important coping strategies for many older adults, particularly in the context of dealing with chronic conditions (Vitorino, Lucchetti, Santos, et al., 2016).

 See ONLINE LEARNING ACTIVITY 12-1: RESOURCES FOR INFORMATION ABOUT SPIRITUALITY AND AGING at http://thepoint.lww.com/Miller8e.

A Student's Perspective

When I interviewed one of the residents, I felt like I got a really good impression of the things he valued most and the exciting experiences in his life. I think the most significant part for me was when we talked about religion. When I asked Mr. E. if he was religious, he answered very politely saying that his parents tried to raise him Catholic but that it was never really him. I then asked if he saw himself as spiritual and he said that he is very spiritual and that he definitely thinks there is something "more" after death. He said that he didn't feel like he needed to go to a church to be a good person. I really connected with this because I was able to see that we have something in common. I also feel very spiritual even though I am not really affiliated with any particular religion.

Erika B.

Wellness Opportunity

Nurses promote wellness by asking older adults about relationships that provide meaning in their lives.

Cultural Considerations

Cultural factors strongly influence the way a person defines and perceives all aspects of psychosocial function. In assessing psychosocial function in older adults, for example, it is essential to recognize that every society has guidelines for determining whether behaviors are healthy or unhealthy (Box 12-1). Many societies, however, do not have the rigid distinctions between health and illness that are part of Western cultures, and concepts, such as mental health, have little meaning in many non-Western societies (Ehrmin, 2016). Cultural perceptions determine all of the following aspects of psychosocial function:

- Definition of mental health and mental illness
- Belief about the causes of mental health and illness
- Expression of symptoms or clinical manifestations of mental health and illness
- Criteria for labeling or diagnosing someone as mentally ill
- Decisions concerning appropriate healer(s)
- Choice of treatment(s) to cure mental illness
- Determination that mental health has been restored after an illness episode
- Relative degree of tolerance for abnormal behavior by other members of society

In some instances, people from diverse cultures may perceive or interpret physical symptoms and their related psychological or emotional components in a manner that is unfamiliar to professionals who do not share the same cultural background. **Culture-bound syndromes**, which also are referred to as folk illnesses, are specific manifestations that are unique to a particular cultural group (Ehrmin, 2016). Examples of these syndromes (which nurses in geriatric care settings may encounter) include the following:

- *Dhat, Jiryan,* in people from India: dizziness, fatigue, weakness, loss of appetite, sexual dysfunction, and feeling of guilt
- *Ghost sickness*, in Navaho Native Americans: weakness, sense of pending doom, loss of appetite, fainting, dizziness, hallucinations, and feeling of suffocation

Box 12-1 Cultural Considerations: Cultural Influences on Psychosocial Function

Cultural Influences on Beliefs About the Cause of Mental Disorders

- In traditional Chinese culture, many diseases are attributed to an imbalance of yin and yang.
- Many Native American groups embrace a belief system in which balance and harmony are essential for mental and physical health.
- For some Hispanics, mental illness may be viewed as a punishment by a supreme being for past transgressions.
- Some African Americans, especially those of circum-Caribbean descent, may attribute the cause of mental illness to voodoo, sorcery, or other spiritual forces.

Cultural Influences on the Manifestations of Mental Illness

- Cultural norms determine whether behaviors, such as any of the following, are viewed as either normal or abnormal: dreams, fainting, visions, trances, sorcery, delusions, hallucinations, intoxication, suicide, speaking in tongues, communicating with spirits, and the use of certain substances (e.g., alcohol, tobacco, peyote, marijuana, and other drugs).
- Posttraumatic stress disorders are relatively common in immigrants and refugees.
- Hispanic older adults define mental health problems as alcohol and other drug abuse.
- Filipino Americans consider forgetfulness and anger to be mental health problems.
- Hispanic, Chinese, and other groups are likely to express psychological distress through physical symptoms.
- Depression may be expressed through physical symptoms, such as pain, headache, or gastrointestinal symptoms.
- Although psychotic disorders (i.e., loss of contact with reality) occur in every society and are characterized by similar primary symptoms (e.g., insomnia, delusions, hallucinations, flat affect, and social or emotional withdrawal), the secondary features (e.g., content and focus) are highly influenced by cultural factors.
- In some groups, guilt and suicidal ideation do not accompany depression.
For some peoples, suicide is an acceptable escape from problems.

Cultural Influences on Stress and Coping

- Cultural factors often create barriers to the use of formal support services by ethnic elders, and these barriers may increase the feelings of burden experienced by caregivers.
- African American families tend to use religion and spirituality to help them cope with caregiving stress, and religious organizations are a major source of social support for them.
- In Chinese families, cultural ideals promoting filial piety, family interdependence, veneration of elderly family members, and acceptance of family caregiving roles may affect the way families experience and cope with stress related to their roles as caregivers.

Source: Andrews, M. M., & Boyle, J. S. (2016). *Transcultural concepts in nursing care* (7th ed.). Philadelphia, PA: Wolters Kluwer/Lippincott Williams & Wilkins.

- *Nervios*, in Latino people: irritability, tearfulness, sleep disturbances, difficulty concentrating, and feeling of vulnerability and emotional distress to stressful life experiences
- *Shenjing*, in Chinese people: depression, anxiety, dizziness, headaches, and sleep and gastrointestinal disturbances.

Professionals and folk or indigenous healers with the same cultural background usually are knowledgeable about

interventions for culture-bound syndromes. Older adults may be reluctant to discuss culture-bound syndromes or folk treatments with health care professionals, especially if the care provider has a different cultural background. The reasons for withholding such information are complex and may include fears that the nurse or other health care provider will disapprove, ridicule, or fail to understand their folk or indigenous healing system. Because of these factors, nurses may consider asking the person's permission to include folk or indigenous healers in discussions about health-related issues. These healers frequently have considerable insight into the cultural and psychosocial aspects of human behavior, and they may be remarkably successful in treating culture-bound syndromes and other disorders that have psychological and emotional components. Because herbal remedies that are sometimes used to treat culture-bound syndromes may interact with prescription or over-the-counter medications, nurses need to make every effort to elicit information about such remedies as part of an assessment (see Chapter 8).

A Student's Perspective

While I was caring for my client, she asked if she could tell me a story. She proceeded to tell me that a few nights earlier, she was lying in bed unable to sleep because of various health issues. All of a sudden, she heard this calm yet intense chant moving down the hall. One of the residents is Native American and recently received news that his nephew had passed away. He was performing a traditional chant in mourning for the loss of a loved one. My client said that the sound was peaceful and soothing as she lay awake in bed. She wished she could have recorded it to play every night. She felt it was special that this man was able to maintain his culture in a place far from home and that people respected his need to express himself in this way. She was very touched—and so was I—as she told me this story. I believe that maintaining one's culture is a part of the healing process and should be respected and upheld.

Eliza T.

Case Study

Mrs. Y. is a 79-year-old native of the Philippines. She moved to an urban area in California to be near her four children, who live in the same state. She had lived in the same town in the Philippines for her entire adult life and had stayed there to care for her husband and her sister, who both required care for chronic conditions. Although she was a much-needed and highly esteemed member of her household in the Philippines, Mrs. Y., like many other immigrants, experienced role reversal when she lost her once-dominant position in the family and became financially dependent on her adult children after her relocation.

Also like many older immigrants from the Philippines, Mrs. Y. had a more active social network before her relocation.

As did many of her peers, Mrs. Y. spoke a dialect and did not speak Tagalog, the language spoken by many younger residents of the Philippines. After her relocation to the United States, her communication and interaction with others became restricted to her extended family because she did not feel confident using her limited English and could not find other speakers of her dialect. To buffer the disequilibrium she felt as a result of her migration, Mrs. Y. sought comfort through prayer and regular attendance at the local Roman Catholic Church. She also began to care regularly for her two daughters' children.

You are the nurse at the local hospital who treated Mrs. Y. in the emergency department after she fractured her wrist. During your assessment, you note that Mrs. Y.'s injury would place a strain on the family because they would temporarily be without their child care provider.

THINKING POINTS

- How would you involve the family members in the discharge plan for Mrs. Y. so that her recovery could be ensured, she would not lose respect, and she would not feel responsible to assume her usual duties until her injury healed and she felt better?
- What problems would you anticipate with communicating with Mrs. Y. in the emergency department? How would you handle these problems?
- What psychosocial repercussions did Mrs. Y.'s move to the United States have? Did she cope with these effectively? Would you have had any other suggestions for helping her to cope?
- How did Mrs. Y.'s culture influence her coping mechanisms?

Case example reprinted with permission from McKenna, M. A. (2012). Transcultural perspectives in the nursing care of older adults. In M. M. Andrews & J. S. Boyle (Eds.), *Transcultural concepts in nursing care* (6th ed., pp. 182–207). Philadelphia, PA: Lippincott, Williams & Wilkins. (Questions that follow the case example were written by Carol A. Miller.)

 ## RISK FACTORS THAT AFFECT PSYCHOSOCIAL FUNCTION

Theories about stress and coping and research about causes of impaired mental health in older adults provide information about risks that can affect psychosocial function. The following factors contribute to high levels of stress and poor coping in older adults:

- Poor physical health
- Impaired functional abilities
- Weak social supports
- Lack of economic resources
- An immature developmental level
- Narrow range of coping skills
- The occurrence of unanticipated events
- The occurrence of several daily hassles at the same time
- The occurrence of several major life events over a short time

In addition, because the ability to determine the potential for change influences one's response to a stressful situation, people who cannot realistically appraise a situation may have more difficulty coping effectively. This is particularly pertinent regarding health and functioning because ageist attitudes and stereotypes may contribute to the false belief that health changes and functional decline are inevitable consequences of aging. Thus, nurses have important roles in teaching older adults about risk factors and potential interventions for health problems. For example, older adults who experience urinary incontinence or difficulties with sexual function may consider these changes to be inevitable consequences of age. Based on this appraisal, they may use passive, emotion-focused coping mechanisms, trying simply to accept the situation. In addition, they are more likely to experience an unnecessary and unfortunate functional impairment and a diminished quality of life. By contrast, if the situation is appraised more accurately as a potentially treatable condition, older adults are more likely to use active, problem-focused coping mechanisms. Even when older adults accurately appraise health problems as changeable, health care professionals also must understand the problem and attempt to find solutions. Thus, both older adults and health care professionals must accurately appraise the situation so they can initiate interventions and achieve wellness outcomes.

Wellness Opportunity

Nurses promote wellness by allowing older adults to function as independently as possible and providing the supports they need, even if this is not as time-efficient as doing things for them.

 ## FUNCTIONAL CONSEQUENCES ASSOCIATED WITH PSYCHOSOCIAL FUNCTION IN OLDER ADULTS

Although negative functional consequences are commonly associated with psychosocial function in older adults, positive functional consequences also occur in older adults. This section reviews loneliness as a negative functional consequence that nurses can address. In addition, cognitive impairment and depression are serious negative functional consequences that are discussed in Chapters 14 and 15, respectively. Resilience in later life, which is a topic that currently is receiving much attention in gerontological literature, is discussed in this section as a positive functional consequence.

Loneliness

Older adults frequently experience feelings of **loneliness**, which is defined as a feeling of emptiness or a lack of satisfying human relationships that is not alleviated by being around other people. Older adults are particularly vulnerable to experiencing loneliness because of the many losses associated with aging, including loss of health, spouse, friends, and social status. In addition to widowhood, life events of older adulthood that increase the risk for loneliness include retirement, death of friends, relocation to new environments, and health-related problems (e.g., serious illness, significant vision or hearing impairment). Studies indicate that loneliness increases the risk for all of the following: depression, cognitive decline, functional decline, impaired sleep, poor physical health, and increased mortality (Shankar, McMunn, Demakakos, et al., 2017; Zhong, Chen, Tu, et al., 2017; Zhou, Wang, & Fang, 2017). These negative consequences can be alleviated, or at least diminished, through interventions to improve and expand social networks for older adults (Domenech-Abella, Lara, Rubio-Valera, et al., 2017; Petersen, Kaye, Jacobs, et al., 2016).

Resilience

During the early 2000s, gerontologists began studying the concept of **resilience** in older adults, and currently this topic is of great interest in relation to psychosocial wellness. Resilience is defined as the "capacity to adjust to challenges, persevere in the face of hardship, maintain a chosen course of action or pursue desired goals despite the presence of stressors that threaten to disrupt the status quo" (Brown & Frahm, 2016). This definition includes the following dimensions:

- Recovery: the ability to return to the prior state of functioning after experiencing a traumatic event
- Resistance: the capacity to maintain baseline functioning throughout a stressful or traumatic event
- Reconfiguration: reforming baseline thoughts, beliefs, and behaviors in response to a stressor, which may ultimately enhance one's ability to endure future traumatic events

A recent nursing review of research found that resilience is a multidimensional process that can be improved during later adulthood, leading to reduced depression and increased happiness and well-being (MacLeod, Musich, Hawkins, et al., 2016). Interventions that support the development of resilience in later life focus on maintaining optimal health and functioning, providing social supports, and encouraging activities that provide a sense of purpose in life (Aldwin & Igarashi, 2016). Nurses have many opportunities to promote resilience through the interventions discussed in this chapter and throughout the text.

PATHOLOGIC CONDITION RELATED TO PSYCHOSOCIAL FUNCTION: ALCOHOL ABUSE

Alcohol abuse is only one component of the broader topic of substance abuse, which generally also includes misuse of opioids, marijuana, and prescription and nonprescription drugs. This chapter covers alcohol abuse by older adults because alcohol is the substance most commonly abused by that group. It is beyond the scope of this text to address substance abuse comprehensively; however, please note that much of the information about alcohol abuse also relates to abuse of other substances. In addition, Online Learning

Activity 12-2 includes information related to substance misuse and alcohol use disorders in older adults.

See ONLINE LEARNING ACTIVITY 12-2: RESOURCES FOR INFORMATION ABOUT SUBSTANCE MISUSE AND ALCOHOL USE DISORDERS IN OLDER ADULTS at http://thepoint.lww.com/Miller8e.

National surveys indicate that between 7% and 14% of adults age 65 and older report alcohol abuse, dependence, binge drinking, or at-risk use of alcohol dependence (Tampi, Tampi, & Durning, 2016). In addition, recent data point to a trend toward increasing prevalence of all of the following behaviors among adults aged 50 and older: increased overall use of alcohol, more incidences of past-month binge drinking, and increased alcohol abuse disorders (Han, Moore, Sherman, et al., 2017). Some older adults who abuse alcohol are long-term users, whereas others are late-onset users who have started using alcohol excessively. Older adults are likely to abuse alcohol for any of the following reasons: boredom, loneliness, stress reduction, continuation of long-term social patterns, or management of pain or sleep problems. Many of these reasons are associated with conditions common during older adulthood, such as depression, poor health, and decreased social supports (Loscalzo, Sterling, Weinstein, et al., 2017). Alcohol abuse needs to be addressed through interprofessional collaboration, with nurses having an essential role in identifying older adults who would benefit from interventions. Nurses can use the information in Box 12-2 as a guide to addressing the needs of older adults who are at risk for alcohol-related health problems.

Diversity Note

More than one-fifth of lesbian, gay, and bisexual (LGB) older adults report high-risk drinking behaviors. This disproportionately high rate may be linked to social contexts and drinking norms for LGB women and to discrimination-related stress for LGB men (Bryan, Kim, & Frederiksen-Goldsen, 2017).

NURSING ASSESSMENT OF PSYCHOSOCIAL FUNCTION

Because psychosocial function encompasses a broad range of social, cognitive, and emotional aspects of functioning that are intertwined, the assessment of psychosocial function is addressed comprehensively in a separate chapter. Readers are directed to Chapter 13 for a thorough review of nursing assessment of psychosocial function.

NURSING DIAGNOSIS

The nursing diagnoses of Situational Low Self-Esteem (or Risk for) are applicable in relation to some of the

E B P   **Box 12-2 Evidence-Based Practice: Alcohol Use Among Older Adults**

Unique Considerations Related to Alcohol Use Among Older Adults

- Older adults have higher sensitivity and higher blood concentrations with lower consumption of alcoholic beverages.
- Even healthy older adults are more susceptible to adverse effects of alcohol due to age-related changes in metabolism.
- The risk for adverse effects can increase significantly in older adults who have pathologic conditions (e.g., effects on cognitive functions in the presence of dementia or depression, effects on balance in the presence of mobility or neurologic problems).
- Alcohol may interact with medications to increase the risk of adverse effects.

Health Consequences of At-Risk Drinking[a]

- Increased risk of immediate serious health consequences including falls, accidents, depression, self-neglect, cognitive impairment
- Increased risk of serious long-term chronic conditions including diabetes, depression, cognitive impairment, liver disorders, and cardiovascular disease
- Exacerbation of medical conditions, such as diabetes
- Interactions with medications

Barriers to Identification and Treatment of Alcohol Abuse in Older Adults

Nurse Barriers
- False attribution of symptoms (e.g., falls, forgetfulness) to pathological conditions

[a]At-risk drinking is defined as more than one drink per day or more than three drinks on one occasion, where one drink = 12 ounces of beer, 4 to 5 ounces of wine, or 1.5 ounces of distilled spirits.

- Common misperception that drinking is infrequent among older adults
- Perception that drinking is a harmless pleasure that should be overlooked in older adults
- Erroneous assumption that interventions are not worthwhile or effective for older adults

Patient Barriers
- Shame about substance abuse
- Social and cultural stigma associated with substance abuse
- Perception of alcohol abuse and mental health issues as private matters that should be managed without professional help
- Perception that seeking treatment is a sign of weakness

Nursing Considerations for Assessment and Interventions

- Realize that alcohol abuse problems are often unrecognized in older adults.
- Communicate empathy and a nonjudgmental attitude.
- Avoid terms like "alcoholic."
- State the purpose of questions about substance abuse and link them to health and safety.
- Identify older adults who are problem drinkers by using the following evidence-based tool: The Short Michigan Alcoholism Screening Instrument – Geriatric Version (SMAST-G) (available at www.consultgerirn.org).
- If a screening tool or assessment information identifies at-risk drinking behaviors, initiate a discussion about health risks.
- Ask the older adult about actions he or she might consider to address identified problems.
- As appropriate, initiate referrals for further evaluation and management (e.g., advanced practice nurses, mental health professionals, comprehensive geriatric assessment programs).

psychosocial adjustment issues of older adulthood. Situational Low Self-Esteem is defined as "development of a negative perception of self-worth in response to a current situation" (Herdman & Kamitsuru, 2018, p. 274). Related factors might be the internalization of ageist attitudes, the loss of roles or financial security, the need for a change to a more dependent living arrangement, and chronic illnesses that affect one's abilities and role identities.

If the nursing assessment identifies threats to the older person's sense of control, an appropriate nursing diagnosis is Powerlessness (or Risk for). This is defined as "the lived experience of lack of control over a situation, including a perception that one's actions do not significantly affect an outcome" (Herdman & Kamitsuru, 2018, p. 343). Common related factors for older adults are forced retirement, loss of the ability to drive a vehicle, lack of involvement in decision making, chronic conditions that cause progressive functional declines (e.g., dementia), and institutional constraints, such as lack of privacy and the need to follow schedules that do not meet the needs of the individual.

Social Isolation is defined as "aloneness experienced by the individual and perceived as imposed by others and as a negative or threatening state" (Herdman & Kamitsuru, 2018, p. 455). A closely related nursing diagnosis is Impaired Social Interaction, defined as "insufficient or excessive quantity or ineffective quality of social exchange" (Herdman &

Kamitsuru, 2018, p. 301). These nursing diagnoses can be used when making referrals for community resources to improve social supports for older adults.

Another nursing diagnosis that might be applied to the psychosocial needs of older adults is Ineffective Coping, which is defined as the "inability to form a valid appraisal of the stressors, inadequate choices of practiced responses, and/or inability to use available resources" (Herdman & Kamitsuru, 2018, p. 327). Other nursing diagnoses that might be applicable with regard to specific aspects of psychosocial function include Chronic Sorrow, Grieving, Relocation Stress Syndrome, Spiritual Distress, and Stress Overload. The diagnosis of Readiness for Enhanced Spiritual Well-Being is applicable for addressing older adults' sense of meaning and purpose. This wellness diagnosis is defined as "a pattern of experiencing and integrating meaning and purpose in life through connectedness with self, others, art, music, literature, nature, and/or a power greater than oneself, which can be strengthened" (Herdman & Kamitsuru, 2018, p. 365).

Wellness Opportunity

Readiness for Enhanced Coping and Readiness for Enhanced Resilience are wellness nursing diagnoses that are applicable for many older adults who are experiencing psychosocial stress.

PLANNING FOR WELLNESS OUTCOMES

Wellness outcomes related to psychosocial function focus on stress reduction, enhanced coping skills, and improved quality of life. When planning wellness outcomes pertinent to Situational Low Self-Esteem (or Risk for) or Readiness for Enhanced Self-Concept, nurses can apply any of the following Nursing Outcomes Classification (NOC) terminology: Psychosocial Adjustment—Life Change; Self-Esteem; Adaptation to Physical Disability; Body Image; Grief Resolution; Personal Autonomy; Depression Level; and Quality of Life.

Outcomes for older adults who experience Powerlessness include Hope, Personal Autonomy, and Participation in Health Care Decisions. Outcomes related to the nursing diagnosis of Social Isolation include Loneliness Severity, Social Support, Social Involvement, Leisure Participation, and Personal Well-Being.

When nurses plan care for older adults with nursing diagnoses of Impaired Adjustment, Ineffective Coping, or Readiness for Enhanced Coping, any of the following NOC terms may be pertinent: Psychosocial Adjustment—Life Change; Acceptance: Health Status; Adaptation to Physical Disability; Coping; Decision Making; Knowledge: Health Resources; Personal Well-Being; and Stress Level.

Wellness Opportunity

Hope and Quality of Life would be appropriate NOC terms when nurses direct care toward improving psychosocial wellness.

NURSING INTERVENTIONS TO PROMOTE HEALTHY PSYCHOSOCIAL FUNCTION

Nurses have many opportunities to promote healthy psychosocial function during the usual course of caring for older adults. For example, they can incorporate communication techniques and other interventions to enhance self-esteem, promote a sense of control, and address spiritual needs. They also can use life review and reminiscence interventions, especially in home and long-term care settings. In addition to incorporating interventions in usual care, nurses promote psychosocial wellness by facilitating referrals for social supports. In some settings, nurses can implement group interventions, such as healthy aging classes, to help older adults cope effectively with the life events of older adulthood.

The following Nursing Interventions Classification terms relate to interventions discussed in this chapter: Active Listening; Coping Enhancement; Decision-Making Support; Emotional Support; Grief Work Facilitation; Hope Inspiration; Presence; Religious Ritual Enhancement; Reminiscence Therapy; Resiliency Promotion; Role Enhancement; Self-Esteem Enhancement; Socialization Enhancement; Spiritual Growth Facilitation; Spiritual Support, Support System Enhancement; and Teaching: Group.

In addition to the interventions reviewed in this chapter, interventions that improve functional abilities promote psychosocial wellness because of the close relationship between physiologic and psychosocial aspects of health and function. Nurses can apply information discussed in all chapters in Part 4 of this text to promote independent functioning of older adults, which, in turn, are interventions for improving many aspects of psychosocial function.

Enhancing Self-esteem

Self-esteem enhancement is an essential component of nursing care for older adults because self-esteem is an important coping resource and a factor that influences well-being. Self-esteem is the emotional component of self-concept and is based on one's perceptions of other people's opinions about oneself. Good self-esteem is a characteristic that is associated with being happier, healthier, less anxious, more independent, more self-confident, and more effective in meeting environmental demands than people with low self-esteem. Chapter 13 includes information on assessing self-esteem, whereas this chapter focuses on nursing interventions that enhance self-esteem, with emphasis on addressing factors that threaten it (e.g., dependence, devaluation, depersonalization, and powerlessness).

Many factors that are threats to self-esteem are associated with staff and environments of institutional settings and can be addressed through relatively simple nursing interventions. This is particularly important in environments such as long-term care settings where the caregiving environment affects virtually every aspect of daily life for the residents. For instance, in institutional settings, it is important to identify environmental or other factors that can be modified to promote a sense of control and minimize or eliminate a threat to self-esteem, as in the following examples:

- Ensuring easy access to usual assistive devices (walkers, eyeglasses, hearing aids)
- Providing as much privacy as possible
- Asking about food preferences and ensuring as much choice as possible
- Asking open-ended questions, such as, "Is there anything that we can do to help you manage better while you're here?"
- Asking, "Is there anything you're worried about that I can help you with?"
- Ensuring that staff members address persons by their preferred names
- Involving older adults as much as possible in decisions that affect them

Threats to self-esteem also arise when caregivers promote unnecessary dependence for their own convenience. For example, using incontinence products in beds and telling a dependent person to wet the bed because it is easier to change the disposable pad than to assist with toileting is a tremendous blow to the person's self-esteem.

Because self-esteem depends to some extent on the perceived appraisal of significant others, it is important to avoid communicating even subtle messages that may be perceived as ageist. For example, a remark such as "You certainly look good for 85 years old," although said with good intentions, can reinforce ageist attitudes. Such a statement may subtly communicate the message that when you are old, you generally do not look good. In contrast, a statement such as the following might enhance an older person's self-esteem: "At 85 years old, you must have a lot of wisdom. Can you share a bit of that wisdom with me?" Nonverbal communication also can influence the person's perception of self-worth. For example, a simple action like walking past an older person sitting in a hallway without acknowledging his or her presence may be perceived as an indicator that the nurse does not value the older person. Even though the nurse had not intended to communicate a negative message, this action may adversely affect that older person's self-esteem. Thus, nurses must keep in mind that the perception of their actions is often more important than their intent, and they must use verbal and nonverbal messages to communicate feelings of positive regard whenever possible.

For dependent older adults, the negative impact of disability and functional impairments on self-esteem is heightened by behaviors of others that convey attitudes of **infantilization** (i.e., treating an adult in a way that is similar to the way infants are treated). For example, remarks such as "He acts just like a baby" or "Now, now, dear, let's be a good girl," convey infantilization. The term **elderspeak**—also called "baby talk"—describes speech that is modified when addressed to older adults, usually by younger adults. Elderspeak is characterized by short sentences, slow speech, simple words, exaggerated intonation, high and variable pitch and volume, and inappropriately intimate terms of endearment. This type of communication is demeaning and patronizing, and it can have serious negative consequences, such as resistance to care and negative vocalizations in people with dementia (Williams, Perkhounkova, Herman, et al., 2016). Moreover, it reflects ageist attitudes and negative and inaccurate stereotypes (Gendron, Welleford, Inker, et al., 2016). Thus, nurses need to monitor their communication with older adults to ensure that they avoid inappropriate terminology and elderspeak. Box 12-3 summarizes nursing interventions for enhancing self-esteem in older adults.

Wellness Opportunity

Nurses can enhance self-esteem by pointing out an older adult's positive qualities during routine care activities.

Promoting a Sense of Control

Having a sense of control is a factor that significantly affects psychosocial wellness because studies indicate that higher levels of perceived mastery are associated with benefits such as better physical, cognitive, and psychological health

---

Box 12-3 Nursing Interventions to Promote Self-Esteem

Communication Techniques

- Acknowledge person by using their preferred names and titles.
- When talking with older people, use the same tone of voice you use for your colleagues.
- Provide positive feedback for individual accomplishments, even in daily self-care tasks that require effort.
- Focus conversations on persons' strengths and positive attributes rather than on their limitations. (e.g., for people who have physical impairments, focus on nonphysical attributes, such as personality characteristics or interpersonal relationships.)
- When negative functional consequences are attributed to old age, offer an alternative explanation and identify a contributing factor that is amenable to change. (e.g., when older people attribute weakness "simply" to being old, remind them that they are recovering from hip surgery and should expect to improve with therapy.)
- Be cautious about communicating ageist attitudes, even inadvertently, in conversations.

Verbal Communication to Observe for and Avoid

- Do not use names or phrases that reflect ageist attitudes (e.g., "little old lady," "dirty old man"), even in jest.
- Do not raise your voice except when necessary to facilitate communication with someone who has impaired hearing.
- Do not use terms that are associated with babies (e.g., *diapers*, *baby food*).
- Do not use *we* or *us* unless the term is accurate (e.g., do not say "Let's take our medicine now").
- Do not use the term *senile*.

Nonverbal Communication Techniques and Additional Nursing Actions

- When labeling clothing, put the person's name in an inconspicuous place.
- Use actions consciously to communicate positive regard (e.g., recognize the presence of someone as you walk past).

(Duan-Porter, Hastings, Neelon, & Van Houtven, 2017; Helvik, Bjorklof, Corazzini, et al., 2016; Lee, 2016). Thus, nurses address psychosocial needs of older adults with interventions that promote a sense of control and that involve older adults in decisions. Nursing interventions to promote a sense of control for older adults include involving them as much as possible in organizing their care activities and providing information about their plan of care.

Many studies have confirmed the importance of modifying the way people perceive and explain events, shifting attention to factors that can be changed or controlled. In the classic study by Rodin and Langer (1980), whenever a nursing home resident attributed a problem to being old, the staff provided another explanation and identified a causative factor that was amenable to change. For instance, when residents attributed feelings of fatigue to being old, they were reminded that they were awakened at 5:30 AM (Rodin & Langer, 1980). Rodin and Langer's research laid the groundwork for the current emphasis on caring for older adults in ways that support autonomy and involvement in decision making. Nurses can find opportunities to challenge older adults' perceived lack of control and rephrase the situation in a context that is empowering. For example, they can help older adults develop problem-focused coping mechanisms rather than passively, and sometimes inaccurately, accepting the negative functional consequences of aging.

Nursing interventions also address factors that can threaten perceived control, such as lack of privacy and loss of individuality, which commonly occur in institutional settings. Nurses can show respect for privacy by knocking on bedroom doors and asking permission before entering, by closing doors when privacy is desired, by asking permission before pulling bed curtains open, and by being careful about moving personal belongings without permission from the older person. Encouraging the person to have personal belongings and to arrange these belongings in whatever fashion is desired also shows concern for individuality.

Wellness Opportunity

Nurses show concern for individuality by asking an older adult about a family photograph or greeting card that is in view.

Involving Older Adults in Decision Making

Older people are frequently left out of the decision-making process, even for those decisions that most profoundly affect their lives, such as moving to a long-term care facility. This lack of involvement occurs for a variety of reasons, related both to the older adult and to the decision makers. Some of the barriers within the older adult may be dementia, depression, long-term passivity regarding decisions, or hearing impairments or other communication barriers. Some of the barriers within the decision makers that may thwart the decision-making process include stereotypes of older people as incompetent, perceptions that the older adult is not interested in or capable of making decisions, and an unwillingness to deal with the older person's anticipated resistance to the desired outcome.

Many of the reasons for excluding older adults from the decision-making process are related to the attitudes of the family and of professional caregivers, so one nursing intervention is to challenge these attitudes. For example, in acute care settings, nurses facilitate communication between older patients and their primary care provider to ensure that the older person is included in all decisions about medical treatment and discharge plans. In long-term care settings, nurses have numerous opportunities to involve older adults in decisions about their daily care, medical interventions, and discharge plans. In home settings, nurses can work with family members and older adults to ensure that the latter are involved in decisions about their care and that their rights are respected. In any setting, nurses may have to remind health care professionals, as well as family members and other caregivers, that although people may gain rights by virtue of being a certain age, they do not lose their rights just because they reach a certain age. For additional discussion of the role of nurses in decisions regarding long-term care for people with dementia, refer to Chapter 9.

Other aspects of decision making that can be addressed in nursing interventions are one's verbal interactions and choice of terminology. With regard to verbal communication, health care professionals often talk *about* older adults when in their presence rather than directing communication *to* them and focusing the conversation *on* them. This is especially common when family members or other caregivers are discussing situations with a nurse or other professional and the conversation takes place in the presence of the older person without directly involving him or her. Whenever appropriate, it is important to include older adults in conversations when the topic is directly related to them. However, if older adults cannot participate directly, make sure that the conversations takes place out of hearing distance. Another strategy is to ask the older person's permission to discuss his or her situation with family member or caregivers and then report back to the older person, in language that the person can understand, about any discussions that take place or decisions that are made or pending.

With regard to terminology, the phrase "nursing home placement" is commonly used in reference to an older adult's admission to a nursing home. This term denotes passivity on the part of the older adult—it is closer to the terminology used when objects are placed on a shelf than to words normally used in reference to human beings. An alternative approach that communicates a greater sense of control is to refer to an "admission" to a nursing home. This approach indicates that certain criteria have been met and that an active decision has been made to determine whether the person meets these criteria. Equally important, nurses must ensure that older adults are, in fact, actively involved in the decision-making process, rather than passively being "placed." Nurses can help older adults and their families with decisions about long-term care by helping them assess their situation and by correcting misinformation and providing accurate information about specific resources and the range of services available (as described in Chapter 6).

Addressing Role Loss

Meaningful roles (e.g., spouse, caregiver, volunteer) are important determinants of feelings of worth, efficacy, and self-esteem. Participating in volunteer work is an excellent way of providing social interaction and a sense of purpose. The Experience Corps, which involves older adults building on their experiences and volunteering to meet unmet needs of elementary school children, is a win–win situation that helps older adults feel productive (Gruenewald, Tanner, Fried, et al., 2016). Research reviews have identified the following positive health effects associated with volunteering: improved functioning, longer life expectancy, increased social interaction, and increased well-being and self-rated health (Detollenaere,

Willems & Baert, 2017; Rogers, Demakakos, Taylor, et al., 2016; Tabassum, Mohan, & Smith, 2016). Participation in volunteer activities also is associated with reduced risk for cognitive impairment and cardiovascular disease (Burr, Han, & Tavares, 2016; Infurna, Okun, & Grimm, 2016). In addition to helping older adults develop new roles, nurses can focus on past and current achievements as an intervention for enhancing self-esteem. This is especially important for older adults who depend on others and who have limited opportunities for feeling a sense of accomplishments.

> ### Wellness Opportunity
>
> Nurses can ask older adults about their accomplishments in areas, such as work and family, and give positive feedback about meaningful roles.

Encouraging Life Review and Reminiscence

Life review and reminiscence are two closely related processes that are used to promote psychosocial health in older adults. Butler (2001) describes life review as a progressive return to consciousness of past experiences, particularly unresolved conflicts, for re-examination and reintegration. If the reintegration process is successful, the process gives new significance and meaning to life and prepares the person for death by alleviating fear and anxiety (Butler, 2001). Positive effects of life review include accepting one's mortality, righting of old wrongs, taking pride in accomplishments, gaining a sense of serenity, and feeling that one has done one's best (Butler, 2001). Nurses have used a life-story review group to improve mild to moderate depression in community-living older adults (Chan, Leong, Heng, et al., 2014).

Reminiscence is based on the same theoretical framework as life review; however, it can be done outside the life review process, and it is more informal and less intense. Another difference is that life review addresses both pleasant and unpleasant issues of the past, whereas reminiscence focuses primarily on pleasant and positive experiences. Reminiscence therapy as a nursing intervention is the recall of past events, feelings, images, and memories that are associated with comfort, pleasure, and pleasant experiences. As a group therapy, the reminiscence group is one of the most widely used interventions for older adults, including those with mild cognitive impairment and mild to moderate dementia. Nurses have many opportunities to incorporate principles of reminiscence during the usual course of care, for example, by asking about pleasant memories of holidays.

> ### Technology to Promote Wellness in Older Adults
>
> A mobile application to promote reminiscence, which was tested in a long-term care facility, may be effective in improving well-being for people with memory loss, especially when used in partnership with a support person (e.g., a caregiver or family member) (Hamel, Sims, Klassen, et al., 2016). Nurses can encourage families of people with dementia to find information about this Alzheimer's Reminiscence Memory Game at http://moaitechnologies.com/memorymatters

A Student's Perspective

Performing a life review on anyone from a time other than your own is an interesting experience. I found it to be an amazing opportunity to sit down with Mrs. B. and for her to open up to a 20-year-old girl that she had met only the week before. Within the first few minutes, she talked about her husband and I watched the tears roll down her face. This became the most significant part of our interview because I was able to understand how exposed she was allowing herself to be. It also made me realize how open the elderly can be in reminiscing about their lives and how important this topic is for them to share. It amazed me how just starting a conversation with an older person could bring so much emotion and joy at the exact same time.

The interview with Mrs. B. has affected my approach to older adults in clinical practice. I believe that a life review can be done on a daily basis while working with clients. This way, you can get to know each person on a personal level in order to provide individualized care. Each time you see a patient, you could continue the conversation and develop a relationship that benefits not only the client, but also yourself. I have learned that by showing interest in a person's life, you can allow them to discuss a significant part of who they have become, which is something they do not get to do on a daily basis.

Jillian B.

Fostering Social Supports

Nurses have many opportunities to foster the development of social networks for older adults, and this is an effective intervention for social isolation. Social isolation is likely to occur because of any of the following factors that commonly occur in older adulthood:

- Hearing impairments and other communication barriers
- Chronic illnesses that limit activity or energy
- Lack of social opportunities because of caregiving responsibilities
- Mobility limitations, including the inability to drive a vehicle
- Mental or psychosocial impairments that interfere with relationships
- Loss of spouse, friends, or family through death, illness, or physical distance

Thus, nursing interventions that address these risk factors (e.g., improved mobility or sensory function) are also likely to have the positive consequence of improved social supports.

In long-term care settings, nurses can foster positive social interactions in group settings, such as dining and activity rooms. Sometimes, a very simple intervention, such as positioning chairs (including wheelchairs) so that people can interact with each other, can significantly influence social contacts. Whenever possible, room assignments in long-term care settings should be directed toward facilitating positive social interactions. In addition, nurses can facilitate referrals for social and therapeutic activities in long-term care facilities.

In home settings, nurses can identify community resources, such as volunteer visitor and meal programs, to decrease social isolation. Support and education groups that primarily focus on coping with a chronic illness (e.g., stroke clubs, or better breathing groups) also provide excellent opportunities for social contact and the development of friendships with people who are in similar situations. For people who are socially isolated because of caregiving responsibility, caregiver support groups can enhance coping abilities and provide social support.

In any setting, nurses can encourage older adults to participate in structured group activities to enhance their well-being. Electronic networks can be particularly helpful for older adults who are socially isolated due to functional impairments, transportation issues, or geographic distance. For example, internet-based social network platforms can be used to decrease loneliness, strengthen intergenerational ties, expand one's social network, and maintain connections with family and friends (Cornwell & Schafer, 2016). Selected nursing interventions to promote psychosocial wellness are described in Box 12-4.

Wellness Opportunity

Nurses can talk with older adults about the benefits of support groups and provide a list of local resources that address specific needs of older adults and their caregivers.

Addressing Spiritual Needs

Addressing spiritual needs of patients is within the scope of nursing, as exemplified in the following interventions that are commonly included in nursing care:

- Intentionally communicating caring and compassion
- Facilitating reminiscence
- Honoring a person's integrity
- Providing active and passive listening
- Caring for someone who feels hopeless
- Arranging for participation in religious services
- Encouraging or facilitating participation in activities such as prayer and meditation
- Making referrals for spiritual care

Box 12-4 Nursing Interventions to Promote Psychosocial Wellness

Facilitating Maximum Independence

- Make sure that the person has access to all necessary assistive devices and personal accessories (e.g., wigs, canes, dentures, walkers, and hearing aids).
- Allow enough time for the person to perform tasks at her or his own pace, and avoid unnecessary dependence that results from an overemphasis on time efficiency.
- Make sure that the environment has been adapted as much as possible to compensate for sensory losses and other functional impairments.

Promoting a Sense of Control

- Make a conscious effort to involve older adults in decisions regarding their care, both in small daily matters and in major health care concerns.
- Ask about likes and dislikes and try to address personal preferences.
- Whenever possible, allow persons to choose between two alternatives, even if the options are in a very narrow range (e.g., "Would you prefer to wear the yellow sweater or the pink one today?").
- Ensure as much privacy, or perceived privacy, as possible.
- Knock on the door and ask for permission before entering a bedroom, even in institutional settings.
- Allow as much expression of individuality as possible in the personal environment (e.g., use personal furniture when possible and display family pictures in full view).
- Make sure that the call light is accessible for people who are confined.
- Do not talk about someone in his or her presence as if he or she does not exist.
- Avoid referring to nursing home *placement*. Refer instead to an *admission*, and include the person in the decision-making process.

Addressing Role Loss

- Identify new roles for people and acknowledge those past and present roles that are viewed positively.

- Encourage participation in reminiscence groups and other group therapies.
- Find opportunities to create meaningful roles, such as helper or assistant, by involving older adults in useful tasks, such as folding laundry.
- When older adults volunteer to assist others, acknowledge their contribution with a remark such as, "You certainly help us a lot when you help take Mrs. Smith to the dining room in her wheelchair."
- Acknowledge an older adult's nonphysical assets and attributes, such as family relationships or a good sense of humor.
- Focus on positive relationships by acknowledging or asking about the receipt of flowers, greeting cards, and other visible signs of concern expressed by others.
- Ask older adults about their responsibilities as parents, grandparents, or roommates and point out their positive contributions.
- Ask older adults about family photographs, initiate a discussion of positive relationships, and remind them that others care about them (e.g., encourage them to talk about their grandchildren and great-grandchildren).
- Ask older adults about accomplishments in areas such as work, family, hobbies, and volunteer activities.
- Respond with comments such as, "You must be proud of your children," or "You certainly have accomplished a lot."

Fostering Social Supports

- Use interventions to address hearing impairments and other communication barriers (see Chapter 16).
- Encourage participation in group activities.
- For people in wheelchairs, especially those who cannot move independently, position the chair in a way that promotes social interaction.
- For nursing home residents, plan table and room arrangements in a way that fosters social relationships.

Despite acknowledgment that interventions to address spiritual needs are well within the scope of nursing, many nurses are uncomfortable with providing spiritual care. Nursing interventions to address the spiritual needs of older adults need to be individualized and offered only if the person is receptive to the interventions. In addition, nurses need to be nonjudgmental about religion and spirituality and avoid imposing their personal beliefs. Moreover, because cultural factors significantly influence a person's spirituality and religious beliefs, interventions must be culturally sensitive.

A spiritual nursing intervention that is acceptable to all patients and relatively easy to implement during usual care is **presence.** Presence, which is considered a basic element of spiritual care, simply requires that nurses attend fully during all interactions with their patients. Presence is viewed as synonymous with core nursing concepts, such as caring, healing, empathy, support, and nurturance (du Plessis, 2016).

In addition to addressing spiritual needs as a routine part of psychosocial nursing care, nurses often address spiritual needs during times of spiritual distress. For example, older adults are likely to express spiritual needs when they are coping with the loss of a significant relationship or dealing with news about a serious or terminal illness. Older adults who are caregivers for others, especially a spouse, are likely to express spiritual needs in relation to decisions about the care of the other person. For example, they may experience feelings of guilt about not being able to meet the needs of a dependent loved one or feelings of "playing God" with regard to decisions about mentally incompetent loved ones. In these circumstances, the provision of support, information, and reassurance from a nurse who has dealt with these decisions in professional experiences may be an effective counseling intervention. At times, information from the primary care provider may be helpful in alleviating spiritual distress associated with end-of-life decisions or decisions about long-term care. In these cases, the nurse may be able to facilitate communication between the primary care provider and the family to alleviate the spiritual distress. Some nursing interventions that address spiritual needs of older adults are listed in Box 12-5.

See ONLINE LEARNING ACTIVITY 12-3: ARTICLE ABOUT PRESENCE AS A NURSING INTERVENTION at http://thepoint.lww.com/Miller8e.

Teaching About Managing Stress in Daily Life

Nurses have important roles in teaching older adults, as well as caregivers, about managing stress in daily life as an intervention for promoting psychosocial wellness. Although stress management is often overlooked, it is an essential aspect of health promotion for people of all ages. Nurses can encourage and demonstrate the use of simple relaxation techniques, such as deep breathing, during the usual course of caring for older adults and talking with caregivers. Nurses also can encourage participation in individual and group activities that are effective for reducing stress, such as yoga, meditation, and tai chi.

Box 12-5 Nursing Interventions to Address Spiritual Needs

Therapeutic Communication Interventions

- Use verbal and nonverbal communication to establish trust and convey empathic caring.
- Use active supportive listening.
- Convey nonjudgmental attitudes.
- Communicate respect for individuality.
- Provide a supportive presence.
- Be open to expressions of feelings, such as fear, anger, loneliness, and powerlessness.
- Honor a person's integrity.
- Support the person in his or her feeling of being loved by others and by a higher power (e.g., God, Allah, Jehovah).
- Encourage verbalization of feelings about meaning of illness.
- Provide positive feedback about faith, courage, sense of humor, and other such feelings and experiences.
- Encourage discussion of events and relationships that provide spiritual support.

Actions to Foster Religious and Spiritual Activities

- Facilitate referrals for visits from religious care providers and sources of spiritual care (clergy, rabbis, church members, spiritual directors).
- Facilitate participation in religious services or activities (e.g., tapes, readings, videos, observations of "holy days").
- Assist with obtaining requested religious items (books, music, statues).
- Provide quiet and private time for individual spiritual or religious activities (e.g., prayer, reflection, meditation, guided imagery).
- Provide necessary support for religious rituals (e.g., lighting candles, receiving communion, praying the rosary).
- Encourage participation in relaxing and enjoyable activities (art, music, nature).

Interventions for Specific Circumstances

- Provide support and care during times of suffering.
- Assist in the process of dying.
- Assist a person who is fearful of the future.
- Provide care for the person who feels hopeless.
- Facilitate reconciliation among family members.
- Encourage participation in support groups.

Box 12-6, Tips on Managing Stress in Daily Life, can be given to older adults and caregivers as a teaching tool.

 Technology to Promote Wellness in Older Adults

An NIH-funded study at Oregon Health & Science University found that internet-based Mindfulness Meditation Interventions were effective for improving daily meditation practice in the older adult participants (mean age: 76.2 years) (Wahbeh, Goodrich, & Oken, 2016).

Promoting Wellness Through Healthy Aging Classes

When older adults need assistance in coping with specific functional consequences or when they need education to

Box 12-6 Tips on Managing Stress in Daily Life

Recognize the Different Types of Stressors

- Events are stressful according to the degree to which they have an emotional impact and are perceived as desirable and controllable.
- Even events that are desirable, such as holidays and births and weddings of grandchildren, can be stressful.
- When stress cannot be alleviated, it is important to manage your perception of, and emotional responses to, the situation.
- Use problem-focused strategies to cope with situations that can be changed.

Coping Strategies for Situations That Cannot Be Changed

- Develop an attitude of acceptance, reframe your perspective, and focus on what you can learn from this.
- Acknowledge and express feelings, even those that are unpleasant, such as grief, anger, and sadness.
- Talk with someone and accept their caring and understanding; communicate to them that you do not expect to change the situation but appreciate an opportunity to express feelings.
- Foster supports for social, emotional, and spiritual enrichment (e.g., friends, family, pets, hobbies, groups).
- Identify and use healthy ways of releasing tension and expressing emotions (e.g., physical activity, actions that lead to a sense of accomplishment).
- Engage in distracting activities, especially those that are pleasurable, health enhancing, and spiritually enriching.
- Use relaxation methods, such as meditation, yoga, progressive relaxation.

- Express feelings and develop insights through activities, such as journaling and self-talk.
- Seek guidance from counselors or health care professionals.

Problem-Focused Coping Strategies

- Time pressures: evaluate demands, determine priorities, and plan a schedule for the most important things; include time for activities that relieve stress.
- Set realistic limits and become comfortable telling others what the limits are.
- Seek advice and reliable information from friends, family, or professionals who can assist with developing a problem-solving plan.
- Adapt the environment so it is most conducive to your current needs.

Strategies to Avoid

- Smoking
- Excessive eating or drinking (including alcohol or caffeine)
- Inappropriate use of medications or recreational drugs
- Inaccurately or inappropriately directing anger or emotions toward others
- Actions that are harmful to people, animals, or the environment

Adapted with permission from Miller, C. A. (2013). Wellness activity tool for stress management. In C. A. Miller (Ed.), *Fast facts for health promotion in nursing: Promoting wellness in a nutshell* (pp. 61–62). New York: Springer.

---

clarify myths and misunderstandings about age-related changes, individual counseling may be the best intervention. When older adults need counseling about psychosocial adjustments, however, educational groups may be more effective. Nurses often are involved with establishing and leading support and educational groups for caregivers. Common themes that nurses can address in groups include use of resources, coping with losses, and promoting optimal functioning.

An example of a nurse-led group intervention that allows for sharing of experiences among peers is the healthy aging class, developed by this author and used successfully during two decades in a variety of settings with older adults at various functional levels. This model is based on the belief that older adults who are beginning to recognize age-related physical and psychosocial changes or who are already dealing with such changes can benefit from sharing their experiences with their peers. Nurses can use this model, which is described in detail, to enhance the coping skills of older adults who are adjusting to any of the challenges of older adulthood.

Goals

Goals for older adults who participate in healthy aging classes follow:

- Recognize the impact of common age-related physical and psychosocial changes.

- Support and encourage any effective coping mechanisms already being used.
- Develop new skills that could be effective for coping with current stressors.
- Obtain information that will facilitate problem-focused coping mechanisms for stressful situations that are amenable to change.
- Provide an opportunity for the sharing of similar experiences with peers.

Setting

Nurses in any setting can initiate healthy aging classes, but long-term care institutions are perhaps the most conducive setting for the following reasons:

- Nurses have many opportunities to establish and lead groups.
- Residents of long-term care facilities provide a captive audience from which to select group members.
- Residents of long-term care institutions usually are not acutely ill, and they are dealing with psychosocial adjustments that are readily identified.
- Residents of long-term care settings have in common at least one major life event, which is a temporary or permanent move to a more dependent setting.

Community settings also are conducive to successful healthy aging classes, but nurses may have to be more creative in gathering the group members. Nurses who provide health services or education programs for adults in senior centers or assisted-living facilities might be able to establish ongoing healthy aging classes as part of their responsibilities. In these settings, a healthy aging class may be an efficient, as well as effective, way of providing health education using a format that has the additional advantage of enhancing coping mechanisms.

In acute care settings, nurses usually do not plan and implement group therapies, but in rehabilitative settings, nurses may have the opportunity to initiate healthy aging classes. In psychiatric units, often there are enough older adults among the patient population to warrant the implementation of healthy aging classes as a form of group therapy.

Membership Criteria

The primary criteria for group membership are that the person be willing to acknowledge age-related changes and be capable of acquiring insight into his or her adjustment to these changes. This author has led groups ranging from highly functional older adults in community settings to seriously impaired older adults in a hospital-based medical geropsychiatric unit. Group members may be coping with similar psychosocial stresses, but this is not necessarily a criterion for participation. For example, a healthy aging class can comprise older adults who all have some degree of depression or who are coping with a particular stressful event, such as widowhood. An ideal group includes members who are coping with various life events commonly associated with older adulthood and who are motivated to learn effective coping styles.

The group works best if the membership is stable and closed, but this is not always possible. A disadvantage of an open group is that it is very difficult to develop cohesiveness. If the membership is open and changing, the leader must be more directive, and the group as a whole will not be able to establish ongoing priorities for discussion topics. In addition, with changing membership, the leader has to focus more attention on the exchange of information about group members at the beginning of each session.

Size of Group and Length, Duration, and Frequency of Sessions

Although group size can range from 5 to 12 members, the ideal is about 8 members. Groups can be either ongoing or time-limited. When the membership is changing, such as in acute or rehabilitative settings, sessions can be an ongoing mode of therapy. In long-term care or community settings, it is best to schedule group meetings for a predetermined length of time, such as 8 to 10 weeks, and allow for changes in membership at the end of each period. One-hour sessions are held at weekly intervals, at a consistent time and place. In community settings, it can be helpful to convene the groups in conjunction with a meal program because participants will already have social relationships. As in institutional settings, a community center offers an audience from which to select

the group members. Other potential community-based sites include assisted-living facilities and group settings, such as adult care homes (also called board-and-care homes).

Criteria for and Responsibilities of Group Leaders

One nurse can lead group sessions, but it is often helpful to have a co-leader who has had social service training. An older adult who has made a positive psychosocial adjustment and who can serve as a role model also can be a good co-leader. The nurse must be able to clarify myths and misunderstandings about age-related changes and be skilled in group dynamics. As with the reminiscence group, the healthy aging class is not an intense psychotherapy session; therefore, the group leader is not required to be specially trained in mental health. To lead a healthy aging class, however, a good understanding of both the physiologic and psychosocial aspects of aging is essential.

The primary responsibilities of the group leaders are to facilitate the discussion of psychosocial adjustments of older adulthood and to provide feedback and clarification to the members. As with other groups, the leader must ensure that all members have an opportunity to participate and that the members attend to the identified topic. The leaders also must ensure that the group reaches some conclusions before the end of each session so that members leave with a feeling of accomplishment relating to at least one psychosocial challenge of older adulthood.

Format

As in all educational groups, the leader begins with an explanation of the purpose of the group and an introduction of the leaders and members. The leader also reviews the details of the sessions, such as their length, the duration of the group, the role of the leader, and the expectations of the members. After addressing questions and introductory material, the leader introduces the concepts of life events and adjustments to the challenges of older adulthood. The leader can use a statement similar to the following: "Throughout life, certain events are likely to occur that affect us emotionally. These events may involve our health, our personal relationships, the place where we live, our job or career responsibilities and opportunities, or other events that require an adjustment on our part. These are called major life events, and they often occur at certain points of life. To begin our discussion today, let's look at some of the major life events that are likely to occur in younger adulthood, around the age of 20 to 30 years." The group then identifies various life events, such as finding a job, moving from the family home, finding a partner, and starting a family. The leader then asks members to identify life adjustments that are likely to occur between 30 and 50 years of age.

After the members have identified these life events, the leader emphasizes that one purpose of the healthy aging class is to identify effective ways of addressing the challenges inherent in the life events of older adulthood. The term *challenges* is used to communicate an active mode of addressing issues. The leader may want to discuss the phrase "challenges of older adulthood" and allow the group members to comment on what they see as challenges in their lives. As the members identify the life events of older adulthood, the leader writes the events on a board or paper so that all the members can see the list. The leader can then ask about life events that the members think they are likely to experience in the next few years. As events are identified, the members are also asked to identify the consequences of the events that require an adjustment. Examples of these life events and consequences have been discussed earlier in this chapter, and they are summarized in Figure 12-1. If group members do not identify all the life events, the leader may ask about a certain event, such as coping with one's own or a spouse's retirement. This discussion should continue until all the events and consequences in Figure 12-1 have been identified.

If the group is ongoing and has a stable membership, the leader may devote the majority of the first meeting to this discussion. The leader should emphasize that the rest of the meetings will be devoted to discussions of the identified issues and that the first meeting will set the stage for future sessions. If the group is open and has a changing membership, the leader may need to be more directive during this first phase to limit the time spent on this topic. With changing membership, this initial identification of issues would be limited to the first 20 to 30 minutes. The group can then discuss coping mechanisms for one specific issue during the latter half of the meeting.

After the issues are identified, the leader summarizes the discussion, referring to the list of challenges written for the members to see. The members then share ideas about coping strategies that they have found to be helpful in adjusting to these changes. The leader may begin this part with a statement such as, "Now that we've identified the challenges of older adulthood, let's look at what things are helpful in responding to these challenges. I'd like each of you to share with the group one thing you do to help yourself face difficult challenges." After members have identified general coping mechanisms, the leader can suggest that the group choose one specific life event of older adulthood and discuss coping mechanisms that are helpful for addressing this challenge. Examples of coping strategies that might be discussed in relation to specific life events are summarized in Table 12-1. As these coping strategies are identified, they should be written on a surface for all to see, and members should be encouraged to relate their personal experiences.

As the cohesiveness and trust level among members increase, particularly in closed groups, the sharing of experiences may become very open and revealing. The task of the leader, then, is to keep the discussion focused on appropriate coping mechanisms. In cohesive groups with highly functional members, the leader might have an opportunity to discuss the difference between emotion-focused and problem-focused mechanisms. The depth of discussion will depend on the degree of group cohesiveness and trust, the functional level of the members, and the comfort level and willingness of the leader to deal with the identified issues.

During the last 10 minutes of each session, the leader should attempt to bring the discussion to some closure on at least one issue. This may be accomplished by summarizing the issues and coping mechanisms that were identified. In open groups, the leader would end by encouraging those members who do not return to the group to look at coping mechanisms for their own specific issues, either

TABLE 12-1 Coping Strategies for the Psychosocial Challenges of Older Adulthood	
Psychosocial Adjustment	**Coping Strategy**
Ageist stereotypes	Develop a firm self-identity, challenge the myths, question any behaviors that are based on age-determined expectations
Retirement	Develop new skills, use time for hobbies and personal pursuits, become involved with meaningful volunteer activities
Reduced income	Take advantage of discounts for seniors
Declining physical condition	Maintain good health practices (nutrition, health exercise, rest)
Functional limitations	Adapt the environment to ensure safety and optimal functional status, take advantage of assistive devices and equipment, accept help when necessary
Changes in cognitive skills	Take advantage of educational opportunities, enroll in classes, keep mentally stimulated, join a discussion group, use the library, avoid dwelling on the things you cannot do and focus on your abilities. Take advantage of increased potential for wisdom and creativity
Death of spouse, friends, and family members	Allow yourself to grieve appropriately, take advantage of opportunities for group or individual counseling and support, establish new relationships, renew old friendships, cherish the happy memories of the past, realize new freedoms
Relocation from family home	Look into the broad range of options for housing, appreciate the relief from the responsibilities of home ownership, take advantage of new services and opportunities for socialization
Other challenges to mental health	Maintain a sense of humor, use stress-reduction techniques, learn assertiveness skills, participate in support groups

by themselves or with a friend or confidant(e). For ongoing groups, the leader would end the session by facilitating agreement about the issues that will be discussed during the next session. The leader also can encourage members to think about the identified issues in the interim.

EVALUATING THE EFFECTIVENESS OF NURSING INTERVENTIONS

Nurses evaluate the effectiveness of interventions for older adults with Self-Concept Disturbance by determining the extent to which older adults express positive views of themselves. Another measure of effective nursing care is that older adults no longer verbalize ageist attitudes. Nursing care of older adults who express a sense of Powerlessness is evaluated by the extent to which they become involved in decisions that affect them and the degree to which they express feelings of control over their lives. Nurses evaluate care for older adults with Ineffective Individual Coping by observing behaviors that reflect the use of a variety of coping strategies (see Table 12-1). For example, an older adult might learn to use problem-focused coping strategies for a situation he or she previously viewed as hopeless and unchangeable.

Case Study

Mr. P. is 86 years old and was recently admitted to a nursing facility for long-term care. His medical diagnoses are diabetes, glaucoma, retinopathy, and dementia of Alzheimer type. Mr. P. lived with his wife until 6 months ago, when she died after a brief illness. After her death, he needed help with all his activities of daily living, and his daughter arranged home care assistance for 6 hours a day. About 1 month ago, he started getting up and wandering outside at night. Once, he wandered off at 3:00 AM, and the police had to take him home. After this episode, he was afraid to be alone, and he agreed to go to a nursing facility because he could not afford to pay for 24-hour assistance at home.

During the first week in the nursing facility, Mr. P. was cooperative with the staff and sociable with the other residents. He was resistant to the morning schedule of getting up at 6:00 AM, but he passively complied when the staff firmly directed him. His daughter visited him daily and accompanied him to social and recreational activities with other residents. Mr. P. has been in the nursing facility for 10 days, and he is becoming very resistant to staff efforts to get him dressed for breakfast. When he attends group activities, he is disruptive, yelling about being a hostage in a monastery. Mr. P. tells and eating breakfast in the dining room at 7:30 AM other residents that he was tricked into coming to this place and that the only reason he has to stay is because his daughter has taken over his house and is living there with her family. He frequently paces up and down the corridors and says he has to find his daughter to take him home because his wife is sick and she needs him to take care of her. You walk with him in the hallway, and he says, "I don't know why they keep me locked up here. I can't do anything like I used to do at home. It's like a monastery where you have to get up in the middle of the night and they make you get cleaned up and eat breakfast when it's still dark out."

NURSING ASSESSMENT

Your nursing assessment shows that Mr. P. needs supervision in all activities of daily living because of poor vision and memory impairment. He needs some assistance with personal care, but he can dress himself if staff set his clothes out for him. When Mr. P. was admitted to the nursing facility, he was assigned to the "night-shift wakers" group, which means that the night shift is responsible for waking him and getting him ready for breakfast by 7:30 AM. The night-shift nursing assistants help him with showering, shaving, and dressing.

During the admission interview, Mr. P.'s daughter, Jane, said that his typical morning routine at home was to get up around 8:30 AM and get dressed independently, using the clothes that were set out for him by the home health aide. He ate breakfast around 9:30 AM and then spent the day "working on his papers." Jane, who lives out of town, would call her father four times a week. When Jane talked with him on the phone, he always told her how busy he was working on his papers. Although Jane was paying all his bills from a joint bank account, Mr. P. would spend hours and hours with bill stubs, old bank statements, and an inactive checking account, thinking he was paying his bills.

Jane was staying at her father's house for the 2 weeks before his admission and for 1 week after admission to the nursing facility. She plans to return to town for a couple of days every other month and will visit her father at those times. The only nearby relative is a sister-in-law who comes to visit Mr. P. every 2 weeks.

NURSING DIAGNOSIS

You use the nursing diagnosis of Powerlessness related to relocation to a nursing facility and lack of control over activities of daily living. You select this diagnosis, rather than Impaired Adjustment or Ineffective Individual Coping, because Mr. P. focuses on a theme of loss of control. Your assessment identifies several factors that contribute to his powerlessness, and you address these factors in your nursing care plan.

NURSING CARE PLAN FOR MR. P.

Expected Outcome	Nursing Interventions	Nursing Evaluation
Mr. P. will feel he has greater control over his morning schedule	• Take Mr. P. off the "night-shift wakers" list and allow him to sleep until 8 AM • Allow Mr. P. to wear his pajamas and robe to breakfast and to shower, bathe, and dress after breakfast	Mr. P. will no longer verbalize feelings of being locked up in a monastery or a prison
Mr. P. will function as independently as possible.	• The staff will set out Mr. P.'s clothing and allow him to dress himself • The staff will give Mr. P. positive feedback for dressing himself	Mr. P. will dress himself with minimal supervision Mr. P. will perform his personal care activities at a pace that is comfortable for him
Mr. P. will engage in a familiar activity that gives him a meaningful role	• Ask Jane to send a set of bill stubs, old bank statements, and the inactive checkbook so that Mr. P. can do his "work" • Encourage Mr. P. to "work with his papers" in the activity room, where he can interact with other residents • Give Mr. P. positive feedback when he interacts with other residents • Compliment Mr. P. about doing his paperwork	Mr. P. will resume his former routine of working with his papers and will interact with other residents

Chapter Highlights

Life Events: Age-Related Changes Affecting Psychosocial Function (Figure 12-1)

• Life events are the major changes that occur during the life cycle and significantly affect daily life.
• Life events commonly experienced by older adults are ageist attitudes, retirement, relocation, chronic illness and functional impairments, decisions about driving a vehicle, widowhood, and death of family and friends.

Theories About Stress and Coping in Older Adults

• Sources of stress for older adults are major life events, daily hassles, and chronic stressors.
• Older adults are more likely to use emotion-focused coping styles that involve management of thoughts and feelings.
• Social supports are an important resource for coping in older adults.
• Nurses facilitate effective coping in older adults through interventions that improve their functional abilities.

Factors That Influence Psychosocial Function in Older Adults

• Religion and spirituality are increasingly important resources for older adults.

• Cultural factors influence definitions and perceptions of all aspects of psychosocial functioning (Box 12-1).
• Culture-bound syndromes are culturally specific disorders associated with psychosocial characteristics of a particular group.

Risk Factors That Affect Psychosocial Function

• Physical, functional, and psychosocial health significantly affect coping skills.
• The ability to accurately appraise a situation affects psychosocial function.
• Learned helplessness results when uncontrollable events reinforce the idea that future events will also be uncontrollable.

Functional Consequences Associated With Psychosocial Function in Older Adults

• Negative functional consequences include anxiety, loneliness, depression, and cognitive impairment.
• Older adults also experience emotional well-being (e.g., joy, happiness, satisfaction, purpose in life, and sense of mastery).
• Gerontologists are currently investigating the concept of resilience in older adults, which is defined as the ability to bounce back and recover physical and psychological health in the face of adversity.

Pathologic Condition Related to Psychosocial Function: Alcohol Abuse

- Between 7% and 14% of adults age 65 years and older report alcohol abuse, dependence, binge drinking, or at-risk use of alcohol
- Nurses have essential roles in identifying older adults who are at risk for alcohol-related problems and facilitating referrals for further evaluation and treatment (Box 12-2)

Nursing Assessment of Psychosocial Function

- Refer to Chapter 13.

Nursing Diagnosis

- Situational Low Self-Esteem (or Risk for)
- Powerlessness
- Social Isolation
- Ineffective Coping
- Readiness for Enhanced Coping
- Readiness for Enhanced Resilience

Planning for Wellness Outcomes

- Psychosocial Adjustment: Life Change
- Adaptation to Physical Disability
- Personal Autonomy
- Self-Esteem
- Quality of Life

Nursing Interventions to Promote Healthy Psychosocial Function

- Enhancing self-esteem: improving functioning, using verbal and nonverbal communication, avoiding infantilization and elderspeak
- Promoting a sense of control: providing information, rephrasing events, addressing threats such as lack of privacy and loss of individuality
- Involving older adults in decision making: challenging attitudes, facilitating communication, using verbal and nonverbal communication techniques
- Addressing role loss: identifying meaningful roles
- Encouraging life review and reminiscence
- Fostering social supports
- Addressing spiritual needs: communicating caring and compassion, instilling hope, referring for spiritual care, encouraging participation in religious activities
- Leading Healthy Aging classes

Evaluating the Effectiveness of Nursing Interventions

- Positive self-perceptions
- Involvement in decisions
- Effective coping strategies

Critical Thinking Exercises

1. Take a sheet of paper and draw two vertical lines to make three equal columns. Think of someone you know in your personal life or professional practice who is 80 years old or older. In the left column, list three or more life events that this person has experienced in later adulthood. In the center column, describe the impact of the life event on the person's daily life. In the right column, list the coping mechanisms the person has used to deal with the life event. You can guess at the information, as needed, to complete the information in the center and right columns.

2. Think of a recent life event in your own life and answer the following questions: How close in time was the life event to other stressful events in your life? What impact did the life event have, and what were the manifestations of stress in your life (e.g., in your work, your health, your personal life, your relationships with other people)? What coping mechanisms did you use? Were the coping mechanisms effective? What coping mechanisms would you like to develop to prepare yourself for older adulthood?

3. You are asked to lead a 1-hour discussion titled "Mental Health and Aging" for a group of 10 people at a senior citizen center. Describe your approach to this topic. What would be your goals for the class? How would you involve the participants? What visual aids would you use?

 For more information about topics discussed in this chapter, be sure to check out the interactive Online Learning Activities and other helpful resources at http://thepoint.lww.com/Miller8e.

REFERENCES

Aldwin, C., & Igarashi, H. (2016). Coping, optimal aging, and resilience in a sociocultural context. In V. L. Bengston & R. A. Stettersten (Eds.), *Handbook of theories of aging* (3rd ed., pp. 551–576). New York: Springer Publishing Company.

Andrews, M. M., & Boyle, J. S. (2012). *Transcultural concepts in nursing care* (6th ed.). Philadelphia, PA: Wolters Kluwer/Lippincott Williams & Wilkins.

Andrews, M. M., & Boyle, J. S. (2016). *Transcultural concepts in nursing care* (7th ed.). Philadelphia, PA: Wolters Kluwer/Lippincott Williams & Wilkins.

Aneshensel, C., Harig, F., & Wight, R. (2016). Aging, neighborhoods, and the built environment. In L. K. George & K. F. Ferraro (Eds.), *Handbook of aging and the social sciences* (8th ed., pp. 315–335). Boston, MA: Elsevier Academic Press.

Baars, J. (2016). Aging: Learning to live a finite life. *Gerontologis*. Doi: 10.1093/geront/gnw089

Barry, L., & Byers, A. (2016). Risk factors and prevention strategies for late-life depression and mood disorders. In K. Warner Schaie & S. L. Willis. *Handbook of the Psychology of Aging* (8th ed., pp. 410–424). Boston: Elsevier Academic Press.

Bellingtier, J., & Neupert, S. Negative aging attitudes predict greater reactivity to daily stressors in older adults. *Journals of Gerontology: Psychological Sciences*. [Epub] Doi: 10.1093/geronb/gbw086

Bock, O., & Akpinar, S. (2016). Performance of older persons in a simulated shopping task is influenced by priming with age stereotypes. *PLoS One, 11*(9), e0160739.

Brown, L., & Frahm, K. (2016). The impact of disasters: Implications for the well-being of older adults. In L. K. George & K. F. Ferraro (Eds.), *Handbook of aging and the social sciences* (8th ed., pp. 357–374). Boston, MA: Elsevier Academic Press.

Bryan, A., Kim, H.-J., & Frederiksen-Goldsen, K. (2017). Factors associated with high-risk alcohol consumption among LBG older adults: The roles of gender, social support, perceived stress, discrimination, and stigma. *Gerontologist, 57*, S95–S104.

Burkhardt, M. A., & Nagai-Jacobson, M. G. (2016). Spirituality and health. In B. M. Dossey & L. Keegan (Eds.), *Holistic nursing: A handbook for practice* (6th ed., pp. 135–163). Boston, MA: Jones & Bartlett.

Burr, J. A., Han, S. H., & Tavares, J. L. (2016). Volunteering and cardiovascular disease risk: Does helping others get "under the skin?" *Gerontologist, 56*, 937–947.

Butler, R. N. (2001). Life review. In M. D. Mezey (Ed.), *The encyclopedia of elder care* (pp. 401–402). New York: Springer Publishing Co.

Cahill, K., Giandrea, M., & Quinn, J. (2016). In L. K. George & K. F. Ferraro (Eds.), *Handbook of aging and the social sciences* (8th ed., pp. 271–291). Boston, MA: Elsevier Academic Press.

Carpentieri, J. D., Elliott, J., Brett, C., et al. (2017). Adapting to aging: Older people talk about their use of selections, optimization, and compensation to maximize well-being in the context of physical decline. *Journals of Gerontology: Social Sciences, 72*, 351–361.

Chan, M. P., Leong, K. S., Heng, B. L., et al. (2014). Reducing depression among community-dwelling older adults using life-story review: A pilot study. *Geriatric Nursing, 35*(2), 105–110.

Cornwell, B., & Schafer, M. (2016). Social networks in alter life. In L. K. George & K. F. Ferraro (Eds.), *Handbook of aging and the social sciences* (8th ed. pp. 181–201). Boston, MA: Elsevier Academic Press.

Detollenaere, J., Willems, S., & Baert, S. (2017). Volunteering, income and health. *PLos One, 12*(3), e0173139.

Domenech-Abella, J., Lara, E., Rubio-Valera, M., et al. (2017). Loneliness and depression in the elderly: The role of social network. *Social Psychiatry and Psychiatric Epidemiology, 52*(4), 381–390.

Duan-Porter, W., Hastings, S. N., Neelon, B., et al. (2017). Control beliefs and risk for 4-year mortality in older adults: A prospective cohort study. *BioMed Central Geriatrics, 17*(13). Doi: 10.186/s12877-016-0390-3.

Du Plessis, E. (2016). Presence: A step closer to spiritual nursing care. *Holistic Nursing Practice, 30*, 47–53.

Ehrmin, J. T. (2016). Transcultural perspectives in mental health nursing. In M. M. Andrews & J. S. Boyle (Eds.), *Transcultural concepts in nursing care* (7th ed., pp. 272–316). Philadelphia, PA: Lippincott Williams & Wilkins.

Falk, D. (2016). The psychology of death and dying in later life. In K. Warner Schaie & S. L. Willis (Eds.), *Handbook of the psychology of aging* (8th ed., pp. 475–489). Boston, MA: Elsevier Academic Press.

Federal Interagency Forum on Aging-Related Statistics. (2016). *Indicator 19: Respondent-assessed health status. Older Americans 2015: Key indicators of well-being*. Washington, DC: Government Printing Office.

Gendron, T. L., Welleford, E. A., Inker, J., et al. (2016). The language of ageism: Why we need to use words carefully. *Gerontologist, 56*, 997–1006.

Gruenewald, T., Tanner, E., Fried, L., et al. (2016). The Baltimore experience corps trial: Enhancing generativity via intergenerational activity engagement in later life. *Journals of Gerontology: Psychological Sciences, 71*, 661–670.

Hagood, E. W., & Greunewald, T. L. (2016). Positive versus negative priming of older adults' generative value: Do negative messages impair memory? *Aging and Mental Health*. [Epub]. Doi: 10.1080/13607863.2016.1239063.

Hamel, A., Sims, T., Klassen, D., et al. (2016). Memory Matters: A mixed-methods feasibility study of a mobile aid to stimulate reminiscence in individuals with memory loss. *Journal of Gerontological Nursing, 42*(7), 15–24.

Han, B. H., Moore, A. A., Sherman, S., et al. (2017). Demographic trends of binge alcohol use disorders among older adults in the United States, 2005–2014. *Drug and Alcohol Dependency, 170*, 198–207.

Helvik, A. S., Bjorklof, G. H., Corazzini, K., et al. (2016). Are coping strategies and locus of control orientation associated with health-related quality of life in older adults with and without depression? *Archives of Gerontology and Geriatrics, 64*, 130–137.

Herdman, T., & Kamitsuru, S. (Eds.). (2018). *NANDA International Nursing Diagnoses Definitions and Classification, 2018–2020* (11th ed., pp. 34–44). New York: Thieme Publishers.

Hicks, S., & Siedlecki, K. (2016). Leisure activity engagement and positive affect partially mediate the relationship between positive views on aging and physical health. *Journals of Gerontology: Psychological Sciences, 72*(2), 259–267.

Holmes, T. H., & Rahe, R. H. (1967). The social readjustment rating scale. *Journal of Psychosomatic Research, 11*, 213–218.

Infurna, F. J., Okun, M. A., & Grimm, K. J. (2016). Volunteering is associated with lower risk of cognitive impairment. *Journal of the American Geriatrics Society, 64*, 2263–2269.

Krause, N., & Hayward R. D. (2016). Religion, health, and aging. In L. K. George & K. F. Ferraro (Eds.), *Handbook of aging and the social sciences* (8th ed., pp. 251–270). Boston, MA: Elsevier Academic Press.

Lee, P. L. (2016). Control beliefs level and change as predictors of subjective memory complaints. *Aging and Mental Health, 20*, 329–335.

Loscalzo, E., Sterling, R. C., Weinstein, S. P., et al. (2017). Alcohol and other drug use in older adults: Results form a community needs assessment. *Aging Clinical and Experimental Research*. [Epub] Doi: 10.1007/s40520-016-0718-z.

MacLeod, S., Musich, S., Hawkins, K., et al. (2016). The impact of resilience among older adults. *Geriatric Nursing, 37*, 266–272.

Marquet, M., Missotten, P., & Adam, S. (2016). Ageism and overestimation of cognitive difficulties in older people: A review. *Geriatric Psychology and Neuropsychatry, 14*, 177–186.

Mazerolle, M., Regner, I., Barber, S. J., et al. (2016). Negative aging stereotypes impair performance on brief cognitive tests used to screen for predementia. *Journals of Gerontology B: Journals of Psychological Sciences and Social Sciences*. [Epub] Doi: 10.1093/geronb/gbw083.

McKenna, M. A. (2012). Transcultural perspectives in the nursing care of older adults. In M. M. Andrews & J. S. Boyle (Eds.), *Transcultural concepts in nursing care* (6th ed., pp. 182–207). Philadelphia, PA: Lippincott Williams & Wilkins.

Miller, C. A. (2013). Wellness activity tool for stress management. In C. A. Miller (Ed.), *Fast facts for health promotion in nursing: Promoting wellness in a nutshell* (pp. 61–62). New York: Springer.

Morrow-Howell, N., & Greenfield, E. (2016). In L. K. George & K. F. Ferraro (Eds.), *Handbook of aging and the social sciences* (8th ed., pp. 293–313). Boston, MA: Elsevier Academic Press.

Nelson, T. D. (2016). Promoting healthy aging by confronting ageism. *American Psychologist, 71*, 276–282.

Perrig-Chiello, P., Spahni, S., Hopflinger, F., et al. (2016). Cohort and gender differences in psychosocial adjustment to later-life widowhood. *Journals of Gerontology: Social Sciences, 71*, 765–774.

Petersen, J., Kaye, J., Jacobs, P. et al. (2016). Longitudinal relationship between loneliness and social isolation in older adults: Results from the cardiovascular health study. *Journal of Aging and Health, 28*, 775–795.

Rodin, J., & Langer, E. (1980). Aging labels: The decline of control and the fall of self-esteem. *Journal of Social Issues, 36*(2), 12–29.

Rogers, N. T., Demakakos, P., Taylor, M. S., et al. (2016). Volunteering is associated with increased survival in able-bodies participants of the English longitudinal study of ageing. *Journal of Epidemiology and Community Health, 70*, 583–588.

Selye, H. (1956). *The stress of life*. New York: McGraw-Hill.

Shankar, A., McMunn, A., Demakakos, P., et al. (2017). Social isolations and loneliness: Prospective associations with functional status in older adults. *Health Psychology, 36*, 179–187.

Tabassum, F., Mohan, J., & Smith, P. (2016). Association of volunteering with mental well-being. *BMJ Open, 6*(8), e011327.

Tampi, R., Tampi, D., & Durning, M. (2016). Substance use disorders in late life: A review of current evidence. *Healthy Aging Research*, *4*. Doi: 10.12715/har.2015.4.27

Uchino, B., Ong, A., Queen, T., et al. (2016). Theories of social support in health and aging. In V. L. Bengston & R. A. Stettersten (Eds.), *Handbook of theories of aging* (3rd ed., pp. 235–258). New York: Springer Publishing Company.

Vitorino, L. M., Lucchetti, G., Santos, A. E., et al. (2016). Spiritual religious coping is associated with quality of life in institutionalized older adults. *Journal of Religion and Health*, *55*, 549–559.

Wahbeh, H., Goodrich, E., & Oken, B. S. (2016). Internet-based mindfulness meditation for cognition and mood in older adults: A pilot study. *Alternative Therapies in Health and Medicine*, *22*, 44–53.

Wang, M., & Shi, J. (2016). Work, retirement and aging. In K. Warner Schaie & S. L. Willis. *Handbook of the Psychology of Aging* (8th ed., pp. 340–358). Boston: Elsevier Academic Press.

Weiss, D. (2016). On the inevitability of aging: Essentialist beliefs moderate the impact of negative age stereotypes on older adults' memory performance and physiological reactivity. *Journals of Gerontology: Psychological Sciences and Social Sciences*. [Epub] Doi: 10.1093/geronb/gbw087.

Westera, D. A. (2017). *Spirituality in Nursing Practice*. New York: Springer Publishing Company.

Westra, B. L., Paitich, N., Ekstrom, D., et al. (2013). Getting on with living life: Experiences of older adults after home care. *Home Healthcare Nurse*, *31*(9), 493–501.

Williams, K., Perkhounkova, Y., Herman, R., et al. (2016). A communication intervention to reduce resistiveness in dementia care: A cluster randomized controlled trial. *Gerontologist*. [Epub] Doi.10.1093/geront/gnw047.

Zhong, B.-L., Chen, S.-L, Tu, X., et al. (2017). Loneliness and cognitive function in older adults: Findings from the Chinese longitudinal healthy longevity Survey. *Journals of Gerontology: Social Sciences*, *72*, 120–128.

Zhou, Z., Wang, P., & Fang, Y. (2017). Loneliness and the risk of dementia among older Chinese adults: gender differences. *Aging and Mental Health*, *17*, 1–7.

chapter **13**

Psychosocial Assessment

LEARNING OBJECTIVES

After reading this chapter, you will be able to:

1. Describe the purpose, scope of, and procedure for a psychosocial assessment of older adults.

2. Describe communication techniques that are helpful for conducting a psychosocial assessment.

3. Describe how to assess each of the following specific components of mental status: physical appearance, motor function, social skills, response to the interview, orientation, alertness, memory, and speech and language characteristics.

4. Explain how to perform a nursing assessment of skills involved with decision making and executive function in older adults.

5. Describe how to assess each of the following components of affective function: mood, anxiety, self-esteem, depression, happiness, and well-being.

6. Discuss distinguishing characteristics of delusions, hallucinations, and illusions as they relate to the underlying conditions common in older adults.

7. Explain how to perform a nursing assessment of the following aspects of social supports: social network, barriers to services, and economic resources.

8. Explain how to perform a nursing assessment of older adults' spiritual needs including factors that cause spiritual distress as well as those that promote spiritual wellness.

circumstantiality	hallucinations
confabulation	illusions
decision making	insight
delusions	memory
executive function	mental status assessment
Geriatric Anxiety Inventory (GAI)	orientation
	social supports

P sychosocial assessment is a complex and challenging, but essential, aspect of nursing care for older adults. Although psychosocial impairments are often attributed to factors relating to normal aging or to untreatable conditions, a careful psychosocial assessment can identify the underlying cause(s) of mental changes, many of which can then be reversed or addressed through interventions. This chapter supplements the information about cognitive function discussed in Chapter 11 and psychosocial function discussed in Chapter 12. In addition, it complements the assessment information in other chapters of this text, particularly the chapters on elder abuse (Chapter 10), delirium and dementia (Chapter 14), and depression (Chapter 15).

 OVERVIEW OF PSYCHOSOCIAL ASSESSMENT OF OLDER ADULTS

In contrast to physical and functional assessment procedures, which are viewed as routine measures to identify the causes of troublesome symptoms, psychosocial assessment procedures tend to be perceived as formal psychological tests that analyze personality traits or identify the need for psychiatric treatment. Consequently, health care professionals may overlook the psychosocial component of assessment or relegate

KEY TERMS

abstract thinking	anxiety
affect	aphasia
alertness	attention

it to the realm of mental health professionals. However, an assessment of psychosocial function is an essential component of holistic nursing care, which addresses the body–mind–spirit needs of older adults.

This chapter focuses on those aspects of psychosocial function that are pertinent to caring for older adults from a wellness perspective. This comprehensive perspective is like the emergency cart that is available in every hospital unit. The cart stands ready at all times and is equipped with any item needed to handle medical emergencies. When a serious medical problem arises, health care professionals quickly pull the cart to the patient's bedside and select the needed items. Similarly, nurses must have access to an array of skills for assessing psychosocial function as the need arises. In a few situations, their entire array of skills will be called into play, but in most situations, only a few of the examination tools will be necessary. Nurses can use the material in this chapter to "fill their mental status assessment carts," so they can use appropriate tools for each situation.

The first sections of this chapter cover the purposes of, scope of, and procedures for a psychosocial assessment and are applicable to nursing care of all older adults. The second major section reviews aspects of communication and cultural considerations in relation to a psychosocial assessment. Each of the following components, which nurses would selectively assess depending on the individual situation, is discussed in separate sections: mental status, decision making and executive function, affective function, contact with reality, and social supports.

Purposes of the Psychosocial Assessment

From a wellness perspective, the purposes of psychosocial assessment include the following:

- Detecting asymptomatic or unacknowledged health problems at an early stage
- Identifying signs or symptoms of psychosocial dysfunction (e.g., anxiety, depression, memory problems, change in mental status)
- Identifying stressors and other risk factors that affect cognitive, emotional, or social function
- Obtaining information about the person's usual personality, coping mechanisms, and cognitive abilities
- Identifying social supports and other coping resources that could be supported or strengthened
- Identifying the older adult's personal goals for psychosocial wellness

As with other types of assessment, nurses use this information to plan interventions that are based on realistic expectations.

Older adults who experience a change in their mental status need a comprehensive assessment by an interprofessional team to assure that underlying causes are identified and addressed. A common mistake is to label the changes as "normal for the person's age." This is not only unfair to the older adult but can be detrimental, particularly if

a treatable underlying condition is overlooked, or appropriate interventions to improve functional abilities are neglected. As should be clear from the discussion of cognitive function in Chapter 11, age-related cognitive changes are rarely brought to the attention of health care professionals. For example, an older adult would be unlikely to make the following complaint: "I know I can learn new information, but I don't seem to be able to comprehend information as quickly as I used to." When older adults experience mental changes, every effort should be made to identify the underlying cause rather than simply attribute the changes to age.

Scope of the Psychosocial Assessment

An important part of a psychosocial assessment is identifying the unique meaning of life events, with particular attention on identifying any effects on health. Initial questions can focus on events that occurred many years ago. For example, a question such as "What kind of work did you do?" may prompt a discussion of feelings about retirement. Because changes in living arrangements can precipitate feelings of loss, a non-threatening question such as "What were the circumstances of your moving here?" might lead to further discussion of the meaning of the living arrangement for that person. People who have experienced the loss of a pet may be reluctant to acknowledge the depth of their feelings and they need to know that they will not be judged. Because pets may be particularly significant for older adults, it is appropriate to include at least one question about pets in the psychosocial assessment of older adults.

Questions to assess the meaning of medical conditions and functional limitations are an essential component of the psychosocial assessment because coping with health changes is a common and challenging task for many older adults. Nurses also try to identify the person's concerns about the functional consequences that are likely to be associated with illness and disability. For example, older adults with diabetes may be less interested in knowing how the pancreas functions than in learning to cope with the attendant visual impairment or their fear of increasing dependence on others. Therefore, rather than focus the assessment on medical diagnoses, ask a broader question such as "If you had to rate your health on a scale of 0% to 100%, what rating would you give it today?" After the person responds to this question, ask follow-up questions, such as "What would have to be changed for you to feel 100% healthy?" or "What rating would you have given yourself a year ago?" Answers to these questions can assist in establishing realistic and person-centered goals for interventions.

During a psychosocial assessment, nurses might hear information that is contrary to their own values or cultural expectations, such as the following examples:

- Expressions of racial prejudice, including use of derogatory labels
- Attitudes of extreme passivity about decisions involving the patient's care

- Situations in which older adults are abused or exploited by friends, family, or others
- Attitudes that are judgmental about women or other groups or not in accordance with the nurse's beliefs

When dealing with these types of situations, it helps to be aware of one's own feelings and to address them accordingly. Although it is essential to communicate a nonjudgmental attitude during interactions with patients and clients, it also is important to acknowledge their feelings. For instance, if the person describes an episode of extreme exploitation and expresses feelings of anger about the situation, the nurse can show empathy and understanding with a statement such as "That sounds like a terrible situation to have been in." Nurses also need to consider that some of the information they obtain may involve legal or ethical issues that require further action. For example, information about recent or ongoing abuse or exploitation may necessitate a referral for further investigation, as discussed in Chapter 10.

Procedure for the Psychosocial Assessment

Nurses obtain psychosocial assessment information by interviewing older adults and their caregivers and by observing older adults in their environments. Opportunities for performing psychosocial assessments vary in different health care settings and much of the assessment information is obtained informally during the course of providing care. In acute care settings, nurses perform an assessment at the time of admission to establish a baseline for planning nursing care. Although the initial nursing assessment focuses on the patient's immediate physical needs, nurses should not overlook the psychosocial assessment, because it often provides clues to the causes of existing medical problems. Thus, as soon as the patient's condition is medically stable, nurses assess psychosocial issues as an important component of holistic care and discharge planning. In long-term care settings, psychosocial assessment information is usually discussed during interdisciplinary care conferences. In home settings, nurses have unique opportunities to obtain valuable psychosocial assessment information by observing the older adult in his or her personal environment.

In addition to interviewing and observing older adults, it often is appropriate to obtain information from other sources. For example, when the older person's cognitive function is compromised, it is essential to obtain information from family members and others who can provide a reliable history of the mental changes. In long-term care settings, nursing assistants—the health care workers who spend the most time with residents—are an important source of psychosocial information. Although nursing assistants are not routinely included in team discussions when psychosocial problems are addressed, nurses can obtain information from them and incorporate it in the care plans.

The tools for an effective psychosocial assessment are a trusting relationship, a listening ear, an intuitive mind, a

Box 13-1 Self-Assessment of Attitudes About Psychosocial Aspects of Aging

What Is My Level of Comfort in Discussing Psychosocial Issues With Older Adults?

- How comfortable am I discussing emotional, cultural, spiritual, and psychosocial subjects?
- Are there certain topics with which I am uncomfortable (e.g., death, suicide, alcoholism, sexuality, spirituality, terminal illness, abusive relationships)?
- Does the person's age influence my degree of comfort (e.g., Am I more comfortable discussing certain topics with someone who is in their 30s than with someone who is in their 90s)?
- Does the person's gender influence my degree of comfort?
- To what groups of older adults do I find it easy or difficult to relate?
- How do I feel about older adults who are living in nontraditional relationships?

When I Was Growing Up...

- How were older adults in my family treated?
- What did I observe about the treatment of older adults in society?
- How were people with mental or emotional disorders viewed?
- What language was used to describe aging, old age, and older adults with altered mental function?
- What words did my family use, and what was the connotative meaning of the words used, to describe older adults? Was it positive, negative, or mixed?

What Experiences Have I Had With Older Adults...

- From different racial, ethnic, religious, and socioeconomic backgrounds?
- With functional impairments or mental, psychological, or emotional disorders?

sensitive heart, and good communication skills. Because psychosocial issues may involve topics that are considered private, older adults may feel threatened by psychosocial assessment questions, particularly if they are trying to cover up cognitive deficits. Nurses, also, may be uncomfortable with assessing spirituality and other psychosocial aspects, so it is important to reflect on one's own attitudes and identify areas of discomfort (Williams, Voss, Vahle, et al., 2016). Box 13-1 can be used as a guide to self-assessment related to psychosocial assessment of older adults.

A Student's Perspective

My experience interviewing Mr. M. was an amazing one. I learned a lot about older adults and also about my interview technique. I think several of my techniques helped Mr. M. feel more comfortable and at ease. I told him if he felt uncomfortable answering any questions, he should feel free to pass and that did not happen once. I started asking him easy questions about his job and things like that. Then I moved into more personal questions related to his childhood and whether he thought it had been easy or difficult. I thought he might not remember a lot of that time in his life, but he told me many stories from when he was younger. He also had a lot of pride in the work that he did as a middle-aged adult when he was foreman in a factory.

Another technique I used was to allow him to wander away from the "path" of the question that I had asked him, because I didn't want him to feel conformed to answer the specific question. By using this technique, I learned much more about him than the scope of my original question, and it also gave him time to tell me things at his own pace. I could also tell what information he valued as important and what he found more private.

Erin H.

Begin a psychosocial assessment by explaining the purpose in relation to a nursing goal, with a statement like one of the following:

- "I'd like to ask you some questions about your interests so we can plan for your care while you're here at the nursing facility."
- "I'd like to ask some questions so we can make the best plans for follow-up after you leave the hospital."
- "I'd like to ask some questions about how you've been managing things at home so we can identify any community services that may be helpful to you."

An effective approach is to ask social questions, such as where the person was born and grew up. Although health care professionals may believe that it is unprofessional to talk about themselves, offering a little information about their own family or pets, for instance, may help to establish a framework of mutual interest. Sharing information about ethnic background also can be an effective and nonthreatening way of obtaining information about possible cultural influences.

If formal mental status assessment tools are to be used, they can be introduced after the older adult is more comfortable with discussing psychosocial issues. Because questions about memory can be very threatening, the topic might be introduced as follows: "I notice you have a hard time remembering dates. Have you noticed any other problems with your memory? Is it okay with you if I ask some questions about your memory?" If no evidence of cognitive impairment is evident, but other people have expressed concern about the person's memory, a statement such as the following might be used: "Your daughter is concerned that you don't remember to keep appointments. Have you noticed any problems with your memory? Is it okay with you if I ask some questions about your memory?"

COMMUNICATION SKILLS FOR PSYCHOSOCIAL ASSESSMENT

Just as nurses use a stethoscope and other tools for assessing physical function, nurses use communication techniques as an essential tool for establishing a trusting relationship and obtaining pertinent information about psychosocial function.

Box 13-2 Barriers to Effective Communication With Older Adults

Situational Barriers

- Different primary languages of speaker and listener
- Too much information being exchanged at one time
- More than one person communicating at one time
- Environmental noise, particularly for people who have impaired hearing or use hearing aids

Barriers Associated With the Older Adult

- Vision or hearing impairments
- Neurologic conditions that affect skills related to concentration, language, information processing, language skills (e.g., anxiety, aphasia, dementia, mild cognitive impairment)
- Physical discomfort (e.g., pain, thirst, hunger, fatigue, bladder fullness, or uncomfortable temperatures)

Barriers Associated With the Person Who Is Communicating

- Rapid or inarticulate speech
- Obstructive mannerisms (e.g., covering one's mouth or turning one's head away)
- Minimizing the person's feelings
- Giving false reassurances
- Offering trite responses (e.g., "Why cry over spilled milk?")
- Changing the subject to avoid sensitive issues
- Jumping to conclusions
- Using elderspeak or inappropriate titles (e.g., "dear" or "honey")

Nurses frequently need to address communication barriers that arise from several sources: the older adult, the situation itself, and the person who is communicating, as listed in Box 13-2. It also is imperative to avoid communication that conveys infantilization, as discussed in Chapter 12. In addition, cultural differences can create communication barriers that are very challenging. For example, foreign-born people who have a condition that affects their cognitive function may revert to their native language, even if they previously spoke English well. In these situations, family members may be able to facilitate communication, or it may be appropriate to use interpreters, as discussed in Chapter 2.

When discussing psychosocial issues, it is important to establish a private and comfortable environment and use interventions to improve hearing and vision. Box 13-3 describes strategies for enhancing communication with older adults, with details specific to a psychosocial assessment.

Nurses have many opportunities to identify psychosocial issues by listening for pertinent concerns and asking appropriate questions to obtain further information. For example, consider the case of Mrs. P. who, during an admission interview, gave the following response to a question about where she lives:

I moved to Sunnybrook Retirement Village after my last stroke. I couldn't stay in my own home, because the bedrooms were on the second floor. The doctor told me I had to live where I could get help, and my daughter didn't want me with her. Now that I've fallen and broken my wrist, I'm not sure what the doctor will tell me. My daughter doesn't want to be bothered with me.

Box 13-3 Strategies to Enhance Communication With Older Adults

General Strategies

- Arrange for face-to-face positioning.
- Ensure as much privacy as possible.
- Provide good lighting, and avoid background glare.
- Eliminate as much background noise as possible.
- Compensate as much as possible for vision or hearing impairments (e.g., make sure the person is using eyeglasses and hearing aid, if appropriate).
- Address physical needs and concerns about comfort.
- Begin contact with an exchange of names and, if appropriate, a handshake.
- Use culturally appropriate titles of respect, such as Señor, Señora, Señorita, Mr., Mrs., Ms., Dr., Reverend, Elder, Bishop, and so forth.
- Pronounce names correctly, and if in doubt, ask the older adult to say his or her name.
- Avoid linguistic messages that may convey bias or inequality.
   - Avoid slang expressions and never use pejorative or derogatory terms to refer to ethnic, racial, religious, or any other groups.
- Use touch purposefully and with awareness of individual preferences.
- Be aware of cultural differences that influence the perception and interpretation of verbal and nonverbal communication.

Strategies Specific to a Psychosocial Assessment

- Explain the purpose of the psychosocial assessment in relation to a nursing goal; then, begin with questions about remote, nonthreatening topics.
- Maintain good eye contact.
- Be comfortable using silence.
- Use attentive listening skills.
- Use open-ended questions.
- Encourage the person to elaborate on information with statements such as "and then what happened?"
- Ask how the person felt about or responded to a situation.
- Periodically clarify the messages.
- Remain nonjudgmental in your responses, but show appropriate empathy.
- Ask formal mental status questions, or the most threatening questions, toward the end of the interview.
- Gain the person's permission before asking formal assessment questions regarding memory and other cognitive abilities.

A Student's Perspective

*When I conducted a functional assessment, I found some communication techniques were therapeutic, whereas others were not. One barrier that I encountered was the difficulty of understanding my client, because he did not have any teeth, and therefore, it was difficult for him to pronounce his words. Also, there was limited privacy, and the client seemed to be distracted by other people in the room. Another barrier was that I found myself looking down at the paper as opposed to maintaining consistent eye contact. To combat these barriers, it would be important to provide more privacy and to minimize distractions. Also, because the client was difficult to understand, it would be important to ask for clarification about anything that was unclear. In addition, it is important to remember that a lack of eye contact is nontherapeutic. In order to improve on communication techniques, it is important to realize any barriers, identify ways to combat them, and think about what to do differently in the next situation. A helpful way to combat barriers is to remember the communication model of SOLER: **S**it facing the client, **O**bserve an open posture, **L**ean toward the client, **E**stablish and maintain intermittent eye contact, and **R**elax.*

Brittany D.

This response gives clues to several potential issues, which the nurse can explore with any of the following questions:

- "What do you miss most since you moved?"
- "You mentioned that your daughter didn't want you living with her. Is that something you had hoped you could do?"
- "Do you worry that the doctor will suggest that you go to a nursing home?"
- "Do you see your daughter as often as you'd like?"

Answers to these questions might uncover psychosocial concerns that need to be addressed as a part of discharge planning.

When communicating about psychosocial issues, it is important to periodically clarify the messages. One clarification technique is to repeat part of a prior answer when asking further questions. For example, saying to Mrs. P., "You mentioned that your daughter doesn't want you living with her...," gives feedback about what the nurse heard and leads into further questions about underlying feelings. Feedback can also be helpful when discrepancies between verbal and nonverbal communication are observed. For example, Mrs. P. might begin to cry and clench her fists as she says, "My daughter has her own life to worry about. I can take care of myself. It doesn't bother me that I can't live with her." A statement such as "You look awfully sad. Are you sure it doesn't bother you?" might lead to an acknowledgment of feelings such as anger, rejection, and loneliness.

Another important aspect is to consider the effects of nonverbal communication, which can be strongly influenced by cultural factors. For example, touch, handshaking, eye contact, and facial expressions can be used effectively to enhance communication, but they also can create barriers if they are misinterpreted. In addition, it is important to consider each person's "comfort zone," which is the physical space required for the person to feel at ease when communicating with others. This space is categorized as *intimate distance* (0 to 18 in), *personal distance* (1.5 to 4 ft), and *social distance* (4 to 12 ft). Cultural factors can influence all these aspects of nonverbal communication, as described in Box 13-4.

Box 13-4 Cultural Considerations: Cultural Influences on Communication

Touch

- Cultural groups that are likely to be most comfortable with physical touch are Jews, French, Spanish, Italians, Indonesians, and Latin Americans.
- Cultural groups that are likely to be uncomfortable with touch are British, Chinese, Germans, Hindus, Muslims, and North Americans.
- Asians may believe that it is disrespectful to touch the head, because it is thought to be a source of the person's strength.
- Vietnamese view the human head as the seat of life and highly personal; they may feel anxious if touched on their head or shoulders; if any orifice of the head is invaded, they may fear these procedures could provide an escape for the essence of life.
- Mexican Americans and Native Americans may view touch as a means for healing, preventing harm, or removing an evil spell.

Touch Between Men and Women

- Cultural groups that do not allow physical touch between men and women outside the home include Bosnians, Mexicans, Middle Easterners, Muslims, and Somalis.
- In many Hispanic and Middle Eastern cultures, male health care providers may be prohibited from touching or examining part or all of the female body.
- In some Asian cultures, touching between persons of the same sex (but not between those of the opposite sex) is common and acceptable.

Hand Shaking

- It is appropriate to greet Amish clients with a smile and a handshake.
- Middle Eastern women may not shake hands with men.
- Asian women may not shake hands with each other or with men.
- Native Americans may interpret vigorous handshaking as an aggressive action and are offended by a firm, lengthy handshake.

Eye Contact

- People from some Asian, Hispanic, Hindu, Hmong, Indochinese, Appalachian, Middle Eastern, and African American cultures may consider direct eye contact impolite, immodest, or aggressive, and they may avert their eyes when talking with health care professionals or, if female, when talking with men.
- Native Americans may direct their eye contact to the floor during conversations as an indication that they are paying close attention to the speaker.
- Hispanic cultures dictate appropriate deferential behavior in the form of downcast eyes toward others on the basis of age, sex, social position, economic status, and position of authority (e.g., elders expect respect from younger people).
- Cultural groups that are likely to maintain steady eye contact during conversations include Arabs, European Americans, Greeks, and Turks.
- Some cultural groups (e.g., Bosnians) maintain eye contact between women but not between men and women.

Facial Expression

- Italians, Jews, Hispanics, and African Americans smile readily and use many facial expressions along with words and gestures to communicate pain, happiness, or displeasure.

Perception of Personal Space

- Cultural groups that are likely to have a closer range for personal distance include Arabs, Hispanics, Greeks, Japanese, Iranians, East Indian, Latin Americans, and Middle Easterners.
- British, Canadians, Irish, and European North Americans are likely to require the most personal space.
- Men usually like to have larger personal space than women.

Source: Andrews, M. M., & Boyle, J. S. (2016). *Transcultural concepts in nursing care* (7th ed.). Philadelphia, PA: Wolters Kluwer; Purnell, L. D. (2013). *Transcultural health care: A culturally competent approach* (4th ed.). Philadelphia, PA: F. A. Davis Co.

A Student's Perspective

My communication with patients is something that I am always aware of. I have continued to learn something new each week. Silence during a conversation is something that is always uncomfortable for me. When talking with my client last week, I was trying to get a better sense of his level of family support. I began by asking him if he had any children. He indicated that he had two daughters, but they lived in Florida. Normally I would have had a follow-up question for this response, but I decided to give the client some time to see if he would expand on his original response. It was an awkward few minutes—okay, it was probably just a few seconds that seemed like minutes—but he did open up tremendously. He went on to explain to me that he felt like they have abandoned him since their mother passed away. He began to tear up as he went on to explain that he has grandchildren he has only seen in pictures on Christmas cards. I was able to talk with him about his feelings about these issues and offer him some encouragement. Had I chosen to guide the conversation I would have most likely never had this opportunity. I continue to enjoy confronting uncomfortable communication situations so that I can overcome them and foster better therapeutic communication between myself and clients.

Amanda A.

 MENTAL STATUS ASSESSMENT

A **mental status assessment** is an organized approach to collecting data about a person's psychosocial function. The mental status assessment is very broad in scope, so this section focuses on cognitive abilities, and other aspects of psychosocial function (i.e., affective function, contact with reality, and social supports) are discussed in the following sections. Indicators of psychosocial function that are addressed in this section on a mental status assessment are physical appearance, psychomotor behavior, social skills, orientation, alertness, memory, and speech characteristics. Mental status assessments are performed by various health care professionals, with each discipline specializing in various components. For example, psychiatrists are skilled in assessing affective and cognitive components, whereas social workers are skilled in assessing family relationship components. In the framework of this text, nurses assess the aspects of psychosocial function that most directly influence the day-to-day activities of older adults.

Mental Status Screening Tools

Screening tools have been used in clinical settings since the 1970s to identify the need for further assessment. Nursing protocols recommend a two-step process for assessing mental status: (1) screening to determine the presence or absence of cognitive impairment and (2) more comprehensive evaluation, as necessary, based on screening outcome (Heeren, Flamaing, Tournoy, et al., 2016). In addition to identifying the need for further evaluation, screening tests are performed periodically to assess progression of cognitive changes in people with dementia and other neurodegenerative disorders (Grossman & Irwin, 2016). Clinical settings generally incorporate a mental status screening tool or basic mental status assessment items in electronic health records. Table 13-1 delineates commonly used screening tools. The Mini-Mental State Examination (MMSE) has been the most commonly used tool; however, a current trend in geriatric settings is to use the Montreal Cognitive Assessment (MoCA) tool because of its improved ability to screen for mild cognitive impairment as well as dementia (Ciesielska, Sokolowski, Mazur, et al., 2016). In recent years, health care practitioners began using a short form of the MoCA (called the s-MoCA) as an easy-to-use and evidence-based tool, with a scoring system that can be compared directly to the MMSE (Larner, 2017; Roalf, Moore, Mechanic-Hamilton, et al., 2017). Online Learning Activity 13-1 provides links to the MoCA and helpful information about using these screening tools in clinical settings with older adults. Keep in mind that the purpose of these tools is simply to identify indicators of altered mental status; they do not provide a broad or in-depth perspective on psychosocial function, as is presented in this chapter. In addition, Chapters 14 and 15 provide information about screening tools for delirium and depression. Nurses have essential roles in facilitating referrals for comprehensive neuropsychological evaluations when they identify any indicators of impaired mental status, as discussed in this chapter.

See ONLINE LEARNING ACTIVITY 13-1: EVIDENCE-BASED INFORMATION ABOUT SCREENING TOOLS FOR IDENTIFYING COGNITIVE IMPAIRMENT IN OLDER ADULTS at http://thepoint.lww.com/Miller8e.

Technology to Promote Wellness in Older Adults

Studies indicate that as a way of improving access to mental status assessment in rural areas, or when it is difficult to bring the person to a clinical setting, direct-to-home videoconferencing is effective for neuropsychological assessment for people with cognitive impairment (Lindauer, Seelye, Lyons, et al., 2017; Wadsworth, Galusha-Glasscock, Womack, et al., 2016).

Physical Appearance

Physical appearance is readily observed and reveals many aspects of psychosocial function. Clothing, grooming, cosmetics, and hygiene provide many clues to psychological function, but they are only clues, and questions must be asked before any conclusions are drawn. For example, the presence of body odor, poor hygiene, and tattered clothing may be associated with any of the following conditions: depression, incontinence, impaired cognitive abilities, limited financial resources, overwhelming caregiving responsibilities, impaired vision or sense of smell, or lack of access to or inability to use bathing facilities.

Motor Function, Body Language, and Psychomotor Behaviors

Assessment of motor function, which includes posture, movement, and body language, can provide clues to broader aspects of psychosocial function. For example, a shuffling, staggering, or uncoordinated gait could indicate neurologic deficits secondary to a disease process or adverse effects from alcohol or medications. Gait disturbances, as well as

TABLE 13-1	Tools Commonly Used to Screen for Cognitive Impairment
Tool	**Features**
Folstein Mini-Mental State Examination (MMSE)	Assesses orientation, memory, attention, abilities to name, follow verbal and written command, write a sentence spontaneously, and copy a complex polygon. Maximum of 30 points
Mini-Cog with Clock Drawing Test	Assesses cognitive function, memory, language comprehension, visual–motor skills, and executive function
4AT	Assigns a numerical value to the following items: alertness, attention, acute change or fluctuation, ability to state age, date of birth, current location, and current year
AD8: The Washington University Dementia Screening Test	Uses eight items to assess changes in memory, orientation, judgment, and function, as compared to previous levels
Montreal Cognitive Assessment (MoCA)	Includes 30 items assessing short-term memory recall, visuospatial abilities, three-dimensional cube copy, and executive functions
One-Minute Verbal Fluency for Animals	Tests ability to name as many animals as he or she can in 1 minute
Blessed Memory Test	Tests ability to recall five-item name and address

other abnormal movements, are possible signs of tardive dyskinesia or extrapyramidal symptoms. Evidence of tardive dyskinesia raises the question of past or present use of psychotropic medications (discussed in Chapter 8) and may give clues to psychiatric history.

Body language also provides clues to affective illnesses. Slouching and head hanging are common manifestations of withdrawal and depression. Poor eye contact, particularly looking at the floor, may be indicative of depression. As with all aspects of assessment, it is important to consider that cultural factors can influence the type and amount of eye contact that is considered to be appropriate (refer to Box 13-4).

Psychomotor behaviors are part of the mental status assessment, because the ability to purposefully carry out simple motor skills is highly influenced by cognitive status. For example, observations of how someone navigates and avoids obstacles in the environment provide clues to the person's judgment and awareness of the environment. Nurses can assess psychomotor behaviors by asking the person to perform a simple activity of daily living (e.g., combing hair) and observing the person's ability to comprehend and perform the request.

Another assessment component is observations related to abnormal psychomotor function, such as extreme slowness or agitation. Depression is usually associated with slowed psychomotor function, but excessive activity can be a symptom of agitated depression. Agitation can also be a symptom of an adverse medication effect or an indicator of a physiologic disturbance (e.g., dehydration, electrolyte imbalance) or a pathologic condition (e.g., pneumonia, urinary tract infection), particularly in older adults with dementia.

Social Skills

Assessment of social skills provides information about many aspects of psychosocial function. For example, friendly and cooperative people with good conversational skills may use social skills to hide their cognitive deficits, particularly if they are motivated to do so. By contrast, people with long-standing patterns of hostility, social isolation, poor social skills, and a lack of ambition may be less motivated to perform well. In addition, people sometimes use the following social skills to cover up cognitive deficits: humor, evasiveness, leading the conversation, and making up answers to questions. Some older adults with dementia maintain very good social skills, even in the later stages of dementia when other skills have long since declined. Nurses also need to be aware of cultural factors that influence social skills and consider the cultural context of the relationship between the interviewer and the interviewee.

Response to the Interview

The older adult's initial response to the interview, as well as changes that occur during the interview, can provide important assessment information. For example, an older adult may initially be very receptive to the questions but may become defensive or sarcastic when he or she is uncomfortable with the line of questioning. In addition, nurses assess the amount of time and effort expended in answering questions. This is particularly important when trying to differentiate between dementia and depression because cognitively impaired people may exert great effort in responding to questions, but depressed people may lack energy or motivation to answer correctly. Thus, two people may score the same on a formal mental status questionnaire, but one may miss the questions because of dementia and the other may miss them because of depression. When nurses suspect that lack of motivation is a reason for incorrect or missing answers, they might clarify this by asking, "Is it that you don't know the answers or that you just don't feel like answering the questions?"

Nurses may encounter attitudes of resistance and defensiveness for a variety of reasons. A person who is depressed may be apathetic and may not want to expend the energy to answer the questions. A cognitively impaired person may be angry, hostile, or defensive, particularly if he or she is trying to hide or deny cognitive deficits. A person who has always been reclusive or suspicious may be unwilling to answer questions or may feel very defensive. Assessing the person's underlying attitude is as important as assessing the accuracy of responses to questions.

Assessing for **confabulation**, which is the process of making up information, is difficult when the nurse does not know the correct information. For example, questions about the person's place of birth or childhood experiences are not effective for assessing cognitive function unless the accuracy of the answers can be confirmed. People with mild cognitive changes may use confabulation to conceal memory loss. **Circumstantiality** involves the use of excessive details and roundabout answers in responding to questions.

Finally, nurses assess all information in relation to the person's usual personality traits. For example, highly sociable people might always use humor, whereas talkative people might naturally use circumstantiality. The use of humor and circumstantiality by people who are normally quiet and serious might indicate a great effort to cover up cognitive deficits. On the other hand, people who are normally quiet and withdrawn may be perceived falsely as being depressed. Nurses can obtain information about a person's usual personality by asking a question such as "Would you describe what you were like when you were 40 years old?" Family members and caregivers who have known the person for a long time are good sources of information about lifelong personality characteristics. Box 13-5 summarizes guidelines for assessing physical appearance, motor function, social skills, and responses to the interview in relation to the person's psychosocial function.

Orientation

Orientation to person, place, and time is the indicator of mental status that is most routinely assessed and

Box 13-5 Guidelines for Assessing Physical Appearance, Motor Function, Social Skills, and Response to the Interview

Observations Regarding Physical Appearance and Motor Function

- What is the person's apparent age in relation to his or her chronologic age?
- How do the following factors reflect psychological function: hygiene, grooming, clothing, cosmetics?
- Does the person's physical appearance provide clues to dementia or depression or to other impairments of psychosocial function?
- What do the person's gait, posture, and body language indicate about his or her psychological function?
- Is there any evidence of tardive dyskinesia or other adverse medication effects?
- How does the person maneuver in the environment, and what does this reflect regarding judgment, vision, and other skills?

Observations Regarding Social Skills and Response to the Interview

- What are the person's lifelong patterns of social skills, and how do these influence the assessment process?
- How do the person's social skills influence the interviewer's interpretation of other aspects of psychosocial function?
- Is the person motivated to answer questions?
- What is the person's attitude about the interview?
- If the person does not answer the questions, or gives incorrect answers, is it because of inability, cultural factors, or lack of motivation?
- Does the person use any of the following in an attempt to hide possible cognitive deficits: humor, sarcasm, avoidance, evasiveness, confabulation, circumstantiality, or leading the conversation?
- Does the person manifest any of the following characteristics: anger, hostility, resistance, defensiveness, or suspiciousness?
- Do the person's underlying attitudes reflect his or her usual personality, or are they manifestations of cognitive or affective disturbances?

documented. Often, however, orientation is viewed as the primary indicator of cognitive function, rather than as one small piece of a larger picture. For example, the following questions are the gold standard for assessing orientation: "What is your name?" "Where are you?" and "What time is it?" Based on the accuracy of each answer, the person is then labeled as "oriented times one," "oriented times two," or "oriented times three." The superficial use of orientation questions and the subsequent labeling of the person as oriented times one, two, or three ignores important considerations, such as:

- Are any environmental clues available to the person to orient him or her to the time or place?
- Has the person been at the institution long enough to have learned its name?
- If the person cannot state the exact name of the facility, can he or she describe the type of facility it is or its general location?

- Do sociocultural factors influence the person's response to these questions?
- Can the person name familiar people, such as a spouse or children, even if he or she cannot state his or her own name?
- If the person cannot give specific names of other people, can he or she describe the correct role of the other person?
- If the person cannot state the exact time, can he or she give the general time of day?
- Does the person have medical problems that interfere with cognition?
- Is the person taking medications that can influence mental function?

A good assessment extends beyond the three classic questions and describes levels of orientation that are meaningful for the person in a particular setting. For example, the following description is far more useful than simply noting that the person is "oriented times one":

Mrs. S. could state her name but did not remember the name of this hospital. She could not give her daughter's name but was able to introduce her daughter to me without stating her name. She thought that the month was December because of the Chanukah decorations in her room. She could not state the time because she did not have her watch with her, but she thought that it was afternoon because lunch had recently been served.

If the nurse had used only the standard questions of "What is your name?" "Where are you?" and "What time is it?" Mrs. S. would be judged to be "oriented times one." Most health care providers, after reading the results of that assessment, would have assumed that Mrs. S. had serious cognitive impairment, particularly if she were 85 years of age or older. Mrs. S.'s actual responses, however, reflected various cognitive skills involved in organizing information, making associations, and using judgment. The more detailed description shows that Mrs. S. is probably quite a logical person who has not yet learned the name of the hospital and who might have some temporary memory impairment because of anxiety, medications, or acute medical problems.

Alertness and Attention

Besides orientation, level of **alertness** is the mental status indicator that health care providers most frequently assess and document. Level of alertness is measured along a continuum, which includes stupor, drowsiness, somnolence, intermittent alertness/drowsiness, and hyperalertness. An important aspect of assessing the person's level of alertness is the identification of any factors that can either increase or decrease alertness, with particular attention to those factors that can be addressed. For example, excessive daytime drowsiness can be associated with any of the following factors: medical problems, electrolyte imbalances, adverse medication effects (e.g., narcotics, anticholinergics, psychoactive medications), depression, dementia, excessive alcohol intake, or lack of sleep at night because of a variety of reasons (e.g., caregiver responsibilities).

As a mental status indicator, attention describes the ability to focus on a task, filter out distractions, and sustain focus as needed to complete a task. This is an essential, but often overlooked, indicator of altered mental status particularly as a key indicator of delirium (De, Wand, Smerdely, et al., 2016; Hendry, Quinn, Evans, et al., 2016). Asking an older adult to recite the months of a year backwards is a simple test of attention that can help identify delirium (Adamis, Meagher, Murray, et al., 2016; Leonard, O'Connell, Williams, et al., 2016). As with other aspects of psychosocial assessment, attention skills are one piece of a large puzzle that is put together to provide a broader picture of mental status.

Memory

Formal memory testing assesses the person's memory, that is, recall of remote events, recent past events, and immediate memory, which is further divided into retention, recall, and recognition. Nurses can assess memory during regular conversations because all verbal communication depends to some degree on memory function. Nurses pay particular attention to assessing memory in relation to activities that are important in daily life, such as remembering to pay bills, take medications, and shop for groceries. This assessment is made in relation to the expectations and demands of the person's usual environment. For example, if the person lives alone and manages finances independently, the ability to pay bills is quite important. By contrast, if the person lives with a daughter and her family, remembering the birth dates of grandchildren may be an important memory task.

Assessment of memory is particularly challenging because older adults who are depressed may perceive their memory skills as more impaired than they are in reality and may even exaggerate their deficits (Hill, Mogle, Wion, et al., 2016). In contrast to this situation, older adults with dementia may have little or no awareness of their memory deficits, or they may deny memory problems as a self-protective response. Thus, the answer to the question, "Do you ever have trouble remembering things?" may reveal more about the person's perception of memory than about his or her actual memory function. Although this question may be quite useful in identifying any concerns that the older adult might have, it is not necessarily useful for assessing memory function.

It also is important to assess the person's use of memory aids by posing a question such as "Is there anything you do to help you remember appointments or other things?" Assessment of the extent to which the person depends on memory aids is useful in setting goals and planning for improved memory function. For example, if the person's memory function is barely adequate and is based heavily on memory aids, then the potential for further improvement is minimal. By contrast, if the person has some memory deficits but does not use any memory aids, then the potential for improvement increases. Observations about the use of memory aids may also provide clues to unacknowledged memory deficits. For example, if the person denies problems with memory, but repeatedly refers to written notes during an interview, then he or she may be compensating for an impaired memory. In this situation, the person is quite willing to use memory aids but is unwilling to acknowledge the need for such aids. Box 13-6 summarizes guidelines for nursing assessment of orientation, alertness, and memory and includes examples of appropriate questions for assessing the different types of memory.

Speech and Language Characteristics

Speech and language characteristics provide important information about many aspects of psychosocial function,

---

 Box 13-6   Guidelines for Assessing Orientation, Alertness, and Memory

Interview Questions to Assess Orientation

Note: Examples of direct questions are identified by quotation marks to distinguish them from the questions that are answered indirectly through observations.

- *Person:* "What is your name?" "What is your wife's name?" If names can't be given, can the person describe roles?
- *Place:* "What is your address?" "What is the name of this place?" "What kind of place is this?" "What is the name of this city?" "What is the name of this state?"
- *Time:* "What time is it?" "What day of the week is today?" "What month and date is it today?" "What season is it?"

Observations to Assess Alertness

- What is the person's level of alertness on the following continuum: hyperalert, alert, drowsy, somnolent, stuporous?
- Does the person's level of alertness fluctuate? If so, is there any pattern to the fluctuations?
- Are there physiologic factors that might influence the person's level of alertness, such as medical conditions or effects of chemicals or medications?
- Are there psychosocial factors that might influence the person's level of alertness, such as anxiety, depression, nighttime caregiving responsibilities, or any other factor that might disrupt nighttime sleep?

Interview Questions to Assess Memory

- *Remote events:* "Where were you born?" "Where did you go to grade school?" "What was your first job?" "When were you married?"
- *Recent past events:* "Do you live with anyone?" "Do you have any grandchildren?" "What are the names of your grandchildren?" "When was the last time you went to the doctor?"
- *Immediate memory, retention:* State three unrelated words and ask the person to repeat the information, both immediately and again after 5 minutes.
- *Immediate memory, general grasp and recall:* Ask the person to read a short story and then to summarize the information presented in the story.
- *Immediate memory, recognition:* Ask a multiple-choice question and then ask the person to choose the correct answer.

such as the ability to organize and communicate thoughts. In addition, a good assessment of language skills helps the nurse to identify words and language patterns that are most appropriate for use with an older person. Because speech and language skills are highly dependent on cultural, educational, and socioeconomic factors, it is important to consider these influences, particularly when assessing foreign-born older adults. During verbal interactions, nurses can assess speech and language characteristics, such as the ones delineated in Box 13-7.

Aphasia is a communication disorder that is associated with neurologic conditions such as stroke or vascular dementia. Expressive aphasia occurs when comprehension abilities are not affected but word retrieval or word-finding abilities are impaired. Receptive aphasia occurs when verbal and comprehension abilities are impaired but some language skills are retained. Global aphasia, which is a combination of receptive and expressive aphasia, results from more extensive neurologic damage and is manifested by inconsistent and poorly controlled language skills.

Calculation and Higher Language Skills

Reading, writing, spelling, and arithmetic are calculation and higher language skills that are assessed as indicators of cognition. As with assessments of other indicators, the person's education, occupation, and other influencing factors must

be considered. Nurses can informally assess these skills in relation to how the person performs important daily activities. For example, for an older adult who lives alone, an assessment of the ability to pay utility bills and use money to purchase groceries is more valuable than a measurement of mathematical skills using a psychometric test. Likewise, a person's ability to read the daily newspaper or the markings on a thermostat may be a more valid gauge of functional ability than a score on a formal reading test.

Written health education materials can be used to assess reading and comprehension skills informally. For example, when collecting a urine sample, the nurse can give the person a list of instructions and ask him or her to read the instructions aloud. An observation of how well the person comprehends the instructions provides an assessment of reading and comprehension skills that are important in daily life. Another opportunity for assessing reading comprehension may arise if the person is reading a newspaper and the nurse asks a nonthreatening question such as "What's new in the paper today?" Answers to this question can provide information about the person's interests in outside events and his or her ability to comprehend and remember written information.

Nurses can assess writing and other higher language skills by observing older adults during interactions that pertain to their care. For example, nurses can observe the way an older adult signs his or her name on documents such as permission forms. Nurses can also observe the older adult during

---

 Box 13-7 Guidelines for Assessing Speech Characteristics, and Calculation and Higher Language Skills

Observations to Assess Speech Characteristics

- Is the pace of speech normal, slow, or fast?
- Is the tone of voice suggestive of underlying feelings, such as anger, hostility, or resentment?
- Is the volume abnormally soft or loud?
- Do the sentences flow coherently and smoothly?
- Is there evidence of any problem with integrating speech sounds into words (e.g., neologisms, or phonemic or semantic errors)?
- Do any of the following factors affect the person's speech: dry mouth, poorly fitting dentures, absence of teeth or dentures, alcohol or medication effects, or neurologic or other pathologic processes?
- Does the person exhibit any of the following: agnosia; perseveration; or expressive, receptive, or global aphasia?

Observations and Associated Underlying Conditions

- Slow-paced or excessively brief verbal communication: depression, neurodegenerative disease
- Tone of voice: indirectly expressed feelings such as anger, hostility, and resentment
- Hypophonia (i.e., abnormally low speech volume): depression, physical illness
- Abnormally loud speech volume: impaired hearing or long-term experience communicating with someone who is hearing impaired
- Poor articulation or slurred speech: hearing impairment, ill-fitting dentures, lack of teeth or dentures, neurologic disorder, effects of alcohol or medications

- Incorrect word pronunciation: hearing impairment, cognitive deficits, educational and cultural influences
- Semantic errors (i.e., misinterpretation of the meaning of words): hearing impairment, cognitive deficits, educational and cultural influences
- Neologisms (i.e., self-created and meaningless words): dementia, psychotic disorder, repetition of a word that was not heard accurately
- Incoherent speech: dementia, aphasia, psychiatric disorders, alcohol or medication effects
- Perseveration (i.e., a repetitive or stuttering pattern of verbal or written communication) and agnosia (i.e., difficulty finding the correct word or the inability to name an object accurately, particularly if it is unfamiliar): dementia

Observations to Assess Calculation and Higher Language Skills

- What is the person's ability to comprehend written materials encountered in the course of routine activities, such as the daily newspaper or instructions for medications?
- What is the quality of the person's handwriting (e.g., his or her signature)?
- Is the person able to perform mathematical computations necessary for daily activities?

the performance of more complex tasks such as compiling a written medication list or a list of questions to discuss with the primary care provider. Difficulty with writing skills is a common sign of early stages of dementia.

Traditional mental status tests measure calculation with the "serial 7s" test: the person is asked to subtract 7 from 100 and to continue subtracting 7s. Because this test is highly influenced by level of education, it is not necessarily the most appropriate test for older adults. It may be better to ask the older person to add 3 plus 3 and to continue adding 3s. Older adults who are depressed may not answer correctly because they do not want to expend the energy to calculate serial sevens. Older adults who have dementia may be able to perform well on this task if they try hard and if they previously had highly developed mathematical skills. Box 13-7 summarizes the considerations that are important in assessing speech characteristics and calculation and higher language skills.

DECISION MAKING AND EXECUTIVE FUNCTION

Decision making—one of the most important and complex of all cognitive abilities—is an important aspect of psychosocial function because all legally competent older adults, including those with dementia, have the right to be involved in decisions about their care. Determination of competency is a complex issue with many implications not only for older adults and their families and caregivers but also for health care professionals (as discussed in Chapter 9). As an integral part of psychosocial nursing care, nurses assess cognitive skills—including insight, learning, memory, reasoning, judgment, problem solving, and abstract thinking—that are involved with decision making. Although no one assessment tool focuses specifically on decision making, nurses assess this aspect of psychosocial function by observing the abilities of older adults to solve problems during the course of daily activities and by asking pertinent assessment questions.

Abstract thinking is defined as strongly influenced by other factors such as education, personality, and affective state. People who are very anxious or depressed may lack the attention or motivation required to respond to the questions typically used for the assessment of abstract thinking patterns. Similarity questions such as "How are apples and oranges alike?" or "How are a table and chair alike?" are used to assess the person's ability to think abstractly.

During an interview, opportunities for assessing abstract thinking may arise, and the nurse listens for clues to the person's level of abstract versus concrete thinking. The following exchange is an example of an unsolicited opportunity that this author had to assess one older adult's concrete thinking pattern:

Nurse: How did you feel about having to move from your home in Texas to live with your daughter and her family here in Ohio?

Mr. L: I don't know; how would you feel?

Nurse: I'm not sure how I'd feel; that's never happened to me. I'm not in your shoes.

Mr. L: Well, here, put them on (stated emphatically while taking off his shoes to give to the nurse).

One interpretation of Mr. L.'s response is that his thinking pattern is very concrete, rather than abstract.

Nurses assess problem-solving abilities through observations about how older adults meet their needs in a particular situation. For instance, the nurse observes the way older adults use call lights to meet their needs when confined to a bed or the way in which they deal with complex decisions related to discharge planning. Similarly, a very important problem-solving task for an older adult who lives alone may be meeting basic safety needs. Therefore, questions such as "What would you do if you fell at home and could not get up?" or "What would you do if you woke up and smelled smoke?" might be an appropriate way of assessing judgment related to safety. For an older adult who lives in a nursing home, a very important but complex problem-solving task may involve dealing with a disruptive roommate. In this situation, the answer to a question such as "What would you do if your roommate started taking your belongings?" might provide the most pertinent information for assessing problem-solving skills.

Insight is the ability to understand the significance of the present situation. This skill is an important component of the problem-solving process because it establishes a basis for planning care. Level of insight is affected by pathologic changes in the brain and by psychosocial factors, such as feelings, personality, and coping mechanisms. Lack of insight is sometimes labeled as *denial,* which is a defense mechanism that is often used to protect oneself from unpleasant realities. However, when insight is limited because of conditions such as dementia, it is inappropriate and inaccurate to label this as denial; the more appropriate approach is to assess and document the person's level of insight.

Nursing assessment of insight concentrates on those areas of function that are pertinent to the care plan. For example, in assessing the insight of an older adult who has been brought to the hospital with malnutrition and uncontrolled hypertension, the nurse may ask questions such as the following:

- Why did your daughter bring you to the hospital?
- How do you manage with grocery shopping and getting your meals?
- Do you take any medications?
- What are the medications for?
- What kinds of things does your daughter do for you?
- What kind of help do you think you may need when you leave the hospital?

Answers to questions such as these facilitate care planning because they help the nurse assess the person's understanding of the present situation.

When the person has little or no understanding of his or her health situation, the nurse tries to identify the factors that interfere with insight. In the example just described, insight may be absent or limited because of one or more of the following conditions: dementia, depression, mild cognitive impairment, lack of information about the medication regimen, inability to remember information, or fear of losing independence. An essential component of discharge planning is identifying both the level of insight and the factors that interfere with insight. In addition, the nurse attempts to identify factors that may improve the person's insight. If insight is lacking because of denial that stems from exaggerated fears, then alleviating the fears may facilitate insight.

In recent years, health care professionals have recognized the importance of assessing executive function abilities in conjunction with determining a patient's capacity to safely and reliably plan and carry out activities related to daily living. **Executive function** is multifaceted and involves an interrelated set of abilities that enable and drive adaptive and goal-directed activity. Executive function deficits, called executive dysfunction, begin during the earliest stages of dementia and can be present even before memory problems are evident, particularly when the pathologic processes affect the frontal lobe. Indicators of executive function deficits include diminished mental flexibility, limited ability to think abstractly, difficulty with problem solving, decline in ability to conceptualize, diminished ability to adapt to new situations, and difficulty shifting thought processes from one idea to another. People with executive cognitive dysfunction may perform well on the MMSE but still not be able to perform essential daily activities safely and independently. Online Learning Activity 13-2 provides additional information about screening tools nurses can use to identify executive dysfunction, as recommended by the Hartford Institute for Geriatric Nursing.

 ONLINE LEARNING ACTIVITY 13-2 ADDITIONAL INFORMATION ABOUT EVIDENCE-BASED SCREENING TOOLS FOR ASSESSING EXECUTIVE FUNCTION AND DECISION MAKING IN OLDER ADULTS at http://thepoint.lww.com/Miller8e.

Because it is important to assess executive skills in relation to a previous level of function, it may be necessary to ask family members or the person being assessed if they have noticed changes in these abilities in recent years. When families or health care providers have serious questions about the decision-making abilities of an older person, or when a major decision must be made and there is disagreement about it, a more comprehensive assessment using neuropsychological tests may be warranted. For example, if a cognitively impaired older person expresses a strong desire to live alone but family members question the person's ability to function safely, a comprehensive geriatric assessment with emphasis on decision-making and executive function skills will provide useful information.

AFFECTIVE FUNCTION

A person's **affect** refers to his or her mood, emotions, and expressions of emotions. Happiness and sadness are feelings commonly associated with affective states, but all of the following have been identified as *primary affects* (also called *discrete emotions*): joy, awe, hope, fear, pain, rage, pride, guilt, shame, anger, regret, relief, hatred, surprise, interest, boredom, elation, confusion, jealousy, depression, suspicion, frustration, anxiety, bewilderment, amorousness, and lack of feelings.

The components of affective state that are reviewed in this section are general mood, anxiety, self-esteem, depression, and happiness. These five aspects were selected for the following reasons:

- An assessment of general mood assists the nurse in determining appropriate goals based on the person's usual affective state.
- Anxiety is a common factor in older adults that can often be alleviated or minimized through nursing interventions.
- Self-esteem is a major determinant of feelings, particularly depression and happiness.
- Self-esteem is particularly important because older adults face many conditions that threaten their self-esteem.
- Depression and happiness are two primary affects that have been the target of much of the research regarding affective states in older people.

Nursing interventions are directed toward all of these affective components to improve the quality of life of older adults.

Guidelines for Assessing Affective Function

Affective function is assessed both quantitatively and qualitatively in relation to expectations about acceptable expressions of emotions. For example, people are expected to show some expression of sadness when talking about sad events. When the person's expression of feelings is not consistent with the external event, however, the affect is considered inappropriate. Affect is also assessed in relation to the personal meaning and the nearness in time of an event. People are expected to show greater feelings of sadness in response to tragic news than in response to neutral events. Likewise, people are expected to show a deeper affective response soon after experiencing a sad event than they would years after the event occurred.

The depth and duration of affect, which are important considerations in differentiating between dementia and depression in older adults, are also assessed. The affect of depressed people is generally sad and negativistic and is not influenced by external circumstances. By contrast, the affect of people who have dementia fluctuates more and changes in response to distractions. Emotional lability (i.e., emotional instability or fluctuation) occurs with strokes, vascular dementia, vascular depression, and other pathologic conditions that affect certain areas of the brain.

Nonverbal behaviors, such as those indicating anxiety, sadness, and happiness, provide important information about a person's affective state that the person may not offer verbally. For example, despite a person's denial of feeling sad, he or she may exhibit the following nonverbal cues: crying, slouching over, looking at the ground, and having a mournful facial expression. The nurse uses this information as the basis for a leading comment such as "You look like you're feeling sad."

Expressions of emotions are strongly determined by cultural norms and personality characteristics. In most Western societies, crying is more acceptable for women and children than for men and older boys, and showing anger and rage is more acceptable for men than for women. Cultural expectations also influence the way a person expresses feelings in certain circumstances. For example, a person may be expected to cry and loudly proclaim mournful feelings at a funeral but may be prohibited from expressing any feelings in front of strangers or in a public place such as a hospital. Because some emotions, such as anger or depression, are viewed as less acceptable than others, such as happiness, people learn to deny and hide feelings that may be judged as unacceptable. Older adults, particularly, may have learned that certain feelings should not be expressed directly or verbally. Thus, it is particularly important to observe for any indirect or nonverbal cues of anger, depression, and other less socially acceptable feelings.

In assessing the affective state of older adults, it is important to identify the terminology that is most acceptable. Many people will not admit to feeling anxious or depressed because they associate these terms with a serious mental illness or with a socially unacceptable state. Therefore, the nurse begins the assessment of affective state by focusing on feelings that are viewed positively or neutrally. If the person initiates the topic of feeling anxious or depressed, the nurse responds to those feelings and pursues a related line of questioning. In most circumstances, however, it is best to begin with open-ended questions. A simple question such as "How are you feeling today?" when asked with sincerity, is a familiar and comfortable way of eliciting information.

Mood

Mood is closely associated with emotions but differs from them in that it is more pervasive, less intense, and longer lasting. People are usually quite comfortable describing their mood as either bad or good and are more likely to offer information about their mood than their emotions. Thus, during a mental status examination, a question such as "How would you describe your usual mood?" may be perceived as less threatening than the question "How do you feel most of the time?" Nonverbal behaviors provide many clues about a person's mood and may be more accurate than verbal responses as an indicator of affective state. Joy, anger, anxiety, sadness, happiness, and depression are examples of moods that are expressed in nonverbal behaviors in everyday life by most people.

Anxiety

Anxiety is a feeling of distress, subjectively experienced as fear or worry, and objectively expressed through autonomic and central nervous system responses. Mild or moderate anxiety can be beneficial because it motivates protective behaviors, but excessive anxiety is detrimental because it channels personal energy into defensive behaviors. Risk factors for excessive anxiety in older adults include pain, depression, and the presence of three or more medical conditions (Gould, O'Hara, Goldstein, et al., 2016).

In assessing anxiety, nurses must identify the terminology that is most acceptable to the older adult. Words like "worries" and "concerns" are readily understood and usually elicit responses about sources of anxiety. Older adults may talk about "trouble with my nerves" in reference to anxiety. Nurses observe for nonverbal manifestations of anxiety to supplement the information obtained from verbal communication. In any adult, anxiety may be manifested in the following nonverbal ways: pacing, shakiness, restlessness, irritability, fidgeting, diaphoresis, tachycardia, hyperventilation, dry mouth, voice changes, smoking habits, urinary frequency, increased muscle tension, poor eye contact, poor attention span, inability to sit still, changes in eating patterns, rapid or disconnected speech, or repetitive motions of facial muscles or any extremities. Although any of these indicators may be observed in older adults, the presence of mobility limitations or pathologic conditions can interfere with some of them. For example, older adults who are confined to bed cannot pace but may experience subtle changes in eating or sleeping patterns because of anxiety. Older adults may be reluctant to report that they are worried or anxious; instead, they may focus on physiologic symptoms (e.g., pain, fatigue, anorexia, insomnia, or stomach distress).

Because anxiety is always a response to real or perceived threats, the nurse tries to identify sources of anxiety, even though they may not be readily apparent. Potential sources of anxiety (i.e., real or perceived threats) include health, assets, values, environment, self-concept, role function, needs fulfillment, goal achievement, personal relationships, and sense of security. People do not always recognize the source of their anxiety because it may arise from unconscious conflicts, unacknowledged fears, maturational crises, or developmental challenges. Even when people recognize the source of anxiety, they may be reluctant to discuss it, or they may refer to the threat only indirectly. For example, an older adult may have the perception that other people have the power to "put him away" in a nursing home simply because of a slight memory impairment. If the person knows other older adults who have been admitted unwillingly to a nursing home, this fear may be exacerbated. Further anxiety may arise from the person's fear of discussing the subject because of the perception that initiating the topic might precipitate actions leading to nursing home admission. Rather than directly talking about the fears, the person may provide vague clues, for instance: "I felt so sorry for Mildred when her son put her in the nursing home."

Nurses must phrase questions aimed at identifying sources of anxiety in the least threatening way possible. When older adults express concerns about other older people, it may be appropriate to ask questions aimed at determining whether they have the same worries about themselves. For example, in response to the statement, "I felt so sorry for Mildred," the nurse might ask, "Do you ever worry that you'll have to go to a nursing home?" Nurses use open-ended questions that allow for a wide range of answers to identify sources of anxiety that might not otherwise be revealed. For example, nurses in institutional settings can ask, "What is your biggest worry about going home?" or "Do you have any worries about how you'll manage at home after you leave here?" In home settings, the nurse might ask an even broader question such as "Do you have any concerns about the future?" or "What kinds of things do you worry about?" Answers to these questions are usually filled with clues to sources of anxiety and lead to many additional questions.

Anxiety can be caused or exacerbated by physiologic conditions arising from disease processes or the adverse effects of bioactive substances, as in the following examples:

- Herbs, caffeine, nicotine, and medications (both prescription and over-the-counter) can cause anxiety reactions.
- Anxiety may be associated with withdrawal from nicotine or alcohol.
- Pathologic processes that diminish cerebral oxygen, such as pulmonary or cardiovascular diseases, can cause anxiety reactions.
- Endocrine disorders, such as hyperthyroidism, may be manifested primarily by anxiety or other psychosocial symptoms.
- People with dementia may show signs of excessive anxiety when they are experiencing pain or physical discomfort, particularly if their verbal communication skills are impaired.
- Pacing is a commonly observed manifestation of anxiety in ambulatory older adults who have dementia.

Therefore, information about medical conditions and the person's use of herbs, caffeine, and medications is an essential component of the anxiety assessment.

Medications that affect the central or autonomic nervous systems may precipitate or exacerbate anxiety. *Akathisia* is a frequently reported extrapyramidal effect of some neuroleptics that may subjectively or objectively be interpreted as anxiety. Akathisia is defined as an inner sense of restlessness that is worsened by inactivity and is manifested by motor restlessness. It is more common in women and older adults, and it can occur anytime during the course of treatment with psychotropic medications. Therefore, if an older adult who is taking neuroleptics complains of certain feelings, such as "shaking on the inside," the possibility of adverse medication effects must be considered as a cause.

In addition to identifying sources and manifestations of anxiety, it is important to identify appropriate methods for reducing anxiety. Even if the sources of anxiety are not identified or cannot be changed, the experience of anxiety can be addressed through self-care interventions that improve coping. To this end, the nurse asks questions about usual coping methods. Questions such as "What do you do when you have trouble with your nerves?" or "What do you find helpful when your nerves are bad?" can pave the way for a discussion about coping with anxiety. If the person cannot identify effective coping mechanisms, the nurse offers suggestions in a nonjudgmental way and assesses the person's response to them. For example, nurses can ask any of the following questions:

- "Does it help to talk to someone about your worries?"
- "Have you ever tried any relaxation methods when you're nervous?"
- "Do you find that taking a walk helps you when your nerves are bad?"

Figure 13-1 illustrates the **Geriatric Anxiety Inventory (GAI)**, which is an evidence-based screening tool used widely in research and clinical settings for measuring anxiety level in older adults (Dissanayaka, Torbey, & Pachana, 2015; Kneebone, Fife-Schaw, Lincoln, et al., 2016; Ribeiro, Teixeira, Araújo, et al., 2015). This tool has been translated into more than two dozen languages, with consideration of cultural and language nuances. Although the GAI was developed for self-administration, nurses can ask older adults about each of the 20 items and score the tool. A positive response to nine or more items indicates the need for further evaluation. An important role for nurses is to facilitate referrals for further evaluation when symptoms of anxiety are identified by using this screening tool or the assessment guidelines discussed in this chapter.

Self-Esteem

Self-esteem cannot be measured numerically, but nurses can observe for verbal and nonverbal indicators. For example, a statement such as "You're wasting your time on me; you have more important things to do" is a clue to poor self-esteem. Nonverbal indicators of self-esteem include the way people dress, care for themselves, and present themselves to others. Although interpreting behaviors in relation to self-esteem must be done with caution, the following behaviors may be associated with low self-esteem: rigidity, procrastination, unnecessary apologies, lack of confidence, expectations of failure, exaggeration of deficits, disappointment in self, self-destructive behaviors, constant approval-seeking, overemphasis on weaknesses, inability to accept compliments, minimizing personal capabilities, disregarding one's own opinions, inability to form close relationships, inability to accept help from others, and inability to say "no" when appropriate. It may be acceptable to ask some questions, however, particularly about the person's perception of positive qualities.

In addition to observing for indicators of self-esteem, nurses can ask questions that give insight into the older

Please answer the items according to how you've felt in the last week.

Check the column under **Agree** if you mostly agree that the item describes you;
check the column under **Disagree** if you mostly disagree that the item describes you.

	Agree	Disagree
✱ I worry a lot of the time.		
I find it difficult to make a decision.		
I often feel jumpy.		
I find it hard to relax.		
I often cannot enjoy things because of my worries.		
✱ Little things bother me a lot.		
I often feel like I have butterflies in my stomach.		
✱ I think of myself as a worrier.		
I can't help worrying about even trivial things.		
✱ I often feel nervous.		
✱ My own thoughts often make me anxious.		
I get an upset stomach due to my worrying.		
I think of myself as a nervous person.		
I always anticipate the worst will happen.		
I often feel shaky inside.		
I think that my worries interfere with my life.		
My worries often overwhelm me.		
I sometimes feel a great knot in my stomach.		
I miss out on things because I worry too much.		
I often feel upset.		

A score of 9 or more checks in the AGREE column indicates the need for further evaluation.

Items preceded by ✱ are the ones most strongly associated with anxiety in older adults.

FIGURE 13-1 The Geriatric Anxiety Inventory. (Adapted with permission of UniQuest Pty Limited and the creators, Prof Nancy Pachana and Prof Gerard Byrne. Original GAI reference: Pachana, N. A., Byrne, G. J., Siddle, H., et al. (2007). Development and validation of the Geriatric Anxiety Inventory. *International Psychogeriatrics, 19,* 103–114. ©The University of Queensland, 2010. Copyright in the Geriatric Anxiety Inventory is the property of The University of Queensland. All content is protected by Australian copyright law and, by virtue of international treaties, equivalent copyright laws in other countries. The Geriatric Anxiety Inventory may not be reproduced or copied without the prior written permission of UniQuest Pty Limited.)

adult's self-perceptions. For example, a question such as "What is the quality in yourself that other people admire the most?" is nonthreatening. Moreover, this kind of question helps identify strengths that can be supported, and it provides clues to self-esteem. Nursing assessment is also directed toward identifying actual and potential threats to self-esteem, so they can be addressed through interventions, as discussed in Chapter 12.

Because self-esteem is influenced by the person's perception of the opinions held by significant others, it is important to identify who the significant others are for any particular person (e.g., peers; spouse or partner; authority figures; and people in the work, church, and social environments). Culture often defines who adopts the role of the significant other. Some Chinese American older adults, for example, expect their oldest son to look after their affairs and make key decisions about their health and well-being. Widows in some Middle Eastern and African cultures expect one of their husband's brothers to take care of them—an arrangement that fosters social and economic security for women who have lost a spouse. Being cared for by a family member (rather than by strangers) enhances self-esteem for older adults from all cultural backgrounds and increases the likelihood that their needs will be met as they age.

Depression

Depression is discussed as a general component of a psychosocial assessment in this chapter, and it is covered more comprehensively as an aspect of impaired psychosocial function in Chapter 15. Nurses can apply information in this chapter when assessing all older adults and use the information in Chapter 15 as a guide to assessing and caring for older adults who are depressed. Also, because cultural factors strongly influence the ways in which emotions are expressed, cultural considerations related to assessment of depression as described in Chapter 15 (Box 15-4) are pertinent to assessing expressions of emotions.

Nurses assess for depression by identifying verbal and nonverbal cues. Direct questions such as "Are you depressed?" are usually not effective in eliciting information because people may associate the word "depressed" with states of overwhelming grief. Older adults may be more comfortable responding to questions about whether they feel "sad," "blue," or "down in the dumps." Therefore, unless the older adult uses the term "depressed" to describe his or her feelings, other terminology is more likely to elicit an accurate response. As with other aspects of the mental status assessment, it is best to start with open-ended questions, such as "How are you feeling right now?" or "How have you been feeling this week?"

One of the purposes of an assessment of depression is to identify the person's usual patterns of coping with losses. For this reason, the nurse encourages older adults to express their feelings about significant changes in their lives. For instance, when an older adult talks about a change that might be experienced as a loss, nurses can ask nonthreatening questions that might lead to a discussion of feelings, such as "What's it like to live alone after 50 years of being married?" "How is life different since your friend moved away?" "Are there people you miss seeing since you retired?" "Are there any activities you miss doing since you no longer drive?" If the questions do not elicit information about feelings, the nurse can comment on specific feelings that the person is likely to be experiencing. For example, a remark such as "It seems like it would be pretty sad and lonely being here all by yourself after 55 years of marriage" allows the person to agree, disagree, or offer an alternative to the suggested feelings.

Happiness and Well-Being

Happiness in relation to aging is often equated with morale, wellness, contentment, well-being, life satisfaction, successful aging, quality of life, and "the good life." A literature review identified the following dimensions of well-being that can be addressed by health care professionals in relation to aging (Kiefer, 2008):

- Staying active
- Interacting with peers
- Feeling financially secure
- Having a sense of personal autonomy
- Setting personal goals and challenges
- Having positive social interactions
- Developing effective coping strategies
- Participating in exercise and sports activities
- Actively contributing to society through paid or volunteer work

Although nurses cannot address all these dimensions in a psychosocial assessment, they can include a few questions about happiness and well-being so they can identify ways of promoting wellness through nursing interventions. Psychologists sometimes use the following question to assess happiness: "Taking all things together, how would you say things are today—would you say you're very happy, pretty happy, or not too happy these days?" Nurses can ask a similar question such as "If you had to rate your present level of happiness on a scale of 0% to 100%, what rating would you give it?" Nurses can use the person's response as a base for additional questions such as "What would have to change to increase the rating by 10%?" "What kinds of things interfere with your happiness?" "If you could change one thing to be happier, what would it be?" Older adults will usually respond to these questions in a realistic manner, and their answers will provide information for establishing appropriate goals.

Box 13-8 summarizes the considerations involved in assessing components of affective function in older adults.

CONTACT WITH REALITY

Although a certain amount of fantasy is acceptable in everyday patterns of thinking, people are expected to remain in contact with the world around them and to respond appropriately to the same realities that others perceive. People lose contact with reality for numerous reasons including dementia, delirium, psychotic disorders, and a transient denial of a threatening reality. Many of these underlying conditions are treatable; however, when older adults lose contact with reality, they are likely to be labeled as "senile." Thus, because of stereotypes about older people, as well as the broad array of potential causes for loss of contact with reality, the assessment of an older person's contact with reality is particularly challenging.

Loss of contact with reality includes a wide range of behaviors ranging from simple and harmless misperceptions of reality to unyielding delusions or disturbing hallucinations. For example, people who are in the early stages of dementia may actively conceal or refuse to acknowledge memory deficits, and those in later stages of dementia may experience delusions that lead to behaviors that are inappropriate or even dangerous. For instance, if someone believes that his belongings have been stolen, he may report the theft to the police or insist on going out to look for the robber.

Box 13-8 Guidelines for Assessing Affective Function

General Affective Function

- Are the quantity and quality of emotions appropriate for the objective reality?
- What is the depth and duration of emotions regarding a particular event?
- What are the nonverbal cues to the person's affective state?
- How do sociocultural or environmental factors influence the person's expression of emotions?
- What terminology is acceptable to this person, particularly with regard to feelings such as anger, anxiety, and depression?
- Does the person have any pets, or has he or she lost any pets?

Observations and Questions to Assess Mood

- What is the person's usual affective state?
- What are the nonverbal indicators of the person's mood?

Observations and Questions to Assess Anxiety

- What are the nonverbal indicators of anxiety?
- What real or perceived threats are present that might be sources of anxiety for the person?
- Might any of the following factors be contributing to the person's anxiety: caffeine, pathologic conditions, medications, herbs, or interventions by folk or indigenous healers that act on the central or autonomic nervous systems?
- What methods of coping have the person tried, and what have been the effects of these interventions?
- "What kinds of things do you worry about?"
- "Do you have any worries that you'd be willing to discuss with me?"
- "Do you ever have trouble with your nerves?"

Observations and Questions to Assess Self-Esteem

- What verbal and nonverbal cues to self-esteem can be detected?
- What are the factors that influence self-esteem for this person?
- Does the environment present any real or potential threat to self-esteem?
- How are my actions as a nurse influencing the self-esteem of the older adult to whom I relate?
- Are caregiver attitudes and actions, such as infantilization or the promotion of unnecessary dependence, affecting the person's self-esteem?

Observations and Questions to Assess Depression

- What are the verbal and nonverbal cues to depression?
- "Do you ever feel blue or down in the dumps?"
- "How has your life changed since your husband died?"
- "What do you miss the most since you moved from your family home?"

Observations and Questions to Assess Happiness and Life Satisfaction

- How is the person's happiness and life satisfaction influenced by the following: functional abilities, personal relationships, and socioeconomic resources?
- "On a scale of 0% to 100%, how happy would you say you are right now?"
- "If you could change one thing to increase your happiness rating, what would it be?"

Three types of loss of contact with reality are delusions, hallucinations, and illusions, which are defined as follows:

- **Delusions**: Fixed false beliefs that have little or no basis in reality and cannot be corrected by appealing to reason.
- **Hallucinations**: Sensory experiences that have no basis in an external stimulus. Visual and auditory hallucinations are most common, but tactile, olfactory, and gustatory hallucinations also occur.
- **Illusions**: Misperceptions of an external stimulus. They may be mistaken for hallucinations, but differ in having some basis in reality, whereas hallucinations do not.

Just as a fever is one manifestation of a physical illness, loss of contact with reality is one manifestation of an underlying disorder. For example, common manifestations of loss of contact with reality in people with dementia include delusions, hallucinations, misidentification, and false accusations. Certain characteristics of delusions and hallucinations are associated with specific conditions such as delirium, dementia, and depression. In addition, loss of contact with reality typically occurs in combination with other manifestations of an underlying condition. Thus, an astute nursing assessment of contact with reality can provide essential information for identifying underlying causes. Table 13-2 shows distinguishing features of delusions, hallucinations, and illusions, and the following sections address these in relation to associated conditions that are most common in older adults. Chapter 14

discusses neuropsychiatric symptoms of dementia, which occur almost universally in people with dementia.

Delusions

Delusions are a psychological mechanism that helps people preserve their egos, maintain control over threatening situations, and organize information that is difficult to process. Paranoia (i.e., an extreme degree of suspiciousness) is a type of delusion that is common in older adults with dementia, as in the following examples:

- Accusing others of stealing their money or belongings
- Perceiving that they are being cheated, observed, attacked, persecuted, or sexually harassed
- Believing that others are entering their rooms when they are not there and moving things or messing up their belongings

Although the terms *paranoia* and *delusions* are sometimes used interchangeably in geriatric practice and references, this is inaccurate because there are many types of delusions.

In older adults, delusions can arise from pathologic conditions, such as delirium, dementia, depression, and paranoid disorder. Delusions associated with each of these disorders are characterized in unique ways and occur in combination with other manifestations of the underlying condition, as discussed in the following sections. Additional information

TABLE 13-2 Distinguishing Features of Delusions, Hallucinations, and Illusions

Underlying Cause	Accompanying Manifestations	Characteristics
Delirium	Diminished attention, a clouded state of consciousness, and other typical manifestations of delirium; metabolic disturbance, adverse medication effect, or other underlying cause	*Delusions:* Poorly organized, persecutory *Hallucinations:* Vivid, visual, colorful, threatening; accusatory auditory hallucinations induced by alcohol withdrawal *Illusions:* Brief, poorly organized
Dementia	Cognitive impairment (particularly memory deficits); alert level of consciousness. Agitation, anxiety, or wandering may be associated with loss of contact with reality. Neurologic manifestations may accompany hallucinations, particularly when the underlying cause is vascular dementia	*Delusions:* Not fixed, loosely organized, readily changed, or forgotten. Themes may include theft, fears, misidentification of places or people, and spousal infidelity *Illusions:* Occur more commonly than hallucinations; may be partially attributable to environmental factors *Hallucinations:* More often visual than auditory; may be partially attributable to environmental factors
Depression	Typical depressive symptoms including anorexia, lack of energy, sleep disturbances, and weight loss	*Delusions:* Themes may include death, guilt, money, illnesses, self-reproach, gloomy foreboding, diminished self-esteem, and feelings of worthlessness. There may be some basis in reality, but perceptions are exaggerated *Hallucinations:* Typically auditory and derogatory
Paranoid Disorder	Absence of cognitive deficits or affective disorders; long-term social isolation or suspicious personality; may be well hidden for years	*Delusions:* Fixed and well organized; may subside temporarily in different environments. Themes usually involve plots, noises, threats, obscenities, or sexual assaults *Hallucinations:* If present, these are related to the delusional themes

about psychotic symptoms of delirium and dementia is discussed in Chapter 14.

Delusions Associated With Pathophysiologic Conditions

Delusions arising from delirium are only one manifestation of a complex pathologic process that is further characterized by physiologic disturbances, diminished attention, a clouded state of consciousness, and sometimes hallucinations (described in Chapter 14) that subside once the delirium resolves. In addition to being associated with delirium, delusions may be caused by pathologic conditions, such as strokes or dementia. They also can be caused by abuse of or withdrawal from alcohol or drugs. Some of the physiologic disorders that are likely to cause delusions or hallucinations in older adults are listed in Table 13-3.

Delusions Associated With Dementia

Delusions occur commonly in people with dementia. Common delusional themes in people with dementia are theft, abandonment, suspiciousness, spousal infidelity, misidentification of familiar places or people, and loved ones who have died are still alive. Delusions in people with dementia can lead to problematic behaviors, which often are repetitive or even obsessive, as in the following examples:

- Accusing someone of being intent on harming the person
- Perceiving a family member as a stranger
- Believing that a family caregiver is intent on leaving (i.e., abandoning) the person
- Accusing others of stealing things
- Demanding that a family member leave the home that is shared by the person with dementia

- Refusing to let a caregiver or family member provide care because the person with dementia does not trust that person
- Insisting that a spouse or family member is not the person he or she claims to be
- Requesting to go home, even when the person is already at home
- Believing that one's spouse is having an affair
- Looking for a spouse or parent who has been deceased for many years, then grieving when informed that the person is dead
- Refusing to sleep in the same bed or room with spouse
- Believing that strangers are living in the house
- Insisting on leaving because "I need to go take care of the babies."

TABLE 13-3 Physiologic Disorders Causing Delusions or Hallucinations

Type of Disorder	Specific Examples
Metabolic disorders	Uremia, dehydration, electrolyte imbalance
Endocrine disorders	Hypoglycemia, thyroid disorders
Neurologic disorders	Stroke, cerebral trauma, cortical ischemia
Infections	Septicemia, pneumonia, urinary tract infections, subacute bacterial endocarditis
Adverse medication effects	Anticholinergics, anticonvulsants, antidepressants, antiparkinson agents, benzodiazepines, corticosteroids, digitalis toxicity, narcotics
Drug or alcohol abuse or withdrawal	Alcohol, barbiturates, meprobamate

For the person with dementia, delusions of danger, abandonment, and infidelity are associated with more discomfort compared with other delusional themes (Cohen-Mansfield, Cohen, Golander, et al., 2016). Studies suggest that certain delusional themes are associated with pathologic changes in specific brain regions—for example, misidentification delusions are associated with lesions in the right hemisphere and frontal lobe (Boublay, Schott, & Krolak-Salmon, 2016; Darby, Laganiere, Pascual-Leone, et al., 2017; Perini, Carlini, Pomati, et al., 2016).

People with dementia will readily talk about delusions, whereas those who do not have dementia typically withhold or are secretive about information. The challenge in assessing these delusions, however, is to identify the possible reality of the situation. It is imperative to recognize that not all accusations are unfounded just because people have serious cognitive impairments. Before labeling ideas as delusional, assess for any basis in reality because even the most bizarre-sounding assertions may be totally or partially true.

Another consideration is that communication techniques differ for people with psychosis or dementia. For example, the usual psychiatric nursing approach for delusions associated with psychosis is to talk with the client about the delusional thoughts as a problem in his or her life. In contrast, for people with dementia, it is more appropriate to avoid arguing and provide distractions. In addition, it is essential to address underlying feelings of fear, anxiety, and insecurity by providing reassurance. For example, it is usually effective to focus on the present with a reassuring statement, such as "I am staying here with you to make sure everything is OK, so let's have a little snack right now."

Delusions Associated With Depression

Persecutory and other delusions can be a manifestation of a major depression, but they are often overlooked or attributed to other factors, particularly in older adults living in community or long-term care settings. For example, when dementia and depression coexist, delusional thoughts may be attributed to dementia rather than being identified as an indicator of an affective disorder. Likewise, when a person with a paranoid personality becomes depressed, the delusions may be falsely attributed to the personality, particularly if the delusions are persecutory in nature. When delusions arise from depression, other manifestations of depression are usually identified in a thorough depression assessment, as discussed in Chapter 15.

Delusional themes may provide clues to an affective disorder, particularly if the focus is on a recent loss. Therefore, carefully listening to the content of the delusions is essential to an accurate assessment. In depressed older adults, delusional themes often revolve around an exaggerated emphasis on guilt, money, illnesses, self-reproach, gloomy foreboding, diminished self-esteem, or feelings of worthlessness. Although some basis may exist in reality, the feelings of being persecuted and deserving of punishment are grossly exaggerated. The following are some examples of delusions arising from depression:

- Mrs. N. believes that she is responsible for her husband's death; therefore, she believes she does not deserve help for her own illness.
- Mr. A. believes that his Medicare insurance has been canceled as punishment for his not cashing his Social Security check and insists that he cannot go to a doctor because he has no insurance.
- Ms. K. has an unshakable belief that she has undiagnosed cancer and begins to plan for her funeral, even though numerous doctors have not found any disease process.
- Mr. B., who recently had surgery for prostate cancer, is convinced that his house is going to explode from a gas leak and repeatedly calls the gas company to come check it.

Delusions Associated With Paranoid Disorder

Paranoid disorder—also called *paranoid ideation*—refers to a delusional disorder that is not associated with schizophrenia and is characterized by the tendency to view individuals or agencies with suspicion or as having harmful intentions. Factors associated with an increased risk for developing a late-life paranoid disorder include depression, social isolation, pathologic conditions, sensory impairment, and sense of loss of control over the environment. Common themes of paranoid delusions include spies, noises, threats, obscenities, lethal gases, bodily harm, stolen belongings, sexual infidelity or molestation, poisoned food or water, and having people enter living quarters by mysterious means at night. The delusions may occur more often when the person is socially isolated or in a particular environment, such as the home. If the person takes action based on the delusions, such as moving to another apartment or living with a family member, the delusions may subside temporarily.

Many people who have a paranoid disorder function well in the community, with the exception of one or two functional areas that are influenced by the delusions. Sometimes, a delusional state that was previously well hidden may surface when the person is admitted to a long-term care facility, and the staff may think that the problem is new. In other situations, nurses will identify a paranoid disorder on making a home visit or interviewing an older person who has been admitted to the hospital. If the person also suffers from dementia, the delusions may be interpreted mistakenly as evidence of advancing dementia. When this occurs, a recommendation for long-term institutional care may be made when other recommendations might be more appropriate.

Identifying a paranoid disorder in the psychosocial assessment is important so that the symptoms can be alleviated with appropriate interventions. When left unattended or written off as eccentricities, these disorders may progress and seriously disrupt functional abilities. Therefore, when delusions and cognitive impairments coexist, it is essential to determine whether the delusions existed before the dementia and to what extent, if any, they interfered with daily activities. If the delusions are part of a long-term pattern that has not interfered with the person's ability to function in daily life, the person may be able to remain in the community with support services and treatment directed toward the cognitive impairment. When delusions interfere with daily activities, however, medical intervention (e.g., psychotropic medications) may be effective in eliminating the delusions or minimizing their effects so that the person can maintain an independent level of function. When interventions are directed toward both the delusions and the cognitive impairment, the older person may be able to remain independent.

Hallucinations

In older adults, hallucinations are associated with dementia, depression, social isolation, sensory impairment, and physiologic disturbances including adverse medication effects. Visual hallucinations may develop in people with Parkinson disease and dementia with Lewy bodies, and are related not only to the disease but also to the medications (e.g., levodopa) used for treatment (Goldman, 2016; Hanagasi, Tufekcioglu, & Emre, 2017). As with delusions, it is important to identify the underlying cause of hallucinations, because the selection of appropriate interventions depends on an accurate assessment.

Some older adults are aware of—and can describe—their hallucinatory experiences, particularly when hallucinations are caused by the adverse effects of medications (e.g., anticholinergics) or Parkinson disease. However, in many situations, identification of hallucinations is based on astute observations of behaviors such as:

- Reaching out for objects that are not there
- Stepping over objects on the ground that are not visible to others
- Conversing with people who are not there
- Reporting sounds that have no environmental source (e.g., knocking, ringing)

An appropriate assessment technique is to elicit information from family and caregivers with a statement such as "Sometimes people see or hear things that others don't perceive. Do you notice any evidence of that happening to your father?"

Because hallucinations are abnormal sensory experiences, it is essential to assess for environmental influences and to make sure that sensory deficits are compensated for as much as possible. This is especially important for people with dementia because they may have difficulty processing information. For example, an older adult who has dementia and is visually impaired may look at a chair and misperceive it as someone sitting. Similarly, auditory hallucinations are more common in people who have impaired hearing. In these situations, appropriate nursing interventions are implemented to compensate as much as possible for hearing and vision impairments and to facilitate referrals for hearing and vision evaluations.

Hallucinations Associated With Pathophysiologic Conditions

Hallucinations are a common manifestation of delirium and are assessed with the larger context of this complex condition. Hallucinations associated with delirium are characterized as brief, vivid, visual, colorful, threatening, and poorly organized. Occasionally, hallucinations are the earliest sign of delirium, and they may be overlooked or attributed to another condition (e.g., dementia). Visual hallucinations also are symptoms of ophthalmic conditions, such as cataract, glaucoma, or age-related macular degeneration (Bernardin, Schwan, Lalanne, et al., 2017; Waters & Fernyhough, 2017).

Hallucinations arising from drug or alcohol withdrawal may occur during the first days of admission to an acute care setting or in any circumstance in which the person suddenly does not have access to their usual drugs or alcohol. Auditory hallucinations associated with alcohol withdrawal are typically accusatory and threatening, and they are sometimes organized into a complete paranoid system. The detection of alcohol-induced delirium is particularly important in acute care settings because people who are dependent on alcohol are more likely to acknowledge the problem and agree to appropriate interventions when they are in a crisis. The following example illustrates such a situation.

Case Study

Mr. K. is 73 years old and has been caring for his wife, who has Alzheimer disease, for several years. He is a very proud man who has difficulty accepting help. One morning, Mr. K. begins vomiting coffee-ground emesis and is admitted to an acute care setting with the diagnosis of gastrointestinal bleeding. On admission, Mr. K. is very pleasant and expresses concern about his wife's care. The next morning, Mr. K. complains angrily to the nurses about the bars on the windows and is belligerent about the fact that he has been put in jail. He develops additional manifestations of delirium and is treated for alcohol withdrawal.

When the delirium subsides, the nurse initiates a conversation about the care of his wife and asks him how he copes with the responsibility. Mr. K. admits that he has difficulty coping with his and his wife's declining health and his increasing loneliness and responsibilities. He has always been a social drinker, but he has gradually increased his consumption of alcohol to three six-packs of beer a day. As part of the discharge plan, Mr. K. agrees to talk with a sponsor from Alcoholics Anonymous.

Table 13-2 summarizes the physiologic disorders, including some adverse medication effects, which are most likely to cause hallucinations.

Hallucinations Associated With Dementia

Hallucinations and illusions may occur at any time in the course of a dementing illness and are also likely to occur during a transient ischemic attack—a condition associated with vascular dementia. Visual illusions and hallucinations are a key diagnostic indicator of Parkinson disease and dementia with Lewy bodies (Onyike, 2016). When illusions occur, they are often related to environmental conditions that can be modified. For example, poor lighting or reflections from glass or mirrors can cause visual illusions, and background noise can contribute to auditory illusions, particularly for people with hearing aids.

Psychiatric literature usually addresses illusions only with regard to misperceptions of visual or auditory stimuli, whereas an illusion, by definition, is a misinterpretation of any external stimulus. Nurses who care for people with dementia can cite numerous examples of behaviors that fit this broader definition of an illusion, such as the following:

- Mistaking the identity of caregivers, family members, or other familiar people
- Perceiving an object as something other than what it really is
- Taking an object under the mistaken belief that it belongs to them
- Refusing to believe that they are in their home when they really are

These experiences might be labeled as delusions or disorientation, but they are more accurately defined as illusions because they involve a misinterpretation of reality rather than a false perception that has no base in reality.

Hallucinations Associated With Depression

Severely depressed older adults are more likely to experience delusions rather than hallucinations, but visual and auditory hallucinations of deceased loved ones commonly occur during periods of bereavement. Hallucinations associated with depression are likely to be auditory and derogatory, or they may involve visual perceptions of dead people. The following examples are typical of hallucinations arising from depression:

- Ms. C. reports that at night she hears the people in the next apartment saying that she has cancer.
- Mr. T. reports hearing younger men say that he is sexually impotent and that he was not a good provider to his wife (who died within the past year).
- Ms. F. looks down from her second-floor window and sees a man, dressed in black, lying injured on the sidewalk.
- Mr. S. insists that there is a pervasive smell of skunk coming from his basement, and he believes he will be contaminated if he goes downstairs.

Hallucinations Associated With Paranoid Disorder

If hallucinations are a symptom of paranoid disorder, they are likely to be closely related to the theme of the delusions. The following examples are characteristic of hallucinations arising from paranoid states:

- Mr. J. says that he hears people in the next apartment talking about him. These are the same people whom he

believes will come in and steal things when he leaves the apartment.
- Ms. J. reports seeing men observing her when she undresses or takes a bath. Moreover, when she goes to the grocery store, the man at the checkout always offers her money in exchange for sexual favors.

Table 13-3 summarizes the characteristics that distinguish delusions, hallucinations, and illusions according to their underlying causes.

Special Considerations for Assessing Contact With Reality in Older Adults

Assessment of contact with reality presents a special assessment challenge for nurses for a variety of reasons:

- People often try to conceal delusions and hallucinations.
- When delusions and hallucinations arise from social isolation, opportunities for assessment are extremely limited.
- To determine whether a reported experience is delusional, the nurse needs information about the reality, which is difficult to obtain if a reliable and objective observer is not available.
- Even after delusions or hallucinations are identified as such, the underlying factors may be difficult to identify.
- Older adults often have more than one underlying condition, such as a delirium superimposed on a dementia.

Delusions are usually more readily acknowledged than hallucinations, and the most effective tools for assessing delusions are asking leading questions and listening attentively. Most older adults will confide their delusions to a nurse who they perceive as interested, sympathetic, and nonjudgmental, particularly if a trusting relationship has been established. Difficulty arises, however, when nurses hear information that may be interpreted as delusional but, in fact, is based wholly or partially in reality. For example, financial exploitation, violation of rights, and other aspects of elder abuse are not uncommon, particularly in older adults who are cognitively impaired or who live with family members who are psychosocially impaired. When older adults who have cognitive impairments or a lifelong suspicious personality describe abusive or exploitative situations, they are likely to be considered delusional or not to be taken seriously. In these situations, the assessment challenge is to determine what is real, what is distorted, and what is not based at all in reality.

Nurses also consider the potential effects of environmental and interpersonal factors in contributing to delusions, illusions, or hallucinations. For example, the reflection of fluorescent lights on a highly polished floor can produce the illusion of water on the floor, and an older adult might walk around the reflection. Stressful interpersonal relationships may contribute to the development of paranoid ideations, particularly in the context of past or present exploitation or abuse. Another important assessment consideration is whether a lack of assistive devices, such as eyeglasses and hearing aids, is contributing to altered perceptions. For example, if someone usually depends on eyeglasses, contact

Box 13-9 Guidelines for Assessing Contact With Reality

General Principles

- In assessing any loss of contact with reality, the effects of alcohol, medications, and physiologic disturbances must always be considered as potential causative influences.
- People who are not cognitively impaired are usually more reluctant to talk about delusions and hallucinations than people who have dementia.
- When people talk about things that might be delusional, it is important to determine, through information provided by a reliable and objective observer, whether their perceptions have any basis in reality.
- When delusions are initially identified, it is important to determine whether they are of recent onset or have been long-standing but only recently discovered.
- When delusions are identified in someone who has dementia, it is particularly important to consider the influence of treatable causative factors, such as depression or physiologic disturbances.
- People who have dementia are likely to have illusions rather than hallucinations.

- People who are socially isolated are usually quite successful in concealing hallucinations.
- In assessing hallucinations and illusions, it is particularly important to consider the influence of the environment.

Interview Questions to Assess Delusions, Hallucinations, and Illusions

- "Do you have any thoughts that you can't seem to get rid of?"
- "People sometimes have thoughts that they're afraid to talk about because they believe others will think they're 'crazy.' Do you ever have thoughts like that?"
- "Do you sometimes hear voices when you're alone?"
- "Do you sometimes think you see things that other people don't see?"

Nonverbal Clues to Hallucinations

- Extreme withdrawal and isolation
- Contentment with social isolation, particularly if the person previously had many social contacts
- Gestures and other actions that normally occur in response to perceived stimuli

---

lenses, or a hearing aid for adequate visual or auditory function, the absence of these items may contribute to the development of illusions or hallucinations.

During the assessment, nurses consider cultural factors that are likely to influence perceptions of reality and manifestations of mental illness, as discussed in Chapter 12. Religious background is a common cultural factor that can influence the content of delusions or hallucinations. For example, delusions and hallucinations in Irish Catholics are likely to focus on Jesus, a saint, or the Virgin Mary. Similarly, Muslims with African, Near Eastern, or Middle Eastern cultural heritage may focus on the Prophet Mohammed. Box 13-9 summarizes guidelines for assessing an individual's contact with reality.

SOCIAL SUPPORTS

Social supports, which are categorized as *informal* and *formal,* refer to the services provided to address functional and psychosocial needs. Although even the most independent people receive social supports (e.g., emotional support from family and friends), social supports are usually discussed in relation to meeting the needs of people who depend on others in some way for assistance. While friends, family, clergy, neighbors, or coworkers provide informal social support, workers who are paid by the older person or their family or by health and social service agencies or institutions provide formal social support.

Social supports significantly influence psychosocial function in older adults because they affect one's ability to cope with stressful life experiences by buffering them against harmful effects and improving one's physical and emotional well-being. Because the importance of social supports increases in relation to the degree of impairment of the

older adult, it is essential to assess the social supports for any older adults who have conditions that affect their functional abilities. Nursing assessment of social supports identifies not only the resources that are needed, available, or being used to support the highest level of functioning but also the barriers to the use of appropriate resources. Specific aspects of social supports that nurses assess include social network, economic resources, and religion and spirituality. Box 13-10 summarizes important questions and considerations involved in assessing social supports.

Social Network

Nursing assessment of the social network addresses the social supports that are important for day-to-day functioning as well as those that affect the person's quality of life. The nurse can initiate the assessment by asking a broad question such as "Whom do you rely on for help?" The nurse can then ask more specific questions about how the person accomplishes tasks that are most important for day-to-day function. For example, in discussing a follow-up appointment for medical care, the nurse may ask, "How do you get to your doctor appointments?" Because a relationship with a confidant(e) is a significant predictor of quality of life for older adults, at least one question relating to this factor should be posed, such as "Is there anyone you can talk to about your worries?" The answer to this question may also be important if the nurse or health care team is assisting the older adult with a decision about long-term care because the older adult may want the confidant(e) to be involved in the decision-making process. In addition, the response to this question may provide important information about whether the older person has recently experienced a loss, or change in the availability, of a confidant(e).

After identifying existing social networks, the nurse identifies the resources that might be helpful in addressing unmet

Box 13-10 Guidelines for Assessing Social Supports

Interview Questions to Assess Social Supports

- "On whom do you rely for help?"
- "Is there anyone who helps you with grocery shopping? Getting to doctor appointments? Getting prescriptions filled? Managing your money and paying bills?"
- "Is there anyone you can talk to when you have worries or difficulties?"
- "Is there anything you would like help with that you don't have help with now?"
- "Is there anyone in the family who could help with grocery shopping?"
- "Have you ever received information about the transportation services (or meals, or other services) that are available through the senior center?"

Potential Barriers to the Use of Formal Supports

- Unwillingness to acknowledge, or lack of insight to recognize, the need for services
- Expectation that family members will provide the needed care
- Unwillingness to admit that family members cannot or will not provide the needed care
- Lack of financial resources to purchase services, or unwillingness to spend money for services
- Perceived correlation between formal services and "welfare"
- Lack of transportation to access services
- Mistrust of service providers or an unwillingness to allow outsiders into the home

- Bad experiences with service providers or hearsay about the bad experiences of others
- Fear that the home situation will be judged as socially unacceptable, or embarrassment because it is socially unacceptable
- Fear that having outsiders in the house will lead to admission to a nursing home
- Lack of time, energy, or problem-solving ability to obtain information about and select the appropriate services
- Fear that the service will be provided by someone about whom the care recipient holds prejudices
- Language and cultural barriers

Interview Questions to Assess Financial Resources

- "Do you have any money worries?"
- "Do you have any concerns about paying for services that you might need?"
- "Would you like to talk to someone about any financial concerns?"
- "Do you think you can afford the kind of help that your doctor recommended?"
- "Have you received any advice about financial planning for nursing home care?"

Interview Questions to Assess Religious Affiliation

- "Do you belong to any church, synagogue, or mosque?"
- "Are you aware of any programs available at your church, synagogue, or mosque that might be helpful to you?"

---

needs. Such questions as "Do you have any grandchildren or neighbors who could help with shoveling the snow?" are aimed at identifying informal supports that are available but are not currently being used. A question such as "Are you aware that the senior center has a van that takes people to doctor appointments?" is aimed at identifying the person's awareness of formal supports that may not be in use.

Barriers to Obtaining Social Supports

In addition to assessing the number and types of social supports available, nurses try to identify the barriers that interfere with the use of social supports. Many older adults who are eligible for service programs do not use these resources because they view them as costly, impersonal, overly structured, and hard to arrange. Because older adults prefer to receive help from family and friends, negative attitudes about the use of formal social supports may be a source of resistance to their use. Without adequate informal supports, or when conflicts exist between older adults and their informal supports, an increase in dependence can trigger less effective coping mechanisms. The following case study is typical of such a situation.

In addition to some older people's preference for obtaining services from families rather than outside agencies, there are many other barriers to the use of formal services. Fears about outsiders coming into the home rank high among the barriers to the provision of in-home services. Financial

barriers also often exist, either because of an inability or an unwillingness to pay for services. Additional barriers include unwillingness to accept help, lack of knowledge about types of services available, and not knowing where to go for specific services. The identification of these barriers is essential because counseling and educational interventions (e.g., providing information about services that are available) can address many of these issues. Issues that are not amenable to intervention may represent impenetrable barriers to the provision of social supports.

Case Study

Mr. and Mrs. D. are 81 and 79 years old, respectively. They always expected their children to care for them, but the children moved to other cities and visit several times a year. Mr. and Mrs. D. refuse to accept any of the formal services that are available because of their cost, and also because they expect their children to provide the services out of filial responsibility. Furthermore, Mrs. D. cared for her parents when they were old, so she expects her daughter to do the same for her.

Mr. and Mrs. D. frequently call their daughter and son-in-law to complain about their inability to get groceries and go to doctors' appointments. Rather than make use of transportation or other services available from the community, they neglect themselves. During the children's visit over the

Christmas holiday, they find that their parents have not been eating adequately and are not taking their prescribed medications. When they mention these observations to their parents, Mr. and Mrs. D. respond, "If you loved us, you'd be taking care of us, and this wouldn't be happening."

Assessing barriers to support services is particularly challenging because direct questions about these issues often are inappropriate and usually are very threatening. Rather, identification of these barriers is best accomplished by carefully listening to older people and their caregivers and by asking nonthreatening questions. For example, a caregiver might talk about a friend who had a home health aide who did nothing but watch television all day and got paid $18 an hour. In response to this, the nurse might ask, "Do you think that might happen if we arrange for a home health aide to care for your father?" Other attitudinal barriers, such as prejudices, may be identified through statements made by the caregiver about prior experiences.

Economic Resources

Financial issues are generally within the purview of social workers, and nurses usually prefer to avoid discussing money with older adults or their families. In planning for formal services for older adults, however, some assessment of financial assets is necessary, and the nurse is often the health care professional who obtains this information, particularly in home or other community settings. If no long-term care or community-based services are needed, the nurse can forego the financial assessment.

Many older adults and their families are shocked to find out that Medicare does not cover the costs of long-term care, with the exception of skilled care. In addition, people are often appalled by the restrictive definition of skilled care as well as many other restrictions that are applied to determine eligibility for services. Even if a social worker has explained these facts, it is usually the nurse who deals with the related anxiety and other emotional reactions of the older adults and their families. Because nurses are in a position to help older adults and their families address and cope with the financial issues of long-term care, they frequently become involved in assessing the financial resources of the person and family.

It is not always necessary to ask details about monthly income or the exact amount of savings and assets, but questions must be asked about the resources available for the purchase of services. Asking a question such as "Do you have any money worries?" might reveal some anxieties that can be dealt with or allayed through counseling or the provision of accurate information. When the nurse reviews with the older adult or caregiver the services that are available, information also can be provided about the cost of these services, at which time a question such as "Do you think you could afford this kind of help?" can be posed.

RELIGION AND SPIRITUALITY

As discussed in Chapter 12, religion and spirituality become more important in older adulthood, and they are resources that should be identified as part of a comprehensive psychosocial assessment. The person's religious affiliation is assessed as a component of his or her social supports, whereas spirituality is assessed as a separate component of the psychosocial assessment. It is important to recognize that spirituality is an integral component of all humans but not all people identify with a religious affiliation.

Identification of religious affiliation is a simple but important part of the psychosocial assessment, because available religion-based programs for older adults may be perceived as more acceptable than those provided by a public or nonreligious agency. For example, an older Jewish adult might be willing to go to the Jewish Community Center for a senior meal program, and an older Roman Catholic adult might be willing to accept mental health services from Catholic Social Services, but these people might refuse to avail themselves of the same kinds of services when they are offered by another organization. Often, religion-based services are viewed by the older adult as services that they deserve as a reward for years of attendance at or service to a church or synagogue. Although most religion-based programs serve older adults regardless of their religious affiliations, the programs are often perceived as more appropriate if the person is of the same faith.

In addition to being perceived as more appropriate, some religion-based services are not available elsewhere and they are often provided by trained volunteers free of charge. Examples of programs or services that may be available to members of a particular church, synagogue, or mosque include transportation, respite care, peer counseling, chore assistance, friendly visiting, and telephone reassurance. Older adults can also take advantage of any church-, synagogue-, or mosque-based program that is available for people of all ages. The Stephen Ministries, founded in 1975, is an example of a volunteer program that is available in many Christian denominations throughout the United States. This program offers peer counseling and other services provided by volunteers with special training in ministering to older, depressed, shut-in, and grieving persons.

Identification of a specific place of worship is also important because attendance at religious services may be a significant factor in the older adult's social life. For many older adults, particularly those with limited mobility or those who have full-time caregiving responsibilities, attendance at religious services is their only opportunity for social interaction and personal support. Most people who are unable to attend religious services can arrange for home visits by a clergy person or lay minister; indeed, these visits may be the only source of outside contact and emotional support that is acceptable to a home-bound older adult. Moreover, for people who are socially isolated, a visitor from their place of worship may be the only person monitoring the home situation. In these situations, health professionals who are concerned about home-bound older adults may be able to monitor their status through these visitors. The following case study describes a situation in which the nurse's contact with a lay minister was an important part of the discharge plan.

Spirituality is increasingly being recognized as an essential component of well-being for all humans and for older adults in particular, as discussed in Chapter 12. The intent of a spiritual assessment is not to evaluate whether a person is more or less spiritual; rather, the purpose is to identify indicators of spiritual distress, so these can be addressed in holistic care plans. Spiritual distress often occurs in the context of transitions that older adults face, such as needing to move from their homes or making decisions about treatments for serious conditions. Another purpose is to identify sources of strength and meaning in the older adult's life, so these can be supported. Nurses can introduce the topic of spiritual assessment with statements such as "Many people draw on spiritual or religious resources during times of illness and suffering. Is this true for you as well, and if so, can you tell me more about that?" (Westera, 2017, p. 128).

An easy-to-use and evidence-based tool for four domains of spiritual assessment is the FICA, which is an acronym for **F**aith and belief, **I**mportance of beliefs, **C**ommunity for support, and concerns to **A**ddress in care. Online Learning Activity 13-3 provides the link to this tool and additional information about how to use it in clinical settings.

Nurses, like many people, may not be comfortable discussing spirituality, but they can increase their comfort level by recognizing their own feelings and viewing spirituality as a universal human need. It also is helpful to recognize that many of the communication skills used in the course of providing nursing care are also effective for addressing spiritual needs. For example, active listening, intentional presence, and expressions of empathy are effective for providing spiritual care (Burkhardt & Nagai-Jacobson, 2016). Box 13-11 presents guidelines for assessing spiritual needs, and Online Learning Activity 13-3 provides a link to a nursing article describing a study pertinent to the topic of spiritual assessment.

 ONLINE LEARNING ACTIVITY 13-3: ADDITIONAL INFORMATION ABOUT ASSESSMENT OF SPIRITUALITY IN OLDER ADULTS AND AN ARTICLE DESCRIBING A STUDY ABOUT WAYS IN WHICH NURSES ASSESS PATIENTS' SPIRITUAL WELL-BEING at http://thepoint.lww.com/Miller8e.

 Box 13-11 Guidelines for Assessing Spiritual Needs

Guidelines for Nursing Assessment

- Be aware of your own feelings about spirituality, so that you can recognize and respond to the spiritual needs of others.
- Recognize that spiritual needs are a universal human phenomenon. Although not all people experience spiritual distress, all people have spiritual needs and the potential for spiritual growth.
- Recognize that it is within the realm of holistic nursing care to identify and plan interventions for spiritual growth as well as for spiritual distress.
- Convey a nonjudgmental, open-minded attitude when eliciting information about a person's spirituality and religious beliefs.

Questions to Assess Spiritual Health

- "What in your life is meaningful and important?"
- "What do you hope to accomplish in your life?"
- "What do you do that gives you pleasure and satisfaction?"
- "Who are the people you can turn to when you need someone to listen to you or to help you?"
- "Do you believe in a higher being?" (e.g., God, Goddess, Divinity) "How do you describe this being?"
- "Do you participate in any activities (rituals) that foster a connection with a higher being?" (e.g., prayer or other religious activities)
- "What activities are helpful in bringing you inner peace and relieving stress?" (e.g., meditation, walking in the woods)
- "What are your beliefs about death?"
- "Do you see a connection between your body, your mind, your emotions, and your soul?"

- "Is there anything you need or would like to have to support your beliefs and your spiritual needs?" (e.g., Bible, sacred or revered object)
- "Would you like to arrange a visit from a spiritual leader?"
- "Are there any health practices that you would like to consider, even though our society may not consider them to be conventional?" (e.g., therapeutic touch, guided imagery)

Observations/Questions to Assess Spiritual Distress

- During the psychosocial interview, listen for clues to spiritual distress, such as the following: suicidal ideation; anger toward God; inability to forgive others; feelings of hopelessness, uselessness, or abandonment; questions about the meaning of life, losses, or suffering.
- "Are there any conflicts between your beliefs or values and actions that you feel you should be taking?" (e.g., feeling entitled to some time to oneself, which may be in conflict with the demands of caregiving for a spouse)
- "Are there any conflicts between what you believe in and what society or health care professionals are encouraging or suggesting you do?" (e.g., questioning the wisdom of using a feeding tube for a spouse who is chronically and severely impaired and unable to participate in the decision)
- "Do you have any special religious considerations that are not being addressed?" (e.g., dietary practices, observance of religious holidays)
- *For people in institutional settings:* "Is there anything here that interferes with your spiritual needs?" (e.g., noisy environment, lack of privacy)

Case Study

Mr. V. was admitted to the hospital after a syncopal episode that resulted in a minor car accident. On admission, Mr. V. was slightly unkempt and showed some memory deficits, but his self-care abilities improved during his 2-day hospitalization. The nurse suggested that Mr. V. consider home-delivered meals and the use of other community resources, but he refused these services. His situation did not warrant a report to a protective services agency.

The nurse was concerned because Mr. V. lived alone and had no outside contacts other than Ms. C., a lay minister who had visited weekly for 2 years. The nurse asked for and received permission from Mr. V. to contact Ms. C. to inform her of available community services. Ms. C. was grateful for the information and said that she would contact the appropriate agencies if Mr. V.'s condition declined or if he agreed to accept help.

Chapter Highlights

Overview of Psychosocial Assessment of Older Adults

- Psychosocial assessment is a complex process that involves the use of good communication skills, appropriate interview questions, purposeful observations, and relevant assessment tools.
- Nurses can assess their own attitudes to increase their comfort level in performing a psychosocial assessment of older adults (Box 13-1).

Communication Skills for Psychosocial Assessment (Boxes 13-2 to 13-4)

- Barriers to communication are associated with the situation, the older adult, and the person who is communicating.
- Establishing rapport, using touch if appropriate, listening, asking questions, and giving feedback can enhance communication during psychosocial assessment.
- Nurses create an environment for effective communication by speaking face-to-face at eye level, respecting the person's comfort zone, ensuring privacy, eliminating distractions, and facilitating optimal vision and hearing function.
- It is important to be aware of cultural influences on communication, particularly regarding nonverbal communication.

Mental Status Assessment (Boxes 13-5 to 13-7; Table 13-1)

- An assessment of mental status involves an assessment of all of the following: physical appearance, motor function, social skills, response to the interview, orientation, alertness and attention, memory, speech characteristics, and calculation and higher language skills.

Decision Making and Executive Function

- Assessment of cognitive skills, such as executive function, is particularly important for determining the ability of the older adult to participate in decision making.
- Insight, learning, memory, reasoning, judgment, problem solving, and abstract thinking are some of the cognitive skills that are involved with decision making.

Affective Function (Box 13-8)

- An assessment of affective function includes consideration of mood, anxiety, self-esteem, depression, and happiness and well-being.

Contact With Reality (Box 13-9; Tables 13-2 and 13-3)

- Nurses assess contact with reality within the context of behavioral indicators to identify potential underlying causes of any loss of contact with reality.
- Conditions associated with delusions and hallucinations in older adults include dementia, depression, paranoid disorder, and pathophysiologic conditions.

Social Supports (Box 13-10)

- Psychosocial assessment identifies social supports and economic resources, as well as barriers to obtaining services.

Religion and Spirituality (Box 13-11)

- A holistic nursing assessment addresses religious affiliation and spirituality.

Critical Thinking Exercises

1. Complete the psychosocial self-assessment in Box 13-1.
2. Think of several different situations in the past few weeks in which you worked with older adults and answer the following questions:
   - What aspects of psychosocial function did you observe?
   - What questions did you ask that would give you information about their psychosocial function?
   - What information did you obtain about their social supports?
3. Name at least three things you would observe or determine in order to assess each of the following when you are working with older adults: physical appearance, social skills, orientation, alertness and attention, memory, speech characteristics, calculation and higher language skills, decision-making skills, anxiety, self-esteem, depression, and contact with reality.
4. What questions would you ask an older adult to identify social supports and barriers to the use of services?

5. What approach would you use to assess an older adult's spiritual health and identify spiritual distress?

 For more information about the topics discussed in this chapter, be sure to check out the interactive Online Learning Activities and other helpful resources at http://thepoint.lww.com/Miller8e.

REFERENCES

Adamis, D., Meagher, D., Murray, O., et al. (2016). Evaluating attention in delirium: A comparison of bedside tests of attention. *Geriatrics and Gerontology International, 16*, 1028–1035.

Bernardin, F., Schwan, R., Lalanne, L., et al. (2017). The role of the retina in visual hallucinations: A review of the literature and implications for psychosis. *Neuropsychologia, 99*, 128–138.

Boublay, N., Schott, A. M., & Krolak-Salmon, P. (2016). Neuroimaging correlates of neuropsychiatric symptoms in Alzheimer's disease: A review of 20 years of research. *European Journal of Neurology, 23*, 1500–1509.

Burkhardt, M., & Nagai-Jacobson, M. (2016). Spirituality and health. In B. M. Dossey, & L. Keegan (Eds.), *Holistic nursing: A handbook for practice* (7th ed., pp. 135–163). Boston, MA: Jones & Bartlett.

Ciesielska, N., Sokolowski, R., Mazur, E., et al. (2016). Is the Montreal Cognitive Assessment (MoCA) test better suited than the Mini-Mental State Examination (MMSE) in mild cognitive impairment (MCI) detection among people aged over 60? Meta-analysis. *Psychiatria Polska, 50*, 1039–1052.

Cohen-Mansfield, J., Cohen, R., Golander, H., et al. (2016). The impact of psychotic symptoms on persons with dementia experiencing them. *American Journal of Geriatric Psychiatry, 24*, 213–220.

Darby, R. R., Laganiere, S., Pascual-Leone, A., et al. (2017). Finding the imposter: Brain connectivity of lesions causing delusional misidentifications. *Brain, 140*(Pt 2), 497–507.

De J., Wand, A. P., Smerdely, P. I., et al. (2016). Validating the 4A's test in screening for delirium in a culturally diverse geriatric inpatient population. *International Journal of Geriatric Psychiatry,* doi: 10.1002/gps.4615 [Epub ahead of print].

Dissanayaka, N. N., Torbey, E., & Pachana, N. A. (2015). Anxiety rating scales in Parkinson's disease: A critical review. *International Psychogeriatrics, 27*, 1777–1784.

Goldman, J. (2016). Neuropsychiatric issues in Parkinson disease. *Continuum, 22*, 1086–1103.

Gould, C., O'Hara, R., Goldstein, M. K., et al. (2016). Multimorbidity is associated with anxiety in older adults in the Health and Retirement Study. *International Journal of Geriatric Psychiatry, 31*, 1105–1115.

Grossman, M., & Irwin, D. J. (2016). The mental status examination in patients with suspected dementia. *Continuum, 22*, 385–403.

Hanagasi, H. A., Tufekcioglu, Z., & Emre, M. (2017). Dementia in Parkinson's disease. *Journal of Neurologic Sciences, 374*, 26–31.

Heeren, P., Flamaing, J., Tournoy, J., et al. (2016). Assessing cognitive function. In M. Boltz, E. Capezuti, T. Fulmer, & D. Zwicker (Eds.), *Evidence-based geriatric nursing protocols for best practice* (pp. 77–88). New York: Springer Publishing Company.

Hendry, K., Quinn, T. J., Evans, J., et al. (2016). Evaluation of delirium screening tools in geriatric medical inpatients: A diagnostic test accuracy study. *Age & Ageing, 45*, 832–837.

Hill, N. L., Mogle, J., Wion, R., et al. (2016). Subjective cognitive impairment and affective symptoms: A systematic review. *The Gerontologist, 56*(6):e109–e127.

Kiefer, R. A., (2008). An integrative review of the concept of well-being. *Holistic nursing practice, 22*, 244–252.

Kneebone, I. I, Fife-Schaw, C., Lincoln, N. B., et al. (2016). A study of the validity and the reality of the Geriatric Anxiety Inventory in screening for anxiety after stroke in older inpatients. *Clinical Rehabilitation, 30*, 1220–1228.

Larner, A. J. (2017). Short Montreal Cognitive Assessment. *Journal of Geriatric Psychiatry and Neurology, 30*, 104–108.

Leonard, M., O'Connell, H., Williams, O., et al. (2016). Attention, vigilance and visuospatial function in hospitalized medical patients: Relationship to neurocognitive diagnosis. *Journal of Psychosomatic Research, 90*, 84–90.

Lindauer, A., Seelye, A., Lyons, B., et al. (2017). Dementia care comes home: Patient and caregiver assessment via telemedicine. *Gerontologist,* doi: 10.1093/geront/gnw206 [Epub ahead of print].

Onyike, C. U. (2016). Psychiatric aspects of dementia. *Continuum, 22*, 600–614.

Perini, G., Carlini, A., Pomati, S., et al. (2016). Misidentification delusions: Prevalence in different types of dementia and validation of a structured questionnaire. *Alzheimer's Disease and Associated Disorders, 30*, 331–337.

Ribeiro, O., Teixeira, L., Araújo, L., et al. (2015). Predictors of anxiety in centenarians: Health, economic factors, and loneliness. *International Psychogeriatrics, 27*, 1167–1176.

Roalf, D. R., Moore, T. M., Mechanic-Hamilton, D., et al. (2017). Bridging cognitive screening tests in neurologic disorders: A crosswalk between the short Montreal Cognitive Assessment and Mini-Mental State Examination. *Alzheimer's Dementia,* doi: 10.1016/j.jalz.2017.01.015 [Epub ahead of print].

Wadsworth, H. E., Galusha-Glasscock, J. M., Womack, K. B., et al. (2016). Remote neuropsychological assessment in rural American Indians with and without cognitive impairment. *Archives of Clinical Neuropsychology, 31*, 420–425.

Waters, F., & Fernyhough, C. (2017). Hallucinations: A systematic review of points of similarity and difference across diagnostic classes. *Schizophrenia Bulletin, 43*, 32–43.

Westera, D. A. (2017). *Spirituality in nursing practice.* New York: Springer Publishing Company.

Williams, M. G., Voss, A., Vahle, B., et al. (2016). Using the FICA spiritual history tool to assess patients' spirituality. *Nurse Educator, 41*, E6–E9.

chapter 14

Impaired Cognitive Function: Delirium and Dementia

Healthy older adults experience only minor changes in cognitive abilities (as described in Chapter 11), but as people age, they are increasingly likely to experience pathologic conditions that have a major impact on cognitive function. Nurses in all settings frequently care for older adults who have dementia or delirium, which are the two main causes of significant cognitive impairment in older adults. Nurses are responsible for identifying factors that contribute to impaired cognitive functioning in older adults. In addition, nurses and others who care for people with dementia must meet the challenge of preserving as much of the person's dignity and quality of life as possible, despite the serious and progressive losses the person with dementia experiences.

Delirium

OVERVIEW OF DELIRIUM

Although delirium has been documented in patients for centuries, only in recent years have researchers and practitioners addressed delirium as a serious, preventable, treatable, commonly occurring, and often unrecognized condition that disproportionately affects older adults. Delirium is a syndrome that develops over hours or days, fluctuates over the course of the day, and can persist for months. Changes in mental status involve problems with attention and consciousness and several or many additional changes, including altered sleep–wake patterns.

 ### PREVALENCE, RISK FACTORS, AND FUNCTIONAL CONSEQUENCES OF DELIRIUM

Studies indicate that delirium is present in 10% to 31% of medical patients on admission, with an additional 11% to 42% developing delirium after admission (Tullmann, Blevins, & Fletcher, 2016). Delirium also occurs in postacute care settings, residential care facilities, and home settings; however, little evidence-based information is available about delirium in nonhospital settings.

Delirium results from an interaction between *predisposing factors,* which increase the person's vulnerability, and *precipitating factors,* which account for the immediate threat. The most commonly identified predisposing factors include advanced age, dementia, depression, functional dependency, and number of medications. Common precipitating factors include surgery, infections, serious illness, and physical restraints. The risk for developing delirium is highest for people with several predisposing factors in combination with one or more precipitating factors. The risk also is disproportionately high in older adults with dementia, with dementia accounting for 65% of the cases of delirium in hospital settings (Jackson, Gladman, Harwood, et al., 2017; Tomlinson, Phillips, Mohebbi, et al., 2017). Additional risk factors for delirium in hospitalized patients include the following:

- History of delirium
- Higher numbers of chronic diseases
- Medications: anticholinergics, benzodiazepines, corticosteroids, H2-receptor antagonists, meperidine, sedative hypnotics
- Infections
- Metabolic–endocrine disturbances
- Mechanical ventilation

(Arumugam, El-Menyer, Al-Hassani, et al., 2017; Ostremba, Wilczynski, & Szewieczek, 2016; Stroomer-van Wijk, Jonker, Kok, et al., 2016)

Functional consequences include longer hospital stays, increased mortality, increased dependency, short- and long-term functional impairment, long-term cognitive impairment, and higher rates of permanent residency in long-term care facilities (Kosar, Thomas, Inouye, et al., 2017; Paulo, Scruth, & Jacoby, 2017; Slooter, Van De Leur, & Zaal, 2017). Functional consequences are more severe and of longer duration when delirium is superimposed upon dementia (Davis, Muniz-Terrera, Keage, et al., 2017). Consistent evidence from longitudinal studies following hospitalization suggests that greater severity of delirium and poorer predelirium cognitive and physical functioning are conditions associated with worse long-term outcomes (Ciampi, Bai, Dyachenko, et al., 2017; Hshieh, Saczynski, Gou, et al., 2017; Jackson, Wilson, Richardson, et al., 2016). Because functional consequences can be serious, long-term, or irreversible, it is imperative to identify delirium and implement multicomponent interventions as early in the process as possible.

 ## NURSING ASSESSMENT OF DELIRIUM

Because manifestations of delirium are wide ranging and can fluctuate quickly, frequent assessment is imperative for effective detection. In addition, nurses may hold unfounded beliefs that delirium is unimportant, unavoidable, or self-limiting, and these misunderstandings can interfere with assessment and interventions (Coyle, Burns, & Traynor, 2017; Zalon, Sandhaus, Kovaleski, et al., 2017).

Because delirium occurs so commonly in hospitalized older adults and is often unrecognized, routine cognitive screening is essential. The Confusion Assessment Method, first developed in 1990, is the most widely used screening tool to detect delirium in acute care units and long-term care facilities (Tullmann, Blevins, & Fletcher, 2016). This method is based on the following four-point algorithm; the presence of features in points one *and* two, and *either* point three *or* point four, confirms delirium:

1. Acute onset or fluctuating course: change in mental status from baseline or onset of abnormal behaviors that tend to come and go or increase and decrease in severity
2. Inattention: easy distractibility, difficulty focusing, diminished ability to keep track of conversations
3. Disorganized thinking: incoherent, disorganized, rambling, or illogical thinking or conversation
4. Altered level of consciousness: alert (normal), vigilant, lethargic, stupor, or coma

Nurses obtain information through direct observation, patient assessment, and from caregivers. It also is important to ask the older adult about self-observation because some people with delirium can self-report to describe changes in their mental status.

Another assessment consideration is that, in addition to mental status changes, delirium subtypes are categorized according to motor and behavioral manifestation. Three subtypes of delirium are characterized as follows:

- Hyperactive: restlessness, agitation, combativeness, anger, wandering, laughing, swearing, emotional lability, and fast or loud speech
- Hypoactive: lethargy, staring, slowed movement, paucity of speech, and unresponsiveness
- Mixed: fluctuations between hyperactive and hypoactive

Whereas the hyperactive type of delirium occurs more commonly and is more readily recognized, older adults are more likely to experience mixed delirium, with fluctuations between hyperalertness and somnolence. In addition to being more often undiagnosed in older adults, it also is associated with more serious outcomes (Eeles, Davis, & Bhat, 2017).

Nursing Diagnosis and Outcomes

The nursing diagnosis of Acute Confusion is defined as "reversible disturbances of consciousness, attention, cognition and perception that develop over a short period of time, and which last less than 3 months" (Herdman & Kamitsura, 2018, p. 254). Defining characteristics include fluctuation in cognition, consciousness, or psychomotor activity; hallucinations or misperceptions; increased restlessness or agitation; and lack of motivation to initiate or follow through with purposeful or goal-directed behavior.

To address this diagnosis, nurses can use the following Nursing Outcomes Classification (NOC) terms in their care plans: Anxiety Level, Cognition, Cognitive Orientation, Concentration, Comfort Status, Information Processing,

Memory, Neurologic Status, Psychomotor Energy. In addition, the following NOC terms may be applicable to address causative factors: Electrolyte and Acid/Base Balance, Hydration, Infection Severity, Nutritional Status, Risk Control, and Sensory Function.

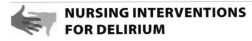

Wellness Opportunity

Nurses can use the NOC Comfort Level in their care plans to holistically address the needs of older adults with delirium.

NURSING INTERVENTIONS FOR DELIRIUM

The complexity of delirium requires a multidisciplinary approach to management, with nurses having a key role in detection, ongoing assessment, and management.

Current emphasis is on implementing multicomponent programs in hospitals for prevention, early detection, and treatment of delirium because outcomes are worse among those with more severe and persistent delirium. This approach requires interprofessional collaboration to address all contributing factors. Ideally, all staff in the hospital or long-term care setting share responsibility for implementing interventions, with nurses having lead roles in directly providing the interventions, initiating referrals as needs are identified, coordinating the care, and maintaining effective communication among all involved. Figure 14-1 illustrates a flow that identifies key components of care for patients with delirium based on assessment of changes in mental status and identified needs according to physiologic conditions, safety, and comfort. Table 14-1 provides an overview of some of the interventions and identifies the team members who

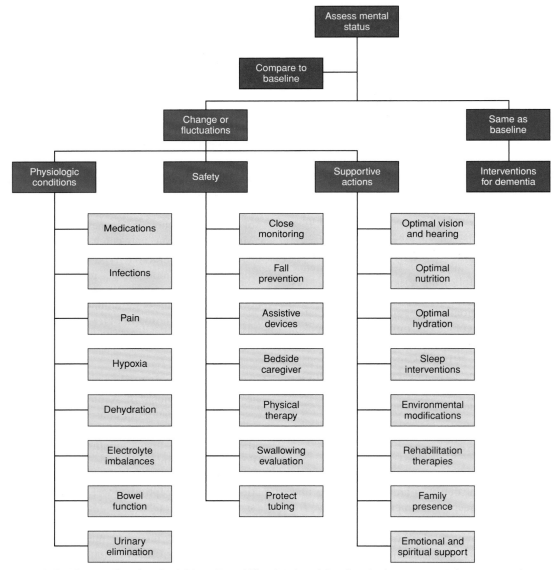

FIGURE 14-1 Flowchart for delirium. (From Miller, C. A. (2012). *Fast facts for dementia care: What nurses need to know in a nutshell.* Used with permission from Springer Publishing Company.)

TABLE 14-1 Interventions for Delirium and Professionals Responsible for Interprofessional Collaboration

Intervention	Lead Responsibility for Interprofessional Collaboration
Optimal management of all medical conditions	Medical, nursing, rehabilitation, pharmacy
Avoidance or discontinuation of medications that are associated with higher risk for delirium	Medical, nursing, pharmacy (see Chapter 8)
Pain management	Medical, nursing (see Chapter 28)
Promotion of adequate sleep and rest	Nursing (see Chapter 24), medical, environmental modifications by all staff, professionals qualified to provide complementary and integrative health care
Early and aggressive ambulation	Rehabilitation therapists, nursing, medical
Prevention of falls	Nursing, rehabilitation, all support staff (see Chapter 22)
Optimal nutrition	Registered dietitian, dietary staff, nursing staff
Prevention of aspiration for those at risk	Speech-language therapist, registered dietitian, nursing (see Chapter 18)
Provision of aids to orientation with correct information (e.g., clock, calendar, white board)	Nursing, all staff
Frequent verbal orientation and explanation of current activities	Nursing, all staff
Access to personal aids to improve sensory function (e.g., clean eyeglasses, hearing aids with working batteries)	Nursing, social services, all staff (see Chapters 16 and 17)
Prevention of pressure injuries for those at risk	Nursing, registered dietitian, medical (See chapter 23)
Maintenance of good bowel function	Nursing, medical, registered dietitian (See Chapter 18)
Maintenance of urinary elimination	Nursing, medical (See Chapter 19)
Psychological and spiritual support	Nursing, social services, chaplain (see Chapters 12 and 13)
Appropriate level of cognitive and social stimulation	Nursing, social services, occupational therapy
Family caregiver support and presence	Nursing, social services, all staff
Environmental support (e.g., noise reduction, maintenance of normal day–night lighting pattern, access to familiar objects	Nursing, all staff

are primarily involved with implementation of the care plan. It is important to recognize that lead team members are identified for each intervention; however, these interventions require shared responsibility among all staff, even including housekeeping. Additional points related to care of older adults with delirium are:

- Patients with delirium may benefit from comprehensive geriatric assessment or consultation with specialized geriatric health professionals, such as advanced practice nurses, geriatricians, geropsychiatrists, or geriatric neurologists.
- Comprehensive and interprofessional planning needs to be done to ensure effective transitions in care.
- Comprehensive and interprofessional planning needs to address discharge needs, including the need for follow-up and on-going evaluation and management.
- Staff education needs to be done for all staff on an ongoing basis.

The following Nursing Interventions Classification (NIC) terms are examples of interventions that can be used in care plans for Acute Confusion: Anxiety Reduction, Behavior Management, Cognitive Stimulation, Delirium Management, Energy Management, Environmental Management,

Fluid/Electrolyte Management, Hallucination Management, Medication Management, Mood Management, Nutrition Management, Pain Management, Reality Orientation, Sedation Management, and Surveillance: Safety.

Wellness Opportunity

Nursing interventions to holistically address the needs of older adults during confusional states include use of a Calming Technique, Emotional Support, Music Therapy, Presence, and Touch.

See **ONLINE LEARNING ACTIVITY 14-1: ADDITIONAL INFORMATION AND CASE STUDY VIDEO ABOUT NURSING CARE OF OLDER ADULTS WITH DELIRIUM** at **http://thepoint.lww.com/Miller8e**

Dementia

OVERVIEW OF DEMENTIA

Dementia is one of the most multifaceted topics discussed in this textbook, with evidence-based information rapidly emerging from many clinical, scientific, social, and ethical perspectives. This overview section provides background information that is relevant to current understanding of dementia, and the remainder of this chapter applies the information to clinical practice.

Two considerations need to be addressed in relation to evidence-based information about dementia. First, it is important to recognize that recent developments in neuroimaging techniques have led to major improvements in the diagnosis of dementia, but many of these diagnostic methods are not widely available outside of research centers. Similarly, although many clinical trials of interventions for dementia are in progress, these are available only in research studies. Second, when reading media reports about products for the prevention of cognitive decline or about purported breakthroughs in the diagnosis or treatment of dementia, it is imperative to ascertain the source of evidence related to these claims. Recognize that some claims are based on biased studies supported by manufacturers. Even information that is based on scientifically sound research may be discounted after longitudinal studies are carried out. Nurses need to keep up to date on research by obtaining information from reliable sources, such as the ones listed in the Online Learning Activities in this chapter. In addition, nurses have essential roles in teaching older adults about obtaining information from reliable sources, as discussed in the section on nursing interventions.

TERMINOLOGY TO DESCRIBE DEMENTIA

An understanding of impaired cognitive function is complicated by the many terms that are used interchangeably—and sometimes inaccurately—to describe dementia. Recent research has greatly improved the ability of clinicians to diagnose and treat different types of dementia, but it has also brought about a confusing proliferation of dementia-related terminology. Perhaps more than any other terms used in reference to older adults, those associated with cognitive impairment are the most misused, misunderstood, and emotionally charged. The following are some of the terms commonly used in reference to cognitive impairment in older adults: confusion, dementia, senility, Alzheimer's disease, small strokes, memory problems, and organic brain syndrome. Different terms are more or less acceptable to different people and the selection of a term is often based on emotional preferences or lack of accurate information. Because cognitive impairment is an emotionally charged subject, it is imperative to use the most appropriate term based on an understanding of the underlying causes for the impairment and an assessment of what term is most acceptable to the older adult and his or her care partners.

Medical references to dementia can be traced back to 1906, when a German physician, Alois Alzheimer, described neuritic plaques in the autopsied brain of a woman who was 55 years old at the time of her death and had experienced cognitive and behavior changes for about 5 years before her death. Building on earlier studies, Alzheimer concluded that cognitive impairment in *younger* adults was caused by neuritic plaques; whereas cognitive impairment in *older* adults was due to hardening of the arteries. During the 1960s, this viewpoint was challenged when autopsy studies led to the conclusion that the neuropathologic changes of Alzheimer's disease represent a single disease process, regardless of the age at onset. During the 1970s, the term "multi-infarct dementia" was used to describe dementias of cerebrovascular origin. It is now understood that many pathologic processes cause dementia, as discussed in the section on Types of Dementia. Scientists and clinicians also recognize that vascular and neurodegenerative pathologic changes frequently coexist in people over the age of 75, which is the age group when over 70% of dementia cases occur (Dichgans & Leys, 2017; Perneczky, Tene, Attems, et al., 2016; Raz, Knoefel, & Bhaskar, 2016).

In clinical settings, dementia is the medical term that includes a group of brain disorders characterized by a gradual decline in cognitive abilities (e.g., memory, understanding, judgment, decision-making, communication) and changes in personality and behavior. Because Alzheimer's disease is a type of dementia that occurs most commonly and has the longest history of recognition, *Alzheimer's disease* and *dementia* are sometimes used interchangeably, although this is not always accurate. Because the term "dementia" is closely associated with the uncomplimentary use of the term "demented," a phrase, such as "a person with dementia," is more appropriate when referring to the medical syndrome of impaired cognitive function.

An additional point must be emphasized regarding the term *dementia*. Dementia is not a single disease but a group of diseases, and each type is associated with a different cause and unique combination of manifestations. Additional considerations that complicate the use of terms related to impaired cognitive function are as follows:

- Two or more types of dementia can develop at the same time or sequentially
- Commonly available diagnostic techniques cannot always determine the type of dementia
- Terms may be used inaccurately even by health care professionals
- Because the ability to differentiate between types of dementia is still in early stages, many of the studies on Alzheimer's disease have included subjects with other types of dementia

In this chapter, the term *dementia* is used except when the information is pertinent to a particular type. The text refers to Alzheimer's disease when a source used that term; however, it is important to recognize that many of the citations on Alzheimer's disease refer to dementia in the broader sense.

TYPES OF DEMENTIA

The current approach to diagnosing dementia in usual clinical settings can be likened to the approach taken to diagnosing an infection. An infection is a generic diagnosis indicating the presence of a constellation of signs and symptoms (e.g., malaise, elevated temperature), but it does not indicate the causative factor. As additional information is collected, the specific type of infection is identified (e.g., pneumonia, urinary tract infection, bacterial, viral), and sometimes, more than one infection is discovered. Until the specific causative agent is identified, generic measures are taken (e.g., antipyretics, broad-spectrum antibiotics). After the specific causative agent is identified (e.g., through culture and sensitivity tests), the infection is treated with very specific antimicrobial agents. At all stages, comfort measures are used.

Analogously, dementia is an umbrella diagnosis indicating a constellation of signs and symptoms (e.g., memory impairment, personality changes), but during the early stages there rarely are clear indicators of the specific types of dementia. In many cases, neuropsychologic testing is required to distinguish patterns of change that are associated with either normal aging or pathologic processes during the early stages. As the condition progresses and more signs and symptoms develop, one or more causative factors may be identified. However, there is no diagnostic equivalent of a "culture and sensitivity" test for dementia, so it is difficult to distinguish between the different types of dementia. Thus, diagnosis of specific types of dementia is based on clinical observations, history of risk factors, and information from currently available diagnostic methods.

Based on current scientific literature, the four most commonly recognized types of dementia are Alzheimer's disease, vascular dementia, Lewy body dementia, and frontotemporal dementia. It is important to recognize that there are significant overlaps in manifestations of the different types of dementia, and during the early stage it is often difficult to determine if cognitive changes are due to normal aging or pathologic processes. Observations during the course of the dementia provide clues to the underlying pathologic processes, but it is often difficult, or even impossible, to distinguish one type of dementia from another. Moreover, older adults often have more than one type of dementia, which is called *mixed dementia*. Clinically relevant information about each of the four most common types of dementia is reviewed in this section and the rest of this chapter presents information about functional consequences, assessment, and interventions applicable to all types. Table 14-2 describes the distinguishing features of the four most common types of dementia.

 GLOBAL PERSPECTIVE

The World Health Organization projects that from 2015 to 2050 the numbers of people living with dementia will increase as follows according to region: slightly less than twofold in Europe, slightly more than twofold in North America, threefold in Asia, and fourfold in Latin America. These projected variations in prevalence are associated primarily with population aging (World Health Organization, 2016).

Alzheimer's Disease

Alzheimer's disease accounts for 60% to 80% of the cases of dementia (Alzheimer's Association Report, 2017) and, as already discussed, is the type of dementia with the strongest research base. Hallmark pathologic characteristics of Alzheimer's disease are as follows:

- Loss of neurons
- Atrophy of large cortical neurons
- Loss of synaptic connections between neurons
- Accumulation of neuritic plaques and neurofibrillary tangles
- Abnormal deposits of a protein fragment called beta-amyloid, which is formed from the breakdown of a larger protein called amyloid precursor protein
- Abnormal clusters of a protein called tau

TABLE 14-2 Distinguishing Features of Common Types of Dementia		
Type	**Onset and Course**	**Typical Manifestations**
Alzheimer disease	Insidious onset; diagnosis often made retrospectively; slowly progressive over 5–10 years, with accelerated decline associated with concomitant conditions (e.g., heart failure, delirium)	Early cognitive changes, usually but not always involving memory loss. Gradual loss of other cognitive abilities (e.g., decision-making, language) and communication skills. Gradual onset of behavior and personality changes (e.g., depression, irritability, agitation, indifference)
Vascular dementia	Abrupt onset due to cumulative effects of small strokes OR sudden onset if related to major stroke. History of vascular risks (e.g., stroke, hypertension). Irregular course OR improvement is possible depending on causative factors	Manifestations consistent with area of brain that is affected: aphasia, memory impairment, apathy, depression, emotional lability, and sensory-motor deficits (e.g., hemiparesis, gait disturbances, hemisensory loss, urinary incontinence)
Lewy body dementia	Insidious onset with a progressive decline in cognitive, behavioral, and motor symptoms; manifestations similar to Parkinson's disease	Significant cognitive impairment; fluctuating levels of cognition; parkinsonism; hallucinations; sleep disturbances; loss of postural stability; highly sensitive to neuroleptic medications
Frontotemporal dementia	Gradual onset often between the ages of 45 and 64; family history common; progressive decline in functioning	Early and progressive changes in behavior, motor abilities, or speech-language skills. Memory impairments occur later during the course of the disease

Preclinical AD

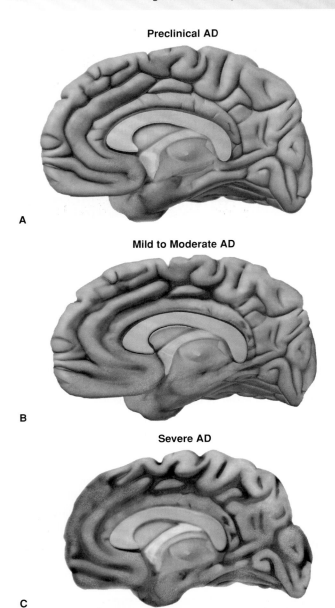

A

Mild to Moderate AD

B

Severe AD

C

FIGURE 14-2 (**A**) During preclinical Alzheimer disease, subtle degenerative changes begin to occur, and the person develops mild cognitive impairment. (**B**) In mild to moderate stages of Alzheimer disease, pathologic changes affect the areas of the brain that control memory, language, and reasoning. (**C**) In the severe stage of Alzheimer disease, pathologic changes cause significant atrophy in many areas. (Courtesy of the National Institute on Aging/National Institutes of Health.)

The gradual progression of brain atrophy is correlated with stages of Alzheimer's, from preclinical to severe, as illustrated in Figure 14-2.

In 2011, the National Institute on Aging and the Alzheimer's Association published the first major update on diagnostic guidelines for Alzheimer's since 1984. These guidelines, which are similar to those published by the International Working Group on Alzheimer's disease, define Alzheimer's disease as a neurologic condition that begins with a preclinical stage and progresses to clinical diagnosis of dementia. Box 14-1 presents evidence-based information from these guidelines and additional pertinent research information about Alzheimer's disease (Alzheimer's Association, 2017).

Vascular Dementia

Vascular dementia refers to cognitive impairment, ranging from mild to severe, that is caused by the death of nerve cells in the regions nourished by the diseased vessels. Underlying pathologic processes include clinical stroke (e.g., hemorrhage or occlusion of blood vessels) or subclinical vascular brain injury (e.g., lacunar strokes of the small arteries). Although vascular dementia has been viewed as a distinct type of dementia, reviews of recent studies indicate that cerebrovascular damage most often occurs concurrently with the neuropathologic changes of Alzheimer's disease (Gorelick, Counts, & Nyenhuis, 2016; Love & Miners, 2016). Manifestations of vascular dementia range from mild to severe and vary according to the progression of the disease and the onset of concurrent conditions. Factors that are strongly associated with increased risk for vascular dementia include stroke, hypertension, hypercholesterolemia, obesity, diabetes, and atrial fibrillation. Vascular dementia is considered the most preventable type because primary interventions can be implemented to decrease risks for stroke and cardiovascular disease, as discussed in Chapter 20 (Mijajlovic, Pavlovic, Brainin, et al., 2016; Smith, 2016). Table 14-2 provides information about the onset, course, and typical manifestations of vascular dementia.

Lewy Body Dementia

Lewy body dementia is part of a group of disorders called Lewy body disease, which also includes Parkinson's disease and Parkinson's disease with dementia. The hallmark pathologic characteristic of Lewy body disease is the presence of abnormal proteins (i.e., Lewy bodies) in the brain that eventually damage the neurons and affect all the following: cognitive abilities, motor function, sensory function, sleep patterns, and autonomic function. Clinically it is difficult to differentiate between Lewy body dementia and Alzheimer's disease because they have overlapping features and often occur together. Features that are more characteristic of dementia with Lewy bodies (compared with Alzheimer's disease) include more pronounced fluctuations in attention and cognition, disorganized speech, excessive daytime sleepiness, prolonged periods of staring into space, spontaneous motor manifestations of parkinsonism, and visual hallucinations as an early and recurrent manifestation (Gomperts, 2016; Murphy & Leverenz, 2017). Also, longitudinal studies indicate that Lewy body dementia causes a more rapid cognitive decline (Kramberger, Auestad, Garcia-Ptacek, et al., 2017; Rongve, Soennesyn, Skogseth, et al., 2016). Table 14-2 lists distinguishing features of Lewy body dementia.

People with Lewy body dementia are highly sensitive to medications with anticholinergic properties and they can

---

Box 14-1 Alzheimer Disease (AD) in the United States: Facts, Figures, and Overview

Prevalence and Incidence of AD

- In 2016, 10% of people age 65 years and 32% of those age 85 years and older had AD.
- In 2016, there was one new case every 66 seconds; in 2050, there will be one new case every 33 seconds.
- AD is more common among older Hispanics and African Americans than white older adults, which may be due to higher prevalence of health conditions such as diabetes and cardiovascular disease in those groups.

Consequences of AD

- AD is the fifth leading cause of death in adults age 65 years and older.
- Between 2000 and 2014, the death rate from AD increased by 89%.
- AD is a leading condition contributing to disability and poor health.
- At age 80, 75% of people living with dementia will be cared for in a nursing home, compared with only 4% of the others at the same age.

Stages of AD as Proposed by 2011 Criteria of the National Institute on Aging and the Alzheimer's Association

- *Preclinical AD:* Pathologic changes begin 20 years or more before the onset of symptoms; this stage cannot be diagnosed in usual clinical settings, but is being used for research purposes.
- *Mild cognitive impairment (MCI) due to AD:* Measurable changes in cognitive abilities that are noticeable to the person affected and to people who have frequent contact with the person; cognitive changes do not significantly affect the person's everyday activities.
- *Dementia due to AD:* Memory, thinking, and behavioral symptoms that impair the person's ability to function in daily life.

Manifestations of AD

- Memory loss that disrupts daily life
- Challenges in planning or solving problems

- Difficulty completing familiar tasks at home, at work, or at leisure
- Confusion with time and place
- Trouble understanding visual images and spatial relationships
- Changes in language or writing skills
- Misplacing things and losing the ability to retrace steps
- Impaired judgment
- Withdrawal from work or social activities
- Changes in mood and personality

Factors That Increase the Risk for AD

- Increased age
- Family history of people who have a first-degree relative with AD (i.e., parent or sibling)
- Inheriting the APOE-$_E$4 gene from one or both parents
- Risks for cardiovascular disease: smoking, obesity, diabetes, hypertension, hypercholesterolemia
- Traumatic brain injury

Factors That Decrease the Risk for AD

- Physical activity
- Diet that is low in saturated fats and rich in vegetables and vegetable-based oils
- Higher levels of education, which help build a "cognitive reserve"
- Engaging in social and cognitive activities

Consequences for Families and Caregivers

- Significantly increased demands on caregivers, with AD caregivers providing an average of 21.9 hours of care per week
- Family caregivers provide care for a long duration, with 57% providing care for 4 or more years
- High levels of stress and poor emotional health (e.g., 30% to 40% of AD caregivers reported depression, compared with 5% to 17% of adults of the same age who are not caregivers)

Source: Alzheimer's Association Report. (2017). *Alzheimer's & Dementia, 13,* 325–373.

---

develop extreme, idiosyncratic, or fatal reactions to even low doses of neuroleptic medications (Gomperts, 2016). For example, sedatives or antipsychotics may cause parkinsonism, hallucinations, agitation, or extreme somnolence. Thus, anticholinergic medications, including over-the-counter products, should be avoided, and if they are used, doses should be minimal, and patients should be observed carefully for adverse effects. Another clinically important characteristic is that people with Lewy body dementia may decompensate rapidly and significantly when they have a medical condition (e.g., minor infection) or when their environment is changed.

Frontotemporal Dementia

Frontotemporal dementia describes a spectrum of heterogenous neurodegenerative disorders involving the frontal or temporal lobes, or both. Pick's disease was first identified as a type of frontotemporal dementia in 1892, and in recent years, frontotemporal dementia has been recognized as a major cause of young-onset dementia. Frontotemporal dementia represents the leading cause of early-onset dementia, with symptoms beginning as early as 30 years. Frontotemporal dementia accounts for approximately 20% of cases of dementia (Finger, 2016; Pang & Miller, 2017).

Manifestations of frontotemporal dementia vary widely according to the order in which the frontal or temporal lobes of the brain are affected. Types of frontotemporal dementia as classified by symptoms are as follows:

- Behavioral and personality manifestations: apathy, disinhibition, emotional lability, changes in behavior and personality, and diminished concentration, attention, reasoning, judgment
- Language decline: loss of abilities related to speaking, writing, and language comprehension
- Motor function: falls, gait changes, movement disorders, muscle rigidity, difficulty with tasks involving fine motor skills

Diagnosis of frontotemporal dementia is difficult because manifestations vary widely and overlap with those of other types of dementia or with psychiatric disorders such as bipolar disorder (Baez, Pinasco, Roca, et al., 2017; Fernández-Matarrubia, Matías-Gulu, Cabrera-Martín, et al., 2017). People with frontotemporal dementia are often misdiagnosed as having a psychiatric illness because of their younger age, better performance on usual cognitive tests, and lack of insight. Because of its early onset and prominent and difficult-to-manage behavioral manifestations, frontotemporal dementia is associated with significant stress and financial burden for spouses and other care partners.

A consideration related to management is that usual medications for dementia (i.e., cholinesterase inhibitors or memantine) are not effective for frontotemporal dementia; however, there is some evidence that some antidepressants (e.g., citalopram, fluoxetine, and trazodone) may be effective for managing symptoms (Pang & Miller, 2017). In addition, because usual nonpharmacologic management strategies for dementia, such as redirecting the person, have limited effectiveness, nurses need to be creative in developing individualized care plans. For example, nurses can facilitate and coordinate an interdisciplinary team approach, including all the following: speech-language therapists to address speech, language, and swallowing problems; physical and occupational therapists to address progressive motor decline; and social workers and mental health professionals to address behavioral and emotional components.

FACTORS ASSOCIATED WITH RISK FOR DEMENTIA

Risks for dementia vary by type. For Alzheimer's disease and vascular dementia, advanced age and cardiovascular factors (e.g., diabetes, obesity, hypertension, hyperlipidemia) are associated with increased risk (Alzheimer's Association, 2017; Yaffe & Al Hazzouri, 2017). Genetic factors are the focus of much research, with different genetic factors being associated with each type of dementia. Although research is in very early stages, Alzheimer's disease is the type of dementia with the most conclusive evidence. For Alzheimer's disease, abnormalities on chromosomes 1, 14, 19, and 21 have been identified for several subtypes.

From a wellness perspective, it is important to recognize not only the factors that increase the risk for dementia but also those that protect against cognitive impairment. Cognitive reserve, as discussed in Chapter 11, is a factor that consistently has been identified as delaying the onset of dementia symptoms through the protective effect of higher education (Matthews, 2017). In recent years, researchers and policy makers have increasingly emphasized the importance of addressing modifiable risk factors as an intervention for preventing dementia. A consistent conclusion of studies related to risks for dementia is that behaviors and interventions that are effective for preventing cardiovascular disease (as discussed in Chapter 20) and promoting overall health are also associated with delaying the onset

of Alzheimer's disease and other types of dementia (as discussed in Chapter 11) (Barone, Gustafson, Crystal, et al., 2016; Santos, Snyder, Wu, et al., 2017).

Wellness Opportunity

Nurses can teach all adults that engaging in social, mental, and physical activity is a risk-free way of promoting cognitive wellness and may also prevent dementia.

 ## FUNCTIONAL CONSEQUENCES ASSOCIATED WITH DEMENTIA IN OLDER ADULTS

Functional consequences related to Alzheimer's disease have been studied since the 1950s, but research on the unique manifestations of different dementias is in very early stages. Many functional consequences are common to all the dementias, and as the disease progresses, manifestations of all types of dementia become more similar. It is important to recognize, however, that during all stages and in all types of dementia, functional consequences vary tremendously among individuals because of unique personality characteristics, coexisting conditions (e.g., depression, functional impairments), and other influences. Because dementia involves progressive loss of function over a long period, it has broad functional consequences in all aspects until the end of the person's life. It also necessarily involves serious and long-term consequences for all the people who live with or have relationships with the person with dementia. In the following sections, the topic of functional consequences is addressed in relation to stages of dementia, self-awareness, and personal experiences of the person with dementia, and effects on family and others who are close to the person with dementia.

Stages of Dementia

In the mid-1980s, an American psychiatrist, Reisberg, proposed a seven-stage model for describing the functional consequences of Alzheimer's disease. Reisberg's staging schema, which has been updated and refined, is referred to as the Global Deterioration Scale/Functional Assessment Staging, or GDS/FAST. The GDS/FAST, as delineated in Table 14-3, is widely used as an evidence-based tool for determining the progression of Alzheimer's disease from early to terminal stages. According to this framework, the diagnosis of Alzheimer's disease is made retrospectively because it is based on a progression of manifestations. Although this staging system was developed three decades ago, it is consistent with current information confirming a preclinical stage and progressing to a terminal stage.

Self-Awareness of People With Dementia

People with dementia are often perceived as having little or no awareness of, or insight into, their cognitive deficits and

TABLE 14-3 Global Deterioration Scale/Functional Assessment Staging (GDS/FAST) of Alzheimer's Disease

Stage	Effects on Functioning
1: Normal adult	No deficits or complaints
2: Age-associated memory impairment	Deficits consistent with normal aging (i.e., no objective findings, difficulty with word finding, forgets location of objects)
3: Mild cognitive impairment	Some deficits in performing complex tasks, particularly in demanding social and employment settings; diminished organizational skills; deficits noted by others for the first time
4: Mild dementia	Diminished ability to perform complex tasks (e.g., meal planning, financial management); decreased knowledge of current and recent events; flattened affect and withdrawal from challenging situations
5: Moderate dementia	Obvious cognitive deficits; unable to manage complex daily tasks without some supervision or assistance; difficulty remembering names of familiar people
6: Moderately severe dementia	Increasingly obvious cognitive deficits (e.g., disorientation, significant short-term memory impairment); personality and emotional changes (e.g., anxiety, delusions) Loss of abilities in the following order: a. Difficulty putting clothing on properly without assistance b. Unable to bathe independently c. Unable to handle all aspects of toileting (e.g., does not wipe properly) d. Occasional or frequent urinary incontinence e. Occasional or frequent fecal incontinence
7: Severe dementia	Progressive loss of all verbal and psychomotor abilities: a. Verbal abilities limited to six or fewer different words b. Verbal abilities limited to a single intelligible word c. Unable to walk without assistance d. Unable to sit without assistance e. Unable to smile f. Unable to hold up head independently

Source: Reisberg, B. (1986). Dementia: A systematic approach to identifying reversible causes. *Geriatrics, 41*(4), 30–46.

limitations. This perception has led to labeling people with dementia as being "in denial." It also underlies inaccurate statements about people with dementia, such as "If they can ask if they have Alzheimer's disease, then they don't have it." **Anosognosia**, which is the diagnostic term for poor insight or lack of awareness, may lead to dangerous behaviors and affect the ability of the person with dementia to live independently (Parrao, Brockman, Bucks, et al., 2017). Anosognosia is assessed by having the person who is being evaluated and a family member or caregiver independently answer questions related to the person's behaviors and daily activities (e.g., repetitive talking, indicators of forgetfulness, lack of interest in usual activities). Assessment of self-awareness needs to be based on information from both the person with dementia and an observer, such as a family member or caregiver. Studies indicate that self-ratings of people with dementia may be more accurate than assessments based solely on information from a family member or caregiver (Martyr & Clare, 2017).

Programs emphasizing the provision of person-centered care are based on the premise that even when awareness of cognitive deficits is limited, people with dementia maintain emotional awareness and are capable of expressing their needs. Studies of the feelings and experiences of individuals with dementia provide important insight into their expressed needs as described in boxes throughout this chapter with direct quotes from people with dementia. Box 14-2 summarizes statements of people with dementia about how they are perceived by others.

Personal Experiences and Emotional Responses of People With Dementia

During the early stages, only the individual with dementia and people who live, work, or have close contact with the person notice the initial changes, such as impaired judgment and short-term memory. When the changes are noticed, numerous explanations may be applicable, and the deficits may be attributed to such factors as depression or the occurrence of a major life event (e.g., retirement, widowhood). People in the early stages of dementia may withdraw from complex tasks as a way of protecting themselves from the effects of diminishing cognitive abilities. For example, employed people may retire without acknowledging cognitive impairments as the reason. People who do not have to perform complex intellectual or psychomotor tasks may be able to conceal or compensate for the cognitive losses until the deficits seriously interfere with activities of daily living (ADLs). As the disease progresses, however, the person with dementia is less able to cover up the changes, and people with less intimate contact will begin to question the underlying cause of the deficits.

- "It would be nice if a lot of people had more understanding and appreciate what you have got. I was in town, and this other lady started laughing because of the way I was trying to struggle to talk and that started to make me feel uncomfortable; I thought if only she understood, then perhaps she wouldn't stand there and laugh."
- "If you say to someone, 'Can you wait a couple of minutes; I've got dementia and I want to explain,' they look at you and think there is nothing wrong with you; you should not be able to talk. Then again, you get some who say 'HOW-ARE-YOU?' and you think, 'Grr, I'm not that bad.'"
- "It's as though that's it, you are dribbling and nodding, and that's the picture of Alzheimer's. But we are all sitting here and talking perfectly normally. We have got Alzheimer's of some form; we are not nodding and dribbling."
- "I'm trying to guard that I don't get looked down on. I don't want the feeling of being back in first grade or whatever… of going in the other direction, of decreasing instead of improving, and I have inward anger."
- "Everybody I have met has been absolutely amazed that (a) I can still talk and still think, and (b) I have a diagnosis of dementia. They do not understand it."
- "No one really understands how hard it is to live life like this, so people tend to trivialize how you feel, patronize you, and make out that they feel the same way."
- "Written off as being devoid of feelings and needs… It was clear to me that my dementia negated the things that I said. It was very painful."
- "It has been proven by thousands of early-stage people with dementia to be capable and intelligent beings just moving a little slower."

Source: Alzheimer's Society (2008); Alzheimer's Society (2010); Beard and Fox (2008); Beard, Knauss, and Moyer (2009); Clare, Rowlands, and Quin (2008).

Common emotions and behaviors of people with dementia include loss, fear, shame, anger, sadness, anxiety, frustration, loneliness, depression, uncertainty, sense of uselessness, self-blame, diminished affect, and withdrawal from challenging activities. Studies find that people with dementia want to understand their illness; maintain their personal identity; retain their functional independence; and maintain their quality of life through health, relationships, and positive coping (Powers, Dawson, Krestar, et al., 2016). During the later stages of dementia, emotional responses are altered, but they are not absent. As dementia progresses, the person is likely to express emotions nonverbally and behaviorally. Thus, two important responsibilities of caregivers are to encourage and interpret nonverbal communication, which becomes the primary mode of communication during later stages of dementia.

It also is imperative to acknowledge that the personhood of each individual who has dementia is always present and needs to be addressed in every interaction. Although dementia has long been associated with a "loss of self," a recent study stated that "personhood can be understood as increasingly concealed rather than lost" (Smebye & Kirkevold,

2013, p. 29). This perspective highlights the responsibility of nurses and all who provide care to acknowledge and discover the underlying personhood of each person who has dementia. In this and the following sections of this chapter, the experiences of people with dementia are described in boxes to illustrate the unique ways in which dementia affects individuals and their care partners. Box 14-3 describes the experiences and feelings of people with dementia about the earliest changes and their diagnoses.

- "I knew my brain wasn't what it used to be because I've always remembered that I gave birth to my girls and one time I thought, 'I can't remember what their birthday is.'"
- "To sing a song that I have sung 100 times before to music I have heard 100 times before and I'm standing there thinking, 'What the hell am I doing here and what am I going to sing?' This started to happen more and more, and when you are out on the stage on your own and you don't know what you are doing, it is a terrifying prospect."
- "If I was getting dressed in the morning, I would put my clothes on, and I would guarantee you there was at least a pair of trousers, a shirt, or a hat and coat—and it had all gone on upside down, back to front."
- "I'm still the same person I've always been. It's just that now I'm *me* with Alzheimer's. I am still loving and caring, and I still have feelings, and I would like to think that I haven't changed in myself."
- "Although I was expecting it by then, the words were still devastating to hear."
- "I feel like I still have enough intelligence to be a person and not just someone you pat on the head as you go by… It's devastating, and it takes away your sense of self. I feel like I'm still a person and my wants and desires should at least be considered before decisions are made."
- "The angst and anger that I went through during the diagnostic process. I could have actually gone and thumped people."
- "It was as if the thunderclouds had been taken away because they had given an answer to me why I was treating my family so like a louse that I was."
- "I was relieved really that what I was trying to convince people had been verified."
- "I think the word Alzheimer's puts a fear in you, like cancer does."
- "It is a really frightening thing when no one can tell you how fast you will deteriorate. It is hard to get across how that feels, but it gnaws at you continually, and each day you wonder what faculty will be lost next."
- "It is quite strange because dementia seems to hit people in very different ways. There are little threads of commonality in it, but everyone is affected in a slightly different way."
- "I think I have a very different view about how long I'll be around, or when life will come to an end, or when I'll be incompetent, than I did before the diagnosis. No question."
- "I certainly think that it's important to let family be aware of one's problems. Not to the extent of complaining and complaining, but this is what it is, and I have to deal with that. I wouldn't deny it ever."

Source: Alzheimer's Society (2008); Alzheimer's Society (2010); Beard and Fox (2008); Beard, Knauss, and Moyer (2009); Clare, Rowlands, and Quin (2008).

A Student's Perspective

There is a woman at my nursing home who has severe dementia, to the point where she often is not very kind to the nurses, PTs, OTs, and other staff. For most of our clinical rotation, I only heard reports of her being angry and sometimes insulting. This can be comical at times, and we all know not to take it personally because we know her attitude is a result of her disease. Understanding the chance I was taking, I went to talk to her during breakfast because she was just staring off into space. Kneeling at her eye level and placing my hand on her shoulder, I began by asking how her morning was. She complained about the cold weather and about how aggressive the OTs were in dressing her. I let her vent, I made some positive remarks, and I complimented her on how beautiful she looked that day.

As I rose to my feet to leave her a few minutes later, she reached for my arm and said, "You're such a sweetheart; you're so kind." My first internal reaction was to be blown away! I had never heard of this woman delivering compliments! But throughout the rest of the day, I couldn't keep the smile off my face. This encounter helped me realize that this woman's beautiful personality is still with her and will always be a part of her. Yes, right now it's being masked most of the time by her dementia, but she still has feelings of kindness and a desire for happiness that fight past her disease every once in a while. I'm just glad I got to be part of that moment and discover that she's still there and needs to be treated like it always. One day she'll have the opportunity and power to express her thanks for those who showed her love and patience.

Shannon H.

Wellness Opportunity

Nurses holistically address psychosocial needs by recognizing that individuals vary significantly in their emotional responses, but people with dementia never lose the ability to respond to others.

Behavioral and Psychological Symptoms of Dementia

Significant behavioral disturbances, called **behavioral and psychological symptoms of dementia (BPSD)** (also called *neuropsychiatric symptoms*), occur during all stages of dementia in nearly all people with dementia (Onyike & Rabins, 2017). Some examples of BPSD are as follows:

- Agitation: abnormal level of verbal, vocal, or motor activity (e.g., aggression, screaming)
- Psychiatric symptoms: delusions, hallucinations
- Personality changes, disinhibition
- Mood disturbances: apathy, depression, euphoria, emotional lability
- Aberrant motor movements: pacing, rummaging, wandering
- Changes in sleep, eating, appetite
- Hypersexual behavior: inappropriate statements, sexually aggressive actions, masturbation in public places

The BPSD most commonly reported by nurses in long-term care facilities are verbal aggression and behaviors (e.g., swearing, screaming, calling out, repetitive verbalizations); aggressive physical behaviors; resident-to-resident aggression; physically agitated behaviors; resistance-to-care behaviors; and inappropriate social and sexual behaviors (Davison, McCabe, Bird, et al., 2017). When BPSD or increased confusion or restlessness becomes worse or occurs primarily in the early evening, this is called **sundowning**. Factors that are associated with sundowning include fatigue, overstimulation (including environmental overstimulation), adverse medication effects, fear of darkness, and altered circadian rhythm. Functional consequences of BPSD include concomitant functional decline, admission to a residential facility, increased caregiver burden, and faster cognitive decline (Canevelli, Valletta, Trebbastoni, et al., 2016; Toot, Swinson, Devine, et al., 2017).

Aggression and agitation are types of BPSD that are strongly associated with serious functional consequences, including distress and reduced quality of life for the person with dementia and for those who are care partners and increased risk for being admitted to a hospital or long-term care setting. Conditions associated with physical and verbal aggressive behavior include depression, psychosis, poor physical health, severe cognitive impairment, inability to communicate about unmet needs, and environmental conditions. Conditions associated with agitation include pain; overstimulation; social isolation; disruption of usual routines; and unmet physical needs related to sleep, thirst, hunger, fatigue, or elimination. Evidence-based models of care emphasize that the first step in managing aggressive behaviors is identifying the precipitating conditions and addressing underlying causes (Curyto, McCurry, Luci, et al., 2017; Desai, Wharton, Struble, et al., 2017).

Although BPSD occurs in almost all people with dementia, these symptoms vary widely and none of these behaviors occurs in all people with dementia. Also, manifestations of BPSD change during the course of the illness in each person and many resolve as dementia progresses. It is not unusual for one or more manifestation of BPSD to resolve at the same time that new ones develop. Because of the wide variability in these symptoms, many people, including health care professionals, hold stereotypes or misunderstandings about BPSD. Remarks such as, "I know he doesn't have Alzheimer's disease because he doesn't hallucinate," or "I know she doesn't have Alzheimer's disease because she's not violent," reflect a false belief that certain difficult behaviors are an inevitable consequence of dementia. Similarly, a question such as "Can you tell if my mother will be the 'nice kind' or the 'mean kind' as her Alzheimer's gets worse?" indicates the need for accurate information about BPSD. Another consideration is that spouses and other family members may have difficulty distinguishing between long-term personality patterns and behaviors arising from dementia. This is especially challenging when the person with dementia has a history of dysfunctional behaviors (e.g., alcohol abuse, anger management) or unhealthy relationships.

A serious consequence of these misunderstandings is that the symptoms are misinterpreted and causative factors are not addressed. Responsibilities of nurses include dispelling myths and misunderstandings and helping caregivers identify triggers. In addition, it is important to avoid terminology that perpetuates misunderstandings, such as the commonly used term "refuses to. . . ." Table 14-4 summarizes some common misperceptions and related facts about dementia-associated behaviors.

A major nursing responsibility is to look for contributing causes and implement strategies to prevent BPSD or minimize the effects of these behaviors. Common contributing causes include pain, fatigue, physical discomfort, environmental conditions, changes in routine, overstimulation, or lack of stimulation. It also is imperative to recognize that behavioral manifestations in people with dementia can be caused, at least in part, by delirium superimposed on dementia, as discussed in the Delirium section. Strategies for addressing behavioral symptoms are discussed in the section on nursing interventions.

Another nursing responsibility, which is consistent with a person-centered approach to care, is to identify the feelings and experiences that the person with dementia is attempting to communicate through his or her behavior. Results of a study by Dupuis and colleagues (2012) suggest that professionals replace the concept of challenging behavior with the term *responsive behavior* in people with dementia. This approach emphasizes that behaviors are meaningful and "moves us away from judging behaviors to *understanding meaning in actions* and responses. It means moving away from a focus on dysfunction, deficit and decline, to recognizing, valuing and believing in the continued abilities of persons with dementia to express their experiences and act in purposeful, meaningful and even intentional ways" (Dupuis, Wiersma, & Loiselle, 2012), p. 170).

Effects for Family and Others Who are Close to the Person With Dementia

In addition to the functional consequences that directly affect the person with dementia, caregivers and families of people with dementia also experience significant consequences. The term *care partners* is sometimes used in this chapter instead of *caregivers* to denote that the person with dementia is viewed as a *partner in the process* rather than a *passive recipient*, especially during mild and even moderate stages. This phrase also emphasizes that care of people with dementia requires the *partnership* of many personal and professional support people working together to address this complex situation. The term *caregiver* is used in reference to the needs of family members and supports people who are most directly affected, particularly during moderate or severe stages. Caregiver also is used when citing a reference that uses that term.

People with dementia require ongoing support and assistance from their spouses, families, friends, and other unpaid care providers. Because unpaid care providers have essential and long-term roles that vary throughout the course of dementia, they are considered "invisible second patients" (Fletcher, 2016; Sanders, 2016). Commonly identified needs of caregivers focus on management of the person with dementia and the personal health of the caregiver, as in the following examples:

- Information and knowledge
- Management of daily care
- Management of functional impairments (e.g., incontinence, mobility problems)
- Dealing with the care recipient's emotions and behaviors
- Management of BPSD
- Formal care assistance
- Informal care assistance
- Management of safety issues
- Dealing with the changing relationship between care partner and care recipient
- Caregiver's physical and psychological needs
- Management of caregiver's daily life
- Dealing with financial and social effects

(McCabe, You, & Tatangelo, 2016; Steiner, Pierce, & Salvador, 2016). It is beyond the scope of this text to fully address this complex topic; however, nursing responsibilities related to

---

TABLE 14-4 Misperceptions and Realities About Dementia-Associated Behaviors

Misperceptions of Behaviors	Realities
"He refuses to …"	He has no idea about what is offered; needs to do something else before agreeing to the activity; wants to feel he has a choice; may not have ability to carry out the activity.
"She fights me when I …"	She may be experiencing pain or discomfort, which is exacerbated by activity; she may not understand the activity.
"He denies any problem."	The person may not have insight, awareness, or ability to understand.
"There's no reason for him to act that way."	There usually is a triggering event or an unmet need and the behavior is a way to cope, adapt, respond, or express a need.
Manipulative, deliberate actions to get attention.	The person probably does not have enough insight or intent to be manipulative; may be the only way the person is able to express needs.
Nothing to do to prevent the behavior.	Care partners can be proactive in identifying and addressing triggers.
Interventions that were effective in the past will be effective now.	If usual interventions no longer work, be flexible, creative, and try something else; use a "trial and error" approach by trying variations of interventions that worked.

Adapted from Miller, C. A. (2012). *Fast facts for dementia care: What nurses need to know in a nutshell.* Used with permission from Springer Publishing Company.

addressing needs of caregivers are discussed in Chapter 27. Also, nurses can teach caregivers using the information in this chapter related to care of people with dementia.

NURSING ASSESSMENT OF DEMENTIA IN OLDER ADULTS

Dementia is a complex syndrome that usually involves a long and fluctuating course that progresses to a terminal phase. Thus, assessment is an ongoing process that focuses on identifying conditions that cause negative consequences during the course of dementia. It also is important to identify and address conditions that interfere with the assessment of dementia.

Factors That Influence the Assessment of Dementia

Attitudes, myths, and lack of information are risk factors that can interfere with an appropriate assessment of, and interventions for, dementia. In recent years, tremendous progress has been made in understanding and identifying causes of impaired cognitive function; however, many older adults and their families and care partners still view serious cognitive impairments as an expected and normal concomitant of aging. When this happens, treatable conditions are likely to be overlooked, and older adults are denied the appropriate interventions for managing their conditions. Even in the absence of curative treatments, many interventions are effective in delaying the progression of the condition, managing symptoms, assisting with long-term planning, and improving quality of life for the person with dementia and his or her care partners.

Cultural factors that influence perceptions about aging and illness can significantly affect both the evaluation and treatment of dementia. For example, some cultural groups accept cognitive impairment as "normal aging," whereas others view dementia-related behaviors as shameful.

Wellness Opportunity

Nurses have many opportunities to teach older adults and their care partners about the importance of evaluating any significant changes in cognitive function.

Initial Assessment

With the exception of delirium and poststroke dementia, manifestations of cognitive impairment develop and progress slowly, and an assessment is often delayed until the changes significantly interfere with normal functioning. Because progressive cognitive impairment is a very complex phenomenon, the assessment process generally is multidisciplinary, requiring input from primary care providers, psychiatrists, nurses, social workers, and rehabilitation therapists. Members of the assessment team must work with the family and other care partners to obtain information and determine the appropriate level of involvement of the cognitively impaired person with regard to discussing assessment results and planning care. The major nursing focus is to determine the person's level of function, to identify the factors that affect the person's level of function, and to identify the person's response to his or her illness. Frequently, the nurse serves as the team leader and is responsible for coordinating information and facilitating communication among team members and with the older adult and his or her family or other care partners. Nurses can use Box 14-4 as a guide for assessing progressive cognitive impairments in older adults.

Ongoing Assessment of Consequences

Because dementia is a progressive condition that commonly coexists with other conditions, all people with dementia require ongoing assessment of all of the following:

- Changes in cognitive and psychosocial function related to the dementia (e.g., a decline in cognitive abilities, the onset of anxiety or depression)
- Changes in mental status related to concurrent conditions (e.g., delirium due to a medical condition or adverse medication effects)
- Changes in functional abilities
- Causes of behavioral changes related to treatable conditions (e.g., anxiety, physical discomfort, environmental factors)

A major goal of ongoing assessment is to identify factors that interfere with the person's level of functioning or quality of life, so that interventions can be initiated to alleviate these contributing factors. Even though dementia is a progressive condition that gradually affects all levels of functioning, some of the changes that occur are caused by concurrent conditions rather than by the dementia itself. Thus, ongoing assessment to identify all factors that affect level of functioning is essential. Another goal of ongoing assessment is to identify the person's strengths and limitations in order to plan individualized interventions to improve the person's functioning and quality of life. One way of assessing strengths and weaknesses is to inquire about the ways in which dementia has affected daily living and how the person has coped with, or adjusted to, these changes. Box 14-5 summarizes some statements of people with dementia about ways of coping and daily living.

Nurses can use Table 14-3 as a guide to assessing the progression of dementia from early to later stages. In addition, the following nursing assessment guides are pertinent to aspects of functioning that are affected in people with dementia:

- Chapter 7, functioning and safety
- Chapter 8, medications
- Chapter 12, psychosocial function
- Chapter 15, depression

Box 14-4 Assessing Progressive Cognitive Impairment in Older Adults

General Principles

- Assessment of impaired cognitive function is a long-term process.
- Even though the person with impaired cognitive function may not be a reliable reporter, his or her perceptions should be an integral part of the assessment and the accuracy of information should be validated.
- The feelings of the person with cognitive impairment should be assessed and acknowledged.
- Health care professionals must respect the person's rights and ask permission before obtaining information from others, including family members.
- Do not assume that the family has drawn accurate conclusions about events of the past (e.g., family members may state that the person retired and then showed cognitive deficits when, in reality, the person retired because of an inability to cope with job demands).

Focus of the Assessment

- The primary purpose of the assessment is to identify the causes of the cognitive impairment.
- An assessment of a person with impaired cognitive function is multidisciplinary and includes the following components: complete medical history and physical examination including a review of all medications; a functional assessment; a comprehensive psychosocial and formal mental status assessment; and an assessment of environmental and caregiver influences, with particular emphasis on those factors that affect safety and functional abilities.

- The assessment includes an interview with caregivers, family members, and other people who can describe the progression of the manifestations of impairment.
- Information about lifelong patterns of personality, coping, and performance characteristics is considered in relation to the person's current functional level.
- It may be necessary to ask probing questions to help family members recognize clues to cognitive deficits retrospectively.

Considerations in Assessing Risk Factors Contributing to Impaired Cognitive Function

- Never assume that all cognitive impairments and behavioral manifestations stem from a dementing illness.
- Because risk factors can either cause the initial cognitive impairments or develop later, causing additional impairments, they must be reassessed periodically.
- The following categories of risk factors must be assessed, both initially and on an ongoing basis: depression, physiologic alterations, functional impairments, adverse medication effects, and environmental and psychosocial influences.
- Early in the assessment, ensure that vision and hearing impairments are compensated for as much as possible and that the environment does not interfere with the person's performance (e.g., as possible, make sure the person is using eyeglasses and a hearing aid if needed, and make sure the lighting is optimal).
- A priority is to identify and treat those factors that are reversible before deciding on a long-term management plan.

Box 14-5 Lived Experiences: Coping and Daily Living With Dementia

About Ways of Coping

- "I think it is alright to allow yourself a bit of time to focus on the pain and fear. That is only human; but it is important to move away from the sad focus and not let it consume you."
- "I try to be more patient with myself and forgive myself."
- "Staying busy doing what I love to do really keeps me going and gets me through. I'm in two support groups; I have weekly mandolin lesions; I do a weekly men's meditation class with daily homework; I'm reading about consciousness and healing that supports my living in the now and taking care of my spirit."
- "I think as long as I can make decisions, I can still go out and sail a boat. Sailing is all about making decisions. If you're racing a yacht, just about every 3 minutes you've got to make a decision and I have some fantastic crew on my boat who are always going to guide me."
- "We have this problem and we can't change that, but we can improve our lives by not letting it just bring us unhappiness 24 hours a day."
- "Usually I just slow down, and reset my expectations. Expecting that you can be who you used to be is just a recipe for pain and sadness."
- "I need to have the knowledge that I'm doing what I can. Because oftentimes it's so subtle, and I curse it every now and then and that helps."
- "I ask people not to expect me to remember to do things."
- "Ahh! I have a great lack of ease with not remembering things. Oh God, it drives me crazy… but we have to accept what we cannot change."

About Day-to-Day Living

- "Tomorrow I'll have little memory of today, and this makes living today like pushing the rock up the hill knowing it will roll back."
- "Inertia is a serious problem with me, and sometimes I seem glued to my chair. Likely it's just that it's so much effort to get myself organized to do things, that I'm mentally exhausted before I even start."
- "I streamline everything and get rid of everything I don't use very often. Keeping the house clutter free helps to minimize the time necessary to find misplaced items."
- "I try to find ways to compensate. For example, I now use a GPS to help me from getting lost when I drive."
- "My brother-in-law removed all my cabinet doors in my kitchen so I can see all my food in my pantry when I walk into my kitchen."
- "I do the shopping, and my wife does these beautiful lists and they're in order of where everything is in the shop."
- "I think it would be better if I did not drive; and actually mentally, it is much better that I make that decision than somebody makes that decision for me. Psychologically, it is very good that I am actually in a position where they said, 'OK you can drive,' and just left it at that, and I turned around and said, 'Well, thanks very much, but I am actually not going to drive.'"

Source: Alzheimer's Society (2008); Alzheimer's Society (2010); Beard and Fox (2008); Beard, Knauss, and Moyer (2009); Clare, Rowlands, and Quin (2008); Fetherstonhaugh, Tarzia, and Nay (2013).

- Chapter 16, hearing
- Chapter 17, vision
- Chapter 18, pain
- Chapter 19, urinary function
- Chapter 22, fall risk
- Chapter 25, sleep and rest

Online Learning Activity 14-2 provides links to resources for assessing aspects of functioning in people with dementia.

 See ONLINE LEARNING ACTIVITY 14-2: EVIDENCE-BASED TOOLS FOR ASSESSING ASPECTS OF FUNCTIONING IN PEOPLE WITH DEMENTIA at http://thepoint.lww.com/Miller8e

> **Wellness Opportunity**
>
> Nurses promote wellness by identifying factors that support optimal functioning rather than focusing only on those that are problematic.

NURSING DIAGNOSIS

Although the nursing diagnosis of Chronic Confusion may describe the overall condition of an older adult, it does not describe the multidimensional foci of care that nurses typically address when caring for older adults with dementia. Numerous nursing diagnoses are applicable to the broad range of functional consequences associated with dementia, such as any of the following: Fear, Anxiety, Risk for Compromised Human Dignity, Impaired Memory, Impaired Social Interaction, Self-Esteem Disturbance, and Ineffective Coping. When dementia affects a person's functional abilities, applicable nursing diagnoses include Wandering, Imbalanced Nutrition, Urinary Incontinence, Self-Care Deficit, Impaired Verbal communication, Risk for Falls, Risk for Injury, Disturbed Sensory Perception, and Disturbed Sleep Pattern.

Nursing diagnoses also address the needs of caregivers because much of the care of people with dementia focuses on helping the family and other caregivers address the day-to-day needs and issues of the person with dementia. Nursing diagnoses that might be used to address caregiver needs include Stress Overload, Compromised Family Coping, and Caregiver Role Strain (or Risk for Caregiver Role Strain). During the later stages of dementia, the nursing diagnosis Anticipatory Grieving may be appropriate, particularly for spousal caregivers.

> **Wellness Opportunity**
>
> Readiness for Enhanced Coping is a wellness nursing diagnosis that nurses can apply for people with dementia as well as their caregivers.

PLANNING FOR WELLNESS OUTCOMES

During all stages of dementia, nursing care is directed toward promoting the highest level of functioning, while also supporting the highest quality of life. Nurses can apply the following NOC terminology to address the needs of people with dementia: Agitation Level, Cognition, Cognitive Orientation, Comfort Status, Communication, Coping, Leisure Participation, Memory, Mood Equilibrium, Nutritional Status, Quality of Life, Self-Care Status, Sleep, Social Interaction Skills, and Symptom Control.

When friends, family members, or paid caregivers care for the person with dementia, nurses plan outcomes to promote caregiver wellness. In the early stages of dementia, the foremost needs of care partners might be for information about the disease and about resources that address the changing needs of the person with dementia and all those involved. As the dementia progresses, caregivers are likely to need emotional support and practical assistance. Some NOC terms that are pertinent to caregivers include Anxiety Level, Caregiver Emotional Health, Caregiver Lifestyle Disruption, Caregiver–Patient Relationship, Caregiver Physical Health, Caregiver Role Endurance, Caregiver Stressors, and Caregiver Well-Being.

> **Wellness Opportunity**
>
> Hope is an NOC that would be applicable when nurses plan wellness outcomes to address body–mind–spirit needs of both people with dementia and their caregivers.

NURSING INTERVENTIONS TO ADDRESS DEMENTIA

Information about interventions to address dementia is evolving at a rapid pace, and research by nurses and other health care professionals is shedding light on appropriate interventions for managing the functional consequences. Many interventions, such as reassurance for anxiety and confusion and redirection for unsafe or inappropriate behaviors, are applicable to all people with dementia and are individualized according to specific manifestations. Similarly, health promotion interventions, such as exercise and nutrition, are applicable for primary and secondary prevention in all people with dementia. In most health care settings, interventions primarily focus on management of BPSD, as discussed in the section on Interventions for Dementia-Related Behaviors. Online Learning Activity 14-3 provides a link to resources for information about evidence-based interventions for BPSD. A major consideration about interventions for dementia is that nurses have key roles in planning and implementing interventions, but effective care for people with dementia requires consistent and significant input from many health care professionals and other care partners. Thus, it is imperative to address nursing interventions in the context of comprehensive, multidisciplinary, and person-centered approach to the complex issues related to dementia.

See ONLINE LEARNING ACTIVITY 14-3:
PODCAST ABOUT COMPLEX CARE NEEDS
OF OLDER ADULTS WITH DEMENTIA at
http://thepoint.lww.com/Miller8e

Examples of NIC terminology that may be applicable to caring for people with dementia include Active Listening, Activity Therapy, Anxiety Reduction, Behavior Management, Calming Technique, Dementia Management, Elopement Precautions, Emotional Support, Environmental Management, Exercise Promotion, Fall Prevention, Humor, Memory Training, Milieu Therapy, Music Therapy, Presence, Reality Orientation, Reminiscence Therapy, Self-Care Assistance, Spiritual Support, and Touch. Nurses can use the following NIC terms when they address caregiver needs: Anticipatory Guidance, Caregiver Support, Consultation, Coping Enhancement, Counseling, Decision-Making Support, Humor, Referral, Respite Care, Relaxation Therapy, Spiritual Growth Facilitation, and Teaching.

> **⬤ Wellness Opportunity**
>
> Hope Inspiration is a NIC that nurses address when they help people with dementia and their caregivers to identify a positive meaning for their situation.

Teaching About Medications for Dementia

In 1993, the U.S. Food and Drug Administration (FDA) approved the first medication for the treatment of Alzheimer's disease and by 2001 three additional cholinesterase inhibitors had been approved: donepezil (Aricept), rivastigmine (Exelon), and galantamine (Razadyne, formerly called Reminyl). These three cholinesterase inhibitors have become standard treatment for *mild to moderate* Alzheimer's disease. In 2003, memantine (Namenda) became the first medication approved for treatment of *moderate to severe* Alzheimer's disease. The physiologic action of this medication, which differs from that of cholinesterase inhibitors, blocks the neural toxicity associated with excess release of glutamate. These four drugs can reduce symptoms and slow the rate of decline in some patients with dementia, but they do not modify the underlying pathology. Reviews of research emphasize the importance of individualizing the selection and dose of medications, frequently assessing for adverse effects, and including nonpharmacologic interventions as integral parts of care plans (Gomoll, Sanders, & Caserta, 2014). The usual pharmacologic approach is to begin a cholinesterase inhibitor before or during the moderate stage of dementia and to add memantine during the moderate or later stages. The most common adverse effects of cholinesterase inhibitors are nausea, vomiting, diarrhea, weight loss, and loss of appetite. Adverse effects of memantine include dizziness, headache, constipation, and increased confusion.

It is important to recognize that in 2017, no disease-modifying drug was available in the United States, despite intense and ongoing research related to the development of drugs for dementia during the past several decades (Tsai & Cummings, 2017). Also, the FDA has approved new forms and doses of the four drugs currently available, but no new drug has been approved since 2003. Current recommendations of the Alzheimer's Association and other major organizations emphasize the importance of nonpharmacologic interventions for promoting wellness and preventing decline in people with dementia, as discussed in the following sections.

Nonpharmaceutical Interventions for Promoting Wellness in People With Dementia

As anyone who has cared for a person with dementia knows, interventions must be highly individualized and frequently modified. An intervention that works for one person may not work for others, and interventions that are effective one day will not necessarily be effective the next day. A dominant theme of research and practice is the implementation of person-centered interventions that are based on a comprehensive and ongoing assessment of the person's unique and changing needs.

One way in which nurses promote wellness for people with dementia is by addressing concerns that improve quality of life. Dementia can affect all the following aspects of quality of life for people with dementia: health, independence, self-determination, social interaction, financial security, psychological well-being, security and privacy, religion and spirituality, and being of use or giving meaning to life. An essential intervention for promoting wellness is to pay careful attention to the verbal and nonverbal ways in which the person with dementia communicates his or her needs and feelings. Box 14-6 provides statements of people with dementia about their needs and quality of life.

> **💡 Technology to Promote Wellness in Older Adults**
>
> There is increasing interest in the development and use of robotic assistants for functional and social assistance for people with dementia, as in the following examples:
>
> - "Paro" is a social robot in the form of a cuddly white seal that has been used for individual and group therapy in nursing homes and geropsychiatric programs in Japan and Europe since 2003 and in the United States since 2009. Paro has sensors for touch, light, sound, motion, and temperature. In the United States, Paro is classified as an FDA-approved biofeedback device for treating dementia-related symptoms (Petersen, Houston, Qin, et al., 2017). Studies have shown the following positive effects on patients: reduced stress, increased social interaction, improved sense of well-being, and decreased behavioral symptoms of dementia (Joranson, Pedersen, Rokstad, et al., 2016; Lane, Noronha, Rivera, et al., 2016; Liang, Piroth, Robinson, et al., 2017). Information about Paro is available at ttp://www.parorobots.com/index.asp.
> - Studies in Australia found that Sophie and Jack, two baby-face robots, were effective for providing sensory enrichment, positive social engagement, and entertainment (Chu, Khosla, Khaksar, et al., 2017).

Box 14-6   Lived Experiences: Needs and Quality of Life

About Needs

- "Just explain it a bit more, like when he said, 'I will refer you to the memory clinic,' you know, another two or three sentences. I just want to put you in the picture as to what will go on there, what it's for, what the setup is."

- "My independence is really important to me, and I know if someone came in and started telling me how I should run things or do things, I would certainly retaliate and not conform to anything they would want to do."

- "As you have been diagnosed, there should be a follow-up with information on what you have got, how do you cope with it, what to look for, what's gonna happen."

About Quality of Life

- "Quality of life is living with your family—your circle of friends and family."

- "Friendship is good. Very important to have friends."

- "Oh there's nothing better than peace and quiet to be happy and comfortable, but if you ain't got peace, you're upset, and when you've got peace and quiet, you don't have anything in the mind."

- "To feel safe. I've lived here for about 2 years and feel secure and safe. No accidents. This is important."

- "I want to keep my own environment… because I am familiarized with it."

- "It's not just the environment in the house, it's when you go out… in the bank, environment in the shops you go into, or restaurant is another environment, which you have got to overcome."

- "I think your physical health is very important because even though I've got problems in myself, with my brain through my vascular dementia, I feel that if you have got your physical fitness then it still gives you that form of independence that you can still do things. Like I can still go to the bathroom and shave, where if you haven't got good health and you start having problems as well, it must be horrendous."

Source: Alzheimer's Society (2008); Alzheimer's Society (2010); Fetherstonhaugh, Tarzia, and Nay (2013).

Another way of promoting wellness for people with dementia is through interventions that support the person's strengths and individuality during all stages of dementia by providing person-centered care, as described in the following sections. Nurses also promote wellness through interventions that support optimal levels of functioning because at least some of the functional decline associated with dementia can be categorized as **excess disability**, which is defined as limitations that are beyond what is to be expected. As an example, when caregivers provide unnecessary assistance with tasks such as eating or dressing, people with dementia may lose their ability for self-care sooner than if they had performed the tasks with the necessary direction from caregivers. Another major focus is on nonpharmacologic interventions to improve functioning and quality of life for people with dementia and their care partners, as described in Table 14-5. Nurses can facilitate referrals for these interventions,

---

TABLE 14-5   Research on Nonpharmacologic Interventions for People With Dementia

Intervention or Review of Studies	Results	References
Aromatherapy with a mixture of lemongrass and eucalyptus oils, delivered by two methods: hand massage, and indirect inhalation during sleep via air humidifier	Residents with moderate to severe dementia showed reduced agitation compared with the control group.	Turten Kaymaz and Ozdemir (2017)
Aromatherapy massage on the person's neck, shoulders, and arms with a mixture of lavender and orange oils once weekly for 8 weeks	Residents with dementia showed reduced agitation and depression compared with the control group.	Yang, Wang, and Wang (2016)
Systematic reviews focusing on nonpharmacologic interventions for dementia-related behaviors	Music-based interventions are effective for managing many behavioral symptoms of dementia.	Goris, Ansel, and Schutte (2016); Milan-Calenti, Lorenzo-Lopez, Alonso-Bua, et al. (2016)
Comprehensive literature review of music therapy for dementia	Music therapy is effective for deducing anxiety and disruptive behavior and may also improve depression and quality of life.	Zhang, Cai, An, et al. (2017)
Personalized interactive systems for laptops or portable devices that are programmed with music, photos, movies, and messages for individual self-directed activity	The Memory Box system, which participants used for a mean daily running time of 2.6 hours, was effective for improving quality of life and decreasing anxiety and depression in nursing home residents with dementia.	Davison, Nayer, Coxon, et al. (2016)
Review of 12 studies of provision of a doll to people with moderate to late stage dementia	Doll therapy was effective for alleviating behavioral and psychological symptoms and improving overall well-being.	Ng, Ho, Koh, et al. (2017)
Reviews of studies on sensory stimulation as interventions for reducing sleep disturbances	Bright light therapy is effective for improving sleep in people with dementia	Dimitriou and Tsolaki (2017)

which are particularly important during early and moderate stages of dementia. These interventions address aspects of functioning and quality of life, but they are not necessarily applicable to addressing dementia-related behaviors, which are discussed in a separate section.

GLOBAL PERSPECTIVE

The Alzheimer's Society in Great Britain encourages participation of people with dementia and their care partners in a popular program called "Singing for the Brain." Studies indicate that this program is beneficial in all of the following ways: improved memory function, social inclusion and support, shared experiences, positive impact on relationships, lifting of the spirits, and acceptance of the diagnosis (Osman, Tischler, & Schneider, 2016). Although this dementia-specific program is not currently available in the United States, nurses can encourage older adults with dementia and their care partners to explore resources for participating in singing groups.

Wellness Opportunity

Nurses holistically address behavioral symptoms by trying to identify nonpharmacologic interventions that improve quality of life for the person with dementia and his or her caregivers.

Improving Safety and Function Through Environmental Modifications

Environmental modifications are important interventions for people with dementia because environmental factors profoundly affect their safety, functioning, and quality of life.

Current emphasis is on the influence of all of the following aspects of the total physical and psychosocial environment:

- Sounds
- Floor surfaces
- Colors and color contrast
- Lighting (e.g., glare, shadows, brightness)
- Design and placement of exits and bathrooms
- Living things (e.g., plants, birds, fish, pets)
- Furniture (seating, placement, heights of tables and chairs)
- Safety devices (e.g., rails, grab bars)
- Provisions for privacy and social interaction
- Items that improve comfort and hominess (e.g., decorative items, textured items, meaningful personal belongings)
- Absence of potentially harmful items (e.g., clutter, obstacles, sharp knives, cleaning solutions, and other potentially toxic products)

Box 14-7 summarizes environmental interventions and techniques to address safety and independence in ADLs.

GLOBAL PERSPECTIVE

Cities, town, and villages in over 30 countries across the world are working toward making their communities "dementia friendly" by creating public environments that enable people with dementia to function independently with supports (Lin, 2017). In the United States, dementia-friendly communities are available in some residential settings (described in Chapter 6); however, larger scale efforts are beginning through organizations such as Dementia Friendly America (www.dfamerica.org).

Box 14-7 Environmental Adaptations and Techniques for Improving Safety and Functioning in People With Dementia

General Environmental Modifications

- Modify the environment to compensate as much as possible for sensory deficits and other functional impairments. (Refer to interventions in Chapters 16 to 19 and 22.)
- Use clocks, calendars, daily newspapers, and simple written cues for orientation (e.g., day, date, names, place, and events).
- Use simple pictures, written cues, or color codes for identifying items and places (e.g., toilet, bedroom).
- Use simple written cues to clarify directions for operating radios, televisions, appliances, and thermostats (e.g., on, off, directional arrows).
- Place pictures of familiar people in highly visible places, but use nonglossy pictures and nonglare glass in picture frames.
- Turn lights on as soon as, or before, it gets dark.
- Use nightlights, or leave dim lights on during the night.
- Provide adequate environmental stimuli while avoiding overstimulation.

Techniques to Ensure Safety

- Make sure the person carries some form of identification, along with the phone number of someone to call.
- Adapt the environment for safety (e.g., use alarm devices on doors to prevent wandering).
- Keep the environment uncluttered.
- Keep medications, cleaning solutions, and any poisonous chemicals in inaccessible places.

- Enroll the person in a protective program, such as the Safe Return program sponsored by the Alzheimer's Association.

Techniques to Facilitate Independent Performance of Activities of Daily Living

- Keep all activities as simple and routine as possible.
- Establish routines that allow for maximum independence and the least amount of frustration.
- While keeping the routines as consistent as possible, recognize that they will have to be changed as the person's level of function changes.
- Lay out one set of clothing in the order in which the items are to be donned.
- If the person needs assistance with hygiene, use matter-of-fact statements such as "It's time for your bath."
- Arrange personal care items, such as grooming and hygiene aids, in a visible and uncluttered place, in the order in which the items are to be used.
- Leave a toothbrush on the bathroom sink with toothpaste already on it.
- Establish an individualized toileting plan that allows for maximum independence but minimal risk for incontinence episodes.
- Offer finger foods and nutritious snacks if the person will not sit at the table to eat a meal.

Communicating With Older Adults With Dementia

Verbal and nonverbal communication techniques are widely recognized as essential interventions for people with dementia throughout the entire course of the disease. Nurses need to pay particular attention to the effects of touch, facial expressions, tone of voice, and body language on communication. Box 14-8 summarizes techniques for facilitating communication with people with dementia. These techniques are general guidelines, and it is important to adapt communication to the particular needs of each person with dementia.

See ONLINE LEARNING ACTIVITY 14-4: ARTICLE ABOUT PROVIDING PERSON-CENTERED CARE AND ADDRESSING SPIRITUAL NEEDS OF OLDER ADULTS LIVING WITH DEMENTIA at http://thepoint.lww.com/Miller8e

Interventions for Dementia-Related Behaviors

Health care professionals increasingly recognize that dementia-related behaviors reflect an attempt to communicate needs that the person may not consciously recognize and cannot express verbally. Thus, nurses must direct their interventions toward the underlying needs of the person with dementia. Hall and Buckwalter (1987) proposed a theoretical framework for addressing dementia-related behaviors called the *progressively lowered stress threshold* (PLST) model. Briefly stated, this model posits that dysfunctional behaviors indicate a progressive lowering of the stress threshold which, in turn, interferes with the person's functioning and ability to interact with the environment. Common stressors associated with dysfunctional episodes are fatigue; change of environment, routine, or caregiver; misleading stimuli or inappropriate stimulus levels; internal or external demands that exceed functional capacity; physical stressors (e.g., pain, illness, depression); and affective response to loss. The goal of nursing care, then, is to maximize the person's function by relieving stressors that cause excess disability. The choice of interventions is based on an ongoing assessment of anxiety "as a barometer to determine how much activity and stimuli the anxious person can tolerate at any point during their illness. As anxious behaviors occur, activities and environmental stimuli are modified and simplified until the anxiety disappears" (Hall & Buckwalter, 1987, p. 403). This approach (summarized in Box 14-9) is highly individualized; from a nursing perspective, it is analogous to adjusting insulin doses for people with diabetes according to serum glucose levels. It is widely used in long-term care settings and also can be taught to caregivers in home settings. A randomized controlled trial found that PLST-based interventions in home settings resulted in decreased depression, decreased caregiver burden, and increased quality of life for family caregivers (Soylemez, Kucukguclu, & Buckwalter, 2016).

Box 14-8 Facilitating Communication With People Who Have Dementia

Verbal Communication

- Adapt your level of communication to the abilities of the person with dementia.
- Simplify sentences according to the person's ability to process information.
- Present only one idea at a time.
- Allow enough time for processing.
- Avoid infantilization (e.g., do not talk baby talk or use a demeaning or condescending tone of voice).
- Assist with word finding (e.g., supply missing words, repeat the person's sentence with the correct word).
- Avoid shaming the person (e.g., do not emphasize deficits).
- Paraphrase what the person says, and ask for clarification about the meaning.
- If the person does not understand a statement, repeat the statement using the same words, or simplify the wording.
- Do not argue with the person, unless it is a matter of safety.
- Avoid complex or sarcastic humor.
- Use positive statements (i.e., avoid using statements containing the word "don't" or other negative commands).
- Involve the person with decisions to the best of his or her ability by offering simple and concrete choices (e.g., "Do you want chicken or steak?" rather than "What do you want to eat?").
- Do not ask questions that you know the person cannot answer correctly.
- Do not test the person's memory unnecessarily.
- Listen to the feelings the person is trying to express and respond to the feelings, rather than the statement.
- When discussing activities of daily living, avoid statements, such as "You need a bath now," which may be interpreted as judgmental.

Nonverbal Communication

- Attract and maintain the person's attention (e.g., through eye contact, pleasant facial expressions).
- Use a relaxed and smiling approach.
- Reinforce verbal communication with appropriate nonverbal communication (e.g., demonstrate what you are asking the person to do).
- Use simple pictures rather than written cues.
- Use appropriate touch for communication (e.g., to gain the person's attention or reinforce feelings of concern), unless the person responds negatively to touch.
- Be aware of your own nonverbal communication.
- Keep in mind that your nonverbal cues will probably communicate more than your spoken words and will not necessarily be interpreted correctly.
- Closely observe all nonverbal cues exhibited by the person, particularly those that express feelings.
- Assume that all nonverbal expressions of the person with dementia are attempts to communicate needs or feelings.

Box 14-9 Nursing Interventions for People With Dementia Based on the Progressively Lowered Stress Threshold Model

- Maximize safety by modifying the environment to compensate for cognitive losses.
- Control any factors that increase stress, such as fatigue; physical stressors; competing or overwhelming stimuli; changes in routine, caregiver, or environment; and activities or demands that exceed the person's functional ability.
- Plan and maintain a consistent routine.
- Implement regular rest periods to compensate for fatigue and loss of reserve energy.
- Provide unconditional positive regard.
- Remain nonjudgmental about the appropriateness of all behaviors except those that present threats to safety.
- Recognize individual expressions of fatigue, anxiety, and increasing stress and intervene to reduce stressors as soon as possible.
- Modify reality orientation and other therapeutic interventions to incorporate only that information needed for safe function.
- Use reassuring forms of therapy, such as music and reminiscence.

Source: Hall, G. R., & Buckwalter, K. C. (1987). Progressively lowered stress threshold: A conceptual model for care of adults with Alzheimer's disease. *Archives of Psychiatric Nursing,* 1, 399–406.

Box 14-10 summarizes statements of people with dementia about their lived experiences related to needing help from others and being part of a support group.

Decisions about the use of psychotropic medications for dementia-related disruptive behaviors are complex for several reasons. First, because dementia-related behaviors are often precipitated by modifiable factors, including medical conditions, environmental influences, and adverse medication effects (e.g., anticholinergic medications), initial interventions should always address any contributing factors. For example, if behaviors are due to the adverse effects of medications, initial interventions focus on eliminating or reducing the dose. Second, there is always a risk that medications will further interfere with function and perhaps even cause serious harm, such as further reduction in cognitive function or increased risk for falls. A third consideration is whether the behaviors justify the risks associated with medications. Bothersome or socially inappropriate behaviors may best be ignored or tolerated than treated with medications. However, if the behavior is unsafe, uncomfortable, or interferes with the function of the person with dementia or the rights or safety of others, then pharmaceutical intervention may be appropriate, but only if other interventions are not successful. In any situation, health care professionals should view behavior-modifying medications as one component of a comprehensive management plan that addresses the complex nature of dementia-related behaviors.

Although antipsychotics have been used for the management of dementia-related behaviors for many decades, there are increasing concerns about serious adverse effects and lack of effectiveness in people with dementia. Concerns about safety of so-called first-generation antipsychotics (e.g., haloperidol) led to increased use of newer antipsychotics (called atypical antipsychotics), including olanzapine (Zyprexa), quetiapine (Seroquel),

---

Box 14-10 Lived Experiences: Experiences and Feelings About Needing Help From Others and Being Part of a Support Group

About Needing Help From Others

- "When the day comes that I have got to start asking for help and if that independence is taken away, then I would like to think that I could still be consulted and still have some say in my independence."
- "It is very beneficial, when I am unable to verbalize what I want, for my wife to display multiple options and allow me to choose one."
- "If all else fails, I rely on my partner and my family to come up with solutions I cannot solve."
- "I think it would be nice if people gave you the courtesy of time to finish what you are trying to say."
- "You can't do what you want. You have to ask. So you have to adjust your schedule to someone else's. I guess the best word for it is that it is somewhat humiliating to be in that position when you're used to running your own life."
- "I'm slower at making decisions, and I'm slower on purpose. And I talk to more people about it before I would do it. I'm quite dependent on my wife because I can't do most things independently any more."
- "Before I'd take a walk around the block rather than blow my stack. By the time I got back, my feet hurt so much that I quit worrying about what I was mad about. Now my husband will go with me, and that doesn't do it."

About Being Part of a Support Group

- "Since it is difficult to maintain my old social networks, I reach out to others online through e-mail groups and chat rooms for people with dementia. These can be real life savers some days."

- "It is that bit of extra that you know these people are having the same problems and *really* understand."
- "I commiserate with my friends going through the same things."
- "When I've gotten real down, it seems as though my failure in things I do is exaggerated many times. I feel as though my power has been lost to do anything about it. I feel hopeless and helpless. Thank God for my chat group sticking with me to crawl out."
- "I participate in the group in hopes that people with dementia will begin to be treated with more respect and dignity and to help others recognize how much coping we must do to accomplish even simple things throughout a normal day."
- "I have always been a person who has wanted to make a difference in the world, and through the group, I feel I have been able to change a small part of the way some people think about early-stage dementia."
- "Let's work together to change paradigms about what persons with dementia can and can't do. Don't limit us—help us push the envelopes of our new abilities."
- "The benefits to me personally are so important, as I can still feel that I am a valuable contributing member of society, even though I'm 'cognitively disabled.'"
- "Today I have met people who are in very much the same boat as I am with things they can and can't do, so for me it's a relief to find that there are others in the same boat."

Source: Alzheimer's Society (2010); Beard and Fox (2008); Beard, Knauss, and Moyer (2009); Clare, Rowlands, and Quin (2008); Fetherstonhaugh, Tarzia, and Nay (2013).

and risperidone (Risperdal). Current evidence-based guidelines indicate that neuroleptic medications should be avoided because they are associated with serious adverse effects and have little to no benefit for treating dementia-related behaviors (Allers, Dörks, Schmiemann, et al., 2017; Forlenza, Loureiro, Pais, et al., 2017).

Current emphasis is on nonpharmacologic approaches to addressing dementia-related behaviors, based on a person-centered approach. Reviews of over 200 articles published between 2004 and 2016 recommended that multimodal interventions be used, including any of the following:

- Personalized social interaction (i.e., meaningful and individualized one-to-one social interaction)
- Regular physical activity
- Occupational activities
- Music therapy
- Aromatherapy
- Prophylactic pain management
- Bright light therapy
- Cognitive rehabilitation
- Caregiver supportive interventions

(Fessel, Mann, Miyawaki, et al., 2017; Forlenza, Louriero, Pais, et al., 2017; Travers, Brooks, Hines, et al., 2016).

Smith, Schultz, Seydel, et al. (2013) describe a major 3-year project funded by the Agency for Healthcare Research and Quality that culminated in the development of an evidence-based algorithm and guidelines related to treating problem behaviors in nursing home residents without the use of antipsychotic medications (see Box 14-11

Box 14-11 Nondrug Management of Problem Behaviors and Psychosis in Dementia

Step 1: Assess and Treat Contributing Factors

FOCUS on one behavior at a time
- Note how often, how bad, how long, and document specific details
- **Ask:** What is really going on? What is causing the problem behavior? What is making it worse?

IDENTIFY what leads to or triggers problems
- **Physical:** pain, infection, hunger/thirst, other needs?
- **Psychological:** loneliness, boredom, nothing to do?
- **Environment:** too much/too little going on; lost?
- **Psychiatric:** depression, anxiety, psychosis?

REDUCE, ELIMINATE things that lead to or trigger the problems
- Treat medical/physical problems
- Offer pain medications for comfort or to help cooperation
- Address emotional needs: reassure, encourage, engage
- Offer enjoyable activities to do alone, 1:1, small group
- Remove or disguise misleading objects
- Redirect away from people or areas that lead to problems
- Try another approach; try again later
- Find out what works for others; get someone to help

DOCUMENT outcomes
- If the behavior is reduced or manageable, go to Step 3
- If the behavior persists, go to Step 2

Step 2: Select and Apply Interventions

CONSIDER retained abilities, preferences, resources
- Cognitive level
- Physical functional level
- Long-standing personality, life history, interests
- Preferred personal routines, daily schedules
- Personal/family/facility resources

DEVELOP a Person-Centered plan
- Adjust caregiver approaches
- Adapt/change the environment
- Select/use best evidence-based interventions tailored to the person's unique needs/interests/abilities

ADJUST your approach to the person
- **Personal approach:** cue, prompt, remind, distract; focus on person's wishes, interests, concerns; use/avoid touch as indicated. <u>Do not</u> try to reason, teach new routines, or ask to "try harder"

- **Daily routines:** simplify tasks and put them in a regular order; offer limited choices; use long-standing patterns and preferences to guide routines and activities
- **Communication style:** simple words and phrases; speak in short sentences; speak clearly; wait for answers; make eye contact; monitor tone of voice and body language
- **Unconditional positive regard:** <u>do not</u> confront, challenge, or explain misbeliefs (hallucinations, delusions, illusions); accept belief as real to the person; reassure, comfort, and distract

ADAPT or CHANGE the environment
- **Eliminate things that lead to confusion:** clutter, TV, radio, noise, people talking; reflections in mirrors/dark windows; misunderstood pictures or decor
- **Reduce things that cause stress:** caffeine; extra people; holiday decorations; public TV
- **Adjust stimulation:** if overstimulated–reduce noise, activity, and confusion; if understimulated (bored)–increase activity and involvement
- **Help with functioning:** signs, cues, pictures help way-finding; increase lighting to reduce misinterpretation
- **Involve in meaningful activities:** personalized program of 1:1 and small group or large group as needed
- **Change the setting:** secure outdoor areas; decorative objects; objects to touch and hold; home-like features; smaller, divided recreational and dining areas; natural and bright light; spa-like bathing facilities; signs to help way-finding

SELECT and USE evidence-based interventions
- Work with the team to fit the intervention to the person
- Check care plan for additional information
- Contact supervisor with problems/issues

Step 3: Monitor Outcomes and Adjust Course as Needed
- Track behavior problems using rating scale(s)
- Assure adequate "dose" (intensity, duration, frequency) of interventions
- Adapt/add interventions as needed to get the best possible outcomes
- Make sure all people working with the person understand and cooperate with the treatment plan and are trained as needed

Reprinted with permission from Carnahan, R., Smith, M., Reist, J., et al. (2012). Improving antipsychotic appropriateness in dementia patients. *Portal of Geriatrics Online Education.* Available from: http://www.pogoe.org/productid/21209. Also available at: https://igec.uiowa.edu/ia-adapt

for more information). Online Learning Activity 14-5 provides a link to additional evidence-based resources from this project and other major initiatives addressing problem behaviors in people with dementia.

 See ONLINE LEARNING ACTIVITY 14-5: ADDITIONAL INFORMATION ABOUT IMPROVING ANTIPSYCHOTIC APPROPRIATENESS IN PATIENTS WITH DEMENTIA at http://thepoint.lww.com/Miller8e

Considerations for Non-Alzheimer's Dementia

As already mentioned, more information is available for Alzheimer's disease than for other types of dementia. However, information specific to other types of dementia is increasingly becoming available, particularly for Lewy body dementia, as in the following considerations that pertain to nursing care:

- Use anticholinergic medications (e.g., antipsychotics and benzodiazepines) with caution, and only in very low doses.
- Assess for physiologic disorders at the first sign of changes in behavior, because people with Lewy body dementia decompensate more when they have a medical condition.
- Assess for signs of autonomic nervous system dysfunction affecting swallowing, digestion, blood pressure, temperature regulation, and bowel and bladder control.
- Consider referrals for occupational and physical therapy because movement and balance disorders occur early in the disease.

A consideration related to vascular dementia is that management of cardiovascular risk factors (e.g., lipids, blood pressure, lifestyle interventions) is an integral part of the treatment plan.

General Principles of Nursing Interventions in Different Settings

In recent years, there has been increasing implementation of multifaceted models of care for people with dementia in long-term care settings, including assisted living and nursing facilities. Many nursing facilities have specially designed dementia special care units and some assisted living facilities are designed specifically for the care of people with dementia. Essential features of these units for cognitively impaired residents include environmental modifications, family involvement, individualized care plans, dementia-specific activity programs, and specially trained and selected staff. Some nursing homes incorporate these features into all nursing care units and address the individualized needs of the residents. Long-term residential facilities typically address the needs of people who are in moderate to severe stages of dementia, although some residents are in the early stages. Box 14-12 summarizes statements of people with moderate to severe dementia in a residential care home about their experiences.

Older adults with dementia are frequently admitted to acute care settings for evaluation and treatment of medical or behavioral problems that are superimposed on the dementia. Consequently, nurses in hospital settings usually deal not only with the acute illness but also with the dementia-related behaviors, which are exacerbated by the medical problem, the hospital environment, the unfamiliar caregivers, and the

---

Box 14-12 Lived Experiences: People With Moderate to Severe Dementia in Residential Care Homes

I Still Am Somebody

- "I can remember all those things, and they come back. And I know I can't do them now, but if I think about them, I'm sort of living them again, so that's really nice."
- "Well, I ebb and flow a bit because I'm older and I've had heart trouble for years, so I think, really, I do ever so well. I've got no complaints at all."
- "I used to do a lot. I may get back to it, and particularly if we get a nice Spring sort of thing, it might be better for me."
- "I'm thankful for what I can do, you know what I mean? I won't give in."

Nothing's Right Now

- "Don't lose me, will you? Please don't lose me."
- "Things you like to remember, you can't remember, and things that you can remember easily drift away in front of you."
- "I don't know what's the matter with me and why people don't talk to me much. I feel to be an outsider."
- "I don't know whether I'm stuck here for the rest of my life or what's happening really."
- "I'm frightened; please help me to know."
- "Nobody wants me. I mean, that's the case, nobody does. If I was wanted by anybody, I could be quite useful. But nobody knows that I want a job."

I'm All Right; I'll Manage

- "I wouldn't say it was as good as home at a place like this. You're just one of a number—group—who are pretty well in a similar position, but you do your best and give as much help. I've been sorting books out all morning."
- "It's not as nice as I'd like it to be, but I have to be satisfied with small things these days."
- "I haven't got to do any shopping, I haven't got to cook any meals, and that's a lot, isn't it? You've gotta get used to it, haven't you?"
- "I never thought I'd come to a place like this, but I'm quite happy."
- "I've got a pal; she helps me out."

It Drives Me Mad

- "I'd rather be doing something, yes, although there's not a lot I can do… I'm capable of doing."
- "I get bored here. They go to sleep and I feel like throwing something at them, because they… nobody talking or nobody goes walking. You've gotta do something, haven't you, to help you go through? Because it wasn't the things I've been used to. They just sit here; it drives me mad."
- "I want to be free… or die. I don't mind dying, but I don't want to be coddled here."

Source: Clare, Rowlands, Bruce, et al. (2008); Clare, Rowlands, and Quin (2008).

change in routines. Thus, nurses in acute care settings face a tremendous challenge in caring for people with dementia.

One of the most important initial interventions is to involve at least one of the older adult's usual caregivers in planning and implementing an individualized care plan for the cognitively impaired person. Although the person with dementia is likely to exhibit different behaviors in the hospital than at home, it is crucial to identify interventions that were effective in the home environment. Because people with moderate to severe dementia may not be able to express their needs verbally, nurses need to obtain information from family caregivers who understand how the person expresses his or her needs. During the admission process, nurses may save a lot of time and frustration by interviewing the caregivers about specific methods that help or hinder care. Figure 14-3 illustrates a form that can be used to obtain helpful information from family caregivers. Information about this form and additional information related to care of hospitalized patients with dementia are available through the link to Nurses Improving Care for Healthsystem Elders in Online Learning Activity 14-6.

See ONLINE LEARNING ACTIVITY 14-6: ADDITIONAL INFORMATION ABOUT CARING FOR HOSPITALIZED PATIENTS WITH DEMENTIA at http://thepoint.lww.com/Miller8e

Another strategy for addressing the needs of patients who have dementia is to involve one of the person's usual caregivers in care tasks such as feeding or to ask him or her to provide a familiar presence during the hospitalization. Despite a need for respite from caregiving responsibilities, family and other caregivers may be willing to provide assistance and guidance. This may be particularly helpful during the first few days of hospitalization, and with patients who are particularly difficult to manage. Assessment and intervention tools for addressing the needs of hospitalized people with dementia, including cost-free videos demonstrating the application of these tools, are available at the websites listed in Online Learning Activity 14-6.

Addressing Needs of Caregivers

In all settings, a major role of nurses is to work with family members or paid caregivers to provide appropriate interventions that focus on improving functioning for the person with dementia, alleviating the burden for the caregivers, and improving quality of life for all. An intervention that might be most effective, as well as efficient, is to encourage caregivers' participation in educational or support groups, which often are led or coled by nurses. The number of groups addressing the needs of caregivers is increasing rapidly, and information about these groups is available from the Alzheimer's Association or local hospitals. Nurses also can encourage caregivers to purchase one of the many caregiver guides that

are available in bookstores or through the Internet and other resources.

In addition to educating caregivers about specific management problems, nurses in community settings must be ready to discuss resources for medical care, home services, and other community-based services for people with dementia and their caregivers. As the number and range of services increase, it is becoming more and more difficult to keep up to date on the resources in one's own community. Although nurses cannot be expected to know all the details about all available community services, they should know generally about the services available. A good rule of thumb is to suggest that caregivers call the local area agency on aging and the local Alzheimer's Association because these organizations serve every part of the United States. Online Learning Activity 14-7 provides links to resources for caregivers of people with dementia.

Technology to Promote Wellness in Older Adults

WeCareAdvisor is an interactive evidence-based tool for a tablet, smartphone, or desktop designed to guide caregivers of people with dementia through individualized strategies to manage BPSD (Kales, Gitlin, Stanislawski, et al., 2017). This app is based on development of an NIH-funded evidence-based approach to addressing BPSD, called the DICE process, which stands for **D**escribe, **I**nvestigate, **C**reate, and **E**valuate. Nurses can encourage caregivers to explore information about this tool at http://www.programforpositiveaging.org/wecareadvisor.

See ONLINE LEARNING ACTIVITY 14-7: RESOURCES FOR CAREGIVERS OF PEOPLE WITH DEMENTIA at http://thepoint.lww.com/Miller8e.

EVALUATING THE EFFECTIVENESS OF NURSING INTERVENTIONS

Nurses can evaluate the care of people with dementia according to the extent to which they receive necessary supports and maintain their dignity and quality of life. Because a decline in function is an inherent part of dementia, nursing care is evaluated on an ongoing basis as the person's condition changes and in relation to appropriate and changing goals. Nurses evaluate the degree to which quality of life is maintained by obtaining feedback about life satisfaction, which people in the early and middle stages of dementia usually can express verbally or nonverbally. For example, nurses can evaluate the extent to which the person enjoys or participates in meaningful activities and interactions. As dementia progresses, it becomes more difficult to obtain this kind of information, and nurses rely more on feedback from caregivers and their own judgment. During the later stages of dementia, measures of quality of life focus more on comfort and basic physical needs. Throughout the dementia course,

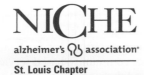

nicheprogram.org

Author: Maggie Murphy-White, MA, Alzheimer's Association St. Louis Chapter
Series Editor: Marie Boltz, PhD, RN, Managing Editor: Scott Bugg

NEED TO KNOW FOR PATIENTS & FAMILIES

Family Caregiver Report

Family Members, use this form to share information with staff about how your loved one is normally, when they are not sick or in crisis. Encourage patient involvement in the development of this information as much as possible. This information will help staff understand and provide for your loved one's needs.

Name: _____What does he/she preferred to be called?_____

Where does he/she live?_____Alone? Or with?_____

Does he/she become upset? Yes No How does he/she show this? _____

What triggers this?_____ What makes he/she feel comfortable?_____

In general, what helps he/she cope (for example, religion, music, certain people)? _____

What fluids or simple foods does he/she enjoy? _____

Would he/she like chaplain to visit? Yes No What other religious/spiritual activity would he/she desire? _____

What is his/her normal bedtime routine (for example, dentures in/out, call to family, a prayer, etc.)?_____

_____

What kind of work did he/she do? _____

What are his/her interests or hobbies? _____

What else can you tell us that will help us care for him/her? Strengths/Challenges? _____

_____

Does he/she normally need help...	Always	Sometimes	Never	Don't Know	Details
Understand where he/she is?					
Follow directions?					
Tell others what he/she needs?					
Tell others when he/she is in pain?					
Wear a hearing aid?					
Wear glasses?					
Have dentures?					
Using the bathroom?					
Walking?					
Getting out of bed?					
With bathing, brushing teeth, etc.?					
Dressing?					
Eating?					

Is there anything else you want the staff to know about him/her? _____

Name & relationship of person completing this form: _____

FIGURE 14-3 A form that can be used to obtain helpful information from family caregivers. (Used with permission from Murphy-White, M. (2013). *NICHE need to know: Dementia transition series.* St. Louis Chapter: Nurses Improving Care for Healthsystem Elders & Alzheimer's Association. © 2013 NICHE All rights reserved. The information contained in this tool is provided for informational purposes only.)

care can be evaluated by the extent to which the person is free from pain, fear, and anxiety.

Another evaluation consideration is the extent to which the needs of caregivers are met. One evaluation criterion is whether caregivers express satisfaction with their own quality of life, despite the demands of the situation. Other criteria may be a caregiver's attendance at support groups and his or her use of resources to assist with or guide care.

Case Study

Mrs. D. is 85 years old and lives with her 86-year-old husband in an apartment complex for the elderly. Two years ago, Mrs. D. was diagnosed with Alzheimer's disease, but she was able to participate in her usual activities until the past year. Now she is neglecting her personal care and is unsafe during meal preparation.

When Mrs. D. wakes up several times nightly to go to the bathroom, she sometimes goes to the apartment door rather than returning to the bedroom. Mr. D. worries that she will leave in the middle of the night. This disrupts his sleep because he maintains a state of constant vigilance. Mr. D. has called a home care agency requesting home health aide (HHA) assistance, and you are the nurse responsible for the initial assessment and for working with the HHAs.

NURSING ASSESSMENT

During your initial assessment, you find that Mrs. D. is pleasant and receptive but has little insight into her need for help. She acknowledges that her doctor told her she has "a memory problem" but reports that this problem doesn't affect her daily life, except that her husband has to remind her about things like turning the stove off after cooking meals. She acknowledges being lonely and says she misses being able to read books and talk to people. Mrs. D. takes donepezil (Aricept) and vitamin E and is otherwise physically healthy.

With regard to ADLs, Mrs. D. has not taken a bath or shower in several months, and she gets very angry if Mr. D. suggests that she take one. She gets confused about her clothing and sometimes wears her underwear over her regular clothes or wears a skirt and slacks at the same time. She insists on doing the meal preparation, but she is not safe while using the stove and gets confused about ingredients in recipes (e.g., she has used salt instead of sugar). Mrs. D. has always done the laundry and housekeeping, but in the past months, she "made a lot of mistakes," such as using powdered milk for laundry detergent.

Mr. D. reports feeling very stressed about the full-time responsibilities of caring for his wife. This stress has escalated in the past month because he no longer feels he can leave her alone. Mrs. D. "shadows" him and feels very insecure if he is out of her sight for more than a few minutes. Mr. D. took her everywhere with him for the past year, but in the last few months, this has become increasingly difficult. For example, when they are grocery shopping, Mrs. D. gets very impatient and pushes the cart into other people. Then, while they are waiting in the checkout line, she insists on taking one of each of the nearby tabloids and magazines, and she creates a scene if Mr. D. doesn't buy them for her.

Mr. D. confides that he expected to be able to care for his wife at home "until the end," but now he has doubts about his ability to keep her at home. He perceives her as "senile" and feels he should be able to meet her needs. There are no nearby family members who can help with her care, but his son and daughter have offered to help pay for some services. Mr. D. is aware of support groups offered by the Alzheimer's Association, but he has not attended any because he cannot leave his wife alone. When asked about his health, Mr. D. says, "I see the doctor for my arthritis and heart problems, but I get along okay, except that I'm supposed to have cataract surgery, and I don't know how I'll manage to get that done."

NURSING DIAGNOSIS

Your nursing diagnosis for Mrs. D. is Altered Thought Processes related to the effects of dementia. You use the nursing diagnosis of Caregiver Role Strain for Mr. D. because you recognize the need to address Mr. D.'s problems. Your immediate goal is to arrange for supportive services and assistance with Mrs. D.'s care because this will improve the quality of life for both Mr. and Mrs. D., and it will alleviate some of the caregiver stress for Mr. D. A long-term goal is to arrange for respite services, so Mr. D. can undergo cataract surgery. You also recognize the need for educational and support services for Mr. D.

NURSING CARE PLAN FOR MR. AND MRS. D.

Expected Outcome	Nursing Interventions	Nursing Evaluation
Mrs. D. will function at her highest level of independence	• Work with Mr. D. to identify ways to improve Mrs. D.'s ability to function safely and independently in performing ADLs (For instance, Mr. D. can involve Mrs. D. in selecting an outfit to wear and can set out the clothing in the order in which it should be donned.) • Arrange for an HHA to work with Mrs. D. and assist her with complex tasks such as laundry, housekeeping, and meal preparation • Teach the HHA to assume an "assistant" and "friend" role by providing only subtle supervision and minimal direct help with activities such as laundry	• Mrs. D. will perform ADLs and instrumental ADLs with minimal assistance

(continued)

NURSING CARE PLAN FOR MR. AND MRS. D. *(Continued)*

Expected Outcome	Nursing Interventions	Nursing Evaluation
Mrs. D.'s quality of life will be maintained	• Work with Mr. D. and the HHA to identify activities that are interesting, satisfying, and intellectually stimulating (e.g., "word find" games) • Explore the possibility of Mrs. D. attending an adult day care program for group activities • Support Mrs. D. in carrying out familiar roles and meaningful activities	• Mrs. D. will continue to engage in activities that are satisfying
Mr. D. will use sources of support to alleviate caregiver-related stress	• Arrange the HHA's schedule to enable Mr. D. to attend caregiver support groups and educational programs • Help Mr. D. in identifying one activity per week that he could do to promote his own well-being (e.g., going to lunch with a friend) • Provide HHA assistance for 4-hour periods to allow Mr. D. time for grocery shopping and pursuing his own interests • Provide Mr. D. with information about the "Caregiver Connection Hot Line" at the Alzheimer's Association, and suggest that he join this telephone support network	• Mr. D. will verbalize feelings of being able to cope effectively with caregiver responsibilities • Mr. D. will participate in one activity per week focused on his own needs and interests

THINKING POINTS

- Use the GDS/FAST in Table 14-3 to assess Mrs. D.'s stage of dementia.
- What would you identify as Mr. D.'s needs as a caregiver?
- What health education information would you plan for Mr. D.?
- What approaches would you suggest for Mr. D. and home care workers for communicating with Mrs. D.?
- What challenges would you anticipate having to address as you provide ongoing supervision of the HHA and continue to work with Mr. and Mrs. D.?

Chapter Highlights

Delirium

Overview of Delirium

- Delirium is a serious, preventable, treatable, commonly occurring condition and is often unrecognized in older adults.
- Delirium results from an interaction between predisposing factors such as dementia and advanced age, and precipitating factors such as surgery and infections.

Prevalence, Risk Factors, and Functional Consequences of Delirium

- Delirium occurs commonly in all health care settings.
- Functional consequences include decline in functioning, increased mortality, and permanent residency in long-term care facilities.

Nursing Assessment of Delirium

- The Confusion Assessment Method is an evidence-based tool for confirming the diagnosis of delirium based on the following: acute onset or fluctuating course, inattention, disorganized thinking, and altered level of consciousness.
- Nurses obtain information through direct observation and patient assessment and from caregivers.
- Delirium subtypes according to motor and behavioral subtypes are hyperactive, hypoactive, and mixed.

Nursing Diagnosis and Outcomes

- The nursing diagnosis of Acute Confusion is applicable for delirium
- Applicable NOC includes Cognition, Concentration, Comfort Status, and Neurologic Status

Nursing Interventions for Delirium

- Interventions for delirium must be interdisciplinary and multifaceted to address the underlying factors (Figure 14-1, Table 14-1).

Dementia

Overview of Dementia

- Dementia is a medical term that includes a group of brain disorders characterized by a gradual decline in cognitive abilities and changes in personality and behavior.

Terminology to Describe Dementia

- Many terms are used interchangeably—and not always accurately—to describe dementia.
- Two or more types of dementia can develop at the same time or sequentially.
- Commonly available diagnostic techniques cannot always determine the type of dementia.

Types of Dementia

- Current medical literature addresses four main types of dementia as Alzheimer's disease, vascular dementia, Lewy body dementia, and frontotemporal dementia (Figure 14-1, Table 14-2).

Factors Associated With Dementia (Box 14-1, Table 14-2)

- Risk factors for Alzheimer's disease include family history, genetic factors, diagnosis of mild cognitive impairment, and traumatic brain injury.
- Factors that decrease the risk for Alzheimer's disease include physical activity, healthy diet, higher educational level, and engagement in social and cognitive activities.

Functional Consequences Associated With Dementia

- Dementia progresses through stages involving cognitive and functional decline (Table 14-3).
- Self-awareness and personal experiences of people with dementia vary significantly (Boxes 14-2 and 14-3).
- Examples of BPSD include agitation, personality changes, mood disturbances, repetitive movements, and changes in sleep and eating.
- Nurses need to recognize and address misperceptions about behaviors in people with dementia (Table 14-4).
- Families and others who are close to the person with dementia experience numerous functional consequences of caregiving.

Nursing Assessment of Dementia

- The initial assessment of cognitive impairment is complex and based on multidisciplinary assessment of all aspects of health and functioning (Box 14-4).
- Assessment is an ongoing process involving assessment of stages and all aspects of health and functioning (Table 14-3, many other chapters in this text).
- Ongoing assessment of consequences also includes attention to the emotional experiences of the person with dementia (Box 14-5).

Nursing Diagnosis

- Nursing diagnoses for the person with dementia include Chronic Confusion, Anxiety, Impaired Memory, Risk Falls, Self-Care Deficit, Disturbed Sleep Pattern, Imbalanced Nutrition, Wandering, Urinary Incontinence.
- Nursing diagnoses to address needs of caregivers include Family Coping and Caregiver Role Strain (or Risk for), Anticipatory Grieving.

Planning for Wellness Outcomes

- NOC for the person with dementia: Agitation Level, Cognition, Cognitive Orientation, Comfort Status, Communication, Memory, Mood Equilibrium, Nutritional Status, Self-Care Status, Sleep, Symptom Control.
- NOC for caregivers: Anxiety Level, Caregiver Emotional Health, Caregiver Physical Health, Caregiver Stressors, Caregiving Endurance Potential.
- For both the person with dementia and his or her caregivers: Coping, Quality of life.

Nursing Interventions to Address Dementia

- Nurses have important roles in teaching older adults and their caregivers about medications for slowing the progression of dementia.
- Nurses use nonpharmacologic interventions to promote wellness and improve quality of life for people with dementia (Box 14-6, Table 14-5).
- Environmental modifications are effective for improving safety and functioning (Box 14-7).
- It is important to adapt communication techniques for people with dementia (Box 14-8).
- The PLST model is an evidence-based approach to addressing dementia-related behaviors (Box 14-9).
- It is important to recognize feelings of people with dementia about their lived experiences of needing help from others and being part of a support group (Box 14-10).
- Nonpharmacologic interventions can be used to address problem behaviors in people with dementia (Box 14-11).
- It is important to recognize the feelings of people with moderate to severe dementia about needing care in a residential care home (Box 14-12).
- Nursing interventions to address needs of caregivers include the following: encouraging participation in educational or support groups, teaching about management of dementia-associated behaviors, and facilitating referrals for community services.

Evaluating the Effectiveness of Nursing Interventions

- Effectiveness of nursing interventions is evaluated as the person's condition changes and in relation to appropriate and changing goals.
- Nurses evaluate the degree to which quality of life is maintained by obtaining feedback about life satisfaction from people with dementia and their caregivers.

Critical Thinking Exercises

1. Define each of the following terms, and describe the relevance of each term according to our current understanding of impaired cognitive function: senility, organic brain syndrome, hardening of the arteries, delirium, dementia, and Alzheimer's disease.

2. Describe how you would explain the distinguishing features of Alzheimer's disease, vascular dementia, Lewy body dementia, and frontotemporal dementia to the family of someone who asks about the types of dementia.

3. You are working in a nursing clinic at a senior center. How would you respond to the following questions, posed by a 74-year-old woman: "I've been having memory problems lately, but I know it's not Alzheimer's, because I haven't done anything really stupid. What do you think I should do? My friend takes a supplement and says that helps her a lot, and I was thinking of trying that. Do you know how much of it I should take?"

4. You are planning an in-service program to nursing home staff about medications used in the treatment of dementia and the management of dementia-related behaviors. What information would you present?

 For more information about topics discussed in this chapter, be sure to check out the interactive Online Learning Activities and other helpful resources at http://thepoint.lww.com/Miller8e

REFERENCES

Allers, K., Dörks, M., Schiemann, G., et al. (2017). Antipsychotic drug use in nursing home residents with and without dementia: Keep an eye on the pro re nata medication. *International Journal of Clinical Psychopharmacology, 32*(4), 213–218.

Alzheimer's Association Report. (2017). 2017 Alzheimer's disease facts and figures. *Alzheimer's & Dementia, 13*, 325–373.

Alzheimer's Society. (2008). *Dementia: Out of the shadows.* London: Alzheimer's Society.

Alzheimer's Society. (2010). *My name is not dementia: People with dementia discuss quality of life.* London: Alzheimer's Society.

Arumugam, S., El-Menyar, A., Al Hassani, A., et al. (2017). Delirium in the intensive care unit. *Journal of Emergency Trauma and Shock, 10*, 37–46.

Baez, S., Pinasco, C., Roca, M., et al. (2017). Brain structural correlates of executive and social cognition profiles in behavioral variant frontotemporal dementia and elderly bipolar disorder. *Neuropsychologia*, 2017 Feb 17. doi: 10.1016/j.neuropsychologia.2017.02.012.

Barone, F., Gustafson, D., Crystal, H., et al. (2016). First translational "Think Tank" on cerebrovascular disease, cognitive impairment and dementia. *Journal of Translational Medicine, 14*, 50.

Beard, R. L., & Fox, P. J. (2008). Resisting social disenfranchisement: Negotiating collective identities and everyday life with memory loss. *Social Science & Medicine, 66*, 1509–1520.

Beard, R. L., Knauss, J., & Moyer, D. (2009). Managing disability and enjoying life: How we reframe dementia through personal narratives. *Journal of Aging Studies, 23*, 227–235.

Canevelli, M., Valletta, M., Trebbastoni, A., et al. (2016). Sundowning in dementia: Clinical relevance, pathophysiological determinants, and therapeutic approaches. *Frontiers in Medicine, 3*, 73.

Chu, M. T., Khosla, R., Khaksar, S. M., et al. (2017). Service innovation through social robot engagement to improve dementia care quality. *Assistive Technology, 29*, 8–18.

Ciampi, A., Bai, C., Dyachenko, A., et al. (2017). Longitudinal patterns of delirium severity scores in long-term care settings. *International Psychogeriatrics, 29*, 11–17.

Clare, L., Rowlands, J., Bruce, E., et al. (2008). The experience of living with dementia in residential care: An interpretative phenomenological analysis. *The Gerontologist, 48*(6), 711–720.

Clare, L., Rowlands, J. M., & Quin, R. (2008). Collective strength: The impact of developing a shared social identity in early-stage dementia. *Dementia, 7*(1), 9–30.

Coyle, M. A., Burns, P., & Traynor, V. (2017). Is it my job? The role of RNs in the assessment and identification of delirium in hospitalized older adults. *Journal of Gerontological Nursing, 43*(4), 29–37.

Curyto, K., McCurry, S., Luci, K., et al. (2017). Managing challenging behaviors of dementia in veterans. *Journal of Gerontological Nursing, 43*(1), 33–43.

Davis, D. H., Muniz-Terrera, G., Keage, H. A., et al. (2017). Association of delirium with cognitive decline in late life: A neuropathologic study of 3 population-based cohort studies. *JAMA Psychiatry, 74*, 244–251.

Davison, T., McCabe, M., Bird, M., et al. (2017). Behavioral symptoms of dementia that present management difficulties in nursing homes. *Journal of Gerontological Nursing, 43*(2), 34–43.

Davison, T., Nayer, K., Coxon, S., et al. (2016). A personalized multimedia device to treat agitated behavior and improve mood in people with dementia: A pilot study. *Geriatric Nursing, 37*, 25–29.

Desai, A., Wharton, T., Struble, L., et al. (2017). Person-centered primary care strategies for assessment of and interventions for aggressive behaviors in dementia. *Journal of Gerontological Nursing, 43*(2), 9–17.

Dichgans, M., & Leys, D. (2017). Vascular cognitive impairment. *Circulation Research, 120*, 573–591.

Dimitriou, T. D., & Tsolaki, M. (2017). Evaluation of the efficacy of randomized controlled trials of sensory stimulation interventions for sleeping disturbances in patients with dementia: A systematic review. *Clinical Interventions in Aging, 12*, 543–548.

Dupuis, S. L., Wiersma, E., & Loiselle, L. (2012). Pathologizing behavior: Meanings of behaviors in dementia care. *Journal of Aging Studies, 26*, 162–173.

Eeles, E., Davis, D., & Bhat, R. (2017). Delirium. In H. M. Fillit, K. Rockwood, & J. B. Young (Eds.). *Brocklehurst's textbook of geriatric medicine and gerontology* (8th ed., pp. 426–432). Philadelphia, PA: Elsevier.

Fernández-Matarrubia, M., Matías-Guiu, J. A., Cabrera-Martín, M. N., et al. (2017). Different apathy clinical profile and neural correlates in behavioral variant frontotemporal dementia and Alzheimer's disease. *International Journal of Geriatric Psychiatry*, doi: 10.1002/gps.4695.

Fessel, M. M., Mann, M., Miyawaki, C. E., et al. (2017). Multi-component interventions and cognitive health: A scoping review. *Journal of Gerontological Nursing, 43*(5), 39–48.

Fetherstonhaugh, D., Tarzia, L., & Nay, R. (2013). Being central to decision making means I am still here!: The essence of decision making for people with dementia. *Journal of Aging Studies, 27*, 143–150.

Finger, E. (2016). Frontotemporal dementias. *Continuum, 22*, 464–486.

Fletcher, K. (2016). Dementia: A neurocognitive disorder. In M. Boltz, E. Capezuti, T. Fulmer, & D. Zwicker (Eds.). *Evidence-based practice protocols for best practice* (5th ed., pp. 233–250). New York: Springer Publishing.

Forlenza, O., Loureiro, J., Pais, M., et al. (2017). Recent advances in the management of neuropsychiatric symptoms in dementia. *Current Opinion in Psychiatry, 30*, 151–158.

Gomoll, B. P., Sanders, B. D., & Caserta, M. T. (2014). Psychopharmacologic treatments for Alzheimer disease and related dementias. *Psychopharm Review, 49*(1), 9–16.

Gomperts, S. (2016). Lewy body dementias: Dementia with Lewy bodies and Parkinson disease dementia. *Continuum, 22*, 435–463.

Gorelick, P., Counts, S., & Nyenhuis, D. (2016). Vascular cognitive impairment and dementia. *Biochimica et Biophysica Acta, 1862*, 860–868.

Goris, E. D., Ansel, K. N., & Schutte, D. L. (2016). Quantitative systematic review of the effects of non-pharmacological interventions on reducing apathy in persons with dementia. *Journal of Advanced Nursing, 72*(11), 2612–2628.

Hall, G. R., & Buckwalter, K. C. (1987). Progressively lowered threshold: A conceptual model for care of adults with Alzheimer's disease. *Archives of Psychiatric Nursing, 1*, 399–406.

Herdman, T., & Kamitsura, S. (Eds). (2018). *NANDA International Nursing Diagnoses Definitions and Classification, 2018–2020* (11th ed., pp. 34–44). New York: Thieme Publishers.

Hshieh, T. T., Saczynski, J., Gou, R. Y., et al. (2017). Trajectory of functional recovery after postoperative delirium in elective surgery. *Annals of Surgery, 265*, 647–653.

Jackson, T. A., Gladman, J. R., Harwood, R. H., et al. (2017). Challenges and opportunities in understanding dementia and delirium in the acute hospital. *PLOS Medicine, 14*(3), e1002247.

Jackson, T., Wilson, D., Richardson, S., et al. (2016). Predicting outcome in older hospital patients with delirium: A systematic literature review. *International Journal of Geriatric Psychiatry, 31*, 392–399.

Joranson, N., Pedersen, I., Rokstad, A. M., et al. (2016). Change in quality of life in older people with dementia participating in Paro-activity: A cluster-randomized controlled trial. *Journal of Advanced Nursing, 72*, 3020–3033.

Kales, J., Gitlin, L., Stanislawski, B., et al. (2017). WeCareAdvisorTM: The development of a caregiver-focused, web-based program to assess and manage behavioral and psychological symptoms of dementia. *Alzheimer's Journal*, [Epub] doi: 10.1097/WAD.0000000000000177.

Kosar, C. M., Thomas, K. S., Inouye, S. K., et al. (2017). Delirium during postacute nursing home admission and risk for adverse outcomes. *Journal of the American Geriatrics Society*, [Epub] doi: 10.1111/jgs.14823.

Kramberger, M. G., Auestad, B., Garcia-Ptacek, S., et al. (2017). Long-term cognitive decline in dementia with Lewy bodies in a large multicenter, international cohort. *Journal of Alzheimer's Disease, 57*(3), 787–795.

Lane, G. W., Noronha, D., Rivera, A., et al. (2016). Effectiveness of a social robot, "Paro," in a VA long-term care setting. *Psychological Services, 13*, 292–299.

Liang, A., Piroth, I., robinson, H., et al. (2017). A pilot randomized trial of a companion robot for people with dementia living in the community. *Journal of the American Medical Directors Association*, [Epub] Doi: 10.1016/j.jamda.2017.05.019.

Lin, S. Y. (2017). "Dementia-friendly communities and being dementia friendly in healthcare settings. *Current Opinion in Psychiatry, 30*, 145–150.

Love, S., & Miners, J. (2016). Cerebrovascular disease in ageing and Alzheimer's disease. *Acta Neurology, 131*, 645–658.

Martyr, A., & Clare, L. (2017). Awareness of functional ability in people with early-stage dementia. *International Journal of Geriatric Psychiatry*, [Epub] doi: 10.1002/gpa.4664.

Matthews, B. (2017). Alzheimer's disease. In B. L. Miller, & B. F. Boeve (Eds.). *The Behavioral Neurology of Dementia* (2nd ed., pp. 123–142). Cambridge, UK: Cambridge University Press.

McCabe, M., You, E., & Tatangelo, G. (2016). Hearing their voice: A systematic review of dementia family caregivers' needs. *Gerontologist, 56*, e70–e88.

Mijajlovic, M., Pavlovic, A., Brainin, M., et al. (2016). Post-stroke dementia – a comprehensive review. *BioMed Central Medicine*, doi: 10.1186/s12916-017-o779-7.

Milan-Calenti, J., Lorenzo-Lopez, L., Alonso-Bua, B., et al. (2016). Optimal nonpharmacological management of agitation in Alzheimer's disease: Challenges and solutions. *Clinical Interventions in Aging, 11*, 175–184.

Miller, C. A. (2012). *Fast facts for dementia care: What nurses need to know in a nutshell.* New York: Springer.

Murphy, R., & Leverenz, J. (2017). The Lewy body dementias. In B. L. Miller, & B. F. Boeve (Eds.). *The behavioral neurology of dementia* (2nd ed., pp. 278–300). Cambridge, UK: Cambridge University Press.

Ng, Q. X., Ho, C. Y., Koh, S. S., et al. (2017). Doll therapy for dementia sufferers: A systematic review. *Complementary Therapy in Clinical Practice, 26*, 42–46.

Onyike, C., & Rabins, P. (2017). Neuropsychiatry of dementia. In B. L. Miller, & B. F. Boeve (Eds.). *The behavioral neurology of dementia* (2nd ed., pp. 9–18). Cambridge, UK: Cambridge University Press.

Osman, S., Tischler, V., & Schneider, J. (2016). "Singing for the Brain": A qualitative study exploring the health and well-being benefits of singing for people with dementia and their carers. *Denmentia, 15*, 1326–1339.

Ostremba, I., Wilczynski, K., & Szewieczek, J. (2016). Delirium in the geriatric unit: Proton-pump inhibitors and other risk factors. *Clinical Interventions in Aging, 11*, 397–405.

Pang, S., & Miller, B. (2017). Frontotemporal dementia. In B. L. Miller, & B. F. Boeve (Eds.). *The Behavioral Neurology of Dementia* (2nd ed., pp. 143–155). Cambridge, UK: Cambridge University Press.

Parrao, T., Brockman, S., Bucks, R., et al. (2017). The structured interview for insight and judgment in dementia: Development and validation of a new instrument to assess awareness in patients with dementia. *Alzheimer's & Dementia, 7*, 24–32.

Paulo, M., Scruth, E., & Jacoby, S. (2017). Dementia and delirium in the elderly hospitalized patient. *Clinical Nurse Specialist, 31*, 66–69.

Perneczky, R., Tene, O., Attems, J., et al. (2016). Is the time ripe for new diagnostic criteria of cognitive impairment due to cerebrovascular disease? Consensus report of the International Congress on Vascular Dementia working group. *BioMed Central Medicine, 14*, doi: 10.1186/s12916–016–0719-y.

Petersen, S., Houston, S., Qin, H., et al. (2017). The utilization of robotic pets in dementia care. *Journal of Alzheimer's Disease, 55*, 569–574.

Powers, S. M., Dawson, N. T., Krestar, M. L., et al. (2016). "I wish they would remember that I forget:" The effects of memory loss on the lives of individuals with mild-to-moderate dementia. *Dementia (London), 15*, 1053–1067.

Raz, L., Knoefel, J., & Bhaskar, K. (2016). The neuropathology and cerebrovascular mechanisms of dementia. *Journal of Cerebral Blood Flow & Metabolism, 36*, 179–186.

Rongve, A., Soennesyn, H., Skogseth, R., et al. (2016). Cognitive decline in dementia with Lewy bodies: A 5-year prospective cohort study. BMJ Open, doi: 10.1136/bmjopen-2015–010357.

Sanders, A. (2016). Caregiver stress and the patient with dementia. *Continuum, 22*, 619–625.

Santos, C., Snyder, P., Wu, W. C., et al. (2017). Pathophysiologic relationship between Alzheimer's disease, cerebrovascular disease, and cardiovascular risk: A review and synthesis. *Alzheimer's & Dementia, 7*, 69–87.

Slooter, A. J., Van De Leur, R. R., & Zaal, I. J. (2017). *Delirium in critically ill patients. Handbook of Clinical Neurology, 141*, 449–466.

Smebye, K. L., & Kirkevold, M. (2013). The influence of relationships on personhood in dementia care: A qualitative, hermeneutic study. *BioMed Central Nursing, 12*(1), 29.

Smith, E. (2016). Vascular cognitive impairment. *Continuum, 22*, 490–509.

Smith, M., Schultz, S. K., Seydel, L. L., et al. (2013). Improving antipsychotic agent use in nursing homes: Development of an algorithm for treating problem behaviors in nursing homes. *Journal of Gerontological Nursing, 39*(5), 24–35.

Soylemez, B., Kucukguclo, O., & Buckwalter, K. (2016). Application of the Progressively Lowered Threshold Model with community-based caregivers. *Journal of Gerontological Nursing, 42*, 44–54.

Steiner, V., Pierce, L., & Salvador, D. (2016). Information needs of family caregivers of people with dementia. *Rehabilitation Nursing, 41*, 162–169.

Stroomer-van Wijk, A., Jonker, B. W., Kok, R. M., et al. (2016). Detecting delirium in elderly outpatients with cognitive impairment. *International Psychogeriatrics, 28,* 1303–1311.

Tomlinson, E. J., Phillips, N. M., Mohebbi, M., et al. (2017). Risk factors for incident delirium in an acute general medical setting: A retrospective case-control study. *Journal of Clinical Nursing, 26,* 658–667.

Toot, S., Swinson, T., Devine, M., et al. (2017). Causes of nursing home placement for older people with dementia: A systematic review and meta-analysis. *International Psychogeriatrics, 29,* 195–208.

Travers, C., Brooks, D., Hines, S., et al. (2016). Effectiveness of meaningful occupation interventions for people living with dementia in residential aged care: A systematic review. *JBI Database of Systematic Reviews and Implementation Reports,* doi: 10.11124/JBISRIR-2016–003230.

Tsai, P. H., & Cummings, J. (2017). Treatment of Alzheimer's disease. In B. L. Miller, & B. F. Boeve (Eds.). *The behavioral neurology of dementia* (2nd ed., pp. 415–424). Cambridge, UK: Cambridge University Press.

Tullmann, D. F., Blevins, C., & Fletcher, K. M. (2016). Delirium: Prevention, early recognition, and treatment. In M. Boltz, E. Capezuti, T. Fulmer, & D. Zwicker (Eds.). *Evidence-based practice protocols for best practice* (5th ed., pp. 251–261). New York: Springer Publishing.

Turten Kaymaz, T., & Ozdemir, L. (2017). Effects of aromatherapy on agitation and related caregiver burden in patients with moderate to severe dementia: A pilot study. *Geriatric Nursing,* [Epub] doi: 10.1016/j.gerinurse,2016.11.001.

World Health Organization. (2016). The epidemiology and impact of dementia: Current state and future trends. Available at www.who.int/mental_health/neurology/dementia/en

Yaffe, K., & Al Hazzouri, A. Z. (2017). Epidemiology and risk factors for dementia. In B. L. Miller, & B. F. Boeve (Eds.). *The behavioral neurology of dementia* (2nd ed., pp. 44–56). Cambridge, UK: Cambridge University Press.

Yang, Y. P., Wang, C. J., & Wang, J. J. (2016). Effect of aromatherapy massage on agitation and depressive mood in individuals with dementia. *Journal of Gerontological Nursing, 42,* 38–46.

Zalon, M., Sandhaus, S., Kovaleski, M., et al. (2017). Hospitalized older adults with established delirium. *Journal of Gerontological Nursing, 43,* 33–40.

Zhang, Y., Cai, J., An, L., et al. (2017). Does music therapy enhance behavioral and cognitive function in elderly dementia patients? A systematic review and meta-analysis. *Ageing Research Review, 35,* 1–11.

chapter 15

Impaired Affective Function: Depression

Healthy older adults are no more likely than younger adults to experience depression; however, depression commonly occurs in older adults with chronic conditions or functional impairments. Theories are evolving to explain causes of depression in these older adults. Unrecognized and untreated depression leads to serious consequences, including functional decline, poor quality of life, and increased morbidity and mortality. Nurses have important roles in addressing late-life depression by applying evidence-based guidelines for assessment and interventions for older adults who are depressed. Nurses also have important roles in addressing the risk for suicide in older adults.

DEPRESSION IN OLDER ADULTS

Although psychiatric references describe many types of depression, which are also called *mood disorders*, the two types most commonly discussed in relation to older adults are major depression (also called major depressive disorder) or subthreshold (also called minor, subclinical, or nonmajor) depression. Diagnostic criterion for *major depression* includes depressed mood and/or loss of interest or pleasure along with at least five of the following signs and symptoms: weight loss, appetite change, sleep disturbances, observable, psychomotor agitation or retardation (i.e., slowness), fatigue or loss of energy, feeling worthless or excessively guilty, cognitive impairment, and recurrent thoughts of death or suicide. In addition, a defining characteristic of major depression is that it noticeably interferes with usual functioning and is associated with significantly diminished quality of life. Minor depression is characterized by these same signs and symptoms, but they are not as severe and their effects on functioning and quality of life are not as serious.

Late-life depression refers to the onset of depression after age 65. Although manifestations differ only slightly in older adults, causative factors are more complex and it often occurs concomitantly with other conditions. In addition, late-life depression is associated with more serious consequences

Addressing Depression in Older Adults

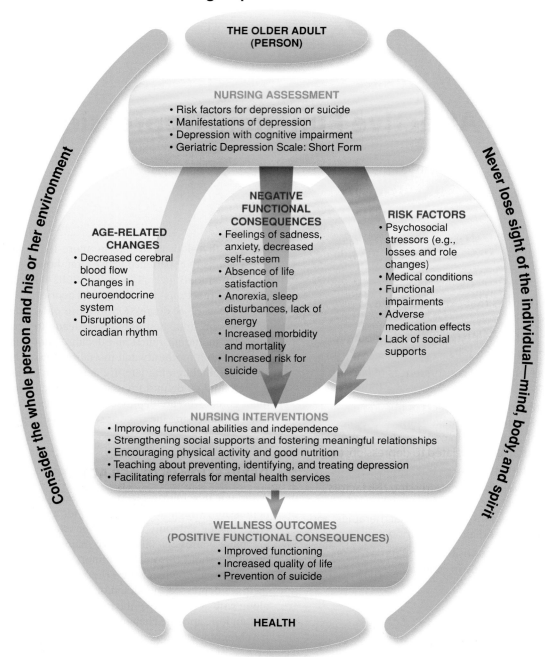

THE OLDER ADULT (PERSON)

NURSING ASSESSMENT
- Risk factors for depression or suicide
- Manifestations of depression
- Depression with cognitive impairment
- Geriatric Depression Scale: Short Form

AGE-RELATED CHANGES
- Decreased cerebral blood flow
- Changes in neuroendocrine system
- Disruptions of circadian rhythm

NEGATIVE FUNCTIONAL CONSEQUENCES
- Feelings of sadness, anxiety, decreased self-esteem
- Absence of life satisfaction
- Anorexia, sleep disturbances, lack of energy
- Increased morbidity and mortality
- Increased risk for suicide

RISK FACTORS
- Psychosocial stressors (e.g., losses and role changes)
- Medical conditions
- Functional impairments
- Adverse medication effects
- Lack of social supports

NURSING INTERVENTIONS
- Improving functional abilities and independence
- Strengthening social supports and fostering meaningful relationships
- Encouraging physical activity and good nutrition
- Teaching about preventing, identifying, and treating depression
- Facilitating referrals for mental health services

WELLNESS OUTCOMES (POSITIVE FUNCTIONAL CONSEQUENCES)
- Improved functioning
- Increased quality of life
- Prevention of suicide

HEALTH

Consider the whole person and his or her environment

Never lose sight of the individual—mind, body, and spirit

and it is often unrecognized and undertreated. Much of the current research focuses on the relationships between late-life depression and chronic conditions that are common in older adults, such as pain, stroke, dementia, and cardiovascular disease. Estimates of prevalence of late-life depression range from 5% to 16% in community settings and from 50% to 54% for residents of long-term care facilities (McKenzie & Harvath, 2016; Jerez-Roig, de Oliveira, de Lima Filho, et al., 2016).

THEORIES ABOUT LATE-LIFE DEPRESSION

Late-life depression is multifaceted because it is associated with many interacting conditions and circumstances that commonly occur in or affect older adults. Gerontologists currently are exploring the complex and bidirectional relationship between depression and concomitant conditions, including dementia, cardiovascular disease, and cerebrovascular disease. Although no single theory can explain why older adults are likely to become depressed, theories can help explain causative factors from various perspectives.

Psychosocial Theories

Psychosocial theories focus on the impact of loss as well as the buffering effects of social supports and the social network in protecting against depression. These theories address psychosocial factors that can increase the risk for developing late-life depression such as any of the following:

- Ageism
- Loss of social roles
- Lower socioeconomic status
- Early experiences including impoverishment and childhood trauma
- Recent social stressors including stressful life events
- Inadequate social network (e.g., no spouse/partner, few friends, small family network)
- Diminished social interaction
- Poor social integration (e.g., unstable environment, lack of strong religious affiliation)

The **learned helplessness theory** addresses depression in the context of the following four areas: cognitive, motivational, self-esteem, and affective-somatic. According to this theory, depression occurs when people expect bad things to happen, believe they can do nothing to prevent them, and perceive that the events result from internal, stable, and global factors. This theory would explain the occurrence of depression in older adults who are in situations over which they have little control. The learned helplessness theory supports the use of nursing interventions directed toward improving self-efficacy and a sense of control over one's environment.

The **cognitive triad theory** is a psychosocial theory based on the premise that people appraise themselves by the "cognitive triad" of their self-image, their environment or experiences, and their future. According to this theory, depression is caused not by adverse events themselves but by distorted perceptions that impair one's ability to appraise oneself and the event in a constructive manner. Depressed people judge these three realms as lacking some features that are necessary for happiness. Examples of negative appraisals are feelings of worthlessness, interpretations of neutral events as bad, and unrealistic feelings of hopelessness. The second element of the cognitive triad theory involves schemas, which are internalized assumptions that influence one's thoughts, feelings, and behaviors. Depressed people typically hold negative assumptions that lead to faulty conclusions. For instance, a depressed person might believe, "I must not be important because the nurse didn't stop to see me." The third component of this theory is the influence of certain logical errors such as personalization, minimization, magnification, and overgeneralization. This theory underlies cognitive-behavioral therapy, which helps depressed people address their dysfunctional thought processes.

Theories About Depression and Medical Conditions

Biologic theories about late-life depression investigate the relationships among aging, depression, and changes in the brain, nervous system, and neuroendocrine system. These theories explore links between depression and inflammatory mechanisms or changes in the neuroendocrine system. For example, the link between depression and cardiovascular disease may be due to increased activity in the hypothalamic–pituitary–adrenal axis caused by stress (Halaris, 2017). Also, there is much current emphasis on the complex and bidirectional relationships between depression and medical conditions, such as dementia, cerebrovascular disease, and cardiovascular disease (Lohman, Dumenci, & Mezuk, 2016). Other biologic theories address anatomic changes (e.g., lesions in white or deep gray matter), neurophysiologic brain changes (e.g., decreased cerebral blood flow), and disruption of the circadian rhythms (e.g., sleep patterns).

Since the early 2000s, gerontologists have recognized a strong relationship between depression and dementia, with cognitive deficits being both a predictor and consequence of depression (Ismail, Elbayoumi, Fischer, et al., 2017; Mirza, Ikram, Bos, et al., 2017). Examples of hypotheses about the relationship between depression and cognitive changes currently under investigation include the following:

- Older adults may experience an increase in depressive symptoms in response to declines in cognitive abilities (Brailean, Aartsen, Muniz-Terrera, et al., 2017).
- Loss of autonomy and diminished quality of life is the underlying cause of depression in people with dementia (Gomez-Gallego, Gomez-Garcia, Ato-Lozano, 2017).
- Increased risk of dementia associated with depressive symptoms involves two different underlying pathways (Lugtenburg, Zuidersma, Oude Voshaar, et al., 2016).
- Treatment of depression in older adults may delay or even prevent the onset of dementia (Lara, Koyanagi, Domenech-Abella, et al., 2017).

Vascular depression occurs in the context of cerebrovascular disease without evidence or history of major stroke. Although research about vascular depression is in an early stage, studies indicate that the brain changes associated with cerebrovascular disease are strongly linked to the occurrence and worsening of depression in older adults (Kim, Woo, Kang, et al., 2016). One study indicates that the cerebrovascular changes begin in mid-life and progress to symptoms of late-life depression (Scott & Paulson, 2017). Vascular depression is characterized by apathy, functional impairment, psychomotor retardation, and cognitive impairments, including poor insight and executive dysfunction.

Another area of intense investigation is the common co-occurrence of depression and cerebrovascular disease, with stroke being identified as an independent risk factor for depression (Kim, Oh, & Lee, 2017). Poststroke depression affects one-third of stroke survivors at any one time, with highest incidence during the first year (Towfighi, Ovbiegele,

Husseini, et al., 2017). Poststroke depression is most likely to occur in people with greater functional and cognitive impairment and is associated with increased mortality and poor recovery (Karaahmet, Gurcay, Avluk, et al., 2017; Salinas, Ray, Nassir, et al., 2017).

The relationship between depression and cardiovascular disease is another current focus of intense investigation by cardiologists and gerontologists. During the past two decades, researchers have identified all the following links: (1) depression is an independent risk factor for cardiovascular diseases, including hypertension, myocardial infarction, and heart failure; (2) depression is often chronic and recurrent in people with cardiovascular disease; and (3) depression is an independent risk factor for adverse cardiovascular outcomes, including poor recovery and increased mortality (Gathright, Goldstein, Josephson, et al., 2017; van der Wall, 2016).

> ### Wellness Opportunity
>
> From a holistic nursing perspective, it is important to recognize that there are many types of depression, and in older adults particularly, depression is complex and likely to occur concomitantly with dementia and other conditions.

 ## RISK FACTORS FOR DEPRESSION IN OLDER ADULTS

Risk factors that are likely to cause or contribute to depression in older adults include demographic factors and psychosocial influences, medical conditions and functional impairments, and effects of medications and alcohol. Although these factors can increase the risk for depression in people of any age, older adults are more likely than younger people to have one or more of these variables. The following sections discuss each category of risk in relation to older adults. Additional risk factors for depression include cognitive impairments and dementia, as discussed in other sections of this chapter.

Demographic Factors and Psychosocial Influences

Demographic factors and psychosocial influences that are associated with depression in older adults include:

- Female sex
- Personal or family history of depression
- Bereavement, loss of significant relationships
- Loneliness
- Chronic stress
- Recent social stressors
- Stressful social environment
- Loss of meaningful social interaction
- Lack of social supports
- Loss of significant roles
- Current or previous experiences of abuse or neglect
- Being a caregiver (including assuming primary care of a grandchild)

Although losses and stress can be risk factors for depression, social supports (e.g., having at least one close relationship) and effective coping mechanisms can protect older adults from depression and improve recovery. Thus, the stressors alone are not the primary risk factor for depression; rather, it is the combination of stressors and the absence of social supports that increase the risk for depression. Lack of the following sources of social support for older adults is most significantly associated with depression: spouses, family, and friends (Gariepy, Honkaniemi, & Quesnel-vallee, 2016; Suanet & Antonucci, 2017).

Medical Conditions and Functional Impairments

The relationships among medical conditions, functional impairments, and depression are complex and interactive, as in the following examples:

- Depression in medically ill older adults is associated with increased mortality, longer hospitalizations, and extended recovery time.
- Medical illnesses can threaten survival, independence, self-concept, role functions, economic resources, and sense of well-being.
- Disability leads to depression because it causes social isolation, low self-esteem, restricted social activity, strained interpersonal relationships, and loss of perceived control.
- Depression in medically ill older adults can lead to other health problems, such as hip fractures and increased susceptibility to infection.
- Chronic pain is a common cause of depression, and it is sometimes a symptom of depression.
- Depression worsens pain, and pain worsens depression.
- Functional impairment is associated with depression as both a contributing factor and a consequence.
- Nutritional deficiencies can be both a risk factor for and effect of depression.

Box 15-1 lists medical conditions that are strongly linked to an increased risk for depression. Current emphasis is on screening for depression in people with chronic conditions and functional impairments and initiating appropriate treatment. For example, nursing studies attest to the value of screening for depression in patients with stroke or cardiac disease (McIntosh, 2017; Ski, Worrall-Carter, Cameron, et al., 2017).

Effects of Medications and Alcohol

People of any age may experience depression as an adverse medication effect, but older adults are at higher risk because they are likely to take more medications. Medications may be risk factors for depression in the following ways:

- Adverse medication effects can cause a depressive syndrome that improves or disappears when the medication is stopped.
- Adverse medication effects can induce a depression that does not remit when the medications are stopped.

Impaired Affective Function: Depression **CHAPTER 15** 295

 Box 15-1 Medical Conditions Associated With an Increased Risk for Depression

Central Nervous System Disorders

Dementia
Stroke
Parkinson's disease
Tumors
Normal-pressure hydrocephalus

Cardiovascular Conditions

Myocardial infarction
Heart failure

Metabolic and Endocrine Disorders

Diabetes
Hypothyroidism/hyperthyroidism
Renal disease
Liver disease
Adrenal disease

Miscellaneous

Pain
Rheumatoid arthritis
Cancer
Nutritional deficiencies (e.g., iron, folate, vitamin D)

 Box 15-2 Examples of Medications that Can Cause Depression

Analgesics

Indomethacin
Narcotics
Propoxyphene

Antihypertensives and Cardiovascular Agents

Beta-blockers
Clonidine
Digitalis
Guanethidine
Hydralazine
Methyldopa
Reserpine

Antiparkinsonian Agents

Levodopa

Central Nervous System Agents

Alcohol
Barbiturates
Benzodiazepines
Fluphenazine
Haloperidol
Meprobamate
Histamine Blockers
Cimetidine

Steroids

Corticosteroids
Estrogen

Anticancer (Chemotherapeutic) Agents

- Adverse medication effects can simulate a depressive syndrome by causing lethargy, insomnia, and irritability.
- The withdrawal of certain medications, such as psychostimulants, can cause a depressive syndrome.

Depression, as an adverse effect of medications, is usually related to the use of medications, such as those prescribed for chronic conditions and listed in Box 15-2. However, depression can also be an adverse effect of alcohol or drugs that are abused (e.g., benzodiazepines). Moreover, although people of any age may experience adverse effects from alcohol, older people are more sensitive to these adverse effects because of age-related changes. Alcohol and depression have a synergistic relationship: Alcohol causes depression and depression leads to alcohol abuse, which in turn exacerbates the depression.

 FUNCTIONAL CONSEQUENCES ASSOCIATED WITH DEPRESSION IN OLDER ADULTS

Depression has serious functional consequences for people of any age, but for frail and seriously depressed older adults, the effects can be life-threatening. Functional consequences range from a negative impact on well-being and quality of life to the most serious consequence, which is **suicide**, the intentional taking of one's own life. This section discusses the wide range of functional consequences that are associated with depression. Suicide is addressed as a separate topic at the end of this chapter because nurses need to address it not only as the most serious consequence of depression but also as an entity in itself.

Physical Health and Functioning

Studies have identified a decline in physical functioning and a concomitant increase in unmet needs as a serious functional consequence of depression in older adults (Xiang, An, & Heinemann, 2017). Additional functional consequences that affect health and functioning are a high number of physical complaints, perception of worse health, and inability to carry out important life functions, such as managing money or medications. It is important to recognize that some of these consequences, such as the inability to manage money or medications, may be a central factor in preventing the person from living independently. Box 15-3 lists ways in which depression affects physical health and functioning.

Appetite disturbances, particularly anorexia, are among the most common physical complaints of depressed older adults. Sometimes, the depressed person does not complain of anorexia and may even deny the problem, but a caregiver or family member may note that the person is not interested in food and is losing weight. Other gastrointestinal complaints that may be functional consequences of depression include flatulence, constipation, early satiety, and attention to bowels. Any of these disturbances may be attributed to

Box 15-3 Functional Consequences of Late-Life Depression

Impact on Physical Function

Loss of appetite
Weight loss
Digestive system complaints, particularly dysphagia, flatulence, constipation, stomach distress, or early satiety
Insomnia, hypersomnia, frequent awakening, early morning awakening, and other sleep disturbances
Fatigue, loss of energy
Pain, discomfort, dyspnea, general malaise
Slowed or increased psychomotor activities
Loss of libido or other problems with sexual function

Impact on Psychosocial Function

Affect: sad, low, "blue," worried, unhappy, "down in the dumps"
Absence of feelings; feeling numb or empty
Diminished life satisfaction
Low self-esteem
Loss of interest or pleasure
Passivity, lack of motivation to do things
Inattention to personal appearance
Feelings of guilt, hopelessness, self-blame, unworthiness, uselessness, helplessness
Anxiety, worry, irritability
Slowed thinking, poor memory, inability to concentrate, poor attention span, inability to make decisions, exaggeration of any mental deficits
Rumination about past and present problems and failures

or caused by other factors such as medical conditions or adverse medication effects; however, depression must be considered as a possible underlying factor. Sleep changes, chronic fatigue, and diminished energy are additional functional consequences of late-life depression that are likely to be attributed to or caused by other conditions.

Older adults, like seriously depressed people of any age, are likely to experience psychomotor agitation or retardation. **Psychomotor retardation** is manifested as slowed body movements and slowed verbal responses, sometimes to the point of muteness. A monotonous or whispering tone of voice might also be an indicator of psychomotor retardation. Affected people often complain of feeling extremely fatigued and having little or no energy. In contrast to people with psychomotor retardation, people with **psychomotor agitation** present an atypical picture of depression. These people manifest high levels of activity, such as pacing and hand wringing. They may be unable to sit still and may have verbal outbursts, such as shouting. Another activity associated with psychomotor agitation is compulsive behavior, such as frequent toileting or handwashing.

Psychosocial Function and Quality of Life

Depression is inherently characterized by a depressed mood or sad affect, but older adults may not perceive or acknowledge these mood disturbances in themselves. Rather than acknowledging that they are depressed, older adults are more

likely to talk about being "blue" or "down in the dumps." Depressed older people may feel like crying but may not be able to cry or identify the underlying reason for their sadness. Another psychosocial consequence of depression is the absence of life satisfaction even when the person has reasons to feel satisfied.

Anxiety, irritability, diminished self-esteem, and negative feelings about self are some of the more generalized affective consequences of depression. The absence of feelings, or a feeling of emptiness, can also be a functional consequence of depression. A loss of interest in social activities may be the depression-related psychosocial change that is most obvious to others. Similarly, other people are likely to observe that the depressed older person has little or no concern about personal appearance. In addition, the depressed person may be overly or unrealistically worried about illnesses, financial affairs, and family issues.

Cognitive impairments can occur because of depression, and in older adults, these deficits are likely to be viewed as a primary problem rather than as a consequence of another problem. Depressed older adults may, in fact, exaggerate cognitive deficits and make statements about global deficits, such as, "I can't remember anything at all." In particular, they may emphasize memory deficits and attribute these to normal aging when the underlying problem is actually a depression-related difficulty in concentrating. See Box 15-3 for a list of functional consequences of depression that affect psychosocial function.

Late-life depression is strongly associated with diminished quality of life for older adults and their families. Symptoms of depression that affect quality of life are fatigue, sad affect, excessive worry, sleep disturbances, a sense of hopelessness, and loss of interest in social and productive relationships. Other consequences of depression that affect quality of life are unsatisfactory social functioning, lower levels of life satisfaction, and poor perceptions of physical and mental health.

Wellness Opportunity

Because people who are depressed tend to have very low self-esteem, nurses can point out concrete examples of positive qualities that they see in the person.

NURSING ASSESSMENT OF DEPRESSION IN OLDER ADULTS

Whereas Chapter 13 addressed all aspects of psychosocial assessment, this section focuses on the following specific aspects of late-life depression: identifying the unique manifestations of depression in older adults, identifying depression in people with dementia, and using screening tools to identify late-life depression. Assessing the suicide risk in older adults is discussed in the section on suicide. The assessment information in Chapter 13, particularly Box 13-9, can be used with the information in the following sections as a guide for assessing depression in older adults.

TABLE 15-1 Comparison of Depression in Younger and Older Adults

Depressed Younger Adults	Depressed Older Adults
More likely to report emotional symptoms	Report more cognitive and physical symptoms
Sense of hopelessness, uselessness, and helplessness	Apathy; exaggeration of personal helplessness
Negative feelings toward self	Sense of emptiness, loss of interest, withdrawal from social activities
Insomnia	Hypersomnia; early morning awakening
Eating disorders	Anorexia, weight loss
More verbal expressions of suicidal ideation than successful attempts; more passive means of suicide	Less talk about suicide, but more successful attempts and more violent means of suicide

Wellness Opportunity

Nurses can ask a depressed older adult, "Can you think of one thing that we can do to improve your quality of life today?"

Identifying the Unique Manifestations of Depression

Assessment of late-life depression is complicated by a wide array of possible manifestations, as reviewed in the functional consequences section. Moreover, manifestations of depression in older adults may differ from those in younger adults. For example, older adults are less likely to show

affective symptoms (e.g., sadness, crying spells, feeling fearful) and are more likely to have physical complaints (e.g., poor appetite, weight loss, gastrointestinal symptoms, loss of interest in sex) or perceptions of cognitive decline (Schaakxs, Comijs, Lamers, et al., 2017; ZLatar, Muniz, Galasko, et al., 2017). Although it is difficult to generalize about manifestations of depression according to age categories, some conclusions about the differences in younger and older adults are summarized in Table 15-1.

In assessing depression in any cognitively impaired older adult, it is often difficult to distinguish between manifestations of depression and dementia. Table 15-2, which identifies specific features that are most likely to be associated with either dementia or depression, can be used as a guide for nursing assessment to differentiate between these two conditions. It is important to keep in mind that older adults frequently have both depression and dementia, so manifestations will not always be clearly distinguishable.

Cultural factors can influence one's perception of depression, and nurses must consider these, particularly during their assessments. For example, people in diverse cultural groups tend to express symptoms of depression through bodily symptoms, such as pain, headache, and stomach ache (Ehrmin, 2016). Nurses can use the information in Box 15-4 to identify some of the cultural variations in expressions of depression. In addition, nurses need to be aware of and sensitive to the fact that many cultural groups attach a strong stigma to depression and other forms of mental illness. As emphasized in Chapter 2, it is imperative to be aware of cultural influences without making assumptions or applying stereotypes. Thus, nurses need to use appropriate communication techniques when assessing for depression and discussing interventions with older adults and their caregivers.

TABLE 15-2 Distinguishing Features of Dementia and Depression

Parameter	Dementia	Depression
Onset of symptoms	Gradual onset, recognized only by hindsight	Abrupt onset, possibly involving a triggering event
Presentation of symptoms	Unawareness of symptoms, or attribution to nonpathologic causes	Exaggeration of memory problems and other cognitive deficits
Memory and attention	Impaired memory, particularly for recent events; poor attention; strong attempts to perform well	Memory and attention deficits attributable to lack of motivation and inability to concentrate
Emotions	Labile affect that changes in response to suggestions; possible apathy owing to cognitive impairments	Consistent feelings of sadness and being "down in the dumps"; unresponsive to suggestions
Response to questions	Evasive, angry, sarcastic; use of humor, confabulation, or social skills to cover up deficits	Slowed, apathetic, frequent response of "I don't know," with no effort expended
Personal appearance of motivation or diminished self-esteem	Inappropriate dress and actions owing to impaired perceptions and thought processes	Little or no concern about appearance because of lack
Physical complaints	Vague fatigue and weakness; complaints are inconsistent and easily forgotten	Anorexia, weight loss, constipation, insomnia, decreased energy
Neurologic features	Aphasia, agnosia, agraphia, apraxia, perseveration	Complaints of dysphagia without any physical basis
Contact with reality	Denial of reality; illusions more predominant than hallucinations; if present, delusions are aimed at explaining deficits	Exaggerated sense of gloom; possible auditory hallucinations or self-derogatory delusions

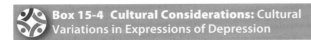

Box 15-4 Cultural Considerations: Cultural Variations in Expressions of Depression

Cultural Group	Common Expressions of Depression
African Americans	Fatigue and somatic complaints
Alaskan Natives/Native Americans	Feeling "heavy" or "out of harmony"
Arabs	Fatigue, sadness, restlessness, hypersomnia; talking about physical complaints protects the person from stigma associated with mental health problems
Chinese Americans	Shameful to discuss; may be called "neurasthenia" (i.e., symptoms produced by social stressors)
Cubans	Attribute symptoms to "nerves," anxiety, or extreme stress; shameful
East Indians	Not clearly recognized as depression but is seen as a sign of spiritual unhappiness
Filipinos	Shameful to discuss; may refer to *Lungknot* (i.e., sadness)
Greeks	Emotional distress is likely to present with somatic complaints such as dizziness and paresthesias
Haitians	The concept of *voudun* attributes depression to being possessed by malevolent spirits or punishment for not honoring protective spirits; depression can be viewed as a hex placed by a jealous or envious individual
Japanese Americans	Because of shame and stigma, emotional distress may be expressed through physical symptoms and may become severe before help is sought
Koreans	Emotions are expressed as physical complaints, including headaches, insomnia, anorexia, lack of energy
Latinos	Use *depression* to convey sadness, grief, or anguish; use *nervios* (nervousness) or *ataque de nervios* (attack of nerves) to describe depressive symptoms
Navajo	*Ghost sickness* describes weakness, fainting, sense of doom, loss of appetite, and preoccupation with death
South Asians	References to *Dil uddas hona*, associated with spiritual unhappiness
People from countries with a recent history of war, violence, or political upheaval	May be associated with posttraumatic stress disorder; feelings of helplessness; memories of war-related brutalities; may be at increased risk for suicide

Source: Ehrmin, J. T. (2016). Transcultural perspectives in mental health nursing. In M. M. Andrews, ., & J. S. Boyle. *Transcultural concepts in nursing care* (7th ed. pp. 272–316). Philadelphia, PA: Wolters Kluwer; Lipson, J. G., & Dibble, S. L. (2005). Culture and clinical care. San Francisco, CA: UCSF Nursing Press; Purnell, L. D. (2013). *Transcultural health care: A culturally competent approach* (4th ed.). Philadelphia, PA: F.A. Davis Co.

Diversity Note

A study of Korean American older adults found high rates of depression, underutilization of mental health services, and an association between depression and not achieving social and material success in America and strained relationships with their children (Lee-Tauler, Lee-Kwan, Han, et al., 2016).

Wellness Opportunity

Nurses respect individual preferences by listening carefully to identify acceptable terminology in older adults who do not want to acknowledge being "depressed."

Using Screening Tools

Concerns about depression being unrecognized and under-treated in older people have stimulated the development of very brief screening tools that health care professionals can use in a variety of settings. The **Patient Health Questionnaire (PHQ-2)** is an evidence-based easy-to-use screening tool that is recommended by major organizations for routine use in clinical settings (Trangle, Gursky, Haight, et al., 2016; Tsoi, Chan, Hirai, et al., 2017). Routine screening involves asking two questions: (1) During the past 2 weeks (or month), have you felt down, depressed, or hopeless? and (2) During the past 2 weeks (or month), have you felt little interest or pleasure in doing things? A positive response to either of these questions warrants further assessment with a formal depression scale.

The **Geriatric Depression Scale: Short Form (GDS-SF)** is an evidence-based screening tool that is widely used across health care settings to detect depression in older adults, including those with cognitive impairment (see Figure 15-1). The tool, which can be administered in 5 to 7 minutes, consists of 15 questions with points allocated for "yes" or "no" answers to specific questions. A systematic review and meta-analysis found that a score of 5 or higher indicated the need for evaluation of depression (Pocklington, Gilbody, Manea, et al., 2016). This tool and related scoring form can be downloaded without cost in English and more than 30 other languages. Online Learning Activity 15-1 provides links to this tool and helpful resources related to this and other screening tools.

See ONLINE LEARNING ACTIVITY 15-1: LINKS TO ADDITIONAL INFORMATION ABOUT ASSESSMENT OF DEPRESSION IN OLDER ADULTS at http://thepoint.lww.com/Miller8e.

NURSING DIAGNOSIS

Because there is no specific nursing diagnosis for depression, the following nursing diagnoses may be applicable: Anxiety, Ineffective Coping, Grieving, Hopelessness, Powerlessness, Social Isolation, Caregiver Role Strain, and Risk for Compromised Resilience. Related factors commonly found in

Geriatric Depression Scale (Short Form)

	Yes	No
1. Are you basically satisfied with your life?	Yes	No
2. Have you dropped many of your activities and interests?	Yes	No
3. Do you feel that your life is empty?	Yes	No
4. Do you often get bored?	Yes	No
5. Are you in good spririts most of the time?	Yes	No
6. Are you afraid that something bad is going to happen to you?	Yes	No
7. Do you feel happy most of the time?	Yes	No
8. Do you often feel helpless?	Yes	No
9. Do you prefer to stay at home rather than go out and do new things?	Yes	No
10. Do you feel you have more problems with memory than most?	Yes	No
11. Do you think it is wonderful to be alive now?	Yes	No
12. Do you feel pretty worthless the way you are now?	Yes	No
13. Do you feel full of energy?	Yes	No
14. Do you feel that your situation is hopeless?	Yes	No
15. Do you think that most people are better off than you are?	Yes	No

Score:___/15   One point for "No" to questions 1, 5, 7, 11, 13
One point for "Yes" to other questions

Normal	3 ± 2
Mildly depressed	7 ± 3
Very depressed	12 ± 2

FIGURE 15-1   Geriatric Depression Scale (short form). (Available at www.stanford.edu/~yesavage/GDS.html.)

older adults are chronic pain, cognitive impairment, medical conditions, functional limitations, financial concerns, social isolation, caregiving responsibilities, multiple social stressors, and loss of significant roles or relationships.

Wellness Opportunity

Nurses can use the wellness nursing diagnosis of Readiness for Enhanced Coping for older adults who are interested in improving their coping skills to address depressive symptoms that are not severe.

PLANNING FOR WELLNESS OUTCOMES

When caring for older adults who are depressed, nurses identify outcomes as an essential part of the planning process. The following Nursing Outcomes Classification terminology is applicable to depressed older adults: Caregiver Emotional Health, Coping, Depression Level, Hope, Knowledge: Depression Management, Self-Esteem, Social Support, and Social Involvement. Suicide Self-Restraint is applicable when care plans address risks for suicide. Specific interventions to achieve outcomes related to depression and suicide are discussed in the following sections.

Wellness Opportunity

Quality of life is a wellness outcome that is achieved by addressing the functional and psychosocial consequences of depression.

NURSING INTERVENTIONS TO ADDRESS DEPRESSION

Although all nurses are responsible for addressing depression in older adults, those who work in community-based and long-term care settings have the most ongoing opportunities to identify manifestations of depression and to request further evaluation and treatment. Nurses in these settings also have many opportunities to implement and evaluate the effectiveness of the interventions discussed in the following sections. In recent years, primary care physicians and nurse practitioners have been the health care professionals evaluating and managing depression, and referrals to psychiatrists and other mental health professionals for depression have become less common. This trend is due to the emphasis on cost-effectiveness and the availability of safer and more effective antidepressant medications. Nursing protocols for depression in elderly patients emphasize the important responsibility of nurses in reducing the negative consequences of depression through early recognition, intervention, and referrals for care (McKenzie & Harvath, 2016).

Nursing Interventions Classification terminology pertinent to interventions for older adults who are depressed includes the following: Caregiver Support, Coping Enhancement, Counseling, Crisis Intervention, Emotional Support, Exercise Promotion, Grief Work Facilitation, Hope Inspiration, Mood Management, Referral, Role Enhancement, Self-Esteem Enhancement, Suicide Prevention, and Teaching: Individual. The next sections review the role of the nurse in planning and implementing interventions for late-life depression.

Alleviating Risk Factors

Nurses promote wellness for depressed older adults by addressing the many risk factors that are well within the realm of nursing, such as functional impairments, adverse medication effects, and excess alcohol use. Many nursing interventions that improve the level of functioning are also effective for alleviating or preventing depression. For example, dementia, sensory impairments, urinary incontinence, and mobility impairments are examples of conditions that can contribute to depression and will respond to nursing interventions (refer to Chapters 14, 16, 17, 19, and 22). Interventions to promote resilience, as discussed in Chapter 12, are another means of preventing and managing depression in older adults (Rutherford, Taylor, Brown, et al., 2017; Wermelinger Avila, Lucchetti, & Lucchetti, 2017).

Wellness Opportunity

Nurses promote wellness by challenging ageist stereotypes that falsely attribute functional impairments to inevitable consequences of aging.

If adverse medication effects are a risk factor for depression, nurses can educate the person about this potential relationship and identify problem-solving strategies to address the adverse effects (as discussed in Chapter 8). For example, if the older person understands that there is a wide array of antihypertensive medications and that not all of them will cause depression, the person can use this information in discussing the problem with his or her primary care provider. Nurses can also reassure the older adult that it is acceptable to initiate this kind of problem-solving discussion with health care practitioners. When the nurse, rather than the patient, is the one who communicates with the primary care provider, the nurse can raise appropriate questions about depression as an adverse medication effect. This problem-solving approach is particularly important when the primary care provider is considering adding an antidepressant medication to a regimen that includes a depression-inducing medication. In these situations, the solution may be to change medications rather than to add another medication and increase the risk for adverse effects.

If excess alcohol use is a risk factor for depression, individual and group interventions can be effective, particularly when the alcohol abuse is a reaction to recent losses. Alcoholics Anonymous (AA) is the most widely used group program for alcoholics of any age, and in some areas, age-homogeneous groups have been established, including some for older adults. Nurses can encourage older adults to initiate contact with AA, or they might directly facilitate the referral if the person agrees to this. Individual and family counseling may also be effective, and nurses can suggest or facilitate referrals for these mental health services.

Improving Psychosocial Function

In any clinical setting, nurses can focus on interventions to promote autonomy, personal control, self-efficacy, and decision making about daily care as an intervention for depression (McKenzie & Harvath, 2016). In addition, interventions to improve overall psychosocial function, as discussed in Chapter 12, are applicable for addressing risk factors for and symptoms of depression. For example, interventions to strengthen social supports and foster meaningful roles are particularly pertinent and relatively easy to implement (Juang, Knight, Carlson, et al., 2017). Nurses have many opportunities to encourage participation in group meal or social programs. Most communities in the United States have some social programs for older adults, and many provide transportation. Many churches and religious organizations also have programs designed to meet the social needs of isolated older adults. Volunteer visitor or phone call programs, for example, are sometimes available to address the needs of people who have difficulty with getting out of the house. Other programs, such as pet therapy or "Adopt-a-Grandparent," are available in some home, community-based, and long-term care settings, and they can be helpful in alleviating loneliness and depression. Nurses can also encourage older adults to maintain social contacts through simple measures such as phone calls.

Involvement in volunteer activities can enhance self-esteem and provide meaningful roles for older adults who are mildly depressed. Nurses can suggest that older adults explore opportunities for volunteer activities through organizations such as the National Senior Service Corps (previously called the Retired Senior Volunteer Program), which is one of many programs in the United States that assist older adults in becoming involved in volunteer activities.

Wellness Opportunity

Nurses promote quality of life by encouraging an older adult to engage in activities that are pleasant and meaningful to that person.

Promoting Health Through Physical Activity and Nutrition

The beneficial effects of exercise as an intervention for depression have been documented in research reviews (Trangle, Gursky, Haight, et al., 2016). Older adults, however, may not view exercise as important, or they may be reluctant to participate in exercise programs because of chronic illnesses such as arthritis. If older adults understand the benefits of exercise for both their physical and mental health, and if an individually tailored program is developed for them, they may be more willing to become involved in exercise programs. In community and long-term care settings, nurses can facilitate the establishment of group exercise programs and encourage depressed older adults to participate in them. In addition to encouraging participation in exercise programs, nurses can encourage participation in many other forms of physical activity. Even in hospital settings, nurses can facilitate referrals to physical, occupational, and recreational therapists as a psychosocial nursing intervention (McKenzie & Harvath, 2016).

Nutrition is an important consideration as an intervention for depression for three reasons. First, depression often negatively affects nutritional status, and this can cause additional negative consequences. Second, good nutrition has a positive effect on mental health and cognitive function. Third, constipation is both a consequence of depression and an adverse effect of some antidepressant medications, and nutritional interventions can be effective in alleviating it. During phases of serious depression, malnutrition can lead to medical problems, which may progress to the point of being life-threatening. When depression is severe enough to lead to malnutrition, the older person must be evaluated for in-patient psychiatric care. Interventions for less severely depressed older people are aimed at maintaining adequate hydration and nutrition and preventing or managing constipation (as discussed in Chapter 18).

> ### Wellness Opportunity
>
> Nurses address the body–mind–spirit interrelationship by incorporating interventions for optimal nutrition as an essential component of care for depressed older adults.

Providing Education and Counseling

Many types of individual and group psychosocial therapies are effective interventions for late-life depression. For example, when multiple stressors challenge the person's coping abilities and contribute to depression, individual or group therapy can be an important intervention for improving the person's psychosocial health and alleviating depression. In addition, nurses provide psychosocial support through holistic nursing interventions such as the following (Helming, 2016):

- Helping older adults identify nonverbalized fears and providing reality-based information to help them evaluate the fear
- Assisting older adults to verbalize emotions by identifying and labeling them so they can communicate more effectively about their emotions and fear
- Providing counseling based on basic psychological theories and concepts
- Encouraging "storytelling" and helping older adults to acknowledge their strengths as well as weaknesses through the power of storytelling
- Facilitating referrals to appropriate mental health services

In addition, good communication skills, such as active listening and expressing empathy, can be effective for addressing sadness about losses. Nurses in home care settings are in a unique position to use psychosocial interventions for depression while they also are addressing needs related to functional impairment, and these can be especially effective for homebound older adults (Groh & Dumlao, 2016).

> ### A Student's Perspective
>
> *The life review interview with Mrs. R. enlightened me for one very simple reason: She loves the life she lived. She has no regrets about her life and said she would change nothing. She is a very positive person, and hearing her outlook at life really got me thinking about the way I want to continue to live my life. It was inspiring to hear her views, and it takes away some of my fears of growing older.*
>
> *The most significant point in the life review interview is actually the same as the most difficult part. We were discussing family, and I wasn't sure if I should ask about her late husband because I didn't know how to bring him up. I finally found a way to ask about him and immediately her eyes filled with tears. She began to describe him and the things they used to do together. It was sad; yet hearing about how much she loved him was touching. She continued to cry as she said he was the best person she ever knew. Without even thinking, I grabbed her hand. As she squeezed my hand, I saw her become more at ease. With just that little action, I feel like I made her feel better. I had no idea that holding someone's hand could have such a powerful effect.*
>
> *Molly D.*

Nurses need to be sufficiently familiar with psychosocial therapies that are commonly used for depressed older adults, so they can encourage or facilitate referrals for these interventions. Types of psychosocial therapies that are effective for depression in older adults, either as individual or as group therapies, include the following:

- Cognitive-behavioral therapy, which involves cognitive restructuring and behavioral activation
- Problem-solving to address problems related to social engagement, relationships, mood, and health
- Supportive therapy, which involves evaluating the person's strengths and weaknesses and facilitating choices that improve coping abilities
- Life review and reminiscence, which helps people re-experience meaningful events of their lives
- Bibliotherapy, which uses books and articles to enhance coping skills or assist the person in identifying and reducing dysfunctional thought processes.

Reviews of literature have identified reminiscence therapy, social relationships, and intergenerational interactions as effective evidence-based psychosocial interventions for depressed older adults (Simning & Simons, 2017; Willis, 2016).

Support and self-help groups also can improve psychosocial function and alleviate depression in older adults who are coping with life events, such as caregiving, widowhood, or grief reactions. Other group models used as interventions for late-life depression include relaxation, art therapy, focused imagery, and creative movement. In addition to groups specifically targeted for depression, groups such as the "Healthy Aging Class" (described in

Chapter 12), which are directed at developing coping skills, may be effective in alleviating depression.

Although adult daycare programs are not primarily a group therapy for depressed older adults, they are a commonly available resource for providing structured social and therapeutic activities. Similarly, many community-based senior programs provide opportunities for group meals, exercise, and social interaction, and these can be quite effective in alleviating mild to moderate depression in older adults. Information about these and other group programs for older adults can be obtained from local offices on aging, and nurses can encourage older adults or their caregivers to seek out and take advantage of these programs.

Technology to Promote Wellness in Older Adults

Studies indicate that higher use of social technology (e.g., e-mail, social networking, video/audio communication) among older adults (mean age 84 years in one study and 76 in another) is associated with reduced loneliness, increased well-being, and fewer depressive symptoms (Chopik, 2016; Czaja, Boot, Charness, et al., 2017; Sims, Reed, & Carr, 2016).

Facilitating Referrals for Psychosocial Therapies

Nurses have important roles in facilitating referrals for appropriate psychosocial therapies, particularly for older adults who are seriously depressed. In addition to facilitating referrals for mental health services, nurses often have opportunities to initiate discussion of psychosocial therapies during the course of their usual work with older adults. Interprofessional geropsychiatric and geriatric assessments offer assessment and treatment of late-life depression, and some community mental health centers have programs for depressed older adults. Nurses can either suggest or directly facilitate referrals to these programs. A major consideration with regard to referrals for depression interventions is that there is compelling evidence to support the effectiveness of many psychosocial therapies either alone or in combination with antidepressant medications (McKenzie & Harvath, 2016; Trangle, Gursky, Haight, et al., 2016). Guidelines also emphasize the importance of interprofessional collaboration among all clinicians in addressing depression in older adults, with nurses having essential roles (Crespy, Haitsma, Kleban, et al., 2016).

Wellness Opportunity

Nurses promote wellness when they convince an older person that depression is not a necessary consequence of aging but is a condition that can respond to treatment.

Teaching About Nonpharmacologic Therapies for Depression

In recent years, there has been increasing attention on identifying nonpharmacologic interventions for reducing depressive symptoms, in addition to the psychosocial therapies discussed in the previous section. For example, group music therapy is emerging as an evidence-based intervention for older adults with depression (Werner, Wosch, & Gold, 2017; Zhao, Bai, Bo, et al., 2016). There also is increasing emphasis on mindfulness-based interventions, such as meditation, as effective self-care strategies for management of depression (Creswell, 2017; Khusid & Vythilingam, 2016; Mathur, Sharma, & Bharath, 2016). Studies also support the use of yoga, acupuncture, and tai chi as nonpharmacologic therapies for depression (Chu, Wu, Lin, et al., 2017; Trangle, Gursky, Haight, et al., 2016; Wang, Wang, Liu, et al., 2017).

There has been increasing interest in the use of herbs and other natural remedies for depression. St. John's wort (*Hypericum perforatum*) is widely used in Europe as an antidepressant and is the most commonly used antidepressant in Germany. Since 1998, the National Institutes of Health Office of Alternative Medicine has sponsored randomized, controlled, double-blinded studies in the United States to compare placebo, St. John's wort, and prescription antidepressants. Recent reviews of studies conclude that St. John's wort may be effective for treating mild to moderate depression but is not effective for serious depression (Trangle, Gursky, Haight, et al., 2016). Common side effects include fatigue, headache, photosensitivity, dry mouth, and gastrointestinal effects. St. John's wort is relatively safe, but serious drug interactions can occur with, for example, antidepressants, digoxin, and anticoagulants. This herb is widely available in the United States and is inexpensive, but products are not standardized or regulated for quality, as discussed in Chapter 8.

Light therapy (also called bright-light therapy) is an evidence-based treatment for some types of depression, including those with seasonal patterns, both as a stand-alone intervention and to enhance the effects of antidepressants (Trangle, Gursky, Haight, et al., 2016). Light therapy involves exposure to 5000 to 10,000 lux of bright light for 30 to 60 minutes daily. Nurses can use Box 15-5 as a guide for teaching older adults about interventions that may be helpful for preventing or alleviating depression.

Box 15-5 Health Promotion Interventions Commonly Used for Preventing or Alleviating Depression

- Engage in enjoyable physical activity daily.
- Maintain healthy eating habits.
- Maintain good sleep patterns.
- Seek individual or group counseling to address stressful situations.
- Participate in social activities.
- Engage in meaningful activity, such as volunteer activities.
- If symptoms of depression affect daily functioning or quality of life, seek evaluation and treatment from a primary care practitioner.
- Use stress-reduction interventions, such as relaxation, meditation, mindfulness, yoga, tai chi, or qigong.
- Use creative and expressive activities, such as dance, art, music, and drama.

Antidepressant Medications for Depression in Older Adults

Antidepressants are considered the mainstay of medical management for major depression; however, current evidence indicates that these medications are not significantly better than a placebo for mild or moderate depression (Tangle, Gursky, Haight, et al., 2016). In particular, there are strong recommendations against the use of cyclic antidepressants (i.e., the type that was first developed in the 1950s, with second-generation agents being widely used since the mid-1980s) for older adults (American Geriatrics Society, 2015). Currently, newer types of antidepressants with fewer adverse effects are widely used; however, the American Geriatrics Society Beers Criteria for Potentially Inappropriate Medications list many of these as antidepressants to be used with caution in older adults, including mirtazapine, selective serotonin reuptake inhibitors (SSRIs), and serotonin and norepinephrine inhibitors (SNRIs) (American Geriatrics Society, 2015). Antidepressants that are commonly used for older adults are listed in Table 15-3 according to their classifications, with an asterisk to indicate the ones that are listed in the Beers Criteria.

Clinical guidelines recommend SSRIs as the first-line medications for depression in older adults because there is a strong base of evidence in support of their relative safety, high efficacy, and broad spectrum of action (Tangle, Gursky, Haight, et al., 2016). Although SSRIs are safer than other types of antidepressants, it is important to assess for adverse effects and drug interactions. For example, because SSRIs are metabolized in the liver and some of them are highly bound to plasma protein, SSRIs may interact with other drugs that are metabolized in the liver or are highly protein bound. In addition, it is important to observe for drug interactions, including interactions with over-the-counter products (e.g., nonsteroidal anti-inflammatory drugs or low-dose aspirin) or another drug or dietary supplement that increases serotonin levels in the brain (e.g., meperidine, dextromethorphan, L-tryptophan, St. John's wort). Drug interactions may occur even after an SSRI with a long half-life (e.g., fluoxetine) has been discontinued. Common adverse effects of SSRIs include nausea, vomiting, diarrhea, headache, nervousness, insomnia, tremor, dry mouth, and sexual dysfunction. Withdrawal effects of SSRIs include nausea, tremor, anxiety, dizziness, palpitations, and paresthesias.

In addition to considerations already discussed, concerns related to specific antidepressants listed in Table 15-3 include the following:

- Venlafaxine may cause an increase in blood pressure; mirtazapine can be helpful for stimulating appetite, but it also can be sedating.
- Trazodone and nefazodone are very sedating and may be useful in the treatment of depression with sleep disturbances.
- Bupropion has a stimulating effect, which can sometimes be therapeutic but is contraindicated in people with a seizure disorder.
- It is important to monitor serum sodium levels initially and periodically for older adults taking SSRIs because these antidepressants are associated with increased risk for hyponatremia.

Nursing Responsibilities Regarding Antidepressants

An important nursing responsibility regarding antidepressants is to educate older adults about the primary purpose of these medications, which is to alleviate depressive symptoms so that the person is able to respond to additional interventions such as psychosocial therapy. For older adults who have both depression and dementia, antidepressant medications may improve the affective symptoms so that overall abilities are improved and the person is able to function more effectively and independently.

Nursing responsibilities regarding antidepressant medication therapy include observing for both adverse and therapeutic effects and educating the older adult about the unique aspects of these medication therapies. Another important responsibility is educating older adults about the need for ongoing evaluation and treatment of depression including the monitoring of antidepressant medication use. Older adults who have been diagnosed with major depressive disorder are at high risk for recurrence, and this risk is increased if antidepressant medications are not maintained for at least 6 months. Older adults often want to discontinue medications when their depressive symptoms resolve, and nurses need to teach them about the importance of ongoing antidepressant

TABLE 15-3 Antidepressants Commonly Used for Older Adults

Category	Examples	Trade Names
Selective serotonin reuptake inhibitors (SSRIs)[a]	citalopram escitalopram paroxetine sertraline	Celexa Lexapro Paxil Zoloft
Serotonin–norephinephrine reuptake inhibitors (SNRIs)[a]	duloxetine venlafaxine	Cymbalta Effexor
Serotonin modulators	nefazodone trazodone	Serzone Desyrel
Norephinephrine–dopamine reuptake inhibitors[a]	bupropion	Wellbutrin
Cyclic antidepressants[a]	amoxapine desipramine doxepine imipramine nortriptyline	Asendin Norpramin Sinequan Tofranil Pamelor
Alpha 2-adrenergic receptor antagonist[a]	mirtazapine	Remeron
Newer antidepressants	vortioxetine vilazodone	Brintellix Vibryd

[a]Types listed in the American Geriatrics Society 2015 Updated Beers Criteria for Potentially Inappropriate Medication Use in Older Adults.

Box 15-6 Health Education About Antidepressant Medications

Information to Be Shared With the Older Adult

- Immediate improvement will not be evident, but a fair trial must be given to the medication as long as serious adverse effects are not noticed.
- The fair trial may take as long as 12 weeks, but some positive effects should be noticed within 2 to 4 weeks.
- If one type of antidepressant is not effective, another type may be effective.
- Antidepressants cannot be used on an "as needed" basis.
- Antidepressants should be viewed as part of a comprehensive approach to treating depression, and psychosocial therapies should be considered along with antidepressants.
- Antidepressants can interact with alcohol, nicotine, and other medications, including over-the-counter medications, possibly altering the effects of the medication or increasing the potential for adverse effects.
- It is important to have information about potential adverse effects and drug–drug or food–drug interactions.
- The prescribing health care practitioner should be consulted before discontinuing an antidepressant.
- If postural hypotension occurs, the effects can be minimized through such interventions as changing position slowly and maintaining adequate fluid intake.
- If monoamine oxidase inhibitors are prescribed, certain medications must be avoided, and a low-tyramine diet must be followed (i.e., avoidance of beer, yogurt, red wine, fermented cheese, and pickled foods, as well as excessive amounts of caffeine and chocolate).

Principles Regarding Dosage and Length of Treatment

- Older adults should be started at one-half to one-third the normal adult dose.
- Dosages can be increased gradually until maximal therapeutic levels are reached, while observing for adverse effects.
- Age-related changes may increase the time needed for medication to reach maximal effectiveness.
- A once-daily regimen is a standard dosing schedule for most antidepressants.
- Bedtime administration of an antidepressant may facilitate sleep as a result of the drug's hypnotic effects, but some antidepressants (e.g., fluoxetine) may be better taken in the morning because of side effects such as agitation.
- The length of treatment is usually 6 months for a first-time depression, 1 to 2 years for people with a history of a prior depressive episode, and lifetime maintenance for people with a history of three or more depressive episodes.

therapy and periodic reevaluations after medications are discontinued. This is particularly important because a patient's beliefs about the use of medications affect adherence; therefore, beliefs need to be explored before and during medication therapy. Box 15-6 summarizes guidelines for the nursing responsibilities regarding antidepressant medications.

Teaching About Electroconvulsive Therapy and Neuromodulation Treatments

Electroconvulsive therapy (ECT), which involves the electrical induction of seizures, has been used for decades as a

treatment for severe depressive episodes. With the exception of psychiatric settings, nurses will not be involved with the care of people who are undergoing ECT. Nurses caring for depressed people in any setting, however, need to be aware of evidence-based guidelines for the use of ECT and maintain an open mind about this therapy. In addition, nurses may be in a position to encourage older adults or their caregivers to seek advice about ECT from knowledgeable professionals.

Evidence-based guidelines recommend consideration for ECT in any of the following circumstances (Trangle, Gursky, Haight, et al., 2016):

- Geriatric depression
- When antidepressants are ineffective, not tolerated, or pose significant medical risk
- When any of the following conditions exist: catatonia, severe risk of suicide, depression with psychosis
- When the patient's health is significantly compromised due to depression (e.g., not eating, functional impairment)
- Combination of depression and Parkinson's disease

Studies consistently find that ECT is a rapid, effective, and well-tolerated treatment for major depression in older adults (Dols, Bouchaert, Sineaert, et al., 2017; Kumar, Mulsant, Liu, et al., 2016). Adverse effects (e.g., headache, nausea, disorientation, memory loss, impaired attention, and decreased concentration) are usually transient (Geduldig & Kellner, 2016).

EVALUATING THE EFFECTIVENESS OF NURSING INTERVENTIONS

Nurses evaluate their care of depressed older adults by documenting improved coping skills and diminished manifestations of depression. For example, the person may report diminished feelings of hopelessness and improved appetite and sleep. Another measure reflecting improved quality of life would be the older adult's interest and participation in meaningful activities. Effectiveness of nursing interventions may also be evaluated by whether the older adult has begun taking antidepressant medications and participating in individual or group therapies. Box 15-7 summarizes evidence-based guidelines for nursing assessment and interventions related to depression in older adults.

See **ONLINE LEARNING ACTIVITY 15-2: LINK TO AN ARTICLE ABOUT NURSING ASSESSMENT AND INTERVENTIONS FOR DEPRESSION IN HOMEBOUND OLDER ADULTS** at http://thepoint.lww.com/Miller8e.

SUICIDE IN LATE LIFE

Suicide in late life is often overlooked because older adulthood is associated with passivity and nonviolence, whereas suicide is associated with aggressiveness and violence.

E·B·P Box 15-7 Evidence-Based Practice: Guidelines for Depression in Older Adults

Statement of the Problem

- Depression is highly prevalent in older adults and is not a natural part of aging.
- Depression in older adults tends to be underrecognized, misdiagnosed, and subsequently undertreated.
- Depressive symptoms are associated with higher morbidity and mortality rates in older adults; specific consequences of depression include heightened pain and disability, delayed recovery from illness or surgery, worsening of medical conditions, and suicide.
- Depressive symptoms are more common in older adults who have dementia or more severe or chronic disabling conditions.
- In older adults who are cognitively impaired, depression may be expressed through the following behaviors: repetitive verbalizations, agitated vocalizations, expressions of unrealistic fears, repetitive statements about the occurrence of bad events, exaggerated concerns about health, and verbal and/or physical aggression.
- Nurses are at the front line in the early recognition of depression and the facilitation of mental health services.

Recommendations for Nursing Assessment

- Depression may range in severity from mild symptoms to more severe forms, both of which can persist over longer periods and have serious negative consequences for the older adult.
- Depression can occur for the first time in late life or it can be part of a long-standing affective disorder.
- Recognition of depression in older adults is complicated by the coexistence of medical illnesses, disability, cognitive dysfunction, and psychosocial adversity in older adults.
- The nursing standard of practice for depression in older adults includes the following assessment parameters: identifying risk factors and high-risk groups, using GDS-SF for screening, performing a focused depression assessment on all high-risk groups, obtaining and reviewing medical history and physical/neurologic examination, assessing for medications and medical conditions that may contribute to depression, and assessing cognitive function and level of functioning.

Recommendations for Care

- For severe depression (e.g., GDS 11 or greater), refer for psychiatric evaluation and treatment with medication, psychosocial therapies, hospitalization, or ECT.
- For less severe depression (e.g., GDS score between 6 and 10), refer to mental health services for psychosocial therapies and determination of whether antidepressant therapy is warranted.
- For all levels of depression, develop an individualized plan integrating nursing interventions that address issues such as safety, nutrition, risk factors, health education, social support, pleasant reminiscence, and relaxation therapies.

Recommendations for Patient Teaching

Teach older adults and caregivers about the following:
- Depression is common, treatable, and not the depressed person's fault.
- Adherence to the prescribed treatment regimen, including medications, is imperative to prevent recurrence.
- It is important to be aware of the therapeutic and adverse effects of the prescribed antidepressant.

Source: McKenzie, G., & Harvath, T. (2016). Depression. In E. Capezuti, D. Zwicker, M. Mezey, & T. Fulmer (Eds.), *Evidence-based geriatric nursing protocols for best practice* (4th ed., pp. 211–232). New York: Springer Publishing Co.

In addition, there has been increasing media attention to suicide in teens and young adults, but less attention to suicide in older adults. Despite the lack of attention to suicide in older adults, this issue is a major public health concern that will likely increase in severity as indicated by the following statistics:

- Across groups by age and race, white men aged 85 years and older have the highest suicide rate.
- In 2008, the suicide rate for adults aged 65 and older was more than 30% higher than that of those below age 65.
- There is particular concern about the cohort of adults born between 1946 and 1964 (i.e., "Baby Boomers") because this group consistently had a high rate of suicide during each stage of life development (Conwell & O'Riley, 2013; Crosby, Ortega, & Stevens, 2013; Nadorff, Fiske, Sperry, et al., 2013).

Official data about suicide do not include information about suicidal events that are unreported for reasons such as family efforts to conceal evidence and difficulty determining the true cause of death in medically ill people. Nor do these rates reflect the unrecognized suicidal acts that older adults indirectly or subtly use to take their own lives such as refusal to eat, failure to take medically necessary medications, and other means of self-neglect. Suicide rates and mechanisms vary significantly by sex and ethnicity, as illustrated in Figures 15-2 and 15-3.

Diversity Note

At all ages, and by race and ethnicity, the suicide rates are consistently higher for males than for females.

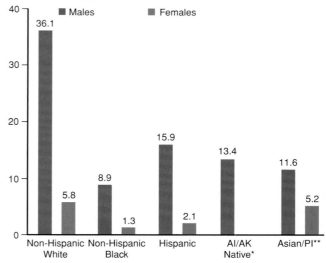

FIGURE 15-2 Suicide rates for people 65 and older in the United States according to race/ethnicity and sex, 2014. Numbers shown are suicide deaths per 100,000 population. *AI/AK Native, American Indian/Alaskan Native; **PI, Pacific Islander. Health USA 2015. Trend Table 30. (Available at *https://www.cdc.gov/nchs/data/hus/hus15.pdf.*)

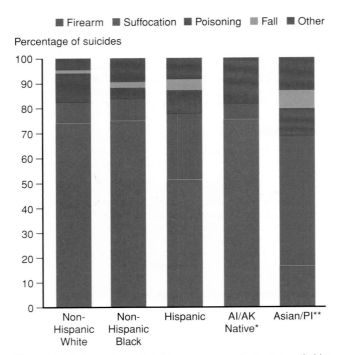

FIGURE 15-3 Percentage of suicides among people 65 years and older in the United States, by race/ethnicity and mechanism, 2005–2009. Numbers shown are suicide deaths per 100,000 population. *AI/AK Native, American Indian/Alaskan Native; **PI, Pacific Islander. (Adapted from Centers for Disease Control and Prevention [2013]. Atlanta, GA.)

Assessing the Risks for Suicide

Nursing assessment of suicide risk is particularly important because most older people give clues, sometimes to many people, about potential suicide. These clues, however, may be subtle, and the person who hears them may not associate them with suicide risk, particularly in older adults. By identifying risk factors, nurses can initiate interventions to prevent suicide. This is particularly important because three-quarters of older people who commit suicide visit their primary care provider within 1 month before the act, but they are not likely to directly express suicidal ideation. Thus, health care providers need to assess for risks and identify those older adults who may be contemplating suicide. The following are some of the more commonly identified risks for suicide in older adults:

- Depression, which may be masked by excessive focus on physical complaints
- Personal or family history of depression
- Past suicide attempts
- Loneliness, limited social support
- Family discord
- Feelings of abandonment
- Recent bereavement
- Presence of chronic or severe pain

Because depression is consistently identified across studies as a risk factor for suicide, it is important to assess for suicidal ideation in any depressed older adult. In addition

to these conditions, factors that are predictive of actual suicide actions include functional limitations, physical pain, psychological pain, and executive dysfunction impairment (Kim, 2016; Klonsky, Qiu, & Saffer, 2017; Rizvi, Iskric, Calati, et al., 2017). It is important to recognize that for every completed suicide among older adults, an estimated 2 to 4 attempts have occurred, whereas for younger adults the ratio can be as high as 200 attempts for every completed suicide (Barry & Byers, 2016). Thus, any history of suicide attempts is a red flag for suicide in older adults.

When risk factors or clues to potential suicide are identified, the nurse must further assess the actual risk for a suicide attempt. This assessment is multilevel, with each level of questions depending on the response to the previous level. Nurses begin the assessment with level-1 questions to determine the presence or absence of suicidal thoughts. Although health care professionals may be reluctant to initiate questions about suicide because they fear that this line of questioning may "put ideas in the person's head," this fear is unfounded. People who do not have suicidal thoughts usually respect the necessity of the questions but do not begin thinking about suicide just because the topic was broached. Even so, rather than beginning with a blunt question such as "Do you ever think about committing suicide?" the nurse can phrase the question in such a way that the person will give clues to his or her intent if it exists but will not be offended by the question if it does not (see Box 15-8 for examples of questions to ask).

Nurses need to recognize that older adults may express a loss of interest in living and may even state that they wish they were dead, but these verbalizations are not necessarily associated with suicidal thoughts. These verbalizations of hopelessness may arise from feelings of being overwhelmed with an illness or stressful situation, and they are not necessarily indicators of a desire to take one's own life. If suicidal thoughts are suspected or identified at level 1, nurses ask level-2 questions, which are aimed at determining the presence or absence of thoughts about self-harm. If the answer to any of these questions is positive, nurses ask level-3 questions, which are very direct and specific because this information is crucial to assessing the immediate risk for suicide. If the person describes a detailed plan and has access to all the necessary implements, the potential for suicide is extremely high. By contrast, if the person has a plan that is vague or that cannot possibly be carried out, the immediate potential for suicide is lower. For example, if the plan involves a gun, but the person does not have a gun and cannot get out of the house, then the chance of a successful suicide is low. By contrast, if the person threatens to consume the bottle of barbiturates that is readily available in the medicine cabinet, then the chance of a successful suicide is quite high. Nurses proceed to level-4 questions to assess the immediacy of the risk when the person has described a plan. When answers to level 3 or 4 are positive, the nurse must plan immediate interventions to deal with the suicide risk. An essential nursing responsibility with regard to level-4

Box 15-8 Guidelines for Assessing Suicide Risk

Risk Factors for Suicide in Older Adults

- Demographic factors: white race, male gender
- Depression, particularly when accompanied by insomnia, agitation, and self-neglect
- Chronic illness with increasing dependence and helplessness; diagnosis of cancer or a terminal illness
- Poor social supports; social isolation, particularly recent isolation
- History of psychiatric illness, particularly major depression
- Onset of major depression within the past year
- Family history of suicide; personal or family history of suicide attempts
- Patterns of impulsive behavior
- Alcohol abuse
- Poor communication skills

Verbal Clues to Suicide Intent

- "Pretty soon you won't have to worry about me."
- "I would be better off dead."
- "I'll make sure I won't be a burden to others."
- Expressions of hopelessness
- Remarks about life being unbearable
- Reflections on the worthlessness of life

Nonverbal Clues to Suicide Intent

- Making a will; giving belongings away; preparing for own funeral
- Serious self-neglect, particularly in people who have no cognitive impairments
- Frequent visits to primary care provider(s)
- Excessive use of medications or alcohol
- Accumulation of prescription medications
- Unusual preoccupation with self and withdrawal from others

Interview Questions to Assess the Immediate Risk of Suicide

- "Do you think that life is not worth living?"
- "Do you think about escaping from your problems?"
- "Do you wish you were dead?"
- "Do you think about harming yourself?"
- "Do you think about ending your life?"
- "Do you have a plan?"
- "What would you do to take your life?"
- "Have you ever started to act on a plan to harm yourself?"
- "Under what circumstances would you act on that plan?"
- "What prevents you from acting on the plan?"

---

questions is to ask what prevents the person from carrying out the plan because this information provides a base for supporting important patient-identified reasons for living.

Nursing Diagnosis and Outcomes

If the nursing assessment identifies risk factors for suicide, an applicable nursing diagnosis would be Risk for Suicide. Related factors would include any risk factors and verbal and nonverbal clues to suicide. An example is an 85-year-old widower who says his life is no longer worthwhile and who makes frequent visits to his doctor for complaints of weight loss and sleep disturbance. Outcomes for older adults at risk for suicide include Suicide Self-Restraint and Personal Safety Behavior.

Nursing Interventions for Preventing Suicide

Nurses do not routinely encounter suicidal older adults, but they need to be prepared to implement immediate interventions whenever they identify a patient at risk. The most important intervention is to seek psychiatric resources and activate referrals to the appropriate protective service agency rather than attempting to deal with potentially suicidal people without the help of specialized resources. All communities have some emergency psychiatric resources, and nurses can follow institutional policies regarding referrals for appropriate services. In any situation, nurses use appropriate communication techniques to address potentially suicidal older adults. In addition, it may be appropriate to assess for accessibility to firearms and educate families and caregivers about firearm safety precautions because 67% of suicides

among older adults occur via firearms (Barry & Byers, 2016; Slovak, Pope, & Brewer, 2016). Some guidelines for working with people who are potentially suicidal are listed in Box 15-9

Box 15-9 Nursing Interventions for People Who Are Potentially Suicidal

Communicating With Someone Who Is Potentially Suicidal

- Be direct and honest; do not be afraid to ask direct questions, such as, "Are you thinking of hurting yourself?"
- Express feelings of concern and confidence.
- Acknowledge the person's feelings of helplessness and hopelessness.
- Encourage the person to talk about the precipitating event, if there is one.
- Emphasize that suicide is only one of several options; then explore other options.
- Emphasize positive relationships; talk about the negative impact of suicide on survivors.
- Maintain a nonjudgmental attitude.
- Make a contract: ask the person to agree to do certain things for limited amounts of time and to call for help if he or she cannot keep the agreement.
- Discuss reasons that the person identifies for not carrying out a suicide plan and find ways to support and strengthen these.
- Discuss the problems openly with the family and caregivers.

Crisis Intervention

- Focus on the immediate precipitating event.
- Reduce the immediate danger by removing the implements, interfering with the plan, and providing constant supervision.
- Obtain psychiatric help; call a suicide hot line, or activate emergency psychiatric services if necessary.

Evaluating the Effectiveness of Nursing Interventions

Nursing care of older adults who are at high risk for self-harm is evaluated by the prevention of harm. Another measure is the degree to which the older adult develops coping skills to deal with the issues that underlie his or her suicidal thoughts. Nurses can also find out whether the older adult obtained suggested mental health services and determine the effectiveness of any referrals that were made.

See ONLINE LEARNING ACTIVITY 15-3: LINKS TO RESOURCES FOR FURTHER INFORMATION ABOUT LATE-LIFE DEPRESSION AND SUICIDE at http://thepoint.lww.com/Miller8e.

Case Study

Mrs. D. is 81 years old. Recently, she was diagnosed with vascular dementia. She lives with her husband, who has diabetes, macular degeneration, and severe arthritis. Mrs. D. had managed all household and financial responsibilities until approximately 1 year ago, when she began having trouble with her memory. Mrs. D. was evaluated at the geriatric assessment program where you work, and she was advised to stop driving and to arrange for some help with complex tasks, such as bill paying and grocery shopping. Two months after the initial evaluation, Mrs. D. returns for follow-up and informs you that she limits her driving to short, daytime trips in familiar areas. When asked about getting help with complex tasks, she states, "I just don't have any energy to make all those calls you suggested. Besides, I don't want anyone else looking at my finances or going to the store for me."

NURSING ASSESSMENT

A mental status assessment indicates that Mrs. D.'s level of cognitive impairment is unchanged since her initial evaluation. She has some deficits in calculation, short-term memory, abstract thinking, problem-solving, and language skills. Your psychosocial assessment reveals that Mrs. D. has a very sad affect and low self-esteem, and she expresses feelings of hopelessness and helplessness. She admits to being overwhelmed with feelings of responsibility for herself and her husband, and she says she feels "paralyzed because there's no light at the end of the tunnel." She scored 11 on the GDS-15.

When you ask about her daily life, Mrs. D. says she spends most of her time at home because she does not have the energy to go out. She admits that she has difficulty falling asleep at night, and she wakes up at around 4 AM and is unable to return to sleep. She naps for a couple of hours in the morning and in the afternoon because "I feel tired all the time, and I can't go out and do things anyway." Her appetite is poor, and in the past 2 months, her weight declined from 140 to 126 pounds (her height is 5'6"). She complains of constipation and "heartburn."

When you ask about meaningful activities, she tells you she no longer goes to her weekly bowling club because it meets in the evening, and she does not want to drive at night. She has also given up her church activities (Thursday discussion club and Sunday service) because she does not want to inconvenience anyone by having them drive her. She feels it is "demeaning to have to tell my friends that I need a ride." She used to enjoy reading, but she has not felt like going to the library, and she is not interested in any of the books she has at home.

NURSING DIAGNOSIS

You use the nursing diagnosis of Ineffective Individual Coping, related to depression and declining cognitive abilities. Evidence comes from Mrs. D.'s sad affect, low self-esteem, loss of interest in activities, feelings of hopelessness and helplessness, inability to address her problems effectively, and a GDS-15 score indicative of depression. Physical manifestations are her poor appetite, weight loss, sleep disturbances, and complaints about constipation and heartburn.

Expected Outcome	Nursing Interventions	Nursing Evaluation
Mrs. D. will be able to identify her coping patterns	• Ask Mrs. D. to describe her prior experiences in dealing with her husband's illness • Help Mrs. D. to identify coping strategies that have been helpful in the past	• Mrs. D. will recognize and acknowledge the coping strategies that have been helpful in the past

NURSING DIAGNOSIS (Continued)

Expected Outcome	Nursing Interventions	Nursing Evaluation
Mrs. D. will learn about depression and be encouraged to obtain further evaluation of her depression	• Talk with Mrs. D. about her signs and symptoms of depression, emphasizing the fact that depression is a treatable condition • Discuss the relationship between depression and the inability to cope effectively with stressful situations • Ask Mrs. D. if she is willing to see a geropsychiatrist, or talk to her primary care practitioner for further evaluation and treatment • Explain that antidepressant medications can be very effective when combined with counseling	• Mrs. D. will follow through with an appointment with a geropsychiatrist or talk with her primary care practitioner
Effective coping strategies for addressing Mrs. D.'s declining abilities will be identified	• Discuss with Mrs. D. several options for ongoing support and counseling to assist her in coping with her declining abilities (e.g., the "Something for You" support group for people with memory loss; or individual counseling sessions with the social worker who is affiliated with the geriatric assessment program) • Emphasize the importance of developing short-term goals that can be addressed through problem-solving (e.g., suggest that Mrs. D. begin to address her lack of meaningful activities by going to the library for reading material)	• Mrs. D. will attend one support group on a trial basis and talk with you about the experience at her next appointment in 1 month • Mrs. D. will make an appointment for counseling with the social worker • Mrs. D. will participate in one meaningful activity each week for the next month.

THINKING POINTS

- What risk factors are likely contributing to Mrs. D.'s depression?
- What further assessment information would you obtain?
- What questions on the GDS-15 (Figure 15-1) do you think would be indicative of depression for Mrs. D.?
- What additional interventions would you suggest for Mrs. D.?

Chapter Highlights

Depression in Older Adults

- Signs and symptoms of depression in older adults are on a continuum of severity from major depression to sub-threshold depression.
- Depression is characterized by depressed mood and/or loss of interest, along with additional manifestations, including weight loss, appetite change, sleep disturbances, psychomotor agitation or retardation, fatigue, cognitive impairment, feeling worthless or excessively guilty, and recurrent thoughts of death or suicide.
- Late-life depression refers to the onset of depression after the age of 65 years.

Theories About Late-Life Depression

- Psychosocial (e.g., learned helplessness, cognitive triad)
- Theories about the interrelationship between depression and pathologic conditions (e.g., dementia, cerebrovascular disease, cardiovascular disease)

Risk Factors for Depression in Older Adults

- Demographic and psychosocial
- Medical conditions and functional impairment (Box 15-1)
- Effects of alcohol and medications (Box 15-2)

Functional Consequences Associated With Depression in Older Adults (Box 15-3)

- Physical health and functioning
- Psychosocial function and quality of life

Nursing Assessment of Depression in Older Adults

- Unique manifestations in older versus younger adults (Table 15-1)
- Differentiating between dementia and depression (Table 15-2)
- Cultural variations in expressions of depression (Box 15-4)
- Screening tools (Figure 15-1)

Nursing Diagnosis

- Readiness for Enhanced Coping
- Ineffective Coping
- Hopelessness
- Caregiver Role Strain
- Risk for Compromised Resilience

Planning for Wellness Outcomes

- Coping
- Hope
- Caregiver Emotional Health
- Depression Level

Nursing Interventions to Address Depression

- Alleviating risk factors (addressing functional limitations, teaching about adverse effects of medications and excessive alcohol)
- Improving psychosocial function (social supports, meaningful activities)
- Promoting health through physical activity and nutrition
- Providing education and counseling (individual and group psychosocial interventions)
- Facilitating referrals for psychosocial therapies
- Teaching about nonpharmacologic therapies (Box 15-5)
- Antidepressant medications (Table 15-3, Box 15-6)
- Teaching about ECT and neuromodulation treatments

Evaluating the Effectiveness of Nursing Interventions (Box 15-7)

- Improved coping skills
- Fewer manifestations of depression
- Expressed feelings of improved quality of life
- Effective use of appropriate mental health services

Suicide in Late Life

- Suicide rates and mechanisms (Figures 15-2 and 15-3)
- Nursing assessment of suicide risk (Box 15-8)
- Nursing diagnosis and outcomes
- Nursing interventions for preventing suicide (Box 15-9)
- Evaluating effectiveness of interventions

Critical Thinking Exercises

1. Think of an older adult in your personal life or professional practice who is or has been depressed. What are (were) the risk factors in that person's situation that might play (have played) a part in the depression?
2. Describe at least four cultural variations in the way depression might be expressed.
3. What assessment observations would you make and what questions would you ask to differentiate between dementia and depression in older adults?
4. Develop a case example of someone who is potentially suicidal and who would require all four levels of suicide assessment. Describe how you would phrase the questions for each of the levels.
5. Describe a teaching plan for an 84-year-old woman for whom Paxil, 10 mg daily, has been prescribed.

 For more information about the topics discussed in this chapter, be sure to check out the interactive Online Learning Activities and other helpful resources at http://thepoint.lww.com/Miller8e.

REFERENCES

American Geriatrics Society. (2015). American Geriatrics Society 2015 Updated Beers Criteria for potentially inappropriate medication use in older adults. *Journal of the American Geriatrics Society, 63,* 2227–2246.

Barry, L. C., & Byers, A. L. (2016). Risk factors and prevention strategies for late-life mood and anxiety disorder. In K. W. Schaie & S. L. Willis (Eds.), *Handbook of the Psychology of Aging* (8th ed., pp. 409–417). Boston, MA: Elsevier.

Brailean, A., Aertsen, M. J., Muniz-Terrera, G., et al. (2017). Longitudinal associations between late-life depression dimensions and cognitive functioning: A cross-domain latent growth curve analysis. *Psychological Medicine, 47,* 690–702.

Chopik, W. J. (2016). The benefits of social technology use among older adults are mediated by reduced loneliness. *Cyberpsychology, Behavior and Social Networking, 19,* 551–556.

Chu, I. H., Wu, W. L., Lin, I. M., et al. (2017). Effects of yoga on heart rate variability and depressive symptoms in women: A randomized controlled trial. *Journal of Alternative and Complementary Medicine, 23*(4):310–316.

Conwell, Y., & O'Riley, A. (2013). The challenge of suicide prevention in later life. In H. Lavretsky, M. Sajatovic, & C. F. Reynolds, III (Eds.), *Late-life mood disorders* (pp. 206–219). Oxford: Oxford University Press.

Crespy, S., Van Haitsma, K., Kleban, M., et al. (2016). Reducing depressive symptoms in nursing home residents: Evaluation of the Pennsylvania Depression Collaborative Quality Improvement Program. *Journal for Healthcare Quality, 38,* e76–e88.

Creswell, J. D. (2017). Mindfulness interventions. *Annual Review of Psychology, 68,* 491–516.

Crosby, A. E., Ortega, L., & Stevens, M. R. (2013). Suicides: United States, 2005–2009. *Morbidity and Mortality Weekly Report, Supplement, 62(3),* 179–183. Available at www.cdc.gov.

Czaja, S., Boot, W. R., Charness, N., et al. (2017). Improving social support for older adults through technology: Findings from the PRISM randomized controlled trial. *Gerontologist.* [Epub] doi: 10.1093/geront/gnw249.

Dols, A., Bouckaert, F., Sienaert, P., et al. (2017). Early- and late-onset depression in late life: A prospective study on clinical and structural brain characteristics and response to electroconvulsive therapy. *American Journal of Geriatric Psychiatry, 25,* 178–189.

Ehrmin, J. T. (2016). Transcultural perspectives in mental health nursing. In M. M. Andrews, & J. S. Boyle (Eds.), *Transcultural concepts in nursing care* (7th ed. pp. 272–316). Philadelphia, PA: Wolters Kluwer.

Gariépy G., Honkaniemi, H., & Quesnei-Vallee, A. (2016). Social support and protection from depression: Systematic review of current findings in Western countries. *British Journal of Psychiatry, 209,* 284–293.

Gathright, E. C., Goldstein, C. M., Josephson, R. A., et al. (2017). Depression increases the risk of mortality in patients with heart failure: A meta-analysis. *Journal of Psychosomatic Research, 94,* 82–89.

Geduldig, E. T., & Kellner, C. H. (2016). Electroconvulsive therapy in the elderly: New findings in geriatric depression. *Current Psychiatry Reports, 18.* doi: 10.1007/s11920-016-0674-5.

Gomez-Gallego, M., Gomez-Garcia, J., & Ato-Lozano, E. (2017). The mediating role of depression in the association between disability and quality of life in Alzheimer's Disease. *Aging & Mental Health, 21,* 163–172.

Groh, C., & Dumlao, M. (2016). Depression in home-based care: The role of the home health nurse. *Home Healthcare Now, 34,* 360–368.

Halaris, A. (2017). Inflammation-associated co-morbidity between depression and cardiovascular disease. *Current Topics in Behavioral Neuroscience, 31,* 45–70.

Helming, M. B. (2016). Relationships. In B. M. Dossey & L. Keegan (Eds.), *Holistic nursing: A handbook for practice* (6th ed., pp. 479–499). Boston, MA: Jones & Bartlett Publishers.

Ismail, Z., Elbayoumi, H., Fischer, C. E., et al. (2017). Prevalence of depression in patients with mild cognitive impairment: A systematic review and meta-analysis. *Journal of the American Medical Association: Psychiatry, 74,* 58–67.

Jerez-Roig, J, de Oliveira, N. P., de Lima Filho, B. F., et al. (2016). Depressive symptoms and associated factors in institutionalized elderly. *Experimental Aging Research, 42,* 479–491.

Juang, C., Knight, B., Carlson, M., et al. (2017). Understanding the mechanisms of change in a lifestyle intervention for older adults. *Gerontologist.* [Epub] doi: 10.1093/geront/gnw152.

Karaahmet, O. Z., Gurcay, E., Avluk, O. C., et al. (2017). Poststroke depression: risk factors and potential effects on functional recovery. *International Journal of Rehabilitation Research, 40,* 71–75.

Khusid, M. A., & Vythilingam, M. (2016). The emerging role of mindfulness meditation as effective self-management strategy. Part 1: Clinical implications for depression, post-traumatic stress disorder, and anxiety. *Military Medicine, 181,* 961–968.

Kim, M., Oh, G. J., & Lee, Y. H. (2017). Association between stroke status and depression in a community setting: The 2014 Korean National Health and Nutrition Examination Survey. *Journal of Clinical Neurology, 13,* 55–61.

Kim, S., Woo, S. Y., Kang, H. S., et al. (2016). Factors related to prevalence, persistence, and incidence of depressive symptoms in mild cognitive impairment: Vascular depression construct. *International Journal of Geriatric Psychiatry, 31,* 818–826.

Kim, S. H. (2016). Suicidal ideation and suicide attempts in older adults: Influences of chronic illness, functional limitations, and pain. *Geriatric Nursing, 37,* 9–12.

Klonsky, E., Oiu, T., & Saffer, B. (2017). Recent advances in differentiating suicide attempters from suicide ideators. *Current Opinion in Psychiatry, 30,* 15–20.

Kumar, S., Mulsant, B. H., Liu A. Y., et al., et al. (2016). Systematic review of cognitive effects of electroconvulsive therapy in late-life depression.*American Journal of Geriatric Psychiatry, 24,* 547–565.

Lara, E., Koyanagi, A., Domenech-Abella, J., et al. (2017). The impact of depression on the development of mild cognitive impairment over 3 years of follow-up: A population-based study. *Dementia and Geriatric Cognitive Disorders, 43,* 155–169.

Lee-Tauler, S. Y., Lee-Kwan, S. H., Han, H., et al. (2016). What does depression mean for Korean American elderly? A qualitative follow-up study. *Psychiatry Investigation, 13,* 558–565.

Lohman, M., Dumenci, L., & Mezuk, B. (2016). Depression and frailty in late life: Evidence for a common vulnerability. *Journals of Gerontology: Journal of Psychological Sciences and Social Sciences, 71,* 630–640.

Lugtenburg, A., Zuidersma, M., Oude Voshaar, R. C., et al. (2016). Symptom dimensions of depression and 3-year incidence of dementia: Results from the Amsterdam Study of the Elderly. *Journal of Geriatric Psychiatry and Neurology, 29,* 99–107.

Mathur, S., Charma, M. P., & Bharath, S. (2016). Mindfulness-based cognitive therapy in patients with late-life depression: A case series. *International Journal of Yoga, 9,* 168–172.

McIntosh, C. (2017). A depression screening protocol for patients with acute stroke: A quality improvement project. *Journal of Neuroscience Nursing, 49,* 39–48.

McKenzie, G. L., & Harvath, T. A. (2016). Late-life depression. In M. Boltz, E. Capezuti, T. Fulmer, & D. Zwicker (Eds.), *Evidence-based geriatric nursing protocols for best practice* (5th ed. pp. 211–232). New York: Springer Publishing.

Mirza, S. S., Ikram, M. A., Bos, D., et al. (2017). Mild cognitive impairment and risk of depression and anxiety: A population-based study. *Alzheimer's Dementia, 13,* 130–139.

Nadorff, M. R., Fiske, A., & Sperry, J. A., et al. (2013). Insomnia symptoms, nightmares, and suicidal ideation in older adults. *Journals of Gerontology: Psychological Sciences and Social Sciences, 68*(2), 145–152.

Pocklington, C., Gilbody, S., Manea, L., et al. (2016). The diagnostic accuracy of brief versions of the Geriatric Depression Scale: A systematic review and meta-analysis. *International journal of geriatric psychiatry, 31*(8), 837–857

Rizvi, S., Iskric, A., Calati, R., et al. (2017). Psychological and physical pain as predictors of suicide risk: Evidence from clinical and neuroimaging findings. *Current Opinion in Psychiatry, 30,* 159–166.

Rutherford, B., Taylor, W., Brown, P., et al. (2017). Biological aging and the future of geriatric psychiatry. *Journals of Gerontology: Biological Sciences and Medical Sciences, 72,* 343–352.

Salinas, J., Ray, R. M., Nassir R., et al. (2017). Factors associated with new-onset depression following ischemic stroke: The Women's Health Initiative. *Journal of the American Heart Association, 6*(2). [Epub] doi: 10.1161/JAHA.116.003828.

Schaakxs, R., Comijs, H. C., Lamers, F., et al. (2017). Age-related variability in the presentation of symptoms of major depressive disorder. *Psychological Medicine, 47,* 543–552.

Scott, R., & Paulson, D. (2017). Cerebrovascular burden and depressive symptomatology interrelate over 18 years: Support for the vascular depression hypothesis. *International Journal of Geriatric Psychiatry.* [Epub] doi:10.1102/gps.4674.

Simning, A., & Simons, K. V. (2017). Treatment of depression in nursing home residents without significant cognitive impairment: A systematic review. *International Psychogeriatrics, 29,* 209–226.

Sims, T., Reed, A. E., & Carr, D. C. (2016). Information and communication technology use is related to higher well-being among the oldest-old. *Journals of Gerontology: Psychological Sciences and Social Sciences.* [Epub] doi: 10.1093/geronb.gbw130.

Ski, C. F., Worrall-Carter, L., Cameron, J., et al. (2017). Depression screening and referral in cardiac wards: A 12-month patient trajectory. *European Journal of Cardiovascular Nursing, 16,* 157–166.

Slovak, K., Pope, N., & Brewer, T. (2016). Geriatric case managers' perspectives on suicide among community-dwelling older adults. *Journal of Gerontological Social Work, 59,* 3–15.

Suanet, B., & Antonucci, T. C. (2017). Cohort differences in received social support in later life: The role of network type. *Journals of Gerontology: Journal of Psychological Sciences and Social Sciences, 72*(4), 706–715.

Towfighi, A., Ovbiagele, B., El Husseini, N., et al. (2017). Poststroke depression: A scientific statement for healthcare professionals from the American Heart Association/American Stroke Association. *Stroke, 48,* e30–e43.

Trangle, M., Gursky, J., Haight, R., et al. (2016). Institute for clinical systems improvement: Health care guideline: Adult depression in primary care. Retrieved from www.icsi.org.

Tsoi, K. K., Chan, J. Y., Hirai, H. W., et al. (2017). Comparison of diagnostic performance of two-question screen and 15 depression screening instruments for older adults: Systematic review and meta-analysis. *British Journal of Psychiatry.* [Epub] doi: 10.1192/bjp.bp.116.186932.

Van der wall, E. E. (2016). Cardiac disease and depression: A direct association? *Netherlands Heart Journal, 24,* 485–497.

Wang, Z., Wang, X., Liu, J., et al. (2017). Acupuncture treatment modulates the corticostriatal reward circuitry in major depressive disorder. *Journal of Psychiatric Research, 84,* 18–26.

Wermelinger Avila, M. P., Lucchetti, A., L., & Lucchetti, G. (2017). Association between depression and resilience in older adults: A systematic review and meta-analysis. *International Journal of Geriatric Psychiatry, 32*(3), 237–246.

Werner, J., Wosch, T., & Gold, C. (2017). Effectiveness of group music therapy versus recreational group singing for depressive symptoms of elderly nursing home residents: Pragmatic trial. *Aging and Mental Health, 21,* 147–155.

Willis, M. (2016). *Literature review for the non-pharmacological treatment of geriatric depression.* Thesis submitted to the Kent State University Honors College, May, 2016.

Xiang, X., An, R., & Heinemann, A. (2017). Depression and unmet need for assistance with daily activities among community-dwelling older adults. *Gerontologist.* [Epub] doi: 10.1093/geront/gnw262.

Zhao, K., Bai, Z. G., Bo, A., et al. (2016). A systematic review and meta-analysis of music therapy for older adults with depression. *International Journal of Geriatric Psychiatry, 31,* 1188–1198.

Zlatar, Z. Z., Muniz, M., Galasko, D., et al. (2017). Subjective cognitive decline correlates with depression symptoms and not with concurrent objective cognition in a clinic-based sample of older adults. *Journals of Gerontology: Journal of Psychological Sciences and Social Sciences.* [Epub] doi: 10.1093/geronb/gbw207.

part **4**

Promoting Wellness in Physical Function

Unfolding Patient Stories: Sherman "Red" Yoder · Part 3

Recall from Parts 2 and 3 Sherman "Red" Yoder, an 80-year-old male with insulin-dependent diabetes and a foot wound. During the assessment the home health nurse discovers that he is having urgency incontinence and often avoids fluids, especially before driving 20 miles to have coffee with friends. How can urinary incontinence affect Red's quality of life? What age-related changes and conditions can increase the potential for urinary incontinence? What further assessments and interventions can be incorporated in the nursing plan of care to promote urinary wellness?

Care for Red and other patients in a realistic virtual environment: **vSim** *for Nursing* (thepoint. lww.com/vSimGerontology). Practice documenting these patients' care in DocuCare (thepoint.lww.com/ DocuCareEHR).

Unfolding Patient Stories: Henry Williams · Part 1

Henry Williams, age 69, is a retired rail system engineer who has chronic obstructive pulmonary disease (COPD), which is exacerbated by frequent respiratory infections. In addition to COPD, what age-related alterations and risk factors can affect his respiratory function? What nursing interventions and education can promote Henry's respiratory wellness? What resources could the nurse suggest to Henry to improve self-management of COPD? (Henry Williams' story continues in Part 5.)

Care for Henry and other patients in a realistic virtual environment: **vSim** *for Nursing* (thepoint. lww.com/vSimGerontology). Practice documenting these patients' care in DocuCare (thepoint.lww.com/ DocuCareEHR).

chapter 16

Hearing

LEARNING OBJECTIVES

After reading this chapter, you will be able to:

1. Describe age-related changes that affect hearing.
2. Identify risk factors that affect hearing wellness.
3. Discuss the functional consequences that affect hearing wellness.
4. Conduct a nursing assessment of hearing, with emphasis on identifying opportunities for health promotion.
5. Identify nursing interventions to promote hearing wellness for older adults by addressing risk factors that interfere with hearing.

KEY TERMS

assistive listening device
auditory rehabilitation
cerumen
cochlear implants
conductive hearing loss
hearing aid
impacted cerumen
mixed hearing loss
noise-induced hearing loss (NIHL)
otosclerosis
presbycusis
sensorineural hearing loss
tinnitus

Performance of many important daily activities—including communicating, protecting oneself from danger, and enjoying music, voices, and sounds—is highly dependent on good hearing. In older adults, age-related changes combine with risk factors to affect hearing wellness. This chapter addresses the functional consequences associated with hearing in older adults and discusses nursing assessment and interventions related to promoting hearing wellness in older adults.

AGE-RELATED CHANGES THAT AFFECT HEARING

Auditory function depends on a sequence of processes, beginning in the three compartments of the ear and ending with the processing of information in the auditory cortex of the brain. Sounds are coded according to intensity and frequency. Intensity, or amplitude, reflects the loudness or softness of the sound and is measured in decibels (dB). Frequency, which is measured in cycles per second, or hertz (Hz), determines whether the pitch is high or low. Sound intensity and frequency may be altered if certain risk factors come into play. Even in the absence of risk factors, normal age-related changes affect frequency, causing hearing problems for many older adults.

External Ear

Hearing begins in the external or outer ear, which consists of the pinna and the external auditory canal (Figure 16-1). These cartilaginous structures localize sounds so the source can be identified. The auditory canal is covered by skin and lined with hair follicles and cerumen-producing glands. The function of **cerumen**, or earwax, is to cleanse, protect, and lubricate the ear canal. Age-related processes that interfere with the normal processes of expelling cerumen include an increased concentration of keratin, the growth of longer and thicker hair (especially in men), and thinning and drying of the skin lining the canal. These changes cause cerumen to be drier and more difficult to expel, thereby increasing the potential for cerumen to accumulate and block the canal.

Middle Ear

The tympanic membrane is a transparent, pearl-gray, slightly cone-shaped layer of flexible tissue that separates the outer and middle ear. Its primary functions are to transmit sound

Promoting Hearing Wellness in Older Adults

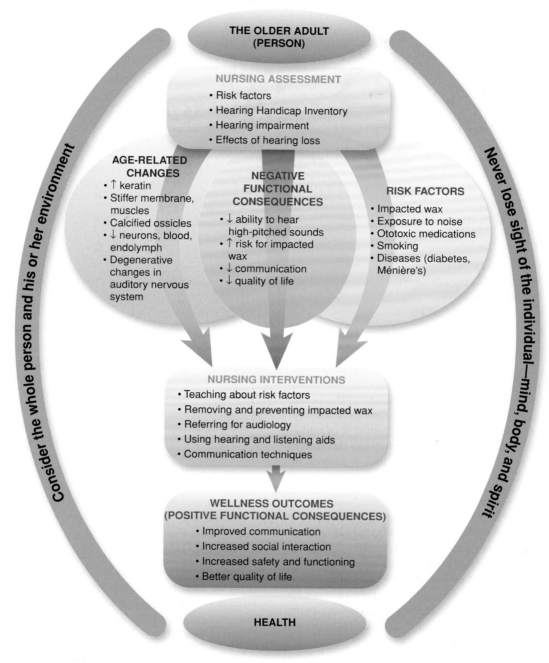

THE OLDER ADULT (PERSON)

NURSING ASSESSMENT
- Risk factors
- Hearing Handicap Inventory
- Hearing impairment
- Effects of hearing loss

AGE-RELATED CHANGES
- ↑ keratin
- Stiffer membrane, muscles
- Calcified ossicles
- ↓ neurons, blood, endolymph
- Degenerative changes in auditory nervous system

NEGATIVE FUNCTIONAL CONSEQUENCES
- ↓ ability to hear high-pitched sounds
- ↑ risk for impacted wax
- ↓ communication
- ↓ quality of life

RISK FACTORS
- Impacted wax
- Exposure to noise
- Ototoxic medications
- Smoking
- Diseases (diabetes, Ménière's)

NURSING INTERVENTIONS
- Teaching about risk factors
- Removing and preventing impacted wax
- Referring for audiology
- Using hearing and listening aids
- Communication techniques

WELLNESS OUTCOMES (POSITIVE FUNCTIONAL CONSEQUENCES)
- Improved communication
- Increased social interaction
- Increased safety and functioning
- Better quality of life

HEALTH

Consider the whole person and his or her environment

Never lose sight of the individual—mind, body, and spirit

energy and protect the middle and inner ear. With increased age, collagenous tissue replaces the elastic tissue, resulting in a thinner and stiffer eardrum. Sound vibrations pass through the tympanic membrane to the three auditory ossicles: the malleus, incus, and stapes. These bones act as a lever and transmit sound vibrations across the air-filled middle ear, through the oval window, and into the fluid-filled inner ear. Sound transmission depends on the frequency of each sound and is best for the middle-frequency range of normal voices and less effective for low- and high-frequency sounds.

Age-related calcification of the ossicles can interfere with the transfer of sound vibrations from the tympanic membrane to the oval window.

The middle ear muscles and ligaments respond to loud noises to protect the delicate inner ear and filter out auditory distractions originating from one's own voice and body movements. With increased age, degenerative changes in the middle ear muscles and ligaments interfere with this protective response and diminish the elasticity of the tympanic membrane.

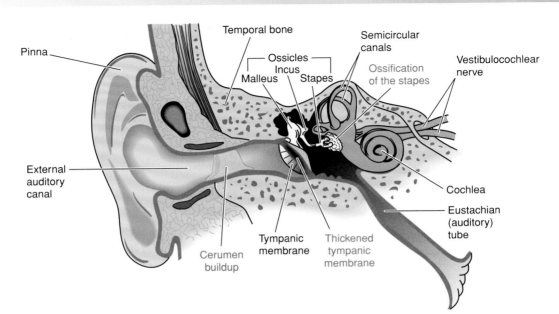

FIGURE 16-1 The ear. Age-related changes in structures of the ear, indicated with red labels, can affect hearing in older adults.

Inner Ear

In the inner ear, vibrations are transmitted to the cochlea, where they are converted to nerve impulses and coded for intensity and frequency. Nerve impulses stimulate the eighth cranial nerve and send the auditory message to the brain. Age-related changes of the inner ear include loss of sensory hair cells, reduction of blood supply, diminution of endolymph production, decreased basilar membrane flexibility, degeneration of spiral ganglion cells, and loss of neurons in the cochlear nuclei.

Auditory Nervous System

Functions of the auditory nervous system include localizing sound direction, fine-tuning auditory stimuli, and transferring information from the primary auditory cortex to the auditory association area. The auditory nervous system is affected by all the following age-related changes: degenerative changes in the inner ear, narrowing of the auditory meatus from bone apposition, diminished blood supply, and central nervous system changes.

 ## RISK FACTORS THAT AFFECT HEARING WELLNESS

In addition to the age-related changes that affect hearing, factors associated with lifestyle, heredity, environment, medications, impacted cerumen, and disease conditions can cause hearing loss. A major focus of research is on modifiable conditions, such as smoking and exposure to noise, which can be addressed through health promotion interventions. For example, smoking is associated with increased prevalence of bilateral hearing impairment beginning at age 30 (Change, Ryou, Jun, et al., 2016). Researchers also are exploring potential interrelationship between two or more risk factors. For example, people who are genetically predisposed to hearing loss may be more susceptible to the damaging effects of noise exposure or ototoxic medications. Because age-related changes increase the risk for hearing loss, it is especially important to identify modifiable risk factors in older adults so that those risks can be addressed. Most likely, some hearing loss attributed to age-related changes actually results from risk factors, such as exposure to noise or ototoxic substances. Box 16-1 summarizes some factors that interfere with hearing wellness, either alone or in combination.

Exposure to Noise

A commonly occurring risk factor for hearing loss is prolonged or intermittent exposure to noise, which can be viewed as both a lifestyle choice and an environmental factor. Although age-related changes account for a greater amount of hearing loss than occupational noise exposure, **noise-induced hearing loss (NIHL)** is an important preventable type of hearing loss. Short-term exposure to noise causes temporary hearing loss, and prolonged exposure causes permanent hearing loss due to gradual destruction of sensory cells in the inner ear. Many occupational and leisure activities are associated with an increased risk for NIHL, with several of the most common ones identified in Box 16-1. Exposure to toxic chemicals in the workplace or the environment is another risk factor for hearing loss that has been under investigation since the 1990s, with current research focusing on metals, solvents, asphyxiants, and pesticides/herbicides. Although the National Institute for Occupational Safety and Health enforces safety standards for workplace

Box 16-1 Risk Factors for Impaired Hearing

Genetic predisposition
Increased age
Male gender
White race
Impacted cerumen
Occupational exposure to noise—examples of occupations:
  Military workers
  Farmers
  Miners
  Construction workers
  Musicians
Recreational exposure to noise—examples:
  Listening to music using earphones or sound systems at high
    volumes
  Hunting or target shooting
  Riding all-terrain vehicles or motorcycles
  Operating power tools (e.g., chain saws, leaf blowers, drills)
Exposure to toxic chemicals in the workplace or the environment—
  examples:
  Heavy metals (e.g., lead, mercury)
  Solvents

Asphyxiates
Pesticides/herbicides
Carbon monoxide
Fuels
Smoking of nicotine products
Ototoxic medications
  Aminoglycosides (e.g., gentamicin, neomycin)
  Aspirin and other salicylates
  Cisplatin and other chemotherapeutic agents
  Hydroxychloroquine
  Loop diuretics (e.g., bumetanide, furosemide)
  Macrolides (e.g., erythromycin, clarithromycin)
  Quinine
  Quinolones (e.g., ciprofloxacin, ofloxacin)
Medical conditions—examples:
  Diabetes
  Hypertension
  Cardiovascular disease
  Ménière disease

conditions that pose risks for hearing loss, it is important to consider that many older adults were exposed to harmful work environments before these standards were established. Because the effects of NIHL and age-related changes are cumulative, the hearing loss may not be noticed until later adulthood. For US military veterans, tinnitus and hearing loss are the two most prevalent causes of service-connected disability, affecting veterans of all ages and sometimes not occurring until years after active service (National Academy of Sciences, Engineering, & Medicine, 2016). Figure 16-2 illustrates the noise levels of various activities. Sounds louder than 80 to 85 dB are considered potentially ototoxic.

**See ONLINE LEARNING ACTIVITY 16-1:
HOW LOUD IS TOO LOUD?
at http://thepoint.lww.com/Miller8e**

Impacted Cerumen

Impacted cerumen (also called impacted wax) is common in older adults as a leading cause of hearing loss, particularly in nursing home residents. Age-related changes, which make the cerumen dryer and more concentrated, increase the risk of impaction. In addition to causing hearing loss, impacted cerumen can cause pain, otitis, tinnitus, dizziness, fullness, or coughing. Cerumen accumulation is preventable and treatable and, most important, it is readily amenable to nursing interventions (as discussed later in this chapter in the section on Impacted Cerumen), which lead to improved hearing.

Adverse Effects of Medications and Treatments

Ototoxic effects of quinine and salicylates were first observed more than a century ago. More recently, health care

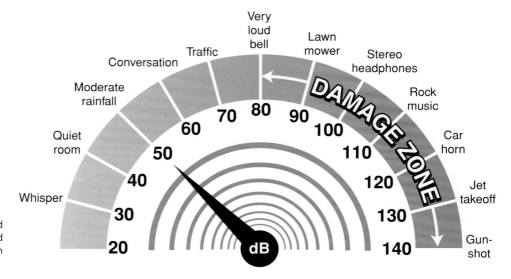

FIGURE 16-2 Noise levels associated with common activities are measured in decibels (dB). Sounds louder than 80 dB are potentially harmful to ears.

Unfolding Case Study

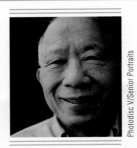

Photodisc V/Senior Portraits

Part 1: Mr. H. at 60 Years of Age

Mr. H. is 60 years old and owns a small home-remodeling business. He has been a carpenter for 38 years, but in the past 9 years, he has spent most of his time in the office, managing his business. He enjoys hunting and fishing on weekends. He has smoked two packs of cigarettes a day since he was 16 years old. His wife has been telling him she thinks he hears only what he wants to hear. Mr. H. admits that he turns the television volume up louder than he used to but denies having any "real hearing problem."

THINKING POINTS

- What age-related changes and risk factors contribute to Mr. H.'s hearing loss?
- Describe the hearing loss that Mr. H. is likely to be experiencing.

- What environmental conditions will contribute to Mr. H.'s hearing difficulty?

professionals have recognized the ototoxic effects of certain medications, such as the ones listed in Box 16-1. In addition, hearing loss is being addressed as an adverse effect of cancer treatments, including platinum-based chemotherapy, radiation for head and neck cancers, and surgery involving the ear and auditory nerve (Landier, 2016; Waissbluth, Peleva, & Daniel, 2016). Although age alone does not increase the risk for ototoxicity, older adults are more likely to have conditions that increase the risk for medication-related ototoxicity, such as renal failure, dehydration, and potentiation between two ototoxic medications, such as furosemide and aminoglycoside antibiotics. Although ototoxicity is potentially reversible, medications may be overlooked as a causative factor if the hearing loss is mistakenly ascribed to inevitable and irreversible degenerative changes.

Disease Processes

Otosclerosis is a hereditary disease of the auditory ossicles that causes ankylosis of the footplate of the stapes to the oval window. Although otosclerosis usually begins in youth or early adulthood, the hearing loss may not be detected until middle or later adulthood when age-related changes compound the disease-related changes. Otosclerosis primarily causes a conductive hearing loss, but older adults are likely to also experience significant sensorineural hearing loss that is beyond the expected age-related changes (Ishai, Halpin, Shin, et al., 2016). Ménière disease and acoustic neuromas are auditory system diseases that commonly cause hearing impairment.

Medical conditions and systemic diseases that can cause or contribute to hearing impairment include diabetes, hypertension, meningitis, hypothyroidism, lipid disorders, head injury, high fevers, Paget disease, renal failure, cardiovascular disease, and viral infections (e.g., measles and mumps).

Wellness Opportunity

Modifiable and preventable risk factors for hearing loss include noise, medications, and impacted cerumen.

FUNCTIONAL CONSEQUENCES AFFECTING HEARING WELLNESS

In 2014, 33% of people between the ages of 65 and 74 years and 47% of those 75 years and older had a hearing loss (National Center for Health Statistics, 2016). Figure 16-3 illustrates the percentage of older adults reporting a hearing loss by age, sex, race, and Hispanic origin. Hearing impairment is most common in people who have one or more of the risk factors previously discussed.

Hearing impairment is categorized according to the site of impairment as follows:

- **Conductive hearing loss** results from abnormalities of the external and middle ear that interfere with sound conduction.
- **Sensorineural hearing loss** is caused by abnormalities of the sensory and neural structures of the inner ear, which usually are age related or noise induced.
- **Mixed hearing loss** involves both conductive and sensorineural impairments.

Diversity Note

In the United States, higher prevalence of hearing loss is associated with the following characteristics: older age, male sex, white race, American Indian, or Alaska Native (National Center for Health Statistics, 2016).

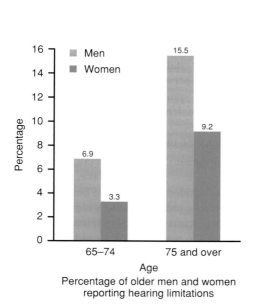

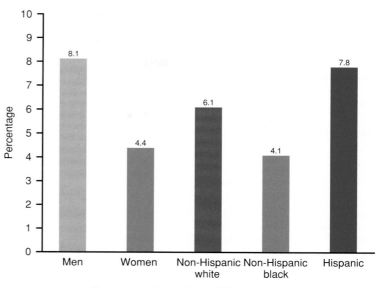

FIGURE 16-3 Percentage of older adults with hearing impairment, by age, sex, race and Hispanic origin, and degree of limitation in 2014. (From National Center for Health Statistics. (2016). *Health, United States, 2015*. Trend Table 44, Hearing Limitations among adults aged 18 and over, by selected characteristics: United States, Selected Years 1997–2014. Washington DC: U. S. Government Printing Office; Federal Interagency Forum on Aging-Related Statistics. (2016). *Older Americans 2015: Key indicators of well-being*, Indicator 22, Tables 22a & 22c, Percentage of people age 65 and over with a disability, by race and Hispanic origin and functional domain, 2014.)

Effects on Communication

Accurate comprehension of speech depends on speech pace, sound frequencies, environmental noise, and internal auditory function. Hearing acuity for high-frequency tones normally begins to decline in early adulthood, and by the age of 30 years for men and 50 years for women, there is some decline in hearing sensitivity at all frequencies.

 Global Perspective

Globally, hearing loss has been identified as the fifth leading cause of years lived with disability (National Academies of Sciences, Engineering, and Medicine, 2016).

Speech comprehension is most directly influenced by the frequency of *phonemes*, the smallest units of sound. Each phoneme in a word has a different frequency; generally, vowels have lower frequencies and consonants have higher frequencies. Although most word phonemes have lower-range frequencies, sibilant consonants (those that have a whistling quality, such as *ch, f, g, s, sh, t, th,* and *z*) have higher-range frequencies. Because the earliest and most universal age-related changes affect one's ability to code higher-frequency sounds, older adults typically have difficulty understanding words that are rich in consonants (Kalaiah, Thomas, Bhat, et al., 2016).

Presbycusis is the age-related hearing loss that has been described as "the most prevalent neurodegenerative disease and number one communication disorder of our aged population" (Frisina, Ding, Zhu, et al., 2016, p. 2018). Presbycusis typically begins in the fourth decade, but the sharpest increase in prevalence occurs after the tenth decade (Wattamwar, Qian, Otter, et al., 2016). Presbycusis usually occurs in both ears, but the degree of impairment in each ear can vary. An early functional consequence of presbycusis is the loss of ability to hear high-pitched sounds and sibilant consonants. When high-pitched sounds are filtered out, words become distorted and jumbled and sentences become incoherent. For example, someone with presbycusis might interpret a sentence like "I think she should go to the store" as "I wish we could go to the show." This characteristic, known as *diminished speech discrimination,* is influenced by the speaker's rate of speech: rapid, slow, or slurred speech patterns make it increasingly difficult for the older person to discern words. As the hearing loss progresses, explosive consonants, such as *b, d, k, p,* and *t,* also become distorted.

Background noise and environmental conditions, such as echoing or poor acoustics, interfere with the ability of older adults to understand speech, even in the absence of a significant hearing loss (Vermeire, Knoop, Boel, et al., 2016). Thus, older adults in a hospital or long-term care facility, for example, may be particularly sensitive to background noises to which the staff may have become accustomed.

A conductive hearing loss is characterized by a reduced intensity of sounds and difficulty hearing vowels and low-pitched tones. In contrast to presbycusis, all sound frequencies are heard equally once the sound threshold is reached,

TABLE 16-1 Functional Consequences of Age-Related Changes Affecting Hearing

Structure	Change	Consequence
External Ear	• Longer, thicker hair • Thinner, drier skin • Increased keratin	Potential for impacted cerumen and subsequent impaired sound conduction
Middle Ear	• Diminished resiliency of tympanic membrane • Calcified, hardened ossicles • Weakened and stiff muscles and ligaments	Impaired sound conduction
Inner Ear and Nervous System	• Diminished neurons, endolymph, hair cells, and blood supply • Degeneration of spiral ganglion and arterial blood vessels • Decreased flexibility of basilar membrane • Degeneration of central processing systems	*Presbycusis:* diminished ability to hear high-pitched sounds, especially in the presence of background noise

and background noise does not interfere as much with speech comprehension. Often there is a history of otosclerosis, perforated eardrum, or other ear diseases. In older adults, impacted cerumen is a common contributing factor. Depending on the causative factor, conductive hearing loss occurs in one or both ears (see Table 16-1 for a summary of the functional consequences of age-related changes affecting hearing).

 See ONLINE LEARNING ACTIVITY 16-2: THROUGH THE EARS OF OLDER ADULTS at http://thepoint.lww.com/Miller8e

Effects of Hearing Loss on Overall Wellness

Adequate hearing is a primary component of communication that enables people to enjoy humor, appreciate music, obtain information, relate to others, and respond to threats. Thus, hearing deficits inevitably affect safety, functioning, and quality of life in many ways. Reviews of studies have identified all the following functional consequences of hearing loss in older adults:

- Diminished cognitive function
- Functional decline
- Loneliness, isolation, and diminished participation in social activities
- Diminished emotional vitality, defined as a high level of happiness and sense of personal mastery and low levels of anxiety and depressive symptoms
- Increased prevalence of depression
- Decreased autonomy
- Increased dependence on others

(Cardin, 2016; Fortunato, Forli, Guglielmi, et al., 2016; Sung, Li, Blake, et al., 2016).

It is important to consider the effects of hearing loss on cognitive function because reduced auditory input may affect performance on mental status evaluations (Hume & Young, 2016). Nurses also need to consider that people with hearing loss may refrain from answering questions or give inaccurate responses because they are unable to comprehend the questions. Poor performance on tests of cognitive abilities can mistakenly lead to a perception that the person has cognitive impairments or dementia when, in fact, the person has a hearing loss.

In addition to having a negative influence on the quality of life, hearing deficits can affect the safety and functioning of older adults. For example, people with hearing impairments are likely to be less responsive when warning signals are sounded for fires, ambulances, and other emergencies. Besides creating actual safety hazards, the hearing deficit can lead to fear and anxiety about personal safety.

Negative societal attitudes about aging and hearing loss can result in a doubly negative effect on the person who is old as well as hard of hearing. The older person may be reluctant to acknowledge a hearing deficit, choosing to limit opportunities for communication rather than face the stigma associated with hearing impairments. These attitudes and accompanying behaviors can contribute to additional psychosocial consequences such as loneliness, depression, and even more social isolation.

Wellness Opportunity

Nurses can initiate conversations that reflect positive and nonjudgmental attitudes about aging and hearing loss.

Unfolding Case Study

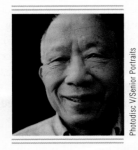

Photodisc V/Senior Portraits

Part 2: Mr. H. at 69 Years of Age

Mr. H. is now 69 years old and has been retired for several years. He spends several days a week hunting and fishing seasonally. He also spends time in his basement making small pieces of furniture and doing other woodworking. He continues to smoke but has cut down to one pack per day. His wife and he attend the weekly "lunch bunch" group at the local senior center where you are the nurse. They make an appointment to talk with you because Mrs. H. is concerned about her husband's hearing. Mr. H., who blames his problem on "old age," refuses to have an evaluation for a hearing aid because he does not think an aid would do any good and "besides, it would stick out like a sore thumb."

Part 2: Mr. H. at 69 Years of Age (*Continued*)

THINKING POINTS

- What factors contribute to Mr. H.'s hearing loss?
- What environmental and other conditions might make the hearing loss worse?

- What myths or misunderstandings are likely to influence Mr. H.'s perception of his hearing problem and potential interventions for it?

QSEN APPLICATION

QSEN Competency	Knowledge/Skill/Attitude	Application to Mr. H. When He Is 69 Years Old
Patient-centered care	(K) Integrate understanding of multiple dimensions of patient-centered care	Identify Mr. H.'s misunderstandings about hearing loss and hearing aids and use a nonjudgmental approach to provide correct information
	(K) Discuss principles of effective communication	Encourage Mrs. H. to verbalize her concerns directly to Mr. H. during your meeting so these can be addressed and misinformation can be corrected
	(S) Elicit patient values, preferences, and expressed needs	
	(A) Value seeing health care situations "through patients' eyes"	

PATHOLOGIC CONDITION AFFECTING HEARING: TINNITUS

Tinnitus is the persistent sensation of ringing, roaring, blowing, buzzing, or other types of noise that do not originate in the external environment. In the United States, 14.3% of adults aged 60 to 69 years experience tinnitus, and about 90% of people with tinnitus also have hearing loss (Al-Swiahb & Park, 2016). Tinnitus is a symptom of an underlying condition, such as impacted cerumen, otosclerosis, or Ménière disease. Most often, it occurs in conjunction with sensorineural hearing loss. A primary responsibility of nurses is to encourage people who have tinnitus to discuss this symptom with their primary care practitioners to identify reversible or serious causes. A referral to a specialist is especially important if tinnitus is unilateral, bothersome, or accompanied by hearing loss.

See ONLINE LEARNING ACTIVITY 16-3: THROUGH THE EARS OF SOMEONE WHO HAS TINNITUS at http://thepoint.lww.com/Miller8e

Wellness Opportunity

Nurses can teach people who have tinnitus about the exacerbating effects of conditions—including smoking cigarettes and drinking alcoholic or caffeinated beverages—that can be addressed through self-care actions.

NURSING ASSESSMENT OF HEARING

Nursing assessment of hearing is aimed at identifying the following:

- Factors that interfere with hearing wellness
- Actual hearing deficit

- Impact of any hearing deficits on safety and quality of life
- Opportunities for improving hearing wellness
- Barriers to implementing interventions

Each of these factors is important in helping older adults and their caregivers compensate for hearing deficits. Assessment is accomplished through interviewing, observing behavioral cues, and administering hearing tests.

Interviewing About Hearing Changes

Use interview questions, such as the ones in Box 16-2, to acquire information about (1) present and past risk factors, (2) the person's awareness and acknowledgment of a hearing impairment, (3) the psychosocial impact of any hearing deficit, and (4) attitudes that might influence health promotion interventions. Begin with questions about family history of hearing impairments and a personal history of prolonged exposure to loud noises. Identification of ototoxic medications as a risk factor can be included as part of the hearing assessment or as part of the medication history.

If the older adult does not initiate a discussion of hearing problems, ask direct questions, such as "Do you think you have a hearing loss?" If the nursing assessment identifies behavioral cues indicative of a hearing deficit but the person denies having a hearing problem, attempt to elicit further information by asking questions such as "I notice you turn your left ear toward me. Is your hearing better in that ear?" If a hearing loss is present, assess related functional consequences by asking about changes in social activities or ability to function independently because of difficulty hearing.

Box 16-2 Guidelines for Assessing Hearing

Questions to Identify Risk Factors for Hearing Loss

- Do you have a family history of hearing loss or deafness?
- Have you been exposed to loud noises in your job or leisure activities?
- Do you have a history of any of the following: diabetes, hypothyroidism, Ménière disease, or Paget disease?
- What medications do you take? (Refer to Box 16-1 to identify potentially ototoxic medications.)
- Have you ever had impacted wax in your ears?

Questions to Assess Awareness and Presence of Hearing Deficit

- Do you have any trouble with your hearing?
- Have you noticed any change in your ability to understand conversations or hear words?
- Are you bothered by any noises in your ears, such as ringing or buzzing?

Questions to Ask if Hearing Loss is Acknowledged

- How long have you noticed a hearing loss?
- Do you notice differences in hearing in your left ear versus your right ear?
- Has there been a progressive loss, or did the hearing problem begin suddenly?
- Describe your hearing difficulty.
- Are there any conditions, such as noisy environments or particular voices or sounds that especially interfere with your hearing?
- Does your hearing loss interfere with your ability to communicate with others, either individually or in groups?
- Are there any activities that you would like to do but feel you cannot because of hearing problems?

- Have you ever had, or thought about having, an evaluation for a hearing aid?
- Have you ever tried using a hearing aid?

Questions to Identify Opportunities for Education About Disease Prevention and Health Promotion

- Does the person engage in any activities that expose him or her to loud noises, such as woodworking or lawn mowing? If so, does he or she understand the importance of wearing ear protectors?
- If the person has a history of impacted wax, does he or she take preventive measures?
- Does the person smoke cigarettes or live in a household with a smoker? If so, does the person realize that this is a risk factor for hearing loss?
- What are the person's attitudes about hearing loss?
- Is hearing loss considered normal and untreatable?
- Is a hearing aid considered to be a stigma?
- If the person is resistant to an audiologic evaluation, what are the barriers? (e.g., Are there financial or transportation limitations that interfere with obtaining a hearing aid?)
- Does the hearing loss contribute to a sense of isolation, depression, paranoia, or low self-esteem?
- What are the person's usual communication opportunities, and how does the hearing loss influence these usual patterns? (For instance, does the person live in an environment where it is important to be able to use the phone?)
- Does the person live in a noisy environment and find relief in the hearing impairment?
- If the person lives in an environment where group activities are a large part of daily activities, does the person want to participate in these activities?

Wellness Opportunity

Nurses address the whole person by including questions about the impact of a hearing loss on his or her quality of life.

Another assessment aspect for older adults with hearing loss is to identify their attitudes and perceptions about hearing aids and other interventions. Common barriers to use of hearing aids include all the following:

- Perception that hearing aids are of little use
- Concerns about cost
- Difficulty arranging for evaluations
- Lack of transportation for appointments
- Embarrassment about the visibility of hearing aids
- Lack of manual dexterity necessary for use of smaller hearing aids

Another assessment consideration is that the person may not be motivated toward improved communication and may even prefer social isolation or limited opportunities for communication. It is also important to consider whether a desire to avoid opportunities for communication may be associated with dementia, depression, close relationships, or living arrangements.

The Hearing Handicap Inventory for the Elderly (HHIE-S) is a 10-item questionnaire that can be administered to older adults in approximately 5 minutes to assess the presence and functional consequences of hearing loss (Figure 16-4). This tool has been widely used since the early 1980s and is recommended by the Hartford Institute for Geriatric Nursing as a valid and reliable tool for measuring social and emotional effects of hearing loss.

Wellness Opportunity

Nurses promote self-care by asking an older adult to use the HHIE-S and then reviewing the results of this assessment to identify goals.

Observing Behavioral Cues

Behavioral cues related to hearing loss provide important information about the presence of a hearing impairment, the psychosocial consequences of any such impairment, and the person's attitudes about assistive devices. If the older adult denies a hearing deficit that has been noticed by others, behavioral cues can be an important source of assessment information. Denial of a hearing deficit can be rooted in lack of awareness of the impairment because of gradual onset or, if the older person is socially isolated, can be caused by

ITEM	YES (4 pts)	SOMETIMES (2 pts)	NO (0 pts)
Does a hearing problem cause you to feel embarrassed when you meet new people?	_____	_____	_____
Does a hearing problem cause you to feel frustrated when talking to members of your family?	_____	_____	_____
Do you have difficulty hearing when someone speaks in a whisper?	_____	_____	_____
Do you feel handicapped by a hearing problem?	_____	_____	_____
Does a hearing problem cause you difficulty when visiting friends, relatives, or neighbors?	_____	_____	_____
Does a hearing problem cause you to attend religious services less often than you would like?	_____	_____	_____
Does a hearing problem cause you to have arguments with family members?	_____	_____	_____
Does a hearing problem cause you difficulty when listening to TV or radio?	_____	_____	_____
Do you feel that any difficulty with your hearing limits or hampers your personal or social life?	_____	_____	_____
Does a hearing problem cause you difficulty when in a restaurant with relatives or friends?	_____	_____	_____

RAW SCORE_____ (sum of the points assigned each of the items)

INTERPRETING THE RAW SCORE
   0 to 8 = 13% probability of hearing impairment (no handicap/no referral)
   10 to 24 = 50% probability of hearing impairment (mild–moderate handicap/refer)
   26 to 40 = 84% probability of hearing impairment (severe handicap/refer)

FIGURE 16-4 The screening version of the Hearing Handicap Inventory for the Elderly (HHIE-S). (Reprinted with permission from Wolters Kluwer, publisher of *Ear and Hearing*.)

a paucity of opportunities for communication. Feelings of embarrassment or misconceptions that the hearing loss is an inevitable and untreatable consequence of aging can also contribute to denial. Box 16-3 lists behavioral cues that the nurse should observe as part of the hearing assessment.

Using Hearing Assessment Tools

Nurses assess hearing by using an otoscope to examine the ear and a tuning fork to check hearing. The purpose of the otoscopic examination is to identify impacted cerumen and other factors that can interfere with hearing, whereas

 Box 16-3 Guidelines for Assessing Behavioral Cues Related to Hearing

Behavioral Cues to a Hearing Deficit
- Inappropriate or no response to questions, especially in the absence of opportunities for lip reading
- Inability to follow verbal directions without cues
- Short attention span, easy distractibility
- Frequent requests for repetition or clarification of verbal communication
- Intense observation of the speaker
- Mouthing of words spoken by the speaker
- Turning of one ear toward the speaker
- Unusual physical proximity to the speaker
- Lack of response to loud environmental noises
- Speech that is too loud or inarticulate

- Abnormal voice characteristics, such as monotony
- Misperception that others are talking about him or her

Behavioral Cues About Psychosocial Consequences
- Uncharacteristic avoidance of group settings
- Lack of interest in social activities, especially those requiring verbal communication or those that the person enjoyed in the past (e.g., bingo, card games)

Behavioral Cues About Assistive Devices
- Not using a hearing aid that has been purchased
- Failure to obtain batteries for a hearing aid
- Expression of embarrassment about using assistive devices

Box 16-4 Guidelines for Otoscopic and Tuning Fork Assessment

Using the Otoscope to Assess Factors That Could Interfere With Hearing

- Hold the otoscope upside down, resting your hand on the person's head to stabilize the instrument
- Before inserting the speculum, pull the earlobe up and back, while tilting the person's head slightly back and toward the opposite shoulder
- If cerumen has accumulated to the point of interfering with the examination or occluding the canal, follow the cerumen removal procedure described in the section on Nursing Interventions
- Normal otoscopic findings in older adults include the following:
  - ◆ Small amount of cerumen
  - ◆ Pinkish-white epithelial lining, no redness or lesions
  - ◆ Pearl-gray tympanic membrane, which is less translucent than in younger adults
  - ◆ Light reflex anteroinferiorly from the umbo
  - ◆ Visible landmarks

Using the Tuning Fork to Detect Hearing Impairment

- Use a tuning fork with frequencies of 512 to 1024 Hz
- Hold the tuning fork firmly at the stem
- Strike the fork against the palm of your hand, or strike the fork with a rubber reflex hammer, to set it in motion

Weber Test

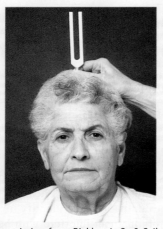

Reprinted with permission from Bickley, L. S., & Szilagyi, P. G. (2009). *Bates' guide to physical examination and history taking* (10th ed.). Philadelphia, PA: Lippincott Williams & Wilkins.

Procedure: Place the tip of a vibrating tuning fork at the center of the person's forehead or on the top of the person's head. Ask where they hear the sound and whether it is louder in one ear than in the other.
Normal finding: The sound from the tuning fork is heard equally in both ears.
Abnormal finding: The sound from the tuning fork is heard better in one ear, indicating a possible hearing loss.

Rinne Test

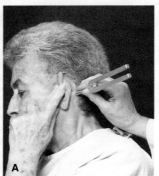 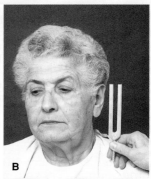

Reprinted with permission from Bickley, L. S., & Szilagyi, P. G. (2009). *Bates' guide to physical examination and history taking* (10th ed.). Philadelphia, PA: Lippincott Williams & Wilkins.

Procedure: Mask one ear, then place a vibrating tuning fork on the mastoid process of the opposite ear until the person indicates that the sound from the vibrations can no longer be heard. Then, quickly place the tuning fork in front of the ear canal with the top near the ear canal.
Normal finding: The duration the tuning fork vibrations can be heard over the ear canal is approximately twice as long as the time it can be heard over the mastoid bone.
Abnormal finding: The length of time the tuning fork vibrations are heard in front of the ear is shorter than twice as long as the time it can be heard when placed on the mastoid process. In such a case, the person should undergo further tests for impaired hearing.

---

the purpose of the tuning fork test is to detect hearing impairments and to differentiate between conductive and sensorineural losses. Box 16-4 describes the procedure for performing a nursing assessment of hearing using the otoscope and tuning fork. A handheld audioscope is another assessment tool that is recommended in nursing guidelines; however, this tool is not as widely available as an otoscope or tuning fork. When a hearing deficit is identified, the nurse can recommend that further evaluation be conducted at a speech and hearing center or by a specialized physician, such as an otolaryngologist.

See ONLINE LEARNING ACTIVITY 16-4: ARTICLE WITH CASE SCENARIOS ABOUT NURSING ASSESSMENT AND INTERVENTIONS FOR HEARING LOSS at http://thepoint.lww.com/Miller8e

NURSING DIAGNOSIS

A nursing assessment might identify an actual hearing deficit or risk factors for impaired hearing. To emphasize the goal of promoting wellness, use the diagnosis of

Readiness for Enhanced Communication, defined as "a pattern of exchanging information and ideas with others, which can be strengthened" (Herdman & Kamitsuru, 2018, p. 262). If psychosocial consequences are identified, pertinent nursing diagnoses might include Anxiety, Impaired Social Interaction, Ineffective Coping, and Risk for Loneliness. When the hearing impairment is severe and uncompensated to the point that the person does not function safely, then Risk for Injury might be an applicable nursing diagnosis.

Wellness Opportunity

Nurses can use the wellness nursing diagnosis of Readiness for Enhanced Communication for older adults who are willing to explore possibilities for improving their hearing through health promotion interventions.

PLANNING FOR WELLNESS OUTCOMES

When risk factors for hearing loss are identified, an appropriate Nursing Outcomes Classification (NOC) label is Risk Control: Hearing Impairment, defined as personal actions to understand, prevent, eliminate, or reduce threats, to hearing function. Two NOC labels applicable to older adults who are experiencing hearing loss are Hearing Compensation Behavior and Sensory Function: Hearing. Additional NOC labels that are related to the functional consequences of hearing loss are Communication, Depression Level, Leisure Participation, Loneliness Severity, Personal Safety Behavior, Social Involvement, and Social Interaction Skills. Nursing interventions to achieve these outcomes are discussed in the following section.

Wellness Opportunity

Quality of Life is a wellness outcome that is achieved through nursing interventions that improve communication for older adults with impaired hearing.

NURSING INTERVENTIONS FOR HEARING WELLNESS

Nursing interventions to promote hearing wellness for older adults focus on preventing hearing loss, helping older adults compensate for hearing deficits, and using communication methods that facilitate optimal communication. Specific interventions to achieve these goals are discussed in detail in the following sections. Use any of the following pertinent Nursing Interventions Classification labels in care plans: Communication Enhancement: Hearing Deficit, Ear Care, Environmental Management: Safety, Environmental Management: Risk Protection, Health Education, Health Screening, Health System Guidance, or Risk Identification.

Wellness Opportunity

Nurses can emphasize that even though interventions to prevent hearing loss ideally begin early in life, it is never too late to begin protecting ears from noise.

Promoting Hearing Wellness for All Older Adults

For all older adults, it is important to correct the misperception that hearing loss is an inevitable and inconsequential effect of growing older. Emphasize that all people can take actions to protect their hearing and teach older adults

---

Unfolding Case Study

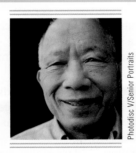

Photodisc V/Senior Portraits

Part 2: Mr. H. at 69 Years of Age *(Continued)*

Recall that Mr. H. is a 69-year-old participant in activities at the local senior center where you are the nurse. You are meeting with Mr. and Mrs. H. to discuss Mrs. H.'s concerns about her husband's hearing problem.

THINKING POINTS

- Which of the questions and considerations in Boxes 16-2 and 16-3 would you use in assessing Mr. H.?
- Would you involve Mrs. H. in any part of the assessment? If so, how would you involve her?

- What health promotion advice would you give Mr. H. at this time?

> ## Box 16-5 Health Promotion Teaching About Hearing
>
> ### Prevention of Hearing Loss
>
> - Limit your exposure to loud noise.
> - Use ear protectors whenever you are exposed to loud noise.
> - Quit smoking.
>
> ### Early Detection and Treatment of Hearing Loss
>
> - Ask your primary care practitioner to evaluate for medical conditions that cause hearing loss.
> - Have your ears checked for impacted wax.
> - Use interventions to prevent impacted wax if this has been a problem.
> - Obtain evaluation for hearing loss.
> - Obtain professional recommendations for a hearing aid, assistive hearing device, or auditory rehabilitation services.
> - Consider using amplifying devices (e.g., for phones, radios, doorbells) or sound substitution devices (e.g., flashing lights, closed-captioned television) as needed for safety and improved quality of life.
> - Take advantage of available assistive listening devices in public places (e.g., churches, theaters, government buildings).

about the exacerbating effects of two risk factors, such as noise and age-related changes. For example, many older adults engage in recreational or occupational activities that can cause NIHL, and they may not realize that age-related changes increase their susceptibility to developing a hearing loss. Similarly, teaching about smoking as a risk factor for hearing loss may encourage older adults who smoke to quit. Use Box 16-5 to teach older adults about health promotion actions they can take to prevent or address hearing loss.

Nurses have important roles in teaching about the importance of engaging in self-assessment to identify hearing deficits. Studies suggest that self-assessment is more important than audiometry as a first step in seeking help for hearing problems (Carson, 2016; Mick & Pichora-Fuller, 2016). Online Learning Activity 16-5 provides links to resources for self-assessment, including access to the HHIE-S (illustrated in Figure 16-4), which can be used as an evidence-based self-assessment tool. Nurses also can encourage older adults to take advantage of free audiology screenings, which are widely available. Whenever a nursing assessment identifies an actual or probable hearing loss, interventions focus on appropriate referrals for further evaluation, as discussed in the section on compensating for hearing deficits.

See ONLINE LEARNING ACTIVITY 16-5: RESOURCES FOR HEALTH PROMOTION ABOUT HEARING at http://thepoint.lww.com/Miller8e

Preventing and Alleviating Impacted Cerumen

Nurses promote hearing wellness through interventions and health education aimed at alleviating or preventing hearing impairment caused by impacted cerumen. Clinical practice guidelines emphasize the importance of all health care professionals assessing for impacted cerumen and teaching patients about proper ear hygiene (Schwartz, Magit, Rosenfeld, et al., 2017). Box 16-6 summarizes current evidence-based recommendations for patient teaching and direct interventions related to impacted cerumen. Keep in mind that monitoring and referrals are essential nursing interventions for older adults who have recurrent episodes of impacted cerumen, especially for those who use hearing aids.

Compensating for Hearing Deficits

When providing care for older adults with hearing loss, nurses can encourage the use of Hearing Health Care Professionals, as described in Box 16-7. Interventions for hearing loss include sound amplification with assistive listening devices or hearing aids, surgical interventions, and auditory rehabilitation. Nursing interventions should focus on a referral for medical and audiology evaluations. Sometimes the nursing interventions also need to address barriers to obtaining a hearing aid, as discussed in the section on hearing aids.

Assistive Listening Devices

Any device that amplifies sounds for individual or group communication is categorized as an **assistive listening device**, as in the following examples:

- A stethoscope is an assistive listening device commonly used by health care workers.
- Megaphones and microphones are used for group communication.
- Closed-captioned televisions, which include all TVs manufactured since the 1990s, substitute visual cues for auditory cues.
- A personal listening system, which consists of a small, battery-powered amplifier and headphones, can be used easily in any setting.
- A small amplifying device can be attached to a telephone receiver.
- Some cell phones are designed to accommodate people who use hearing aids or need amplification. Visual stimuli, such as flashing lights, can be used as a signal for a doorbell.
- Vibratory stimuli can be used as a substitute for an alarm clock.

Advantages of assistive listening devices over hearing aids include lower cost (usually) and the ability to share a device among several people. In addition, these devices are less intrusive than hearing aids and do not require as much manual dexterity. Figure 16-5 shows several examples of devices that can be used to enhance communication with someone who is hard of hearing. Nurses can teach older adults and their caregivers about using assistive listening devices as a substitute for, or as an adjunct to, hearing aids. Many public places, including churches, theaters, and government buildings, provide portable assistive listening devices, and hearing-impaired people can ask about the availability of such devices.

EBP Box 16-6 Evidence-Based Practice: Guidelines for Impacted Cerumen

Statement of the Problem

- Cerumen is normally expelled from the ear canal by a self-cleaning mechanism, but excessive or impacted cerumen occurs in high-risk populations, such as older adults, people who are cognitively impaired, and people who use hearing aids.
- Impacted cerumen affects between 19% and 65% of patients over 65 years old and is often underdiagnosed and undertreated.
- Hearing aids and ear plugs can stimulate the cerumen glands, leading to excessive cerumen production.
- Impacted cerumen can cause hearing loss; diminished cognitive function; and symptoms such as pain, itching, tinnitus, cough, dizziness, and sensation of fullness.
- Cerumen impaction may interfere with hearing aid performance by reducing the intensity of sound, changing the resonance properties of the ears, or causing feedback and poor fitting.
- If cerumen impaction causes symptoms or interferes with hearing, it should be removed.
- Older adults, especially those who are cognitively impaired, may be unaware that they have a cerumen impaction potentially impairing their hearing or that removal of the impaction may improve their hearing; they may even rate their hearing ability as good or fair.

Recommendations for Nursing Assessment

- Arrange for or perform an otoscopic examination whenever any of the following manifestations occur: hearing loss, ear pain, tinnitus, cough, or vertigo.
- Arrange for or perform an otoscopic examination at intervals of 3 to 12 months for older adults who use hearing aids.

Recommendations for Patient Teaching

Teach older adults and caregivers about the following measures:
- Reduce the risk of developing impacted cerumen by using cerumenolytic agents prophylactically.
- Do not insert cotton-tipped applicators or any other foreign object in ear canals.
- Make sure that hearing aids are properly cleaned and cared for.
- If you have an increased risk for cerumen impaction, have your ears cleaned and checked by a qualified health care practitioner every 6 to 12 months.

Use of Cerumenolytic Agents

- Cerumenolytics are wax-softening agents that disperse the cerumen and reduce the need for other interventions.

- Types of cerumenolytics are water based (e.g., water, saline, cerumenex, docusate sodium, hydrogen peroxide, sodium bicarbonate), oil based (e.g., almond oil, mineral oil, olive oil), and nonwater, nonoil based (e.g., Debrox, Audax).
- Studies comparing two or more cerumenolytic agents indicate that any type of cerumenolytic is better than no treatment, but no particular agent is more effective than others.

Interventions for Cerumen Impaction

- The goal of clearing the cerumen is to alleviate symptoms or improve hearing; this does not necessarily involve the removal of all cerumen.
- Impacted cerumen is removed cautiously by qualified professionals by a variety of methods, including irrigation, cerumenolytic agents, and manually with a specialized instrument.
- Instillation of cerumenolytic agents 15 minutes or for several days prior to the removal improves the success of the treatment.
- Ear irrigation should not be performed on patients with a history of ear surgery or those who have any abnormality of the ear canal or a nonintact tympanic membrane; it should be used cautiously in patients with diabetes.
- Patients may be taught to self-irrigate with a bulb syringe; however, jet irrigators should not be used for self-care.
- Interventions for preventing recurrence include irrigation with bulb syringe and regular use of cerumenolytic agents or alcohol or hydrogen peroxide drops.

Potentially Harmful Interventions

- Cotton-tipped swabs should not be used because they can cause further impaction and other complications; they may even be the cause of the original impaction.
- Daily use of olive oil drops or sprays.
- Home use of oral jet irrigators and cotton-tipped swabs is associated with increased risk of damage to the ear canal.
- Ear candling (also called ear coning or thermos-auricular therapy) is a commonly used alternative practice for cerumen removal. Research indicates that ear candling is not effective and is associated with considerable risks, including burns, otitis externa, tympanic membrane perforation, and conductive hearing loss.

Source: Schwartz, S. R., Magit, A. E., Rosenfeld, R. M., et al. (2017). Clinical Practice Guideline (Update) Earwax (Cerumen Impaction). *Otolaryngology – Head and Neck Surgery, 156,* S1–S29.

Box 16-7 Guide to Hearing Care Professionals

Otolaryngologist

Otolaryngologists are licensed doctors of medicine or osteopathy who are trained in the medical and surgical management of disorders of the ear, nose, throat, and related structures of the head and neck.

Otologist

Otologists are a subspecialty with further training in conditions affecting hearing. Services include:
- Diagnosis and management of disorders of the ear, including hearing loss, tinnitus, ear infections, ear pain, and ear-related balance disorders

Audiologist

Audiologists are certified professionals who are licensed in the state in which they practice. Audiology professional and accreditation

organizations, and most state licensure laws, require a minimum of a master's degree in audiology, and in some states, a doctoral degree in audiology (Au.D.). Audiology services include:
- Diagnosis and treatment of disorders of hearing and balance
- Assessment of type and degree of hearing loss
- Prescription and fitting of hearing aids and assistive listening devices
- Provision of hearing rehabilitation services
- Counseling regarding communication strategies

Hearing Instrument Specialist or Hearing Aid Specialist

Hearing Instrument Specialists or *Hearing Aid Specialists* are hearing health professionals who are licensed in each state, with some states requiring certification. Services include:
- Prescription of hearing aids
- Ongoing management of hearing aids

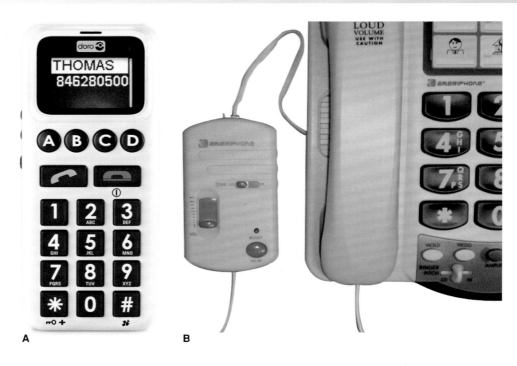

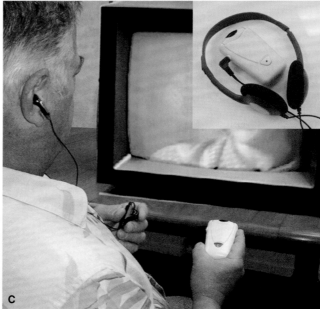

FIGURE 16-5 A. Cell phone with amplification, large keypad, two-way speakerphone, and vibrating ringer alert. **B.** Easy-to-use in-line phone amplifier. **C.** Personal sound amplifier with volume control, swiveling microphone, and lightweight earbud headphones. (Reprinted with permission from ActiveForever.com)

Hearing Aids

A hearing aid is a battery-operated device that consists of an amplifier, a microphone, and a receiver. Because of many recently evolving technologic advances, selection of hearing aids has become increasingly complex. Figure 16-6 illustrates commonly available types according to style.

Although it is impossible to know about all the available types of hearing aids, it is important to teach older adults about general principles related to selection of hearing aids. For example, federal law requires that a medical evaluation be performed before the sale of a hearing aid; however, this requirement can be waived by fully consenting adults. Thus,

an essential teaching point is stressing the importance of obtaining an initial evaluation by a qualified hearing care professional, so reversible causes of hearing loss are identified and the most appropriate interventions are initiated.

Despite the major improvements during recent decades, only 67% to 86% of adults who would benefit from a hearing aid actually use one (National Academies of Sciences, Engineering, and Medicine, 2016). Nurses can address negative attitudes and have a positive effect on the use of hearing aids by helping older adults to explore the many options for amplification, as described in Box 16-8. When working with older adults in residential or other institutional

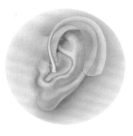

Behind-the-ear (BTE)

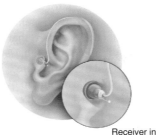

"Mini" BTE

Receiver in
ear canal

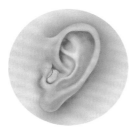

In-the-ear (ITE)

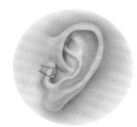

Completely-in-canal (CIC)

FIGURE 16-6 Examples of four types of hearing aids.

settings, teach about the most effective use of hearing aids in different circumstances. For example, encourage the older adult to use the aid for one-on-one conversations but to remove it in the dining area or other large social areas where there is a lot of background noise. Promote realistic expectations with regard to hearing aids by explaining that hearing aids do not restore normal hearing but do improve communication and the quality of life.

Nurses must be familiar enough with hearing aids to assist older adults and their caregivers with their use and care. Although audiologists provide initial instructions about the use and care of hearing aids, these instructions may have to be reviewed or revamped as dependency needs and caregiver roles change. For example, when older adults are in a hospital or nursing home, nursing staff usually provide assistance with use of and care for hearing aids. Likewise, nurses in home settings may have to teach caregivers about hearing aids if the older adult's needs change. Use information in Box 16-8 as a guide to teaching about the selection and care of hearing aids.

Diversity Note

Blacks and Mexican Americans with hearing loss were 58% and 78% less likely, respectively, to use hearing aids than whites (Nieman, Marrone, Szanton, et al., 2016).

Auditory Rehabilitation

Auditory rehabilitation (also called aural or audiologic rehabilitation) refers to services that improve communication

Box 16-8   Guide to the Selection and Care of Hearing Aids

Guidelines for Selecting a Hearing Aid

- Obtain a medical evaluation to identify treatable causes of hearing loss before being evaluated for a hearing aid.
- Obtain initial information about hearing aids from a speech and hearing center or consumer organizations, rather than primarily from a hearing aid dealer who sells only one kind of device.
- During the initial evaluation, obtain information about various types of hearing aids and services for people with hearing loss.
- Ask about audiology rehabilitation programs to improve communication skills and adjustment to hearing loss.
- If financial limitations are a concern, check with the Audient Alliance for Accessible Hearing Care, which is a national nonprofit organization that provides access to quality hearing aids and audiology care for people with limited incomes.
- Recognize that there are many types and styles of hearing aids, which vary significantly in their features and cost; it is important to consider more than one type:
  - Hearing aid styles include behind-the-ear, in-the-ear, in-the-canal, completely-in-the-canal, and mini-behind-the-ear.
  - Considerations for selection of style include features and cost of the aid and personal preferences related to aesthetics and manual dexterity.
  - Levels of technology, from simplest to most complex, are standard analog, programmable analog, entry level digital, advanced digital, and premium digital.
  - Available features of prescribed hearing aids include feedback cancellation, directional microphones, multiple channels, battery indicator, and wax protection systems.
  - Disposable hearing aids are the least expensive (usually under $100) and are designed as a one-size-fits-all; they are discarded after the built-in battery is exhausted; they also are the least individualized.

Guidelines for Care of a Hearing Aid

- Keep a fresh battery available but do not purchase batteries more than 1 month in advance.
- Turn off the hearing aid before changing the battery.
- Remove the battery or turn off the aid when not in use.
- Clean the aid weekly, using warm, soapy water for the earmold and a toothpick or pipe cleaner for the channel.
- Never use alcohol on the earmold because this will cause drying and cracking.
- Check the earmold for cracks or scratches.
- Avoid extreme heat, cold, or moisture.
- Avoid exposure to chemicals, such as hairspray or permanent solutions.
- Avoid dropping the aid on a hard surface; when handling it, keep it over a soft or padded surface.

for people who are hearing impaired. Auditory rehabilitation programs, which are designed to help people learn to live with hearing loss, provide the following services: counseling, education, amplification aids, and communication skills. Although auditory rehabilitation programs can improve cognitive and social function in older adults, rates of utilization are low, and these programs are not widely available (National Academy of Sciences, Engineering, and Medicine, 2016). Nurses play an important role in discussing such programs with older adults and their caregivers and suggesting referrals for comprehensive evaluations by

I
P
C

a speech-language pathologist. Speech and hearing centers, which are often affiliated with medical centers or universities, are good sources of information about auditory rehabilitation programs. Information is also available through Internet resources, such as the American Speech-Language-Hearing Association.

 Technology to Promote Wellness in Older Adults

In addition to teaching about hearing aids and assistive listening devices, nurses can suggest the use of a broad range of technology-based products that are available for improving safety and quality of life for people with a hearing loss, as in the following examples:

- Wearable or portable notification system that connects with devices in the home (e.g., phone, doors, windows, motion sensors, smoke or carbon monoxide detectors) to provide alert via vibration, flashing lights, or amplified sound
- Apps for ipads, smartphones, or portable devices that provide captioning for video programs or audio–video programs, such as FaceTime or Netflix
- Vibrating watches or alarm clocks
- Flashing lights and amplifiers for cell phones
- Flashing lights for weather alerts

The following websites include information about such products:

- ADCO Hearing Products, www.adcohearing.com
- Alexander Graham Bell Association for the Deaf, www.agb.org
- Harris Communications, www.harriscommunications.com
- Hearmore Products for Independent Living, www.hearmore.com
- MaxiAids, www.maxiaids.com

Cochlear Implants

A **cochlear implant** is a small, complex electronic device that consists of an external portion, which is magnetically held in place behind the ear, and an internal component, which is surgically implanted under the skin. Cochlear implants bypass damaged portions of the ear and stimulate the auditory nerve, sending signals directly to the brain. The Food and Drug Administration approved these medical devices for use in adults in the 1980s and for use in children in 2000. Since 2005, the Centers for Medicare and Medicaid have been expanding the criteria for having cochlear implants covered by health insurance.

Currently, there is much evidence to support consideration of cochlear implants for older adults. A study of cochlear implants in patients age 75 and older found that all patients experienced significant improvements in speech perception and concluded that age should not be a limitation for surgery (Wong, Moran, & O'Leary, 2016). Studies also have found that patients aged 65 to 86 years with serious sensorineural hearing loss who subsequently get cochlear implants experienced improved communication, higher quality of life, and improved performance on cognitive testing (Aimoni, Ciorba, Hatzopoulos, et al., 2016; Cosetti, Pinkston, Flores, et al., 2016; Rohloff, Koopmann, Wei, et al., 2017). Based on current evidence, it is important to encourage older adults to explore options for surgical interventions when hearing loss is not adequately improved with other interventions.

When caring for older adults with cochlear implants, nurses need to document information about the external component and ensure that the device is not lost. Another nursing implication is that some implanted hearing devices are affected by or interfere with magnetic resonance imaging (MRI), so it is essential to obtain information about compatibility if an MRI is being considered.

 See ONLINE LEARNING ACTIVITY 16-6: EXPLORING OPTIONS FOR HEARING AIDS, AMPLIFIERS, AND COCHLEAR IMPLANTS at http://thepoint.lww.com/Miller8e

Communicating With Hearing-Impaired Older Adults

Good communication techniques are essential in assisting older adults to compensate for hearing deficits. The primary functional consequence of presbycusis is a diminished acuity for high-frequency sounds, which is exacerbated by fast-paced speech and environmental noise. Therefore, communication interventions are directed toward improving the clarity of words, slowing the rate of speech, and eliminating environmental noise and distractions. Verbal techniques that enhance auditory communication should be augmented by nonverbal techniques, such as body language and written communication, as described in Box 16-9. Nurses can apply

Box 16-9 Techniques for Communicating With Hearing-Impaired People

- Stand or sit directly in front of, and close to, the person.
- Talk toward the better ear, but make sure your lips can be seen.
- Make sure the person pays attention and looks at your face.
- Address the person by name, pause, and then begin talking.
- Speak distinctly, slowly, and directly to the person.
- Do not exaggerate lip movements because this will interfere with lip reading.
- Avoid chewing gum, covering your mouth, or turning your head away.
- If the person does not understand, repeat the message by using different words.
- Avoid or eliminate any background noise.
- Avoid raising the volume of your voice; rather, try to lower the tone while still speaking in a moderately loud voice.
- Keep all instructions simple and ask for feedback to assess what the person heard.
- Avoid questions that elicit simple yes or no answers.
- Keep sentences short.
- Use body language that is congruent with what you are trying to communicate.
- Demonstrate what you are saying.
- Use large-print written communication and pictures to supplement verbal communication.
- Make sure only one person talks at a time; arrange for one-on-one communication whenever possible.
- If the hearing-impaired person normally wears eyeglasses to improve vision, make sure the eyeglasses are clean.
- Provide adequate lighting so that the person can see your lips; avoid settings in which there is glare behind or around you.

these techniques and use this box for teaching caregivers how to improve communication with hearing-impaired people. In recent years, increased attention has been directed toward planning or modifying environments to diminish background noise and to improve the ability of people to hear. Although some noise control modifications, such as using window draperies, are relatively simple and can be applied to many settings, other measures, such as selection of building materials, need to be implemented while environments are being designed.

Unfolding Case Study

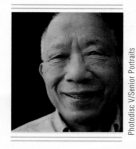

Photodisc V/Senior Portraits

Part 3: Mr. H. at 83 Years of Age

Mr. H. is now 83 years old and has been a widower for 1 year. He has given up hunting and woodworking because he developed Parkinson disease 11 years ago and cannot manage the necessary fine motor movements. He continues to fish seasonally, play poker monthly, and smoke one pack of cigarettes per day. In addition to Parkinson disease, he has hypertension and coronary artery disease. He still lives in his own home and attends the local senior center for meals and social activities three times a week. His hearing loss has progressed to the point that he has difficulty with phone conversations and has to turn the television up loud. He cannot hear the doorbell. At the senior center, participants avoid conversations with him because he has difficulty hearing.

You are the nurse at the senior center, and you see him during the weekly "wellness clinic" for blood pressure checks. One week, he tells you that his daughter is upset with him because he never answers his phone when she calls, and she cannot have a decent phone conversation with him. She lives in another state and worries about him. She has offered to pay for a hearing aid evaluation for him, but he has told her, "Those things stick out like a sore thumb and they don't do any good anyway. I can hear anything I want to hear and there's a lot I don't care to hear, so why should you spend a lot of money for something that I won't use." He asks your opinion about this and is wondering whether he should at least get a checkup to pacify his daughter. He expects he will be told that nothing can be done and that his daughter will have to be satisfied with the situation.

THINKING POINTS

- Which information in Box 16-2 would be most pertinent to obtain at this time?
- What myths and misunderstandings influence Mr. H.?
- What nursing diagnosis would you apply to Mr. H.?
- Which information in Boxes 16-5 and 16-6 would be pertinent to this situation?
- What health promotion teaching would you do to address Mr. H.'s resistance to having his hearing evaluated?

- What additional health promotion advice would you give?
- Because you usually see Mr. H. weekly, you can develop a long-term teaching plan. How would you establish priorities for immediate and long-term goals?

QSEN APPLICATION

QSEN Competency	Knowledge/Skill/Attitude	Application to Mr. H.
Patient-centered care	(K) Examine common barriers to active involvement of patients in their own health care processes	Use assessment boxes and the HHIE-S (Figure 16-4) to help identify and address Mr. H.'s resistance to obtaining a hearing evaluation
	(S) Elicit patient values, preferences, and expressed needs	Emphasize the importance of obtaining a medical evaluation to identify reversible causes of hearing impairment
	(A) Value seeing health care situations "through patients' eyes"	
Evidence-based practice	(S) Base individualized care plan on patient values, clinical expertise, and evidence	Provide a list of reliable and noncommercial sources of information about hearing loss (see Online Learning Activity 16-5 on the Point) and encourage him to obtain information and an evaluation

EVALUATING EFFECTIVENESS OF NURSING INTERVENTIONS

Nurses observe compensatory behaviors of hearing-impaired older adults to evaluate the effectiveness of interventions, as indicated by the following:

- Improved ability to communicate
- Effective use of hearing aids and amplification devices
- Increased participation in social activities
- Environmental modifications to eliminate background noise
- Participation in auditory rehabilitation program

Evaluation of effectiveness of interventions varies in different health care settings. For example, nurses in short-term settings provide health education as part of a discharge plan that includes information about resources for hearing evaluations. Evaluation of the effectiveness of this intervention is based on the patient's positive response to the nurse's suggestions, but the nurse is not likely to know whether the person followed through with the referral and had beneficial outcomes. In home, community, and long-term care settings, nurses address long-term goals by facilitating referrals for audiology services. In these settings, the evaluation of interventions is based on the person's use of additional resources to improve communication abilities.

 See ONLINE LEARNING ACTIVITY 16-7: EVIDENCE-BASED PRACTICE at http://thepoint.lww.com/Miller8e

Unfolding Case Study

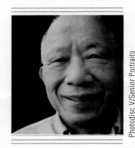

Photodisc V/Senior Portraits

Part 4: Mr. H. at 89 Years of Age

Mr. H. is an 89-year-old widower who has had Parkinson disease for 17 years. Presbycusis is listed as an additional diagnosis on his medical record. He is being admitted to a nursing home because his condition has declined to the point that his daughter, Ms. D., can no longer manage his care in her home, where he has lived for several years. He is medically stable but needs assistance in all activities of daily living.

NURSING ASSESSMENT

During the admission interview, you notice that Mr. H. has difficulty hearing your questions and that he frequently asks his daughter to give the requested information. He shows no significant cognitive deficits, but he seems to have difficulty understanding verbal communication. When you ask about any hearing impairment, Ms. D. tells you that her father has used hearing aids for 5 years and has been reevaluated periodically at a speech and hearing center. Two months ago, he obtained new hearing aids, but wears them only for one-on-one conversations with her. Because of Mr. H.'s tremors and difficulty with fine motor movements, Ms. D. cares for his hearing aids and assists with their insertion and removal.

Ms. D. has encouraged her father to wear his hearing aids during family gatherings, but he says the noise from small children is too annoying. Except for family gatherings, Mr. H. has very few opportunities for social interaction, and he has become more and more withdrawn. He used to enjoy playing poker, but has not played in several years because all of his friends have died. Now he spends much of his time watching closed-captioned television programs. Ms. D. hopes that her father will respond to the opportunities for social interaction provided at the nursing home and that his quality of life will improve.

NURSING DIAGNOSIS

In addition to nursing diagnoses related to Mr. H.'s chronic illness and self-care deficits, you identify a nursing diagnosis of Impaired Social Interaction related to the effects of hearing loss. You select this as a nursing diagnosis because Mr. H.'s hearing impairment has already been evaluated and sound amplification devices are available to him.

NURSING CARE PLAN FOR Mr. H.

In your care plan, you address the psychosocial consequences of Mr. H.'s hearing impairment. Your nursing care is directed toward improving his social interaction through the use of available devices and through other communication techniques that will enhance his social interaction skills.

NURSING CARE PLAN FOR Mr. H. *(Continued)*

Expected Outcome	Nursing Interventions	Nursing Evaluation
Mr. H. will develop effective communication techniques for resident–staff interactions	• During the initial interview, talk with Mr. H. and Ms. D. about the importance of good verbal communication with staff; emphasize the need for the staff to get to know Mr. H. so his needs can be addressed • Ask Mr. H. to wear his hearing aids during all one-on-one interactions with staff • Use effective communication techniques when talking with Mr. H. (as in Box 16-9) • Make sure all staff members provide appropriate assistance with insertion and removal of Mr. H.'s hearing aids • Include hearing aid maintenance as part of the daily responsibilities of the nursing aide	• Mr. H. will wear his hearing aids during all one-on-one conversations with staff • Mr. H. will report satisfactory verbal interactions with the staff • Mr. H.'s hearing aids will be maintained in good operating condition
Mr. H. will engage in social interaction with one other resident	• During the initial care plan conference, identify several other residents who might converse with Mr. H. • Ask the staff to encourage one-on-one conversations between Mr. H. and the selected resident (e.g., suggest that they watch closed-captioned television programs together) • Ask Mr. H. to wear his hearing aids during one-on-one interactions with residents • Provide assistance with inserting and removing hearing aids as needed • Provide a quiet environment for one-on-one conversations with other residents	• Mr. H. will wear his hearing aids at least once daily for a conversation with one other resident
Mr. H. will engage in small group activities with other residents	• During the first monthly care review conference, ask the activities staff to invite Mr. H. to a poker game with three other residents in the small group room • Make sure that environmental noise is controlled as much as possible	• By the second month in this facility, Mr. H. will participate in weekly poker games with three other residents

THINKING POINTS

• What nursing responsibilities would you have with regard to addressing Mr. H.'s hearing impairment? How would you work with other staff to implement the care plan described in the concluding case example?
• What are some of the advantages and disadvantages of hearing aids in a long-term care setting? How would you address the disadvantages?

• How would you involve Ms. D. in the care plan to address Mr. H.'s hearing impairment?
• If Mr. H. were in an acute care setting, how would you address his hearing problem?

Chapter Highlights

Age-Related Changes That Affect Hearing (Figure 16-1; Table 16-1)

• External ear: thicker hair, thinner skin, increased keratin
• Middle ear: less resilient tympanic membrane, calcified ossicles, stiffer muscles and ligaments
• Inner ear and auditory nervous system: fewer neurons and hair cells, diminished blood supply, degeneration of spiral ganglion and central processing systems
• Auditory nervous system: degenerative changes in auditory nerve and central nervous system

Risk Factors That Affect Hearing Wellness (Figure 16-2; Box 16-1)

• Genetic predisposition to otosclerosis
• Exposure to noise

- Impacted cerumen
- Ototoxic medications: aminoglycosides, aspirin, loop diuretics, quinine
- Disease processes: otosclerosis, Paget disease, Ménière disease

Functional Consequences Affecting Hearing Wellness (Figure 16-3; Table 16-1)

- Presbycusis: diminished ability to hear high-pitched sounds, especially in the presence of background noise
- Predisposition to impacted cerumen
- Psychosocial consequences: depression, social isolation, decline in cognitive function, increased dependency, diminished quality of life

Pathologic Condition Affecting Hearing: Tinnitus

- Tinnitus: persistent sensation of noises that do not originate in the external environment

Nursing Assessment of Hearing (Figure 16-4; Boxes 16-2 to 16-4)

- Screening tool: HHEI-S
- Past and present risk factors (e.g., use of ototoxic medications, noise exposure, family history of otosclerosis)
- Attitudes about hearing aids if impairment is present
- Impact of hearing impairment on communication and quality of life
- Behavioral cues to impaired hearing
- Otoscopic examination for impacted cerumen
- Tuning fork tests for hearing

Nursing Diagnosis

- Readiness for Enhanced Communication
- Additional diagnoses related to functional consequences of hearing loss: Anxiety, Impaired Social Interaction, Ineffective Coping, Risk for Injury, and Risk for Loneliness

Planning for Wellness Outcomes

- Improved communication
- Increased social interactions
- Improved quality of life
- Increased safety and functioning

Nursing Interventions for Hearing Wellness (Figures 16-5 and 16-6; Boxes 16-5 to 16-8)

- Health promotion teaching to address modifiable risk factors: smoking, exposure to noise, use of ototoxic medications
- Removing and preventing impacted cerumen
- Promoting referrals for appropriate professional services
- Using assistive listening devices
- Teaching about the use and care of a hearing aid
- Communicating with hearing-impaired older adults

- Compensating for hearing deficits by using hearing devices and hearing aids

Evaluating Effectiveness of Nursing Interventions

- Improved communication
- Use of appropriate amplification aids
- Appropriate environmental modifications
- Increased participation in social activities

Critical Thinking Exercises

1. Describe presbycusis and explain the functional consequences of this condition as it affects the everyday life of an older adult.
2. What risk factors would you consider in an 83-year-old person who complains of recent problems with hearing?
3. What advice would you give to someone who asks you about a brochure she received from a hearing aid company that offers free hearing screenings describing a new high-powered hearing aid? The person has trouble hearing but has never had an evaluation.
4. Describe at least 10 ways in which you can adapt your communication for a hearing-impaired person.
5. Find at least one resource (*not* a hearing aid dealer) in your community that you could recommend to an older adult who needs a hearing evaluation.
6. Visit at least three Internet sites that provide educational materials about hearing impairment, and choose the one you think would be best for obtaining health information brochures.

 For more information about the topics discussed in this chapter, be sure to check out the interactive Online Learning Activities and other helpful resources at http://thepoint.lww.com/Miller8e

REFERENCES

Aimoni, C., Ciorba, A., Hatzopoulos, S., et al. (2016). Cochlear implants in subjects over age 65: Quality of life and audiological outcomes. *Medical Sciences Monitor, 22,* 3035–3042.

Al-Swiahb, J., & Park, S. N. (2016). Characterization of tinnitus in different age groups: A retrospective review. *Noise & Health, 18,* 214–219.

Cardin, V. (2016). Effects of aging and adult-onset hearing loss on cortical auditory regions. *Frontiers in Neuroscience, 10,* 199.

Carson, A. J. (2016). The decision-making spiral in seeking help for hearing problems. *The Hearing Journal, 69,* 28, 30, 32.

Chang, J., Ryou, N., Jun, H., et al. (2016). Effect of cigarette smoking on hearing impairment: Data from a population-based study. *PLOS One,* doi: 10.1371/journal.pone.0146608.

Cosetti, M. K., Pinkston, J. B., Fiores, J., et al. (2016). Neurocognitive testing and cochlear implantation: Insights into performance in older adults. *Clinical Interventions in Aging, 11,* 603–613.

Fortunato, S., Forli, F., Guglielmi, et al. (2016). A review of new insights on the association between hearing loss and cognitive decline in ageing. *Acta Otorhinolaryngology Italy, 36,* 155–166.

Frisina, R., Ding, B., Zhu, X., et al. (2016). Age-related hearing loss: Prevention of threshold declines, cell loss and apoptosis in spiral ganglion neurons. *Aging, 8*(9), 2081–2086.

Herdman, T., & Kamitsura, S. (Eds). (2018). *NANDA International Nursing Diagnoses Definitions and Classification, 2018-2020.* (11th ed., pp. 34-44). New York: Thieme Publishers.

Humes, L. E., & Young, L. A. (2016). Sensory-cognitive interactions in older adults. *Ear & Hearing, 37*, 52S–61S.

Ishai, R., Halpin, C., Shin, J., et al. (2016). Long-term incidence and degree of sensorineural hearing loss in otosclerosis. *Otology & Neurotology, 37*, 1489–1496.

Kalaiah, M. K., Thomas, D., Bhat, J. S., et al. (2016). Perception of consonants in speech-shaped noise among young and middle-aged adults. *Journal of International Advanced Otology, 12*, 184–188.

Landier, W. (2016). Ototoxicity and cancer therapy. *Cancer, 122*, 1647–1658.

Mick, P., & Pichora-Fuller, K. (2016). Is hearing loss associated with poorer health in older adults who might benefit from hearing screening? *Ear & Hearing, 37*, e194–e201.

National Academies of Sciences, Engineering, & Medicine. (2016). *Hearing health care for adults: Priorities for improving access and affordability.* Washington, DC: National Academies Press.

National Center for Health Statistics. (2016). *Health, United States, 2015.* Washington, DC: U. S. Government Printing Office.

Nieman, C., Marrone, N., Szanton, S., et al. (2016). Racial-ethnic and socioeconomic disparities in hearing health care among older Americans. *Journal of Aging & Health, 28*, 68–94.

Rohloff, K., Koopman, M., Wei, D., et al. (2017). Cochlear implantation in the elderly: Does age matter? *Otology & Neurotology, 38*, 554–559.

Schwartz, S. R., Magit, A. E., Rosenfeld, R. M., et al. (2017). Clinical Practice Guideline (Update) Earwax (Cerumen Impaction). *Otolaryngology – Head and Neck Surgery, 156*, S1–S29.

Sung, Y. K., Blake, C., Betz, J., et al. (2016). Association of hearing loss and loneliness in older adults. *Journal of Aging & Health, 28*, 979–994.

Verveire, K., Knoop, A., Boel, C., et al. (2016). Speech recognition in noise in younger and older adults: Effects of age, hearing loss, and temporal resolution. *Annals of Otology Rhinology & Laryngology, 125*, 297–302.

Waissbluth, S., Peleva, E., & Daniel, S. J. (2016). Platinum-induced ototoxicity: A review of prevailing ototoxicity criteria. *European Archives of Otorhinolaryngology, 274*(3), 1187–1196.

Wattamwar, K., Qian, Z., Otter, J., et al. (2016). Increases in the rate of age-related hearing loss in the older old. *JAMA Otolaryngology Head & Neck Surgery,* doi: 10.1001/jamaoto.2016.2661.

Wong, D. J., Moran, M., & O'Leary, S. J. (2016). Outcomes after cochlear implant in the very elderly. *Otology & Neurotology, 37*, 46–51.

chapter 17

Vision

LEARNING OBJECTIVES

After reading this chapter, you will be able to:

1. Describe age-related changes that affect vision.

2. Identify risk factors that can affect visual wellness.

3. Discuss the functional consequences that affect visual wellness.

4. Describe three pathologic conditions that cause vision impairments in older adults.

5. Conduct a nursing assessment of vision, with emphasis on identifying opportunities for health promotion.

6. Identify nursing interventions to facilitate visual wellness in older adults by addressing risk factors that interfere with vision.

KEY TERMS

accommodation

acuity

age-related macular degeneration (AMD)

cataracts

color perception

depth perception

diabetic retinopathy

glare

glaucoma

low-vision aids

ophthalmologist

optician

optometrist

presbyopia

visual field

visual impairment

vision rehabilitation

Because important daily activities—including communicating, enjoying visual images, and maneuvering in the environment—are highly dependent on eyesight, visual impairments can profoundly affect a person's safety, functioning, and quality of life. Although age-related changes and risk factors affect visual wellness, nurses have an array of interventions to assist older adults in maintaining optimal visual function. This chapter addresses functional consequences affecting vision in older adults and focuses on the role of nurses in assessing vision and helping older adults achieve visual wellness.

AGE-RELATED CHANGES THAT AFFECT VISION

Visual function depends on a sequence of processes, beginning with the perception of an external stimulus and ending with the processing of neural impulses in the cerebral cortex. Age-related changes affect all the structures involved in visual function; however, in the absence of disease processes, these gradual changes have only a subtle impact on the daily activities of the older person. Age-related changes in the structures of the eye are illustrated in Figure 17-1 and summarized in this section.

Eye Appearance and Tear Ducts

During early stages, age-related changes in the appearance of the eye and eyelids do not interfere with visual function, but they may progress to the point of requiring interventions. For example, drooping of the upper eyelid initially is a cosmetic issue, but if it progresses to the point of interfering with vision, a minor surgical intervention might be appropriate. Table 17-1 summarizes age-related changes in appearance and tear ducts and the associated effects on visual function.

The Eye

The *cornea* is a translucent covering over the eye that refracts light rays and provides 65% to 75% of the focusing power of the eye. As the eye ages, the cornea becomes opaque and yellow, interfering with the passage of light to the retina. Other corneal changes, such as the accumulation of lipid deposits, can cause an increased scattering of

Promoting Visual Wellness in Older Adults

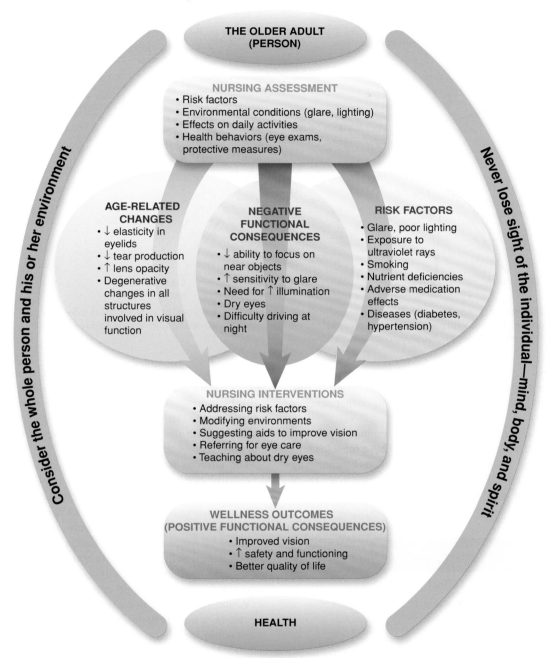

THE OLDER ADULT (PERSON)

NURSING ASSESSMENT
- Risk factors
- Environmental conditions (glare, lighting)
- Effects on daily activities
- Health behaviors (eye exams, protective measures)

AGE-RELATED CHANGES
- ↓ elasticity in eyelids
- ↓ tear production
- ↑ lens opacity
- Degenerative changes in all structures involved in visual function

NEGATIVE FUNCTIONAL CONSEQUENCES
- ↓ ability to focus on near objects
- ↑ sensitivity to glare
- Need for ↑ illumination
- Dry eyes
- Difficulty driving at night

RISK FACTORS
- Glare, poor lighting
- Exposure to ultraviolet rays
- Smoking
- Nutrient deficiencies
- Adverse medication effects
- Diseases (diabetes, hypertension)

NURSING INTERVENTIONS
- Addressing risk factors
- Modifying environments
- Suggesting aids to improve vision
- Referring for eye care
- Teaching about dry eyes

WELLNESS OUTCOMES (POSITIVE FUNCTIONAL CONSEQUENCES)
- Improved vision
- ↑ safety and functioning
- Better quality of life

HEALTH

Consider the whole person and his or her environment

Never lose sight of the individual—mind, body, and spirit

---

light rays and have a blurring effect on vision. In addition, age-related changes in the curvature of the cornea influence the refractive ability.

The *lens* consists of concentric and avascular layers of clear, crystalline protein. Because the lens has no blood supply, it depends on the aqueous humor for metabolic and support functions. New layers are continually formed peripherally and the old layers are compressed inward toward the center, where they eventually become absorbed into the nucleus. This process gradually increases the size and density

of the lens, causing a tripling of its mass by 70 years of age. Thus, the lens gradually becomes stiffer, denser, and more opaque. These age-related changes decrease responsiveness of the lens and increase the diffusion of light rays, resulting in fewer rays reaching the retina. These changes do not affect all wavelengths equally; rather, the most detrimental effect occurs with the shorter blue and violet wavelengths.

The *iris* is a pigmented sphincter muscle that dilates and contracts to control pupillary size and regulate the amount of light reaching the retina. With increasing age, the iris

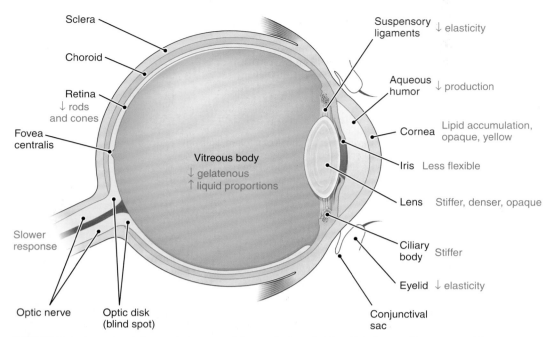

FIGURE 17-1 Age-related changes in structure of the eye, indicated with red labels, can affect vision in older adults. (Adapted with permission from Cohen B.J. (2015). Memmler's the human body in health and disease [13th ed.]. Philadelphia, PA: Lippincott Williams & Wilkins.)

becomes less flexible and the *pupil* becomes smaller. These changes interfere with the ability to respond to low levels of light and reduce the amount of light that reaches the retina.

The *ciliary body* is a mass of muscles, connective tissue, and blood vessels surrounding the lens. These muscles regulate the passage of light rays through the lens by changing the shape of the lens. Primary functions of the ciliary body are production of aqueous fluid and control of the ability

to focus. Because of age-related changes, muscle cells are replaced with connective tissue, and the ciliary body gradually becomes smaller, stiffer, and less functional. With advanced age, diminished secretion of aqueous humor interferes with the nourishment and cleansing of the lens and cornea.

The *vitreous* is a clear, gelatinous mass that forms the inner substance and maintains the spherical shape of the eye. With increasing age, the gelatinous substance shrinks, causing a proportionate increase in the liquid portion. Because of these changes, the vitreous body pulls away from the retina, resulting in symptoms such as floaters, blurred vision, distorted images, or light flashes. In addition, these changes can cause light to scatter more diffusely through the vitreous, reducing the amount of light reaching the retina.

Visual stimuli are transformed into neural impulses in the *retina*, which is composed of rods and cones. Rods are responsible for vision under low light, and cones, which require high levels of light, are responsible for **color perception** and **acuity** (i.e., the ability to detect details and discern objects). Rods are distributed throughout the peripheral retina and cones are concentrated in the central and most sensitive part of the macula, called the *fovea*. Although the number of cone cells diminishes with increasing age, the loss is primarily in the periphery rather than the fovea, and the effects are minimal. The number of rod cells also declines, but the remaining rods increase in size and maintain their ability to capture light. Additional age-related changes in retinal structures include accumulation of lipofuscin, and thinning and sclerosis of the blood vessels and pigment epithelium.

TABLE 17-1 Effects of Age-Related Changes in Appearance and Tear Ducts

Age-Related Changes	Effect
Loss of orbital fat, decreased elasticity of eyelid muscles, accumulation of dark pigment around the eyes	Enophthalmos = appearance of sunken eyes Blepharochalasis = drooping of upper eyelid, which can eventually impair vision
Relaxation of lower eyelid	Ectropion = lower eyelid falls away from conjunctiva, causing decreased lubrication Entropion = lower eyelid becomes inverted and eyelashes irritate the cornea
Accumulation of lipids in outer part of the cornea	Arcus senilis (also called corneal arcus) = development of yellow or gray-white ring around the iris
Narrowing of tear duct opening, reduced production of tears	Dry eye syndrome = excessive tearing, watery eyes, irritation, and inflammation

The Retinal–Neural Pathway

Photoreceptor cells converge in the ganglion cells of the optic nerve. Neurosensory information is passed from the optic nerve, through the thalamus, to the visual cortex. Age-related changes affecting these neurons result in slower processing of visual information.

EFFECTS OF AGE-RELATED CHANGES ON VISION

Visual acuity begins to decrease in adults by the age of 50, even in the absence of any other factors. However, despite the universal prevalence of age-related vision changes, most older adults can perform their usual activities by using low-vision aids and modifying their environments. Visual impairment, which is defined as vision loss that cannot be corrected by eyeglasses or contact lenses alone, ranges from mild impairment to blindness. Mild visual impairments are caused by normal age-related changes, but they are significantly exacerbated by environmental conditions such as glare and poor lighting. These mild visual impairments are illustrated in Figure 17-2 and discussed in the following sections; consequences of more significant visual impairments are discussed in the Pathologic Conditions Affecting Vision section.

Loss of Accommodation

Presbyopia is the loss of accommodation, which is the ability to focus clearly and quickly on objects at various distances. Presbyopia is an initial and universal age-related vision change, which progresses during older adulthood at

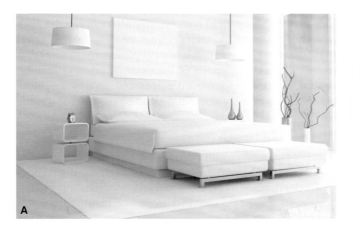

A

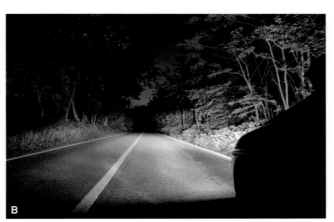

B

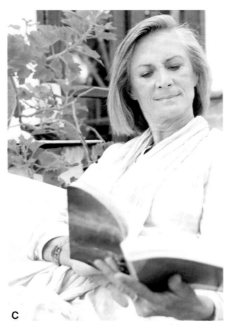

C

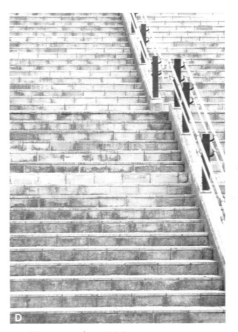

D

FIGURE 17-2 Mild visual impairments include (**A**) reduced contrast sensitivity, (**B**) increased sensitivity to glare and difficulty with night driving, (**C**) increased lighting requirements and decreased ability to focus close up, and (**D**) decreased ability to judge depth perception. (All images from shutterstock.com; copyrights: A (archideaphoto), B (ollyy), C (MJTH), and D (Sakarin Sawasdinaka.)

varying rates. This vision change is caused by degenerative changes in the lens and the ciliary muscle. Functionally, accommodative changes gradually extend the near point of vision, which is the closest point at which a small object can be seen clearly. A typical example of the effects of presbyopia is the need to hold reading materials farther from the eye to focus clearly on the print.

Diminished Acuity

Visual acuity, which is measured against a normal value of 20/20, is assessed by using a Snellen chart. Age-related ocular changes that affect acuity include decreased pupillary size, increased diffusion of light in the cornea and lens, opacification of the lens and vitreous, and loss of photoreceptor cells in the retina. Because of these changes, the amount of light reaching the retina gradually diminishes.

External conditions, such as size and movement of the object and the amount of light reflected off an object, also influence acuity. Because poor illumination compounds the effects of age-related ocular changes, older people require more illumination to see objects clearly. In addition, because visual acuity is more limited for moving objects, it becomes more impaired with increasing speed of the object. These changes in visual acuity can particularly affect night-driving competence.

Delayed Dark and Light Adaptation

The ability to respond to both dim and bright light begins to decline during early adulthood and diminishes more markedly after age 60. This decline is associated with decreased retinal illumination caused by age-related changes in the lens, pupil, retina, and retinal–neural pathways. As a result, the older adult requires more time to adapt to dim lighting when moving from a brighter to a darker environment. For instance, when entering a darkened movie theater, an older person needs extra time to adapt to the changes in lighting before proceeding to a seat. Another consequence is that an older person responds more slowly to lights, such as headlights, and requires more time to recover from exposure to glare and bright lights.

Increased Glare Sensitivity

Glare is experienced when light is reflected from shiny surfaces, when the light is excessively bright or inappropriately focused, or when bright light originates from several sources at once, as in the following examples:

- Bright fluorescent lights in a grocery store reflecting on the clear plastic covering over food products in a white case
- Glass-covered directories in brightly lit shopping malls, particularly when the contrast between the letters and the background is poor
- Facing the sun, especially at sunrise or sunset or in combination with snow
- Driving in the rain or snow

Beginning in the fifth decade, age-related changes increase a person's sensitivity to glare and the time required to recover from glare. Glare sensitivity is influenced primarily by opacification of the lens; however, it is affected also by age-related changes in the pupil and vitreous. Effects on vision include diminished contrast of the viewed object, difficulty discerning details, and blinding effects. In practical terms, these changes can significantly affect the person's ability to read signs, see objects, drive at night, and maneuver safely in bright environments. In many modern buildings and shopping malls, the bright lights, large windows, and highly reflective floors generate glare that can lead to accidents and inaccurate perceptions.

Reduced Visual Field

A visual field is an oval-shaped area encompassing the total view that people perceive while looking straight ahead. The scope of the visual field narrows slightly between the ages of 40 and 50 years and then declines steadily. Functionally, the visual field is important when people engage in tasks that require a broad perception of the environment and moving objects. Walking in crowded places and driving a vehicle are examples of activities that depend on the field of vision.

Diminished Depth Perception

Depth perception is the visual skill responsible for locating objects in three-dimensional space, judging differences in the depth of objects, and observing relationships among objects in space. Factors that influence depth perception include age-related changes, prior perceptual experiences of the observer; movement of the observer's head or body; and characteristics of the object, such as size, distance, texture, brightness, and shading. Older adults experience diminished depth perception, making it more difficult to use objects effectively and maneuver safely in the environment.

Altered Color Vision

Pigments in the retinal cones absorb light in the red, blue, or yellow ranges of the spectrum. Because color perception is influenced by the type and quantity of light waves reaching the retina, age-related changes that interfere with retinal illumination can influence accurate color perception. Opacification and yellowing of the lens interferes most directly with shorter wavelengths, causing an altered perception of blues, greens, and violets. Low levels of illumination and other environmental factors also interfere with color perception.

Functionally, altered color perception is manifested as a relative darkening of blue objects and a yellowed perception of white light. Accurate color perception is not essential in all daily activities, but it is important, for instance, in differentiating between medications that are similar in color, especially those in the blue–green and yellow–white ranges. In addition, altered color perception can interfere with the detection of spoiled food.

TABLE 17-2 Consequences of Age-Related Changes on Vision	
Changes	**Consequences**
• Corneal yellowing and increased opacity • Changes in the corneal curvature • Increase in lens size and density • Sclerosis and rigidity of the iris • Decrease in pupillary size • Atrophy of the ciliary muscle • Shrinkage of gelatinous substance in the vitreous • Atrophy of photoreceptor cells • Thinning and sclerosis of retinal blood vessels • Degeneration of neurons in the visual cortex	• Diminished acuity • Slower response to changes in illumination • Increased sensitivity to glare • Narrowing of the visual field • Diminished depth perception • Altered color perception • Distorted perception of flashing lights • Slower processing of visual information

Slower Visual Information Processing

Age-related changes of the retinal–neural pathway affect the accuracy and efficiency of visual information processing. Thus, older adults generally need more time to process visual information, but the effects are minimal when tasks are familiar. Table 17-2 summarizes age-related vision changes and their effects on vision.

 See ONLINE LEARNING ACTIVITY 17-1: THROUGH THE EYES OF OLDER ADULTS at http://thepoint.lww.com/Miller8e.

 RISK FACTORS THAT AFFECT VISUAL WELLNESS

Lifestyle, nutritional, and environmental factors—including both immediate and long-term conditions—exacerbate age-related vision changes and interfere with visual wellness, as in the following examples:

● Poor nutrition, cigarette smoking, and exposure to sunlight increase the risk for the development of eye diseases.
● Long-term exposure to sunlight exacerbates the effects of age-related changes to increase the risk for eye diseases.
● Warmer environmental temperatures are associated with an earlier age of onset for presbyopia and cataracts.
● Environmental conditions, such as wind, sunlight, low humidity, and secondhand smoke, can cause dry eyes.
● Environmental conditions, such as lighting and color contrast, affect visual function in many ways.

Wellness Opportunity

Poor lighting and exposure to sunlight are risk factors that can readily be addressed through simple self-care practices.

Chronic conditions can adversely affect visual function in various ways. People with dementia or Parkinson disease experience vision changes, which are associated not only with the structures of the eye, but also with the visual-perceptual processes (Pal, Biswas, Pandit, et al., 2016; Weil, Schrag, Warren, et al., 2016). Visuospatial changes and visual hallucinations are common with Lewy body dementia and are considered a distinguishing characteristic early in the course of the disease (Armstrong, 2016). People with diabetes are at increased risk for developing cataracts, glaucoma, and diabetic retinopathy. Studies indicate that 65% of stroke survivors experience poststroke visual impairment, but assessment of vision is often overlooked (Hanna, Hepworth, & Rowe, 2016; Sand, Wilhelmsen, Naess, et al., 2016).

The following medications are associated with potential adverse effects on vision: nonsteroidal anti-inflammatory

Unfolding Case Study

Part 1: Mrs. F. at 60 Years of Age

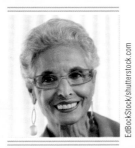

Mrs. F. is 60 years old and has used "readers" (reading glasses) for 15 years but has never needed glasses for anything other than reading and sewing. She recently noticed that she has trouble reading the glass-enclosed directory at the shopping mall. She works in an office building with an atrium that has skylights, and she has trouble reading the signs on the doors.

THINKING POINTS

● What age-related factors contribute to the vision changes that Mrs. F. notices?
● What environmental factors are likely to contribute to Mrs. F.'s difficulty when she is in the shopping mall or at work?

● When Mrs. F. is in her home environment, what tasks might be more difficult because of age-related vision changes?

agents (e.g., aspirin), anticholinergics, phenothiazines, amiodarone, sildenafil, alpha blockers (e.g., doxazosin mesylate), and oral or inhaled corticosteroids. Medications that can cause or contribute to dry eyes include estrogen, diuretics, antihistamines, anticholinergics, phenothiazines, beta blockers, and antiparkinson agents. Systemic anticoagulants can precipitate intraocular hemorrhage in people with pre-existing macular degeneration.

 FUNCTIONAL CONSEQUENCES AFFECTING VISUAL WELLNESS

Disease processes, as discussed in the section on Pathologic Conditions Affecting Vision, are the most common cause of serious visual impairments in older adults. Visual impairments are categorized as "functional" when acuity is 20/50 or worse, as "low vision" when it is between 20/70 and 20/200, and as "blindness" when it is 20/400 or worse. Trouble seeing, even with corrective lenses, affects 13.5% of people aged 65 and over with a higher prevalence among lower-income older adults (National Center for Health Statistics, 2016). Figure 17-3 illustrates differences among subgroups of older adults by age, sex, and poverty level. The following sections describe the functional consequences that are associated with the types of visual impairments that are most likely to occur in older adults.

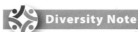 **Diversity Note**

There is a disproportionately higher prevalence of vision impairments and blindness among certain population groups in the United States.
- Uncorrectable visual impairment and blindness: African Americans
- Glaucoma and diabetic retinopathy: Hispanics and African Americans
- AMD: non-Hispanic whites
- Cataract: similar rates across groups until age 70, when rates increase faster for whites
- Untreated cataract as a cause of blindness: individuals of African ancestry
- Diabetic retinopathy: Hispanics beginning at age 50, with highest differences after age 75

(National Academies of Sciences, Engineering, and Medicine, 2016; Varma, Vajaranant, Burkemper, et al., 2016).

Effects on Safety, Function, and Overall Health

Because visual impairments are associated with many aspects of safety and functioning, people who are visually impaired are likely to be more dependent in their activities of daily living. Age-related vision changes most directly influence the following activities:

- Getting outside
- Driving a vehicle

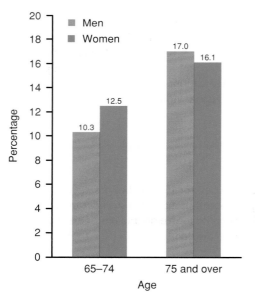

Percentage of older men and women reporting vision limitations

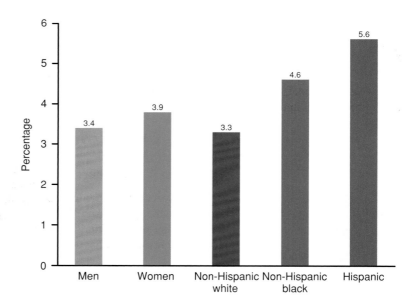

Percentage of people age 65 and over reporting disability due to impaired vision by sex, race, and Hispanic origin

FIGURE 17-3 Percentage of older adults with vision impairment, by age, sex, race, and Hispanic origin, and degree of limitation in 2014. (Source: National Center for Health Statistics. (2016). *Health, United States, 2015.* Trend Table 43, Vision Limitations among adults aged 18 and over, by selected characteristics: United States, Selected Years 1997–2014. Washington, DC: U.S. Government Printing Office; Federal Interagency Forum on Aging-Related Statistics. (2016). *Older Americans 2015: Key Indicators of Well-Being,* Indicator 22, Tables 22a & 22c, Percentage of people age 65 and over with a disability, by race and Hispanic origin and functional domain, 2014.)

- Shopping for groceries
- Going up and down stairs
- Maneuvering safely in dark or unfamiliar environments
- Seeing markings on clocks, radios, thermostats, appliances, and televisions
- Reading newspapers, directories, small-print signs and posters, and labels on food items and medication containers

Most of these activities are affected not only by alterations in visual skills but also by environmental conditions, such as glare and lighting.

The National Academies of Sciences, Engineering, and Medicine issued a major report in 2016 calling for action to address vision loss as a major public health problem. This report emphasized that "the health consequences associated with vision loss extend well beyond the eye and visual system" (National Academies of Sciences, Engineering, and Medicine, 2016, p. 3-1). The following are some of the consequences of visual impairment that studies have identified:

- Higher prevalence of falls, injuries, and fractures
- Higher prevalence of chronic health conditions
- Higher mortality rates, possibly due to accidents and falls
- Impaired ability to self-manage chronic conditions
- Diminished participation in family, social, and community activities
- Poor quality of life
- Increased risk of being admitted to a long-term care facility

Effects on Quality of Life

Age-related vision changes develop gradually and often go unnoticed for many years. As the changes progress and interfere with usual activities, older adults may withdraw from activities rather than acknowledge a vision problem or adjust to the changes. Older adults with impaired vision commonly experience anxiety, depression, and lower levels of psychological well-being, particularly when the visual loss causes functional limitations (Chen & Lu, 2016; Diniz-Filho, Abe, Cho, et al., 2016; van Nispen, Vreeken, Comijs, et al., 2016).

One's usual lifestyle, living environment, and support systems are determinants of the psychosocial consequences of vision changes. Good visual skills are more important for people who live alone or who provide care for others than they are for people who live with, or have frequent contact with, others who have good vision. Also, psychosocial consequences, such as social isolation, will be minimized if visually impaired people can modify their living environment to compensate for age-related vision impairments (Cimarolli, Boerner, Reinhardt, et al., 2017). By contrast, people who live in institutional settings may experience relatively greater negative consequences because of their inability to alter environmental conditions.

Some older adults who notice declines in vision develop fears that negatively affect their quality of life. For example, people may mistakenly fear going blind if they think they have a serious and progressive disease when, in reality, they have a treatable condition. Fear of blindness may be based on myths, inaccurate information, or the experiences of friends who have serious visual impairments. Negative or hopeless attitudes about vision changes can deter the older person from acknowledging the problem or seeking help. Fear of falling is another source of anxiety associated with impaired vision. Inaccurate depth perception can lead to frequent bumping into objects, and the older adult may feel insecure and unsafe, even in familiar environments. If the person has experienced falls or tripping, or knows someone who suffered a fracture as a result of falling, the fears may be magnified.

Wellness Opportunity

Nurses assess the impact of vision impairment on the whole person so they can address fears, anxieties, and other responses that affect quality of life.

Effects on Driving

Vision changes can significantly affect driving skills and exert a profound impact on older adults, their families, and the society. Because driving is associated with considerable safety and independence concerns for drivers and their families—and because unsafe drivers place others at risk—there has been intense and increasing interest in the effects of vision changes on the driving skills of older adults. Visual dimensions that influence driving abilities are near vision, visual search, dynamic vision, contrast sensitivity, and visual processing speed. Consequences of visual impairment with regard to driving include the following:

- Slower dark and light adaptation creates problems when driving in and out of tunnels and when driving at night on streets with variable lighting.
- Decreased peripheral vision interferes with the wide visual field that is important for avoiding collisions.
- Decreased acuity interferes with the perception of moving objects, especially fast-moving vehicles.
- Diminished accommodation and acuity create problems when the older adult tries to read dashboard indicators after focusing on the road.
- Glare interferes with the perception of objects and is heightened by rainy, snowy, or sunny conditions.
- Bright sunlight shortly after sunrise or before sunset can significantly interfere with the perception of red and green traffic lights because of increased sensitivity to glare.
- If the car has tinted windows, the diminished illumination further interferes with visual skills.

In recent years, gerontologists and clinicians have been focusing attention on identifying variables that affect driving in older adults, and many studies address visual skills as an important factor. For example, studies indicate that older drivers with glaucoma may experience difficulty with night driving and changing lanes (Blane, 2016; Wood, Black, Mallon, et al., 2016). A comprehensive literature review found consistent evidence that cataract negatively affects safe driving and that driving improves after cataract surgery (Agramunt, Meuleners, Fraser, et al., 2016).

> ### Wellness Opportunity
>
> Nurses need to be aware of the far-reaching implications of the ability to drive not only on safety of the individual and others but also on independence and the quality of life.

PATHOLOGIC CONDITIONS AFFECTING VISION

Chronic conditions that interfere with visual wellness occur very commonly in older adults, so nurses have important roles in detecting and managing these conditions. Health promotion interventions are particularly important with conditions such as glaucoma because interventions can prevent vision impairment. However, this condition is often undiagnosed so the interventions are not implemented in a timely manner. Among older adults, the most common pathologic eye conditions are cataracts, AMD, glaucoma, and diabetic retinopathy (Figure 17-3; Table 17-3).

Cataracts

Cataracts are a leading and reversible cause of visual impairment, affecting approximately 50% of people aged 80 years and older. Cataracts are caused by the progression of age-related changes in the lens that begin in middle adulthood and eventually can progress to total opacification. As cataracts develop, the normally transparent lens becomes cloudy, transmission of light to the retina is diminished, and vision is impaired. In addition to being caused by age-related changes, risk factors include systemic disease, medications, and environmental factors, as summarized in Table 17-3. Overall, the most modifiable and preventable risk factors for cataracts are cigarette smoking and exposure to sunlight.

> **GLOBAL PERSPECTIVE**
>
> Statistics about worldwide prevalence of blindness are as follows:
> - 82% of blind people and 65% of those who are visually impaired are 50 years and older
> - Cataract is the leading cause of blindness, accounting for more than half of the cases
> - Two-thirds of people who are blind are women; this holds true for both developed and developing countries
> - Higher prevalence rates and lack of access to cataract surgery are the major factors associated with blindness in women in low- and middle-income countries
>
> (Herren & Kohanim, 2016; Iroku-Malize & Kirsch, 2016; Zetterberg, 2016)

Cataracts usually occur in both eyes, but they do not necessarily progress bilaterally at the same rate. Types of cataracts are as follows:

- *Nuclear:* most common type, begins in the center of the lens
- *Cortical:* begins in the periphery and progresses inward
- *Subcapsular:* begins in the posterior lens, progresses more rapidly than other types

In their early stages, cataracts do not necessarily affect visual acuity, but as they progress, they cause difficulty performing activities such as reading and night driving (see Figure 17-4 and Table 17-3).

TABLE 17-3 Common Disease Conditions Affecting Vision

Condition	Risk Factors	Symptoms	Management
Cataract	Advanced age, exposure to sunlight, smoking, obesity, diabetes, malnutrition, trauma or radiation to the eye or head, long-term use of corticosteroids	Dim or blurred vision, increased sensitivity to glare, decreased contrast sensitivity, double vision, seeing halos around bright lights, diminished color perception	Initially managed with changes in corrective lenses Surgical removal of lens followed by implantation of an intraocular lens
Age-related macular degeneration (AMD)	Advanced age, non-Hispanic white ethnicity, family history of AMD, smoking, obesity, exposure to sunlight	**Initially:** Loss of central vision, faces or straight lines appear wavy, blurred vision **Advanced form:** Progressive loss of vision	Smoking cessation, nutritional interventions, visual rehabilitation programs Medical or surgical treatments for wet type
Glaucoma	Advanced age, family history of glaucoma, diabetes, eye injuries, regular or long-term use of corticosteroids	**Chronic:** Slow onset, diminished vision in dim light, increased sensitivity to glare, decreased contrast sensitivity, diminished peripheral vision **Acute:** Sudden onset, intense pain, blurred vision, halos around lights, nausea, and vomiting	**Chronic:** Medical therapy with prescription eye drops **Acute:** Immediate treatment with medications, followed by surgery
Diabetic retinopathy	Obesity, hyperglycemia, hypertension, dyslipidemia	Blurred, hazy, spotted, or fluctuating vision; impaired color vision; floaters	Laser (photocoagulation) treatments; intravitreal injections of medications; vitrectomy

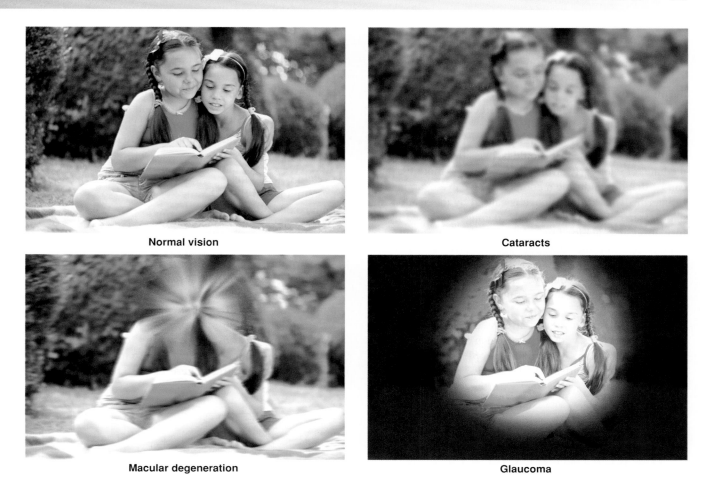

Normal vision

Cataracts

Macular degeneration

Glaucoma

FIGURE 17-4 Examples of normal vision, vision with cataracts, vision with age-related macular degeneration, and vision with glaucoma (Unmodified image from shutterstock.com; copyright: Olesya Feketa.)

When visual acuity declines to the point that it affects the person's safety or the quality of life and provides a reasonable likelihood of improved vision, cataract surgery is usually recommended. An optometrist or an ophthalmologist can diagnose cataracts, but only an ophthalmologist can perform cataract surgery, which is the most commonly performed operation in the United States today. In recent years, major advances have occurred not only in techniques for removal of cataracts but also for correction of other visual problems during the surgery. The surgical procedure is done with local anesthesia, takes less than 1 hour, and has a very low rate of complications. If the person needed corrective lenses before the surgery, the surgeon can insert an intraocular lens that mimics the natural focusing ability of the eye and results in improved vision, with little or no need for additional correction. Cataract surgery has a very low rate of complications and high rates of positive outcomes, including improved overall safety and function (Mönestam, 2016). For example, studies have found that cataract surgery is associated with reduced risk for fractures and accidents (National Academies of Sciences, Engineering, and Medicine, 2016).

Nurses have an important role in dispelling myths and providing accurate information about cataract surgery. Important points to emphasize include the following:

● Advances in surgical techniques for cataract surgery have significantly improved both the process and the outcome of cataract surgery.
● Cataract surgery has an extremely high success rate in significantly improving safety, functioning, and the quality of life.
● It is important to seek reliable information and obtain periodic evaluations from eye care professionals, rather than simply tolerate a loss of vision because of cataracts.

Wellness Opportunity

Nurses promote responsible decision making by encouraging older adults and their caregivers to find reliable information about cataract surgery.

Age-Related Macular Degeneration

Age-related macular degeneration (AMD) is the leading cause of severe vision loss and blindness in people 60 years and older in developed countries (Taylor, 2016). Risk factors associated with AMD are listed in Table 17-3. Early in the disease, deposits of yellow by-products of retinal pigment, called *drusen,* build up in the macula, which is the area in the middle of the retina where visual acuity is the best. Traditionally, the condition has been classified as either *dry type,* which accounts for 80% to 90% of cases, or *wet (exudative) type.* Current clinical guidelines emphasize that AMD is a single type of disease that should be classified as early, intermediate, or late. Early AMD has few or no symptoms, but it can be diagnosed during a comprehensive eye examination. In intermediate AMD, damage is caused by the death of the photoreceptors; in late AMD, the damage is caused by the formation of new blood vessels in the choroid, followed by hemorrhage into the subretinal space. AMD does not necessarily affect both eyes, and if it develops in both eyes, it may not affect both equally. Also, AMD does not always progress, especially if interventions are initiated during the early stage.

When AMD progresses, it affects central vision and significantly interferes with activities such as reading, driving, watching television, recognizing people, and performing many self-care activities (see Table 17-3 and Figure 17-4).

At all stages, the primary treatment goal is to reduce the risk of further vision loss, and all people with AMD require close follow-up by an ophthalmologist to monitor the progression of the condition.

Nurses have important roles in addressing modifiable risk factors, such as smoking and nutrition. An evidence-based intervention for prevention of AMD progression is the daily use of a nutritional supplement that contains all the following:

- Vitamin C 500 mg
- Vitamin E 400 IU
- Zinc oxide 80 mg
- Cupric oxide 2 mg
- Beta carotene 15 mg *or* lutein 10 mg and zeaxanthin 2 mg

This is often referred to as the AREDS formula, named after the Age-Related Eye Disease Study. Additional nursing interventions include teaching about the importance of ongoing evaluations by ophthalmologists and encouraging participation in vision rehabilitation programs to learn the most effective ways of compensating for declining vision. People with AMD are usually taught to test their eyes daily by using the Amsler grid (Figure 17-5) so they will be aware

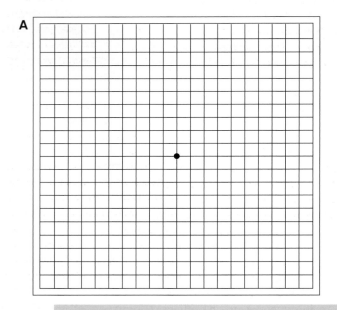

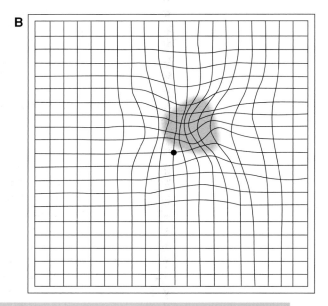

Instructions for Use

1. Tape this page at eye level where light is consistent and without glare.
2. Put on your reading glasses and cover one eye.
3. Fix your gaze on the center black dot.
4. Keeping your gaze fixed, try to see if any lines are distorted or missing.
5. Mark the defect on the chart.
6. TEST EACH EYE SEPARATELY.
7. If the distortion is new or has worsened, arrange to see your ophthalmologist at once.
8. **Always** keep the Amsler grid the **same distance** from your eyes each time you test.

FIGURE 17-5 Amsler grid. (**A**) People with age-related macular degeneration (AMD) use the Amsler grid to perform a simple daily test for sudden changes in their condition. (**B**) This is what the Amsler grid might look like to someone with AMD. (Part A: Reprinted with permission from American Macular Degeneration Foundation, 1-888-MACULAR, www.macular.org.)

of sudden changes. In long-term care settings and for older adults with memory problems, nurses may have to provide daily reminders or assistance with performing this task.

> **Wellness Opportunity**
>
> Nurses holistically address needs of people with AMD by encouraging them to explore support groups and educational services associated with a sight center.

Glaucoma

The term glaucoma refers to a group of eye diseases in which the ganglion cells of the optic nerve are damaged by an abnormal buildup of aqueous humor in the eye. *Aqueous humor* is a clear fluid that is produced in the anterior chamber of the eye and normally maintains eye pressure between 10 and 20 mm Hg. If the fluid cannot flow out of the anterior chamber of the eye through the channel between the iris and the cornea, it accumulates and pushes the optic nerve into a cupped or concave shape. The resulting damage to the optic nerve causes a loss of peripheral vision. If left untreated, the damage can progress to blindness.

> **Diversity Note**
>
> In African Americans, glaucoma occurs five times more often, leads to blindness six times more commonly, and develops an average of 10 years earlier, compared with other groups (Glaucoma Research Foundation, n.d.)

Chronic (open-angle) glaucoma, which accounts for as much as 90% of cases of glaucoma in the United States, occurs when the drainage canals become clogged. This condition has an insidious onset and affects vision when the optic nerve becomes damaged. Early signs include increased intraocular pressure, poor vision in dim lighting, and increased sensitivity to glare. If the condition progresses, manifestations include headaches, "tired eyes," impaired peripheral vision, a fixed and dilated pupil, the perception of halos around lights, and frequent changes in the prescription for corrective lenses. Chronic glaucoma usually occurs in both eyes, but it can begin in only one eye and does not necessarily progress at the same rate in both eyes. Because chronic glaucoma progresses slowly and causes little or no visual impairment in the early stage, annual assessments of intraocular pressure are necessary to detect the condition before visual impairments occur. Chronic glaucoma is most commonly managed with medications, but surgical treatment options include laser surgery and other types of eye surgery. Medication management commonly includes one or more of the following types of prescription eye drops: miotics, prostaglandins, beta blockers, adrenergic agonists, and carbonic anhydrase inhibitors.

Normal-tension glaucoma is another type of glaucoma that occurs in older adults. With this type of glaucoma, the intraocular pressure is within the normal range, but the optic nerve is damaged and the visual field is narrowed (see Figure 17-4). This condition is often managed with the same medications and surgical approaches that are used for chronic glaucoma.

Acute (closed-angle) glaucoma is caused by a sudden complete blockage of the flow of aqueous humor. This condition has an abrupt onset in one or both eyes and should be considered a medical emergency. People with acute glaucoma present with increased intraocular pressure, severe eye pain, clouded or blurred vision, dilation of the pupil, and nausea and vomiting. This condition can be precipitated by medications that cause pupil dilation, such as anticholinergics. Immediate treatment with medications is usually effective for acute attacks, but surgical intervention is often needed.

Health education for older adults with glaucoma focuses on the importance of adhering to ongoing medication routines and regularly being evaluated by their eye care practitioner. If older adults with glaucoma are admitted for institutional care, nurses need to ensure that prescribed eye drops are administered as ordered. In home care situations, nurses may need to develop a plan for administering eye drops on a daily or more frequent basis. If an older adult has memory problems, establishing a routine for administering eye drops can be quite challenging. Many times, complicated eye drop regimens can be simplified by working with the eye care practitioner to decrease the number of eye drops that are necessary or to prescribe a longer-acting medication that can be administered less frequently.

> **Wellness Opportunity**
>
> Nurses promote self-care by teaching people with glaucoma to be aware of prescription and over-the-counter medications that can exacerbate glaucoma.

Diabetic Retinopathy

Diabetic retinopathy refers to pathologic changes that cause leakage of the blood vessels in the retina in people with diabetes. Because of the significantly increasing prevalence of diabetes, diabetic retinopathy has become the leading cause of new cases of blindness among adults in the US and worldwide (National Academies of Sciences, Engineering, and Medicine, 2016; Stewart, 2016). During the earliest stage, called nonproliferative diabetic retinopathy, microaneurysms form in the retina and leak fluid, causing macular edema. Vision changes are minimal during this stage, but the condition can be diagnosed with a comprehensive eye examination. With progression to the proliferative stage, new blood vessels begin to form in the retina and leak blood into the vitreous. Complications of proliferative diabetic retinopathy include retinal detachment and the development of glaucoma. Diabetic retinopathy can progress to total blindness if not treated effectively. Risk factors and treatments are summarized in Table 17-3. An important nursing implication is that good control of diabetes is essential for preventing the progression of diabetic retinopathy. Studies supported by the National Institutes of Health indicate that better glycemic control can

Unfolding Case Study

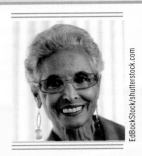

EdBookStock/shutterstock.com

Part 2: Mrs. F. at 72 Years of Age

Mrs. F. is now 72 years old and has been retired for several years. You are the nurse at her local senior center, and she makes an appointment to see you. Mrs. F.'s medical history indicates that she has smoked a pack of cigarettes a day for 40 years and has been taking medications for hypertension and arthritis for 5 years. During a recent medical checkup, her doctor said he thought she had early cataracts, but he told Mrs. F. that he felt it was too early to do anything about them. She has never had an eye examination, other than what her regular doctor does periodically. When asked about her symptoms, Mrs. F. tells you that she sometimes feels like there is a film over her eyes and she has trouble seeing when she is outside on sunny days. Mrs. F. says that she never liked wearing sunglasses and hopes she will not have to start wearing them now. She has recently purchased stronger reading glasses, and these help a little with reading and sewing.

THINKING POINTS

- What factors likely contributed to the development of Mrs. F.'s cataracts?
- When Mrs. F. is driving during the day, what difficulties might she notice because of vision changes? Because of environmental conditions?

- When Mrs. F. is driving at night, what difficulties might she notice because of vision changes? Because of environmental conditions?
- When Mrs. F. is in her home, what changes in visual abilities might she notice because of cataracts?

QSEN APPLICATION

QSEN Competency	Knowledge/Skill/Attitude	Application to Mrs. F.
Evidence-based practice	(K) Describe how the strength and relevance of available evidence influence the choice of intervention	Teach Mrs. F. about evidence-based interventions for preventing the development and progression of cataracts (i.e., quitting smoking and protecting eyes from sunlight)
	(S) Base individualized care plan on patient values, clinical expertise, and evidence	Explore with Mrs. F. whether she is willing to wear broad-brimmed hats when out in the sun because she states that she doesn't like wearing sunglasses
	(A) Value evidence-based practice as integral to determining the best clinical practice	

significantly reduce the progression of diabetic retinopathy in people with diabetes (Action to Control Cardiovascular risk in Diabetes Follow-On Eye Study Group, 2016).

See ONLINE LEARNING ACTIVITY 17-2: ARTICLE ABOUT ASSESSMENT AND INTERVENTIONS FOR AGE-RELATED CONDITIONS IN HOME CARE SETTINGS at http://thepoint.lww.com/Miller8e.

NURSING ASSESSMENT OF VISION

Nursing assessment of vision is aimed at identifying the following:

- Factors that interfere with visual wellness
- Vision problems

- The impact of vision changes on safety, independence, or the quality of life
- Opportunities for promoting visual wellness
- Barriers to implementing interventions

Nursing assessment of visual function is not a substitute for an examination by an eye care specialist. Whereas the purpose of an examination by an eye care specialist is to detect and initiate appropriate treatment of vision problems, the goal of the nursing assessment is to assist the older adult in minimizing the negative consequences of vision changes. Nursing assessment also aims at identifying modifiable risk factors that can be addressed through health promotion. Nurses assess visual abilities by interviewing the older adult (or caregivers of dependent older adults), by observing the older adult's ability to perform activities of daily living, and by testing the older adult's visual skills.

Box 17-1 Guidelines for Assessing Vision

Questions to Assess Awareness and Presence of Vision Impairment

- Have you noticed any changes in your vision during the past few years?
- Do you experience any uncomfortable symptoms, such as dry eyes?
- Do you have difficulty managing any of your usual activities because you have trouble seeing? (Consider asking about the following: sewing, reading, driving, grooming, hobbies, preparing meals, watching television, managing money, writing letters, using the telephone, using dials on appliances, shopping for groceries, and going up and down stairs.)
- Have you ever tripped or fallen because you had trouble seeing?
- Have you stopped doing any activities because of vision problems? (e.g., have you stopped driving at night because of difficulty seeing?)
- Are there things you would do if you could see better?

Questions to Ask If Vision Loss is Acknowledged

- When did you first notice a loss of vision or a change in your ability to see?
- Have the changes been gradual, or did you notice sudden changes at any particular time?
- How would you describe the changes in your ability to see?

- Have you noticed pain, blurred vision, burning or itching, halos around lights, intolerance to bright light, a difference between day and night vision, or spots or flashing lights in front of your eyes?
- What kind of medical evaluation and care, if any, have you had for this problem?

Questions to Identify Opportunities for Education About Disease Prevention and Health Promotion

- When was the last time you had your eyes checked?
- Where do you go for eye care?
- Have you ever had your eyes checked for cataracts, glaucoma, and other eye conditions?
- What do you think about going for regular checkups for glaucoma and other eye problems?

Questions to Identify Risk Factors for Vision Loss

- When you spend time outdoors in the sun, do you use sunglasses or a hat to protect your eyes from bright light?
- Do you smoke cigarettes?
- Do you have a history of diabetes or hypertension?
- Do you have a family history of glaucoma or macular degeneration?
- What medications do you take?

Interviewing About Vision Changes

Nurses use interview questions to elicit the following information: past and present risk factors for vision impairment, the person's awareness of any vision changes, the impact of these changes on daily activities and the quality of life, and the person's attitudes about interventions (Box 17-1). The interview begins with direct questions about the person's awareness of any changes in vision. If the person acknowledges a visual impairment, nurses elicit additional details about the onset and progression of vision changes. Nurses also ask about symptoms that cause discomfort or that indicate the possible presence of disease processes.

Nurses then ask about the impact of vision changes on the person's usual or desired activities. If the person has acknowledged vision changes, nurses can ask specific questions about how these changes have influenced usual activities. If the person is not aware of vision changes, nurses inquire about any difficulties performing complex activities, such as driving, shopping, and meal preparation. Questions about leisure interests are incorporated into the interview to obtain information about the psychosocial consequences of vision impairments. Although the older adult may not associate lifestyle changes with vision impairments, questions about changes in hobbies and leisure activities can help nurses identify the need for interventions to improve visual wellness. Because poor vision increases the risk for falls, especially tripping-related falls, nurses ask about a history of tripping, falling, and near-falling.

Wellness Opportunity

Nurses assess the impact of vision changes on the person's relationships with other people as one aspect of the quality of life.

Identifying Opportunities for Health Promotion

Nurses identify opportunities for health promotion by asking about the person's usual eye care practices and about factors that can interfere with visual wellness. Information about the source, frequency, and dates of the person's eye examinations is particularly useful for planning health promotion interventions that address the early detection of eye disease. Nurses also listen for indicators of myths or misunderstandings that should be addressed through health education. If the person has cataracts, glaucoma, or another chronic condition affecting vision, nurses ask questions to ascertain the person's self-care practices and attitude toward eye examinations and disease management. If no visual impairment is reported, nurses assess attitudes about early detection of treatable conditions.

Last, identification of modifiable risk factors provides an opportunity for health education because there is increasing evidence that prevention of eye disease is a public health concern. For example, analysis of the longitudinal results of Nurses' Health Study emphasizes that age-related eye disease can be prevented through interventions directed toward smoking cessation, maintenance of a healthy weight, prevention of diabetes, and a diet rich in fruits and vegetables (Kang, Wu, Cho, et al., 2016). If the older person is likely to spend time outdoors in sunny climates, nurses ask about exposure to sunlight. Placing this question toward the end of the interview sets the stage for health education about protective measures, such as the use of sunglasses.

Wellness Opportunity

Nurses pave the way for teaching about self-care by assessing attitudes about preventive and protective activities, such as obtaining eye examinations and wearing sunglasses.

Observing Cues to Visual Function

Reliable information about a person's visual function can be obtained simply by being observant. For example, nurses can observe for any abnormalities of the eyelids, such as serious eyelid lag, that might interfere with visual wellness. Nurses can detect other, more subtle indicators of impaired vision by observing the person's appearance and ability to perform daily activities. Finally, community-based nurses may have opportunities to observe older adults in their usual environments to assess their functioning and conditions that can affect visual abilities. When assessments cannot be performed in the person's usual environment, nurses can ask the older person and caregivers for information about the person's abilities in the home setting.

It is also important to identify environmental conditions that might influence visual performance, either positively or negatively. An example of a positive influence might be the presence of good lighting and color contrast. Some negative influences, such as glare from fluorescent lights reflecting on highly polished floors, are more likely to exist in an institutional setting than a home setting. Another factor to consider is whether the person is using corrective lenses, which may not be available during the assessment. Box 17-2

 Box 17-2 Guidelines for Assessing Behavioral and Environmental Cues Related to Visual Performance

Behavioral Cues

- Is clothing spotted, soiled, or mismatched, in contrast to a former pattern of neatness and sense of style?
- Is makeup applied in heavy quantities, in contrast to the usual manner of application?
- Does the person rely heavily on nonvisual cues in performing usual activities, especially maneuvering in the environment (e.g., using the hands to find objects or to probe for obstacles)?

Environmental Cues

- What kind of lighting is used for various tasks? If the lighting is not adequate, can adjustments be made to improve the person's visual abilities?
- Does the person try to economize at home by using dim lights or no lights at all? If so, does this interfere with visual abilities or safe functioning?
- Where does the person usually sit in relation to light sources? Does glare from a window interfere with vision? Do shadows from lamps interfere with vision? Do overhead lights cause glare? Are light bulbs of sufficient wattage?
- What are the sources of light on stairways and hallways?
- Is there sufficient color contrast in the following areas: walls and floors; stairs and landings; furniture; eating utensils and place settings; cooking utensils and counter tops; markings and background on appliance dials?
- Are nightlights used in hallways and bathrooms?

summarizes behavioral and environmental cues related to visual function.

Using Standard Vision Tests

Nurses can assess vision by using both formal and informal tests. Before testing, however, eliminate sources of glare, make sure the testing materials have good color contrast,

Unfolding Case Study

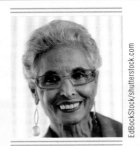

EdBockStock/shutterstock.com

Part 2: Mrs. F. at 72 Years of Age (Continued)

Recall that you are the nurse at the senior center in Mrs. F.'s neighborhood. During a recent visit, the 72-year-old Mrs. F. told you that she feels like there is a "film" over her eyes, and she has trouble seeing when she is outside on sunny days. Several months ago, Mrs. F.'s doctor told her that she has "early cataracts," but she has had no further evaluation.

THINKING POINTS

- Which questions from Box 17-1 would you ask Mrs. F. at this time?
- What sort of information might you be able to glean from behavioral or environmental cues about Mrs. F.'s ability to see? (see Box 17-2.)

- Would assessing Mrs. F.'s vision by using vision-screening tests be appropriate? (see Box 17-3.) If so, which tests would you perform?
- What health promotion education would you give Mrs. F. at this time?

Box 17-3 Guidelines for Using Vision-Screening Tests

Using the Snellen Chart to Assess Distance Acuity

- Position the chart 20 ft away from the person, at eye level.
- If space does not permit a 20-foot distance, the distance between the person and the chart should be either 15 or 10 ft, with final measurements adjusted for distance. Alternatively, a scaled-down Snellen card can be used, if available.
- If the person usually wears corrective lenses, test the corrected vision.
- Ask the person to start reciting the letters in the line that can be read most easily; then ask him or her to read as many letters as possible in the lines directly below that line.
- Document the findings for each eye by noting the figure at the end of the last line on which at least half of the letters were read correctly.
- The upper figure denotes the distance of the person from the chart, whereas the lower figure denotes the distance from the chart at which a person with normal vision would be able to read the line (i.e., a vision measurement of 20/50 indicates that the person being tested can see things at a distance of 20 ft that a person with normal vision would be able to see at a distance of 50 ft).
- Normal Snellen chart test results for older adults are as follows:
  - A corrected vision of 20/20 is considered to be normal.
  - If a distance of 10 ft is used, the corrected vision should be 10/10.
  - The average corrected vision for older adults ranges from 20/20 to 20/50.

Performing the Confrontation Test to Assess Peripheral Vision

- Sit directly across from the older person, about 2 ft away.
- Cover your left eye and have the examinee cover his or her right eye.

- Instruct the examinee to focus on your right eye while you focus on the examinee's left eye.
- Fully extend your right arm midway between you and the examinee.
- While holding a pencil, slowly move your right hand, with the fingers wiggling, from the outer periphery toward the center, testing visual fields from top to bottom.
- While maintaining continuous eye contact, ask the examinee to report the point at which the pencil is visualized.
- Repeat these steps, covering your right eye and the examinee's left eye and using your left arm.
- Normal confrontation test results for older adults: the pencil in your hand should be seen simultaneously by both you and the older person in all quadrants.

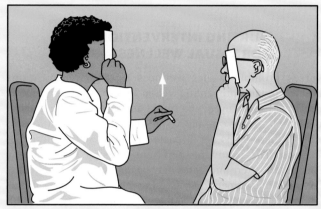

Performing the confrontation test.

and place a light source above the person's head to provide good lighting while avoiding shadows. If the person normally wears corrective lenses, make sure that they are clean and in place. Test each eye separately, using an appropriate eye cover; avoid using a hand as a cover. Box 17-3 describes the Snellen chart for distance acuity and the Confrontation Test for peripheral vision, which nurses can use in clinical settings. Any of the following methods can be used as an informal test of vision:

- Ask the person to read a newspaper or other printed material of various type sizes.
- Ask the person to read a line or two of a form that needs to be signed and observe the person's ability to find the signature line.
- Provide written educational materials and ask the person to read a specific part, such as a phone number.
- Have the person look out a window or down a hallway and describe certain details, such as the words on a sign.

These tests supplement information obtained through interviewing and observations, as described earlier. The purpose of nursing assessment of vision is to provide information that is useful for planning care and identifying the need for further evaluation, but it is not a substitute for a complete eye examination.

 See **ONLINE LEARNING ACTIVITY 17-3: ASSESSMENT IN PRACTICE** at **http://thepoint.lww.com/Miller8e.**

NURSING DIAGNOSIS

Based on the nursing assessment, the nurse might identify actual vision impairment or risk factors for impaired vision. If the visual impairment interferes with the older adult's safety, quality of life, or performance of activities of daily living, any of the following nursing diagnoses can be used to address these functional consequences: Anxiety, Self-Care Deficit, Risk for Injury, Impaired Social Interaction, and Readiness for Enhanced Self-Care.

Wellness Opportunity

The wellness nursing diagnosis of Readiness for Enhanced Knowledge: Improved Vision would be applicable for older adults who are willing to explore interventions that improve their vision.

PLANNING FOR WELLNESS OUTCOMES

When older adults experience vision impairments or have risk factors that affect visual functioning, nurses identify wellness outcomes as an essential part of the planning process. The Nursing Outcomes Classification (NOC) that most directly relates to interventions to improve vision for older adults is Sensory Function Status. In addition, nurses can use any of the following NOCs to describe the effectiveness of interventions to improve vision: Coping, Self-Care: Activities of Daily Living, Self-Care: Instrumental Activities of Daily Living, Stress Level, Knowledge: Personal Safety, and Fall Prevention Behavior. Specific interventions to achieve these outcomes are discussed in the following section.

Wellness Opportunity

Quality of life is a wellness outcome that is achieved through nursing interventions that improve visual function.

NURSING INTERVENTIONS FOR VISUAL WELLNESS

Nurses promote visual wellness through interventions directed toward preventing vision loss, promoting comfort measures for dry eyes, and implementing or teaching about methods to foster optimal visual function. Interventions to achieve these goals are discussed in detail in the following sections. The following pertinent Nursing Interventions Classification terminologies may be applicable to care plans: Coping Enhancement, Dry Eye Prevention, Eye Care, Environmental Management: Safety, Health Education, Health Screening, Risk Identification, and Fall Prevention.

Health Promotion for Visual Wellness

Health promotion interventions focus on maintaining vision at an optimal level by compensating for any visual deficits and identifying any treatable conditions at an early stage. Another important aspect of health promotion is addressing modifiable risk factors, such as smoking and exposure to sunlight. In addition, nurses can teach about nutritional interventions to promote eye health. Box 17-4 summarizes teaching points related to promoting eye health for all older adults. For older adults with visual impairment, nurses have important responsibilities related to self-management of chronic eye disease, such as teaching about optimal control of diabetes for people with diabetic retinopathy and adherence to prescribed medications for people with glaucoma.

In providing health education, it may be helpful to review the differences between opticians, optometrists, and ophthalmologists and provide information about health insurance coverage for these services, as detailed in Box 17-5.

Wellness Opportunity

Nurses promote self-care by encouraging older adults and their families to obtain information from reliable resources.

Box 17-4 Health Promotion Teaching About Visual Wellness

Prevention and Early Detection of Disease

- Minimize exposure to sunlight by using broad-brimmed hats and close-fitting sunglasses with UV-absorbing lenses.
- Have eyes examined annually or more frequently if you notice a change in vision; make sure the examination checks for glaucoma, cataracts, and retinal disease.
- Use the appropriate eye care practitioner (ophthalmologist, optometrist, and optician) as described in Box 17-5.
- Because smoking is a risk factor for many eye diseases, quit smoking.
- Maintain optimal control of hypertension, diabetes, and other chronic conditions.

Nutritional Considerations

- Include foods high in lutein, such as fruits, corn, spinach, green leafy vegetables, and egg yolks.
- Lutein supplements of 10 mg/day are safe and may be effective in preventing cataracts and AMD.
- People who have macular degeneration or risk factors for this condition are encouraged to take a daily supplement containing the following: 500 mg vitamin C, 400 IU vitamin E, 15 mg beta carotene (same as 25,000 IU of vitamin A), 80 mg zinc oxide, and 2 mg cupric oxide (copper). However, people who smoke are advised to avoid beta carotene because it can increase the risk of developing lung cancer.

See ONLINE LEARNING ACTIVITY 17-4: RESOURCES FOR HEALTH EDUCATION at http://thepoint.lww.com/Miller8e.

Comfort Measures for Dry Eyes

If pertinent, simple measures to relieve dry eyes can be discussed. Use of over-the-counter artificial tears or ocular lubricants, especially before reading or engaging in other activities that require frequent eye movements, will usually relieve symptoms. People who use eye drops more frequently than every 3 hours should be advised to use preservative-free solutions to prevent any adverse effects from the preservatives. Other comfort measures, such as applying cold compresses or wearing wraparound glasses, are designed to prevent evaporation of tears. Maintenance of adequate environmental humidity, especially during the winter months or in dry climates, also decreases evaporation of eye moisture and adds to eye comfort. People who experience discomfort from dry eyes should avoid irritants, such as smoke and hairspray, and adverse environmental conditions, such as hot rooms and high wind. People who are bothered by dry eyes and are taking a medication that might exacerbate the discomfort should be encouraged to discuss the problem with their primary care practitioner.

Environmental Modifications

Simple environmental modifications can improve the older person's safe performance of activities of daily living,

Box 17-5 Guide to Eye Care Practitioners

Ophthalmologist

An **ophthalmologist** is a licensed doctor of medicine (MD) or osteopathy (DO) who is trained to diagnose and treat diseases and conditions of the eye. Ophthalmologic services include:

- Comprehensive eye examinations
- Diagnosis of eye diseases and disorders of the eye
- Prescription medications for eye problems (e.g., glaucoma)
- Eye surgery and postoperative care (e.g., cataracts)
- Laser treatments (e.g., retinopathy)
- Prescriptions for eyeglasses and contact lenses
- Prescriptions for low-vision aids
- Referrals for low-vision aids and training
- Medical referrals for diseases of the body that affect the eyes

Optometrist

An **optometrist** is a licensed doctor of optometry (OD), not a physician, who is trained to examine eyes, screen for common eye problems, and prescribe eye exercises or corrective lenses. Optometrists use pharmaceutical agents for diagnosis and treatment of diseases of the eye and related structures. Additional services, such as the performance of laser surgery, vary according to state regulations. Optometric services include:

- Comprehensive eye examinations
- Eye refractions to determine the need for corrective lenses
- Prescriptions for eyeglasses, contact lenses, and low-vision aids
- Vision therapy to improve certain skills, such as tracking and focusing the eyes
- Referrals for low-vision aids and training
- Referrals to physicians for surgery, medication, or further evaluation
- Diagnosis of eye disorders (in some states)
- Postoperative care (in some states)

Optician

An **optician** is an eye care practitioner who is trained to fit, adjust, and dispense eyeglasses and contact lenses that have been prescribed by an optometrist or ophthalmologist. In many states, opticians are licensed. They do not perform eye examinations or refractions, and they cannot prescribe corrective lenses or medications.

Box 17-6 Considerations for Optimal Illumination

- Older adults need at least three times as much light as younger people do.
- Older adults function best in environments with bright, broad-spectrum, nonglaring, indirect sources of light.
- Sources of illumination should be placed 1 to 2 ft away from the object to be viewed.
- The amount of light decreases fourfold when the distance is doubled.
- Flickering light, such as that generated by a single fluorescent tube, will cause fatigue and decreased visual performance.
- Light bulbs should be kept clean.
- Increased illumination has a greater positive effect on impaired vision than it does on normal vision.
- A gradual decrease in illumination from foreground to background is better than sharp contrasts in lighting.
- Moderate overhead lighting can be used to enhance brighter foreground lighting and prevent sharp contrasts.
- To reduce glare from reading material, place the light source to the left side of right-handed readers and to the right side of left-handed readers.
- Avoid glossy paper for reading materials.

commonly used temperature setting, and the older adult can be instructed to turn the dial above or below the matching dots for higher or lower settings.

Architectural designs and institutional constraints may limit the extent of environmental adaptations that nurses can implement, especially in institutional settings. In most settings, however, nurses can improve the visual abilities of older adults by using appropriate colors to enhance contrast, by using curtains to control light and glare, and by placing chairs in positions that enhance illumination and avoid glare. Nurses have many opportunities to teach older adults and their caregivers about environmental modifications that can be used to compensate for deficits in visual skills and to improve safety, as described in Box 17-7. These environmental modifications can be implemented to improve visual function for all people.

Low-Vision Aids

People with visual impairments can improve their safety and quality of life by using **low-vision aids** to enhance contrast, improve focus, improve lighting, or enlarge images (Box 17-8). Low-vision aids are most beneficial when used in conjunction with environmental modifications. For example, magnifiers are most effective when combined with measures that improve illumination and control glare. Low-vision aids are widely available in stores, through catalogs, or at local sight centers. In addition, everyday items, if used advantageously, can serve as low-vision aids. For example, household lamps placed in the correct position and equipped with the right wattage bulb can also serve as low-vision aids. Nurses can use information presented in Boxes 17-6 and 17-9 to teach about effective use of lights and magnification.

thereby reducing risks of falls and accidents. Because older adults require more light for adequate vision, proper nonglare lighting is the single most important—as well as the easiest and the least costly—intervention to improve visual function (Box 17-6). Optimal illumination depends on both the quality and the quantity of lighting. For example, selection of broad-spectrum fluorescent lights and daylight-simulating lamps may be particularly beneficial in compensating for age-related vision changes.

Another important consideration in adapting the environment for optimal visual function is color contrast. Appliances and other items, such as ovens, irons, radios, thermostats, and televisions, may be difficult to use because of poor color contrast around the control mechanisms. Modifications can easily be made to improve the older person's ability to use these items safely and accurately. For example, two dots of red nail polish can be used to mark a designated and

Box 17-7 Environmental Adaptations for Improving Visual Performance

Illumination, Glare Control, and Dark/Light Adaptation

- Position a 60- or 75-watt soft-white light bulb above and close to the head of the older person.
- Use a clear plastic shower curtain, rather than solid colors or printed curtains, for the tub or shower.
- Use light-colored, sheer curtains to eliminate glare from windows.
- Place nightlights in hallways and bathrooms, or keep a high-intensity flashlight at the bedside.
- Use illuminated light switches.
- Provide good lighting in stairways and hallways.
- Use illuminated or magnifying mirrors.

Color Contrast

- Use brightly colored tape or paint on the edges of stairs, especially on the top and bottom steps.
- Use light-colored and dark-colored cutting boards to contrast with dark and light foods.
- Use contrasting, rather than matching, colors for china, place-mats, and napkins.
- Use a toilet seat that contrasts with the bathroom walls and floor. Use colored bars of soap on white sinks and tubs.
- Use utensils with brightly colored handles.

- Place pillows of contrasting colors on stuffed furniture.
- Use decorative or lighted plates over light switches and wall sockets; avoid switch plates that blend in with the wallpaper or paint.
- Place decorative items of contrasting colors, such as plants and ceramics on tables, to provide cues to depth, especially on light-colored furniture that is in a room with light-colored walls.
- Use brightly colored grooming utensils, such as combs, brushes, and razors.
- Use pens with black ink rather than blue ink.

General Adaptive Measures and Environmental Modifications

- Do not rearrange furniture without informing or showing the older person.
- Advise older adults to pause in doorways when going from light to dark rooms (or vice versa) to allow time for their eyes to adjust to the light change.
- Teach older people to use their hands and feet as probes to feel for curbs, steps, edges of chairs, and the like.
- When walking with an older person, stop when necessary to allow a change in focus from near to far and from light to dark.

Technology to Promote Wellness in Older Adults

Nurses can teach older adults and their caregivers about newer technology-based products that are widely available to support independent function for people who are visually impaired, as in the following examples:

- Talking prescription labels and medication reminders
- Talking scales, thermometers, and blood pressure monitors
- Cell phones, tablets, and other mobile technology adapted for visual impairments
- Accessible computers
- Appliances (e.g., stoves, microwaves, washers, dryers, dishwashers) adapted for visual impairments
- Online shopping and banking accessibility

The American Foundation for the Blind (www.afb.org) provides comprehensive and up-to-date information about products that are accessible for people with visual impairments, including reviews and information about where to obtain products. The website also includes a special section for older adults and free access to a monthly magazine called *AccessWorld*.

Vision Rehabilitation

Vision rehabilitation services are multifaceted and include any of the following interventions to help people with low vision:

- Teaching about adaptive strategies for safety and independence in activities of daily living
- Training by orientation and mobility specialists
- Training in the use of low-vision aids
- Guidance on home and environmental modifications
- Information about local resources and support
- Counseling

If a comprehensive vision rehabilitation program is not available, occupational therapists are a good resource for older adults with limited vision. For example, health insurance may cover an occupational therapist visit for a home assessment when visual impairments increase the risk for falls. Use of vision rehabilitation services are associated with the following positive functional consequences: improvements in vision-related functioning, increased social participation, improved quality of life, and decreased levels of depression and emotional distress (Cimarolli, Casten, Rovner, et al., 2016; Draper, Feng, Appel, et al., 2016; Nollett, Bray, Bunce, et al., 2016).

See **ONLINE LEARNING ACTIVITY 17-5: LIVING BETTER AT HOME: VIDEOS AND ARTICLES** at http://thepoint.lww.com/Miller8e.

Wellness Opportunity

Nurses promote self-care for people who are visually impaired by facilitating referrals to local vision rehabilitation services and encouraging older adults and their families to use these resources.

Providing Vision-Friendly Teaching Materials

Although written materials are often difficult to read—even for people who do not have significant visual impairment—there are many relatively simple ways to develop vision-friendly teaching materials, as in the following examples:

- Use a photocopy machine to convert regular-print materials into large-print materials.

Box 17-8 Low-Vision Aids for Improving Visual Performance

Enlargement Aids

- Microscopic spectacles
- Handheld or standing magnifiers

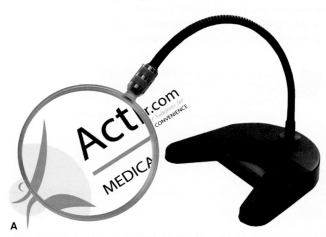

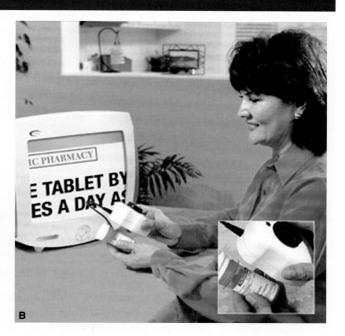

Examples of low-vision aids. (**A**) A combination of high-intensity lamp and magnifier.

- Binoculars and handheld or spectacle-mounted telescopes
- Magnifying sheets
- Field expanders for diminished peripheral vision
- Large-print books, magazines, and newspapers
- Photocopy machines or printers to enlarge print
- Telephones with enlarged letters and numbers, or a pad with enlarged letters and numbers designed to fit over rotary-dial or push-button phones
- Large numbers on rulers, playing cards, and other items
- Thermometers with good color coding and enlarged numbers
- Large-eye sewing needles

Illumination Aids

- High-intensity lights
- Gooseneck lamps
- Floor or table lamps with three-way light bulbs

Contrast Aids

- Use of broad-tipped felt markers in dark, yet bright, colors and colored construction paper for making signs
- Red print on a yellow background or white letters on a green background
- Reading and signature guides (typoscopes)
- Clip-on yellow lenses

Glare Control Aids

- Sunglasses with UV-absorbing lenses
- Sun visors and broad-brimmed hats
- Nonglare (antireflective) coating on eyeglasses
- Yellow and pink acetate sheets
- Pinhole occluders

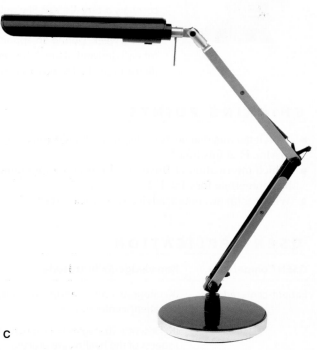

A handheld digital magnifier (**B**) that works with any television to magnify print. A versatile lamp (**C**) that uses an energy-efficient high-definition tube bulb for good contrast and brightness. (Photographs reprinted with permission from ActiveForever.com.)

Box 17-9 Guidelines for Using Magnifying Aids

Using a Handheld Magnifier

- Begin by holding the magnifier close to the reading material.
- Slowly move the magnifier toward the face until the image totally fills the lens.
- For optimal focus, move the magnifier back toward the print about a distance of 2 cm.

Using a Stand Magnifier

- Rest the stand flat against the reading material.
- Do not move the stand.

Using a Spectacle-Mounted Magnifier

- Begin with the reading material close to the nose.
- Slowly move the material away until it becomes clear.

- Use large font and plain text (e.g., Arial, Helvetica, Times New Roman).
- Avoid italics, underline, and all caps.
- Use strong contrast: black on white or pale-colored paper.
- Avoid yellow or pale colors on colored background.
- Do not use glossy finished paper.
- Avoid placing text over graphics, photos, or illustrations.
- Use generous spacing and margins.

See ONLINE LEARNING ACTIVITY 17-6: DEVELOPING VISION-FRIENDLY TEACHING MATERIALS at http://thepoint.lww.com/Miller8e.

Unfolding Case Study

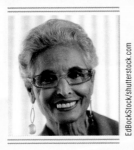

EdBockStock/shutterstock.com

Part 3: Mrs. F. at 81 Years of Age

Mrs. F. is now 81 years old. She had cataract surgery and an intraocular lens implanted in her left eye when she was 76 years old, and in her right eye when she was 77. Her vision was good until a year ago, when she developed macular degeneration. She knows this condition will be progressive, but she continues to drive and live alone. Her current medical conditions are arthritis, hypertension, and coronary artery disease. She quit smoking several years ago after she was hospitalized for coronary artery disease. You are the nurse at the senior care center where Mrs. F. comes for lunch several times a week. During an appointment with you, Mrs. F. confides that she is terrified of becoming totally blind and of losing her independence. Her grandmother went blind several years before she died and she had to go to a long-term care facility.

THINKING POINTS

- Which nursing diagnosis or diagnoses would you apply to Mrs. F. at this time?
- Which information in Boxes 17-4 through 17-9 might be appropriate for Mrs. F.?
- What health promotion advice would you give?

- Would you suggest any referrals for information or community resources?
- What interventions would address Mrs. F.'s fear of becoming blind and losing her independence?

QSEN APPLICATION

QSEN Competency	Knowledge/Skill/Attitude	Application to Mrs. F.
Patient-centered care	(K) Integrate understanding of multiple dimensions of patient-centered care	Take time to listen to Mrs. F. express her fears and concerns and help her identify her strengths and supports
	(K) Describe strategies to empower patients in all aspects of the health care process	Reassure Mrs. F. that there are many options available to help her remain as independent as possible, and these were not available when her grandmother had to move to a long-term care facility
	(S) Provide patient-centered care with sensitivity and respect for diversity of the human experience	
	(A) Value seeing health care situations "through patients' eyes"	
Teamwork and collaboration	(K) Recognize contributions of other individuals and groups in helping patient achieve health goals	Encourage Mrs. F. to contact the local sight center about their services and emphasize that their goal is to help people with vision loss to remain independent
	(S) Integrate the contributions of others who play a role in helping patient achieve health goals	

Maintaining and Improving the Quality of Life

As discussed earlier, the psychosocial consequences of impaired vision can be quite significant for older adults. Many of the interventions that help older adults compensate for visual deficits and function at their highest level will also improve their quality of life and address the psychosocial consequences of impaired vision. The use of appropriate reading glasses and good environmental lighting may enable the older adult to read books, newspapers, and magazines. Subsequently, their quality of life may improve because they experience satisfying social interactions and increased intellectual stimulation. Nurses also encourage participation in support and educational groups because these interventions serve an important role in improving the quality of life for people with significant or progressive vision loss.

Promoting Caregiver Wellness

When caring for someone who is visually impaired, it is important to address the needs of the spouse, family, and others who provide care and support. A primary intervention in these circumstances is to provide information about the many helpful resources available locally and through Internet sites. Caregivers of people who have dementia or other conditions that cause dependency may benefit from information about normal age-related vision changes, so they can take appropriate actions to detect eye disease and promote optimal vision. Nurses can use Box 17-10 for teaching caregivers and encouraging the use of helpful resources.

EVALUATING EFFECTIVENESS OF NURSING INTERVENTIONS

Nurses observe compensatory behaviors of visually impaired older adults to evaluate the effectiveness of interventions for Disturbed Sensory Perception: Visual. The following are indicators of successful interventions:

- Use of corrective lenses and low-vision aids to achieve the best possible visual function
- Adaptations of the environment for safety and improved visual function (e.g., bright, nonglare lighting, good color contrast)
- Expressed feelings of safety in relation to visual function
- Maximum independence in activities such as dressing, personal care, using appliances, and managing medications
- Expressed feelings of improved quality of life, despite visual impairments

Effectiveness of interventions to improve independence is evaluated by assessing and reassessing the older adult's abilities before and after interventions. When interventions address the psychosocial impact of visual impairment, observe the extent to which the person's quality of life and the ability to participate in enjoyable activities

---

Box 17-10 Caregiver Wellness: Vision and Aging

Normal Vision Changes in Older Adults

- Difficulty focusing on near objects, such as small print
- Increased sensitivity to glare
- Decreased contrast sensitivity
- Slower adaptation to changes in lighting
- Diminished depth perception
- Altered color perception
- Difficulty driving at night

Conditions Associated With Visual Impairment

- Lighting that is too dim or causes glare
- Eye diseases: cataracts, glaucoma, retinopathy, macular degeneration
- Conditions that increase the risk for eye disease: cigarette smoking, poor nutrition, exposure to sunlight, effects of some medications, family history of eye disease
- Chronic diseases that increase the risk for impaired vision: diabetes, hypertension, neurologic disease

Actions to Promote Vision Wellness

- Facilitate annual comprehensive eye examination, and immediately if a significant change in vision occurs
- Seek timely, professional, and ongoing advice about medical or surgical interventions for eye diseases (e.g., cataracts, glaucoma, macular degeneration)
- Recognize the importance of interventions for vision impairments as essential actions to improve safety, functioning, and quality of life
- Discuss concerns about driving with primary care practitioner and request appropriate professional evaluation
- Assure good nutrition
- Protect eyes from sunlight
- Provide good nonglare lighting
- Facilitate the use of low-vision aids

Resources for Support, Information, and Low-Vision Aids

American Foundation for the Blind, www.afb.org
EyeSmart, www.aao.org/eye-health
Lighthouse Guild, www.lighthouseguild.org
National Eye Institute, www.nei.nih.gov/healthyeyes
Prevent Blindness America, www.preventblindness.org
VisionAware, www.visionaware.org

---

is improved. For example, better lighting and the use of audiobooks or large-print books may enable someone to enjoy reading again. Nurses evaluate the effectiveness of health education interventions according to the person's expressed intent to follow through with the recommended referral or course of action. In home, community, and long-term care settings, nurses may be able to facilitate referrals for vision screening or other vision care services. In these settings, effectiveness of interventions is evaluated by obtaining feedback from older adults or their caregivers about the actual use of suggested resources.

 See ONLINE LEARNING ACTIVITY 17-7:
EVIDENCE-BASED PRACTICE
at http://thepoint.lww.com/Miller8e.

Unfolding Case Study

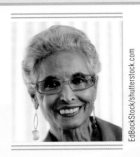

Part 4: Mrs. F. at 86 Years of Age

Mrs. F. is now 86 years old and is recovering from a recent fractured hip, which occurred when she fell while getting out of bed to go to the bathroom. After a brief hospitalization for surgical repair of the fractured hip and a 2-week period of skilled rehabilitation, Mrs. F. was referred to a home care agency for therapy, assessment, monitoring of her medical status, and evaluation of her ability to manage at home.

In addition to AMD, Mrs. F.'s current medical diagnoses include arthritis, hypertension, coronary artery disease, and heart failure. Mrs. F.'s medical conditions had been stable for several years, but during her hospitalization for the fractured hip, she was started on oxygen and her medications were changed. Current medications are furosemide 40 mg daily, digoxin 0.125 mg daily, and enalapril 10 mg twice daily. A 2-g sodium diet has been prescribed, and she has been discharged with an order for oxygen per nasal cannula at a rate of 2 L/min, as needed.

Before her accident, despite the visual limitations from AMD, Mrs. F. had lived alone in her own home, but her daughter has become increasingly concerned about her mother's safety. Now Mrs. F.'s daughter is convinced that her mother should not remain in her own home but should instead move to an assisted-living facility. Mrs. F. is adamant in her desire to stay in her own home and says the only reason she fell and broke her hip was because she was rushing to get to the bathroom. She says she has learned a lesson and will not hurry when she gets up at night. Furthermore, she says, she gave up driving to satisfy her daughter last year—now she is to give up her home, too? Mrs. F.'s daughter is staying with her mother for a few weeks until her mother regains her mobility to the point of independence. The daughter hopes that in the interim, she will be able to convince her mother to move to an assisted-living facility. You are the home care nurse working with Mrs. F. in her home.

NURSING ASSESSMENT

During your initial nursing assessment, you determine that Mrs. F. is motivated to regain her mobility and manage her medical conditions, but she has difficulty reading small-print instructions because of poor vision. When you review Mrs. F.'s medications with her, you observe that she cannot read the labels on the bottles. You also observe that Mrs. F. keeps her medications on the shelf above the kitchen counter, where the lighting is very dim. When you review the proper use of the oxygen, you notice that she has difficulty seeing the markings on the flow meter. Her daughter has been helping her with these regimens, but Mrs. F. hopes to perform these activities independently so she can remain in her own home.

Mrs. F. tells you that she is not concerned about falling because she walks slowly and carefully when she gets up during the night to go to the bathroom. She now uses a walker and says she feels safe. Her daughter expresses concern about her mother managing the oxygen and the walker when going to the bathroom. Mrs. F. uses the oxygen when she sleeps and her daughter is skeptical about her ability to get to the bathroom without rushing.

You observe that the hallway between the bedroom and bathroom is dark and that the bedroom has an overhead light but no bedside lamp. The bathroom has a narrow doorway, and the toilet is at the other side of the sink. You assess the home for safety and determine that the pathways are clear and there is good lighting on the stairway and in the living areas. You identify no additional risks (e.g., throw rugs) to Mrs. F.'s safe mobility, but you do have concerns about Mrs. F.'s ability to navigate safely to the toilet with a walker.

When questioned about her vision problems, Mrs. F. gives her history of successful cataract surgery and a diagnosis of AMD at the age of 80 years. Although her ophthalmologist has told her that her vision will get worse and that he can't do anything about it, she has talked with friends who say they are getting treatments. He had mentioned that the local sight center provides some rehabilitation services for people with low vision, but he told her that those services are mostly for "younger blind people." She is concerned also that the sight center will suggest she purchase items that cost a lot of money, which she would not be able to afford. She says her daughter got her a subscription for the large-print *Reader's Digest,* which she enjoys, and that she is not interested in reading the newspaper because she watches the news on television. She has an appointment to see her eye doctor next month.

Part 4: Mrs. F. at 86 Years of Age (Continued)

NURSING DIAGNOSIS

In the absence of a nursing diagnosis that directly addresses sensory perception, you apply the nursing diagnosis of Ineffective Health Management to address the effects of visual impairment on Mrs. F.'s safety and management of medical conditions. Supporting evidence for this diagnosis can be found in Mrs. F.'s inability to read labels, instructions, or the flow meter markings, and the environmental factors that contribute to unsafe mobility. This diagnosis prompts you to include a long-term goal of encouraging further evaluation and management of the visual impairments. In addition, the nursing diagnoses of Anxiety, Self-Care Deficit, and Risk for Injury might also be applicable to address the functional consequences of Mrs. F.'s visual impairments.

NURSING CARE PLAN FOR MRS. F.

Expected Outcome	Nursing Interventions	Nursing Evaluation
Mrs. F. will manage her medication regimen accurately and independently	• Print simplified medication instructions on large index cards by using black felt-tip marker • Use colored dots to match pill bottles with instruction cards • Establish a medication management system by using pill organizer boxes with markings that are bold and have good color contrast • Teach Mrs. F. how to fill the pill boxes weekly, using the index cards you prepared for her • Suggest that Mrs. F. fill the pill boxes at the kitchen table during daylight hours while using overhead light	• Mrs. F. will demonstrate that she can accurately fill the pill boxes • Mrs. F. will take her medications correctly • Mrs. F.'s daughter will observe that her mother follows the prescribed regimen
Mrs. F. will self-administer oxygen as needed	• Use a copy machine to enlarge the small-print instructions for the oxygen equipment • Place a colored dot at the 2-L mark on the flow meter • Keep the oxygen tank in a well-lit location and suggest using a flashlight to help illuminate the flow meter setting	• Mrs. F. will demonstrate a safe and independent operation of the oxygen equipment • Mrs. F.'s daughter will observe that her mother administers her oxygen correctly
Mrs. F. will be able to use a commode safely and independently	• Ask Mrs. F. to use a bedside commode during the night; emphasize the importance of preventing another fall • Work with physical and occupational therapists to (1) evaluate the feasibility of installing grab bars or other devices that will assist Mrs. F. in safely using the toilet, (2) identify a safe way for Mrs. F. to use the bathroom during the daytime, (3) teach Mrs. F. to transfer between the bed and commode for nighttime use, (4) teach her to empty the bedside commode • Place a lamp on the nightstand and make sure that Mrs. F. can turn it on easily while in bed. Teach Mrs. F. to turn the bedside lamp on and sit at the edge of the bed for a few minutes before getting up at night	• Mrs. F. will demonstrate that she can safely use the bathroom during the day and a bedside commode at night • Mrs. F. will be able to empty the commode independently • Mrs. F. will have no further falls in the bathroom
Mrs. F. will compensate as much as possible for her progressive visual loss	• Educate Mrs. F. and her daughter about the services provided at the local sight center for people with low vision; emphasize that these services address the needs of older adults and people with recent and progressive visual loss. The services are for anyone with low vision, and there are many low-vision aids available to improve the visual function of people with macular degeneration • Suggest that Mrs. F. ask her eye doctor for a referral to the sight center when she sees him next month • Include Mrs. F.'s daughter in the discussion about these services, and ask her to assist with following through once a referral is obtained	• Mrs. F. will make and keep an appointment for an initial evaluation at the sight center • Mrs. F. will use low-vision aids to improve visual function

(continued)

Part 4: Mrs. F. at 86 Years of Age *(Continued)*

THINKING POINTS

- How would you address concerns about Mrs. F. living alone? What aspects of her safety and quality of life would you consider?
- How would you use any of the boxes in this chapter for health promotion teaching?
- What additional nursing diagnoses and outcomes would you identify for Mrs. F.?

- What additional interventions and referrals would you consider for Mrs. F.?
- Identify at least one resource in your community that might provide help or information for Mrs. F. Call that agency to obtain information about their services.

QSEN APPLICATION

QSEN Competency	Knowledge/Skill/Attitude	Application to Mrs. F.
Patient-centered care	(K) Integrate understanding of multiple dimensions of patient-centered care	Recognize that the concerns and needs of Mrs. F. and her daughter are not the same and facilitate a conversation with both of them
	(K) Examine nursing roles in assuring coordination, integration, and continuity of care	Obtain permission from Mrs. F. and her daughter to have the social worker from your home care agency visit to talk with both of them about options for care (e.g., home care assistance, home-delivered meals)
	(S) Elicit patient values, preferences, and expressed needs	
	(S) Provide patient-centered care with sensitivity and respect for diversity of the human experience	Emphasize that the social worker can assist them with making decisions about a plan of care that is mutually acceptable
	(S) Assess own level of communication skill in encounters with patients and families	
	(A) Value seeing health care situations "through patients' eyes"	
Teamwork and collaboration	(K) Recognize contributions of other individuals and groups in helping patient achieve health goals	Provide care coordination for all health care professionals involved with Mrs. F.'s care, including physical and occupational therapists, social workers, and respiratory supply company
	(K) Describe impact of own communication style on others	
	(S) Integrate the contributions of others who play a role in helping patient achieve health goals	Encourage Mrs. F. and her daughter to call the sight center and request that a low-vision specialist make a home visit to assess the need for low-vision aids and teaching about safe and independent functioning

Chapter Highlights

Age-Related Changes That Affect Vision (Figure 17-1; Tables 17-1 and 17-2)

- Changes in appearance include arcus senilis, loss of orbital fat, and diminished elasticity of eyelid muscles
- Diminished tear production
- Degenerative changes affect all structures of the eye, the retinal–neural pathway, and the visual cortex of the brain

Effects of Age-Related Changes on Vision (Figure 17-2)

- Diminished ability to focus clearly on objects at various distances

- Diminished ability to detect details and discern objects
- Slower adaptive response to changes in lighting
- Increased sensitivity to glare
- Narrowed visual field
- Diminished depth perception
- Altered color perception so objects look darker and whites appear more yellowed
- Diminished ability to perceive flashing lights
- Slower processing of visual information

Risk Factors That Affect Visual Wellness

- Environmental factors: glare, sunlight, poor lighting, low humidity
- Lifestyle factors: poor nutrition, cigarette smoking

- Chronic conditions: diabetes, hypertension, Alzheimer or Parkinson disease
- Adverse medication effects: estrogen, corticosteroids, anticholinergics, beta blockers, antiparkinson agents

Functional Consequences Affecting Visual Wellness (Figure 17-3)

- Presbyopia (diminished ability to focus on near objects)
- Need for three to five times more light than previously
- Difficulty with night driving
- Increased risk for unsafe mobility and falls
- Increased difficulty in performing usual activities

Pathologic Conditions Affecting Vision (Figures 17-4 and 17-5; Table 17-3)

- Cataracts
- AMD
- Glaucoma

Nursing Assessment of Vision (Boxes 17-1 to 17-3)

- Vision-screening tests
- Risk factors that affect vision
- Influence of vision changes on performance of activities of daily living
- Attitudes about eye examinations and preventive measures
- Attitudes regarding use of low-vision aids

Nursing Diagnosis

- Readiness for Enhanced Knowledge: Improved Vision
- Diagnoses that address the functional consequences of visual impairment include the following: Anxiety, Ineffective Coping, Self-Care Deficit, Risk for Injury, Impaired Social Interaction, Readiness for Enhanced Coping, and Readiness for Enhanced Self-Care

Planning for Wellness Outcomes

- Improved visual function
- Increased safety
- Improved independence in activities of daily living
- Improved quality of life

Nursing Interventions for Visual Wellness (Boxes 17-4 to 17-9)

- Prevention and detection of eye disease
- Comfort measures for dry eyes
- Environmental modifications (e.g., optimal illumination)
- Low-vision aids

Evaluating Effectiveness of Nursing Interventions

- Use of corrective lenses and other aids that improve vision
- Environmental adaptations for optimal safety and visual function

- Improved independence in daily activities
- Expressed feelings of improved quality of life in relation to visual function

Critical Thinking Exercises

1. Describe presbyopia and explain the functional consequences of this condition in the everyday life of an older adult.
2. What environmental factors are likely to interfere with the visual function of older adults?
3. Describe the specific effects of glaucoma, cataracts, or AMD on one's ability to see a television program.
4. How would you assess the visual abilities of an older adult?
5. Explain the differences between opticians, optometrists, and ophthalmologists.
6. List at least 10 adaptations that might be implemented to improve the visual function of older adults.

 For more information about the topics discussed in this chapter, be sure to check out the interactive Online Learning Activities and other helpful resources at http://thepoint.lww.com/Miller8e.

REFERENCES

Action to Control Cardiovascular Risk in Diabetes Follow-On Eye Study Group. (2016). Persistent effects of intensive glycemic control on retinopathy in type 2 diabetes in the Action to Control Cardiovascular Risk in Diabetes (ACCORD) Follow-on Study. *Diabetes Care, 39,* 1089–1100.

Agramunt, S., Meuleners, L. B., Fraser, M. L., et al. (2016). Bilateral cataract, crash risk, driving performance, and self-regulation practices among older drivers. *Journal of Cataract and Refractive Surgery, 42,* 788–794.

Armstrong, R. A. (2016). Visual signs and symptoms of corticobasal degeneration. *Clinical & Experimental Ophthalmology, 23,* doi: 10.1111/cxo.12429.

Blane, A. (2016). Through the looking glass: A review of the literature investigating the impact of glaucoma on crash risk, driving performance, and driver self-regulation in older drivers. *Journal of Glaucoma, 25,* 113–121.

Chen, X., & Lu, L. (2016). Depression in diabetic retinopathy: A review and recommendation for psychiatric management. *Psychosomatics, 57,* 465–471.

Cimarolli, V. R., Boerner, K., Reinhardt, J. P., et al. (2017). A population study of correlates of social participation in older adults with age-related vision loss. *Clinical Rehabilitation, 31,* 115–125.

Cimarolli, V. R., Casten, R. J., Rovner, B. W., et al. (2016). Anxiety and depression in patients with advanced macular degeneration: Current perspectives. *Clinical Ophthalmology, 10,* 55–63.

Diniz-Filho, A., Abe, R., Cho, H., et al. (2016). Fast visual field progression is associated with depressive symptoms in patients with glaucoma. *Ophthalmology, 123,* 754–759.

Draper, E., Feng, R., Appel, S., et al. (2016). Low vision rehabilitation for adult African Americans in two settings. *Optometry and Vision Science, 93,* 673–682.

Hanna, K. L., Hepworth, L. R., & Rowe, F. (2016). Screening methods for post-stroke visual impairment: A systematic review. *Disability Rehabilitation,* doi: 10.1080/09638288.2016.1231846.

Herren, D. J., & Kohanim, S. (2016). Disparities in vision loss due to cataracts in Hispanic women in the United States. *Seminars in Ophthalmology, 31,* 353–357.

Iroku-Malize, T., & Kirsch, S. (2016). Eye conditions in older adults: Cataracts. *Family Physician Essentials, 445,* 17–23.

Kang, J., Wu, J., Cho, E., et al. (2016). Contribution of the Nurses' Health Study to the epidemiology of cataract, age-related macular degeneration, and glaucoma. *American Journal of Public Health, 106,* 1684–1689.

Mönestam, E. (2016). Long-term outcomes of cataract surgery: A 15-year results of a prospective study. *Journal of Cataract & Refractive Surgery, 42,* 19–26.

National Academies of Sciences, Engineering, and Medicine. (2016). *Making eye health a population health imperative: Vision for tomorrow.* Washington, DC: The National Academies Press.

National Center for Health Statistics. (2016). *Health, United States, 2015.* Washington, DC: U.S. Government Printing Office.

Nollett, C., Bray, N., Bunce, C., et al. (2016). High prevalence of untreated depression in patients accessing low-vision services. *Ophthalmology, 123,* 440–441.

Pal, A., Biswas, A., Pandit, A., et al. (2016). Study of visuospatial skill in patients with dementia. *Annals of the Indian Academy of Neurology, 19,* 83–88.

Sand, K., Wilhelmsen, G., Naess, J., et al. (2016). Vision problems in ischaemic stroke patients: Effects on life quality and disability. *European Journal of Neurology, 23* Suppl 1, 1–7.

Stewart, M. (2016). Treatment of diabetic retinopathy: Recent advances and unresolved challenges. *World Journal of Diabetes, 7,* 333–341.

Taylor, H. R. (2016). The global issue of vision loss and what we can do about it: Jose Rizal Medal 2015. *Asia Pacific Journal of Ophthalmology, 5,* 95–96.

van Nispen, R., Vreeken, H., Comijs, H., et al. (2016). Role of vision loss, functional limitations and the supporting network in depression in a general population. *Acta Ophthalmology, 94,* 76–82.

Varma, R., Vajaranant, T., Burkemper, B., et al. (2016). Visual impairment and blindness in adults in the United States: Demographic and geographic variations from 2015 to 2050. *JAMA Ophthalmology, 134,* 802–809.

Weil, R., Schrag, A., Warren, J., et al. (2016). Visual dysfunction in Parkinson's Disease. *Brain: A Journal of Neurology,* doi: 10.1093/brain/aww175.

Wood, J., Black, A., Mallon, K., et al. (2016). Glaucoma and driving: On-road driving characteristics. *PLOS One,* doi: 10.1371/journal.pone.0158318.

Zetterberg, M. (2016). Age-related eye disease and gender. *Maturitas, 83,* 19–26.

chapter 18

Digestion and Nutrition

KEY TERMS

constipation	malnutrition
dehydration	Mini Nutritional Assessment (MNA)
dysphagia	
food insecurity	olfaction
gustatory function	xerostomia

Digestion of food and maintenance of nutrition are influenced to a small degree by age-related gastrointestinal changes and to a large degree by risk factors that affect most older adults. Although older adults can easily compensate for age-related changes in the digestive tract, they have more difficulty compensating for the many factors that interfere with their ability to obtain, prepare, and enjoy food. This chapter discusses age-related changes and functional consequences in relation to digestion, eating patterns, and nutritional requirements.

AGE-RELATED CHANGES THAT AFFECT DIGESTION AND EATING PATTERNS

Age-related changes affect the senses of smell and taste and all the organs of the digestive tract. Studies have concluded that the gastrointestinal tract has a vast functional reserve, and aging itself is not the primary cause of digestive problems in the elderly (Gidwaney, Bajpai, & Chokhavatia, 2016). Older adults are likely to experience disorders of the gastrointestinal tract because of commonly occurring conditions, as discussed in the section on Risk Factors that Affect Digestion and Nutrition.

Smell and Taste

The senses of taste and smell affect food enjoyment, and both these senses decline in older adults because of a combination of age-related changes and risk factors. **Olfaction** (i.e., the ability to smell odors) depends on the perception of odorants by the sensory cells in the nasal mucosa and on central nervous system processing of that information. The ability to detect and identify odors is best between the ages of 30 and 40 years, then it gradually declines, which is only partially attributable to age-related changes. The U.S. National Health and Nutrition Examination Survey (NHANES) reported prevalence rates for self-reported impaired sense of smell as follows: 4.2% for adults aged 40 to 49, 12.7% for those aged 60 to 69, and 39.4% for adults aged 80 years and older (Hoffman, Rawal, Li, et al., 2016). One current focus of research is determining whether diminished olfactory function is an early diagnostic marker for neurodegenerative diseases, such as Parkinson disease and Alzheimer disease (Devanand, 2016; Liang, Ding, Zhao,

Promoting Digestive and Nutritional Wellness in Older Adults

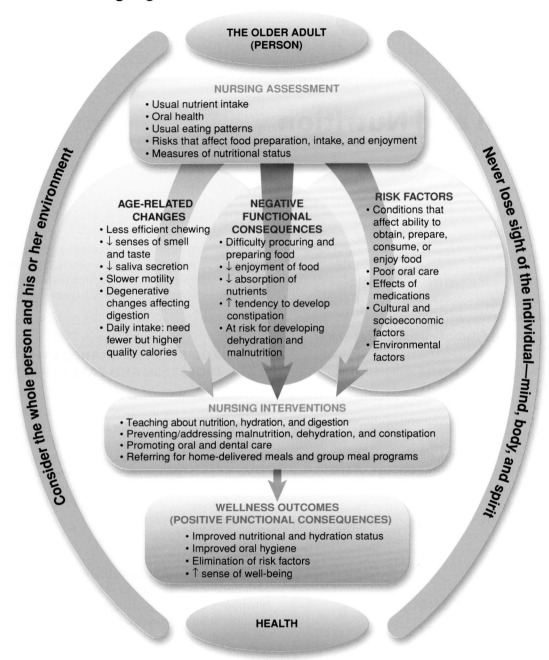

THE OLDER ADULT
(PERSON)

NURSING ASSESSMENT

- Usual nutrient intake
- Oral health
- Usual eating patterns
- Risks that affect food preparation, intake, and enjoyment
- Measures of nutritional status

AGE-RELATED CHANGES

- Less efficient chewing
- ↓ senses of smell and taste
- ↓ saliva secretion
- Slower motility
- Degenerative changes affecting digestion
- Daily intake: need fewer but higher quality calories

NEGATIVE FUNCTIONAL CONSEQUENCES

- Difficulty procuring and preparing food
- ↓ enjoyment of food
- ↓ absorption of nutrients
- ↑ tendency to develop constipation
- At risk for developing dehydration and malnutrition

RISK FACTORS

- Conditions that affect ability to obtain, prepare, consume, or enjoy food
- Poor oral care
- Effects of medications
- Cultural and socioeconomic factors
- Environmental factors

NURSING INTERVENTIONS

- Teaching about nutrition, hydration, and digestion
- Preventing/addressing malnutrition, dehydration, and constipation
- Promoting oral and dental care
- Referring for home-delivered meals and group meal programs

WELLNESS OUTCOMES (POSITIVE FUNCTIONAL CONSEQUENCES)

- Improved nutritional and hydration status
- Improved oral hygiene
- Elimination of risk factors
- ↑ sense of well-being

HEALTH

Consider the whole person and his or her environment

Never lose sight of the individual—mind, body, and spirit

et al., 2016; Ottaviano, Frasson, Nardello, et al., 2016). Conditions that can lead to impaired olfaction include smoking or chewing tobacco, viruses, poor oral health, periodontal disease, nasal sinus disease, trauma, and medications (e.g., diuretics and antidepressants). Thus, although decline in olfactory function occurs more commonly with increasing age, there is evidence that it may be at least partly preventable (Schubert, Fischer, Pinto, et al., 2017).

The ability to taste, called **gustatory function**, depends primarily on receptor cells in the taste buds, which are located on the tongue, palate, and tonsils. Characteristics of taste sensation are measured according to the ability to perceive the intensity of flavors and to identify specific flavors. Diminished taste sensation is common in older adults, with increased prevalence in those who are age 80 or older and those who have chronic conditions (Correia, Lopez, Wroblewski, et al., 2016; Ogawa, Uota, Ikebe, et al., 2016). Common causes of taste disorders are head trauma, radiation, upper respiratory tract infections, medical conditions (e.g., diabetes or hypothyroidism). Recent studies indicate that gustatory function declines gradually in people with Alzheimer disease as the condition progresses (Sakai, Ikeda, Kazui, et al., 2016).

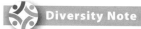
Diversity Note

Throughout life, both the senses of smell and taste are better in women than in men, and these differences increase during later adulthood (Ogawa, Uota, Ikebe, et al., 2017).

Oral Cavity

Digestion begins when food enters the mouth and is acted on by the teeth, saliva, and neuromuscular structures responsible for mastication. Age-related changes in the teeth and support structures influence digestive processes and food enjoyment. With increased age, the tooth enamel becomes harder and more brittle, the dentin becomes more fibrous, and the nerve chambers become shorter and narrower. Because of these age-related changes, the teeth are less sensitive to stimuli and more susceptible to fractures. These changes, along with decades of abrasive and erosive action, also cause a gradual flattening of the chewing cusps. The bones supporting the teeth of older adults diminish in height and density, and teeth may loosen or fall out, particularly in the presence of pathologic conditions (e.g., periodontal disease).

Saliva and the oral mucosa play important roles in digestion. Age-related changes of the oral mucosa include loss of elasticity, atrophy of epithelial cells, and diminished blood supply to the connective tissue. These changes can be exacerbated by conditions common in older adults (e.g., chronic disease, vitamin deficiencies), making the oral mucosa more friable and susceptible to infection and ulceration. Diminished muscle strength is an age-related neuromuscular change that can have a small effect on mastication and swallowing. In the absence of risk factors, however, healthy older adults will not experience significant swallowing problems (as discussed in the Dysphagia section later in this chapter).

Saliva is essential for chewing, swallowing, and maintenance of a moist oral mucosa. Saliva facilitates digestion by supplying digestive enzymes, regulating oral flora, cleansing the taste buds, lubricating the soft tissue, and preparing food for chewing. Although significant hyposalivation (i.e., decreased salivary flow) is not an inherent age-related change, about one-third of older adults experience **xerostomia** (i.e., decreased salivation and uncomfortable dry mouth) because of risk factors (Baer & Walitt, 2017). The most common causes of xerostomia in older adults are chronic conditions (e.g., Sjögren syndrome, malnutrition, renal dialysis), radiation to the head and neck, and adverse medication effects. Xerostomia affects nutrition and gastrointestinal function because it is associated with all the following (Gil-Montoya, Silvestre, Barrios, et al., 2016; Tanasiewicz, Hildebrandt, & Oberszytn, 2016):

- Altered chewing, swallowing, speaking
- Dry, cracked lips
- Burning sensation in mouth and lips
- Dry mucous membrane
- Diminished taste, especially for bitter and salty flavors
- Dental caries and increased plaque
- Gingivitis and periodontitis

Esophagus and Stomach

The second phase of digestion occurs when a combination of propulsive and nonpropulsive waves propels food through the pharynx and esophagus into the stomach. In older adults, the esophagus stiffens and peristaltic waves decrease. After passing through the esophageal sphincter, food enters the stomach, where gastric enzymes liquefy it and gastric action transforms it into chyme. Although reduced gastric acid secretions are sometimes attributed to age-related changes, studies indicate that this reduction is caused primarily by atrophic gastritis or prolonged use of proton pump inhibitors (Soenen, Rayner, Jones, et al., 2016). Consequences of reduced gastric acid include malabsorption of increased bacterial overgrowth in the intestinal tract and malabsorption of iron, calcium, and vitamin B_{12} (Schubert, 2016). Slowing of gastric emptying is an age-related change that can lead to anorexia and inadequate energy intake.

Intestinal Tract

After the chyme passes into the small intestine, digestive enzymes from the small intestine, liver, and pancreas convert the food substances into nutrients. A process of segmentation moves the chyme backward and forward, facilitating the digestion of food and the absorption of nutrients through the villi in the walls of the small intestine. Age-related degenerative changes in the small intestine do not significantly affect digestive functions; however, they may affect immune function and absorption of some nutrients, such as folate, calcium, and vitamins B_{12} and D.

After nutrients are absorbed in the small intestine, the chyme passes into the large intestine, where water and electrolytes are absorbed and waste products are expelled. Age-related changes in the large intestine include reduced secretion of mucus and decreased elasticity of the rectal wall. Although these age-related changes do not significantly affect motility of feces through the bowel, they may predispose the older person to constipation.

Liver, Pancreas, and Gallbladder

The liver assists digestion by producing and secreting bile, which is essential for utilizing fats. It also plays an important role in metabolizing and storing medications and nutrients. With increasing age, the liver becomes smaller and more fibrous, and blood flow to the liver decreases by approximately one-third. However, some of these changes may be pathologic, rather than age related, in origin. Despite any age-related or pathologic changes, the liver has an enormous regenerative and reserve capacity, which allows it to compensate for such changes without significantly affecting digestive function.

A primary digestive function of the pancreas is the secretion of enzymes essential for metabolizing glucose, neutralizing acids in the chyme, and breaking down fats, proteins, and carbohydrates in the small intestine. Degenerative age-related changes in the pancreas increase the susceptibility of older adults to the development of type 2 diabetes.

Age-related changes that affect the gallbladder and biliary tract include diminished bile acid synthesis, widening of the common bile duct, and increased secretion of cholecystokinin, a peptide hormone that contracts the gallbladder and relaxes the biliary sphincter. These age-related changes can increase the susceptibility of older adults to the development of cholelithiasis (gallstones).

NUTRITIONAL REQUIREMENTS FOR HEALTHY AGING

Good nutrition is widely recognized as a major component of healthy aging, as evidenced by the statement that "accumulating data strongly indicate that nutrition is the most important intervention for the promotion of health and the prevention of the great majority of age-associated chronic diseases" (Bertozzi, Tosti, & Fontana, 2017, p. 14). Nutritional deficiencies—which increase the risk for frailty, poor functioning, and pathologic conditions—occur commonly in older adults, as discussed in the section on Risk Factors that Affect Digestion and Nutrition. This section focuses on current recommendations and research related to nutritional requirements for healthy aging.

The Dietary Guidelines Advisory Committee (2015) and the National Academies of Sciences, Engineering, and Medicine (2016) have published reports that cite specific concerns related to nutrients of particular importance to older adults, as summarized in Box 18-1. In addition to the concerns summarized in Box 18-1, current emphasis is on overall dietary patterns and diet quality in relation to healthy aging and chronic diseases that are common in older adults (Milte & McNaughton, 2016). Following are examples of

---

E·B·P | **Box 18-1 Evidence-Based Practice: Nutrients of Particular Importance to Older Adults**

Protein

- Protein deficiency is associated with loss of muscle tissue and increased risk for sarcopenia and frailty
- Current recommended dietary allowance for protein (i.e., .8 g/kg/day) is the same for all adults, without consideration of increased age
- Many recent studies indicate that daily protein intake of 1.2 to 1.5 g/kg is safe for older adults and is beneficial in preserving muscle mass
- A substantial percentage of older adults do not meet current recommended protein intake

Fiber

- Dietary fiber is essential for maintaining colonic functioning
- There is increasing evidence suggesting that fiber is important for preventing coronary heart disease, colorectal and other cancers, type 2 diabetes, and obesity
- Average intake of dietary fiber is half the recommended levels

Folate

- Important for cognitive function, DNA methylation, and preventing high levels of homocysteine
- Some older adults do not meet the RDA, others exceed the upper limit and get too much of synthetic folic acid from fortified foods (e.g., cereals) and supplements
- Excess intake of folate can mask vitamin B_{12} deficiencies, which can cause neurologic deterioration
- Women ages 71 and older tend to have insufficient folate from foods

Vitamin D

- Inadequate Vitamin D intake increases the risk for osteoporosis, neurologic conditions, cardiovascular disease, and other chronic diseases
- Inadequate exposure to sunlight

Calcium

- Low intake of calcium affects many systems, including the skeletal, cardiovascular, and neurologic systems
- Inadequate dietary intake of calcium is common in older adults

Magnesium

- Important for maintaining normal blood pressure
- Low intake associated with diabetes
- Major shortfall in older population

Potassium

- Potassium is considered a "nutrient of public health concern" because of its critical roles in muscle function, cardiac function, and regulation of blood pressure
- Underconsumption of potassium occurs across all groups, but is of particular concern for older adults because of their increased risk for cardiovascular disease

Zinc

- Zinc deficiency occurs commonly in older adults and leads to anorexia, impaired immune function, delayed wound healing, and smell and taste disturbances

Sodium

- Overconsumption of sodium is considered a "nutrient of public health concern" because of its association with adverse health events, such as hypertension

Saturated Fat

- Adults aged 50 and older are the group at highest risk for adverse effects of excessive intake of saturated fats
- Overconsumption of dietary fats is associated with increased risk for cardiovascular disease

Sources: National Academies of Sciences, Engineering, and Medicine. (2016). *Meeting the Dietary Needs of Older Adults: Exploring the Impact of the Physical, Social, and Cultural Environments, Workshop Summary.* Washington, DC: National Academies Press, doi: 10.17226/23496; Dietary Guidelines Advisory Committee (2015). Scientific report of the 2015 Dietary Guidelines Advisory Committee. Washington, DC: U.S. Department of Agriculture; Pisano, M., & Hilas, O. (2016). Zinc and taste disturbances in older adults: A review of the literature. *Consultant Pharmacist: The Journal of the American Society of Consultant Pharmacists, 31,* 267–270; Witard, O. C., McGlory, C., Hamilton, D. L., et al. (2016). Growing older with health and vitality: a nexus of physical activity, exercise and nutrition. *Biogerontology, 17,* 529–546.

recent studies that addressed dietary patterns associated with healthy aging:

- Diets rich in omega-3 fatty acids, such as those found in fish, are important for promoting healthy aging and preventing age-associated chronic conditions (Casas-Agustench, Cherubini, & Andres-Lacueva, 2017; Cederholm, 2017).
- The Mediterranean-style diet is considered the "gold standard" for healthy aging and increased life expectancy (Bihuniak, Ramos, Huedo-Medina, et al., 2016; Martínez-González & Martin-Calvo, 2016; Struijk, Guallar-Castillón, Rodríguez-Artalejo, et al., 2016).
- Studies have found the following specific health benefits associated with the Mediterranean diet for older adults: less atrophy of brain tissue (Luciano, Corley, Cox, et al., 2017), prevention of cardiovascular disease (Martínez-González, 2016), and lower risk of hip fracture (Byberg, Bellavia, Larsson, et al., 2016).
- Increased intake of whole grains and fiber-rich food is associated with successful aging and reduced all-cause mortality (Gopinath, Flood, Kifley, et al., 2016; Kim & Je, 2016; Li, Zhang, Tan, et al., 2016).
- Diets rich in plant-based and unprocessed foods are associated with reduced risk for diabetes, hypertension, obesity, cardiovascular disease, and neurodegenerative diseases (Anderson & Nieman, 2016).
- The following changes would better align the diet quality of older Americans with dietary guidelines: increased intake of whole grains, vegetables and legumes, fat-free and low-fat milk products, and foods and beverages that are lower in sodium and have fewer calories from solids, fats, and added sugars (Federal Interagency Forum on Aging-Related Statistics, 2016).

An additional recommendation related to dietary patterns for older adults is that caloric intake be gradually reduced beginning between the ages of 40 and 50 years. This decrease in caloric intake requires a proportionate increase in the quality of calories (nutritional density) to meet minimal nutritional requirements.

 RISK FACTORS THAT AFFECT DIGESTION AND NUTRITION

Certain behaviors and common disease processes are likely to interfere with nutrition and digestion in older adults. Some detrimental behaviors, such as limiting fluid intake and avoiding fresh fruit, may be based on myths and misconceptions. Although these conditions can create risks for people at any age, they occur more commonly in older adults, and the potential for harm is much greater than in other age groups because of the cumulative effects of risk factors and age-related changes. Risk factors affect every phase of digestion and nutrition, and they can significantly influence eating patterns and nutritional intake. Functional and cognitive impairment is a risk factor that is closely associated with inadequate nutritional intake in older adults in all settings. Risks that can

cause specific nutrient deficiencies are listed in Table 18-1, along with the related functional consequences.

Conditions Related to Oral Care

Oral health influences nutritional status because it affects chewing, eating, swallowing, speaking, and social interaction. Until recently, being edentulous (i.e., having no natural teeth) was so common among older people that it has been inaccurately viewed as a normal consequence of aging. Although the percentage of older adults who are edentulous is gradually diminishing, 25% of older adults aged 75 to 84 and 31% of those aged 85 or older have no natural teeth (Federal Interagency Forum on Aging-Related Statistics, 2016).

Older adults who have natural teeth often have inadequate dental care, periodontal disease, and other pathologic conditions that occur with increasing frequency in later years. In addition, because preventive dental care is a recent trend, older adults may falsely believe that they should visit a dentist only when a toothache does not respond to home remedies. Some factors that contribute to inadequate dental care include low income, less education, lack of transportation, lack of dental insurance, high cost of dental services, more pressing health concerns, and inaccessibility of services.

Inadequate oral care, as indicated by greater bacterial plaque and gingival bleeding, is common in older adults who are cognitively impaired (Gil-Montoya, Sánchez-Lara, Carnero-Pardo, et al., 2017). For people with dementia, daily oral care, prevalence of dental problems, and frequency of professional dental care are conditions that gradually worsen as the degree of cognitive impairment increases. Adverse effects of poor oral health include malnutrition, dehydration, periodontal disease, respiratory infections (e.g., pneumonia and aspiration pneumonia), joint infections, cardiovascular disease, poor glycemic control in diabetes, and increased risk of stroke and heart attack. Because oral health is pertinent to nutrition and digestion, nursing responsibilities are discussed in the sections on Promoting Oral and Dental Health.

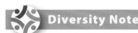 **Diversity Note**

Older African Americans, American Indians, and Alaska Natives are more likely than white Americans to have greater tooth loss.

Wellness Opportunity

Nurses promote wellness by exploring reasons why older adults do not obtain dental care so that these barriers can be addressed.

Functional Impairments and Disease Processes

Functional impairments are strongly associated with poor nutrition, particularly regarding dependence on others for assistance with eating. For example, impaired mobility or vision can interfere with the ability to procure and prepare food. In community settings, the extent to which functional

TABLE 18-1 Causes and Consequences of Nutrient Deficiencies

Nutrient	Possible Causes of Deficiency	Functional Consequences of Deficiency
Calories	Anorexia, depression, mental or physical impairments	Weight loss, lethargy, edema, anemia
Protein	Lack of teeth or dentures, anorexia, depression, dementia, high alcohol or carbohydrate consumption	Poor tissue healing, hypoalbuminemia, reduced protein binding of drugs
Fat	Neomycin, phenytoin, laxatives, alcohol, colchicine, cholestyramine	Inability to absorb vitamins A, D, E, and K
Vitamin A	Mineral oil, neomycin, alcohol, cholestyramine, aluminum antacids, liver disease	Dry skin and eyes, photophobia, night blindness, hyperkeratosis
Thiamine (B_1)	High consumption of alcohol or caffeinated tea, pernicious anemia, diuretics	Neuropathy, muscle weakness, heart disease, dementia, anorexia
Riboflavin (B_2)	Malabsorption syndromes, chronic diarrhea laxative abuse, alcoholism, liver disease	Cheilitis, glossitis, photophobia, blepharitis, conjunctivitis
Niacin (B_3)	Poor dietary patterns, diarrhea, cirrhosis, alcoholism	Dermatitis, stomatitis, diarrhea, dementia, depression
Pyridoxine (B_6)	Diuretics, hydralazine	Dermatitis, neuropathy
Folate (B_9)	Anticonvulsants, triamterene, sulfonamides, alcohol, smoking	Macrocytic anemia, elevated levels of homocysteine
Vitamin B_{12}	Malabsorption syndrome, H_2-receptor blockers, proton pump inhibitors, colchicine, oral hypoglycemics, potassium supplements, vegetarian diet	Pernicious anemia, weakness, dyspnea, glossitis, numbness, dementia, depression
Vitamin C	Aspirin, tetracycline, lack of fruits and vegetables in diet	Lassitude, irritability, anemia, ecchymosis, impaired wound healing
Vitamin D	Phenytoin, mineral oil, phenobarbital, sunlight deprivation	Muscle weakness and atrophy, osteoporosis, fractures
Vitamin E	Malabsorption syndromes	Peripheral neuropathy, gait disturbance, retinopathy
Vitamin K	Mineral oil, warfarin sodium (Coumadin), antibiotics, cholestyramine, phenytoin	Ecchymosis; hemorrhage involving the gastrointestinal, urinary, or central nervous system
Calcium	Phenytoin, aluminum-based antacids, laxatives, tetracycline, corticosteroids, furosemide, high intake of fiber or caffeine	Osteoporosis, fractures, low back pain
Iron	Achlorhydria; neomycin; aspirin; antacids; low intake of animal protein; high consumption of fiber, caffeine, or tannic acid (contained in some teas)	Anemia, weakness, lassitude, pallor
Magnesium	Alcohol, diuretics, diarrhea, bulk-forming laxatives	Cardiac arrhythmias, neuromuscular and central nervous system irritability, disorientation
Zinc	Penicillamine, aluminum-based antacids, bulk-forming laxatives, high consumption of fiber	Poor wound healing, hair loss
Potassium	Laxatives, furosemide, antibiotics, corticosteroids, diarrhea	Weakness, cardiac arrhythmias, digitalis toxicity
Water	Diuretics, laxatives, immobility, incontinence, diarrhea	Dry skin and mouth, dehydration, constipation
Fiber	Poor dietary patterns	Constipation, hemorrhoids

impairments affect nutrition depends to a large degree on the availability of social supports, such as family, friends, or agencies that assist with providing food.

Pathologic processes increase the risk for nutritional and digestive consequences in many ways. For example, vitamin B_{12} deficiency, which is more common with increasing age, can interfere with absorption of nutrients. Pathologic conditions also can interfere with appetite and enjoyment of food in many ways. For example, infections, hyperthyroidism, hypoadrenalism, and heart failure are associated with anorexia, and chronic obstructive pulmonary disease is associated with both decreased appetite and increased energy expenditure. Dementia and other neurodegenerative disorders often have serious negative effects on eating and nutrition related to procuring and preparing food, remembering to eat, and chewing and swallowing food.

Dysphagia

Dysphagia (i.e., difficulty during any phase of the swallowing process) is a functional impairment that can significantly affect chewing, digestion, nutritional status, and safe and effective swallowing. Prevalence of dysphagia in different settings is reported at the following rates: between 16% and 40% of independent older adults, 44% to 47% of those in acute care settings, and 60% of long-term care residents (Baijens, Clave, Cras, et al., 2016; Wirth, Dziewas, Beck, et al., 2016). In addition to interfering with swallowing, dysphagia increases the risk for malnutrition, dehydration, aspiration, and aspiration pneumonia. Using screening tools in clinical settings is an essential first step toward identifying swallowing problems so further evaluation and treatment can be initiated to prevent serious consequences (Heijnen, Speyer, Bulow, et al., 2016; Wakabayashi & Matsushima, 2016). Because nurses caring for older adults are responsible for assessment and interventions related to this common problem, Box 18-2 provides an overview of the topic, including recommendations for nursing assessment and interventions. Figure 18-1 illustrates an evidence-based screening tool for swallowing problems, and Online Learning Activity 18-1 provides links to additional information about dysphagia.

 See ONLINE LEARNING ACTIVITY 18-1: EVIDENCE-BASED TOOL FOR PREVENTING ASPIRATION IN OLDER ADULTS WITH DYSPHAGIA at http://thepoint.lww.com/Miller8e.

Medication Effects

Medications, nutritional supplements, and herbal preparations can create risk factors for impaired digestion and inadequate nutrition through their effects on digestion, eating patterns, and utilization of nutrients. More than 250 medications have potential adverse effects on the absorption, metabolism, and excretion of nutrients, as in the following examples:

- Broad-spectrum antibiotics can alter intestinal flora and impair nutrient synthesis.
- Medications and vitamins that are similar in chemical structure may compete at sites of action, thus altering their excretion pattern.
- Some medications bind to particular ions and form compounds that cannot be absorbed (e.g., tetracycline can bind to iron and calcium).
- Diuretics can interfere with the transport of water, sodium, glucose, and amino acids.

Table 18-2 lists other examples of medications and the related adverse effects on digestion and nutrition. Additional food, herb, and medication interactions are discussed in Chapter 8.

TABLE 18-2 Potential Effects of Medications on Digestion and Nutrition

Medication Examples	Potential Effect on Digestion and Nutrition
Digoxin, theophylline, fluoxetine, antihistamines	Anorexia
Anticholinergics, narcotics, calcium channel blockers; iron-aluminum-, and calcium-based antacids	Constipation
Cimetidine, laxatives, antibiotics, cardiovascular drugs, cholinesterase inhibitors	Diarrhea, nausea, vomiting
Nonsteroidal anti-inflammatory drugs (NSAIDs), aspirin, corticosteroids	Gastric irritation
Phenytoin, nifedipine, diltiazem, cyclosporine	Gum hyperplasia
Anticholinergics, potassium-depleting medications	Paralytic ileus
Bulk-forming agents when taken before meals, anticholinergics	Early satiety
Potassium supplements, NSAIDs, bisphosphonates, prednisone	Dysphagia
Anticholinergics, antihistamines, diuretics, muscle relaxant agents, opioids, psychoactive drugs	Xerostomia
Mineral oil, cholestyramine	Diminished absorption of vitamins A, D, E, and K
Anticonvulsants	Diminished storage of vitamin K, decreased absorption of calcium
Aluminum- or magnesium-based antacids	Diarrhea; decreased levels of calcium, fluoride, and phosphorus
Ampicillin, amoxicillin, cephalosporins, clindamycin	Clostridium difficile diarrhea
Products containing sodium bicarbonate	Sodium overload, water retention
Gentamicin and penicillin	Hypokalemia
Tetracyclines	Diminished absorption of zinc, iron, calcium, and magnesium
Neomycin	Diminished absorption of fat, iron, lactose, nitrogen, calcium, potassium, and vitamin B_{12}
Aspirin	Gastrointestinal bleeding; decreased levels of iron, folate, and vitamin C
Corticosteroids	Increased need for calcium, phosphorus, B vitamins, and vitamins C and D
Beta-carotene supplements	Vitamin E deficiency

Box 18-2 Evidence-Based Practice: Dysphagia

Dysphagia as a Risk for Aspiration

- Dysphagia is defined as impairment of any part of the swallowing process.
- Aspiration, defined as the misdirection of oropharyngeal secretions or gastric content into the larynx and lower respiratory tract, is a common and serious consequence of dysphagia.
- Diminished muscle strength and function, reduced tissue elasticity, and impaired dental status are common conditions that increase the risk for dysphagia in older adults.
- Dysphagia is common in older adults with neurologic conditions, including stroke, dementia, multiple sclerosis, and Parkinson disease.
- In addition to neurologic conditions, the following factors can increase the risk of dysphagia: frailty, altered mental status, and certain medications (e.g., anesthetics, anticholinergics, sedatives, psychotropics, antihistamines, amiodarone).
- Dysphagia increases the risk of malnutrition, dehydration, aspiration, and aspiration pneumonia.

Recommendations for Nursing Assessment

- Speech–language pathologists are responsible for performing comprehensive swallowing assessments, but nurses are responsible for identifying patients/residents who are at risk for dysphagia.
- The EAT-10 (Figure 18-1) is an evidence-based screening tool to identify the need for further evaluation.
- Nursing assessment includes questions about difficulty with chewing or swallowing, avoidance of certain foods or beverages, sensation of food being stuck in throat, inability to handle secretions, voice changes, and so forth.
- Nursing assessment includes the following observations: level of consciousness, voluntary cough, voice quality, and control of secretions.
- Perform a water-swallowing test: have the person drink 3 oz of water without interruption; the person passes the test if he or she does not stop, choke, or have a wet-sounding voice quality during the test or for 1 minute after.
- Signs and symptoms of dysphagia include drooling, coughing during meals, voice changes following meals, gurgling sounds in

the throat, upper respiratory tract infection, wet lung sounds, or packing food in the cheeks.
- Signs and symptoms of aspiration pneumonia include delirium, fever, chills, elevated respiratory rate, pleuritic chest pain, and respiratory crackles.

Recommendations for Nursing Interventions

- Appropriate management of dysphagia requires an interdisciplinary team approach, which includes speech–language pathologists, dietary professionals, primary care practitioners, and all levels of nursing staff.
- Speech–language pathologists are the health care professionals who usually assume primary responsibility for recommendations, but nurses are responsible for initiating the referrals in a timely manner and implementing interventions.
- Speech–language pathologists may recommend the following strategies: adaptive equipment, muscle-strengthening exercises, postural adjustments (e.g., chin-down or chin-tuck maneuver), swallow maneuvers, diet modification (e.g., altered viscosity, thickened liquids).
- Additional interventions include resting for 30 minutes before eating, sitting upright, allowing at least 30 minutes for eating or assisted feeding, alternating small amounts of solid and liquid foods, and minimizing distractions.
- Good oral care is imperative for all patients with dysphagia because it is associated with a lower incidence of pneumonia.

Sources: Baijens, L., Clave, P., Cras, P., et al. (2016). European Society for Swallowing Disorders - European Union Geriatric Medicine Society white paper: oropharyngeal dysphagia as a geriatric syndrome. *Clinical Interventions in Aging, 11,* 1403–1428; Brodsky, M. B., Suiter, D. M., Gonzalez-Fernandez, M., et al. (2016). Screening accuracy for aspiration using bedside water swallow tests: A systematic review and meta-analysis. *Chest, 150,* 148–163; Campbell, G., Carter, T., Kring, D., & Martinez, C. (2016). Nursing bedside dysphagia screen: Is it valid? *Journal of Neuroscience Nursing, 48,* 75–79; Carrion, S., Roca, M., Costa, A., et al. (2017). Nutritional status of older patients with oropharyngeal dysphagia in a chronic versus acute clinical situation. *Clinical Nutrition,* doi: 10.1016/j.cinu.2016.07.009 [Epub ahead of print]; Wirth, R., Dziewas, R., Beck, A. M., et al. (2016). Oropharyngeal dysphagia in older persons - from pathophysiology to adequate intervention: a review and summary of international expert meeting. *Clinical Interventions in Aging, 11,* 189–208.

Lifestyle Factors

Alcohol and smoking can alter an older person's nutritional status in several ways. Alcohol has a high caloric content but low nutrient value, so it provides empty calories. In addition, it interferes with the absorption of the B-complex vitamins and vitamin C. Alcoholism is often unrecognized and undertreated in older adults and may be a common contributing factor to nutritional disorders. Smoking diminishes the ability to smell and taste food and it also interferes with absorption of vitamin C and folic acid.

Psychosocial Factors

Psychosocial factors are likely to affect an older person's appetite and eating patterns. Studies indicate that the main social factors contributing to anorexia and poor nutritional status in older adults are socioeconomic inequality, social isolation, and living alone (Kucukerdonmez, Varli, & Koksal, 2017; Landi, Calvani, Tosato, et al., 2016). A change in mealtime companionship, as may occur through loss or disability of a spouse, can have a negative impact on eating

patterns. When older adults have established a long-term pattern of preparing meals for family and spouse, it may be especially difficult for the older adult to adjust to purchasing, preparing, and eating food for just one person. Similarly, older adults who have never participated in the purchase or preparation of foods may have great difficulty assuming these tasks after the loss of a spouse or other person who performed these tasks. If the older adult depends on others for assistance in procuring food, any factors that limit the availability of support resources may affect the older adult's ability to obtain food.

Stress and anxiety affect digestive processes through their influence on the autonomic nervous system. Although stress-related effects on digestion are not unique to older adults, any alteration of the autonomic nervous system may compound age-related effects that otherwise would not have much effect. Older adults who are depressed are likely to experience anorexia and loss of interest in food, leading to malnutrition (Sanford, 2017). Confusion, memory problems, and other cognitive deficits may significantly interfere with eating patterns and the ability to prepare food.

EAT-10:
A Swallowing Assessment Tool

**Nestlé
NutritionInstitute**

LAST NAME	FIRST NAME	SEX	AGE	DATE

OBJECTIVE:

EAT-10 helps to measure swallowing difficulties.
It may be important for you to talk with your physician about treatment options for symptoms.

A. INSTRUCTIONS:

Answer each question by writing the number of points in the boxes.
To what extent do you experience the following problems?

1 **My swallowing problem has caused me to lose weight.**

0 = no problem
1
2
3
4 = severe problem

6 **Swallowing is painful.**

0 = no problem
1
2
3
4 = severe problem

2 **My swallowing problem interferes with my ability to go out for meals.**

0 = no problem
1
2
3
4 = severe problem

7 **The pleasure of eating is affected by my swallowing.**

0 = no problem
1
2
3
4 = severe problem

3 **Swallowing liquids takes extra effort.**

0 = no problem
1
2
3
4 = severe problem

8 **When I swallow food sticks in my throat.**

0 = no problem
1
2
3
4 = severe problem

4 **Swallowing solids takes extra effort.**

0 = no problem
1
2
3
4 = severe problem

9 **I cough when I eat.**

0 = no problem
1
2
3
4 = severe problem

5 **Swallowing pills takes extra effort.**

0 = no problem
1
2
3
4 = severe problem

10 **Swallowing is stressful.**

0 = no problem
1
2
3
4 = severe problem

B. SCORING:

Add up the number of points and write your total score in the boxes.
Total Score (max. 40 points)

C. WHAT TO DO NEXT:

If the EAT-10 score is 3 or higher, you may have problems swallowing efficiently and safely. We recommend discussing the EAT-10 results with a physician.

Reference: The validity and reliability of EAT-10 has been determined.
Belafsky PC, Mouadeb DA, Rees CJ, Pryor JC, Postma GN, Allen J, Leonard RJ. Validity and Reliability of the Eating Assessment Tool (EAT-10). Annals of Otology Rhinology & Laryngology 2008;117(12):919-924.

www.nestlenutrition-institute.org

FIGURE 18-1 The EAT-10: A Swallowing Assessment Tool. Copyright Nestec 2009. (Reprinted with permission from Nestlé Nutrition Institute. Available at www.nestlenutrition-institute.org)

Cultural Influences

Ethnic background, religious beliefs, and other cultural factors strongly influence the way people define, select, prepare, and eat food and beverages. Cultural factors also can influence eating patterns and selection of food in relation to health status. For example, some Asian and Hispanic people may classify foods, beverages, and medicines as hot or cold, and they may select a particular food on the basis of their belief that their illness would respond to warm, hot, cool, or cold types of remedies. According to this health belief model, illnesses are caused by an imbalance between hot and cold, and so must be treated with substances that have the opposite characteristics. The characteristics of "hot" and "cold" are not related to temperature of the food but are culturally defined by different groups.

Culturally based dietary customs usually are not detrimental for healthy older adults, and in fact can be healthier than typical American diets as in the following examples (Commodore-Mensah, Ukonu, Obisesan, et al., 2016; Melina, Craig, & Levin, 2016; Oldways Nutrition Exchange, 2016):

- Traditional African diets, which are high in fiber and low in fat calories, may play a role in decreasing the risk for colon cancer. Traditional African diets have little added sodium and may decrease the risk for hypertension.
- Traditional Latin American diets may contribute to longer life expectancy and lower rates of heart disease among Hispanics in the United States.
- Vegetarian diets (which are associated with many cultures and religious groups) are associated with decreased prevalence of obesity, hypertension, ischemic heart disease, type 2 diabetes, and certain types of cancer.
- Longer length of stay in the United States for immigrants is associated with increased risk for chronic illness. This is due in part to dietary acculturation to readily available Western-type foods.

Box 18-3 summarizes some of the food patterns that are associated with major cultural and religious groups in the United States. As emphasized in Chapter 2, it is imperative to consider that individual older adults vary in their eating patterns and may not adhere to the patterns of their cultural group.

Nurses address culturally influenced eating patterns in the context of health promotion related to older adults' dietary patterns. For example, the Four Winds Nutrition Guide was developed by Kibbe Conti, a Lakota Indian who is a

---

 Box 18-3 Cultural Considerations: Cultural Influences on Eating Patterns

African Americans

- "Soul food" is common, particularly in the southern United States.
- Common main courses: wild game, fried fish and poultry, pork and all parts of the pig
- Common vegetables and side dishes: corn, rice, okra, greens, legumes, tomatoes, hot breads, sweet potatoes
- Methods of food preparation: stewing, barbecuing, and frying with lard or salt pork
- Low consumption of milk
- Low calcium dietary intake

Asian Americans: Southwest Cuisines (India, Pakistan, Sri Lanka, and Burma)

- Common foods: flat bread, kebabs, rice, wheat, barley, beans, lamb, goat, fish
- Common spices: peppers, chili, cloves, curry, garlic, ginger
- According to Hinduism, cows are used only for their milk

Asian Americans: Northeast Traditions (China, Korea, Japan)

- Common foods: rice, wheat, pork, eggs, chicken, soybean products, and a variety of vegetables
- Methods of food preparation: stir-frying with lard, peanut oil, or sesame oil; seasoning with garlic, ginger, soy sauce, and sesame seeds
- Beverages: green tea; rare use of milk products

Asian Americans: Southeast Style (Thailand, Cambodia, Vietnam, Indonesia)

- Common foods: rice, noodles, pork, eggs, chicken, soybean products, and a variety of vegetables
- Methods of food preparation: quick stir-frying combined with steaming or boiling, supplemented with discrete spices and seasoning (e.g., citrus, basil, cilantro, mint)

Hispanic Americans

- Common foods: eggs, beans, rice, corn, tomatoes, fish, pork, poultry, tacos, tortillas, squash, sweet potato, mango, avocado, pineapple
- Frying is the common method of food preparation
- Beverages: herbal teas, milk in hot beverages, coffee with large amounts of milk and sugar

American Indians

- May be influenced by tribal culture, geographic location, and availability of natural resources
- Corn, squash, and beans are considered the three staples; greens, berries, pumpkins, rice, and wild game also are commonly used
- Herbs play a strong role in food preparation and healing
- Traditionally have obtained foods from their natural environments; however, they have experienced loss of many of these natural assets
- Current efforts focus on restoring access to healthy foods through a comprehensive approach to strengthening food production and reclaiming and restoring native food systems
- May depend on commodity foods provided by the U.S. Department of Agriculture

Religious Influences

- Some groups of Jews follow prescribed rules for preparing and serving foods (e.g., they eat only kosher meat and poultry and do not eat shellfish or any pork products).
- Mormons do not drink tea, coffee, or alcohol.
- Hindus may be vegetarians.
- Seventh-Day Adventists may be lacto-ovo-vegetarians.
- Many Catholics do not eat meat on Ash Wednesday or Good Friday.

Registered Dietician, to teach healthy eating patterns based on traditional food paradigms. The model, which is illustrated in Figure 18-2, is adapted by tribal nations to encourage good choices for healthy beverages and good sources of proteins, fruits, vegetables, and grains within specific cultural contexts (National Academies of Sciences, Engineering, and Medicine, 2016). Online Learning Activity 18-2 provides links to resources related to dietary patterns of culturally diverse groups as well as to information about initiatives to address broader issues, such as lack of access to affordable and culturally appropriate foods.

 See ONLINE LEARNING ACTIVITY 18-2: RESOURCES RELATED TO DIETARY PATTERNS OF CULTURALLY DIVERSE GROUPS at http://thepoint.lww.com/Miller8e.

Socioeconomic Influences

A person's past and present economic status also influences food choices. If nutrient intake has been inadequate because of long-standing financial limitations, the progressive effects of poor nutrition may precipitate new problems in older adults, especially in combination with disease conditions

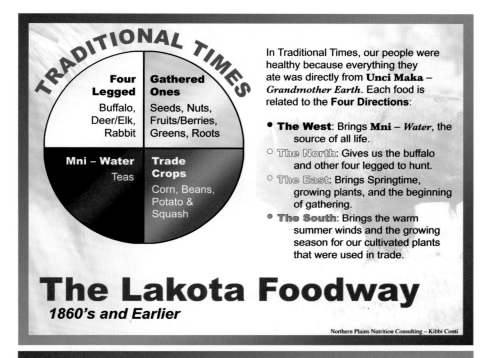

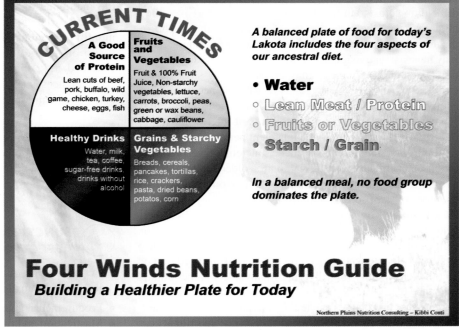

FIGURE 18-2 The *Four Winds Nutrition Guide*. (Copyright 2002. Kibbe Conti, Northern Plains Nutrition Consulting. Reprinted with permission.)

and age-related changes. People with limited finances usually have a narrower selection of foods than do people with higher incomes. Lower socioeconomic status, including educational level, is also associated with lack of dental care and more tooth loss.

Food insecurity, defined as the state of being without reliable access to a sufficient quantity of affordable and nutritious food, affects about 9% of older adults in the United States, with higher prevalence among those who are nonwhite, living alone, and with less than a high school education (Coleman-Jensen, Rabbitt, Gregory, et al., 2016). Food insecurity increases the risk for frailty, chronic conditions, and nutritional deficiencies (Bhargava & Lee, 2016; Perez-Zepeda, Castrejon-Perez, Wynne-Bannister, et al., 2016).

> ### Diversity Note
>
> "Diets of poverty," which are characterized by high fat, high carbohydrate, and low nutrient content, are common among many American Indian groups, as well as other groups with high rates of food insecurity (National Academies of Sciences, Engineering, and Medicine, 2016, p. 81).

> ### Wellness Opportunity
>
> Nurses address cultural needs by identifying food preferences and finding acceptable ways to provide access to these foods.

Environmental Factors

Environmental factors affect the enjoyment of food and the ability to obtain and prepare it. Many barriers to food enjoyment have been identified in the dining environments of long-term care facilities and other institutional settings. Older adults in congregate housing and long-term care facilities may find it difficult to adjust to unfamiliar environments. Moreover, they may not desire the mealtime social interaction that is part of the institutional environment. A noisy or crowded dining room may have a negative impact on food enjoyment and consumption. Such an environment may be particularly stressful for older adults who use hearing aids or who are accustomed to eating alone. The potential outcomes of a move to a new environment include poor nutrition and loss of interest in eating, particularly during the initial adjustment period.

Environmental influences, such as inclement weather conditions, can affect functionally impaired older adults who live in their own homes. For example, older persons who walk to the store or depend on public transportation may be unable or unwilling to obtain groceries in snowy or rainy weather. Likewise, older adults may not be able to tolerate hot or sultry conditions, especially if transportation is not readily available. People who depend on others for transportation or who have difficulty maneuvering in adverse weather conditions are likely to shop for groceries less frequently and to purchase their groceries at smaller convenience stores, where prices are higher and selection is limited. The additional cost

and limited selection may interfere with food intake and lead to nutrient deficiencies. Finally, environmental conditions and packaging trends in the grocery store may create additional difficulties for older people, especially those who are functionally impaired. For example, the combined glare of fluorescent lights; highly polished floors; shiny, clear wrappers; and white freezer cases often make it extremely difficult, if not impossible, for older adults with vision changes to read labels, especially when the print is small and contrasts poorly against the background.

Behaviors Based on Myths and Misunderstandings

Myths and misunderstandings may be detrimental to a person's food intake and behaviors related to bowel function. For example, during the 1950s and 1960s, a widely held belief was that roughage and raw fruits or vegetables were harmful to the older person. It is now known that lack of roughage in the diet and consumption of only cooked fruits and vegetables are eating patterns that contribute to constipation by slowing the transit time of feces through the large intestine. Another commonly held belief is that a daily bowel movement is the norm for good digestive function. Rigid adherence to this standard may, in fact, lead to the unnecessary and detrimental use of laxatives. Advertisements have further reinforced this false belief by implying that daily bowel movements should be attained through medication. Although recent advertising trends emphasize the achievement of healthy bowel patterns through the ingestion of high-fiber food items, the negative impact of long-term beliefs may be difficult to overcome.

Misunderstandings about fluid intake may also interfere with digestion and nutrition. Many older adults reduce the amount of liquids they consume in an attempt to decrease the incidence of urinary incontinence. Fluid intake may also be restricted if functional limitations, such as impaired mobility or manual dexterity, interfere with either the ability to obtain liquids or the ease of urinary elimination. Reduced fluid intake can have a number of detrimental consequences, such as constipation, xerostomia, and diminished food enjoyment.

> ### Wellness Opportunity
>
> Nurses identify myths and misunderstandings about constipation and teach older adults health behaviors that promote healthy elimination patterns.

 FUNCTIONAL CONSEQUENCES AFFECTING DIGESTION AND NUTRITION

Functional consequences affect the following aspects of digestion and nutrition of older adults:

- Procurement, preparation, and enjoyment of food
- Mastication and digestion of food

- Nutritional status
- Psychosocial function

Negative functional consequences occur primarily because of the many risk factors that affect older adults, rather than because of age-related changes alone.

Ability to Procure, Prepare, and Enjoy Food

Activities involved in procuring, preparing, consuming, and enjoying food depend on the skills of cognition, balance, mobility, and manual dexterity, as well as on the five senses. Food procurement depends on getting to the grocery store, pushing a shopping cart, reaching for food items on high shelves, reading the small print on shelves and food packages for cost and nutrition information, and coping with the glare of bright lights, especially in the frozen-food sections. Age-related changes and conditions that may interfere with these activities include vision impairments and any illness, such as arthritis, that limits mobility, balance, or manual dexterity.

Food preparation activities that are likely to be more difficult for older adults include cutting food items, measuring ingredients accurately, carrying food and liquid without spilling, standing for long periods in the kitchen, reaching for items on high shelves and in cupboards, safely using the oven or stove, and reading the temperature controls correctly. Impairments of vision, balance, cognition, mobility, or manual dexterity are likely to cause difficulties in performing these tasks.

Diminished sensory function can affect food enjoyment in all the following ways:

- Inaccurate perception of color, taste, or smell can interfere with appetite and food appeal.
- Diminished gustatory and olfactory sensitivity may lead to excessive use of condiments and seasonings, such as salt and sugar.
- Visual, olfactory, and gustatory impairments may make it difficult to detect spoiled food.

Moreover, food choices are influenced by the condition of the oral cavity and teeth, as well as by the quantity and the quality of natural or replacement teeth.

Wellness Opportunity

Nurses promote wellness through interventions that improve the older adult's independence in procuring and preparing satisfying meals.

Changes in Oral Function

Digestive processes in healthy older adults are not significantly affected by age-related changes, but older adults often have digestive complaints (e.g., heartburn, constipation) caused by commonly occurring risk factors. For example, many negative functional consequences are associated with medications (see Table 18-2). Xerostomia causes negative functional consequences because it can interfere with oral comfort, food enjoyment, and taste sensitivity (Rawal, Hoffman, Bainbridge, et al., 2016). In addition, diminished saliva production makes it more difficult to chew food and increases the susceptibility of the teeth and tongue to bacterial action. Poor oral care increases the risk for gingivitis, oral lesions, dental caries, excessive plaque, periodontal disease, and impaired taste. The functional consequences of being edentulous or using dentures include avoidance of certain foods, decreased chewing efficiency, and increased risk for malnutrition (Zelig, Touger-Decker, Chung, et al., 2016).

Poor Nutritional Status and Weight Changes

Because older adults need fewer calories, a deficiency of essential minerals or vitamins is likely to occur if the quantity of calories is reduced without a corresponding increase in the quality of the food consumed. In addition, risk factors (e.g., medications and pathologic processes) that commonly occur in older adults often cause nutrient deficiencies. For example, iron deficiency is associated with chronic diseases and low socioeconomic status. Specific nutrients that are likely to be deficient in older adults in the United States include fiber, calcium, folate, magnesium, potassium, and vitamins A, C, D, E, and K (National Academies of Sciences, Engineering, and Medicine, 2016). See Table 18-1 for examples of nutrient deficiencies and associated risk factors and functional consequences that are likely to affect older adults.

Age-related changes in body composition and carbohydrate metabolism contribute to gradual weight gains. Throughout life, the proportion of total body water as a percentage of body weight gradually decreases from about 80% of a newborn infant's weight to less than half of an older adult's weight. The proportion of body fat to lean tissue begins to increase at around 30 years of age and leads to disproportionately increased abdominal fat during later adulthood. This pattern of fat distribution is associated with increased risk for diabetes, cardiovascular disease, and other chronic conditions. The gradually increasing prevalence of obesity is a major public health concern for all population groups, but it is most prevalent among older adults between the ages of 65 and 74 years. Even though there is some evidence that the body mass index (BMI) standards should be increased for older adults, abdominal obesity as measured by waist circumference increases the risk for frailty and many serious chronic conditions (Reinders, Visser, & Schaap, 2017).

Malnutrition and Dehydration

Malnutrition (also called undernutrition), which is the intake of nutrients that is less than the amount required to meet daily needs, is common in older adults. Protein-energy malnutrition (i.e., a type of malnutrition that occurs when the intake of calories and protein is less than the amount required) is a type that is of particular concern in geriatric medicine because it leads to loss of bone and muscle mass, and it increases the risk for frailty (Morley & Bauer, 2017). Prevalence of malnutrition varies according to setting, with rates as high as 60% in acute, subacute, and long-term care settings (Cereda, Pedrolli, Klersy, et al., 2016; Edwards, Carrier, & Hopkinson, 2016).

Reviews of studies have identified the following risks for the development of malnutrition in older adults: increased age, frailty, anorexia, dysphagia, constipation, polypharmacy, lower BMI, diminished muscle strength, functional or cognitive impairment, poor or moderate self-reported health status, dependency on others for eating, and loss of interest in life (Chang, 2017; Lahmann, Tannen, & Suhr, 2016; Maseda, Gomez-Caamano, Lorenzo-Lopez, et al., 2016; Moreira, Krausch-Hofmann, Matthys, et al., 2016). Functional consequences of malnutrition in older adults include increased risk for functional and cognitive impairment, slower recovery from illnesses, prolonged length of stay in health care settings, and shorter life expectancy (Naseer, Forssell, & Fagerstrom, 2016; Shakersain, Santoni, Faxen-Irving, et al., 2016).

Dehydration is the depletion of total body water content caused by pathologic fluid losses, diminished water intake, or a combination of these conditions (Mentes, 2016). Dehydration is caused by a combination of risk factors, including polypharmacy, older age, acute and chronic conditions, insufficient fluid intake, and age-related changes (e.g., diminished thirst, decreased renal function, altered body composition). Functional consequences of dehydration include falls, fractures, functional decline, constipation, delayed wound healing, altered mental status, and increased morbidity and mortality (Hooper, Bunn, Downing, et al., 2016; McCrow, Morton, Travers, et al., 2016).

See **ONLINE LEARNING ACTIVITY 18-3: ADDITIONAL INFORMATION AND CASE STUDIES ABOUT NUTRITIONAL DEFICIENCIES, DEHYDRATION, AND UNINTENTIONAL WEIGHT LOSS** at http://thepoint.lww.com/Miller8e.

PATHOLOGIC CONDITIONS AFFECTING DIGESTIVE WELLNESS: CONSTIPATION

Constipation, which is defined as "decrease in normal frequency of defecation accompanied by difficult or incomplete passage of stool and/or passage of excessively hard, dry stool" (Herdman & Kamitsuru, 2018, p. 197), is a pathologic condition associated with digestion that occurs commonly in older adults. The normal frequency for bowel movements, which shows significant individual variation but does not necessarily change with aging, ranges from three times daily to once or twice weekly. Another characteristic is that, persons experience a feeling of incomplete evacuation after a bowel movement.

Although constipation is a common complaint of older adults, it is caused by risk factors rather than age-related changes alone. Slowing of food transit through the gastrointestinal tract may predispose older adults to constipation, but dietary patterns that include adequate fiber and

Unfolding Case Study

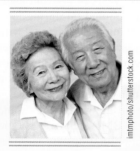

Part 1: Mr. D. at 71 and Mrs. D. at 72 Years of Age

Mr. and Mrs. D., who are 71 and 72 years old, respectively, attend the senior center where you provide monthly group health education sessions and weekly one-on-one "Counseling for Wellness" sessions. Mrs. D. makes an appointment to see you because her bowels get "bound up" and she always feels "bloated." When you ask about her bowel patterns, she reports that she has a bowel movement "about every couple of days" and needs to "sit on the commode for a good half-hour before anything happens." She has taken Milk of Magnesia every night for approximately 20 years, but "it doesn't seem to be of any help anymore." She avoids fresh fruits and vegetables because her mother always told her that canned fruits and vegetables were easier to digest. She rarely eats whole grain foods or foods high in fiber. Her BMI is 25, and she does little walking or exercising because of trouble with arthritis. She takes levothyroxine (Synthroid), 50 μg once daily, and an over-the-counter generic calcium supplement that contains 600 mg calcium carbonate twice daily.

THINKING POINTS

- Identify at least five risk factors that are likely to contribute to Mrs. D.'s constipation.

- Describe how you would begin addressing one of these risk factors in health education.

fluid will compensate for this age-related change. Risk factors common in older adults include functional impairments, depression, pathologic conditions (e.g., endocrine, metabolic, and neurologic disorders), adverse medication effects, laxative abuse, and poor dietary patterns (e.g., inadequate intake of bulk, fiber, and fluid) (Andy, Vaughan, Burgio, et al., 2016; Chokhavatia, John, Bridgemen, et al., 2016; Werth, Williams, & Pont, 2017). Because constipation occurs commonly in older adults, nurses assess for risk factors and initiate health promotion interventions, as discussed in the sections on Nursing Assessment and Nursing Interventions.

NURSING ASSESSMENT OF DIGESTION AND NUTRITION

Nurses assess digestion and nutrition to identify (1) nutritional status and usual eating patterns, (2) risk factors that interfere with optimal nutrition, (3) factors that influence eating patterns, and (4) negative functional consequences of altered digestion or inadequate nutrition. A major purpose of this nursing assessment is to identify opportunities for health promotion interventions.

Interviewing About Digestion and Nutrition

Opportunities for health promotion are identified by asking about the following:

- Usual eating patterns and nutrient intake
- Health behaviors associated with oral care
- Age-related changes and risk factors that affect nutritional needs or digestive processes
- Environmental or social support factors that affect the procurement, preparation, and enjoyment of food
- Symptoms of gastrointestinal dysfunction

Assess the adequacy of nutrient intake by asking older adults to describe foods and beverages consumed during an average day. An effective assessment approach is to begin by asking about the oral cavity and end with questions about bowel elimination, including questions related to risks for constipation and poor nutrition. Box 18-4 summarizes interview questions for a nursing assessment of nutrition and digestion in older adults.

Observing Cues to Digestion and Nutrition

Assess oral health by observing all components of the mouth and oral cavity and pay particular attention to indicators of

---

Box 18-4 Guidelines for Assessing Digestion and Nutrition

Assessing Oral Comfort and Chewing Ability

- Do you have any difficulty with soreness or bleeding in your mouth?
- Do you have any teeth that hurt, are loose, or are sensitive to hot or cold temperatures?
- Do your gums bleed?
- Do you have any problems chewing or swallowing food or liquids? *If yes, ask about particular types of food or liquids that are problematic.*
- Are there foods you avoid because of problems with chewing or swallowing?
- Does your mouth or tongue ever feel dry?

Assessing Dental Care

- How often do you see a dentist?
- When was the last time you had dental care?
- Where do you go for dental care?
- *If the person does not seek dental care at least once per year:* What prevents you from seeing the dentist?
- How do you care for your teeth?
- Do you use dental floss? *If yes:* How often? *If no:* Have you ever been taught to use dental floss?

Assessing Nutritional Needs

- Do you have diabetes, heart disease, or any condition that requires dietary modifications?
- Do you have any food allergies?
- What medications do you take?
- What is your usual daily activity pattern?

Identifying Patterns of Food Procurement

- How do you get your grocery shopping done?
- Do you have any help getting to the store?

- Where and how often do you do your grocery shopping?
- What is your usual food budget?
- Do you have any difficulty getting food because of problems with vision, walking, or transportation?

Identifying Patterns of Food Preparation and Consumption

- Where do you eat your meals?
- With whom do you eat?
- Does anyone help you prepare your meals?
- Do you have any trouble fixing your meals (e.g., difficulty opening containers)?
- Do you have any difficulties getting around your kitchen, using appliances, or reaching the cupboards?
- Have there been recent changes in your eating or food preparation patterns (e.g., loss of eating companion or change in caregiver situation)?

Assessing Patterns of Bowel Elimination

- How often do you have a bowel movement?
- Have you noticed any recent changes in your pattern of bowel movements?
- Do you have any difficulty with your bowel movements? (e.g., do you strain with bowel movements? Or is the stool hard, dry, or difficult to pass?)
- Do you ever have problems with loose stools or diarrhea?
- Do you take laxatives or any other products to help you move your bowels?
- Do you ever have pain or bleeding when you move your bowels?

Box 18-5 Behavioral Cues to Nutrition and Digestion

Observations to Assess Oral Health

- What is the condition of lips, teeth, gums, tongue, and oral mucous membrane?
- Does the person have a sufficient number of teeth and/or use of full or partial dentures?
- How well do dentures fit?
- What are the features of oral care items (e.g., condition of toothbrush, type of toothbrush or denture-cleaning supplies, and use of floss)?

Observations to Assess Eating Patterns

- Does the person seem to enjoy eating meals with others, or does the presence of other people seem to interfere with mealtime enjoyment?
- If the person has dentures, are they worn at meals? If not, why not?
- What are the person's between-meal food and fluid consumption patterns?
- Are enjoyable noncaffeinated liquids readily available for between-meal fluid intake?
- What cultural influences affect the person's food preferences and preparation?

Observations to Assess the Eating Environment

- Do environmental or social influences negatively affect mealtime enjoyment (e.g., a noisy dining room or disruptive mealtime companions)?

- If the person eats alone, is this the best arrangement, or should consideration be given to providing mealtime social interaction?

Cultural Considerations That May Influence Nutrition and Eating Patterns

- What are the usual patterns of meals eaten (e.g., content, frequency, timing)? What is the usual social context of meals?
- Are there any culturally influenced food taboos or preferences? (Refer to Cultural Considerations 18-3.)
- Are there any special foods that are important because of religious or cultural factors? (If yes, are they accessible to the older adult?)
- Are certain foods or beverages avoided or preferred in relation to an illness or chronic condition (e.g., foods or beverages that are considered yin and yang foods)?
- Is there a preference for the temperature of beverages (e.g., use of iced or heated beverages)?
- Is the person's ethnic background likely to increase his or her chance of being lactose intolerant? (Prevalence is highest among Asians, American Indians, and both African and African-American blacks; high among Hispanics; and lowest among whites of northern European descent.)

oral hygiene and the need for dental care. Observe eating patterns and environments for cues to digestion and nutrition, and consider social and cultural factors that influence eating and nutrition. Box 18-5 summarizes observations and cultural considerations that are pertinent to nursing assessment of digestion and nutrition.

Wellness Opportunity

Nurses observe environmental conditions to identify positive or negative effects on eating patterns.

Using Assessment Tools

Assessment tools are used for identifying people at risk for nutritional problems so that preventive and therapeutic interventions can be implemented. The **Mini Nutritional Assessment (MNA)** is an evidence-based tool that has been widely used since 1990 in a variety of settings. A revised short form, called the MNA-SF, was validated in 2009 as a standalone screening tool with six questions to identify people as malnourished, at risk for malnourishment, or normally nourished. The MNA-SF is now widely used in clinical and research settings because of its validation, reliability, ease of use, low cost, acceptability, effectiveness, and availability in many languages (Donini, Poggiogalle, Molfino, et al., 2016; Lera, Sanchez, Angel, et al., 2016; Schrader, Grosch, Bertsch, et al., 2016). This tool is illustrated in Figure 18-3, and additional information and resources are described in

Online Learning Activity 18-4. Because of the high prevalence and serious consequences of nutritional deficits in older adults, routine screening for malnutrition or risks for malnutrition is recommended for all older adults so interventions can be implemented (Artaza-Artabe, Saez-Lopez, Sanchez-Hernandez, et al., 2016; Hamirudin, Chalrton, & Walton, 2016).

See ONLINE LEARNING ACTIVITY 18-4: ASSESSING NUTRITIONAL STATUS IN OLDER ADULTS at http://thepoint.lww.com/Miller8e.

Physical Assessment Related to Nutrition and Hydration Status

Physical assessment of height, weight, and BMI provide information related to the older adult's nutritional status. The BMI is commonly used as an indicator of malnutrition (when it is low) and risk for disease (when it is high). Healthy BMI is between 18.5 and 24.9 lb/in^2 for adults. Although there is no benefit to severe obesity, studies indicate that a BMI between 25 and 30 may have positive effects for adults older than age 65 (Cederholm & Morley, 2016). Thus, it is imperative to consider the BMI in relation to overall health and risk factors, additional assessment findings, and long-term patterns. Also, keep in mind that a high BMI does not eliminate the possibility of risk for malnutrition.

Nurses need to consider individual circumstances in relation to ideal body weight because standardized tables do not

Mini Nutritional Assessment
MNA®

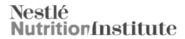

Last name: _____   First name: _____

Sex: _____   Age: _____   Weight, kg: _____   Height, cm: _____   Date: _____

Complete the screen by filling in the boxes with the appropriate numbers. Total the numbers for the final screening score.

Screening

A Has food intake declined over the past 3 months due to loss of appetitie, digestive problems, chewing or swallowing difficulties?
0 = severe decrease in food intake
1 = moderate decrease in food intake
2 = no decrease in food intake ☐

B Weight loss during the last 3 months
0 = weight loss greater than 3 kg (6.6 lbs)
1 = does not know
2 = weight loss between 1 and 3 kg (2.2 and 6.6 lbs)
3 = no weight loss ☐

C Mobility
0 = bed or chair bound
1 = able to get out of bed / chair but does not go out
2 = goes out ☐

D Has suffered psychological stress or acute disease in the past 3 months?
0 = yes   2 = no ☐

E Neuropsychological problems
0 = severe dementia or depression
1 = mild dementia
2 = no psychological problems ☐

F1 Body Mass Index (BMI) (weight in kg) / (height in m²)
0 = BMI less than 19
1 = BMI 19 to less than 21
2 = BMI 21 to less than 23
3 = BMI 23 or greater ☐

IF BMI IS NO AVAILABLE, REPLACE QUESTION F1 WITH QUESTION F2.
DO NOT ANSWER QUESTION F2 IF QUESTION F1 IS ALREADY COMPLETED.

F2 Calf circumference (CC) in cm
0 = CC less than 31
3 = CC 31 or greater ☐

Screening score (max. 14 points)

12 - 14 points: Normal nutritional status
8 - 11 points: At risk of malnutrition
0 - 7 points: Malnourished ☐☐

References
1. Vellas B, Villars H, Abellan G, *et al*. Overview of MNA® - Its History and Challenges. *J Nutr Health Aging*. 2006;**10**:456-465.
2. Rubenstein LZ, Harker JO, Salva A, Guigoz Y, Vellas B. Screening for Undernutrition in Geriatric Practice: Developing the Short-Form Mini Nutritional Assessment (MNA-SF). *J Geront*. 2001;**56A**:M366-377.
3. Guigoz Y. The Mini-Nutritional Assessment (MNA®) Review of the Literature - What does it tell us? *J Nutr Health Aging*. 2006;**10**:466-487.
4. Kaiser MJ, Bauer JM, Ramsch C, et al. Validation of the Mini Nutritional Assessment Short-Form (MNA®-SF): A practical tool for identification of nutritional status. *J Nutr Health Aging*. 2009;**13**:782-788.
® Société des Produits Nestlé, S.A., Vevey, Switzerland, Trademark Owners © Nestlé, 1994, Revision 2009. N67200 12/99 10M
For more information: www.mna-elderly.com

FIGURE 18-3 The Mini Nutritional Assessment (MNA). (From Nestlé Nutrition Institute. Copyright Nestlé, 1994, Revision 2009. Available at www.mna-elderly.com)

Box 18-6 Physical Assessment Findings Related to Digestion and Nutrition

Examination of the Oral Cavity

- Inspect the oral cavity by using a tongue depressor and a light.
- Observe for evidence of oral disease, including pain, lumps, soreness, bleeding, swelling, loose teeth, and abraded areas.
- Note the presence or absence of teeth, dentures, and partial bridges.

Indicators of Nutritional Deficiency

- Lips: dry, fissured, cracked at corners
- Teeth: decayed or missing
- Gums: red, swollen, recessed, spongy or prone to bleeding
- Mucous membranes: dry, ulcerated, inflamed, bleeding, white patches
- Tongue: dry, swollen, reddened, or very smooth

Examination of the Abdomen and Rectum

- Examine the abdomen with the person lying comfortably in the supine position.
- If the person is constipated, perform a rectal examination with the person in the side-lying position

General Physical Assessment Indicators of Malnutrition

- Unintentional weight loss
- Lack of subcutaneous fat
- Diminished muscle strength
- Skin that is dry, rough, or tissue thin
- Edema, especially in the face or lower extremities
- Hair that is dry, dull, thin, brittle, or sparse
- Dry or dull-looking eyes
- Listless, apathetic, or depressed mood

Laboratory Indicators of Possible Nutritional Deficiencies

- Anemia
- Lymphocytopenia
- Low serum ferritin
- Serum 25(OH)D <30 nmol/L (<12 ng/mL)
- Serum albumin level of less than 3.5 g/dL
- Cholesterol levels of less than 160 mg/dL
- Total iron-binding capacity less than 250 mcg/dL

Unfolding Case Study

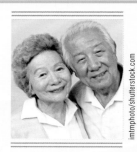

imtmphoto/shutterstock.com

Part 2: Mr. D. at 75 and Mrs. D. at 76 Years of Age

Recall that you are the nurse at the senior center attended by Mr. and Mrs. D., who now are 75 and 76 years old, respectively. During a "Counseling for Health" session, Mrs. D. asks your advice about her gradual unintended weight loss over the past few months. Although Mrs. D. continues to cook meals because her husband enjoys eating, she states that food no longer appeals to her. You notice that her mouth is very dry and her teeth are in poor condition. She had a stroke 2 years ago and recovered well except for some dysphagia and right-sided weakness. Her BMI is 18. She takes an antidepressant and two blood pressure medications but does not know the names of the pills. She asks what she can do about the weight loss.

THINKING POINTS

- What risk factors are likely to be contributing to Mrs. D.'s weight loss?
- Make a list of assessment questions you would use with Mrs. D. Select applicable questions from Box 18-4 and list any additional questions that you would use for further assessment.
- What would you ask Mrs. D. to do to provide additional assessment information so that you can plan some teaching interventions?

QSEN APPLICATION

QSEN Competency	Knowledge/Skill/Attitude	Application to Mrs. D. When She is 76 Years of Age
Patient-centered care	(K) Integrate understanding of multiple dimensions of patient-centered care	Identify the many interacting factors (including physical and psychosocial conditions) that are likely to contribute to Mrs. D.'s unintentional weight loss
	(S) Elicit patient values, preferences, and expressed needs	
	(S) Provide patient-centered care with sensitivity and respect for diversity of the human experience	Use a nonjudgmental approach to explore potential reasons for Mrs. D.'s poor oral care and depression

necessarily provide the most realistic or appropriate goal for older adults. Unintentional weight loss is calculated by subtracting current weight from usual weight and dividing that by the usual weight—for example, (160 lb–120 lb)/160 lb = 40 lb/160 lb, or a 25% weight loss. An unintentional weight loss of more than 5% of body weight in 1 month or more than 10% in 6 months is considered a significant indicator of poor nutrition. In long-term care facilities, unintentional weight loss is an indicator of quality of care provided by the facility.

Although screening tools are useful for identifying risk factors for malnutrition, a comprehensive and interdisciplinary approach is necessary for diagnosing and addressing nutritional deficits, malnutrition, or dehydration. Laboratory data can provide clues to nutrition-related problems, even before any clinical signs are evident; however, test results must be evaluated in relation to a person's overall health status. Box 18-6 summarizes information about physical assessment indicators and laboratory values that are especially important in assessing the nutritional status of older adults. Additional indicators of nutrient deficiencies are listed in Table 18-1 in the column describing functional consequences.

NURSING DIAGNOSIS

The nursing assessment may identify problems related to nutrition, digestion, or oral health. If nutritional deficits are identified, a pertinent nursing diagnosis is Imbalanced Nutrition: Less than Body Requirements, defined as "intake of nutrients insufficient to meet metabolic needs" (Herdman & Kamitsuru, 2018, p. 157). Related factors that may affect older adults include cognitive or functional impairments, medications, anorexia, depression, chewing or swallowing difficulties, social isolation, and inability to procure or prepare food.

If the nursing assessment identifies constipation or risks for constipation, the applicable nursing diagnosis is Constipation. The nursing assessment may also identify certain oral health problems that are common in older adults. These include xerostomia, medication effects, chewing difficulties, periodontal disease, diminished taste sensation, ill-fitting dentures, inadequate oral hygiene, and broken or missing teeth. A relevant nursing diagnosis to address these problems would be Impaired Oral Mucous Membrane. Risk for Aspiration is an appropriate nursing diagnosis for older adults who have any difficulty chewing or swallowing.

Wellness Opportunity

Nurses can use the wellness diagnosis of Readiness for Enhanced Nutrition for older adults who express an interest in improving nutritional patterns.

PLANNING FOR WELLNESS OUTCOMES

Nurses can apply the following Nursing Outcomes Classification (NOC) terms to address risk factors and promote improved nutrition in older adults: Appetite, Bowel Elimination, Knowledge: Diet, Nutritional Status, Oral Health, Self-Care: Oral Hygiene, Sensory Function: Taste and Smell, Swallowing Status, and Weight: Body Mass. NOCs related to Constipation include Hydration, Bowel Elimination, Medication Response, and Symptom Control.

Wellness Opportunity

Knowledge: Health Promotion would be the NOC term for older adults who are ready to improve their nutrition to protect themselves from illness.

 NURSING INTERVENTIONS TO PROMOTE HEALTHY DIGESTION AND NUTRITION

Nurses can apply the following Nursing Interventions Classification terminologies in care plans: Bowel Management, Health Education, Nutrition Management, Nutritional Counseling, Nutritional Monitoring, Oral Health Maintenance, Oral Health Promotion, Referral, Self-Care Assistance, and Weight Management. Nursing interventions to promote healthy digestion and nutrition in older adults include health education about optimal nutrition and disease prevention and direct interventions to eliminate risk factors that interfere with digestion, nutrition, and oral health.

Promoting Optimal Nutrition and Preventing Disease

As already discussed, there is increasing recognition of the role of diet quality as an essential component of disease prevention and healthy aging. Interventions for healthy aging emphasize the inclusion of foods containing antioxidants and other nutrients that may play a protective and preventive role. In analyzing information about nutrients as preventive interventions, distinctions must be made between nutrients obtained from foods and those that are found in supplements. For example, a high dietary intake of a particular nutrient (e.g., carotenoids) may be beneficial in health promotion or disease prevention, but a dietary supplement product with the same nutrient may not necessarily have the same beneficial effects. Thus, nurses need to educate older adults about the importance of obtaining nutrients from food sources rather than relying on dietary supplements.

Nurses teach older adults about basic nutritional requirements, using easy-to-understand educational materials. Current recommendations for older adults, based on national dietary guidelines published, emphasize that older adults need to do the following:

- Increase intake of whole grains, dried peas and beans, all types of fruits and vegetables (especially dark green and orange vegetables).
- Consume fat-free or low-fat dairy products.

Box 18-7   Guidelines for Daily Food Intake for Older Adults

- Select a variety of high-quality foods and avoid "empty calories."
- Choose foods high in fiber.
- Avoid saturated fats; use liquid vegetable oils and soft margarines.

- Drink plenty of liquids without added sugars.
- Use a variety of herbs and spices to reduce the need for added salt and sugar.

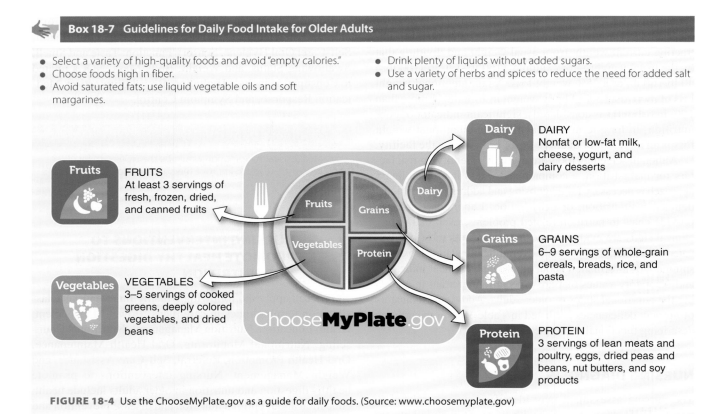

DAIRY
Nonfat or low-fat milk, cheese, yogurt, and dairy desserts

FRUITS
At least 3 servings of fresh, frozen, dried, and canned fruits

VEGETABLES
3–5 servings of cooked greens, deeply colored vegetables, and dried beans

GRAINS
6–9 servings of whole-grain cereals, breads, rice, and pasta

PROTEIN
3 servings of lean meats and poultry, eggs, dried peas and beans, nut butters, and soy products

ChooseMyPlate.gov

FIGURE 18-4   Use the ChooseMyPlate.gov as a guide for daily foods. (Source: www.choosemyplate.gov)

- Replace solid fats with oils, including those in fish, nuts, and seeds.
- Consume less sodium and saturated fat.
- Consume less food and beverages with added sugar, solid fats, and alcohol.
- Reduce caloric intake to maintain healthy weight.

Healthy older adults generally maintain optimal nutritional status through the daily intake of the foods listed in Box 18-7 and illustrated in Figure 18-4.

Interprofessional Collaboration

Nutrition education can be provided on an individual basis or in group settings, perhaps in conjunction with registered dietitians. In health care settings, nurses can facilitate a referral for registered dietitians to provide a more comprehensive assessment of nutritional needs and establish a plan of care aimed at attaining and maintaining optimal nutrition. In community settings, nurses sometimes provide nutrition education to groups of older adults. Nurses making home visits include nutrition education in their health teaching, make referrals for registered dietitian assessment and recommendations, and use available community resources to supplement these interventions. Models of health promotion discussed in Chapter 5 can be applied to working with older adults toward improved nutrition and changes in eating patterns.

Wellness Opportunity

Nurses promote personal responsibility by asking older adults to keep a 7-day diary of food and beverage intake and eating patterns and reviewing this to identify strengths and weaknesses of their diet.

Addressing Risk Factors That Interfere With Digestion and Nutrition

Nursing interventions address functional consequences of age-related changes that affect digestion and nutrition in all older adults. For example, if older adults experience early satiety during meals, they may benefit from eating five smaller meals a day, rather than the customary three meals a day. Similarly, teach older adults to maintain an upright position during eating and for ½ to 1 hour after eating, to compensate for age-related changes in swallowing. When older adults are malnourished or experience difficulties meeting minimal daily nutrient requirements, suggest the use of a high-protein nutritional supplement once or twice daily.

When functional limitations interfere with the activities involved in procuring, preparing, and enjoying food, interventions focus on improving the persons' access to palatable and nutritious meals. For the community-living older adults, this may involve identifying resources that offer assistance in obtaining food. Home-delivered meal programs are widely available to older adults at minimal cost, and group meal programs are available in almost every community through the federally funded National Nutrition Program for the Elderly, established under the Older Americans Act. These programs are effective in reducing nutritional risk for community-living older adults (National Academies of Sciences, Engineering, and Medicine, 2016). In addition to providing inexpensive and nutritionally balanced meals, these programs provide opportunities for social interaction. Local offices on aging may provide assistance with transportation or grocery shopping and are an excellent source of information about group and home-delivered meal programs.

When environmental barriers, such as high cupboards, interfere with older adults' ability to prepare meals safely, environmental modifications can be made. Nurses can apply many of the environmental adaptations suggested in the chapters on vision (see Chapter 17) and mobility (see Chapter 22) to improve the ability of older persons to prepare meals. When older adults have functional impairments, nurses can suggest specially adapted items for improving independence in eating and food preparation, such as the ones illustrated in Figure 18-5.

When older adults need accurate information about preventing constipation, or when other risk factors (e.g., a low-fiber diet) interfere with good bowel function, nursing interventions are directed toward education. Daily use of bran cereals or bran mixed with other foods is a common and effective strategy for preventing constipation. Box 18-8

Box 18-8 Health Education Regarding Constipation

- A bowel movement every day is not necessarily the norm for every adult.
- Each adult has an individual pattern of bowel regularity, with the normal range varying from three times a day to two times a week.
- Include several portions of the following high-fiber foods in your daily diet: fresh, uncooked fruits and vegetables; bran and other cereal products made from whole grains.
- Drink 8 to 10 glasses of noncaffeinated liquid, including fruit juices, every day.
- Avoid laxatives and enemas; instead, use dietary measures to promote good bowel functioning.
- If medication is needed to promote bowel regularity, a bulk-forming agent (e.g., psyllium or methylcellulose) is least likely to have detrimental effects, especially if fluid intake is adequate.
- Do not ignore the urge to defecate; try to respond as soon as you feel the urge.
- Exercise regularly.

identifies some of the foods and other interventions that aid in preventing constipation.

People with dementia are at increased risk for malnutrition and eating problems, as already discussed. Many of the interventions discussed in this chapter are relevant to addressing issues that commonly affect people with dementia; however, it is beyond the scope of this book to discuss this topic in depth. Online Learning Activity 18-5 provides links to resources for addressing mealtime and nutritional issues for people with dementia.

See ONLINE LEARNING ACTIVITY 18-5: EVIDENCE-BASED INFORMATION ABOUT MEALTIME AND NUTRITIONAL ISSUES FOR PEOPLE WITH DEMENTIA at http://thepoint.lww.com/Miller8e.

Wellness Opportunity

Nurses try to find "teachable moments" so they can correct any myths or misconceptions associated with unhealthy eating patterns.

When medications affect nutrition and digestion, nurses, caregivers, or older adults can discuss this problem with prescribing health care practitioners to identify ways of alleviating this risk or addressing the consequences. If over-the-counter medications have a detrimental effect on nutrition or digestion, nurses educate older adults about medication–nutrient interactions and discuss ways of addressing the negative effects. Pharmacists help by suggesting interventions that will compensate for, or minimize, the effects of both prescription and over-the-counter medications on nutrition and digestion. When alcohol consumption interferes with

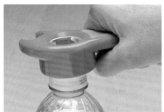
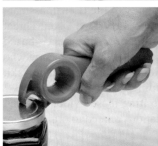
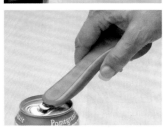
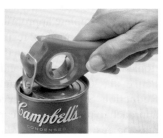
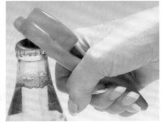

FIGURE 18-5 Adaptive devices. (Reprinted with permission from www.activeforever.com)

nutrition, interventions might address the potential problem of alcoholism, or they may be aimed at compensating for the detrimental effects on nutrition. Nurses can recommend vitamin supplementation for people with a history of alcoholism after a medical evaluation has been performed to identify any underlying conditions, such as pernicious anemia.

Addressing Nutritional Problems in Health Care Settings

In health care settings, nutritional problems are best addressed through a multidisciplinary team approach that includes the roles for health care professionals shown in Box 18-6.

- Geriatric primary care practitioner: addresses medical conditions that affect nutritional and hydration status and eating patterns
- Nurse: addresses all aspects of care related to nutrition and eating; educates direct-care staff about assessment and interventions
- Speech–language therapist: addresses dysphagia
- Rehabilitation therapist: addresses conditions that affect eating; recommends adaptive equipment
- Registered dietician: assesses nutritional status, identifies and addresses risks, establishes nutritional plan of care
- Pharmacist: reviews medications, addresses drug–nutrient interactions
- Social worker: addresses interpersonal relationships and socioeconomic conditions that affect eating and nutrition

Primary responsibilities of nurses include identifying issues that can be addressed by other health care professionals, facilitating referrals, and coordinating care plans. Additional interventions that are within the scope of direct nursing care include providing high-protein nutritional supplements, identifying and arranging to be provided food and mealtime preferences, and arranging for appropriate mealtime assistance.

See ONLINE LEARNING ACTIVITY 18-6: ARTICLE ABOUT NUTRITIONAL INTERVENTIONS FOR FRAIL OLDER ADULTS at http://thepoint.lww.com/Miller8e.

Promoting Oral and Dental Health

Good oral health is increasingly being recognized as an essential component of well-being for older adults (Rouxel, Tsakos, Chandola, et al., 2016). Moreover, good oral care is being addressed as a health promotion intervention for preventing serious conditions such as pneumonia, cardiovascular disease, and systemic inflammatory diseases (Kumar, 2017; Scannapieco & Santos, 2016). Nurses have important responsibilities in implementing interventions to promote oral and dental health for older adults in all settings.

If older adults have avoided dental care because of resignation to poor oral health or a poor understanding of the need for preventive dental care, nurses attempt to change these attitudes through education. Nurses also emphasize the importance of obtaining dental care every 6 months and, if appropriate, facilitate referrals for dental care. For homebound older adults, home dental services are often available, especially in large urban communities. In addition, low-cost dental services and dentures may be available through schools of dentistry. Nurses need to be familiar with local resources, so that they can inform older adults and their caregivers about the dental services that are available in their community. For older adults in any setting, if xerostomia interferes with digestion or nutrition, nurses may suggest or facilitate a referral for a medical evaluation to identify disease processes or medication effects that may be contributing factors.

For independent older adults, nurses provide health education about oral care, including alleviation of dry mouth if this is pertinent, as described in Box 18-9. Older adults who have limited manual dexterity can adapt handles of toothbrushes for ease of use or obtain specially designed brushes to increase the self-care abilities. Nurses can also suggest the use of battery-operated brushes, which are effective, easy to use, and relatively inexpensive. Child-size toothbrushes (manual or automatic) may be easier to use for dependent older adults, especially if access to all their teeth is limited.

Addressing Oral Health Care Needs of Older Adults in Health Care Settings

In health care settings, nursing staff are responsible for providing oral hygiene for patients and residents who cannot initiate or complete appropriate self-care. This is imperative for cognitively impaired residents because maintaining good oral care is an often neglected aspect of care that affects nutritional intake, disease risk, and quality of life (Lee, Plassman, Pan, et al., 2016). The Managing Oral Hygiene Using Threat Reduction Strategies intervention is an evidence-based approach to providing oral care to people with dementia who may be resistant to care (Jablonski-Jaudon, Kolanowski, Winstead, et al., 2016). See Online Learning Activity 18-7 for an excellent video demonstrating these evidence-based nursing strategies. Recommendations related to oral care are described in Box 18-10.

See ONLINE LEARNING ACTIVITY 18-7: EVIDENCE-BASED INFORMATION ABOUT ORAL CARE FOR OLDER ADULTS at http://thepoint.lww.com/Miller8e.

Wellness Opportunity

Nurses promote independence and self-care in oral hygiene by facilitating referrals for occupational therapy for older adults with functional impairments.

Box 18-9 Health Education Regarding Oral Care and Dry Mouth

Health Education Regarding Care of the Teeth and Gums

- Oral care should include daily use of dental floss and twice-daily brushing of all tooth surfaces.
- Use a soft-bristled toothbrush and fluoridated toothpaste.
- If you have any limitations that interfere with your ability to use a regular toothbrush, you may benefit from using an electric or battery-powered brush or a brush with a specially designed handle (available where medical supplies are sold).
- Easy-to-use floss aids are inexpensive and widely available for facilitating dental flossing; they are especially helpful for people with any limitations in manual strength or dexterity, or limited range of motion in the upper extremities.
- Some mouth rinses have cleansing, antimicrobial, and moisturizing effect, but they are used in conjunction with—not instead of—brushing.
- Avoid using alcohol-containing mouthwashes because of their drying effect.
- Because sugar is a major contributing factor to tooth decay, it is important to limit the intake of sugary substances, especially substances that are kept in the mouth for long periods (e.g., gum, hard candy).
- After eating sugar-containing foods, rinse your mouth or brush your teeth.
- Visit a dentist every 6 months for regular oral care.
- If partial or complete dentures are worn, remove them at night, keep them in water, and clean them before placing them back in your mouth.

Health Education Regarding Dry Mouth

- Excessive dry mouth may be caused by medical conditions or medication effects and should be evaluated before symptomatic treatment is initiated.
- Drink at least 10 eight-ounce glasses of noncaffeinated fluid during the day, and drink sips of water at frequent intervals.
- Suck on xylitol-flavored fluoride tablets or sugar-free hard candies to stimulate saliva flow.
- Chew sugar-free gum with xylitol for 15 minutes after meals to stimulate saliva flow and promote oral hygiene.
- Try using one of the many brands of saliva substitutes available at drugstores, but avoid those that contain sorbitol because they can worsen the condition.
- Avoid sucking lozenges containing citric acid because of their detrimental effects on tooth enamel.
- Avoid alcohol, alcohol-containing mouthwashes, and highly acidic drinks (e.g., orange or grapefruit juice) because these tend to exacerbate the condition.
- Avoid smoking because it exacerbates the symptoms and further irritates the oral mucous membranes.
- Pay particular attention to oral hygiene because a dry mouth increases the risk for gum and dental diseases.
- Maintain optimal room humidity, especially at night.

 Box 18-10 Evidence-Based Practice: Oral Health Care for Older Adults

Statement of the Problem

- Oral health is essential for promoting overall health, preventing disease, maintaining speech and alimentary functioning, and preserving quality of life.
- Even though regular oral care is essential for good health, it is often neglected as an aspect of care for older adults.
- Oral hygiene declines as older adults experience cognitive and functional impairments and become increasingly dependent on daily activities.
- Oral problems are not the direct result of aging and can be prevented, or at least detected at an early stage.
- Medications and medical conditions can increase the risk for oral problems, even when good oral care is provided.
- Dental caries and periodontal disease are plaque-related, preventable oral diseases that are likely to develop from poor oral hygiene.
- When untreated, poor oral health can lead to malnutrition, dehydration, pneumonia, cardiovascular disease, joint infections, and poor diabetic control.

Recommendations for Nursing Assessment

- Use an evidence-based assessment tool, such as the Kayser-Jones Brief Oral Health Status Examination, which is available at https://consultgeri.org
- Immediately arrange for a dental evaluation if any of the following occur: enlarged and tender lymph nodes; lips red at corners; discoloration, break in integrity, or any abnormality of any oral tissue that has been present for 2 weeks or more; more than one loose, broken, or missing tooth; redness at borders around teeth; redness or soreness under artificial teeth; fewer than four teeth in either jaw; seven or fewer pairs of teeth in chewing position; dentures missing, not being worn, or damaged.
- Assess self-care ability of older adults related to effective oral care, and involve occupational therapy services as appropriate.

Recommendations for Nursing Interventions

- Use a toothbrush with soft nylon bristles and toothpaste with fluoride.
- Provide oral care (for teeth and dentures) morning, evening, and as needed.
- Brush teeth, dentures, and tongue.
- Plain foam swabs can be used for cleaning oral mucous membrane of an edentulous adult, but they are not as effective as toothbrushes for cleaning teeth.
- Never use lemon–glycerin swabs because they dry the mucous membrane and erode tooth enamel.
- Mouth rinses that contain alcohol dry the mucous membrane and should be diluted in half with water if they are used.
- Use chlorhexidine (e.g., Peridex) only if it is prescribed by a dentist.
- Brush dentures before placing them in a denture cup.
- Arrange for semiannual or annual dental evaluations, or more frequent evaluations if problems are identified.

Additional Recommendations for Nursing Interventions for People With Dementia

- If the person resists oral care, consider that oral pain is the cause of the resistance.
- Develop an individualized oral care plan that includes specific communication techniques, as described in Online Learning Activity 18-7.
- Teach all nursing staff about the individualized care plan and involve family caregivers as appropriate.
- Arrange for more frequent dental examinations if it is difficult to provide adequate oral hygiene.

Sources: O'Connor, L. (2016). Oral health care. In M. Boltz, E. Capezuti, T. Fulmer, & D. Zwicker (Eds.), *Evidence-based geriatric nursing protocols for best practice* (5th ed., pp. 103–110). New York: Springer Publishing Co.; Jablonski-Jaudon, R., Kolanowski, A., Winstead, V., et al. (2016). Maturation of the MOUTh Intervention: From reducing threat to relationship-centered care. *Journal of Gerontological Nursing, 42,* 15–23.

See ONLINE LEARNING ACTIVITY 18-8: RESOURCES FOR HEALTH PROMOTION RELATED TO NUTRITION IN OLDER ADULTS at http://thepoint.lww.com/Miller8e.

EVALUATING EFFECTIVENESS OF NURSING INTERVENTIONS

Nursing care for older adults with Imbalanced Nutrition: Less than Body Requirements is evaluated by determining whether older adults have a daily nutrient intake that corresponds with metabolic needs and by older adults' achieving a body weight within 110% of their ideal body weight. For older adults with constipation, or risks for constipation, evaluation criteria would depend on their verbalizing accurate information about constipation, identifying the factors that contribute to constipation, and reporting that they pass soft stools on a regular basis without any straining or discomfort.

Unfolding Case Study

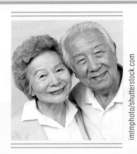

Part 3: Mrs. D. at 76 Years of Age

Mrs. D. returns for a "Counseling for Health" follow-up session with a 7-day diet history and a list of her medications, as you requested. You review the diet history and find that in response to your previous health education about constipation, Mrs. D. now uses whole-wheat bread instead of white, and eats more fresh fruits and vegetables. You assess that her daily intake is only approximately 800 calories, of which pastries account for a high percentage. She rarely eats meat, perhaps because of the poor condition of her teeth. Her medications include levothyroxine (Synthroid) 50 mcg, citalopram (Celexa) 20 mg daily; clonidine (Catapres) 0.2 mg daily; triamterene 37.5 mg or hydrochlorothiazide 25 mg (Dyazide) daily; and 600 mg calcium carbonate twice daily.

THINKING POINTS

- What specific risk factors do you address in your health teaching interventions?
- What health teaching would you give about alleviating risk factors?
- What interventions would you suggest to improve Mrs. D.'s nutrition?
- What interventions would you suggest to address Mrs. D.'s dry mouth (which you noticed during Mrs. D.'s last visit)?
- What health teaching would you provide about oral and dental care?

Unfolding Case Study

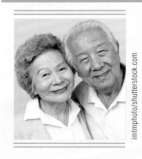

Part 4: Mr. D. at 85 Years of Age

Mr. D. is an 85-year-old widower who was referred for home care after a hospitalization in the Acute Care for the Elderly (ACE) unit for heart failure. During the hospitalization, the geriatric assessment team diagnosed protein-energy malnutrition. Mr. D.'s weight (116 lb) is only 75% of his ideal body weight (155 lb). In addition, laboratory work revealed the following abnormal values: hemoglobin, 10%; hematocrit, 33%; and serum albumin, 3.2 g/dL. Mr. D.'s heart failure is stable, and he ambulates with a walker but is very weak. In addition to orders pertaining to assessment and management of the newly diagnosed heart failure, home care orders include nursing assessment of his home situation, nutrition education, and weight monitoring. The geriatric assessment team in the ACE unit, which included a registered dietitian, recommended that Mr. D. have a daily intake of 1600 calories, including a minimum of 60 g of protein (240 calories). Mr. D. could meet this goal if his daily intake included the minimum number of servings from each food group as listed in Box 18-7.

Part 4: Mr. D. at 85 Years of Age (Continued)

NURSING ASSESSMENT

You are the visiting nurse assigned to perform the initial assessment and develop a care plan. Mr. D. lives alone in a senior high-rise apartment and, until recently, participated in social activities and used the senior transportation service to get to medical appointments and the grocery store. He used to prepare his own meals and shop for his groceries once a week but has not been out of his apartment in the past month because of gradually increasing weakness, shortness of breath, and swelling in his legs. After his health began declining, a neighbor began doing his grocery shopping. Typical meals are toast and coffee for breakfast; canned soup, a lunch meat sandwich, and cookies for lunch; and a Budget Gourmet entrée for supper. Mr. D. says that he never really learned to cook very well but that he got along "well enough for a man my age." He says that he does not particularly enjoy the convenience foods that he eats but states, "They sure are easy to fix, even if they are boring." Mr. D. acknowledges that he has thought about going to the daily noon meal offered at a nearby church but has not followed through because "the senior van doesn't go there, but it does go to the grocery store. Besides, I'm never very hungry because food just doesn't interest me the way it used to when I had Magda's good Hungarian cooking." Mr. D. reports a gradual weight loss of approximately 50 lb since his wife died 2 years ago. He says that he was too heavy when his wife used to do the cooking, so he is not concerned about his weight loss. He has full dentures but has not used them for the past year because they are loose and uncomfortable. He has not done anything about his dentures because he manages to chew soft foods and his dentist retired several years ago.

NURSING DIAGNOSIS

One of the nursing diagnoses that you address in your home care plan is Altered Nutrition: Less than Body Requirements, related to social isolation, declining health, ill-fitting dentures, and lack of enjoyment of food. You also question whether depression may be a contributing factor. Evidence comes from his low body weight, laboratory data consistent with poor nutritional status, and his descriptions of his eating and food preparation patterns.

NURSING CARE PLAN FOR MR. D.

Expected Outcome	Nursing Interventions	Nursing Evaluation
Mr. D. will state what his daily needs are for each food group	• Give Mr. D. a copy of Box 18-7 and use it as a basis for teaching about daily nutrient requirements	• Mr. D. will describe an eating pattern that meets his daily nutritional needs

Mr. D. will identify a method for meeting his nutrient needs	• Gain Mr. D.'s permission to arrange for home health aide assistance three times weekly for meal preparation and grocery shopping
	  ◆ Teach about eating smaller meals more frequently
	• Explore with Mr. D. various options for broadening his food selection to improve his nutritional intake (e.g., including dairy products and more fruits and vegetables)
	• Develop a meal plan with Mr. D. that includes foods that he enjoys but are not currently part of his diet
	  ◆ Discuss the nutritional value of these foods and suggest that he add new food items in each of the food group categories in which he is deficient
		• Mr. D. will describe an acceptable plan for meeting his nutritional needs
		• Mr. D. will gain between 0.5 and 1 lb weekly until he reaches the goal of 150 lb

Mr. D. will have his dentures evaluated and modified or replaced	• Discuss with Mr. D. the importance of dentures in chewing efficiency and food enjoyment • Discuss the long-term detrimental effects of lack of dentures • Explore ways of obtaining a dental evaluation	• Mr. D. will chew his food with dentures that fit properly

(continued)

Part 4: Mr. D. at 85 Years of Age (Continued)

THINKING POINTS

- What risk factors are likely to be contributing to Mr. D.'s gradual weight loss during the past?

- What further assessment information would you want to have?

QSEN APPLICATION

QSEN Competency	Knowledge/Skill/Attitude	Application to Mr. D. When he is 85 Years of Age
Patient-centered care	(K) Integrate understanding of multiple dimensions of patient-centered care	Develop individualized plan for improving nutritional intake, as described in care plan
	(K) Examine common barriers to active involvement in patients	Identify barriers to obtaining dentures and address these in care plan
	(S) Elicit patient values, preferences, and expressed needs	
Teamwork and collaboration	(K) Recognize contributions of other individuals and groups in helping patient achieve health goals	Integrate the services of a home health aide to provide assistance with meal preparation, grocery shopping, and transportation for dental appointments
	(S) Integrate the contributions of others who play a role in helping patient achieve health goals	Consider a referral for a registered dietitian consultation to reinforce and support nutrition teaching
		Develop plan for Mr. D. to obtain dentures
Evidence-based practice	(S) Base individualized care plan on patient values, clinical expertise, and evidence	Discuss information in Box 18-7 in the context of Mr. D.'s food preferences and individualized dietary needs
	(A)Value evidence-based practice as integral to determining the best clinical practice	

Chapter Highlights

Age-Related Changes That Affect Digestion and Eating Patterns

- Diminished senses of smell and taste
- Changes in oral cavity
- Degenerative changes in all structures of the gastrointestinal tract

Nutritional Requirements for Healthy Aging

- Current emphasis on overall dietary patterns associated with healthy aging
- Nutrients of particular importance to older adults (Box 18-1)

Risk Factors That Affect Digestion and Nutrition

- Conditions that can lead to nutritional deficiencies (Table 18-1)
- Functional impairments and disease processes
- Dysphagia (Box18-2, Figure 18-1)
- Effects of medications (Table 18-2)
- Effects of alcohol and smoking
- Psychosocial factors (e.g., dementia, depression, loneliness)
- Cultural considerations (Box 18-3, Figure 18-2)
- Socioeconomic influences

- Environmental factors related to institutional or home settings
- Behaviors based on myths and misunderstandings

Functional Consequences Affecting Digestion and Nutrition

- Ability to procure, prepare, and enjoy food
- Changes in oral function
- Poor nutritional status and weight changes
- Malnutrition and dehydration

Pathologic Condition Affecting Digestive Wellness: Constipation

- Constipation

Nursing Assessment of Digestion and Nutrition (Boxes 18-4 to 18-6)

- Usual nutrient intake and eating patterns
- Risks that interfere with any aspect of obtaining, preparing, eating, and enjoying food
- Physical assessment related to nutrition and hydration status
- The MNA tool (Figure 18-3)

Nursing Diagnosis

- Readiness for Enhanced Nutrition
- Imbalanced Nutrition: Less than Body Requirements
- Constipation
- Impaired Oral Mucous Membrane

Planning for Wellness Outcomes

- Improved appetite, nutritional status, oral health, depression level
- Increased knowledge about diet, improved health beliefs about constipation

Nursing Interventions to Promote Healthy Digestion and Nutrition (Figure 18-4; Boxes 18-7 to 18-10)

- Addressing risk factors: functional limitation, environmental factors, medications, alcohol consumption
- Promoting oral and dental health
- Teaching about optimal nutrition

Evaluating Effectiveness of Nursing Interventions

- Daily nutrient intake that corresponds to metabolic needs
- Achieving/maintaining body weight within 110% of ideal body weight for the individual
- Achieving/maintaining regular bowel elimination
- Mr. D. at 85 years

Critical Thinking Exercises

1. Discuss specific ways in which each of the following factors might influence the eating patterns of older adults: depression, medications, sensory changes, cognitive impairments, functional impairments, economic factors, social circumstances, and oral health factors.
2. Describe at least three characteristics of eating patterns for each of the following cultural groups: American Indians, Hispanic Americans, African Americans, and Asian Americans.
3. How would you assess digestion and nutrition for an older adult in each of the following settings: home, long-term care facility, and acute care facility?
4. Outline a health education plan for teaching older adults about constipation. Include the following points: definition of constipation, risk factors for constipation, and interventions to prevent and address constipation.
5. Outline a health education plan for teaching older adults about oral hygiene and dental care.

 For more information about the topics discussed in this chapter, be sure to check out the interactive Online Learning Activities and other helpful resources at http://thepoint.lww.com/Miller8e.

REFERENCES

Anderson, J., & Nieman, D. (2016). Diet quality-the Greeks had it right! *Nutrients, 8,* E636.

Andy, U. U., Vaughan, C. P., Burgio, K. L., et al. (2016). Shared risk factors for constipation, fecal incontinence, and combined symptoms in older U.S. adults. *Journal of the American Geriatrics Society, 64,* e183–e188.

Artaza-Artabe, J., Saez-Lopez, P., Sanchez-Hernandez, N., et al. (2016). The relationship between nutrition and frailty: Effects of protein intake, nutritional supplementation, vitamin D and exercise on muscle metabolism in the elderly: A systematic review. *Maturitas, 93,* 89–99.

Baer, A. N., & Walitt, B. (2017). Sjögren syndrome and other causes of sicca in older adults. *Clinics in Geriatric Medicine, 33,* 87–103.

Baijens, L., Clave, P., Cras, P., et al. (2016). European Society for Swallowing Disorders - European Union Geriatric Medicine Society white paper: oropharyngeal dysphagia as a geriatric syndrome. *Clinical Interventions in Aging, 11,* 1403–1428.

Bertozzi, B., Tosti, V., & Fontana, L. (2017). Beyond calories: An integrated approach to promote health, longevity, and well-being. *Gerontology, 63,* 13–19.

Bhargava, V., & Lee, J. S. (2016). Food insecurity and health care utilization among older adults in the United States. *Journal of Nutrition in Gerontology and Geriatrics, 35,* 177–192.

Bihuniak, J. D., Ramos, A., Huedo-Medina, T., et al. (2016). Adherence to a Mediterranean-style diet and its influence on cardiovascular risk factors in postmenopausal women. *Journal of the Academy of Nutrition & Dietetics, 116,* 1767–1775.

Brodsky, M. B., Suiter, D. M., Gonzalez-Fernandez, M., et al. (2016). Screening accuracy for aspiration using bedside water swallow tests: A systematic review and meta-analysis. *Chest, 150,* 148–163.

Byberg, L., Bellavia, A., Larsson, S. C., et al. (2016). Mediterranean diet and hip fracture in Swedish men and women. *Journal of Bone Marrow Research, 31,* 2098–2105.

Campbell, G., Carter, T., Kring, D., et al. (2016). Nursing bedside dysphagia screen: Is it valid? *Journal of Neuroscience Nursing, 48,* 75–79.

Carrion, S., Roca, M., Costa, A., et al. (2017). Nutritional status of older patients with oropharyngeal dysphagia in a chronic versus acute clinical situation. *Clinical Nutrition, 36,* 1110–1116.

Casas-Agustench, P., Cherubini, A., & Andres-Lacueva, C. (2017). Lipids and physical function in older adults. *Current Opinion in Clinical Nutrition and Metabolic Care, 19,* 1–4.

Cederholm, T. (2017). Fish consumption and omega-3 fatty acid supplementation for prevention or treatment of cognitive decline, dementia or Alzheimer's disease in older adults - any news? *Current Opinion in Clinical Nutrition and Metabolic Care, 20*(2), 104–109.

Cederholm, T., & Morley, J. (2016). Nutrient interface with biology and aging. *Current Opinion in Clinical Nutrition and Metabolic Care, 19,* 1–4.

Cereda, E., Pedrolli, C., Klersy, C., et al. (2016). Nutritional status in older persons according to healthcare setting: A systematic review and meta-analysis of prevalence data using MNA. *Clinical Nutrition, 35,* 1282–1290.

Chang, S. F. (2017). Frailty is a major related factor for at risk of malnutrition in community-dwelling older adults. *Journal of Nursing Scholarship, 49,* 63–72.

Chokhavatia, S., John, E., Bridgeman, M., et al. (2016). Constipation in elderly patients with noncancer pain: Focus on opioid-induced constipation. *Drugs & Aging, 33,* 557–574.

Coleman-Jensen, A., Rabbitt, M., Gregory, C., et al. (2016). *Household food security in the United States in 2015.* Washington, DC: U.S. Department of Agriculture, Economic Research Service.

Commodore-Mensah, Y., Ukonu, N., Obisesan, O., et al. (2016). Length of residence in the United States is associated with a higher prevalence of cardiometabolic risk factors in immigrants: A contemporary analysis of the National Health Interview Survey. *Journal of the American Heart Association, 5,* e004059.

Correia, C., Lopez, K., Wroblewski, K., et al. (2016). Global sensory impairment in older adults in the United States. *Journal of the American Geriatrics Society, 64,* 306–313.

Correia, M., Hegazi, R., Graf, J., et al. (2016). Addressing disease-related malnutrition in healthcare: A Latin American perspective. *Journal of Parenteral and Enteral Nutrition, 40,* 319–325.

Devanand, D. P. (2016). Olfactory identification deficits, cognitive decline, and dementia in older adults. *American Journal of Geriatric Psychiatry, 24,* 1151–1157.

Dietary Guidelines Advisory Committee. (2015). *Scientific report of the 2015 Dietary Guidelines Advisory Committee.* Washington, DC: U.S. Department of Agriculture.

Donini, L. M., Poggiogalle, E., Molfino, A., et al. (2016). Mini-nutritional assessment malnutrition universal screening tool, and nutrition risk screening tool for the nutritional evaluation of older adult nursing home residents. *Journal of the American Medical Directors Association, 17,* e11–e18.

Edwards, D., Carrier, J., & Hopkinson, J. (2016). Mealtime assistance for older adults in hospital settings and rehabilitation units from the perspective of patients, families and healthcare professionals: A mixed methods systematic review. *JBI Database of Systematic Reviews and Implementation Reports, 14,* 261–357.

Federal Interagency Forum on Aging-Related Statistics. (2016). *Older Americans 2015: Key Indicators of Well-Being.* Washington, DC: Government Printing Office.

Gidwaney, N. G., Bajpai, M., & Chokhavatia, S. (2016). Gastrointestinal dysmotility in the elderly. *Journal of Clinical Gastroenterology, 50,* 819–827.

Gil-Montoya, J. A., Sánchez-Lara, I., Carnero-Pardo, C., et al. (2017). Oral hygiene in the elderly with different degrees of cognitive impairment and dementia. *Journal of the American Geriatrics Society, 65*(3), 642–647.

Gil-Montoya, J. A., Silvestre, F. J., Barrios, R., et al. (2016). Treatment of xerostomia and hyposalivation in the elderly: A systematic review. *Medicina Oral, Patología Oral y Cirugía Bucal, 21,* e355–e366.

Gopinath, B., Flood, V., Kifley, A., et al. (2016). Association between carbohydrate nutrition and successful aging over 10 years. *Journals of Gerontology: Biological Sciences & Medical Sciences, 71,* 1335–1340.

Hamirudin, A. H., Charlton, K., & Walton, K. (2016). Outcomes related to nutrition screening in community living older adults: A systematic review. *Archives of Gerontology & Geriatrics, 62,* 9–25.

Heijnen, B., Speyer, R., Bulow, M., et al. (2016). "What about swallowing?" Diagnostic performance of daily clinical practice compared with Eating Assessment Tool-10. *Dysphagia, 31,* 214–221.

Herdman, T., & Kamitsura, S. (Eds.). (2018). *NANDA International Nursing Diagnoses Definitions and Classification, 2018–2020* (11th ed., pp. 34–44). New York: Thieme Publishers.

Hoffman, H. J., Rawal, S., Li, C. M., et al. (2016). New chemosensory component in the U.S. National Health and Nutrition Examination Survey (NHANES): first-year results for measured olfactory dysfunction. *Review of Endocrine & Metabolic Disorders, 17,* 221–240.

Hooper, L., Bunn, D. K., Downing, A., et al. (2016). Which frail older people are dehydrated? The UK DRIE Study. *Journal of Gerontology: Biological Sciences and Medical Sciences, 71,* 1341–1347.

Jablonski-Jaudon, R., Kolanowski, A., Winstead, V., et al. (2016). Maturation of the MOUTh Intervention: From reducing threat to relationship-centered care. *Journal of Gerontological Nursing, 42,* 15–23.

Kim, Y., & Je, Y. (2016). Dietary fibre intake and mortality from cardiovascular disease and all cancers: A meta-analysis of prospective cohort studies. *Archives of Cardiovascular Disease, 109,* 39–54.

Kucukerdonmez, O., Varli, S. N., & Koksal, E. (2017). Comparison of nutritional status in the elderly according to living situations. *Journal of Nutrition, Health & Aging, 21,* 25–30.

Kumar, P. S. (2017). From focal sepsis to periodontal medicine: A century of exploring the role of the oral microbiome in systemic disease. *Journal of Physiology, 595*(2), 465–476.

Lahmann, N. A., Tannen, A., & Suhr, R. (2016). Underweight and malnutrition in home care: A multicenter study. *Clinical Nutrition, 35,* 1140–1146.

Landi, F., Calvani, R., Tosato, M., et al. (2016). Anorexia of aging: Risk factors, consequences, and potential treatments. *Nutrients, 8,* 69.

Lee, K. H., Plassman, B., Pan, W., et al. (2016). Mediation effect of oral hygiene on the relationship between cognitive function and oral health in older adults. *Journal of Gerontological Nursing, 42,* 30–37.

Lera, L., Sanchez, H., Angel, B., et al. (2016). Mini nutritional assessment short-form: Validation in five Latin American cities: SABE Study. *Journal of Nutrition in Health and Aging, 20,* 797–805.

Li, B., Zhang, G., Tan, M., et al. (2016). Consumption of whole grains in relation to mortality from all causes, cardiovascular disease, and diabetes: Dose–response meta-analysis of prospective cohort studies. *Medicine, 95,* e4229.

Liang, X., Ding, D., Zhao, Q., et al. (2016). Association between olfactory identification and cognitive function in community-dwelling elderly: the Shanghai aging study. *BioMed Central Neurology, 16*(1),199.

Luciano, M., Corley, J., Cox, S. R., et al. (2017). Mediterranean-type diet and brain structural change from 73 to 76 years in a Scottish cohort. *Neurology, 88*(5), 449–455.

Martínez-González, M. A. (2016). Benefits of the Mediterranean diet beyond the Mediterranean Sea and beyond food patterns. *BioMed Central Medicine, 14,* 157.

Martínez-Gonzáles, M. A., & Martin-Calvo, N. (2016). Mediterranean diet and life expectancy; beyond olive oil, fruits, and vegetables. *Current Opinion in Clinical Nutrition and Metabolic Care, 19,* 401–407.

Masada, A., Gomez-Caamano, S., Lorenzo-Lopez, L., et al. (2016). Health determinants of nutritional status in community-dwelling older population: the VERISAUDE study. *Public Health Nutrition, 19,* 2220–2228.

McCrow, J., Morton, M., Travers, C., et al. (2016). Associations between dehydration, cognitive impairment, and frailty in older hospitalized patients. *Journal of Gerontological Nursing, 42,* 19–27.

Melina, V., Craig, W., & Levin, S. (2016). Position of the Academy of Nutrition and Dietetics: vegetarian diets. *Journal of the Academy of Nutrition and Dietetics, 116,* 1970–1980.

Mentes, J. (2016). Managing oral hydration. In M. Boltz, E. Capezuti, T. Fulmer, & D. Zwicker. (Eds.) *Evidence-Based Geriatric Nursing Protocols for Best Practice,* pp. 111–124. New York: Springer Publishing.

Milte, C. M., & McNaughton, S. A. (2016). Dietary patterns and successful ageing: a systematic review. *European Journal of Nutrition, 55,* 423–450.

Moreira, N. C., Krausch-Hofmann, S., Matthys, C., et al. (2016). Risk factors for malnutrition in older adults: A systematic review of the literature based on longitudinal data. *Advances in Nutrition, 16,* 507–522.

Morley, J., & Bauer, J. (2017). Nutrition and aging successfully. *Current Opinion in Clinical Nutrition, 20,* 1–3.

Naseer, M., Forssell, H., & Fagerstrom, C. (2016). Malnutrition, functional ability and mortality among older people aged ≥ 60 years: a 7-year longitudinal study. *European Journal of Clinical Nutrition, 70,* 399–404.

National Academies of Sciences, Engineering, and Medicine. (2016). *Meeting the dietary needs of older adults: Exploring the impact of the physical, social, and cultural environments, workshop summary.* Washington, DC: National Academies Press, doi: 10.17226/23496.

O'Connor, L. (2016). Oral health care. In M. Boltz, E. Capezuti, T. Fulmer, et al. (Eds.), *Evidence-based geriatric nursing protocols for best practice* (5th ed., pp. 103–110). New York: Springer Publishing Co.

Ogawa, T., Uota, M., Ikebe, K., et al. (2016). Taste detection of elderly nursing home residents. *Journal of Oral Rehabilitation, 43,* 505–510.

Ogawa, T., Uota, M., Ikebe, K., et al. (2017). Longitudinal study of factors affecting taste sense decline in old-old individuals. *Journal of Oral Rehabilitation, 44,* 22–29.

Oldways Nutrition Exchange. (2016). *The role of traditional diets in a healthy lifestyle.* Available at www.oldways.org.

Ottaviano, G., Frasson, G., Nardello, E., et al. (2016). Olfaction deterioration in cognitive disorders in the elderly. *Aging and Clinical and Experimental Research, 28*, 37–45.

Perez-Zepeda, M. U., Castrejon-Perez, R. C., Wynne-Bannister, E., et al. (2016). Frailty and food insecurity in older adults. *Public Health Nutrition, 19*, 2844–2849.

Pisano, M., & Hilas, O. (2016). Zinc and taste disturbances in older adults: A review of the literature. *Consultant Pharmacist: The Journal of the American Society of Consultant Pharmacists, 31*, 267–270.

Rawal, S., Hoffman, H. J., Bainbridge, K. E., et al. (2016). Prevalence and risk factors of self-reported smell and taste alterations: Results from the 2011–2012 U.S. National Health and Nutrition Examination Survey (NHANES). *Chemical Senses, 41*, 69–76.

Reinders, I, Visser, M., & Schaap, L. (2017). Body weight and body composition in old age and their relationship with frailty. *Current Opinion in Clinical Nutrition, 20*, 11–15.

Rouxel, P., Tsakos, G., Chandola, T., et al. (2016). Oral health-a neglected aspect of subjective well-being in later life. *Journals of Gerontology: Psychological Sciences and Social Sciences,* doi: 10.1093/geronb/gbw024 [Epub ahead of print].

Sakai, M., Ikeda, M., Kazui, H., et al. (2016). Decline of gustatory sensitivity with the progression of Alzheimer's disease. *International Journal of Psychogeriatrics, 28*, 511–517.

Sanford, A. M. (2017). Anorexia of aging and its role for frailty. *Current Opinion in Clinical Nutrition and Metabolic Care, 20*, 554–560.

Scannapieco, F. A., & Cantos, A. (2016). Oral inflammation and infection, and chronic medical diseases: implications for the elderly. *Periodoltology 2000, 72*, 153–175.

Schrader, E., Grosch, E., Bertsch, T., et al. (2016). Nutritional and functional status in geriatric day hospital patients - MNA short form versus full MNA. *Journal of Nutrition in Health and Aging, 20*, 918–926.

Schubert, M. L. (2016). Gastric acid secretion. *Current Opinion in Gastroenterology, 32*, 452–460.

Schubert, C. R., Fischer, M. E., Pinto, A. A., et al. (2017). Odor detection thresholds in a population of older adults. *Laryngoscope,* doi: 10.1002/lary.26457 [Epub ahead of print].

Shakersain, B., Santoni, G., Faxen-Irving, G., et al. (2016). Nutritional status and survival among older adults: an 11-year population-based longitudinal study. *European Journal of Clinical Nutrition, 70*, 320–325.

Soenen, S., Rayner, C., Jones, K., et al. (2016). The aging gastrointestinal tract. *Current Opinion in Clinical Nutrition, 19*, 12–18.

Struijk, E., Guallar-Castillón, P., Rodríguez-Artalejo, F., et al. (2016). Mediterranean dietary patterns and impaired physical function in older adults. *Journals of Gerontology: Medical Sciences,* doi: 10.1093/gerona/glw208 [Epub ahead of print].

Tanasiewicz, M., Hildebrandt, T., & Obersztyn, I. (2016). Xerostomia of various etiologies: A review of the literature. *Advances in Clinical and Experimental Medicine, 25*, 199–206.

Wakabayashi, H., & Matsushima, M. (2016). Dysphagia assessed by the 10-item Eating Assessment Tool is associated with nutritional status and activities of daily living in elderly individuals requiring long-term care. *Journal of Nutrition in Health & Aging, 20*, 22–27.

Werth, B. L., Williams, K. A., & Pont, L. G. (2017). Laxative use and self-reported constipation in a community-dwelling elderly population. *Gastroenterology Nursing, 40*(2), 134–141.

Wirth, R., Dziewas, R., Beck, A. M., et al. (2016). Oropharyngeal dysphagia in older persons - from pathophysiology to adequate intervention: a review and summary of international expert meeting. *Clinical Interventions in Aging, 11*, 189–208.

Witard, O. C., McGlory, C., Hamilton, D. L., et al. (2016). Growing older with health and vitality: a nexus of physical activity, exercise and nutrition. *Biogerontology, 17*, 529–546.

Zelig, R., Touger-Decker, R., Chung, M., et al. (2016). Associations between tooth loss, with and without dental prostheses, and malnutrition risk in older adults. *Topics in Clinical Nutrition, 31*, 232–247.

chapter 19

Urinary Function

The primary function of urinary elimination is the excretion of water and chemical wastes, such as metabolic and pharmacologic by-products, that would become toxic if allowed to accumulate. This process depends on all of the following: renal blood flow, filtering activities within the kidneys, functioning of all muscles in the urinary tract, and nervous system control over voluntary and involuntary mechanisms of elimination. Control of urinary elimination also depends on cognitive, sensory, and ambulatory abilities and on social, emotional, and environmental factors.

Healthy older adults do not experience major functional consequences affecting urinary elimination, but when risk factors are present, which is very common, negative functional consequences are likely to occur. For example, **urinary incontinence**, which is defined as any involuntary leakage of urine, is common among older adults. A risk factor that is especially pertinent to health promotion for older adults is the widely held perception that urinary incontinence is an inevitable and untreatable consequence of aging. Nurses have many opportunities to improve quality of life for older adults by addressing the risk factors that contribute to urinary incontinence.

AGE-RELATED CHANGES THAT AFFECT URINARY WELLNESS

Control of urinary elimination is affected by age-related changes in the kidney, urinary tract, and other body systems. In addition, any age-related change that interferes with the skills involved in socially appropriate urinary elimination can interfere with urinary control. The next two sections review age-related changes that directly or indirectly affect urinary function and control.

Changes in the Kidneys

The complex process of urinary excretion begins in the kidneys with the filtering and removal of chemical wastes from the blood. Blood circulates through the glomeruli, where

Promoting Urinary Wellness in Older Adults

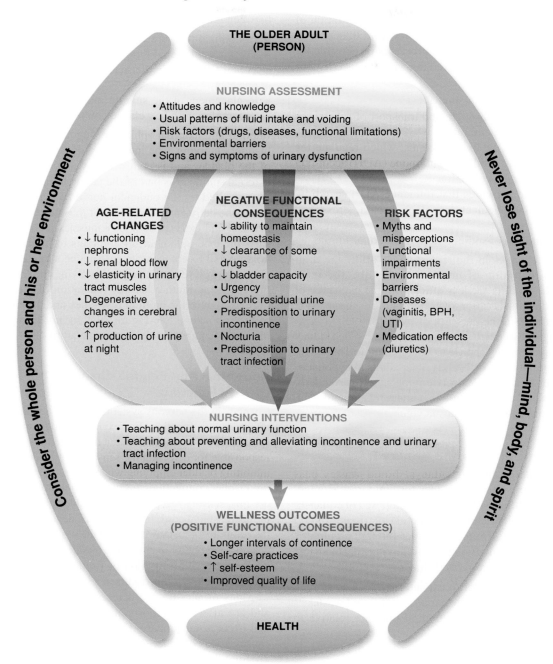

THE OLDER ADULT
(PERSON)

NURSING ASSESSMENT
- Attitudes and knowledge
- Usual patterns of fluid intake and voiding
- Risk factors (drugs, diseases, functional limitations)
- Environmental barriers
- Signs and symptoms of urinary dysfunction

Consider the whole person and his or her environment

Never lose sight of the individual—mind, body, and spirit

AGE-RELATED
CHANGES
- ↓ functioning nephrons
- ↓ renal blood flow
- ↓ elasticity in urinary tract muscles
- Degenerative changes in cerebral cortex
- ↑ production of urine at night

NEGATIVE FUNCTIONAL
CONSEQUENCES
- ↓ ability to maintain homeostasis
- ↓ clearance of some drugs
- ↓ bladder capacity
- Urgency
- Chronic residual urine
- Predisposition to urinary incontinence
- Nocturia
- Predisposition to urinary tract infection

RISK FACTORS
- Myths and misperceptions
- Functional impairments
- Environmental barriers
- Diseases (vaginitis, BPH, UTI)
- Medication effects (diuretics)

NURSING INTERVENTIONS
- Teaching about normal urinary function
- Teaching about preventing and alleviating incontinence and urinary tract infection
- Managing incontinence

WELLNESS OUTCOMES
(POSITIVE FUNCTIONAL CONSEQUENCES)
- Longer intervals of continence
- Self-care practices
- ↑ self-esteem
- Improved quality of life

HEALTH

liquid wastes, called *glomerular filtrate,* pass through Bowman capsule and the renal tubules to the collecting ducts. During this process, substances needed by the body (such as water, glucose, and sodium) are retained, and waste products are excreted in the urine. These functions are important for maintaining homeostasis and excreting many medications. Excretory function, which is measured by the glomerular filtration rate (GFR), depends on the number and efficiency of nephrons and on the amount and rate of renal blood flow.

The kidney increases in weight and mass from birth until early adulthood, when the number of functioning nephrons begins to decline, particularly in the cortex, where the glomeruli are located. This decline continues throughout life, resulting in an approximately 25% decrease in kidney mass by the age of 80 years. Beginning in the fourth decade, renal blood flow and renal function gradually decline at a rate of 1% per year. Although gradual decline of renal function is common in older adults, the rate and extent vary widely, and any *substantial* decline in renal function is associated with other factors, such as physiologic stress due to pathologic conditions.

Renal tubules regulate the dilution and concentration of urine, and subsequent excretion of water from the body, in a diurnal rhythm. The physiologic processes responsible for urine concentration and water excretion are influenced by the following factors:

- The amount of fluid in the body
- Resorption of water through, and transport of substances across, the tubular membrane
- Osmoreceptors in the hypothalamus, which regulate the level of circulating antidiuretic hormone (ADH) according to plasma–water concentration
- Substances and activities that influence ADH secretion, such as caffeine, medications, alcohol, pain, stress, and exercise
- The concentration of sodium in the glomerular filtrate

Degenerative changes in the renal tubules affect the dilution and concentration of urine. Functionally, the renal tubules in older adults are less efficient in the exchange of substances, the conservation of water, and the suppression of ADH secretion in the presence of hypo-osmolality. Age-related changes also decrease the ability of the older kidney to conserve sodium in response to salt restriction. These age-related changes predispose healthy older adults to hyponatremia and other fluid and electrolyte imbalances, particularly in the presence of any condition that alters renal circulation, water or sodium balance, or plasma volume or osmolality.

Changes in the Bladder and Urinary Tract

After being filtered by the kidneys, liquid wastes pass through the ureters into the bladder for temporary storage. The bladder is a balloon-like structure composed of collagen, smooth muscle (called *detrusor*), and elastic tissue. Liquid wastes are eliminated from the bladder through a complex physiologic process involving the following mechanisms, which are affected by age-related changes:

- The ability of the bladder to expand for adequate storage and to contract for complete expulsion of liquid wastes
- The maintenance of higher urethral pressure relative to intravesical pressure
- Regulation of the lower urinary tract through autonomic and somatic nerves
- Voluntary control of urination (micturition) through the cerebral centers

As urine flows into the bladder, the smooth muscle expands without increasing intravesical pressure, and the urethral pressure increases to the point that it is slightly higher than the intravesical pressure. This balance is maintained and urination can be controlled as long as the volume of urine does not rise above about 450 mL in younger adults or about 350 mL in older adults. If the volume rises above this level, or if the detrusor muscle contracts involuntarily, the intravesical pressure will exceed the urethral pressure, and leakage

of urine is likely to occur. In addition to the amount of urine in the bladder, the following factors influence the balance between intravesical and urethral pressure:

- Abdominal pressure
- Thickness of the urethral mucosa
- Tone of the pelvic, detrusor, urethral, and bladder neck muscles
- Replacement of the smooth muscle tissue in the bladder and urethra with less elastic connective tissue

Internal and external sphincters regulate urine storage and bladder emptying. The internal sphincter is part of the base of the bladder and is controlled by autonomic nerves. The external sphincter is part of the pelvic floor musculature and is controlled by the pudendal nerve. When urination takes place, the detrusor and abdominal muscles contract, and the perineal and external sphincter muscles relax. When necessary, the external sphincter contracts to inhibit or interrupt voiding and to compensate for sudden surges in abdominal pressure. Age-related changes involving the loss of smooth muscle in the urethra and the relaxation of the pelvic floor muscles reduce the urethral resistance and diminish the tone of the sphincters. See Figure 19-1 for an illustration of the male and female pelvic floor musculature.

Additional Age-Related Changes That Affect Urinary Function

Changes in the nervous system and other regulatory systems affect urinary function. For example, motor impulses in the spinal cord control urination, but higher centers in the brain are responsible for detecting the sensation of bladder fullness, for inhibiting bladder emptying when necessary, and for stimulating bladder contractions for complete emptying. As the bladder fills, sensory receptors in the bladder wall send a signal to the sacral spinal cord. In older adults, degenerative changes in the cerebral cortex may alter both the sensation of bladder fullness and the ability to empty the bladder completely. Younger adults perceive a sensation of fullness when the bladder is about half full, but this occurs at a later point for older adults.

Many urinary tract structures contain estrogen receptors and are affected by hormonal changes, particularly those that occur at menopause. For example, diminished estrogen causes a loss of tone, strength, and collagen support in the urogenital tissue, which can lead to difficulty controlling urination. Diminished thirst perception is another age-related change that can affect urinary function because underhydration or dehydration can interfere with maintenance of homeostasis, which is necessary for optimal urinary function.

 RISK FACTORS THAT AFFECT URINARY WELLNESS

As with many other areas of functioning, risk factors can affect urinary wellness in many significant ways. Maintaining voluntary control of urination is a fundamental aspect of

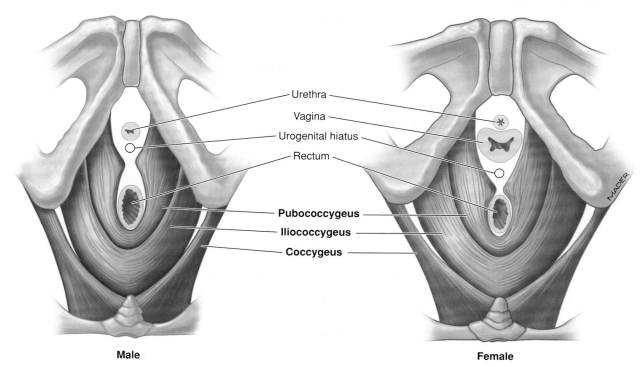

Urethra
Vagina
Urogenital hiatus
Rectum
Pubococcygeus
Iliococcygeus
Coccygeus

Male   **Female**

FIGURE 19-1 Male and female pelvic floor musculature. (Reprinted with permission from Moore, K. L., Agur, A. M., & Dalley, A. F. (2018). *Clinically oriented anatomy* (8th ed.). Philadelphia, PA: Lippincott Williams & Wilkins.)

urinary wellness for older adults that are affected by many risk factors, as discussed in this section.

Misperceptions and Lack of Knowledge

Attitudes based on myths, misperceptions, or lack of knowledge about urinary function can have a detrimental effect on the behavior of older adults and their caregivers. Even though increased age is a risk factor for urinary incontinence, it is a major mistake to perceive incontinence as an inevitable and irreversible consequence of aging. This commonly held misperception can lead to mismanagement of urinary incontinence and serious functional consequences, including significantly decreased quality of life (Xu, Liu, Qu, et al., 2016). Studies in the United States and other countries consistently find that older adults with urinary symptoms often delay seeking help because of embarrassment, lack of knowledge, and the misperception that symptoms are a normal and untreatable consequence of aging (Vethanayagam, Orrell, Dahlberg, et al., 2017).

Diversity Note

Help-seeking for urinary incontinence is lower among black, Latina, and other groups of ethnic minorities in the United States compared to the general population (Duralde, Walter, Van Den Eeden, et al., 2016; Siddiqui, Ammarell, Wu, et al., 2016).

Behaviors of caregivers, based on misperceptions or lack of information, can affect the care of older adults. For instance, if an episode of incontinence occurs soon after an older adult is admitted to an acute-care or long-term care facility, nursing staff may falsely assume that this has been an ongoing symptom. Subsequent behaviors of nursing staff, such as using absorbent products rather than initiating an appropriate care plan, may give the message that voluntary control over urination is not expected. Similarly, caregivers in institutional and home-care settings may promote the use of absorbent products as a substitute for more time-consuming interventions, such as providing assistance with toileting.

Wellness Opportunity

It is important to address one's own misperceptions or ageist perspectives that can interfere with providing evidence-based nursing care to promote urinary wellness.

Fluid Intake and Dietary Factors

Limited fluid intake, which often is perceived as a method of maintaining continence, causes urine to be more concentrated, which leads to increased bladder irritability and subsequent difficulty maintaining continence. In addition, adequate fluid intake is essential for clearance of pathologic organisms from the bladder and prevention of bacteriuria. Some (but not all) studies, have found an association between increased consumption of caffeinated beverages and urinary incontinence (Baek, Song, Lee, et al., 2016; Kosilov, Loparev, Ivanovskaya, et al., 2016). Also, carbonated

TABLE 19-1 Medications That Can Cause Urinary Incontinence

Medication Type	Examples	Mechanism of Action
Diuretics	Furosemide, bumetanide	Increased diuresis can cause urinary urgency, frequency, and polyuria
Anticholinergic agents	Antihistamines, antipsychotics, antidepressants, antispasmodics, antiParkinsonian agents	Decreased bladder contractility and relaxed bladder muscle can cause urinary retention, frequency, and incontinence
Adrenergics (alpha-adrenergic agonists)	Decongestants	Decreased bladder contractility and increased sphincter tone can cause urinary retention, frequency, and incontinence
Alpha-adrenergic blockers	Prazosin, terazosin, doxazosin	Decreased urethral and internal sphincter tone can cause leakage and stress incontinence
Calcium channel blockers	Nifedipine, nicardipine, isradipine, felodipine, nimodipine	Decreased bladder contractility can cause urinary retention, frequency, nocturia, and incontinence
Angiotensin-converting enzyme inhibitors	Captopril, enalapril, lisinopril	Can cause chronic cough, which precipitates or exacerbates stress incontinence
Hypnotics and antianxiety agents	Benzodiazepines	Can interfere with voluntary control over urination by causing sedation, delirium, and cognitive impairments
Alcohol	Wine, beer, liquor	Can interfere with voluntary control over urination by causing sedation, delirium, increased diuresis, and cognitive impairments

beverages, artificial sweeteners, citrus products, and hot peppers are commonly cited as bladder irritants; however, current evidence to support these assumptions is inconsistent.

Medication Effects

Medications influence urinary function in many ways and are common risk factors in the development of urinary incontinence, as delineated in Table 19-1. The following categories of medications are associated with increased risk for urinary incontinence through direct or indirect effects: diuretics, sedatives, antidepressants, antihypertensives, anticholinergics, and cholinesterase inhibitors (Dane, Gatewood, & Peron, 2016; Schneidinger, Umek, & Bohmdorfer, 2016). In addition to causing incontinence through the mechanisms listed in Table 19-1, medications can increase the risk for urinary incontinence through their effects on functional abilities. For example, constipation and altered mental status are adverse effects of medications that can increase the risk for urinary incontinence.

Functional Impairments and Environmental Conditions

Control over urination is affected not only by age-related changes that directly affect urinary function but also by many conditions that affect voluntary control over urination. All the following conditions can affect one's ability to identify and use appropriate toilet facilities in a timely manner:

- Cognition, balance, mobility, coordination, visual function, and manual dexterity
- Identification of a designated receptacle in a private area
- Accessibility and acceptability of toilet facilities
- Ability to get to and use a suitable receptacle

- Amount of time between the perception of the urge to void and the actual need to empty the bladder
- Ability to voluntarily control the urge to void

Functional and cognitive impairments are a major risk factor for the development of incontinence because they can interfere with the ability to recognize and respond to the urge to void in a timely manner. Because older adults have a shorter interval between the perception of the urge to void and the actual need to empty the bladder, any delay in reaching an appropriate receptacle can result in incontinence. Thus, dependency in performing activities of daily living (ADLs) for any reason increases the risk for urinary incontinence. Conditions, such as arthritis or Parkinson disease, may slow the ambulation of older adults as well as their ability to manipulate clothing for toileting. Likewise, dementia and other conditions that impair cognitive abilities can interfere with the timely processing of information that is necessary for maintaining voluntary control over urination.

People with limited mobility or impaired vision encounter many environmental factors that can interfere with their ability to get to accessible toileting facilities in home, public, and institutional settings. Examples of environmental obstacles include stairs, inadequate signage, lack of grab bars, and toilet seats that are too low. Box 19-1 summarizes some environmental risk factors that may contribute to the incidence of incontinence in older adults.

Factors Related to Pathologic Conditions

An increased risk for urinary incontinence is associated with many pathologic conditions including all the following: stroke, arthritis, dementia, delirium, depression, diabetes mellitus, metabolic syndrome, Parkinson disease,

Box 19-1 Environmental Factors That Can Contribute to Urinary Incontinence

- Stairways between the bathroom level and the living or sleeping areas
- A distance to the bathroom that is more than 40 feet
- Living arrangements where several or many people share a bathroom
- Small bathrooms and narrow doors and hallways that do not accommodate walkers or wheelchairs
- Chair designs and bed heights that hinder mobility
- Poor color contrast, as between a white toilet and seat and light-colored floor or walls
- Public settings with poorly visible or poorly color-contrasted signs designating gender-specific bathroom facilities
- Public settings with dim lighting and out-of-the-way bathroom facilities
- Very bright environments, where glare interferes with the perception of signs for bathrooms
- Mirrored walls, which reflect bright lights and create glare

and COPD. In addition, any acute illness or surgical intervention that temporarily limits mobility or compromises mental abilities also represents a risk factor for urinary incontinence. Constipation, fewer than three bowel movements weekly, and fecal impaction are other conditions that increase the risk for urinary incontinence and other urinary tract symptoms.

Neurodegenerative diseases that occur commonly in older adults (e.g., dementia, Parkinson disease, frontal lobe dysfunction) significantly increase the risk for developing urinary incontinence (Buchman, Leurgans, Shah, et al., 2016; Sugimoto, Yoshida, Ono, et al., 2017). Although dementia is strongly associated with urinary incontinence, the relationship between these two conditions is complex, and episodes of incontinence can often be prevented or minimized, particularly during early and middle stages. For example, older adults with dementia may lack the perceptual abilities that are necessary for finding and using appropriate facilities, but they may be able to maintain continence when given appropriate cues and reminders. Even during middle or later stages, caregivers can implement interventions to prevent urinary incontinence (Schumpf, Theill, Scheiner, et al., 2017).

Obesity and larger abdominal circumference is associated with urinary incontinence and urinary tract symptoms (Cagnacci, Palma, Carbone, et al., 2017; de Oliveira, Varella, Angelo, et al., 2016; Gordon, Shorter, Isoldi, et al., 2017). Current smoking is another potentially modifiable risk associated with urinary incontinence (Townsend, Lajous, Medina-Campos, et al., 2017). Other risk factors associated with urinary incontinence that commonly occur in older adults include hearing and/or vision impairment, radiation or surgical treatments for prostate cancer, and residence in a long-term care facility (Dowling-Castronovo & Bradway, 2016). Researchers also are investigating a potential link between vitamin D deficiency and urinary incontinence, with emphasis on its influence on pelvic floor muscle functioning (Kilic,

Kizalarslanoglu, Kara, et al., 2016; Vaughan, Tangpricha, Motahar-Ford, et al., 2016).

Gender-Specific Conditions

Gender-specific conditions of the genitourinary tract commonly occur in older adults and increase the risk for urinary incontinence and other lower urinary tract symptoms. Although these conditions are generally addressed by a gynecologist or urologist, they are discussed in relation to urinary wellness because of their direct effects on control over urination in older men and women.

The term **pelvic floor disorders** (also called pelvic support problems) refers to a group of medical conditions in which a pelvic organ prolapses into the vagina due to weakness or injury involving muscles and connective tissue of the pelvic floor and related structures. These conditions, which sometimes occur together, can involve any of the following structures:

- Urinary bladder (cystocele)
- Bladder and urethra (cystourethrocele)
- Bladder neck (urethrocele)
- Uterus (uterine prolapse)
- Part of the small bowel and peritoneum (enterocele)
- Rectum (rectocele or rectal prolapse)

Sometimes, older women use terms such as "dropped," "sagging," or "fallen" in reference to the involved structure (e.g., "dropped bladder").

In addition to increased age and postmenopausal status, factors that increase the risk for pelvic floor disorders in women include smoking, obesity, surgery, pelvic radiation, genetic predisposition, chronic constipation, high number of vaginal births, and fractures of the pelvis or lower vertebrae. Pelvic floor disorders can lead to urinary frequency and incontinence because these conditions interfere with the complete emptying of the bladder, resulting in residual urine and an increased risk for bacteriuria. Atrophy of the vaginal and trigonal tissue, with subsequent diminished resistance to pathogens, is another condition that can affect urinary wellness in older women because vaginitis and trigonitis can cause urinary urgency, frequency, and incontinence.

Diversity Note

Caucasian women are more likely than African American women to have pelvic organ prolapse.

Benign prostatic hyperplasia (BPH) is a common cause of voiding problems in older men because the enlarged prostate compresses the urethra, which leads to obstruction of the vesical neck. As the condition progresses, the urinary musculature becomes thinner and less elastic and urinary retention occurs, increasing the risk for bacteriuria and infection. Men with prostatic hyperplasia may experience decreased urine flow, incomplete bladder emptying, and urinary urgency and frequency. Eventually, the ureters and kidneys are affected, and hydroureter, hydronephrosis, diminished GFR, and uremia may develop.

 See ONLINE LEARNING ACTIVITY 19-1: CASE STUDY VIDEO DISCUSSING TRANSIENT URINARY INCONTINENCE THAT DEVELOPS DURING HOSPITALIZATION at http://thepoint.lww.com/Miller8e.

 ## FUNCTIONAL CONSEQUENCES AFFECTING URINARY WELLNESS

Despite the many age-related changes in the urinary tract, the elimination of wastes is not significantly affected in healthy, nonmedicated older adults. However, with any unusual physiologic demands, such as those that occur with medications or disease conditions, older adults are likely to experience functional consequences affecting homeostatic mechanisms and urinary control. The most significant functional consequences are those that affect patterns of urinary elimination and predispose older adults to incontinence. When incontinence occurs, additional functional consequences, particularly psychosocial effects, can be quite serious. This section reviews functional consequences that are related to overall renal function and the control over urination.

Effects on Renal Function

Functional consequences related to renal function in healthy older adults include impaired absorption of calcium, a predisposition to hyponatremia and hyperkalemia, and a diminished ability to maintain fluid and electrolyte balance and to correct pH imbalances. In addition, urine is more concentrated because the kidneys become less responsive to ADH. Because of these changes, older adults will more readily develop dehydration, volume depletion, and other fluid and electrolyte imbalances under conditions of physiologic stress (e.g., surgery, infection, fever-producing illness, or excessive fluid loss).

Diminished renal function contributes to the increased incidence of drug interactions and adverse medication reactions in older adults. These age-related changes are most likely to affect water-soluble medications that are highly dependent on GFR (e.g., digoxin, cimetidine, and aminoglycoside antibiotics) or renal tubular function (e.g., penicillin and procainamide). Unless medication doses are adjusted to account for age-related changes in GFR and renal tubular function, excretion may be delayed and toxic substances are likely to accumulate. These adverse medication effects can significantly impair physical and mental abilities and have profound functional consequences, as discussed in Chapter 8.

Effects on Voiding Patterns

Because of age-related changes, the bladder of the older adult has a smaller capacity, empties incompletely, and contracts during filling. Thus, older adults experience shorter intervals between voiding, and they have less time between the perception of the urge to void and the actual need to empty the bladder. Older adults often describe this by saying, "When you gotta go, you gotta go." Another consequence is that the bladder retains residual urine after voiding, causing symptomatic or asymptomatic bacteriuria and predisposing older adults to UTIs.

Age-related changes in the diurnal production of urine cause a shift in voiding pattern to more urinary output at night than during the day. Prevalence of nocturia (i.e., the need to void one or more times during the night) increases with age, with more than half of older adults voiding at least once during the night (Kim, Moon, & Kim, 2016). Nocturia is a common symptom of many urinary tract disorders and it also occurs with systemic conditions such as endocrine disorders, heart failure, renal insufficiency, and certain medications, such as diuretics. Functional consequences of nocturia include disturbed sleep, increased risk for falls, and decreased quality of life (Andersson, Anderson, Holm-Larsen, et al., 2016; Kim, Bang, Kim, et al., 2017; Shao, Wu, Hsu, et al., 2016).

Urinary Incontinence

As already emphasized, urinary incontinence is not inevitable with aging, but it occurs more commonly in older adults due to a combination of age-related changes and risk factors. Estimated prevalence of incontinence for older adults varies widely due to many factors, including underreporting and inconsistent definitions. A summary of evidence by Dowling-Castronovo and Bradway (2016) cites the following ranges for urinary incontinence among different groups in the United States: community-dwelling adults, 8% to 46%; homebound older adults, 15% to 53%; older adults admitted to acute-care settings, 10% to 42%; and people with dementia, 11% to 90%. In addition, 12% to 36% of hospitalized older adults develop urinary incontinence during the hospitalization.

Urinary incontinence is categorized according to potential for reversibility as transient (also called acute) or established (also called chronic or persistent). Transient urinary incontinence is characterized by recent and sudden onset and is associated with resolvable causes, such as delirium, UTI, medications, constipation, limited mobility, or lack of appropriate assistance with toileting. In cognitively impaired older adults, this type of incontinence is often associated with length of stay in acute- or subacute-care settings (Furlanetto & Emond, 2016). Types of established urinary incontinence include stress, urge, mixed, overflow, and functional. Characteristics of each type are described in Box 19-2.

Overactive bladder (OAB) is a syndrome that is closely associated with urinary incontinence and is now widely

---

Box 19-2 Characteristics of Types of Incontinence

Stress: involuntary leakage of small amounts of urine as a result of an activity that increases intra-abdominal pressure, such as lifting, coughing, sneezing, laughing, or exercising

Urge: involuntary urinary loss soon after perceiving the urge to void

Mixed: involuntary leakage of urine with symptoms of both stress and urge incontinence

Overflow: involuntary loss of urine due to overdistension of the bladder, which may be associated with underactive detrusor muscle or outlet obstruction (e.g., due to BPH)

Functional: involuntary loss of control over urination caused by nongenitourinary factors—for example, due to cognitive or physical impairments

---

recognized due to increasing media attention (such as television advertisements). OAB is characterized by a combination of urinary urgency, increased day and night voiding (with or without urinary incontinence) that results in a negative impact on quality of life for approximately one out of six individuals of all age groups (Truzzi, Gomes, Bezerra, et al., 2016).

Urinary incontinence can negatively affect quality of life through both physical and psychosocial consequences. Physical consequences of incontinence include a predisposition to falls, fractures, pressure ulcers, UTIs, and limitation of functional status. In recent years, health care professionals have drawn attention to incontinence-associated dermatitis, which is an inflammatory condition of the skin that differs clinically and pathologically from pressure ulcers and other skin disorders. Psychosocial consequences associated with urinary incontinence include significantly decreased quality of life, shame or embarrassment, anxiety, depression, social isolation, and loss of self-confidence (Bedretdinova, Fritel, Zins, et al., 2016; Villoro, Merino, Hidalgo-Vega, et al., 2016). Also, urinary incontinence has significant negative effects on sexual functioning that extend to existing and new partners (Felippe, Zambon, Girotti, et al., 2017; Hunter, Nakagawa, Van Den Eeden, et al., 2016; Pakgohar, Sabetghadam, Rahimparvar, et al., 2016). Another consequence is that people who experience episodes of incontinence may become preoccupied with avoiding social stigma by covering up any evidence of wetness or urinary odors.

Negative psychosocial consequences can arise when caregivers communicate infantilizing attitudes and behaviors, such as unnecessarily using incontinence products rather than providing assistance with toileting. These attitudes and behaviors can have a devastating effect on the older adult's dignity and self-esteem. In addition, older adults who do not understand age-related changes may have exaggerated fears of progressive incontinence, triggered by the onset of urgency or frequency. Even in older adults who are not incontinent, the experience of urinary urgency and frequency can cause psychosocial consequences, such as anxiety, restricted activity, feelings of insecurity and powerlessness, and embarrassment about frequent trips to the bathroom.

See ONLINE LEARNING ACTIVITY 19-2:
EVIDENCE-BASED INFORMATION
ABOUT URINARY INCONTINENCE
at http://thepoint.lww.com/Miller8e.

Unfolding Case Study

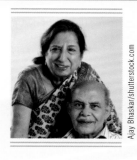

Ajay Bhaskar/shutterstock.com

Part 1: Mr. and Mrs. U. at 69 and 68 Years of Age

Mr. and Mrs. U., who are 69 and 68 years old, respectively, attend the senior center where you provide monthly group health education sessions, weekly blood pressure checks, and one-on-one "Counseling for Wellness" sessions. During a recent health counseling session, Mrs. U. confided that she does not know what to do about her husband's "smelly dribbling" and that she worries that he has prostate problems. She has perceived a strong odor of urine and has noticed yellow stains on his clothing when she does the laundry. Even their children have mentioned the odor to her, but when she tries to discuss it with her husband, he changes the subject. She says that he will not talk with his doctor about it because he "hears so much about prostate cancer, and he's afraid that he has an untreatable condition." She asks your advice about this and asks if you would talk with him when he comes to see you next week. Your next group health education session is entitled "Control of Urine: What's Normal With Aging?" and you plan to have separate group discussions for the men and women. Since Mr. and Mrs. U. usually attend these sessions, you see this as an opportunity to initiate health education about this sensitive topic.

THINKING POINTS

Decide what information you would include in the group session about each of the following topics:

- What can older men (women) expect of their urinary tract?

- What factors increase the risk for having problems with urinary control in older men (women)?

A Student's Perspective

One morning, I was caring for a client who had a Foley catheter. While preparing her to go to breakfast, I noticed there was no cover on her catheter bag and asked her if she had one. My client explained that she once had a cover, but the nurses did not know where it went. I decided to do some searching, which only required my asking the laundry lady, and I discovered that several covers were stored in the linen closet. When I came back to the client's room with the cover, my client was so grateful. She said she had been asking for a long time if she could get another one, but the nurses and aides never cared to search for one. She explained that she doesn't like everyone to be able to see her catheter bag as she rides around the nursing home in her wheelchair. My finding the cover for her catheter bag was a very simple act requiring very little effort, but it showed me the importance of putting a little extra time into the client's care. Although this seemed like a miniscule problem to the nurses, it was a real concern to my client. I hope that as we continue in our nursing careers we remember to do these simple acts, because a seemingly insignificant thing to us can mean the world to a client.

Katrina D.

Wellness Opportunity

Nurses address the person's relationships with others by being sensitive to the psychosocial responses of family caregivers who are dealing with incontinence.

PATHOLOGIC CONDITION AFFECTING URINARY FUNCTION: CATHETER-ASSOCIATED URINARY TRACT INFECTIONS

Catheter-associated urinary tract infections (CAUTIs) are urinary tract infections that develop after an indwelling catheter has been in place for 2 days or more, or within 1 day after the removal of a catheter (Centers for Disease Control and Prevention, 2017). In 2008, the Centers for Medicare & Medicaid Services and major health care organizations began addressing CAUTIs as a preventable health care–associated infection associated with significant negative effects. In recent years, hospitals and nursing facilities have developed and implemented evidence-based protocols to prevent CAUTIs. Currently, national prevention programs that implement a "bundle" of interventions are successfully reducing catheter use and preventing CAUTIs (Bell, Alaestante, & Finch, 2016; Saint, Greene, Krein, et al., 2016). Protocols are interprofessional, with nurses having primary roles related to all aspects of prevention and care, as described in Box 19-3. For example, current protocols for the removal of indwelling catheters in hospitalized patients are increasingly nurse-driven, providing more autonomy for nurses to follow specific criteria rather than relying on physicians' orders (Timmons, Vess, & Conner, 2017). Johnson, Gilman, Lintner, et al. (2016) describe an evidence-based nurse-driven protocol that resulted in a 28% reduction in CAUTI in intensive care units. Online Learning Activity 19-3 provides a link to this article.

Box 19-3 Evidence-Based Practice: Prevention of Catheter-Associated Urinary Tract Infections

Statement of the Problem

- Catheter-associated urinary tract infections (CAUTIs) are considered health care–associated infections, which are often preventable adverse events related to medical care during hospitalization.
- The inappropriate use of indwelling urinary catheters (IUCs) (also called Foley catheters) has been gradually decreasing; however, inappropriate use in hospital settings occurs in patients who are female, older, nonambulatory, and in medical intensive care units.
- IUCs significantly increase the risk for urinary tract infection, delirium, trauma to the genitourinary tissue.
- The risk for developing a CAUTI is directly related to the duration of IUC use, beginning at 48 hours after insertion and increasing at the rate of 5% per day.
- Adherence to recommended infection control measures (as described in the section on Recommendations for Nursing Care) would prevent 20% to 69% of CAUTI.

Recommendations for Nursing Assessment

- Identify appropriate indications for use of an IUC: perioperative care, prolonged surgery, monitoring during surgery or critical illness, major trauma patients, urinary retention or obstruction, urinary bladder irrigation, pressure ulcer management, and comfort care during terminal illness.
- Assess for the following indicators of CAUTI: fever over 38°C, suprapubic tenderness, costovertebral angle pain or tenderness, positive

blood culture with the same organisms as in the urine, and dysuria or urinary frequency if the catheter has already been removed.
- Reassess patients with IUCs at every shift change or at least daily and apply criteria for continuing the use of the catheter.

Recommendations for Nursing Care

- Adhere to criteria and protocols for medically necessary use of IUCs.
- Use alternative methods for urinary elimination in the care plan (e.g., toileting program, collecting devices, and intermittent straight catheterization).
- Recommended care strategies for IUC: select smallest effective size for catheter, use aseptic technique for insertion, provide routine meatal care, prevent reflux, maintain closed system, keep catheter secure in place.
- Nurses have essential roles in ensuring the timely removal of IUCs by frequently reassessing the need for keeping the catheter inserted.

Sources: Gurwitz, J. H., DuBeau, C., Mazor, K., et al. (2016). Use of indwelling urinary catheters in nursing homes: Implications for quality improvement efforts. *Journal of the American Geriatrics Society, 64,* 2204–2209; Thomas, K. (2016). Reduction of catheter-associated urinary tract infections through the use of an evidence-based nursing algorithm and the implementation of shift nursing rounds. *Journal of Wound Ostomy and Continence Nurses, 43,* 183–187;Wald, H. L., Fink, R. M., Makic, M. B. F., & Oman, K. S. (2016). Prevention of catheter-associated urinary tract infection prevention. In M. Boltz, E. Capezuti, R. Fulmer, & D. Zwicker (Eds.), *Evidence-based geriatric nursing protocols for best practice* (5th ed., pp. 363–380). New York: Springer Publishing. Modified version is available online at https://consultgeri.org

See **ONLINE LEARNING ACTIVITY 19-3: ARTICLE ABOUT A NURSE-DRIVEN PROTOCOL FOR REDUCING CAUTIs** at http://thepoint.lww.com/Miller8e.

NURSING ASSESSMENT OF URINARY FUNCTION

Nurses can identify opportunities for health promotion interventions by assessing all of the following aspects of urinary function:

- Risk factors that influence overall urinary function
- Risk factors that increase the potential for incontinence
- Signs and symptoms of any dysfunction involving urinary elimination
- Fears and attitudes about urinary dysfunction
- Psychosocial consequences of incontinence

Assessment information is obtained by reviewing urinalysis results, interviewing older adults and caregivers when appropriate, and observing behaviors and environmental influences.

Talking With Older Adults About Urinary Function

Because urinary elimination is associated with certain social expectations, discussion of this topic may be influenced by a person's attitudes and feelings. People with urinary incontinence often experience stigma, discomfort, and embarrassment. Factors that contribute to the challenge of discussing urinary function include age, gender, or cultural differences; communication barriers such as hearing impairment; and the misperception that urinary problems are an inevitable and untreatable consequence of aging.

Terminology related to urinary elimination presents further difficulties in interviewing older adults. In social settings, people commonly use euphemisms to avoid directly discussing urination (e.g., "I'm going to the powder room," "I'm going to take a leak"). Because of this social context, successful interviewing about urinary elimination and incontinence depends on identifying the terms that are most acceptable to the older adult. If any hearing impairment is present, a term such as "urinate," which is not used in everyday social language, or a one-syllable word like "pee," may be difficult to understand or may be misinterpreted. Although phrases like "use the toilet" and "go to the bathroom" are not specific to urinary elimination, they may prove to be acceptable, particularly if additional questions are asked to distinguish between urinary and bowel elimination. Similarly, the term "incontinence" may be problematic for people who may not be familiar with this term. Older adults are likely to use any of the following words and phrases when referring to urinary incontinence: "accidents," "leaking," "weak kidneys," "bladder trouble," or "trouble holding my water."

Wellness Opportunity

Show respect for older adults by using terms such as "briefs" rather than terms such as diapers, which are associated with infants.

Identifying Opportunities for Health Promotion

Begin a nursing assessment by asking about risk factors and observing the person's responses. If the older adults acknowledge incontinence or "leakage," ask about any actions they have taken and about any effects on their daily activities and social life. Box 19-4 presents interview questions related to urinary elimination. Check other parts of patient records for pertinent information (e.g., use of medications for overactive bladder) and incorporate it into the assessment of urinary elimination. Supplement the assessment interview by obtaining information about the person's patterns of urinary elimination and by assessing environmental factors that may interfere with control over urinary elimination.

A **bladder diary** (also called a bladder record, or voiding or urinary diary) can be used to obtain information about fluid intake, the times of urinations, and other factors that can affect continence (Fig. 19-2). Use the information from the bladder diary to identify potential causes of and interventions for incontinence, particularly in relation to identifying opportunities for health education. Older adults who are cognitively impaired or dependent on others for their care may not be able to keep a bladder diary. In these situations, it is important to obtain information from nursing staff in institutional settings and from caregivers in community-based settings. Box 19-5 summarizes specific observations that may yield important assessment information.

See **ONLINE LEARNING ACTIVITY 19-4: CASE STUDY VIDEO DISCUSSING THE USE OF A BLADDER RECORD FOR ASSESSING URINARY INCONTINENCE** at http://thepoint.lww.com/Miller8e.

Wellness Opportunity

Nurses promote self-care by encouraging older adults to seek further evaluation by qualified health care professionals rather than relying solely on the reported experiences of friends.

Assess home environments for conditions that affect timely access to bathrooms, particularly for people who have a functional impairment or use assistive devices, such as walkers (refer to Box 19-1). Also, assess the environment for safety and assistive devices or their potential benefit to

Box 19-4 Guidelines for Assessing Urinary Elimination

Interview Questions to Assess Risk Factors Influencing Urinary Elimination

- (*Men*) Have you had any surgery for prostate or bladder problems?
- (*Men*) Have you ever been told you had prostate problems? (Or: Do you think you have prostate problems?)
- (*Women*) Have you had any children? (If yes, ask about the number of pregnancies and any problems with childbirth.)
- (*Women*) Have you had any surgery for pelvic, bladder, or uterine disorders?
- (*Women*) Have you had any infections in your vaginal area?
- Do you have any pain, burning, or discomfort when you urinate (pass water)?
- Have you had any urinary tract infections?
- Do you have any chronic illnesses?
- What medications do you take?
- Do you have any problems with your bowels?
- How much water and other liquids do you drink during the day? (Ask for details about timing and the amount of alcoholic, carbonated, and caffeinated beverages consumed.)

Interview Questions to Assess Risk Factors for Socially Appropriate Urinary Elimination

- Do you have any trouble walking or any difficulty with balance?
- Do you have any trouble reading signs or finding restrooms when you are in public places?

Interview Questions to Assess Signs and Symptoms of Urinary Dysfunction

- Do you ever leak urine?
- Do you ever wear pads or protective garments to protect your clothing from wetness?
- Do you ever have difficulty holding your urine (water) long enough to get to the toilet? (Or How long can you hold your urine after you first feel the need to go to the bathroom?)

- Do you have trouble holding your urine (water) when you cough, laugh, or make sudden movements?
- Do you wake up at night because you have to go to the bathroom to urinate (pass water)? (If the response is affirmative, try to differentiate between this symptom and the habit of going to the bathroom after waking up for some other reason.)
- Immediately after urinating (passing your water), does it feel like you have not emptied your bladder completely?
- Do you have to exert pressure during urination to feel like your bladder is being completely emptied?
- (*Men*) When you urinate (pass water), do you have any difficulty starting the stream or keeping the stream going?

Interview Questions If Incontinence Has Been Acknowledged

- When did your incontinence begin?
- What have you done to manage the problem? (Have you cut down on the amount of liquids you drink? Do you empty your bladder at frequent intervals as a precautionary measure?)
- Are there certain things that make the problem worse or better?
- Does it happen all the time, or just at certain times?
- Do you have any pain when you urinate (pass water)?
- (*Women*) Do you feel any pressure in your pelvic area?

Interview Questions to Assess Fears, Attitudes, and Psychosocial Consequences of Incontinence

- Have you ever sought help or talked to a primary care provider or other health care professional about this problem?
- Have you changed any of your activities because you need to stay near a toilet?
- Do you avoid going to certain places because of difficulty holding your urine (water)?

---

the individual, as discussed in the section on Improving Functional Abilities to Help Maintain Continence.

Using Laboratory Information

Data from urinalysis and blood chemistry tests contribute valuable assessment information. A midstream or second-void specimen is the best type of sample for a urinalysis. At the age of 80 years, the normal upper limit for specific gravity is 1.024, and slight proteinuria is normal in older adults. Other than these two variations, the urinalysis results should be within the normal range for healthy older adults. Diagnosis of a UTI is based on results from a dipstick or microscopic examination of a clean-catch urine specimen.

An important assessment consideration is distinguishing between UTI and asymptomatic bacteriuria, which is

---

Box 19-5 Guidelines for Assessing Behavioral Cues to and Environmental Influences on Incontinence

Behavioral Cues

- Does the older adult use disposable or washable pads or products?
- Is there an odor of urine on clothing, floor coverings, or furniture (particularly couches and stuffed chairs)?
- Has the older adult withdrawn from social activities, particularly those held away from home?

Environmental Influences

- Where are the bathroom facilities located in relation to the older adult's usual daytime and nighttime activities?

- Does the person have to go up or down stairs to use the toilet at night or during the day?
- Are there any grab bars or other aids in, near, or on the way to the bathroom?
    - ◆ Is lighting adequate and the pathway uncluttered for safety?
- Would the person benefit from using an elevated toilet seat?
- Does the person use a urinal or other aid to cut down on the number of trips to the bathroom?
- How many people share the same bathroom facilities?
- Is privacy ensured?

Your Daily Bladder Diary

This diary will help you and your health care team figure out the causes of your bladder control trouble. The "sample" line shows you how to use the diary.

Your name: _____

Date: _____

Time	Drinks		Trips to the bathroom		Accidental leaks	Did you feel a strong urge to go?	What were you doing at the time?
	What kind?	How much?	How many times?	How much urine? (circle one)	How much? (circle one)	Circle one	Sneezing, exercising, having sex, lifting, etc.
Sample	Coffee	2 cups	✓✓	sm med lg	sm med lg	Yes (No)	Running
6–7 a.m.				sm med lg	sm med lg	Yes No	
7–8 a.m.				sm med lg	sm med lg	Yes No	
8–9 a.m.				sm med lg	sm med lg	Yes No	
9–10 a.m.				sm med lg	sm med lg	Yes No	
10–11 a.m.				sm med lg	sm med lg	Yes No	
11–12 noon				sm med lg	sm med lg	Yes No	
12–1 p.m.				sm med lg	sm med lg	Yes No	
1–2 p.m.				sm med lg	sm med lg	Yes No	
2–3 p.m.				sm med lg	sm med lg	Yes No	
3–4 p.m.				sm med lg	sm med lg	Yes No	
4–5 p.m.				sm med lg	sm med lg	Yes No	
5–6 p.m.				sm med lg	sm med lg	Yes No	
6–7 p.m.				sm med lg	sm med lg	Yes No	
7–8 p.m.				sm med lg	sm med lg	Yes No	
8–9 p.m.				sm med lg	sm med lg	Yes No	
9–10 p.m.				sm med lg	sm med lg	Yes No	
10–11 p.m.				sm med lg	sm med lg	Yes No	
11–12 midnight				sm med lg	sm med lg	Yes No	
12–1 a.m.				sm med lg	sm med lg	Yes No	
1–2 a.m.				sm med lg	sm med lg	Yes No	
2–3 a.m.				sm med lg	sm med lg	Yes No	

Type and amount of incontinence products used today: _____

Questions to ask my health care team: _____

_____

_____

FIGURE 19-2 Example of a bladder diary. (Adapted from *Let's talk about bladder control for women,* National Kidney and Urologic Diseases Information Clearinghouse. www.kidney.niddk.nih.gov)

characterized by urinalysis results of 105 or more colony-forming units but a lack of localized symptoms, such as dysuria. Asymptomatic bacteriuria is very common in older adults, particularly in long-term care settings and in those with indwelling catheters. An important nursing consideration is that even though the urinalysis shows bacteriuria, treatment for asymptomatic bacteriuria is not warranted and, in fact, may be harmful (Cai, Koves, & Johansen, 2017).

Blood chemistry values that are pertinent to assessment of renal function include the following: electrolyte level, creatinine level, creatinine clearance, nonprotein nitrogen level, and blood urea nitrogen level. In older adults, the serum creatinine may not be an accurate indicator of GFR, but a 24-hour urine collection for creatinine clearance may have greater value as an indicator of renal functioning.

NURSING DIAGNOSIS

Impaired Urinary Elimination is an appropriate nursing diagnosis when nurses identify risks for, or signs or symptoms of, urinary incontinence. Defining characteristics commonly found in older adults include urgency, frequency, nocturia, hesitancy, and incontinence. The following nursing diagnoses might be applicable for negative consequences of urinary incontinence: Anxiety, Social Isolation, Disturbed Sleep Pattern, Impaired Skin Integrity, or Caregiver Role Strain (or Risk for).

Wellness Opportunity

Nurses can use the wellness nursing diagnosis of Readiness for Enhanced Health Management for older adults who are interested in learning self-care practices.

PLANNING FOR WELLNESS OUTCOMES

Nursing care plans are directed toward preventing, minimizing, or compensating for the negative functional consequences that affect urinary elimination. Specific outcomes related to promoting urinary wellness are Fluid Balance, Kidney Function, or Risk Detection. Outcomes for older adults who have urinary incontinence include achieving continence and preventing negative consequences; initial outcomes focus on controlling and alleviating, rather than simply managing, incontinence. The following Nursing Outcomes Classification (NOC) terminology is pertinent to older adults who experience urinary incontinence and related consequences: Urinary Continence, Symptom Severity, Urinary Elimination; Self-Care: Toileting; Health Beliefs: Perceived Control; Immobility Consequences: Physiologic; and Tissue Integrity: Skin.

In addition, any of the following NOCs may be pertinent to caregivers, particularly family members, who are caring for someone with urinary incontinence: Caregiver Stressors; Caregiver Well-Being; Caregiver Performance: Direct Care; Caregiver Lifestyle Disruption; Caregiver Emotional Health; and Caregiver Endurance Potential.

Wellness Opportunity

Quality of life is an outcome that can be achieved for older adults and their caregivers through nursing interventions that are effective in alleviating or managing urinary incontinence.

NURSING INTERVENTIONS TO PROMOTE URINARY WELLNESS

Nurses have numerous opportunities to promote wellness in relation to urinary function, particularly for older adults

Unfolding Case Study

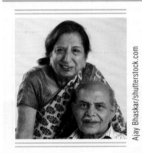

Ajay Bhaskar/shutterstock.com

Part 1: Mr. and Mrs. U. at 69 and 68 Years of Age *(Continued)*

Recall that you are the nurse at the senior center attended by Mr. and Mrs. U. After your class called "Control of Urine: What's Normal With Aging?" Mr. U. schedules an appointment for a Counseling for Wellness session. He tells you that he has a "little dribbling" problem but has ignored it because it did not bother him very much. He has not talked with any doctor about this because he thought it was "to be expected," but now that he attended your session, he thinks that maybe he should have the problem evaluated and wants further information from you. During other health counseling sessions with Mr. U., he has told you that he is taking medications for hypertension and Parkinson disease.

THINKING POINTS

- What risk factors are likely to be contributing to Mr. U.'s problems with urinary control?
- Make a list of assessment questions that you would use with Mr. U. (Use applicable questions from Box 19-4 and any additional questions that might be appropriate.)

- What observations would you make as part of your assessment?
- What would you teach Mr. U. about filling out the bladder diary (see Fig. 19-2)?

who have difficulty maintaining urinary control. For example, nurses can challenge myths about urinary incontinence, address attitudes of resignation, and teach self-care interventions. In addition, nurses have important roles in teaching about medical interventions and suggesting referrals for appropriate evaluation and treatment. The following Nursing Interventions Classifications terminology is pertinent to promoting urinary continence and addressing the associated psychosocial consequences: Biofeedback, Emotional Support, Environmental Management, Fluid Management, Health Education, Pelvic Floor Muscle Exercise (PFME), Prompted Voiding, Referral, Self-Esteem Enhancement, Urinary Bladder Training, Urinary Elimination Management, Urinary Habit Training, and Urinary Incontinence Care.

Promoting Self-Management for Overall Urinary Wellness

Healthy older adults are not significantly affected by age-related kidney changes during normal activities; however, under conditions of physiologic stress, such as exercise, homeostasis can be affected unless the older adult initiates compensatory actions. Thus, an important aspect of health promotion is to teach older adults about self-care actions, such as drinking adequate fluid prior to exercise and avoiding strenuous physical activity in hot or humid conditions. Teach older adults about measures to protect themselves in very hot and humid environments by using fans and air conditioners, maintaining good fluid intake, and avoiding alcoholic, carbonated, and caffeinated beverages. Because older adults with diminished renal function are at increased risk for adverse effects when taking one or more water-soluble medications, dose adjustments may be necessary, as discussed in Chapter 8.

A risk factor that can be alleviated through health education is the false perception of incontinence as an inevitable and irreversible effect of aging. Nurses have important roles in addressing risks for urinary incontinence as an integral aspect of health promotion. For example, interventions for preventing constipation, as discussed in Chapter 18, may improve control over urination. Similarly, health education about the rationale for maintaining adequate fluid intake as a means of preventing incontinence and maintaining good urinary function is a simple but important intervention. Also, explain that because the sensation of thirst diminishes or is absent in older adults, this is not a good indicator of the need for fluids. Box 19-6 summarizes teaching points about health promotion actions for maintaining optimal urinary function and continence.

 Box 19-6 Health Education to Promote Urinary Wellness

Facts About Urinary Control

- Incontinence is not an inevitable age-related change, but it occurs more commonly in older adults due to risk factors.
- Older adults may experience urinary urgency, which means there is a shorter duration between the perception of the urge to void and the actual need to empty the bladder.
- It is normal for older adults to urinate once or twice during the night.
- Conditions that interfere with good urinary control include restricted fluid intake and consuming foods and beverages that irritate the bladder or cause increased urine production.
- If incontinence occurs, a pathologic condition or other influencing factor can usually be identified through a comprehensive evaluation.

Actions to Promote Good Urinary Control

- Avoid foods and beverages that can irritate the bladder (e.g., caffeine, alcohol, artificial sweeteners, and spicy and acidic foods).
- Avoid smoking.
- Maintain ideal body weight and good physical fitness.
- Take steps to prevent constipation (refer to Box 18-8).
- Practice pelvic muscle exercises (refer to Box 19-8).

Improving Functional Abilities to Help Maintain Continence

When incontinence is associated with the inability to reach an appropriate receptacle after perceiving the need to void, interventions are directed toward modifying the environment and improving functional abilities. For instance, an elevated toilet seat, grab bars near the toilet, and grab bars on the walls leading to the toilet may improve the person's safety and ability to maintain urinary continence.

 Interprofessional Collaboration

Physical and occupational therapists can provide recommendations for adapting bathrooms to improve functional abilities to help maintain continence. In addition, physical and occupational therapists may be able to address functional limitations that affect an older adult's ability to maintain continence.

Interventions discussed in chapters on vision (Chapter 17) and mobility (Chapter 22) can address functional limitations that can contribute to incontinence. Box 19-7 lists environmental modifications for preventing incontinence when functional limitations are a contributing factor.

In home and institutional settings, the provision of bedside commodes and privacy can be an effective intervention. If space is limited or privacy cannot be assured, however, bedside commodes may not be acceptable. If environmental adaptations cannot be made, as in public places, older adults are encouraged to become familiar with the location and arrangement of the bathroom facilities before the need to urinate is imminent.

Box 19-7 Environmental Modifications for Preventing Incontinence

Modifications to Enhance Visibility of Facilities

- Use contrasting colors for the toilet seat and surroundings.
- Provide adequate lighting in and near toilet areas, but avoid creating glare.
- Use nightlights in the pathway between the bedroom and bathroom.

Modifications to Improve the Ability to Use the Toilet in Time

- Encourage the use of chairs or beds that are designed to help the person arise unaided after sitting or lying.
- Install handrails in the hallway(s) leading to the bathroom.
- Make sure the pathway to the bathroom is safe and uncluttered.

Modifications to Improve the Ability to Use the Toilet

- Place grab bars at appropriate places to facilitate getting on and off the toilet and to assist men in maintaining their balance when standing at the toilet.
- Use an elevated toilet seat or an over-the-toilet chair to compensate for any functional limitations of the lower extremities.
- If the person has functional limitations involving the upper extremities, clothing for the lower body should feature easy-open closures such as Velcro or elastic waistbands.

Wellness Opportunity

Nurses promote self-care by helping older adults identify ways of improving their functional abilities that can affect urinary control.

Teaching About Pelvic Floor Muscle Exercises

Pelvic floor muscle exercises (PFME) also called pelvic floor muscle training, is an evidence-based self-care practice that is effective as a first-line intervention for men and women with stress, urge, and mixed incontinence, and in women with pelvic organ prolapse (Engberg & Sereika, 2016; Mendes, Rodolpho, & Hoga, 2016; Paiva, Ferla, Darski, et al., 2017). First promoted for postpartum therapy by an American gynecologist named A. H. Kegel, they are now widely used for control of urinary incontinence. The Nursing Intervention Classification of Pelvic Muscle Exercise is defined as "strengthening and training the levator ani and urogenital muscles through voluntary, repetitive contraction to decrease stress, urge, or mixed types of urinary incontinence" (Wilkinson & Barcus, 2017, p. 917). Although there is much evidence that PFME is effective for urinary incontinence and pelvic organ prolapse, this self-care intervention is significantly underutilized in the United States (Lamin, Parrillo, Newman, et al., 2016). There are no contraindications to, or negative effects of, these exercises, which can be initiated by any motivated person who can learn the technique. Nurses can use the information in Box 19-8 to teach older men and women how to perform PFME. A related nursing intervention is to facilitate referrals to physical therapists who are skilled in teaching about these exercises.

Interventions for Continence Training Programs

Continence training is a nursing intervention that can be categorized as (1) methods that are self-directed by motivated and cognitively intact people or (2) methods that are directed by motivated caregivers of cognitively impaired people. The goal of continence training is to achieve a continence interval of 2 to 4 hours between voiding. These intervals will not necessarily be equal and will usually be longer during the night. In self-directed programs, the person hopes to regain voluntary urinary control, whereas in caregiver-directed programs, the caregiver hopes to reduce the episodes

Box 19-8 Instructions for Performing Pelvic Muscle Exercises

Purpose: To prevent the involuntary loss of urine by strengthening the pelvic floor muscles

Frequency: Minimum of 3 sets of 10 contractions/relaxations daily, continued indefinitely

Position: Lying, sitting, walking, or standing with the muscles of your thighs, buttocks, and abdomen relaxed

Results: Most people begin to notice an improvement in urinary control after 3 to 6 weeks, but some will not notice the improvement until several months later

Techniques to Identify the Pubococcygeal Muscle

- Contract the muscle that stops the flow of urine. Do NOT do this regularly when urinating.
- (*Women*) Imagine that you are sitting on a marble and trying to suck it up into your vagina.
- (*Women*) Lie down and insert a finger about three quarters of the way up your vagina. Squeeze the vaginal wall so you feel pressure on your finger and a sensation in your vagina.
- (*Men*) Stand in front of a mirror and try to make the base of your penis move up and down without moving the rest of your body.
- Biofeedback, weighted vaginal cones, or a perineometer (a balloon-like device that is placed in the vagina) can be used to assist in identifying the pubococcygeal muscle and in measuring the strength of the contraction.

Method

- Tighten your pubococcygeal muscle and hold for a period of at least 3 seconds; gradually increase the contraction time by 1 second per week until you can do a 10-second squeeze.
- Relax this muscle for an equal period; rest and take deep breaths between contractions.
- Do 10 sets of a contraction–relaxation cycle (one exercise) three times daily.
- Breathe normally during these exercises and do NOT tighten other muscles at the same time. Be careful not to contract your legs, buttocks, or abdominal muscles while you are contracting your pubococcygeal muscle.
- For each of the daily sessions, vary your position (e.g., perform the exercise while lying down in the morning, standing in the afternoon, and sitting in the evening).

Additional information: You can ask your primary care practitioner for a referral to a physical therapist or continence advisor who can teach you to do these exercises.

of incontinence. Self-directed continence training, alone or in combination with biofeedback or medications, is most successful with urge incontinence.

Although specific techniques vary, essential elements of any continence training program include motivation, an assessment of voiding patterns, an individualized and carefully timed daily fluid intake, timed voiding in the most appropriate place, methods of reinforcing expected behaviors, and ongoing monitoring. During the initial assessment, diaries are used to record times and circumstances of toileting as well as times of and reasons for any episode of incontinence. After the usual voiding pattern is identified, the older adult is encouraged to resist the sensation of urgency and to postpone voiding rather than responding immediately to an urge.

With caregiver-directed methods—often referred to as **prompted voiding** programs—the caregiver uses the initial assessment of voiding patterns to establish a schedule for assisting with voiding. The caregiver gradually increases the interval between voidings until the person can maintain continence for 2 to 4 hours. These methods are most successful when the timed intervals are flexible and are adjusted, based on a good assessment of the person's needs and voiding patterns. Caregiver-directed programs include the use of behavior modification techniques, such as praising the person for staying dry between scheduled trips to the bathroom and self-initiating requests to use the toilet. Box 19-9 identifies some of the terms used for, and the general principles of, continence training programs.

Wellness Opportunity

Nurses promote personal responsibility by encouraging older adults to talk with their primary care practitioner about identifying risk factors for urinary incontinence that can be addressed through self-care measures.

Using Appropriate Continence Aids

When incontinence cannot be alleviated, it can be managed with the use of various aids and equipment, such as incontinence products and collecting devices. When used in conjunction with environmental modifications to increase the accessibility of toilet facilities, such equipment usually has beneficial effects; however, when aids and equipment are used by caregivers as substitutes for other methods of promoting continence, they are beneficial only to the caregiver and are detrimental to the older adult. For example, if protective products are used to manage incontinence, the positive effect for the caregiver may be the ease of care; however, the negative effects for the older adult include the likelihood of skin breakdown and decreased self-esteem. Because continence aids can be beneficial as well as detrimental, they should be used only after careful evaluation of all contributing factors, including needs of family caregivers in home settings.

Selection of the most appropriate products for managing incontinence depends on factors such as cost, convenience, preference, and effectiveness. Economic considerations are particularly important because disposable incontinence

Box 19-9 Continence Training Programs

Goal of Programs

To achieve voluntary control over urination at intervals of 2 to 4 hours

Terminology

Terms used for self-directed programs: bladder drill, bladder training, bladder retraining, bladder exercise, bladder retention exercise
Terms used for caregiver-directed programs: scheduled toileting, routine toileting, prompted voiding, timed voiding, habit training

Method

Step 1: Identify the usual voiding pattern, noting the times of incontinence and information about fluid intake. During the first few days, keep a diary to record the following information at hourly intervals: dry or wet, amount voided, place of voiding, fluid intake, and sensation and awareness of the need to void.
Step 2: Using information from the voiding diary, establish a schedule that allows for emptying of the bladder before incontinence is likely to occur.
Step 3: Provide the equipment and assistance necessary for optimal voiding at scheduled times.
Step 4: Provide 2000 mL of noncaffeinated liquids per day for liquid intake. Consume the largest amounts during the early part of the day, and limit fluid intake at about 2 to 4 hours before bedtime.
Step 5: Gradually increase the length of time between voidings until the interval is 2 to 4 hours long.

products can be quite expensive, particularly if used daily. The initial and periodic cost of reusable products also needs to be considered, as does the time and expense of laundering. Many products are designed specifically for either male or female incontinence. Product absorbency is affected by variables such as size, shape, depth, location, and type of absorbent material (e.g., gel, pulp, polymer). Keep in mind that someone may need several types of products for different activities (e.g., light protection during the day and heavy protection during the night). Ease of use is a major consideration, particularly for people who are independent and can manage incontinence with little or no supervision. "Pull-ups" now provide a convenient alternative to products with adhesive tabs that are difficult to reuse. Box 19-10 lists factors to be considered in selecting and using various types of aids and equipment for managing urinary incontinence. Use Online Learning Activity 19-5 to find information about various products for managing urinary incontinence.

See **ONLINE LEARNING ACTIVITY 19-5: INFORMATION ABOUT PRODUCTS FOR MANAGING URINARY INCONTINENCE** at **http://thepoint.lww.com/Miller8e.**

Teaching About Interventions for Urinary Problems

Nurses are not usually involved with medical or surgical interventions for urinary incontinence, but it is important to be knowledgeable about safe and effective options for

Box 19-10 Considerations Regarding Continence Aids and Equipment

Assessment Considerations

- What are the costs of various disposable and washable products, both initially and over a period of time? (Include the time and expense of laundry when considering costs of washable products.)
- What are the person's preferences? (e.g., is a "brief"- or "pull-up"–style garment more acceptable than a "diaper"-style product?)
- What level of absorbency is appropriate for different circumstances?
- What are the needs and abilities of the caregivers of dependent older adults in home settings? (Can the caregiver manage the tasks involved in toileting?)
- What are the consequences if the incontinence cannot be managed in the home setting? (For example, will the older adult need to be in a long-term care setting?)

Teaching Related to Aids and Equipment

- Many types of external collecting devices are available for men and women (e.g., male or female urinals, condom catheters, retracted penis pouches, and bedside urinals with attached drainage bags).
- An elevated toilet seat with rails can be used to increase safety and transfer mobility.
- Commodes are useful in diminishing the distance between the place of usual activities and toilet facilities.
- A variety of commodes are available and can be selected according to needs and preferences of the dependent person.
- Measures can be taken to ensure privacy and increase social acceptability of commodes (e.g., by placing an attractive screen around the commode).
- Some commodes are attractively designed to resemble normal furniture items.
- A bedpan can be placed on a regular chair—particularly in the bedroom, and removed when not in use.

treatment. A variety of intravaginal or intraurethral devices are available for resolving stress incontinence. For many decades, pessaries have been used as an inexpensive, low-risk, conservative, and evidence-based treatment for pelvic organ prolapse in women (Griebling, 2016; Panman,

Wiegersma, Kollen, et al., 2016). These simple devices are placed in the vagina to support the bladder, compress the urethra, or both. They are available in many sizes and shapes and are individually fitted by a primary care practitioner (Fig. 19-3). Pessaries need to be removed and reinserted at intervals ranging from nightly to once every few months, depending on the type that is used.

In recent years, many urinary control devices have become available or are used in clinical trials for self-insertion into the urethra. For example, urethral bulking agents, collagen gels, and electrical nerve stimulation are therapies that may be effective for OAB and urinary incontinence (Lee, Chermansky, & Damaser, 2016; Losada, Amundsen, Ashton-Miller, et al., 2016; Stewart, Gameiro, Dib, et al., 2016). Other currently available devices for women include urethral plugs; intraurethral catheters with unidirectional valves; and external occlusive devices, which cover the external urinary meatus and provide a watertight seal to prevent leakage. For men, foam-cushioned penile clamps with compression mechanisms are available.

Medications have varying degrees of success for treating incontinence, but their effectiveness depends greatly on identifying and addressing the specific type of incontinence. Medications can also effectively treat an underlying condition that contributes to incontinence (e.g., vaginitis; BPH). When medications are prescribed, nurses are responsible for knowing their expected positive effects as well as their potential adverse effects. Nurses also have important roles in teaching about over-the-counter medications for OAB (which have been available since 2013).

For the control of incontinence, medications that act on the autonomic nervous system are most often used. Alpha-adrenergic agents control stress incontinence by increasing bladder outlet resistance through stimulating receptors at the trigone and internal sphincter. Alpha-adrenergic blocking agents, used either alone or in combination with cholinergic agents, can treat incontinence by decreasing bladder outlet resistance due to BPH (Kim, Sun, Choi, et al., 2017). Antimuscarinic agents are used for urge urinary incontinence and

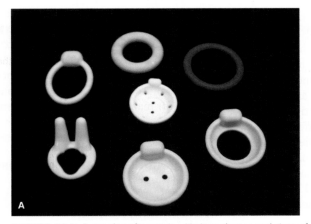

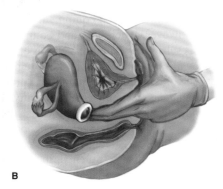

FIGURE 19-3 Examples of pessaries. Various shapes and sizes of pessaries available (**A**) and insertion of one type of pessary (**B**). (**A**, reprinted with permission from Berek, J. S. (2012). *Berek & Novak's gynecology* (15th ed.). Philadelphia, PA: Lippincott Williams & Wikins; **B**, reprinted with permission from Ricci, S. S. (2017). *Essentials of maternity, newborn, and women's health nursing* (4th ed.). Philadelphia, PA: Lippincott Williams & Wilkins.)

OAB because they control the uninhibited or unstable bladder by blocking the transmission of nerve impulses. In recent years, geriatricians have expressed concern about the adverse effects of antimuscarinic agents, because they have the potential to cross the blood–brain barrier and cause adverse effects on the central nervous system. A systematic review and meta-analysis concluded that antimuscarinic agents should be used with caution in older adults due to the increased risk for adverse events (Vouri, Kebodeaux, Stranges, et al., 2017). These medications have the same adverse-effect profile as other anticholinergics, including dry mouth, constipation, blurred vision, and mental changes. People who have glaucoma need to ask their ophthalmologist if they can safely take these drugs. Another nursing implication is that it is important to raise questions about a potential relationship between the onset and worsening of mental changes in anyone taking medications with antimuscarinic action, particularly if the person has dementia or takes other anticholinergic agents.

Interventions for urinary incontinence are developing rapidly. Evidence-based and up-to-date information is available at the websites listed in Online Learning Activity 19-6. Use Box 19-11 to teach about types of options that patients can discuss with a health care professional.

 Technology to Promote Wellness in Older Adults

Nurses can teach women about the FemiScan Home Trainer, which is an interactive program that has been approved by the Food and Drug Administration for treatment of stress and mixed urinary incontinence. The program consists of computer software with a USB interface, a biofeedback device for insertion into the vagina, and a method of providing feedback to the user about correct exercising technique. An 8-week clinical study of 250 women with urinary incontinence aged 54.4+12.7 years who used this interactive program found that 75% considered their symptoms at least 80% improved, with 45% reporting complete subjective cure (Segal, Morse, Sangal, et al., 2016). Men can use the FemiScan Multi Trainer version, which includes an anal probe for biofeedback. Older adults can find information about this home training program for pelvic floor rehabilitation at www.femiscan.com.

 See **ONLINE LEARNING ACTIVITY 19-6: RESOURCES FOR ADDITIONAL INFORMATION ABOUT URINARY WELLNESS AND INCONTINENCE** at http://thepoint.lww.com/Miller8e.

Facilitating Referrals for Treatment

An important nursing role is to encourage older adults who experience urinary incontinence to explore options for treatment rather than only self-managing their symptoms. Thus, nurses facilitate referrals to medical professionals and specialized advanced practice nurses who can perform comprehensive evaluations and prescribe treatments for OAB and urinary incontinence. A resource that is available in many health care settings is a wound, ostomy, and continence nurse (WOCN). Because these nurses have specialized training and certification, they are able to provide expert assessment and management of patients with ostomies, wounds, and urinary and fecal incontinence. Online Learning Activity 19-6 includes a link to the WOCN Association, with information about finding a WOCN by zip code.

Promoting Caregiver Wellness

For caregivers of dependent older adults in home settings, the onset of urinary incontinence often is associated with significant additional stress, particularly in combination with environmental barriers that cannot be modified. Tasks related to incontinence are some of the most difficult, stressful, and time-consuming aspects of caregiving. Caregivers in home settings may feel angry, guilty, frustrated, or inadequate when dealing with incontinence on a daily basis. If the caregiver perceives intentionality on the part of the dependent person in his or her failure to control urination, these feelings will likely be intensified. Nurses play key roles in promoting caregiver wellness by teaching caregivers about the importance of addressing all treatable contributing conditions. Nurses can base their health teaching on the information already discussed in the Nursing Interventions subsections and use Box 19-12 to teach caregivers of older adults who have urinary incontinence.

 Box 19-11 Evidence-Based Practice: Interventions for Urinary Incontinence

Nonpharmacologic Interventions Effective for Men and Women
- Pelvic floor muscle exercises
- Achieving and maintaining healthy weight
- Behavioral techniques: fluid management (i.e., intake of adequate amounts of fluids until several hours before bedtime), timed voiding (i.e., gradually lengthening the interval between urination)

Medical and Surgical Treatment for Men and Women
- Antimuscarinic medications for overactive bladder (pills, patch, gel)
- Biofeedback to enhance performance of pelvic floor muscle exercises through the use of a simple probe placed in the vagina (women) or rectum (men) to measure physiologic processes involved in pelvic muscle contractions

- Neuromodulation (i.e., stimulation of nerves through the use of an implantable device)
- Injection of bulking agent (e.g., collagen, carbon spheres) into tissue around the bladder neck and urethra

Specific for Women
- Vaginal estrogen (cream, tablet, or intravaginal ring)
- Pessary (i.e., ring or other device inserted into the vagina to place pressure on the urethra)
- Surgery for pelvic floor disorders

Specific for Men
- Alpha blockers or 5-alpha-reductase inhibitors for prostate enlargement and bladder outlet obstruction
- Surgical implantation of an artificial urinary sphincter to keep the urethra closed
- Surgical interventions

Box 19-12 Caregiver Wellness: Facts About Urinary Incontinence

- Healthy older adults normally experience the following changes affecting urinary control: diminished bladder capacity, urgency (i.e., shorter interval for maintaining control after perceiving the need to void), and frequency (e.g., voiding once or twice during the night).
- Urinary incontinence (i.e., involuntary loss of urine) occurs more often in older adults, but it is NOT an inevitable or untreatable condition.
- Urinary incontinence ranges from periodic episodes of "leakage" (especially when coughing or laughing) to total inability to maintain control over urination, but causes and treatments for each type differ.
- Stress incontinence is the involuntary loss of small amounts of urine due to activities that increase pressure on the lower abdominal wall, such as coughing, laughing, sneezing, or exercising.
- Urge incontinence is the sudden loss of large amounts of urine soon after feeling the need to urinate.
- Overactive bladder occurs when the bladder muscles contract due to abnormal signals, causing urgency and frequency, and sometimes causing incontinence.
- Never assume that urinary incontinence is irreversible or untreatable—it is not necessarily a condition that should just be tolerated and managed as well as possible.

Conditions That Increase the Risk for Urinary Incontinence

Diseases: dementia, stroke, diabetes, urinary tract infections, Parkinson disease, multiple sclerosis, spinal cord injury
- Conditions: constipation, obesity, limited mobility, cognitive impairment
- Conditions specific to women: pelvic floor disorders, such as prolapsed ("dropped") bladder or uterus, history of vaginal childbirths
- Conditions specific to men: BPH, radiation or surgery for prostate cancer
- Adverse effects of the following types of medications: diuretics, drugs that act on the autonomic nervous system

- Environmental conditions that interfere with the ability to use toileting facility in a timely manner (e.g., inaccessible toilets, toilet seats that are too low, lack of handrails)

Actions to Take to Identify Causes and Treatments for Urinary Incontinence

- Recognize that there are many types of medical, surgical, and minimally invasive treatments for urinary incontinence (see Box 19-7).
- Keep a voiding diary for a few days with information about fluid intake, voiding pattern, and episodes of involuntary loss of urine.
- Talk with your primary care practitioner about a referral for specialized health care professionals, such as a urologist, urogynecologist (for women), or specialized nurse or physical therapist.

Actions to Promote Good Control Over Urination

- Maintain good fluid intake, with the largest amounts being consumed at least several hours before bedtime.
- Avoid or limit foods and fluids that can irritate the bladder or increase the risk for urinary incontinence: caffeine, carbonated beverages, citrus products, alcohol, artificial sweeteners, and spicy foods.
- In addition to using self-management strategies (e.g., pads or briefs for incontinence), it is imperative to obtain a medical evaluation to identify causes and appropriate treatments
- Practice pelvic floor muscle exercises (also called Kegel exercises), which can be effective for alleviating or reducing episodes of urinary incontinence (see Box 19-8).

Resources for Support, Information, and Continence Aids

- National Association for Continence (www.nafc.org).
- American Geriatrics Society Foundation for Health in Aging (www.healthinaging.org).
- Simon Foundation for Continence (http://simonfoundation.org).
- Continence Product Advisor (www.continenceproductadvisor.org).
- Continence Central (www.continencecentral.org).

Unfolding Case Study

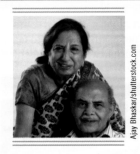

Ajay Bhaskar/shutterstock.com

Part 2: Mr. and Mrs. U. at 73 and 72 Years of Age

Mr. and Mrs. U. are now 73 and 72 years old, respectively, and continue to attend the senior center where you are the nurse.

MR. U.

Mr. U. has been under the care of a urologist for 3 years and has been taking terazosin for prostatic hyperplasia. Until recently, he was able to maintain urinary continence, but lately his Parkinson's has worsened. Then, 1 month ago, he started taking 80 mg of furosemide daily for congestive heart failure. He makes an appointment to ask your advice about incontinence products that would be best for him because "it's just hopeless to get to the toilet on time because our only bathroom is upstairs, and I like to be downstairs during the day." He reports that he limits his fluid intake to 4 cups of liquid daily, which includes 2 cups of black coffee. Because of his Parkinson disease, he has trouble standing at the toilet and usually sits down; however, he is "slow and clumsy" in managing his clothing. His son bought him some "jogging" outfits with elastic waists, but he does not wear them because he prefers to "dress up" when he goes to the senior center, so he wears trousers with belts.

Part 2: Mr. and Mrs. U. at 73 and 72 Years of Age (Continued)

THINKING POINTS WITH REGARD TO MR. U.

- What risk factors are likely to be contributing to Mr. U.'s incontinence, and which factors might be alleviated with interventions?
- What environmental modifications might be helpful in addressing the incontinence?

- What health education would you give about alleviating risk factors?
- What health education would you give about incontinence products?

MRS. U.

Mrs. U. also makes an appointment to see you to discuss her recent problem with incontinence. She tells you that for several years she has been wearing "Lightdays" pads because "I have trouble holding my water whenever I sneeze or cough." In the past few months, she notices that she has to go to the bathroom every hour or two and is reluctant to be away from her house for more than an hour at a time. Her health has been good overall, but her arthritis has been getting worse, and she is very slow moving, particularly when she needs to go up and down stairs. She drinks about 6 cups of liquid daily, consisting mostly of tea and coffee. She has heard some of her friends talking about "those Kegel exercises we had to do when we had our babies."

THINKING POINTS WITH REGARD TO MRS. U.

- What risk factors are likely to be contributing to Mrs. U.'s incontinence?
- What environmental modifications might be helpful in addressing the incontinence?
- What health education would you give about alleviating risk factors?

- What health education would you give about Kegel exercises?
- What health education would you give about incontinence products?

EVALUATING EFFECTIVENESS OF NURSING INTERVENTIONS

Nursing care for older adults with urinary incontinence is evaluated by measuring the extent to which the person can achieve periods of continence that are as long as possible. When older adults attribute incontinence to aging processes, nurses evaluate the effectiveness of their teaching by the degree to which the person verbalizes accurate information and understands the importance of identifying treatable causes. Another measure of the effectiveness of nursing interventions in such cases would be that the person seeks evaluation for his or her incontinence, rather than accept this condition as inevitable.

If incontinence cannot be resolved, nursing care is directed toward managing urinary elimination in such a way as to maintain the dignity of the older adult and to prevent negative consequences. In these situations, the effectiveness of nursing interventions might be measured by the extent to which the person maintains daily activities. For example, if older adults restrict their social activities because of incontinence, a measure of the success of nursing interventions might be that they begin using incontinence products to permit them to be away from their home for 4 hours at a time. For people with total incontinence, a measure of the effectiveness of nursing interventions would be the absence of skin irritation and breakdown.

Unfolding Case Study

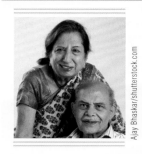

Ajay Bhaskar/shutterstock.com

Part 3: Mrs. U. at 79 Years of Age

Mrs. U., who is now 79 years old, is being transferred to a long-term care facility for rehabilitation after sustaining a hip fracture. An indwelling catheter was inserted before her hip surgery 7 days ago, and it was removed yesterday. She is ambulating with a walker but needs one-person assistance. The discharge summary describes her as incontinent of urine. Mrs. U. hopes to regain her independence in performing ADLs so that she can return to her own home, where she lives with her husband.

(continued)

Part 3: Mrs. U. at 79 Years of Age (Continued)

NURSING ASSESSMENT

During your functional assessment, Mrs. U. tells you she has had "trouble holding her water" since they removed the catheter yesterday. She is quite embarrassed about this and has not discussed it with any other health care practitioner. She says that she had too many other questions to discuss with her orthopedic surgeon and states that the nurses kept a large absorbent pad on her bed so that she would not have to walk to the bathroom. When she went to physical therapy, she used sanitary napkins, which her friend brought to her. She limited her fluid intake to a cup of coffee with each meal and a few sips of water with her pills.

Further assessment of Mrs. U.'s incontinence reveals that, for many years, she has had difficulty with "leaking," particularly when she coughs, sneezes, or exercises. Also, she gets up to urinate about four to five times nightly. It was during one of these trips to the bathroom that she tripped and fractured her hip. She says that she wakes up a lot during the night and goes to the bathroom because she is afraid of wetting the bed. She does not feel the need to urinate every time she wakes up but goes to the bathroom to prevent any leakage. She limits her fluid intake to six glasses per day and does not drink anything after 5 PM. Mrs. U. says, "A few years ago, I started doing Kegel exercises and that helped for a while but I don't bother to do them anymore." She tearfully confides that she thinks that the orthopedic surgeon damaged a nerve in her bladder, which she believes is the reason she has had such little control over urination since the surgery. She thinks that the hospital staff inserted the catheter because she has "weak kidneys." She states, "Before I had this fractured hip, I just had the usual problems holding water like all my friends have, but now it's really bad and I'll probably never be able to hold my water again. I wish you'd just put that tube back in me, so I can go home again and not worry about accidents."

NURSING DIAGNOSIS

In addition to the nursing diagnoses related to Mrs. U.'s impaired mobility, you address her problem with urinary incontinence. In deciding which type of urinary incontinence to include in your nursing diagnosis, you conclude that both Stress Incontinence and Functional Incontinence are appropriate because of the combination of long-term and recent factors that contribute to her incontinence. Your nursing diagnosis is Stress/Functional Incontinence related to limited mobility, recent indwelling catheter, and insufficient knowledge of normal urinary function and pelvic muscle exercises. Evidence for this diagnosis can be found in Mrs. U.'s statements reflecting misconceptions and lack of information, and in her description of current and past problems with incontinence. Evidence is also derived from your observations that she needs one-person assistance for walking and that she uses sanitary napkins and bed pads for urinary incontinence.

NURSING CARE PLAN FOR MRS. U.

Expected Outcome	Nursing Interventions	Nursing Education
Mrs. U.'s knowledge of normal urinary function will increase	• Discuss normal urinary function using a balloon partially filled with water and a simple illustration of the female urinary tract • Emphasize the relationship between adequate fluid intake and continence	• Mrs. U. will be able to describe normal urinary function and the mechanisms involved in maintaining continence.
Mrs. U.'s knowledge about causative factors for incontinence will increase	• Describe age-related changes that contribute to incontinence using the information in Box 19-5 • Discuss the effects of frequent bladder emptying and limited fluid intake on the maintenance of continence • Discuss the relationship between limited mobility and urinary incontinence	• Mrs. U. will describe age-related changes that influence urinary elimination • Mrs. U. will identify risk factors that contribute to her incontinence

NURSING CARE PLAN FOR MRS. U. *(Continued)*

Expected Outcome	Nursing Interventions	Nursing Education
Mrs. U.'s misconceptions about her urinary incontinence will be corrected	• Emphasize that as Mrs. U. regains her mobility, she will regain continence • Emphasize that urinary incontinence is not an inevitable consequence of aging • Explain that the orthopedic surgeon was not operating on or near her bladder or urinary tract • Explain that the Foley catheter probably contributed to her current incontinence, but that this is a temporary situation that will resolve with proper interventions • Emphasize that the nursing home staff will work with her to improve or alleviate her incontinence	• Mrs. U. will state correct information about the relationship between her hip surgery and her incontinence • Mrs. U. will express confidence in regaining urinary control
The factors that contribute to Mrs. U.'s functional incontinence will be eliminated	• Provide a bedside commode for Mrs. U.'s use until she is able to walk to the bathroom without assistance • Work with the physical therapy staff to teach Mrs. U. a proper technique for independent transfer to the commode • The nursing and dietary staff will provide 2000 mL of fluids per day, taking into consideration Mrs. U.'s preferences • The nursing and dietary staff will work with Mrs. U. to schedule her fluid intake at acceptable times of the day with minimal intake in the evening • Talk with Mrs. U. about eliminating the bed pads as soon as she feels confident about maintaining continence	• Mrs. U. will be continent of urine, except for stress incontinence
Mrs. U. will regain full control over urination	• Suggest that Mrs. U. seek a comprehensive assessment of her urinary incontinence • Give Mrs. U. a copy of Box 19-6 as a guide for performing PFME • Emphasize the need to perform PFME on an ongoing basis for the alleviation of stress incontinence • Give Mrs. U. information about health education that may be helpful for her	• Mrs. U. will report a reduction in or elimination of her stress incontinence

THINKING POINTS

- What myths and misunderstandings affect Mrs. U.'s attitude about urinary incontinence?
- What risk factors are contributing to Mrs. U.'s urinary incontinence?
- What additional assessment information would you want to obtain?

(continued)

Part 3: Mrs. U. at 79 Years of Age (Continued)

QSEN APPLICATION

QSEN Competency	Knowledge/Skill/Attitude	Application to Mrs. U.
Patient-centered care	(K) Integrate understanding of multiple dimensions of patient-centered care	Identify the many factors that interact to contribute to Mrs. U.'s current difficulty maintaining urinary continence
	(K) Describe how diverse backgrounds function as a source of values	Provide accurate information to dispel myths and misunderstandings and improve Mrs. U.'s self-efficacy related to urinary control
	(K) Describe strategies to empower patients in all aspects of the health care process	
	(K) Examine common barriers to active involvement of patients in their own health care processes	Use good communication skills to address this sensitive topic
	(S) Provide patient-centered care with sensitivity and respect for diversity of the human experience	Address Mrs. U.'s concerns about being able to return to her own home
	(S) Assess own level of communication skill in encounters with patients and families	
	(S) Communicate care provided and needed at each transition in care	
	(A) Value seeing health care situations "through patients' eyes"	
Teamwork and collaboration	(K) Describe scopes of practice and role of health care team members	Work closely with nursing assistants, dietary staff, and physical and occupational therapists to implement multidisciplinary care plan to address issues that affect Mrs. U.'s ability to maintain urinary continence
	(K) Recognize contributions of other individuals and groups in helping patient achieve health goals	
	(S) Integrate the contributions of others who play a role in helping patient achieve health goals	
Evidence-based practice	(K) Describe how the strength and relevance of available evidence influence the choice of intervention	Base care plan on evidence-based information discussed in this chapter and in Online Learning Activities 19-2 and 19-5
	(S) Base individualized care plan on patient values, clinical expertise, and evidence	
	(S) Read original research and evidence reports related to clinical practice	
	(A)Value evidence-based practice as integral to determining the best clinical practice	

Chapter Highlights

Age-Related Changes That Affect Urinary Wellness

- Kidney: degenerative changes, decreased blood flow, decreased number of functioning nephrons
- Bladder and urinary tract: hypertrophy of bladder muscle, replacement of smooth muscle with connective tissue, relaxation of pelvic floor muscles (Fig. 19-1)
- Voluntary control mechanisms: central nervous system, urinary tract, age-related changes of other systems (e.g., increased postural sway)

Risk Factors That Affect Urinary Wellness

- Misperceptions and lack of knowledge
- Fluid intake and dietary factors
- Medication effects (Table 19-1)

- Functional impairments and environmental conditions (Box 19-1)
- Factors related to pathologic conditions
- Gender-specific conditions (e.g., pelvic floor disorders, BPH)

Functional Consequences Affecting Urinary Wellness

- Effects on renal function: diminished ability to maintain homeostasis, delayed excretion of water-soluble medications, and increased risk of drug interactions and adverse effects
- Effects on voiding patters: changes in diurnal pattern of urine production
- Urinary incontinence (Box 19-2)
- Psychosocial consequences of urinary incontinence

Pathologic Condition Affecting Urinary Function: CAUTIs

- CAUTIs are a preventable infection associated with the use of indwelling catheters (Box 19-3)

Nursing Assessment of Urinary Function (Fig. 19-1; Boxes 19-4 and 19-5)

- Talk with older adults about urinary function (using appropriate terminology)
- Assess usual voiding patterns and influencing factors (Fig. 19-2)
- Identify risk factors for urinary incontinence
- Assess symptoms of impaired urinary elimination
- Be alert to misunderstandings about urinary elimination
- Assess psychosocial consequences of incontinence (e.g., anxiety, depression, social isolation)

Nursing Diagnosis

- Readiness for Enhanced Health Management
- Impaired Urinary Elimination
- Caregiver Role Strain (or Risk for)

Planning for Wellness Outcomes

- Urinary Continence
- Urinary Elimination
- Health Beliefs: Perceived Control
- Caregiver Stressors
- Caregiver Endurance Potential

Nursing Interventions to Promote Healthy Urinary Function (Boxes 19-6 to 19-12)

- Teaching older adults about age-related changes and preventing urinary incontinence
- Promoting self-management for overall urinary wellness
- Improving functional abilities to help maintain continence
- Teaching about PFME

- Interventions for continence training programs
- Using appropriate continence aids
- Teaching about interventions for urinary problems
- Facilitating referrals for treatment
- Promoting caregiver wellness

Evaluating Effectiveness of Nursing Interventions

- Longer intervals of continence
- Accurate understanding of normal urinary function and risks for incontinence
- Self-care practices to promote continence and urinary wellness
- Use of resources for further evaluation of incontinence when appropriate

Critical Thinking Exercises

1. Describe how each of the following age-related changes or risk factors might influence urinary function in older adults: medications; renal function; functional abilities; environmental conditions; altered thirst perception; changes in the urinary tract and nervous system; and myths and misunderstandings on the part of older adults, their caregivers, and health care professionals.
2. What are the psychosocial consequences of urinary incontinence for older adults and their caregivers?
3. Describe how you would address the following statement made by a 74-year-old woman: "Of course I have to wear pads all the time, just like when I was a teenager. I haven't talked to the doctor because I figured this was pretty normal at my age."
4. Describe the nursing assessment, with regard to urinary elimination, for a 75-year-old man and a 75-year-old woman.

 For more information about the topics discussed in this chapter, be sure to check out the interactive Online Learning Activities and other helpful resources at http://thepoint.lww.com/Miller8e.

REFERENCES

Andersson, F., Anderson, P., Holm-Larsen, T., et al. (2016). Assessing the impact of nocturia on health-related quality-of-life and utility: results of an observational survey in adults. *Journal of Medical Economics, 19*, 1200–1206.

Baek, J. M., Song, J. Y., Lee, S. J., et al. (2016). Caffeine intake is associated with urinary incontinence in Korean postmenopausal women: Results from the Korean National Health and Nutrition Examination Survey. *PLoS One, 11*, e0149311.

Bedretdinova, D., Fritel, X., Zins, M., et al. (2016). The effect of urinary incontinence on health-related quality-of-life: Is it similar in men and women? *Urology, 91*, 83–89.

Bell, M., Alaestante, G., & Finch, C. (2016). A multidisciplinary intervention to prevent catheter-associated urinary tract infections using education, continuum of care, and systemwide buy-in. *Ochsner Journal, 16*, 96–100.

Buchman, N. M., Leurgans, S. E., Shah, R. J., et al. (2016). Urinary incontinence, incident Parkinsonism, and Parkinson's disease pathology in older adults. *Journals of Gerontology: Biological Sciences and Medical Sciences,* doi: 10.1093/Gerona/glw235 [Epub ahead of print].

Cagnacci, A., Palma, F., Carbone, M., et al. (2017). Association between urinary incontinence and climacteric symptoms in postmenopausal women. *Menopause, 24,* 77–84.

Cai, T., Koves, B., & Johansen, T. E. (2017). Asymptomatic bacteruria, to screen or not to screen - and when to treat? *Current Opinion in Urology, 27*(2), 107–111.

Centers for Disease Control and Prevention. (2017). *Urinary tract infection (catheter-associated urinary tract infection and non-catheter-associated tract infection and other urinary system infection events.* Available at www.cdc.gov/nhsn/PDFs/pscManual/7pscCauticurrent.pdf.

Dane, K. E., Gatewood, S. B., & Peron, E. P. (2016). Antidepressant use and incident urinary incontinence: A literature review. *The Consultant Pharmacist, 31,* 151–160.

de Oliveira, M. C., Varella, L. R., Angelo, P. H., et al. (2016). The relationship between the presence of lower urinary tract symptoms and waist circumference. *Diabetes, Metabolic Syndrome and Obesity, 9,* 207–211.

Dowling-Castronovo, A., & Bradway, C. (2016). Urinary incontinence. In M. Boltz, E. Capezuti, R. Fulmer, & D. Zwicker (Eds.), *Evidence-based geriatric nursing protocols for best practice* (5th ed., pp. 343–362). New York: Springer. Modified version is available online at http://consultgerirn.org

Duralde, E. R., Walter, L. C., Van Den Eeden, S. K., et al. (2016). Bridging the gap: determinants of undiagnosed or untreated urinary incontinence in women. *American Journal of Obstetrics and Gynecology, 214,* 266, e1–e9.

Engberg, S., & Sereika, S. (2016). Effectiveness of pelvic floor muscle training for urinary incontinence. *Journal of Wound Ostomy & Continence Nursing, 43,* 291–300.

Felippe, M. R., Zambon, J. P., Girotti, M. E., et al. (2017). What is the real impact of urinary incontinence on female sexual dysfunction? A case control study. *Sexual Medicine, 5,* e54–e60.

Furlanetto, K., & Emond, K. (2016). "Will I come home incontinent?" A retrospective file review: Incidence of development of incontinence and correlation with length of stay in acute settings for people with dementia or cognitive impairment aged 65 years and over. *Collegian, 23,* 70–86.

Gordon, B., Shorter, B., Isoldi, K. K., et al. (2017). Obesity with comorbid stress urinary incontinence in women: A narrative review to inform dietetics practice. *Journal of the Academy of Nutrition and Dietetics, 117,* 889–907.

Griebling, T. (2016). Vaginal pessaries for treatment of pelvic organ prolapse in elderly women. *Current Opinion in Urology, 26,* 201–206.

Gurwitz, J. H., DuBeau, C., Mazor, K., et al. (2016). Use of indwelling urinary catheters in nursing homes: Implications for quality improvement efforts. *Journal of the American Geriatrics Society, 64,* 2204–2209.

Hunter, M. M., Nakagawa, S., Van Den Eeden, S. K., et al. (2016). Predictors of impact of vaginal symptoms in postmenopausal women. *Menopause, 23,* 40–46.

Johnson, P., Gilman, A., Lintner, A., et al. (2016). Nurse-driven catheter-associated urinary tract infection reduction process and protocol. *Journal of Nursing Care Quality, 39*(4), 352–362.

Kilic, M. K., Kizilarslanoglu, M. C., Kara, O., et al. (2016). Hypovitaminosis D is an independent associated factor of overactive bladder in older adults. *Archives of Gerontology and Geriatrics, 65,* 128–132.

Kim, J. K., Moon, Y. T., & Kim, K. D. (2016). Nocturia: The circadian voiding disorder. *Investigative and Clinical Urology, 57,* 165–173.

Kim, H. J., Sun, H. Y., Choi, H., et al. (2017). Efficacy and safety of initial combination of an alpha-blocker with an anticholinergic medication in benign prostatic hyperplasia patients with lower urinary tract symptoms: Updated meta-analysis. *PLos One, 12*(1), e0169248.

Kim, S. Y., Bang, W., Kim, M. S., et al. (2017). Nocturia is associated with slipping and falling. *PLoS One, 12*(1), e0169690.

Kosilov, K. V., Loparev, S. A., Ivanovskaya, M. A., et al. (2016) Caffeine as a probable factor for increased risk of OAB development in elderly people. *Current Urology, 9,* 124–131.

Lamin, E., Parrillo, L. M., Newman, D. K., et al. (2016). Pelvic floor muscle training: Underutilization in the USA. *Current Urology reports, 17*(2), 10.

Lee, C., Chermansky, C., & Damaser, M. (2016). Translational approaches to the treatment of benign urologic conditions in elderly women. *Current Opinion in Urology, 26,* 184–192.

Losada, L., Amundsen, C., Ashton-Miller, J., et al. (2016). Expert panel recommendations on lower urinary tract health of women across their life span. *Journal of Women's Health, 25,* 1086–1096.

Mendes, A., Rodolpho, J. R., & Hoga, L. A. (2016). Non-pharmacological and non-surgical treatments for female urinary incontinence: An integrative review. *Applied Nursing Research, 31,* 146–153.

Paiva, L. L., Ferla, L., Darski, C., et al. (2017). Pelvic floor muscle training in groups versus individual or home treatment of women with urinary incontinence: Systematic review and meta-analysis. *International Urogynecology Journal, 28,* 351–359.

Pakgohar, M., Sabetghadam, S., Rahimparvar, S. F., et al. (2016). Sexual function and help seeking for urinary incontinence in postmenopausal women. *Journal of Women and Aging, 28,* 2–8.

Panman, C., Wiegersma, M., Kollen, B., et al. (2016). Effectiveness and cost-effectiveness of pessary treatment compared with pelvic floor muscle training in older women with pelvic organ prolapse: 2-year follow-up of randomized controlled trial in primary care. *Menopause: The Journal of the North American Menopause Society, 23,* 1307–1318.

Saint, S., Greene, M. T., Krein, S. L., et al. (2016). A program to prevent catheter-associated urinary tract infection in acute care. *New England Journal of Medicine, 374,* 2111–2119.

Schneidinger, C. S., Umek, W., & Bohmdorfer, B. (2016). The problem of polypharmacy in female patients with overactive bladder - cross-sectional study in a specialist outpatient department. *Geburtshilfe Frauenheilkd, 76,* 1318–1324.

Schumpf, L., Theill, N., Scheiner, D., et al. (2017). Urinary incontinence and its association with functional physical and cognitive health among female nursing home residents in Switzerland. *BioMed Central Geriatrics, 17,* 17.

Segal, S., Morse, A., Sangal, P., et al. (2016). Efficacy of FemiScan pelvic floor therapy for the treatment of urinary incontinence. *Female Pelvic Medicine & Reconstructive Surgery, 22,* 433–437.

Shao, I. H., Wu, C. C., Hsu, H. S., et al. (2016). The effect of nocturia on sleep quality and daytime function in patients with lower urinary tract symptoms: A cross-sectional study. *Clinical Interventions in Aging, 11,* 879–885.

Siddiqui, N. Y., Ammarell, N., Wu, J. M., et al. (2016). Urinary incontinence and health-seeking behavior among white, black, and Latina women. *Female Pelvic Medicine & Reconstructive Surgery, 22,* 340–345.

Stewart, F., Gameiro, L. F., El Dib, R., et al. (2016). Electrical stimulation with non-implantable electrodes for overactive bladder in adults. *Cochrane Database of Systematic Reviews, 12*:CD010098 doi: 10.1002/14651858.CD010098.

Sugimoto, T., Yoshida, M., Ono, R., et al. (2017). Frontal love function correlates with one-year incidence of urinary incontinence in elderly with Alzheimer disease. *Journal of Alzheimer's Disease,. 56*(2), 567–574.

Tandogdu, Z. & Wagenlehner, F. (2016). Global epidemiology of urinary tract infections. *Current Opinion in Infectious Diseases, 29,* 73–79.

Thomas, K. (2016). Reduction of catheter-associated urinary tract infections through the use of an evidence-based nursing algorithm and the implementation of shift nursing rounds. *Journal of Wound Ostomy and Continence Nurses, 43,* 183–187.

Timmons, B., Vess, J., & Conner, B. (2017). Nurse-driven protocol to reduce indwelling catheter dwell time. *Journal of Nursing Care Quality, 32*(2), 104–107.

Townsend, M. K., Lajous, M., Medina-Campos, R. H., et al. (2017). Risk factors for urinary incontinence among postmenopausal Mexican women. *International Urogynecology Journal, 28*(5), 769–776.

Truzzi, J. C., Gomes, C. M., Bezerra, C., et al. (2016). Overactive bladder – 18 years – Part I. *International Brazilian Journal of Orology, 42,* 188–198.

Vaughan, C. P., Tangpricha, V., Motahar-Ford, N., et al. (2016). Vitamin D and incident urinary incontinence in older adults. *European Journal Clinical Nutrition, 70,* 987–989.

Vethanayagam, N., Orrell, A., Dahlberg, L., et al. (2017). Understanding help-seeking in older people with urinary incontinence: An interview study. *Health and Social Care in the Community, 25,* 1061–1069.

Villoro, R., Merino, M., Hidalgo-Vega, A., et al. (2016). Women with urinary incontinence in Spain: Health-related quality of life and the use of healthcare resources. *Maturitas, 94,* 52–57.

Vouri, S. M., Kebodeaux, C. D., Stranges, P. M., et al. (2017). Adverse events and treatment discontinuations of antimuscarinics for the treatment of overactive bladder in older adults: A systematic review and meta-analysis. *Archives of Gerontology and Geriatrics, 69,* 77–96.

Wald, H. L., Fink, R. M., Makic, M. B., et al. (2016). Prevention of catheter-associated urinary tract infection. In M. Boltz, E. Capezuti, R. Fulmer, & D. Zwicker (Eds.),. *Evidence-based geriatric nursing protocols for best practice* (5th ed., pp. 363–380). New York: Springer Publishing.

Wilkinson, J., & Barcus, L. (2017). *Pearson nursing diagnosis handbook.* (11th ed.). Boston, MA: Pearson.

Xu, D., Liu, N., Qu, H., et al. (2016). Relationships among symptom severity, coping styles, and quality of life in community-dwelling women with urinary incontinence: A multiple mediator model. *Quality of Life Research, 25,* 223–232.

chapter 20

Cardiovascular Function

LEARNING OBJECTIVES

After reading this chapter, you will be able to:

1. Describe age-related changes that affect cardiovascular function.
2. Identify risk factors for cardiovascular disease and orthostatic and postprandial hypotension.
3. Describe the functional consequences of age-related changes and risk factors related to cardiovascular function.
4. Assess cardiovascular function and risks for cardiovascular disease with emphasis on those that can be addressed through health promotion interventions.
5. Teach older adults and their caregivers about interventions to reduce the risk for cardiovascular disease.

KEY TERMS

ambulatory blood pressure monitoring

atherosclerosis

cardiovascular disease

DASH dietary pattern

home blood pressure monitoring

hypertension

lipid disorders

Mediterranean dietary pattern

metabolic syndrome

obesity

orthostatic hypotension

physical inactivity

postprandial hypotension

stepped-care approach

white coat hypertension

The cardiovascular system helps maintain homeostasis by bringing oxygen and nutrients to organs and tissues and by transporting carbon dioxide and other waste products to other body systems for removal. Because the cardiovascular system has a tremendous adaptive capacity, healthy older adults will not experience any significant change in cardiovascular performance because of age-related changes alone. In the presence of risk factors, however, the cardiovascular system is less efficient in performing life-sustaining activities, and serious negative functional consequences can occur. The high prevalence of risk factors among older adults—and the fact that many risk factors can be reduced by health behaviors and preventive interventions—provides numerous opportunities for health promotion. Thus, a major focus of this chapter is on the essential role of nurses in addressing risks for cardiovascular disease.

AGE-RELATED CHANGES AFFECTING CARDIOVASCULAR FUNCTION

As with many aspects of physiologic function, it is difficult to determine whether cardiovascular changes are attributable to normal aging or other factors. Knowledge about distinct age- or disease-related changes in cardiovascular function is confounded by the fact that, until recently, there was no technology to detect asymptomatic pathologic cardiovascular processes. Because some conclusions from earlier studies may have attributed pathologic changes to normal aging, current emphasis is on longitudinal studies of subjects who have been carefully screened for asymptomatic cardiovascular disease. Currently, researchers are exploring the effects of lifestyle and other sociocultural factors that affect cardiovascular function, with emphasis on disease prevention.

Myocardium and Neuroconduction Mechanisms

Age-related changes cause slight atrophy and enlargement of the myocardium, which can interfere with the ability of

Promoting Cardiovascular Wellness in Older Adults

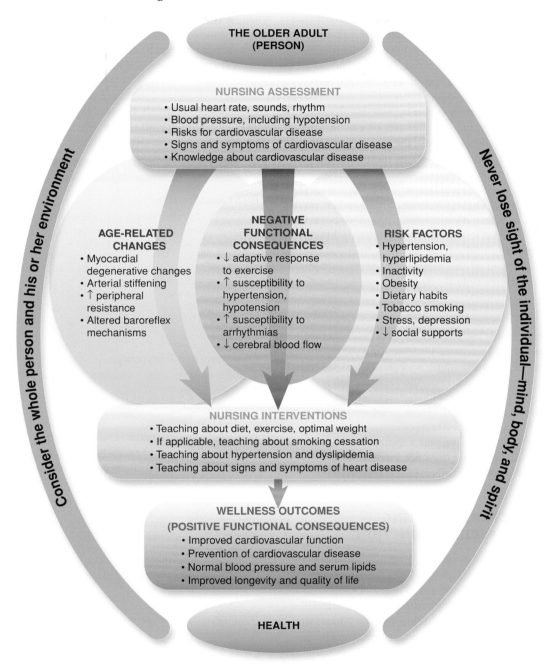

THE OLDER ADULT (PERSON)

Consider the whole person and his or her environment

Never lose sight of the individual—mind, body, and spirit

NURSING ASSESSMENT
- Usual heart rate, sounds, rhythm
- Blood pressure, including hypotension
- Risks for cardiovascular disease
- Signs and symptoms of cardiovascular disease
- Knowledge about cardiovascular disease

AGE-RELATED CHANGES
- Myocardial degenerative changes
- Arterial stiffening
- ↑ peripheral resistance
- Altered baroreflex mechanisms

NEGATIVE FUNCTIONAL CONSEQUENCES
- ↓ adaptive response to exercise
- ↑ susceptibility to hypertension, hypotension
- ↑ susceptibility to arrhythmias
- ↓ cerebral blood flow

RISK FACTORS
- Hypertension, hyperlipidemia
- Inactivity
- Obesity
- Dietary habits
- Tobacco smoking
- Stress, depression
- ↓ social supports

NURSING INTERVENTIONS
- Teaching about diet, exercise, optimal weight
- If applicable, teaching about smoking cessation
- Teaching about hypertension and dyslipidemia
- Teaching about signs and symptoms of heart disease

WELLNESS OUTCOMES (POSITIVE FUNCTIONAL CONSEQUENCES)
- Improved cardiovascular function
- Prevention of cardiovascular disease
- Normal blood pressure and serum lipids
- Improved longevity and quality of life

HEALTH

the heart to contract completely. With less effective contractility, more time is required to complete the cycle of diastolic filling and systolic emptying. In addition, the myocardium becomes increasingly irritable and less responsive to the impulses from the sympathetic nervous system.

The cardiac neuroconduction system also is affected by age-related changes, such as decreased number of pacemaker cells and increased deposits of fat, collagen, and elastic fibers around the sinoatrial node. These age-related changes that occur in healthy older adults affect cardiac performance only under conditions of physiologic stress. Even under physiologically stressful conditions, the heart in healthy older adults is able to adapt, but the adaptive mechanisms may be slightly less efficient.

Vasculature

Age-related changes affect the inner and middle vascular layers of the arteries, with functional consequences varying, depending on which layer is affected. The innermost layer, called the *tunica intima*, prevents clotting by controlling the entry of lipids and other substances from the blood into the artery wall. Degenerative changes of aging that affect the tunica intima increase the vulnerability to atherosclerosis, as discussed in the section on risk factors. The middle layer, called the *tunica media*, provides structural support and controls arterial expansion and contraction. Age-related changes that affect the tunica media include an increase in collagen and a thinning and calcification of elastin fibers. These degenerative changes increase the resistance to blood flow from the heart and contribute to increased systolic blood pressure.

Veins undergo changes similar to those affecting the arteries, but to a lesser degree. Veins become thicker, more dilated, and less elastic with increasing age. Valves of the large leg veins become less efficient in returning blood to the heart. Peripheral circulation is further influenced by an age-related reduction in muscle mass and a concurrent reduction in the demand for oxygen.

Baroreflex Mechanisms

Baroreflex mechanisms are physiologic processes that regulate blood pressure by increasing or decreasing the heart rate and peripheral vascular resistance to compensate for transient changes in arterial pressure. Age-related changes that alter baroreflex mechanisms include arterial stiffening and reduced cardiovascular responsiveness to adrenergic stimulation. These changes cause a blunting of the compensatory response to both hypertensive and hypotensive stimuli in older adults, so the heart rate does not increase or decrease as efficiently as in younger adults.

 ## RISK FACTORS AFFECTING CARDIOVASCULAR FUNCTION

Many factors affect cardiovascular function by increasing the risk for heart disease, which has been the leading cause of death in the United States for a century. **Cardiovascular disease** refers to all pathologic processes that affect the heart and circulatory system including coronary heart disease (also called coronary artery disease), arrhythmias, atherosclerosis, heart failure, myocardial infarction, peripheral vascular disease, venous thromboembolism, stroke, and transient ischemic attacks. Chapter 27 discusses heart failure as a common cardiovascular disease, and this chapter focuses on conditions that can be addressed through health promotion interventions to reduce all types of cardiovascular disease.

Researchers, health planners, and health care providers are concerned about risks for cardiovascular disease not only because of its significant prevalence and mortality rate but also because it poses a heavy economic burden. Most importantly from a wellness perspective, there is mounting evidence that cardiovascular disease is largely preventable through interventions to reduce modifiable risk factors. Thus,

prevention is a major focus of health promotion efforts, including patient education and motivation for behavior change. Modifiable conditions associated with the highest risk for cardiovascular disease are summarized in Box 20-1. These conditions can be addressed through health promotion interventions, as discussed in this chapter and in Chapters 5 (physical inactivity) and 21 (smoking cessation).

Some risk factors, such as age, race, gender, and heredity, cannot be modified, but it is important to consider their influence on the overall risk profile. In recent years, there is

 Box 20-1 Modifiable Risks for Cardiovascular Disease

High Blood Pressure

- Increase of either systolic pressure above 120 mm Hg or diastolic blood pressure above 80 mm Hg is associated with increased risk for coronary heart disease.
- For people aged 50 years and over, more attention is given to increased systolic blood pressure as a major risk factor for cardiovascular disease.
- For people between the ages of 40 and 89, the risk of death from ischemic heart disease and stroke doubles with every increase of 20 mm Hg systolic or 10 mm Hg diastolic blood pressure.

Cholesterol and Triglycerides

- Total cholesterol score is calculated according to the following equation:
- HDL + LDL = 20% of triglycerides
- Ideal total cholesterol is less than 180 mg/dL.

Diabetes

- Adults with diabetes are two to four times more likely to die from heart disease than those without diabetes.
- Ideal fasting blood glucose is less than 100 mg/dL.

Obesity

- Obesity increases the risk for heart disease and stroke.
- Obesity (i.e., body mass index of 30 or higher) is strongly associated with an increased risk for all the following conditions related to cardiovascular disease: diabetes, hypertension, lower HDL cholesterol, higher LDL cholesterol, elevated triglycerides, and triglycerides.

Smoking

- People who smoke are two to four times more likely to develop heart disease than those who do not smoke.
- Stopping smoking cuts the risk for heart disease and stroke in half after 1 year; the risk continues to decline until it is as low as a nonsmoker's risk.

Lack of Physical Activity

- Physical activity can help control blood pressure, blood cholesterol, and diabetes.
- The American Heart Association recommends the following for overall cardiovascular health in adults:
  - At least 30 minutes of moderate-intensity physical activity at least 5 days a week OR at least 25 minutes of aerobic activity at least 3 days a week OR a combination of the two
  - AND moderate high-intensity muscle-strengthening activity at least 2 days a week

increasing recognition that race and gender can affect both the risk for developing cardiovascular disease and the chance of having adverse outcomes. Also, socioeconomic and psychosocial factors, which are particularly relevant to a holistic health promotion approach to care of older adults, also affect the risk profile for heart disease.

Atherosclerosis

Atherosclerosis is a pathologic process in which patchy deposits of lipids and *atherosclerotic plaques* reduce or obstruct blood flow in the arteries. The condition is systemic, but plaque formation may be more concentrated in the coronary or carotid arteries. The development of sophisticated imaging techniques has improved our understanding about the pathophysiology of atherosclerosis since the first theories were proposed during the mid-1970s. It is now understood that atherosclerosis is a pathologic condition that begins during childhood with asymptomatic but identifiable changes and progresses through adulthood.

Atherosclerosis involves a continuum of changes in the arterial wall that develop in the following sequence:

1. During childhood and adolescence: low-density lipoprotein (LDL) cholesterol particles accumulate in the tunica intima and initiate an inflammatory response.
2. During teens and 20s: (a) inflammatory cells accumulate; (b) protective responses are initiated but necrotic debris causes further inflammation; (c) extracellular lipids accumulate in the arterial walls; and (d) a fibrous cap, called a plaque, forms over the necrotic core under the endothelium.
3. After mid-50s: (a) the plaque can become thin and weakened; (b) the plaque is susceptible to rupturing and causing a life-threatening thrombosis; (c) if the plaque does not rupture, it may enlarge and further reduce the arterial lumen; (d) if the plaque occupies more than 40% of the lumen it causes symptoms (e.g., angina); and (e) the pathologic processes within the arterial wall can provoke further plaque formation.

Plaque lesions, which can rupture, remain stable, or continue to grow, are the underlying cause of most cardiovascular disease. When coronary arteries are affected, sudden death is a common consequence. Thus, it is important to identify and address risk factors before patients experience symptoms. All the risk factors described in this section increase the risk for the development and progression of atherosclerosis and consequent cardiovascular disease.

Physical Inactivity

Physical inactivity (also called physical deconditioning) and sedentary behavior are factors that increase the risk for cardiovascular disease in older adults and interfere with their ability to compensate for age-related cardiovascular changes (Carter, Hartman, Holder, et al., 2017; Edwards & Loprinzi, 2017; Hajduk & Chaudhry, 2016). Studies indicate

that amount of physical activity, including leisure time activity, is directly associated with decreased incidence of cardiovascular disease in older adults (Barengo, Antikainen, Borodulin, et al., 2017; Cheung, Moon, Kulick, et al., 2017; O'Donovan, Hamer, & Stamatakis, 2017; Soares-Miranda, Siscovick, Psaty, et al., 2016). Conditions that often occur in older adults and contribute to physical deconditioning include acute illness, a sedentary lifestyle, mobility limitations, any chronic condition that interferes with physical activity, and psychosocial influences, such as depression or lack of motivation.

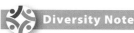

Diversity Note

Physical inactivity increases with increased age and is higher in women than in men and in black and Hispanic adults than in white adults (Mozaffarian, Benjami, Go, et al., 2016).

Tobacco Smoking and Secondhand Smoke

Tobacco smoking is a major avoidable cause of cardiovascular disease, and there is indisputable evidence that all forms of tobacco (i.e., smoking tobacco, using smokeless tobacco products, or exposure to secondhand smoke) increase the risk for cardiovascular disease and mortality, as illustrated by the following research findings (Mozaffarian, Benjamin, Go, et al., 2016):

- Overall mortality for US smokers is three times higher than that for those who have never smoked.
- Current smokers have a two to four times increased risk of stroke compared with nonsmokers or those who have quit for more than 10 years.
- Relative risk ratio for smokers to nonsmokers for developing coronary heart disease was 25% higher in women than in men.
- On average, male and female smokers shorten their life expectancy by 13.2 and 14.5 years, respectively, compared with nonsmokers.
- Nonsmokers exposed to secondhand smoke at home or work increase their risk of developing coronary heart disease by 25% to 30%.

Effects of smoking on the cardiovascular system include acceleration of atherosclerotic processes, increased systolic blood pressure, elevated LDL cholesterol level, and decreased high-density lipoprotein (HDL) cholesterol level. Even short exposures to secondhand smoke increase the risk of a heart attack because of immediate adverse effects on the heart, blood, and vascular systems. These cardiovascular effects are in addition to the effects of nicotine on respiratory function (see Chapter 21) and other aspects of health (e.g., increased risk for development of cataracts and many cancers).

Dietary Habits

Randomized controlled trials confirm that dietary habits can increase many risk factors for cardiovascular disease, including weight, blood pressure, glucose levels, and lipoprotein and triglyceride levels. A review of studies summarized the following findings related to dietary habits and cardiovascular health (Mozaffarian, Benjamin, Go, et al., 2016):

- Replacing saturated fat with polyunsaturated fat reduced cardiovascular risk by 10% for each 5% reduction in energy exchange.
- Each 2% of calories from trans fats was associated with a 23% higher risk of coronary heart disease.
- Intake of 2.5 servings daily of whole grains was associated with a 21% lower risk of cardiovascular disease when compared with 0.2 servings daily.
- When compared with little or no consumption of fish or fish oil, consumption of 1 to 2 servings per week of oily fish was associated with a 35% lower risk of cardiovascular mortality.
- Each daily serving of fruits or vegetables was associated with a 4% lower risk of coronary heart disease and 5% lower risk of stroke.
- Diets rich in potassium and low in sodium were associated with a lower risk of cardiovascular disease, especially stroke.

The section on Nursing Interventions provides teaching information about dietary patterns that are most effective for preventing cardiovascular disease.

Obesity

Obesity, which is defined by body mass index (BMI) 30 kg/m^2 or more, is associated with increased risk for many pathologic conditions including stroke, diabetes, lipid disorders, atherosclerosis, hypertension, and coronary heart disease. In recent years, increasing attention is being paid to abdominal obesity as an independent risk factor for cardiovascular disease. Abdominal obesity (also called central obesity) defined as a waist circumference more than 102 and 88 cm or waist-to-hip ratio of 0.95 and 0.88 for men and women, respectively, can occur even in people with normal BMI. Because abdominal adipose tissue is biologically and metabolically different from subcutaneous fat, it is a risk factor for mortality from cardiovascular disease even among normal-weight women.

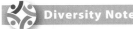

Diversity Note

Overall prevalence of obesity among older adults is 37%, with the highest rates for black women followed by high rates for Hispanic women (Ward, Clarke, Nugent, et al., 2016).

Hypertension

Hypertension is a disease of the cardiovascular system, and it is also an independent risk factor for additional cardiovascular diseases, including coronary artery disease, ischemic stroke, peripheral arterial disease, and heart failure.

Risk factors for the development of hypertension include age, ethnicity, genetic factors, obesity, physical inactivity, sleep apnea, psychosocial stressors, and lower education and socioeconomic status. In addition, dietary patterns that increase the risk for hypertension include high intake of fats and sodium, low potassium intake, and excessive alcohol consumption (Mozaffarian, Benjamin, Go, et al., 2016).

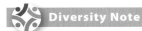

Diversity Note

Prevalence of hypertension in blacks in the United States is among the highest in the world. Additional health disparities include earlier onset, poorer control, and greater morbidity and mortality in blacks compared with whites (Gu, Yue, Desai, et al., 2017; Mozaffarian, Benjamin, Go, et al., 2016).

Lipid Disorders

Lipid disorders (sometimes referred to simply as *cholesterol*) is a broad term that encompasses several abnormalities of lipoprotein metabolism, including low levels of HDL (often referred to as "good cholesterol") and elevated levels of total cholesterol, triglycerides, or LDL (often referred to as "bad cholesterol"). Public awareness of the importance of testing for cholesterol began during the early 1980s, and by the 1990s, there was much scientific support for cholesterol screening for all adults. Since the early 2000s, the American College of Cardiology, the American Heart Association, and the United States Preventive Services Task Force have periodically updated guidelines for the screening and treatment of disorders (refer to the section on Preventing and Managing Lipid Disorders later in the text).

Diversity Note

African Americans and Mexican Americans are less likely than whites to be screened for lipid disorders.

Metabolic Syndrome

Metabolic syndrome (also called *insulin resistance syndrome*) refers to a combination of clinically identifiable conditions, as diagnosed by the presence of at least three of the following five conditions:

- Abdominal obesity, defined as waist circumference of 40 or more inches (102 cm) in men or 35 in (88 cm) in women
- Blood pressure equal to or higher than 130/85 mm Hg
- HDL cholesterol level less than 40 mg/dL in men or equal to or lower than 50 mg/dL in women, or drug treatment for a lipid disorder
- Triglyceride levels of 150 mg/dL or more, or specific treatment for hypertriglyceridemia
- Fasting blood glucose level of 100 mg/dL or more, or drug treatment for increased glucose levels

Although any component of metabolic syndrome is an independent risk factor for cardiovascular disease, the combination of two or more significantly elevates the incidence and severity of all the following: myocardial infarction, heart failure, microvascular dysfunction, impaired cardiac function, and coronary atherosclerosis and calcification (Tune, Goodwill, Sassoon, et al., 2017). Metabolic syndrome also increases the risk for diabetes mellitus, which is another independent risk factor for cardiovascular disease (Dragsbaek, Neergaard, Laursen, et al., 2016).

Psychosocial Factors

Psychosocial factors that are associated with increased risk for developing cardiovascular disease include stress, anxiety, depression, social isolation, poor social supports, and personality characteristics, such as higher anger and hostility indices. Since the mid-1960s, the term "broken heart syndrome" has been used to describe the connection between conditions under which lived experiences trigger cardiac damage and subsequent death (Efferth, Banerjee, & Paul, 2017). Current literature emphasizes that health care professionals should address stress, anxiety, and depression as modifiable risk factors for cardiovascular conditions (Chauvet-Gelinier & Bonin, 2017). Studies have identified the following associations between psychosocial factors and risk for cardiovascular disease:

- A recent review of studies stated that "among typical risk factors for cardiovascular disease, anxiety has emerged as perhaps the most important one" (Allgulander, 2016, p. 14).
- A meta-analysis of studies concluded that anxiety was associated with a 52% increased incidence of cardiovascular disease, independent of traditional risk factors and depression (Batelaan, Seldenrijk, Bot, et al., 2016).
- A meta-analysis of studies related to loneliness and social isolation found that poor social relationships were associated with a 29% increased risk of incident coronary heart disease and a 32% increase in the risk of stroke (Valtorta, Kanaan, Gilbody, et al., 2016).
- Studies have found that anger or emotional upset is associated with increased risk of having an acute myocardial infarction (Smeijers, Mostofsky, Tofler, et al., 2017; Smyth, O'Donnell, Lamelas, et al., 2016; Tully, Harrison, Cheung, et al., 2016).
- Stress and mood disorders are among the conditions that increase the risk for hypertension (DiPilla, Bruno, Taddei, et al., 2016; Ushakov, Ivanchenko, & Gagarina, 2016).
- Depression is a highly prevalent risk factor for incident coronary heart disease (Carney & Freedland, 2017; Liu, Pan, Yu, et al., 2016).

From a preventive perspective, studies indicate that optimism, positive emotions, and a sense of well-being are associated with reduced risk of cardiovascular disease, which may be related to the stress-buffering mechanisms of these characteristics (Avvenuti, Baiardini, & Giardini, 2016; Kim, Hagan, Grodstein, et al., 2017; Sin, 2016). These findings have implications for nursing assessment and interventions that extend to psychosocial aspects of nursing care for older adults, as discussed in the chapters in Part 3 of this text.

Diversity Note

Psychosocial factors, including anger, depression, and stressful events are strongly associated with increased progression of hypertension among African Americans (Ford, Sims, Higginbotham, et al., 2016).

Heredity and Socioeconomic Factors

Heredity plays a significant role in the risk for developing cardiovascular disease. Large population-based studies show a strong link between reported history of premature parental coronary heart disease and cardiovascular disease, including atherosclerosis and myocardial infarction, in offspring (Mozaffarian, Benjamin, Go, et al., 2016). Although inherited conditions cannot be changed, people who are aware of having these risk factors may be more motivated to address modifiable risks.

The relationship between socioeconomic status and cardiovascular disease has been a focus of research for several decades. A Centers for Disease Control and Prevention (CDC) survey of adults found that people with less than a high school level of education were twice as likely as college graduates to have multiple risk factors for cardiovascular disease (Mozaffarian, Benjamin, Go, et al., 2016). Although income and education are not easily modified, it is important to recognize that these conditions influence not only the risk for cardiovascular disease but also the use of preventive and interventional measures. From a holistic perspective, nurses need to consider these factors when planning health education interventions to address individualized needs of older adults.

Risk for Cardiovascular Disease in Women and Minority Groups

Since the 1990s, researchers have been broadening the scope of studies beyond the original focus almost exclusively on middle-aged men. This broadened scope has led to a growing recognition of unique aspects of cardiovascular disease in women and the disproportionate burden of cardiovascular-related death and disability among minority populations. National data show that African Americans have a higher risk of heart disease, more severe hypertension, and lower awareness of cardiovascular symptoms than do whites. In addition, African Americans have the highest age-adjusted death rate for cardiovascular disease, and they are more likely than other groups to have risk factors, such as diabetes, obesity, hypertension, and lipid disorders (Mozaffarian, Benjamin, Go, et al., 2016). Hispanic Americans, American Indians/Alaska Natives, and Native Hawaiians/Pacific Islanders are other groups in which the rate of cardiovascular disease is higher than in whites (American Heart Association, 2016).

Online Learning Activity 20-1 provides links to information about cardiovascular disease in women and minority groups, including links to educational materials developed for non–English-speaking people in the United States.

See ONLINE LEARNING ACTIVITY 20-1: RESOURCES FOR INFORMATION AND EDUCATIONAL MATERIALS FOR WOMEN AND OTHER SPECIFIC GROUPS at http://thepoint.lww.com/Miller8e

FUNCTIONAL CONSEQUENCES AFFECTING CARDIOVASCULAR WELLNESS

Healthy older adults experience no significant cardiovascular effects when they are resting, but when they engage in exercise, their cardiovascular function is less efficient. However, older adults who have risk factors for cardiovascular disease are likely to experience negative functional consequences associated with pathologic processes. This section reviews the functional consequences in older adults who have no risk factors, and the sections on nursing assessment and interventions focus on risk factors that can be addressed to prevent pathologic processes that commonly affect cardiovascular function.

Effects on Cardiac Function

Cardiac output, the amount of blood pumped by the heart per minute, is an important measure of cardiac performance because it represents the heart's ability to meet the oxygen requirements of the body. Although reduced cardiac output is common in older adults, it is associated primarily with pathologic, rather than age-related, conditions. Except for a slight decrease in cardiac output at rest in older women, healthy older adults do not experience any decline in cardiac output.

Effects on Pulse and Blood Pressure

Normal pulse rate for healthy older adults is slightly lower than that for younger adults, but older adults are likely to have harmless ventricular and supraventricular arrhythmias because of age-related changes that affect cardiac conduction mechanisms. Atrial fibrillation—a more serious arrhythmia—commonly occurs in older adults, but this is associated with pathologic conditions (e.g., hypertension, coronary artery disease) rather than with age-related changes. In most populations across the world, there is an age-related linear increase in systolic blood pressure from ages 30 to 40 years, and this change is steeper for women than for men.

Effects on the Response to Exercise

A negative functional consequence that affects cardiovascular performance in healthy older adults is a blunted adaptive response to physical exercise. Physiologic stress, such as that associated with exercise, increases the demands on the cardiovascular system by four to five times the basal level. The adaptive response involves many aspects of physiologic function, including the respiratory, cardiovascular, musculoskeletal, and autonomic nervous systems. The maximum heart rate achieved during exercise is markedly decreased, and the peak exercise capacity and oxygen consumption decline in older adults. Most of this decline is attributable to physical deconditioning and other risk factors, rather than to age-related changes alone.

Unfolding Case Study

Part 1: Mr. C. at 64 Years of Age

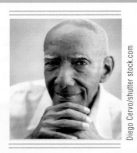

Diego Cervo/shutter stock.com

Mr. C. is a 64-year-old African American who frequently comes to your senior wellness clinic to have you check his blood pressure. He has been taking hydrochlorothiazide, 25 mg, and verapamil, 120 mg, every morning, and his blood pressure ranges between 128/84 and 136/88 mm Hg. Mr. C. sees his primary care provider once a year and obtains additional health care through community resources, such as health fairs. Mr. C.'s 86-year-old mother recently died of a cerebrovascular accident, and his father died in his early 50s of a heart attack. Mr. C. has had hypertension since he was 24, and both of his daughters have high blood pressure as well. Neither Mr. C. nor anyone in the household smokes tobacco. He has low levels of daily physical activity and weighs 210 lb. At a height of 5 ft 8 in his BMI is 32, which is 46 lb above ideal weight. He reports that he "gets winded easily" when walking up or down a flight of steps or when he has to walk "a long distance" (which he defines as the distance across the parking lot to the senior center). He attributes this to "getting old."

THINKING POINTS

- What age-related changes in cardiovascular function is Mr. C. likely to be experiencing?
- What risk factors are likely to be contributing to Mr. C.'s experience of "getting winded?"
- What risk factors does Mr. C. have for cardiovascular disease?
- What further information would you want to obtain for assessing his risk for cardiovascular disease?

Effects on Circulation

Functional consequences also affect circulation to the brain and the lower extremities. For example, age-related changes in cardiovascular and baroreflex mechanisms can reduce cerebral blood flow to some extent in healthy older adults and to a greater extent in older adults who have diabetes, hypertension, lipid disorders, and heart disease. In addition, increased tortuosity and dilation of the veins, along with decreased efficiency of the valves, lead to impaired venous return from the lower extremities. Consequently, older adults are prone to developing stasis edema of the feet and ankles, and they are more likely to develop venous stasis ulcers.

PATHOLOGIC CONDITIONS AFFECTING CARDIOVASCULAR WELLNESS: ORTHOSTATIC AND POSTPRANDIAL HYPOTENSION

Orthostatic and postprandial hypotension are conditions that occur in older adults due to a combination of age-related changes and risk factors. These conditions may be symptomatic or asymptomatic and it clearly is within the realm of nursing to identify hypotension in older adults by assessing lying and standing blood pressure as discussed in the section on Nursing Assessment. Assessing for these conditions is important because orthostatic and postprandial hypotension occur more frequently in older adults and they can lead to serious consequences, including falls and fall-related injuries.

Orthostatic hypotension (also called *postural hypotension*) is a reduction in systolic blood pressure and diastolic blood pressure of at least 20 or 10 mm Hg, respectively, within 2 to 3 minutes of standing after being recumbent for at least 5 minutes. Prevalence of orthostatic hypotension ranges from 8% in community-living older adults to 83% of hospitalized older adults (Gorelik, Feldman, & Cohen, 2016). Orthostatic hypotension is often associated with the risk factors listed in Box 20-2, with increased risk being associated with more than one contributing condition. Conditions that affect autonomic functioning, such as Parkinson disease or dementia with Lewy bodies, are strongly associated with increased risk for orthostatic hypotension (Biaggioni, 2017; Gibbons, Schmidt, Biaggioni, et al., 2016). It is important to recognize that orthostatic hypotension can occur concomitantly with hypertension or orthostatic hypotension, particularly in the older adult population (Chisholm & Applehan, 2017).

Orthostatic hypotension can be asymptomatic (i.e., identified by physical assessment) or it can be accompanied by symptoms such as fatigue, lightheadedness, blurred vision, or syncope upon standing. Whether orthostatic hypotension is symptomatic or asymptomatic, it can affect the safety and quality of life and lead to serious negative functional consequences. For instance, orthostatic hypotension is being addressed as a potentially modifiable cause of falls in

 Box 20-2 Risk Factors for Hypotension

Risks for Orthostatic Hypotension
Pathologic Processes
- Hypertension, including isolated systolic hypertension
- Parkinson disease
- Cerebrovascular disorders
- Diabetes
- Anemia
- Autonomic dysfunction
- Arrhythmias
- Volume depletion (e.g., dehydration)
- Electrolyte imbalances (e.g., hyponatremia, hypokalemia)

Medications
- Antihypertensives
- Anticholinergics
- Phenothiazines
- Antidepressants
- Anti-Parkinson agents
- Vasodilators
- Diuretics
- Alcohol

Risks for Postprandial Hypotension
Pathologic Processes
- Systolic hypertension
- Diabetes mellitus
- Parkinson disease
- Multisystem atrophy

Medications
- Diuretics
- Antihypertensive medications ingested before meals

long-term care residents (Gray-Miceli, Ratcliffe, Thomasson, et al., 2016). In people with Parkinson disease, management of postural hypotension may improve cognition and functional abilities (Centi, Freemna, Gibbons, et al., 2017; Merola, Romagnolo, Rosso, et al., 2016). Current emphasis is on assessing for orthostatic hypotension and initiating interventions, as discussed later in this chapter.

Postprandial hypotension, defined as a systolic blood pressure reduction of 20 mm Hg or more within 2 hours of eating a meal, is common in older adults. Impaired autonomic function is the pathophysiologic mechanism that is responsible for postprandial hypotension. Risk factors associated with increased incidence of postprandial hypotension are constipation, preprandial hypertension, type 2 diabetes, and Parkinson disease (Umehara, Nakahara, Matsuno, et al., 2016). Postprandial hypotension may be asymptomatic or be manifested in any of the following symptoms: falls, nausea, syncope, angina, dizziness, gait changes, light headedness, or visual disturbances (Nair, Visvanathan, & Piscitelli, 2016; Soenen, Rayner, Hones, et al., 2016). It is recommended that nurses assess for postprandial hypotension, even in older adults who are in bed, as an important intervention for reducing the incidence of falls, syncope, strokes, and other complications.

See ONLINE LEARNING ACTIVITY 20-2: INFORMATION ABOUT ORTHOSTATIC HYPOTENSION IN OLDER ADULTS at http://thepoint.lww.com/Miller8e

NURSING ASSESSMENT OF CARDIOVASCULAR FUNCTION

From a wellness perspective, nursing assessment of cardiovascular function focuses on identifying risks for cardiovascular disease and the older adult's knowledge about his or her risk profile because many risks can be addressed through health education interventions. Moreover, when older adults would benefit from improving their health-related behaviors (e.g., nutrition, physical activity), it is important to assess their readiness for changing behaviors, as discussed in Chapter 5. Although assessment of blood pressure does not differ in older and younger adults, it is essential to assess for hypotension in older adults. In addition, nursing assessment needs to consider that older adults may have atypical manifestations of cardiovascular disease (e.g., a heart attack) and they may have risk factors that are unrecognized.

Wellness Opportunity

Nurses address body–mind–spirit interconnectedness by identifying stress-related factors that increase the risk for cardiovascular disease and encouraging the use of stress management methods, such as meditation.

Assessing Baseline Cardiovascular Function

Physical assessment indicators of cardiovascular function (e.g., peripheral pulses and heart rhythm and sounds) are the same for all healthy adults. Keep in mind, however, that older adults are more likely to have chronic conditions that affect cardiovascular function. The following findings are common in older adults, but in the absence of symptoms or other abnormal findings, they usually are not indicative of any serious pathologic process:

- Auscultation of a fourth heart sound
- Auscultation of short systolic ejection murmurs
- Difficulty percussing heart borders
- Diminished or distant-sounding heart sounds
- Electrocardiographic changes such as arrhythmias, left axis deviation, bundle branch blocks, ST-T wave changes, and prolongation of the P-R interval

If a murmur, arrhythmia, or any other unusual finding is detected, it is important to determine whether it reflects a new development, a pre-existing but previously unidentified condition, or a pre-existing condition that has already been evaluated. The nurse asks questions to determine the person's awareness of such abnormal findings. Older adults may use any of the following terms to describe arrhythmias: fluttering, palpitations, skipped beats, extra beats, or flip-flops. During the assessment, ask the older person about a history of arrhythmias before listening to the heart, because asking immediately after auscultation could cause undue concern.

Arrhythmias may be caused by cardiac diseases, electrolyte imbalances, physiologic disturbances, or adverse medication effects; alternatively, they may be harmless manifestations of age-related changes. Likewise, murmurs may be caused by age- or disease-related conditions. Therefore, when murmurs or arrhythmias are detected, their significance is assessed in relation to the person's history as well as in relation to the potential underlying causes. It is also important to find out the date of the person's last electrocardiogram because this may provide baseline information regarding the duration of asymptomatic or unrecognized changes.

Assessing Blood Pressure

Most nurses do not have primary responsibility for medical management of blood pressure, but all nurses are responsible for accurate assessment of blood pressure and for decisions regarding the implications of these findings. Thus, it is important to be familiar with the most current guidelines for detecting hypertension so that health promotion efforts can be directed toward interventions. Despite mounting medical evidence that the identification and management of hypertension has important health benefits, only about half of people with hypertension achieve good control in community settings (Himmelfarb, Hayman, & Worel, 2016). Nurses are in a key position to detect hypertension, provide health education, and refer older adults for further medical evaluation and treatment.

In the early 1970s, the National Heart, Lung, and Blood Institute established the Joint National Committee on Detection, Evaluation, and Treatment of High Blood Pressure, which has developed and periodically updated evidence-based recommendations related to hypertension. The 2014 guideline recommended a goal of 150/90 mm Hg for pharmacologic treatment for adults aged 60 years or older. However, more recent guidelines based on several large-scale longitudinal studies have indicated that a threshold lower than 130 to 140 mm/Hg for systolic blood pressure is associated with a significantly reduced risk of serious adverse effects including stroke, heart disease, and cognitive impairment in older adults (Bangalore, Toklu, Schwartzbard, et al., 2017; Goldstein, Hajjar, Dunn, et al., 2017; Supiano & Williamson, 2017). Currently, major organizations such as the American Heart Association, the American College of Cardiology, and the CDC recommend that targeting a systolic blood pressure well below 140 mm Hg is beneficial in adults between the ages of 60 and 80 years. Goals need to be individualized, with higher target goals being acceptable for older adults who are frail or over the age of 80 years.

Accurately assessing blood pressure in older adults may be more difficult than in younger adults because blood pressure in older adults is more variable and has an increased tendency to fluctuate in response to postural changes and other factors. Another assessment consideration is the common occurrence of white coat hypertension (also called *isolated office hypertension*), which is the phenomenon of blood pressure readings being high only when checked by a health care practitioner. In recent years, home blood pressure monitoring, which is the practice of self-measurement of blood pressure, has been endorsed by national and international guidelines including those posted by the American Heart Association and the Preventive Cardiovascular Nurses Association. Evidence from randomized controlled studies concludes that regular home blood pressure monitoring by patients with hypertension is feasible and is associated with improved outcomes (Banegas, Ruilope, de la Sierra, et al., 2017; Tzourio, Hanon, Godin, et al., 2017).

Ambulatory blood pressure monitoring is another method of both screening for, and monitoring treatment of, hypertension. This method involves the use of a blood pressure cuff and small portable device to measure and record blood pressure at intervals of 15 to 30 minutes during a 24- to 48-hour period. The United States Preventive Services Task Force recommends that ambulatory blood pressure monitoring be used as "the reference standard for confirming the diagnosis of hypertension" (Siu & The U. S. Preventive Services Task Force, 2015, p. 780).

GLOBAL PERSPECTIVE

Ambulatory blood pressure monitoring has been used as a "gold standard" for diagnosing hypertension in many countries in Europe, South Asia, South America, and the African Caribbean for many years (Gill, Haque, Martin, et al., 2017; Grezzana, Moraes, Stein, et al., 2017).

Self-measurement of blood pressure can also be used to detect orthostatic or postprandial hypotension if readings are taken in both sitting and standing positions. In addition to the easy-to-use self-monitoring devices that are widely available, 24-hour blood pressure monitoring devices are increasingly being used to compare in-home readings to in-office measurements (Pigini, Bovi, Panzarino, et al., 2017; Staessen, Li, Hara, et al., 2017). Assessment of blood pressure in older adults is aimed at detecting not only hypertension but also orthostatic and postprandial hypotension, as summarized in Box 20-3.

Technology to Promote Wellness in Older Adults

Mobile devices (e.g., iPads, smartphones) can be used to monitor and track blood pressure using compatible blood pressure cuffs and software apps. Active older adults may view these devices as a convenient way of checking their blood pressure. Smartphone apps also can be used to monitor heart rates to detect atrial fibrillation or other arrhythmias. Older adults who have atrial fibrillation may benefit from using this type of app to help them determine the need for adjustment of medications or reevaluation of the treatment plan. A resource for up-to-date information and reviews about these apps is www.iMedicalApps.com.

Box 20-3   Guidelines for Assessing for Hypotension

For Assessment of Orthostatic Hypotension

- Maintain the person's arm in the same position (either parallel or perpendicular to the torso) during supine and standing positions.
- Obtain initial blood pressure reading after the person has been in a sitting or lying position for at least 5 minutes.
- Obtain second blood pressure reading after the person has been standing for 1 to 3 minutes.

For Assessment of Postprandial Hypotension

- Obtain initial blood pressure reading before a meal.
- Obtain second and third reading at 15-minute intervals after the meal is completed.

Normal Findings

- The normal difference between lying/sitting and standing systolic blood pressure is 20 mm Hg or less after standing for 1 minute.
- The normal difference between lying/sitting and standing diastolic blood pressure is 10 mm Hg or less after standing for 1 minute.

Identifying Risks for Cardiovascular Disease

The assessment of risks for cardiovascular disease, with emphasis on identifying modifiable risk factors, provides a basis for health promotion interventions. Hypertension, lipid disorders, and smoking cessation (discussed in Chapter 21) are important remediable conditions for older adults who have these risks. In addition, obesity, physical inactivity, and certain dietary habits are risk factors that nurses can address through improved health-related behaviors, as discussed in Chapter 5. Nurses can use Box 20-4 as a guide for nursing assessment of risks.

Wellness Opportunity

Nurses promote personal responsibility and self-awareness by teaching older adults to use self-assessment tools to identify their risks for heart disease.

See ONLINE LEARNING ACTIVITY 20-3: EVIDENCE-BASED TOOLS FOR IDENTIFYING RISKS FOR CARDIOVASCULAR DISEASE at http://thepoint.lww.com/Miller8e

Assessing Signs and Symptoms of Heart Disease

Assessment of older adults for heart disease is complicated by the fact that the symptoms often differ from the expected manifestations. For example, older people with angina and acute myocardial infarctions are likely to have more diffuse and milder symptom clusters rather than the classic symptom of chest pain (DeVon, Vuckovic, Ryan, et al., 2017). It also is important to recognize that atypical and subtle manifestations occur more commonly in women than in men and in older adults with comorbidities (Chien, Huang, Huang, et al., 2016;

Box 20-4 Guidelines for Assessing Risks for Cardiovascular Disease in Older Adults

Questions to Identify Risk Factors for Cardiovascular Disease

- Do you have, or have you ever had, any heart or circulation problems (e.g., stroke, angina, heart attack, blood clots, or peripheral vascular disease)? *If yes, ask the usual questions about type of therapy, and so on.*
- What is your normal blood pressure? Have you ever been told that you have high blood pressure, or borderline high blood pressure?
- Do you take, or have you ever taken, medications for heart problems or blood pressure? *If yes, ask the usual questions about type, dose, duration of therapy, and the like.*
- Do you smoke, or have you ever smoked? *If yes, ask additional questions, such as those appropriate for assessing respiratory function; see* Chapter 21.
- Do you know what your cholesterol levels are? When was the last time you had your cholesterol checked?
- Do you have diabetes? When was the last time you had your blood sugar (glucose) level checked and what was the result?
- What is your usual pattern of exercise?

Additional Considerations Regarding Risk Factors

- Calculate BMI and compare the person's ideal weight to his or her present weight.
- Determine usual dietary habits, paying particular attention to the person's intake of sodium, fiber, and types of fat. (This information is usually obtained during the nutritional assessment, as discussed in Chapter 18.)

Manfrini, Ricci, Cenko, et al., 2016; Radovanovic, Pilgrim, Seifert, et al., 2017). Atypical signs and symptoms include weakness, unusual fatigue; nausea; anxiety; shortness of breath; and pain in the jaw, neck, or throat (DeVon, Burke, Vuckovic, et al., 2017). Similarly, heart failure may begin very subtly, with early manifestations of mental changes secondary to the physiologic stress.

An important nursing assessment consideration is that older adults as well as health care professionals are likely to attribute atypical symptoms to other conditions, such as arthritis or indigestion, or even to "normal aging." Therefore, it is important to recognize that complaints about fatigue, digestion, respiration, or musculoskeletal pain in the upper body can be indicators of cardiac disease. Assessment is further complicated by the fact that older adults often have more than one underlying condition that could be responsible for these symptoms. It is not unusual, for example, for an older person to have an esophageal reflux disorder as well as a history of ischemic heart disease. Another consideration is that older adults with functional impairments or limited mobility may not be active enough to experience exertion-related symptoms. Therefore, in addition to focusing on the usual manifestations of cardiovascular function, information about other systems and overall functioning provides pertinent assessment information. In addition, a baseline electrocardiogram is helpful in establishing the possibility of silent or atypical myocardial ischemia.

Assessing Knowledge About Heart Disease

In addition to assessing signs and symptoms, nurses assess the older adult's knowledge about manifestations of heart disease. This is particularly important because immediate medical attention is a major factor in determining outcomes of heart attacks, and all people need to be aware of the warning signs so that they can initiate appropriate help-seeking actions. Thus, it is important to ask at least one question to assess the older adult's knowledge about the signs and symptoms of a heart attack. In addition, include a question about what the person would do and whom they would call if they thought they were experiencing a heart attack. Box 20-5 summarizes the guidelines for assessing cardiovascular function and detecting cardiovascular disease in older adults, emphasizes the assessment components that are unique to older adults, and refers to additional assessment components that apply to adults in general.

Diversity Note

Knowledge of heart attack and stroke symptoms is lacking among adults in the United States and is lowest among older adults, racial minorities, and other groups who are at highest risk for cardiovascular disease.

Box 20-5 Guidelines for Assessing Cardiovascular Function in Older Adults

Questions to Assess for Cardiovascular Disease

- Do you ever have chest pain or tightness in your chest? If yes, ask the usual questions to explore the type, onset, duration, and other characteristics.
- Do you ever have difficulty breathing? If yes, ask the usual questions regarding onset and other characteristics.
- Do you ever feel lightheaded or dizzy? If yes, ask about specific circumstances, medical evaluation, and methods of dealing with symptoms and ensuring safety.
- Do you ever feel like your heart is racing, is irregular, or has extra or skipped beats? If yes, ask about any prior medical evaluation.
- Have you ever been told that you had a heart murmur? If yes, ask about any prior medical evaluation.

Information Obtained During Other Portions of an Assessment That may be Useful in Assessing Cardiovascular Function

- Do you tire easily or feel that you need more rest than is ordinarily required?
- Do you have any symptoms that you think are due to indigestion?
- Do your feet or ankles ever get swollen?
- Do you wake up at night because of difficulty breathing or because of any other discomfort? Have you made any adjustments in your sleeping habits because of difficulty breathing (e.g., do you use more than one pillow or sleep in a chair)?

Interview Questions to Assess for Postural Hypotension

- Do you ever feel lightheaded or dizzy, especially when you get up in the morning or after you've been lying down?
  - If yes: Is this feeling accompanied by any additional symptoms, such as sweating, nausea, or confusion?
  - If yes: Do any of the risks listed in Box 20-2 apply to you?
  - If yes: Ask about any prior medical evaluation.

NURSING DIAGNOSIS

If the nursing assessment identifies risks for cardiovascular disease, a nursing diagnosis of Ineffective Health Maintenance. This diagnosis is defined as "inability to identify, manage, and/or seek help to maintain well-being" (Herdman & Kamitsura, 2018. p. 150). Related factors common in older adults include sedentary lifestyle, hypertension, and insufficient knowledge about preventive measures. For older adults with impaired cardiovascular function, applicable nursing diagnoses include Activity Intolerance and Decreased Cardiac Output. The nursing diagnosis of Risk for Falls may be appropriate for older adults with orthostatic or postprandial hypotension, particularly in the presence of additional risk factors for falls and fractures (e.g., osteoporosis, neurologic disorders, and medication side effects).

Wellness Opportunity

Nurses can use the wellness nursing diagnoses, Readiness for Enhanced Nutrition or Readiness for Enhanced Knowledge, for older adults who are interested in developing heart-healthy dietary habits or learning about health-promoting behaviors to prevent heart disease.

PLANNING FOR WELLNESS OUTCOMES

When older adults have risks for cardiovascular disease, nurses can apply any of the following Nursing Outcomes Classification terminologies to identify wellness outcomes in their care plans: Health Orientation, Health Promoting Behavior, Knowledge: Healthy Diet, Knowledge: Lipid Disorder Management, Risk Control: Tobacco Use, and Weight Loss Behavior. Wellness outcomes for older adults with cardiovascular disease include Self-Management: Cardiac Disease, Circulation Status, Health-Seeking Behavior, and Knowledge: Cardiac Disease Management. Additional outcomes include maintaining blood pressure within the normal range and preventing negative consequences of orthostatic or postprandial hypotension (e.g., falls and fractures).

Wellness Opportunity

Nurses address body–mind–spirit interconnectedness by including stress level as an outcome directed toward reducing the risk for cardiovascular disease.

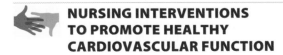

NURSING INTERVENTIONS TO PROMOTE HEALTHY CARDIOVASCULAR FUNCTION

From a wellness perspective, nursing interventions to promote healthy cardiovascular function focus on primary and secondary prevention of cardiovascular disease. These interventions address specific risk factors, such as smoking, hypertension, obesity, and lipid disorders, as well as preventive measures, such as optimal levels of physical activity, heart-healthy dietary patterns, and stress-reduction actions. Although pharmacologic and medical interventions are often used to reduce risk factors, teaching about health promotion actions is a nursing intervention that is appropriate in almost all situations. In addition to addressing risks for cardiovascular disease, nurses can address orthostatic or postprandial hypotension and the related functional consequences, such as falls and fractures.

Nurses can use the following Nursing Interventions Classification terminologies in care plans to promote cardiovascular wellness: Cardiac Risk Management, Coping Enhancement, Counseling, Exercise Promotion, Guided Imagery, Health Education, Meditation Facilitation, Nutritional Counseling, Relaxation Therapy, Self-Responsibility Facilitation, and Teaching: Individual.

Role of Nurses in Teaching About Cardiovascular Disease

In recent years, there is increasing emphasis on preventing cardiovascular disease through interventions for health behavior change, as discussed in Chapter 5. For example, the Heart Health Program is an action-oriented intervention to encourage health behavior change based on the Health Belief Model. This nurse-led intervention promotes heart healthy behavior change in low-income African-American older adults (Menne, Borato, Shelton, et al., 2016). Nurses are taking leading roles in health promotion related to cardiovascular diseases through organizations such as the Preventive Cardiovascular Nurses Association. Online Learning Activity 20-4 provides links to an article about nurse-led models for teaching about prevention of heart disease as well as additional resources. Box 20-6 can be used for health promotion to teach older adults about steps they can take to reduce their risk for cardiovascular disease. Figure 20-1 is an infographic developed by the National Heart, Lung, and Blood Institute that can be used for patient education about addressing the risks for heart disease.

See ONLINE LEARNING ACTIVITY 20-4: JOURNAL ARTICLE AND RESOURCES RELATED TO HEALTH PROMOTION AND CARDIOVASCULAR DISEASE at http://thepoint.lww.com/Miller8e

Addressing Risks Through Nutritional Interventions

Nutritional interventions are particularly important for prevention or management of obesity, hypertension, and lipid disorders. Evidence-based recommendations related to dietary influences on cardiovascular disease support the following dietary patterns for heart health:

- High intake of nuts, fruits, legumes, vegetables, and high-fiber whole grains

Box 20-6 Health Promotion Activities to Reduce the Risks for Cardiovascular Disease

Identification of Risks

- Talk with your primary care practitioner about identifying risks such as diabetes, hypertension, and high cholesterol.

Reduction of Risks

- Work with your primary care practitioner toward optimal management of medical conditions associated with increased risk for cardiovascular disease, such as diabetes, hypertension, or high cholesterol.
- Do not smoke.
- Engage in moderate physical activity for 30 minutes at least 5 days a week.
- Maintain weight within normal limits.
- Avoid breathing secondary smoke and other air pollutants whenever possible.
- Engage in stress management activities such as meditation and yoga.
- Eat heart-healthy foods, as described in the next section.

Heart-Healthy Eating Pattern

- Consume at least 3 to 5 servings of fruits daily, especially the deeply colored ones.
- Consume at least 3 to 5 servings of vegetables daily, especially the deeply colored ones.
- Include 2 to 3 servings of low-fat or nonfat dairy products.
- Choose whole-grain products as sources of carbohydrates and fiber (e.g., rye, barley, oats, whole wheat).
- Aim for at least 25 g of fiber daily.
- Choose only the leanest meats, poultry, fish, and shellfish.
- Avoid foods that are high in calories, trans fats, or refined sugars.
- Use oils that are least saturated (e.g., canola, safflower, sunflower, corn, olive, soybean, and peanut oils) and use margarine that is soft and free of trans fats.
- Limit salt intake to no more than 1500 mg daily.

- Fish, skinless poultry, and plant-based proteins rather than red meats
- Fat-free or low-fat dairy products
- Use of polyunsaturated and monounsaturated fats (e.g., olive oil, oleic acid from vegetable sources) and avoidance of trans fats and saturated fats
- Daily sodium intake limited to 1500 mg or less
- Limited consumption of sugar and sugar-sweetened drinks

(American Heart Association, 2016; Mozaffarian, Benjamin, Go, et al., 2016; Chalvon-Demersay, Azzout-Marniche, Arfsten, et al., 2017).

The **Mediterranean dietary pattern** is widely supported as an evidence-based approach for preventing cardiovascular disease and promoting overall health. The dietary pattern is characterized by higher intakes of fish, poultry, nuts, fruits, legumes, vegetables, and lower intake of red and processed meats. Overall, the Mediterranean dietary pattern involves lower intake of saturated and trans fats, higher intake of monounsaturated and polyunsaturated fats, and complex carbohydrates as the main type of carbohydrates.

The **DASH dietary pattern**, which refers to the *Dietary Approaches to Stop Hypertension,* is an evidence-based eating plan that is promoted by many organizations including the National Institutes of Health and the American Heart Association. This dietary pattern is characterized by high intake of fruits, vegetables, and plant proteins from grains, nuts, and legumes; moderate intake of low-fat or nonfat dairy foods; and low intakes of sodium and animal protein and is widely recognized as a primary and secondary preventive intervention for hypertension. Beneficial effects of DASH-type diets include lowered blood pressure, decreased LDL and triglyceride levels, and lower mortality rates. Studies have confirmed a strong association between a DASH-like diet and reduced incidence of cardiovascular diseases (Mozaffarian, Benjamin, Go, et al., 2016).

Another focus of nutrition-related research is on the potential benefits of foods that are rich in flavonoids (i.e., a polyphenol compound found in plant foods). For instance, there is increasing evidence that tea, cocoa, apples, and extra virgin olive oil have significant cardioprotective effects (e.g., antioxidant, anti-inflammatory, antiplatelet, and vasodilation actions) (Lin, Zhang, Li, et al., 2016; Loffredo, Perri, Nocella, et al., 2017; Lovegrove, Stainer, & Hobbs, 2017).

Addressing Risks Through Lifestyle Interventions

Healthy behaviors that form the foundation of interventions for preventing cardiovascular disease include remaining physically active, managing stress, refraining from smoking, and maintaining ideal body weight. There is strong evidence supporting the importance of physical activity as an intervention for preventing cardiovascular disease and improving life expectancy (Liberman, Forth, Beyer, et al., 2017. For example, a longitudinal study found that incidence of cardiovascular disease was reduced by 58% and 70% in participants who were sufficiently active and highly active, respectively, compared to those who were inactive or insufficiently active (Tambalis, Panagiotakos, Georgousopoulou, et al., 2016). Specific positive effects on cardiovascular function include weight loss; reduced blood pressure; improved overall cardiac function; lower rates of cardiovascular disease; improved lipid, glucose, and triglyceride levels; and decreased risk of developing diabetes and cardiovascular disease. There also is abundant evidence that aerobic exercise is associated with improved cardiovascular health in older adults (Bouaziz, Vogel, Schmitt, et al., 2017). Positive effects of exercise on other aspects of health are noted throughout this text, and nurses can incorporate this information when they teach about the many positive functional consequences of regular physical exercise.

Smoking is a major risk factor for cardiovascular disease, and quitting smoking is the most effective lifestyle change for reducing risk of cardiovascular disease in people who

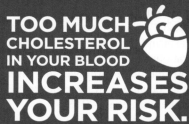

TOO MUCH CHOLESTEROL IN YOUR BLOOD **INCREASES YOUR RISK.**

GET TESTED TO LEARN YOUR TOTAL CHOLESTEROL, GOOD (HDL) AND BAD (LDL) CHOLESTEROL, AND TRIGLICERIDES.

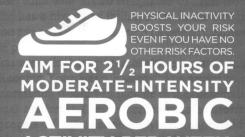

PHYSICAL INACTIVITY BOOSTS YOUR RISK EVEN IF YOU HAVE NO OTHER RISK FACTORS.

AIM FOR 2½ HOURS OF MODERATE-INTENSITY AEROBIC ACTIVITY PER WEEK.

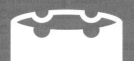

SMOKERS ARE UP TO 6 TIMES MORE LIKELY TO SUFFER HEART ATTACKS.[1] DON'T SMOKE.

VISIT SMOKEFREE.GOV FOR TOOLS TO HELP YOU QUIT.

HEARTTRUTH.GOV

ARE YOU AT RISK FOR **HEART DISEASE?**

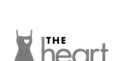

THE heart TRUTH®

A program of the National Institutes of Health

THE HIGHER YOUR BODY MASS INDEX (BMI), THE HIGHER YOUR RISK FOR HEART DISEASE, ESPECIALLY AT BMI GREATER THAN 30.

MAINTAIN A HEALTHY WEIGHT.

HIGH BLOOD PRESSURE GREATLY INCREASES YOUR RISK.

GET TESTED. REDUCE YOUR SODIUM INTAKE. STAY ACTIVE. MAINTAIN A HEALTHY WEIGHT.

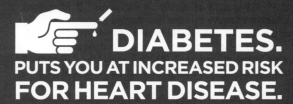

DIABETES. PUTS YOU AT INCREASED RISK FOR HEART DISEASE.

YOU CAN LOWER YOUR RISK BY KEEPING YOUR BLOOD GLUCOSE CLOSE TO THE RECOMMENDED TARGET NUMBERS.[2]

FIGURE 20-1 Example of health promotion material available at the National Heart, Lung, and Blood Institute to teach about reducing the risk for heart disease. Available at https://www.nhlbi.nih.gov/health/educational/hearttruth/downloads/html/infographic-riskfactors/areyouatriskforheartdisease.htm. Footnotes in figure:

[1]National Heart, Lung, and Blood Institute. (2005). *Your guide to a healthy heart*;
[2]Diabetes Prevention Program Research Group. (2002). Reduction in the incidence of type 2 diabetes with lifestyle intervention or metformin. *New England Journal of Medicine, 346*(6), 393–403.

smoke (Chu, Pandya, Salomon, et al., 2016). Benefits of smoking cessation as a secondary prevention intervention begin immediately and are as effective in older adults as they are in younger people. An important nursing responsibility is to provide health education regarding smoking cessation, as discussed in Chapter 21.

Teaching about stress reduction is an important health promotion intervention for reducing risks related to cardiovascular disease. Reviews of studies have found that mind–body therapies such as meditation and tai chi have positive effects on cardiovascular function (Cole, Wijarnpreecha, Chattipakom, et al., 2016; Shi, Zhang, Wang, et al., 2017). In addition, many studies indicate that yoga is effective for primary and secondary prevention of cardiovascular disease, particularly through its effects on blood pressure (Barrows & Fleury, 2016; Cramer, 2016; Kuehn, 2017; Wahlstrom, Rydell-Karlsson, Medin, et al., 2017). Nurses can encourage older adults to participate in mind–body activities, which community- or hospital-based senior centers offer.

Secondary Prevention

When nurses care for older adults who have cardiovascular disease, referrals for secondary prevention programs, such as cardiac rehabilitation, are an important part of care. Evidence-based guidelines recommend cardiac rehabilitation programs as a comprehensive approach to reducing mortality and recurrent cardiovascular events by 20% to 25% (Campkin, Boyd, & Campbell, 2016). Despite this evidence of efficacy and cost-effectiveness, referral and participation rates for cardiac rehabilitation programs are low, especially for older adults and people in minority groups (Schopfer & Forman, 2016; Zhang, Sobolev, Piña, et al., 2017). Although referrals need to be initiated by primary care practitioners, nurses have important roles in encouraging participation when referrals are made. Nurses also can suggest referrals for additional preventive services that address stress management, smoking cessation, or exercise counseling.

Wellness Opportunity

Nurses communicate positive attitudes about aging by talking with older adults about personal responsibility for addressing risks for cardiovascular disease and communicating that it is never too late to incorporate healthy behaviors into daily life.

Low-Dose Aspirin for Primary and Secondary Prevention

Low-dose aspirin is a pharmacologic intervention that has been investigated for the prevention of cardiovascular disease since the early 2000s. Current recommendations of the U.S. Preventive Task Force for adults aged 60 to 69 emphasize that the decision to initiate low-dose aspirin for primary prevention should be made by the individual based on the following: the person's 10-year risk of developing cardiovascular disease and the balance of benefits and harms. No recommendation is made for adults aged 70 years or older because evidence is lacking (National Heart, Lung, and Blood Institute, 2017). A systematic review comparing doses and forms of aspirin for long-term use found that controlled release preparations in doses greater than 100 mg were most effective for prevention of cardiovascular disease; however, this dose was associated with more adverse effects (Lotrionte, Biasucci, Peruzzi, et al., 2016).

Preventing and Managing Hypertension

Although only advanced practice nurses prescribe medications for hypertension, all nurses need to apply current guidelines and recommendations for management of hypertension when caring for older adults. Nursing interventions for people with hypertension include evaluating a patient's response to prescribed medications and teaching about interventions for hypertension. In addition, nurses can promote wellness by teaching about self-care measures for preventing and treating hypertension. This is particularly important because lifestyle interventions—including nutritional interventions, weight loss, physical activity, and stress-reduction techniques—are essential interventions that are within the realm of health promotion.

The stepped-care approach to management of hypertension was introduced in the first JNC report and it has been consistently recommended in subsequent reports. This approach recommends that lifestyle modifications be tried initially, followed by pharmacologic interventions to achieve target blood pressure. Lifestyle interventions that have the most significant impact on hypertension are substantial weight loss and a dietary pattern that includes low-sodium and high-potassium foods. Guidelines from major organizations, such as the American Heart Association and the American College of Cardiology, emphasize that sodium intake of 1500 mg/day or less is associated with greater reductions in blood pressure (Mozaffarian, Benjamin, Go, et al., 2016). Because Americans consume an average daily intake of more than 3000 mg of sodium, nurses have important responsibilities with regard to teaching older adults and their caregivers about sodium intake.

Many medications are used for treating hypertension, and selection of the best medication is based on variables such as therapeutic effectiveness, the presence of concomitant conditions, and avoidance of adverse effects. Current emphasis is on the need for individualized treatment options, particularly for certain groups, such as older adults with multimorbidity, African Americans, and people with chronic kidney disease (Yannoutsos, Kheder-Elfekih, Halimi, et al., 2017). Box 20-7 summarizes guidelines for interventions for hypertension and includes health education information about nutrition and lifestyle interventions. Figure 20-2 illustrates examples of some of the culturally specific health education materials that are available at the National Institutes of Health.

Box 20-7 Guidelines for Nursing Management of Hypertension

Health Promotion Interventions

The following lifestyle modifications are recommended for all people with hypertension:

- Avoidance of tobacco
- Weight reduction when appropriate (i.e., when the person weighs more than 110% of his or her ideal weight)
- 30 to 45 minutes of exercise, such as brisk walking, at least five times weekly
- Limitation of alcohol intake to one drink per day (e.g., 2 ounces of 100-proof whiskey, 8 ounces of wine, or 24 ounces of beer)

The following nutritional interventions are recommended for all people with hypertension:

- Sodium intake limited to 1.5 g daily
- Avoidance of processed foods
- Daily intake of 7 to 8 servings of grains and grain products and 8 to 10 servings of fruits and vegetables

Considerations Regarding the Treatment of Hypertension

- A person's blood pressure should be measured at least three times before making any decisions about treatment.
- Ambulatory or home blood pressure monitoring is recommended for initial and ongoing assessment.
- The safety of antihypertensive agents is improved by carefully selecting the medication, starting with low doses, and changing the medication regimen gradually, in small increments, if necessary.
- The goals of hypertensive treatment are to control blood pressure by the least intrusive means and to prevent cardiovascular morbidity and mortality.
- Treatment is directed toward achieving and maintaining a systolic blood pressure <130/80 mm Hg if this can be achieved without compromising cardiovascular function.
- For older adults with isolated systolic hypertension or systolic blood pressure levels of 140 to 160 mm Hg, lifestyle modifications should be the first treatment step.

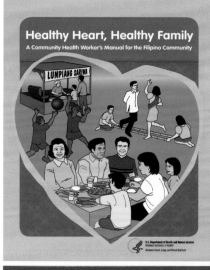

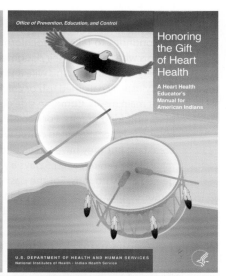

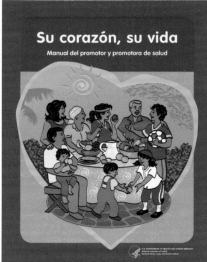

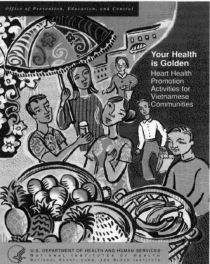

FIGURE 20-2 Examples of culturally specific health education materials that are available from the National Institutes of Health.

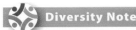

Diversity Note

Studies indicate that calcium blockers, diuretics, and aldosterone blockers are more effective for treatment of hypertension in African Americans, in contrast to beta blockers and angiotensin-converting enzyme (ACE) inhibitors (Brewster, van Montfrans, Ochlers, et al., 2016; Rayner & Spence, 2017).

Wellness Opportunity

Nurses promote personal responsibility for managing hypertension by talking with older adults about self-monitoring of blood pressure.

Preventing and Managing Lipid Disorders

Although nurses usually do not prescribe medications for treatment of lipid disorders, they are responsible for teaching about preventing and managing lipid disorders. This is especially important because statin therapy for primary and secondary prevention of cardiovascular disease is the most common class of medication prescribed in the United States (Miller & Martin, 2016). Currently, there is strong evidence that benefits outweigh the risks in people with any of the following conditions (Egan, Li, White, et al., 2016; Robinson, 2016; Virani, 2016):

- Clinical evidence of atherosclerotic cardiovascular disease
- Primary elevations of LDL cholesterol 190 mg/dL or above

Unfolding Case Study

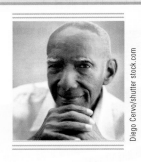

Diego Cervo/shutter stock.com

Part 2: Mr. C. at 70 Years of Age

Mr. C. is now 70 years old and his blood pressure fluctuates between 136/88 and 146/94 mm Hg. He continues to take hydrochlorothiazide, 25 mg, and verapamil, 120 mg, every morning. Mr. C. and his wife live with their daughter and her teenage children. Mr. and Mrs. C. usually do the family grocery shopping, and his wife and daughter prepare the family meals. A diet history reveals that the family usually eats fried fish or chicken about four times a week and pig's feet or ham hocks for the other main meals. Common side dishes are corn, okra, grits, cornbread, sweet potatoes, black-eyed peas, and fried greens. For cooking, the family uses lard, salt pork, or bacon drippings. Their usual beverage is decaffeinated coffee with sugar and cream. The family generally has cereal and toast for breakfast, but they have bacon and eggs on Saturdays and Sundays. Mr. and Mrs. C. eat their noon meal at the senior center 5 days a week. Mr. C.'s BMI is still in the obesity range and he has gradually gained a few pounds. For the past several years, he has participated in the exercise program at the senior center, but gets little additional exercise and continues to complain of "getting winded" when he walks across the parking lot.

THINKING POINTS

- What additional information would you obtain for further assessment of Mr. C.'s cardiovascular status?
- What nutritional and lifestyle interventions would you discuss with Mr. C. regarding his hypertension?

- What teaching materials would you use for health education with Mr. C.?

QSEN APPLICATION

QSEN Competency	Knowledge/Skill/Attitude	Application to Mr. C.
Patient-centered care	(K) Describe how diverse backgrounds function as a source of values	Assess sociocultural factors that influence Mr. C.'s dietary patterns
	(K) Describe strategies to empower patients in all aspects of the health care process	Discuss benefits of weight loss that would have measurable positive effects during daily activities (e.g., improved breathing during mild exertion or walking)
	(S) Elicit patient values, preferences, and expressed needs	
	(S) Provide patient-centered care with sensitivity and respect for diversity of the human experience	

- Diabetes and aged 40 to 75 years
- LDL cholesterol 70 to 189 mg/dL
- Estimated 10-year risk of atherosclerotic cardiovascular disease >7.5%

Although the recommendations are strong for people with those specific conditions, questions remain about the use of statins for primary prevention of cardiovascular disease in women because few longitudinal studies have included women and gender-related differences have not been adequately addressed (Cangemi, Romiti, Campolongo, et al., 2017). In addition, clear guidelines are lacking for statin therapy for in adults age 75 and older without a history of stroke or heart attack (Bibbins-Domingo & U. S. Preventive Services Task force, 2016; Chou, Dana, Blazina, et al., 2016). Current emphasis is on the importance of encouraging patients to discuss statin therapy with their primary care practitioners and engaging in a shared decision-making process (Navar, Stone, & Martin, 2016).

As with treatment of hypertension, nutrition and lifestyle interventions are first-line approaches, with medications (e.g., statins) as the next step if goals are not achieved with nonpharmacologic interventions. Essential nutrition and lifestyle interventions for lipid disorders include dietary modifications, maintenance of ideal body weight, and incorporation of regular exercise in one's daily routine. Nutritional interventions focus on dietary fat intake, with emphasis on higher intake of foods high in polyunsaturated and monounsaturated fats, and avoidance of foods high in saturated fats (Williams & Salter, 2016). Box 20-8 summarizes health education interventions for prevention and management of lipid disorders in older adults.

 See ONLINE LEARNING ACTIVITY 20-5: RESOURCES FOR INFORMATION ABOUT INTERVENTIONS FOR PREVENTION OF CARDIOVASCULAR DISEASE at http://thepoint.lww.com/Miller8e

Preventing and Managing Orthostatic or Postprandial Hypotension

Interventions aimed at preventing orthostatic and postprandial hypotension can be initiated as health measures for older adults who have any of the risk factors listed in Box 20-2. For older adults with symptomatic orthostatic hypotension, interventions to alleviate the problem are important for maintaining quality of life and preventing serious consequences. In addition, nurses address safety issues by implementing interventions that are directed toward preventing falls and fractures, as discussed in Chapter 22.

For older adults with postprandial hypotension, interventions can be implemented around mealtimes. In institutional or home care settings, registered dietitians may be helpful in developing a plan for addressing postprandial hypotension, but in any setting, nurses assume responsibility for health education about interventions. Some interventions that may be effective in reducing postprandial hypotension are low-carbohydrate meals, acarbose, green tea, and agents that delay gastric emptying (e.g., xylose and

---

 Box 20-8 Nutritional Interventions for People With High Cholesterol

Dietary Measures to Promote a Healthy Lipid Profile

- Include foods that are high in fiber content in your daily diet (e.g., whole grains).
- Include soy proteins in your daily diet (e.g., tofu, soy milk).
- Eat a minimum of 2 servings of fatty fish weekly.
- Limit total fat intake to less than 30% of your total daily calorie intake.
- Use nonfat or low-fat dairy desserts.

- Limit consumption of butter or margarine, but margarines that contain stanols are beneficial (e.g., Becanol).
- Use egg whites, omega-3 eggs, or egg substitutes.
- Limit consumption of lean meats to five or fewer 3- to 5-ounce servings per week. Trim fat off meats and the skin off poultry.
- Avoid eating processed meats (e.g., bacon, bologna, sausage, hot dogs).
- Avoid gravies, fried foods, and organ meats.

Guide to Types of Fats

Type of Fat	Sources	Examples	Effect on Lipid Profile
Saturated fatty acids	Animal fats and some vegetable oils (usually solid at room temperatures)	Meat, poultry, butter, and lauric and palm oils	Negative: increases LDL and total cholesterol levels
Trans fatty acids	Vegetable oils that are processed into margarine or shortening	Dairy products, baked goods, and snack foods	Negative: increases LDL cholesterol and lowers cholesterol levels
Monounsaturated fatty acids	Vegetable oils (usually liquid at room temperatures)	Olive, peanut, and canola oils	Positive: decreases LDL level
Polyunsaturated fatty acids	Seafood and vegetable oils (soft or liquid at room temperatures)	Corn, sunflower, safflower, canola, and linoleic oils	Positive: decreases LDL level
Omega-3 fatty acids	Fatty fish	Tuna, salmon, herring, and mackerel	Positive: decreases LDL cholesterol and triglyceride levels

Box 20-9 Education Regarding Orthostatic and Postprandial Hypotension

Preventing and Managing Orthostatic and Postprandial Hypotension

- Maintain adequate fluid intake (i.e., eight glasses of noncaffeinated beverages daily).
- Eat five or six smaller meals daily, rather than large meals.
- Avoid excessive alcohol consumption.
- Avoid sitting or standing still for prolonged periods, especially after meals.

Health Promotion Measures Specific to Orthostatic Hypotension

- Change your position slowly, especially when moving from a sitting or lying position to a standing position.
- Before standing up, sit at the side of the bed for several minutes after rising from a lying position.
- Maintain good physical fitness, especially good muscle tone, and engage in regular, but not excessive, exercise. (Swimming is an excellent form of exercise because the hydrostatic pressure prevents blood from pooling in the legs.)
- Wear a waist-high elastic support garment or thigh-high elastic stockings during the day, and put them on before getting out of bed in the morning.
- Sleep with the head of the bed elevated on blocks.
- During the day, rest in a recliner chair with your legs elevated.
- Take measures to prevent constipation and avoid straining during bowel movements.

- Avoid medications that increase the risk for orthostatic hypotension, particularly if additional risk factors are present (refer to Box 20-2).
- Avoid sources of intense heat (e.g., direct sun, electric blankets, and hot baths and showers) because these cause peripheral vasodilation.
- If taking nitroglycerin, do not take it while standing.

Health Promotion Measures Specific to Postprandial Hypotension

- Minimize the risk for postprandial hypotension by taking antihypertensive medications (if prescribed) 1 hour after meals rather than before meals.
- Eat small, low-carbohydrate meals.
- Avoid alcohol consumption.
- Avoid strenuous exercise, especially for 2 hours after meals.

Safety Precautions if Hypotension Cannot be Prevented

- Reduce the potential for falls and other negative functional consequences of postprandial hypotension by remaining seated (or by lying down) after meals.
- Call for assistance if help is needed with walking.
- Adapt the environment to minimize the risk and consequences of falling (e.g., ensure good lighting, install grab bars, keep pathways clear).

---

the natural food supplement guar gum). Additional interventions are summarized in Box 20-9, which can be used as a tool for educating older adults about orthostatic and postprandial hypotension.

Evaluating Effectiveness of Nursing Interventions

One measure of the effectiveness of health promotion interventions is the extent to which the older adult verbalizes correct information about the risks. Also, the older adult may verbalize intent to change or eliminate the lifestyle factors

that increase the risk of impaired cardiovascular function. For example, the older adult may agree to join an exercise program and follow dietary measures to reduce serum cholesterol levels. Effectiveness of interventions can also be measured by determining the actual reduction in risk factors. For example, the person's serum cholesterol level may decrease from 238 to 198 mg/dL after 6 months of regular exercise and dietary modifications. For older adults with impaired cardiovascular function, nurses evaluate the extent to which the signs and symptoms are alleviated and the extent to which older adults verbalize correct information about managing their condition.

Unfolding Case Study

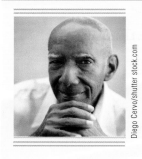

Diego Cervo/shutterstock.com

Part 3: Mr. C. at 74 Years of Age

Mr. C. is now 74 years old and continues to come to the senior wellness clinic for monthly blood pressure checks. He reports that his doctor recently started him on a medication for high cholesterol and told him to "watch my diet," but gave no further information or educational materials about what to do about his cholesterol.

NURSING ASSESSMENT

Mr. C. has no knowledge about the effects of various types of fat and cholesterol and triglyceride levels, and he is unaware that his diet, which he terms "soul food," increases the risk for cardiovascular disease. Although he says that he has heard a lot about "good and bad cholesterol" in the news, he does not know which foods are good or bad. He tries to buy foods that say "no cholesterol" on the label, but says that the labels are too confusing about the different kinds of fats.

Part 3: Mr. C. at 74 Years of Age (Continued)

NURSING DIAGNOSIS

Your nursing diagnosis is Ineffective Health Maintenance related to lack of regular exercise, dietary habits that contribute to hyperlipidemia, and insufficient information about lifestyle factors that increase the risk of cardiovascular disease. Evidence of these risk factors comes from Mr. C.'s inactivity, eating patterns, history of hypertension, and family history of cardiovascular disease. Also, Mr. C. has verbalized insufficient information about the relationship between exercise and cardiovascular function and about dietary measures to control cholesterol.

NURSING CARE PLAN FOR MR. C.

Expected Outcome	Nursing Interventions	Nursing Evaluation
Mr. C.'s knowledge of risk factors for cardiovascular impairment will increase	• Discuss the risk factors for impaired cardiovascular function, using information from Box 20-4 • Emphasize the risk factors that can be addressed through lifestyle modifications (e.g., exercise, weight loss, and dietary measures to control cholesterol levels)	• Mr. C. will be able to describe his risk factors for cardiovascular disease • Mr. C. will identify those risk factors that he can address through lifestyle changes
Mr. C.'s knowledge of the relationship between diet and serum cholesterol levels will increase	• Use teaching materials obtained from the American Heart Association to illustrate the relationship between diet and serum cholesterol levels. Provide a copy of these pamphlets for Mr. C. to take home • Suggest that Mr. C. discuss the information in the pamphlets with his wife and daughter • Ask Mr. C. to bring his wife to the nursing clinic next month so that you can talk with both of them about dietary measures to control cholesterol	• Mr. C. will accurately describe the relationship between food intake and cholesterol levels • Mr. C. will identify family eating habits that contribute to his elevated serum cholesterol level
Mr. C. will modify one dietary habit that contributes to his high cholesterol level	• Work with Mr. C. to make a list of the foods associated with high cholesterol levels (e.g., fried foods, ham hocks, lard, bacon, and eggs) • Give Mr. C. a copy of Box 20-8 and use it to discuss dietary measures to reduce cholesterol • Ask Mr. C. to select one change in dietary habits that will have a positive effect on his cholesterol level (e.g., switching from lard to vegetable oil for frying foods)	• Mr. C. will state that he is willing to change one eating habit that contributes to his high cholesterol level • Next month, Mr. C. will report that he has changed one eating pattern that contributes to high cholesterol levels
Mr. C. will increase his knowledge about the relationship between exercise and cardiovascular function	• Use pamphlets from the American Heart Association to teach about the effects of aerobic exercise on cardiovascular function • Review information about the relationship between exercise and weight	• Mr. C. will describe the beneficial effects of regular aerobic exercise
Mr. C. will begin exercising on a regular basis	• Discuss ways in which Mr. C. can incorporate regular exercise into his daily activities • Invite Mr. C. and his wife to participate in the daily Eldercise program that is offered following the noon meal at the senior center	• Mr. C. will verbalize a commitment to perform 30 minutes of exercise 3 days a week
Mr. C. will eliminate lifestyle factors that increase the risk for cardiovascular disease	• Ask Mr. C. to invite his wife to your monthly appointments so that she can also receive important health education • Identify a plan that will enable Mr. and Mrs. C. to gradually incorporate additional dietary measures aimed at reducing cholesterol into the family meal plans • Identify a plan that will enable Mr. and Mrs. C. to include 30 minutes of exercise five times a week • Discuss weight reduction with Mr. C. and emphasize that dietary modifications and regular exercise are interventions that should facilitate weight loss	• Mr. C.'s total cholesterol level will be 180 mg/dL or less at the end of 6 months • Mr. C. will report that he engages in 30 minutes of exercise five times weekly • Mr. C. will report that he follows the dietary measures presented in Box 20-8 • Mr. C.'s weight will decrease to between 180 and 198 lb, and he will maintain that weight

(continued)

Part 3: Mr. C. at 74 Years of Age (Continued)

THINKING POINTS

- What factors affect Mr. C.'s ability to manage his cardiovascular condition and address his risk factors, and how would you address these factors in your interventions?

- Explore some of the health education listed at the end of this chapter to find teaching tools that would be appropriate for Mr. C.

QSEN APPLICATION

QSEN Competency	Knowledge/Skill/Attitude	Application to Mr. C.
Patient-centered care	(K) Integrate understanding of multiple dimensions of patient-centered care	Help Mr. C. identify one lifestyle change he is willing to address to reduce his risk for cardiovascular disease
	(K) Describe strategies to empower patients in all aspects of the health care process	Talk with Mr. C. about participating with his wife in daily Elder class after they eat lunch at the senior center
	(K) Examine common barriers to active involvement in patients	Ask Mr. C. to invite his wife the next time he comes to the Senior Wellness Clinic, so she can be included in discussions about reducing his risk for cardiovascular disease
	(S) Elicit patient values, preferences, and expressed needs	
	(S) Provide patient-centered care with sensitivity and respect for diversity of the human experience	
Teamwork and collaboration	(K) Recognize contributions of other individuals and groups in helping patient achieve health goals	Use teaching materials from the American Heart Association and the National Institutes of Health, including materials designed specifically for African Americans
	(S) Integrate the contributions of others who play a role in helping patient achieve health goals	
Evidence-based practice	(S) Base individualized care plan on patient values, clinical expertise, and evidence	Use evidence-based information in Box 20-8 to teach about nutritional interventions for people with high cholesterol
	(A) Value evidence-based practice as integral to determining the best clinical practice	

Chapter Highlights

Age-Related Changes That Affect Cardiovascular Function

- Degenerative changes of myocardium and neuroconduction mechanisms
- Degenerative changes of the arteries and veins
- Altered baroreflex mechanisms

Risk Factors Affecting Cardiovascular Function (Box 20-1)

- Atherosclerosis involves pathologic changes of the arteries that begin in childhood and progress through adulthood and predispose older adults to cardiovascular diseases
- Physical inactivity
- Tobacco smoking and secondhand smoke
- Dietary habits
- Obesity (i.e., BMI 30 kg/m^2 or more)

- Hypertension
- Lipid disorders
- Metabolic syndrome
- Psychosocial factors
- Heredity and socioeconomic factors
- Risk for cardiovascular disease in women and minority groups

Functional Consequences Affecting Cardiovascular Wellness

- Effects on cardiac function
- Effects on pulse and blood pressure
- Effects on response to exercise
- Effects on circulation

Pathologic Conditions Affecting Cardiovascular Wellness

- Orthostatic hypotension
- Postprandial hypotension

Nursing Assessment of Cardiovascular Function (Boxes 20-2 to 20-5)

- Baseline cardiovascular function (heart rate, sounds, and rhythm)
- Blood pressure, including hypertension and orthostatic or postprandial hypotension
- Risks for cardiovascular disease, with emphasis on modifiable conditions
- Signs and symptoms of heart disease
- Knowledge about heart disease

Nursing Diagnosis

- Ineffective Health Maintenance
- Activity Intolerance
- Decreased Cardiac Output

Planning for Wellness Outcomes

- Health-Promoting Behaviors
- Risk Control: Cardiovascular Health
- Risk Control: Tobacco Use
- Cardiac Disease Self-Management

Nursing Interventions to Promote Healthy Cardiovascular Function (Figures 20-1 and 20-2, Boxes 20-6 to 20-9)

- Teaching about cardiovascular disease
- Addressing risks through nutritional interventions
- Addressing risks through lifestyle interventions (exercise, heart-healthy diet, optimal body weight, cessation of smoking if applicable)
- Secondary prevention programs for older adults who have cardiovascular disease
- Low-dose aspirin for primary prevention
- Preventing and managing hypertension
- Preventing and managing lipid disorders
- Prevention and management of orthostatic and postprandial hypotension

Evaluating Effectiveness of Nursing Interventions

- Verbalization of correct information about risks
- Reported participation in health promotion interventions (e.g., heart-healthy diet, regular exercise, weight reduction, and smoking cessation when applicable)
- Indicators of cardiovascular function within normal range (e.g., blood pressure, serum lipids)
- If applicable, alleviation of signs and symptoms of cardiovascular disease

Critical Thinking Exercises

1. Discuss how each of the following factors influences cardiovascular function, including orthostatic hypotension: lifestyle, medications, age-related changes, and pathologic conditions.

2. Describe the questions and considerations that you would include in an assessment of cardiovascular function in an older adult who has no complaints of heart problems, but who has a history of falling twice in the past month and who has not been evaluated by a primary care provider in the past year.

3. You are asked to give a health education talk entitled "Keeping Your Heart Healthy" at a senior center. What information would you include in the presentation? What local resources (i.e., specific contact information for agencies or organizations in your area) would you suggest your audience contact for further information? What audiovisual aids would you use? How would you involve the participants in the discussion?

4. You are working in an assisted living facility in which several of the residents have orthostatic hypotension. What would you include in your health education regarding management of orthostatic hypotension?

 For more information about the topics discussed in this chapter, be sure to check out the interactive Online Learning Activities and other helpful resources at http://thepoint.lww.com/Miller8e

REFERENCES

Allgulander, C. (2016). Anxiety as a risk factor in cardiovascular disease. *Current Opinion in Psychiatry, 29*, 13–17.

American Heart Association. (2016). American Heart Association recommendations for physical activity in adults. Available at www.americanheart.org

Avvenuti, G., Baladini, I., & Giardini, A. (2016). Optimism's explicative role for chronic diseases. *Frontiers in Psychology, 7*, Article 295. doi: 10.3389/fpsyg.2016.00295.

Banegas, J. R., Ruilope L. M., de la Sierra, A., et al. (2017). Clinic versus daytime ambulatory blood pressure difference in hypertensive patients: The impact of age and clinic blood pressure. *Hypertension, 69*, 211–219.

Bangalore, S., Toklu, B., Gianos, E., et al. (2017). Optimal systolic blood pressure target after SPRINT insights from a network meta-analysis of randomized trials. *American Journal of Medicine, 130*, 707–719.

Barengo, N. C., Antikainen, R., Borodulin, K., et al. (2017). Leisure-time physical activity reduces total and cardiovascular mortality and cardiovascular disease incidence in older adults. *Journal of the American Geriatrics Society, 65*, 504–510.

Barrows, J. L., & Fleury, J. (2016). Systematic review of yoga interventions to promote cardiovascular health in older adults. *Western Journal of Nursing Research, 38*, 753–781.

Batelaan, N. M., Seldenrijk, A., Bot, M., et al. (2016). Anxiety and new onset of cardiovascular disease: Critical review and meta-analysis. *British Journal of Psychiatry, 208*, 223–231.

Biaggioni, I. (2017). The pharmacology of autonomic failure: From hypotension to hypertension. *Pharmacology Review, 69*, 53–62.

Bibbins-Domingo, K., & U. S. Preventive Services Task Force. (2016). Aspirin use for the primary prevention of cardiovascular disease and colorectal cancer: U.S. Preventive Services Task Force Recommendation Statement. *Annals of Internal Medicine, 164*, 836–845.

Brewster, L., van Montfrans, G., Oehlers, G., et al. (2016). Systematic review: Antihypertensive drug therapy in patients of African and South Asian ethnicity. *Internal and Emergency Medicine, 11*, 355–374.

Bouaziz, W., Vogel, T., Schmitt, E., et al. (2017). Health benefits of aerobic training programs in adults aged 70 and over: A systematic review. *Archives of Gerontology and Geriatrics, 69,* 110–127.

Campkin, L., Boyd, J., & Campbell, D. (2016). Coronary artery disease patient perspectives on exercise participation. *Journal of Cardiopulmonary Rehabilitation and Prevention,* doi: 10.1097/HCR.0000000000000195.

Cangemi, R., Romiti, G. F., Campolongo, G., et al. (2017). Gender related differences in treatment and response to statins in primary and secondary cardiovascular prevention: The never-ending debate. *Pharmacology Research, 117,* 148–155.

Carney, R. M., & Freedland, K. E. (2017). Depression and coronary heart disease. *Nature Reviews: Cardiology, 14,* 145–155.

Carter, S., Hartman, Y., Holder, S., et al. (2017). Sedentary behavior and cardiovascular disease risk: Mediating mechanisms. *Exercise and Sport Science Reviews, 45,* 80–86.

Centi, J., Freeman, R., Gibbons, C. H., et al. (2017). Effects of orthostatic hypotension on cognition in Parkinson disease. *Neurology, 88,* 17–24.

Chalvon-Demersay, T., Azzoul-Mamiche, D., Arfsten, J., et al. (2017). A systematic review of the effects of plant compared with animal protein sources on features of metabolic syndrome. *Journal of Nutrition, 147,* 281–292.

Chauvet-Gelinieer, J. C., & Bonin, B. (2017). Stress, anxiety and depression in heart disease patients: A major challenge for cardiac rehabilitation. *Annals of Physical and Rehabilitation Medicine, 60,* 6–12.

Cheung, Y. K., Moon, Y. P., Kulick, E. R., et al. (2017). Leisure-time physical activity and cardiovascular mortality in an elderly population in Northern Manhattan: A prospective cohort study. *Journal of General Internal Medicine, 32,* 168–174.

Chien, D. K., Huang, M. Y., Huang, C. H., et al. (2016). Do elderly females have a higher risk of acute myocardial infarction? A retrospective analysis of 329 cases at an emergency department. *Taiwan Journal of Obstetrics and Gynecology, 55,* 563–567.

Chisholm, P., & Anpalahan, M. (2017). Orthostatic hypotension – pathophysiology, assessment, treatment, and the paradox of supine hypertension – a review. *Internal Medicine Journal, 47,* 370–379.

Chou, R., Dana, T., Blazina, I., et al. (2016). Statins for prevention of cardiovascular disease in adults evidence report and systematic review for the U. S. Preventive Services Task Force. *Journal of the American Medical Association, 316,* 2008–2024.

Chu, P., Pandya, A., Salomon, J. A., et al. (2016). Comparative effectiveness of personalized lifestyle management strategies for cardiovascular disease risk reduction. *Journal of the American Heart Association,* [Epub] 2016 Mar 195. doi: 10.1161.JAHA.115.002737.

Cole, A. R., Wijarnpreecha, K., Chattipakorn, S. C., et al. (2016). Effects of Tai Chi exercise on heart rate variability. *Complementary Therapies in Clinical Practice, 23,* 59–63.

Cramer, H. (2016). The efficacy and safety of yoga in managing hypertension. *Experimental and Clinical Endocrinology & Diabetes, 124,* 65–70.

DeVon, H., Burke, L., Vuckovic, K., et al. (2017). Symptoms suggestive of acute coronary syndrome: When is sex important? *Journal of Cardiovascular Nursing, 32,* 383–392.

DeVon, H., Vuckovic, K., Ryan, C., et al. (2017). Systematic review of symptom clusters in cardiovascular disease. *European Journal of Cardiovascular Nursing, 16,* 6–17.

DiPilla, M., Bruno, R. M., Taddei, S., et al. (2016). Gender differences in the relationships between psychosocial factors and hypertension. *Maturitas, 93,* 58–64.

Doering, L., McGuire, A., Eastwood, J., et al. (2016). Cognitive behavioral therapy for depression improves pain and perceived control in cardiac surgery patients. *European Journal of Cardiovascular Nursing, 15,* 417–424.

Dragsbaek, K., Neergaard, J., Laursen, J., et al. (2016). Metabolic syndrome and subsequent risk of type 2 diabetes and cardiovascular disease in elderly women: Challenging the current definition. *Medicine, 95,* 36(e4806).

Edwards, M. K., & Loprinzi, P. D. (2017). Combined associations of sedentary behavior and cardiorespiratory fitness of cognitive function among older adults. *International Journal of Cardiology, 229,* 71–74.

Efferth, T., Banerjee, M., & Paul, N. (2017). Broken heart, tako-tsubo or stress cardiomyopathy: Metaphors, meanings and their impact. *International Journal of Cardiology, 230,* 262–268.

Egan, B., Li, J., White, K., et al. (2016). 2013 ACC/AHA cholesterol guideline and implications for healthy people 2020 cardiovascular disease prevention goals. *Journal of the American Heart Association, 5*(e003558). doi: 10.1161/JAHA.116.003558.

Ford, C. D., Sims, M., Higginbotham, J. C., et al. (2016). Psychosocial factors are associated with blood pressure progression among African Americans in the Jackson Heart Study. *American Journal of Hypertension, 29,* 913–924.

Gibbons, C. H., Schmidt, P., Biaggioni, I., et al. (2017). The recommendations of a consensus panel for the screening, diagnosis, and treatment of neurogenic orthostatic hypotension and associated supine hypertension. *Journal of Neurology,* [Epub]. 2017 Jan 3. doi: 10.1007/s00415-016-8375-x.

Gill, P., Haque, M. S., Martin, U., et al. (2017). Measurement of blood pressure for the diagnosis and management of hypertension in different ethnic groups: One size fits all. *BioMed Central Cardiovascular Disorders, 15*(1), 55.

Goldstein, F., Hajjar, I., Dunn, C., et al. (2017). The relationship between cognitive functioning and the JNC-8 guidelines for hypertension in older adults. *Journals of Gerontology: Medical Sciences, 72,* 121–126.

Gorelik, O., Feldman, L., & Cohen, N. (2016). Heart failure and orthostatic hypotension. *Heart Failure Reviews, 21,* 529–538.

Gray-Miceli, D., Ratcliffe, S., Thomasson, A., et al. (2016). Clinical risk factors for orthostatic hypotension: Results among elderly fallers in long-term care. *Journal of Patient Safety,* doi: 10.1097/PTS.0000000000000274.

Grezzana, G. B., Moraes, D. W., Stein, A. T., et al. (2017). Impact of different normality thresholds for 24-hour ABPM at the primary health care level. *Arquivos brasileiros de cardiologia, 108,* 143–148.

Gu, A., Yue, Y., Desai, R. P., et al. (2017). Racial and ethnic differences in antihypertensive medication use and blood pressure control among U. S. adults with hypertension: The National Health and Nutrition examination Survery, 2003 to 2012. *Circulation: Cardiovascular Quality Outcomes,* 2017 Jan. doi: 10.1161/CIRCOUTCOMES.116.003166.

Hajduk, A., & Chaudhry, S. (2016). Sedentary behavior and cardiovascular risk in older adults: A scoping review. *Current Cardiovascular Risk Report,* [Epub] 2016 January. doi: 10.1007/s12170-016-0485-6.

Herdman, T., & Kamitsura, S. (Eds). (2018). *NANDA International Nursing Diagnoses Definitions and Classification, 2018–2020* (11th ed., pp. 34–44). New York: Thieme Publishers.

Himmelfarb, C., Hayman, L., & Worel, J. (2016). How low can we go? Implications of the systolic blood pressure intervention trial for hypertension management. *Journal of Cardiovascular Nursing, 31,* 99–100.

Kim, E. S., Hagan, K. A., Grodstein, F., et al. (2017). Optimism and cause-specific mortality: A prospective cohort study. *American Journal of Epidemiology, 185,* 21–29.

Kuehn, B. M. (2017). Emerging data support benefits of yoga for patients with heart disease. *Circulation, 135,* 398–399.

Liberman, K., Forti, L., Beyer, I., et al. (2017). The effects of exercise on muscle strength, body composition, physical functioning and the inflammatory profile of older adults: A systematic review. *Current Opinion in Clinical Nutrition and Metabolic Care, 20,* 30–53.

Lin, X., Zhang, I., Li, A., et al. (2016). Cocoa flavanol intake and biomarkers for cardiometabolic health: A systematic review and meta-analysis of randomized controlled trials. *Journal of Nutrition, 146,* 2325–2333.

Liu, N., Pan, X. F., Yu, C., et al. (2016). Association of major depression with risk of ischemic heart disease in a mega-cohort of Chinese adults: The China Kadoorie Biobank Study. *Journal of the American Heart Association, 5,* 2016 Dec 21. doi: 10.1161/JAHA.116.004687.

Loffredo, L., Perri, L., Nocella, C., et al. (2017). Antioxidant and antiplatelet activity by polyphenol-rich nutrients: Focus on extra virgin olive oil and cocoa. *British Journal of Clinical Pharmacology, 83*, 96–102.

Lotrionte, M., Biasucci, L. M., Peruzzi, M., et al. (2016). Which aspirin dose and preparation is best for the long-term prevention of cardiovascular disease and cancer? Evidence from a systematic review and network meta-analysis. *Progress in Cardiovascular Disease, 58*, 495–504.

Lovegrove, J. A., Stainer, A., & Hobbs, D. A. (2017). Role of flavonoids and nitrates in cardiovascular health. *Proceedings of the Nutrition Society,* 2017 Jan 19. doi: 10.1017/S0029665116002871.

Manfrini, O., Ricci, B., Cenko, E., et al. (2016). Association between comorbidities and absence of chest pain in acute coronary syndrome with in-hospital outcome. *International Journal of Cardiology, 217*(Suppl), S37–S43.

Menne, H. L., Borato, L., Shelton, E., et al. (2016). Promoting heart health behavior change in a vulnerable older adult population. *Healthy Aging Research, 5*, 11.

Merola, A., Romagnolo, A., Rosso, M., et al. (2016). Orthostatic hypotension in Parkinson's disease: Does it matter if asymptomatic? *Parkinsonism and Related Disorders, 33*, 65–71.

Miller, P. E., & Martin, S. S. (2016). Approach to statin use in 2016: An update. *Current Atherosclerosis Report, 18*, doi: 10.1007/s11883-016-0578-1.

Mozaffarian, D., Benjamin, E., Go, A., et al. (2016). Heart disease and stroke statistics: 2016 update: A report from the American Heart Association. *Circulation, 133*, 447–454.

Nair, S., Visvanathan, R., & Piscitelli, D. (2016). Effects of postprandial blood pressure on gait parameters in older people. *Nutrients, 8*, doi: 10.3390/nu8040219.

National Heart, Lung, and Blood Institute. (2017). Aspirin to prevent first heart attack or stroke. Available at www.nhlbi.gov

Navar, A. M., Stone, N. J., & Martin, S. S. (2016). What to say and how to say it: Effective communication for cardiovascular disease prevention. *Current Opinion in Cardiology, 31*, 537–544.

O'Donovan, G., Hamer, M., & Stamatakis, E. (2017). Relationships between exercise, smoking habit and mortality in more than 100,000 adults. *International Journal of Cancer, 140*, 1819–1827.

Pigini, L., Bovi, G., Panzarino, C., et al. (2017). Pilot test of a new personal health system integrating environmental and wearable sensors for telemonitoring and care of elderly people at home (SMARTA Project). *Gerontology, 63*, 281–286.

Qaseem, A., Wilt, T., Rich, R., et al. (2017). Pharmacologic treatment of hypertension in adults aged 60 years or older to higher versus lower blood pressure targets: A clinical practice guideline from the American College of Physicians and the American Academy of Family Physicians. *Annals of Internal Medicine, 166*, 430–437.

Radovanovic, D., Pilgrim, T., Seifert, B., et al. (2017). Type 2 myocardial infarction: Incidence, presentation, treatment and outcome in routine clinical practice. *Journal of Cardiovascular Medicine, 18*, 341–347.

Rayner, B., & Spence, J. D. (2017). Hypertension in blacks: Insights from Africa. *Journal of Hypertension, 35*, 234–239.

Robinson, J. G. (2016). The future of lipid guidelines. *Current Opinion in Lipidology, 27*, 585–591.

Schopfer, D. W., & Forman, D. E. (2016). Cardiac rehabilitation in older adults. *Canadian Journal of Cardiology, 32*, 1088–1096.

Shi, L., Zhang, D., Wang, L., et al. (2017). Meditation and blood pressure: A meta-analysis of randomized clinical trials. *Journal of Hypertension, 35*, 696–706.

Sin, N. L. (2016). The protective role of positive well-being in cardiovascular disease: Review of current evidence, mechanisms, and clinical implications. *Current Cardiology Reports, 18*, 196.

Siu, A., & The U. S. Preventive Services Task Force. (2015). Screening for high blood pressure in adults: U. S. Preventive Services Task Force Recommendation Statement. *Annals of Internal Medicine, 163*, 778–786.

Smeijers, L., Mostofsky, E., Tofler, G. H., et al. (2017). Anxiety and anger immediately prior to myocardial infarction and long-term mortality: Characteristics of high-risk patients. *Journal of Psychosomatic Research, 93*, 19–27.

Smyth, A., O'Donnell, M., Lamelas, P., et al. (2016). Physical activity and anger or emotional upset as triggers of acute myocardial infarction; The INTERHEART Study. *Circulation, 134*, 1059–1067.

Soares-Miranda, L., Siscovick, D., Psaty, B., et al. (2016). Physical activity and risk of coronary heart disease and stroke in older adults. *Circulation, 133*, 147–155.

Soenen, S., Rayner, C. K., Jones, K. L., et al. (2016). The aging gastrointestinal tract. *Current Opinion in Clinical Nutrition and Metabolic Care, 19*, 12–18.

Staessen, J. A., Li, Y., Hara, A., et al. (2017). Blood pressure measurement anno 2016. *American Journal of Hypertension, 30*, 453–463.

Supiano, M. A., & Williamson, J. D. (2017). Applying the systolic blood pressure intervention trial results to older adults. *Journal of the American Geriatrics Society, 65*, 16–21.

Tambalis, K. D., Panagiotakos, D. B., Georgousopoulou, E. N., et al. (2016). Impact of physical activity category on incidence of cardiovascular disease: Results from the 10-year follow-up of the ATTICA Study (2002-2012). *Preventive Medicine, 93*, 27–32.

Tully, P. J., Harrison, N. J., Cheung, P., et al. (2016). Anxiety and cardiovascular disease: A review. *Current Cardiology Reports, 18*, 120.

Tune, J. D., Goodwill, A. G., Sassoon, D. J., et al. (2017). Cardiovascular consequences of metabolic syndrome. *Translational Research, 183*, 57–70.

Tzourio, C., Hanon, O., Godin, O., et al. (2017). Impact of home blood pressure monitoring on blood pressure control in older individuals: A French randomized study. *Journal of Hypertension, 35*, 612–620.

Umehara, T., Nakahara, A., Matsuno, H., et al. (2016). Predictors of postprandial hypotenstion in elderly patients with de novo Parkinson's disease. *Journal of Neural Transmission, 123*, 1331–1339.

U. S. Preventive Services Task Force. (2016). Statin use for the primary prevention of cardiovascular disease in adults: U. S. Preventive Services Task Force Recommendation Statement. *Journal of the American Medical Association, 316*, 1997–2007.

Ushakov, A. V., Ivanchenko, V. S., & Gagarina, A. A. (2016). Psychological stress in pathogenesis of essential hypertension. *Current Hypertension Review, 12*, 203–214.

Valtorta, N. K., Kanaan, M., Gilbody, S., et al. (2016). Loneliness and social isolation as risk factors for coronary heart disease and stroke: Systematic review and meta-analysis of longitudinal observational studies. *Heart, 102*, 1009–1016.

Virani, S. (2016). The 2013 ACC/AHA cholesterol management guideline: Clearing the confusion from noncontroversial components. *Texas Heart Institute Journal, 43*, 313–314.

Wahlstrom, M., Rydell-Karlsson, M., Medin, J., et al. (2017). Effects of yoga in patients with paroxysmal atrial fibrillation—a randomized controlled study. *European Journal of Cardiovascular Nursing, 16*, 57–63.

Ward, B., Clarke, T., Nugent, C., et al. (2016). *Early release of selected estimates based on data from the 2015 National Health Interview Survey.* Washington, DC: National Center for Health Statistics, Centers for Disease Control and Prevention.

Williams, C., & Salter, A. (2016). Saturated fatty acids and coronary heart disease risk: The debate goes on. *Current Opinion in Clinical Nutrition and Metabolic Care, 19*, 97–102.

Yannoutsos, A., Kheder-Elfekih, R., Halimi, J. M., et al. (2017). Should blood pressure goal be individualized in hypertensive patients? *Pharmacology Research, 118*, 53–63.

Zhang, L., Sobolev, M., Piña, I., et al. (2017). Predictors of cardiac rehabilitation initiation and adherence in a multiracial urban population. *Journal of Cardiopulmonary rehabilitation and Prevention, 37*, 30–38.

chapter 21

Respiratory Function

The primary functions of respiration are to supply oxygen to and remove carbon dioxide from the blood. Adequate respiratory performance is essential to life because all body organs and tissues need oxygen. Healthy, nonsmoking, older adults are able to compensate for age-related changes, but risk factors, such as smoking, anesthesia, and acute or chronic diseases, can impair respiratory function in significant ways.

 AGE-RELATED CHANGES THAT AFFECT RESPIRATORY FUNCTION

As with other physiologic functions, it is difficult to distinguish the effects of age-related changes from those caused by disease processes and external influences, such as environmental factors. Although these influences occur throughout the life span, their cumulative effects become more pronounced in older adults, especially when combined with risk factors. Age-related changes of the respiratory system are summarized in this section and effects of these changes are discussed in the section on Functional Consequences.

Upper Respiratory Structures

The nose and other upper respiratory structures are affected by age-related changes that can affect comfort and function in the following ways:

- Degenerative changes in connective tissue causing the nose to have a retracted columella (the lower edge of the septum) and a poorly supported, downwardly rotated tip
- Diminished blood flow to the nose, causing the nasal turbinates to become smaller
- Thicker mucus in nasopharynx due to degenerative changes in submucosal glands
- Stiffening of trachea due to calcification of cartilage
- Blunted cough and laryngeal reflexes
- Atrophy of the laryngeal nerve endings

Chest Wall and Musculoskeletal Structures

The rib cage and the vertebral musculoskeletal structures are affected by the same kind of age-related changes that affect other musculoskeletal tissue: the ribs and vertebrae become osteoporotic, the costal cartilage calcifies, and the respiratory muscles weaken. Because of these age-related processes, the following structural changes occur: **kyphosis** (i.e., an increased curvature of the spine), shortened thorax,

Promoting Respiratory Wellness in Older Adults

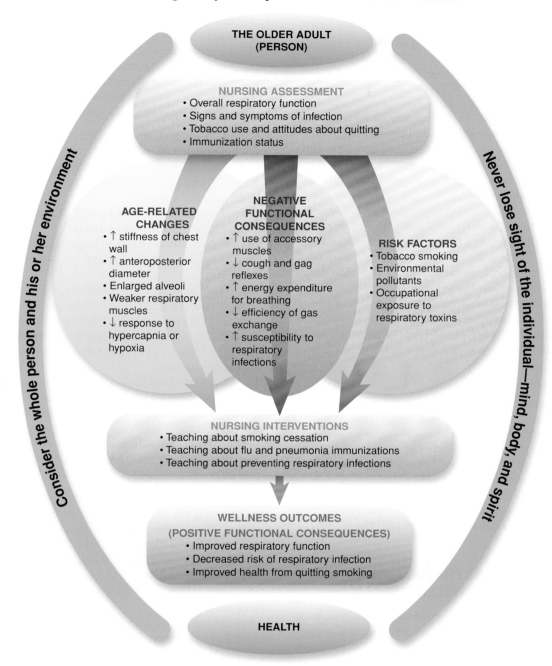

THE OLDER ADULT (PERSON)

NURSING ASSESSMENT
• Overall respiratory function
• Signs and symptoms of infection
• Tobacco use and attitudes about quitting
• Immunization status

AGE-RELATED CHANGES
• ↑ stiffness of chest wall
• ↑ anteroposterior diameter
• Enlarged alveoli
• Weaker respiratory muscles
• ↓ response to hypercapnia or hypoxia

NEGATIVE FUNCTIONAL CONSEQUENCES
• ↑ use of accessory muscles
• ↓ cough and gag reflexes
• ↑ energy expenditure for breathing
• ↓ efficiency of gas exchange
• ↑ susceptibility to respiratory infections

RISK FACTORS
• Tobacco smoking
• Environmental pollutants
• Occupational exposure to respiratory toxins

NURSING INTERVENTIONS
• Teaching about smoking cessation
• Teaching about flu and pneumonia immunizations
• Teaching about preventing respiratory infections

WELLNESS OUTCOMES
(POSITIVE FUNCTIONAL CONSEQUENCES)
• Improved respiratory function
• Decreased risk of respiratory infection
• Improved health from quitting smoking

HEALTH

Consider the whole person and his or her environment

Never lose sight of the individual—mind, body, and spirit

chest wall stiffness, and increased anteroposterior diameter of the chest. Overall, these age-related changes compromise chest wall expansion, and older adults need to expend more energy to achieve respiratory efficiency.

Lung Structure and Function

Even in healthy older adults, lungs become smaller and flabbier, and age-related changes affect the lung parenchyma, which is the part of the respiratory system where gas exchange takes place. Changes that have the most effect on respiratory function are as follows:

• **Ductectasia** (i.e., the alveoli enlarge and their walls become thinner) begins around the age of 20 or 30 years and continues throughout adulthood, resulting in a gradual increase in the amount of anatomic dead space.
• The pulmonary artery becomes wider, thicker, and less elastic.
• The number of capillaries diminishes.

- The pulmonary capillary blood volume decreases.
- The mucosal bed, where diffusion occurs, thickens.

Elastic recoil is the characteristic that keeps the airway open during inspiration by resisting expansion and maintaining a positive pressure across the lung surface. If the airways close prematurely, air is trapped and the lungs cannot expire to their maximum capacity. A combination of age-related changes in the parenchyma and elastic fibers interferes with elastic recoil, which results in early airway closure. Because of this and other age-related changes, gas exchange is compromised in the lower lung regions and inspired air is preferentially distributed in the upper regions. Effects of these changes include decreased arterial oxygen pressure (PaO_2) and changes in airflow rates.

Compensatory changes in respiratory rate are made under conditions of hypercapnia or hypoxia. The response to hypercapnia is initiated by a central chemoreceptor, located in the medulla, whereas the response to hypoxia is initiated by peripheral chemoreceptors, located in the carotid and aortic bodies. Age-related changes reduce the ventilatory response to both hypoxia and hypercapnia, so instead of—or in addition to—experiencing breathlessness or other respiratory symptoms when blood gases are abnormal, older adults are likely to develop mental changes.

Changes in Immune Function

Age-related alterations in the immune system affect respiratory function, even in healthy older adults. For example, diminished immune function leads to an increased susceptibility to pneumonia and other respiratory infections (Brandenberger & Muhlfeld, 2016; Goncalves, Mitchell, & Lord, 2016). In addition, age-related alterations of T cells (i.e., a component of the immune system) are associated with diminished effectiveness of influenza vaccines in older adults (McEldaney, Kuchel, Zhou, et al., 2016).

 ### RISK FACTORS THAT AFFECT RESPIRATORY WELLNESS

For people of any age, tobacco smoking is the single most important risk factor for lung disease and impaired respiratory function. The risks and consequences are both immediate and cumulative. Other risks are mentioned because, particularly for nonsmokers, they can be addressed through health promotion interventions to improve respiratory function. For smokers, however, it is imperative to focus attention on the serious negative consequences of smoking.

Tobacco Use

Tobacco smoking causes detrimental effects through multiple heat and chemical actions on the respiratory system. Harmful physiologic effects on the respiratory system include bronchoconstriction, impaired air flow, inflammation of the mucosa throughout the respiratory tract, and inhibited ciliary action, leading to increased coughing and mucous secretions and diminished protection from harmful organisms. The most serious consequence of smoking is a significantly increased risk of developing cancer, and diseases of the lungs, cardiovascular system, and many other systems. Thus, smoking-related diseases are considered the world's most preventable cause of death. The American Cancer Society (2016a) has cited evidence-based examples of the serious risks and detrimental effects as follows:

- Half of all smokers who continue to smoke will die from smoking-related disease.
- In the United States, tobacco use is responsible for nearly 20% of deaths overall, 30% of all cancer deaths, and 80% of lung cancer deaths.
- Men and women who smoke will shorten their lives by about 12 and 11 years, respectively.
- About two out of three people diagnosed with lung cancer are 65 or older, with the average age at time of diagnosis being 70 years.
- Smoking increases the risk for developing all the following types of cancers: oral cavity, larynx, pharynx, esophagus, lung, liver, kidney, urinary bladder, stomach, pancreas, colon/rectum, uterine cervix, and myeloid leukemia. There is limited evidence of the link between smoking and breast cancer in women.
- Smoking is directly linked to increased risk for COPD, cardiovascular disease, and cerebrovascular disease.
- Smoking is associated with increased risk for all the following conditions: gum disease, tooth loss, delayed wound healing, premature skin aging, cataracts, diabetes, osteoporosis, macular degeneration, peptic ulcers, and rheumatoid arthritis.

Moreover, smoking is associated not only with an increased risk for cancer but also with poorer prognosis and shorter life expectancy after cancer diagnosis (Inoue-Choi, Liao, Reyes-Guzman, et al., 2017; Ordonez-Mena, Schottker, Mons, et al., 2016). Researchers also are identifying links between smoking and impaired cognitive functioning (Campos, Serebrisky, & Castaldelli-Maia, 2016; Toda & Okamura, 2016).

Even though pipes, cigars, and **smokeless tobacco** products (e.g., e-cigarettes, chewing tobacco, nicotine gum) are sometimes viewed as safer than cigarettes, all forms and doses of tobacco are associated with serious health consequences, which are similar to those of cigarette smoking (American Cancer Society, 2016b; O'Malley, 2017). Studies link smokeless tobacco to all the following serious consequences: oral cancer (Awan & Patil, 2016); risk of fatal and nonfatal stroke and ischemic heart disease (Benowitz & Burbank, 2016; Vidyasagaran, Siddiqui, & Kanaan, 2016); and cancers of the mouth, pancreas, pharynx, and esophagus (Sinha, Abdulkader, & Gupta, 2016). As emphasized by the American Cancer Association, "There is no safe way to use tobacco" (American Cancer Society, 2016b). Despite concerns about adverse effects of smokeless tobacco, the use of e-cigarettes as a method of quitting smoking is viewed as "the lesser of 2 harms" (Malais, van der Tempel, Minichiello, et al., 2016; Salloum, Getz, Tan, et al., 2016).

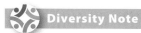

Diversity Note

Prevalence of cigarette smoking among adults in the United States by race/ethnicity in 2014 from highest to lowest: American Indian/ Alaska Natives (29.2%), non-Hispanic whites (18.2%), non-Hispanic blacks (17.5%), Hispanics (11.2%), and Asians (9.5%) (Centers for Disease Control and Prevention, 2016a).

Another potentially detrimental health effect related to smoking that has implications for care of older adults is the potential for altering the effects of medications. Interactions can occur in people who smoke or use nicotine products (including smokeless tobacco) and in people who have recently quit smoking. Interactions can be due directly to the physiologic effects of nicotine or they may be caused by the hydrocarbons in tobacco smoke, which can affect hepatic metabolism of some medications. Additional information and examples of drug–nicotine interactions are discussed in Chapter 8.

Wellness Opportunity

Be aware of opportunities to teach older adults about potential interactions between medications and nicotine products, which are often overlooked.

See ONLINE LEARNING ACTIVITY 21-1: HEALTH DISPARITIES at http://thepoint.lww.com/Miller8e.

Secondhand Smoke and Other Environmental Factors

Secondhand smoke (also called passive smoke or environmental tobacco smoke) is a mixture of smoke that comes from lit tobacco products and smoke that is exhaled by the smoker. Although negative effects of secondhand smoke were viewed with skepticism when they were first reported in the 1964 Surgeon General's Report, increasing evidence indicates that there is no safe level of exposure to secondhand smoke. Secondhand smoke contains more than 7000 chemicals, including about 70 known carcinogens (Centers for Disease Control and Prevention, 2016b). Immediate effects of secondhand smoke include coughing, wheezing, chest tightness, and reduced lung function (Bucheli, Manshad, Ehrhart, et al., 2016; McCormick-Ricket, Canterbury, Ghaffar, et al., 2016). Studies indicate that secondhand smoke is associated with increased risk for all of the following serious conditions:

- Lung cancer
- Cardiovascular disease (e.g., coronary heart disease)

- Stroke
- Atrial fibrillation
- Respiratory illness

(Bastion, Gray, DeRycke, et al., 2016; Centers for Disease Control and Prevention, 2016b; Dixit, Pletcher, Vittinghoff, et al., 2016; Lee, Hong, Lee, et al., 2016; Yang, Wang, Huang, et al., 2016).

Another environmental risk factor that can lead to negative functional consequences is the inhalation of air pollutants. Like the effects of cigarette smoking, the effects of air pollution are cumulative over many years and, therefore, have an increased impact on older adults who have been exposed to air pollutants for as many as eight or nine decades. Occupational exposure to toxic substances is another risk associated with long-term and cumulative consequences. For example, older adults who worked in occupations such as mining and firefighting would not have been protected by regulations that have been enforced under the Occupational Safety and Health Act beginning in the 1970s. In addition, much of the information now available on the harmful effects of certain chemicals was not widely available when these older adults were working. Even though the exposure to harmful substances may have occurred long ago, the signs and symptoms may not manifest until later adulthood. Box 21-1 lists some job categories that are associated with an increased risk for developing respiratory disease.

Additional Risk Factors

Older adults are likely to have additional risks associated with conditions (e.g., obesity or chronic illness) that interfere with their usual ability to obtain adequate physical activity, which is necessary to maintain optimal respiratory function. In addition, even brief periods of bed rest during acute illnesses can increase the risk for developing pneumonia or exacerbate the effects of chronic lung conditions. Kyphosis is associated with compromised pulmonary function and shallow breathing patterns, even in otherwise healthy older

 Box 21-1 Workforces With an Increased Risk for Harmful Respiratory Effects

Firefighters
Miners
Traffic controllers
Shipyard workers
Rubber workers
Aluminum workers
Iron and steel foundry workers
Tunnel and street repair workers
Asbestos workers
Quarry workers
Farmers, agricultural workers, grain handlers
Construction workers
Paper mill workers
Workers exposed to the following: dust, fumes, gases, nickel, arsenic, beryllium, chromium, or radiation

adults (Lorbergs, O'Connor, Zhou, et al., 2017). Lack of vaccinations increases the risk for pneumonia and influenza, as discussed in the section on Preventing Lower Respiratory Infections.

Medications increase the risk for impaired respiratory function in several ways. For example, sedatives and anticholinergic medications can affect upper airway function by drying the mucus. Medications may also influence cough reflexes or cause a persistent dry cough (e.g., angiotensin-converting enzyme inhibitors).

Wellness Opportunity

Recognize the importance of encouraging and assisting patients who are in bed to change position, sit in a chair, and walk as an essential intervention for promoting good respiratory function.

 ## FUNCTIONAL CONSEQUENCES AFFECTING RESPIRATORY WELLNESS

Because of age-related changes, even healthy nonsmoking older adults experience diminished respiratory efficiency and reduced total pulmonary function, as measured with spirometry (Vaz Fragoso, McAvay, Van Ness, et al., 2016). Although this functional consequence is hardly noticeable when older adults are performing their usual activities, under conditions of physiologic stress they are likely to experience dyspnea and fatigue because their respiratory system is less efficient. Degenerative changes of the upper airway structures cause additional minor functional consequences, as delineated in Table 21-1. In summary, healthy older adults expend more energy to achieve the same respiratory efficiency as younger adults, but the overall effects on healthy nonsmoking older people are minimal. Older adults who smoke or have other risk factors experience the same negative consequences as younger adults, but the effects are cumulative and the consequences are more serious.

TABLE 21-1 Functional Consequences of Age-Related Changes Affecting Respiratory Function

Change	Consequence
Degenerative changes affecting nose and upper airway structures	Snoring, mouth breathing, decreased efficiency of cough and gag reflexes, perception of nasal stuffiness
Increased anteroposterior diameter, chest wall stiffness, weakened muscles, and diaphragm	Increased use of accessory muscles, increased energy expended for respiratory efficiency
Enlargement of alveoli, thinning of alveolar walls, diminished number of capillaries	Diminished efficiency of gas exchange, decreased arterial oxygen pressure (PaO_2)
Decreased elastic recoil and early airway closure	Changes in lung volumes, slight decrease in overall efficiency

Increased Susceptibility to Lower Respiratory Infections

Even for healthy nonsmoking older adults, the most important functional consequence related to respiratory wellness is due to a combination of all of the following:

- Age-related changes in the respiratory tract
- Diminished physiologic reserve
- Decreased immune function
- Cumulative effects of exposure to pollution
- The immune system

Because of these age-related risk factors, older adults have higher rates of illness and death due to lower respiratory infections, including influenza and several types of pneumonia. Additional factors that further compromise the ability of some older adults to defend against respiratory infections include frailty, dysphagia, serious illness, limited mobility, and poor oral care. Another complicating factor is the difficulty of diagnosing lower respiratory infections during early stages because the manifestations are subtle and nonspecific, as discussed in the section on Nursing Assessment of Respiratory Function.

Pneumonia in Older Adults

Pneumonia is sometimes classified according to etiology as hospital-acquired, community-acquired, nursing home–acquired, or aspiration. All types are characterized by increased incidence and mortality in older adults, particularly those who have risk factors such as frailty, dehydration, malnutrition, impaired functioning, or compromised immunity. Poor oral care is a risk for all types of pneumonia and is influenced significantly by nursing care for older adults in all health care settings (Kanzigg & Hunt, 2016; Ortega, Sakwinska, Combremont, et al., 2016; Saensom, Merchant, Wara-Aswapati, et al., 2016). Dysphagia is a major risk for aspiration pneumonia and commonly occurs in older adults with conditions such as stroke, dementia, Parkinson disease, and postsurgical care (Ebihara, Sekiya, Miyagi, et al., 2016; Takizawa, Gemmell, Kenworthy, et al., 2016). Nursing interventions for dysphagia are discussed in Chapter 18. Implications related to nursing assessment of, and interventions for, pneumonia are discussed in this chapter.

A Student's Perspective

I was glad to interact with someone who has emphysema and to learn about her struggles and about how care needs to be specialized for her because of her condition. Listening to E. A.'s breath sounds was frightening to me. I knew she was unable to breathe well, but I had no idea it was that obstructed. The struggle and stress her condition puts on her body to breathe is saddening. I really am amazed she is able to function as well as she does with her decreased level of oxygen.

I really enjoyed how talkative E. A. was. I had no problem getting information from her to complete her functional health assessment. It really hit me after I walked out of the nursing home on Friday that she literally talked to me for 3 hours. She was absolutely beside herself just to have someone there to listen and to interact with. I was glad I was able to give that to her. I believe this experience with E. A. will help me in the future to remember to give the emotional care as well as the physical.

In the next week, the things I would like to improve include supporting and promoting E. A. to get up and get dressed. I would like to help her with performing ADLs and help make her morning more worthwhile. I think helping E. A. become a little more productive could also help improve her social interactions. This is an area she needs a lot of help with, and I hope this week I will be able to give her support.

Jenna W.

PATHOLOGIC CONDITION AFFECTING RESPIRATORY FUNCTION: COPD

Chronic obstructive pulmonary disease (COPD) is a term that refers to a group of diseases that cause chronic airflow obstruction and breathing-related problems. The disease is usually progressive and characterized by increasing inflammatory response to noxious stimuli in the airway and lungs (Global Initiative for Chronic Obstructive Lung Disease, 2016). Conditions that increase the risk for developing COPD include smoking (accounting for 85% to 90% of causative factors), exposure to secondary smoke and other air pollutants, increased age, genetic predisposition, low socioeconomic status, and history of significant childhood respiratory disease.

The most common manifestations of COPD are cough, dyspnea, wheezing, and chronic sputum production. Consequences of COPD for older adults include longer and more frequent hospitalizations, an increased risk for being discharged to nursing facilities, and impaired health-related quality of life. Fatigue and frailty are common functional consequences that affect quality of life and disease management for patients with COPD (Kentson, Todt, Skargren, et al., 2016; Lahousse, Ziere, Verlinden, et al., 2016). Older adults with COPD are likely to have several concurrent diseases that increase the complexity of diagnosis, on-going assessment, and management. Cardiovascular disease (i.e., hypertension, heart failure, atrial fibrillation, and ischemic heart disease) represent the most frequent and important diseases coexisting with COPD. Additional diseases that often comorbid with COPD are osteoporosis, infections, anxiety, depression, diabetes, lung cancer, and impaired cognitive function (Global Initiative for Chronic Obstructive Lung Disease, 2016).

An important health promotion implication when caring for older adults with COPD is to encourage participation in programs that support self-management, particularly self-regulation of health behaviors (Chen, Liu, Shyu, et al., 2016; Bal Ozkaptan & Kapucu, 2016). In addition, it is important to encourage participation in physical activity, which is an important intervention for improving symptoms in people with COPD (Torres-Sanchez, Valenza, Cabrera-Martos, et al., 2016). Nurses also can initiate referrals for respiratory therapy and pulmonary rehabilitation, which are essential interventions for patients with COPD, particularly those (such as many older adults) who have functional impairments (Hattab, Albassan, Balaan, et al., 2016; Schroff, Hitchcock, Schurmann, et al., 2016). Smoking cessation and vaccinations for pneumonia and influenza are health promotion interventions discussed in this chapter that are particularly important for older adults with COPD. Box 21-2 summarizes recommendations for nursing assessment and

---

 Box 21-2 Evidence-Based Practice: Nursing Care of Patients With Dyspnea

Statement of the Problem

Dyspnea is the sixth vital sign in people with chronic obstructive pulmonary disease (COPD).

Recommendations for Nursing Assessment

- Assess all the following: vital signs, pulse oximetry, lung sounds, chest wall shape and movement, accessory muscle use, productive or nonproductive cough, peripheral edema, ability to complete a full sentence, level of consciousness
- Assess current level of dyspnea and usual breathing pattern and level of dyspnea, using visual analogue or numeric quantitative scale
- Assess for hypoxemia/hypoxia
- Assess swallowing difficulties
- Identify signs and symptoms of stable and unstable dyspnea and acute respiratory failure
- Screen for COPD in adults older than 40 years who have a history of smoking by asking each patient these three questions: (1) Do you have progressive activity-related shortness of breath? (2) Do you have a persistent cough and sputum production? (3) Do you experience frequent respiratory tract infections?
- Advocate for spirometry testing for patients who have a history of smoking and are older than 40 years
- If inhaler is used, assess self-administration technique

Recommendations for Nursing Interventions

- Acknowledge and accept patient's self-report of dyspnea
- Administer prescribed oxygen therapy, ventilation modalities, and medications (e.g., bronchodilators, corticosteroids, antibiotics, and psychotropics)
- Implement smoking cessation strategies; consider nicotine replacement and other smoking cessation modalities during hospitalization
- Remain with patient during episodes of acute respiratory distress

Recommendations for Teaching Older Adults and Caregivers About Dyspnea

- Prescribed medications, including correct technique for inhaler use
- Administration of oxygen therapy if prescribed
- Strategies for secretion clearance, energy conservation, relaxation techniques, nutrition, and breathing retraining
- Influenza and pneumococcal vaccinations
- Pulmonary rehabilitation and exercise training as appropriate
- Smoking cessation strategies if appropriate
- Disease self-management strategies: action plan, awareness of baseline symptoms and activity level, recognition of factors that worsen symptoms, early recognition of infection or acute exacerbation

Source: Registered Nurses Association of Ontario (RNAO). (2010). Nursing care of dyspnea: The 6th vital sign in individuals with chronic obstructive pulmonary disease. Toronto, ON: RNAO. Document and related resources available at www.rnao.ca.

care for people with dyspnea, which is called the sixth vital sign in people with COPD (Registered Nurses Association of Ontario [RNAO], 2010). Online Learning Activity 21-2 provides links to information and resources about COPD and an article about smoking cessation strategies for patients with COPD.

 See **ONLINE LEARNING ACTIVITY 21-2: RESOURCES RELATED TO COPD, INCLUDING AN ARTICLE ABOUT SMOKING CESSATION STRATEGIES FOR PATIENTS WITH COPD** at http://thepoint.lww.com/Miller8e.

GLOBAL PERSPECTIVE

The Global Initiative for Chronic Obstructive Lung Disease addresses COPD, which is the fourth leading cause of death worldwide, as a public health challenge that is both preventable and treatable. The 2016 report provides up-to-date information about COPD based on frequent reviews of scientific evidence by a panel of international experts. Materials are available at www.goldcopd.org.

NURSING ASSESSMENT OF RESPIRATORY FUNCTION

Although physical examination of overall respiratory function does not differ significantly in older adults, it is imperative to be aware of variations in the manifestations of lower respiratory infections in older adults. Another difference is that older adults may have different life experiences with regard to exposure to environmental toxins and attitudes about tobacco use. From a wellness perspective, nursing assessment of respiratory function focuses on identifying opportunities for health promotion, detecting lower respiratory infections, assessing smoking behaviors, and identifying other risk factors.

Identifying Opportunities for Health Promotion

Nurses interview older adults, or their caregivers, to identify the risk factors that are amenable to health promotion interventions. Because smoking is the risk factor that has the most serious detrimental effects on health, assess the potential for influencing all smokers, even older adults, to quit. Health education is based on assessment information about health-related behaviors, such as quitting smoking and avoiding secondhand smoke, as well as preventive interventions, such as influenza and pneumonia vaccinations. Nurses also assess the attitudes of older adults about these preventive measures, so they can plan appropriate educational approaches. Finally, include questions about overall respiratory function to identify problems that can be addressed in the nursing care plan. Box 21-3 presents an interview format that nurses can use to assess risk factors, overall respiratory function, and opportunities for health education.

Wellness Opportunity

Initiate a discussion about health-promoting behaviors by asking a question such as "What do you do to avoid secondhand smoke?"

Box 21-3 Guidelines for Assessing Respiratory Function

Questions to Identify Risk Factors for Respiratory Problems
- Have you had any respiratory problems, such as asthma, chronic lung disease, pneumonia, or other infections?
- Do you have a family history of chronic lung disease?
- Have you ever worked in a job where you were exposed to dust, fumes, smoke, or other air pollutants (e.g., in mining, farming, or any of the occupations listed in Box 21-1)?
- Have you lived in neighborhoods where there was a lot of pollution from traffic or factories?
- Do you smoke now, or have you ever smoked? (If yes, continue with the questions in Box 21-4.)
- Are you now, or have you been, exposed to passive smoke in home, work, or social environments?

Questions to Identify Opportunities for Education About Disease Prevention and Health Promotion
- Have you ever had a pneumonia vaccination? *If yes,* when was the vaccination administered and has the need for a booster been evaluated if the initial immunization was before the person was 65 years old?
- Do you get annual influenza vaccinations?

Questions to Assess Overall Respiratory Function
- Do you have any problems with breathing?
- Do you have any wheezing?

- Do you have spells of coughing? *If yes,* when do they occur? How long do they last? What brings them on? Are they dry or productive? Does the phlegm come from your throat or lungs? What does the phlegm look like?
- Do you ever have trouble getting enough air during any particular activities or when you lie down at night?
- Have you stopped doing any particular activities because of problems breathing? For example, have you stopped going up or down stairs, or have you limited the amount of walking you do? (For people with mobility limitations, this question might not be relevant.)
- Do you ever have any chest pain or feelings of heaviness or tightness in your chest?
- Do you use more than one pillow at night, or make any other adjustments, because of trouble with breathing?
- Do you wake up at night because of coughing or difficulty with breathing?
- Do you ever feel as though you can't catch your breath?
- Do you have trouble breathing when the weather is hot, cold, or humid?
- Do you tire easily?

Detecting Lower Respiratory Infections

The term *detection* is more accurate than *assessment* with regard to lower respiratory infections because these conditions often present atypically in older adults and treatment may be delayed, increasing the risk for serious complications, including death. Rather than presenting with a cough and purulent sputum, older adults are more likely to have subtler and nonspecific disease manifestations. Even initial chest radiography may not provide accurate diagnostic information. A summary of expert opinion and literature review of manifestations of pneumonia in nursing home residents found that the most important characteristics were fever, dyspnea, tachypnea, decline in overall functioning, and adventitious sounds on auscultation (Hollaar, van der Maarel-Wierink, van der Putten, et al., 2016). In addition, a change in mental status or another alteration in functional status, such as falls or incontinence, may be a major clue to pneumonia. Thus, an important nursing responsibility is to detect nonspecific manifestations of pneumonia and collect additional information. This is essential for ensuring a timely diagnosis and preventing complications.

Assessing Smoking Behaviors

Although smoking affects all people, regardless of age, some aspects of smoking behaviors differ according to age cohorts. The cohort of people born between 1910 and 1930, for example, is the first age group to be exposed to the social pressures that encouraged smoking without knowing about its detrimental effects. Consequently, people who began smoking in the early 1920s, when it became a popular habit for men in the United States, may have smoked for four or five decades before finding out that smoking is harmful. For women in the United States, smoking was not socially acceptable until the mid-1940s. Although the percentage of older adults among current smokers is lower than for other age groups, older smokers may have an outlook reflected in statements such as, "If I've smoked this long and am still alive, why should I quit now?" Also assess the older adult's knowledge about health effects of smoking and benefits related to quitting and attempt to identify misconceptions.

In addition to assessing attitudes and knowledge about smoking, ask about types of nicotine product used and past and current smoking patterns. For example, older adults may be smoking cigarettes that have no filters and higher levels of tar and nicotine. Some older adults, in fact, may still roll their own cigarettes using loose tobacco. In addition, assess the older adult's perception of smoking as a manifestation of his or her rights and autonomy. For example, nursing home residents may view smoking as the one remaining indicator of their former life and the one pleasurable activity that they can control.

Personal attitudes and knowledge about smoking can influence nursing care, especially in relation to older adults. For example, ageism can lead to the view that smoking cessation would not be beneficial for older adults. Similarly,

Box 21-4 Guidelines for Nursing Assessment of Older Adults Who Smoke

Questions to Assess Smoking Behaviors

- How long have you smoked?
- How much do you smoke?
- What do you smoke?
- Have you smoked other types of tobacco in the past?

Questions to Assess Knowledge of the Risk From Smoking

- Do you think there are any harmful effects of smoking for people in general?
- Do you think you are at risk for any harmful effects from smoking?
- Do you think there are any benefits to quitting smoking?

Questions to Assess Attitudes Toward Smoking

- Have you ever thought about quitting smoking?
- Has any health professional ever talked to you about quitting smoking?
- What do you think about the idea of quitting smoking?
- Have you ever tried to quit? *If yes,* what was your experience with the attempt?
- Would you be interested in finding out about quitting smoking now?

although rights of older adults who choose to smoke need to be respected, they should not be excluded from health promotion interventions about smoking based on age alone. Use information in Box 21-4 as a guide to assessing smoking habits, knowledge, and attitudes that are pertinent to developing health promotion interventions.

Wellness Opportunity

To assess smoking behaviors from a whole-person perspective, ask questions about the older adults' knowledge of the detrimental effects of smoking as well as their perception of smoking as an expression of autonomy.

See ONLINE LEARNING ACTIVITY 21-3: THROUGH THE STORIES OF SMOKERS WHO QUIT at http://thepoint.lww.com/Miller8e.

Identifying Other Risk Factors

In addition to assessing tobacco use as a risk factor, identify factors that affect respiratory function, including present and past exposure to secondhand smoke and other respiratory toxins. Occupational exposure to certain harmful substances is particularly important for smokers because the risk of either one of these factors is compounded when the other factor is present. Another consideration is to assess the person's level of activity and identify limitations in mobility or physical activity that can influence the potential improvement in level of activity. If, for example, people have limited mobility because of arthritis, they may not be able to engage in vigorous physical exercise, but they might benefit greatly from water exercises.

Identifying Normal Age-Related Variations

The usual assessment methods of inspection, palpation, percussion, and auscultation are used for all adults, but the following minor variations are common in healthy older adults:

- Slight increase in the normal respiratory rate, which ranges from 16 to 24 respirations per minute
- Increased anteroposterior diameter
- Forward-leaning posture because of kyphosis
- Increased resonance on percussion
- Diminished intensity of lung sounds
- Increased presence of adventitious sounds in the lower lungs

Begin the assessment of respiratory function by observing the person's breathing pattern in different positions, such as walking or sitting. To facilitate auscultation, ask the older adult to sit upright, cough before auscultation, and breathe with his or her mouth open. When observing respirations in a sleeping older adult, assess for brief periods of apnea, which are associated with sleep problems, as discussed in Chapter 24, Sleep and Rest.

Unfolding Case Study

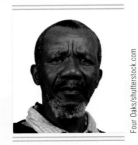

Four Oaks/shutterstock.com

Part 1: Mr. R. at 70 Years of Age

Mr. R. is 70 years old and comes with his wife to the senior center where you provide weekly nursing services. Both Mr. and Mrs. R. smoke one to two packs of cigarettes a day. Mr. R. has mild COPD and Mrs. R. has hypertension and coronary artery disease. Every October, the senior center offers influenza shots for anyone older than 65 years. As you are preparing to give influenza shots, Mr. and Mrs. R. come to you and ask, "Is this the shot that takes care of pneumonia? Our daughter said we should get a pneumonia shot every year, but we don't want a flu shot because our friend says she got the flu from one of those shots and she'll never get a shot again. Can you just give us the pneumonia shot today? We got one from the doctor last year but it's too expensive to get it from him."

THINKING POINTS

- What myths and misunderstandings do Mr. and Mrs. R. express?
- What further assessment questions would you ask?
- What health promotion teaching would you do?

QSEN APPLICATION

QSEN Competency	Knowledge/Skill/Attitude	Learning Activity Related to Mr. R.
Patient-centered care	(K) Integrate understanding of multiple dimensions of patient-centered care	Identify misinformation about flu and pneumonia shots communicated by Mr. and Mrs. R.
	(K) Describe strategies to empower patients in all aspects of the health care process	Use a nonjudgmental approach to provide correct information about flu and pneumonia shots
	(S) Provide patient-centered care with sensitivity and respect for diversity of human experience	
	(A) Value seeing health care situations "through patients' eyes"	
Evidence-based practice	(S) Base individualized care plan on patient values, clinical expertise, and evidence	Use simple patient teaching handouts from a reliable source to provide accurate information about pneumonia and flu shots (e.g., www.cdc.gov)

NURSING DIAGNOSIS

The nursing diagnosis of Ineffective Breathing Pattern would be applicable when the nursing assessment identifies factors that may impair the older adult's respiratory function. If impaired respiratory function interferes with activities of daily living, a nursing diagnosis of Activity Intolerance might be appropriate. A nursing diagnosis of Risk for Infection may be appropriate for debilitated or chronically ill older adults, particularly those who live in group settings where other residents have respiratory infections. For older adults who smoke, use the nursing diagnosis of Ineffective Protection, which is defined as "decrease in the ability to guard self from internal or external threats such as illness or injury" (Herdman & Kamitsuru, 2018, p. 154).

Wellness Opportunity

Use the wellness nursing diagnosis of Readiness for Enhanced Immunization Status when administering immunizations for influenza or pneumonia.

PLANNING FOR WELLNESS OUTCOMES

Wellness-oriented care plans for all older adults address their increased vulnerability to pneumonia and influenza by using NOC labels such as Immune Status, Immunization Behavior, and Risk Control: Communicable Disease. The Nursing Outcomes Classification (NOC) label of Knowledge: Health Behaviors is applicable for older adults who would benefit from health education about quitting smoke, obtaining immunizations, or preventing respiratory infections. A specific and measurable outcome of successful health education might be that older adults obtain immunizations against pneumonia and influenza.

Wellness Opportunity

Nurses promote wellness when their care plans address the immunization status of older adults.

Respiratory Status is the NOC label that is applicable in care plans related to the nursing diagnosis of Ineffective Breathing Pattern. When caring for older adults who smoke, always consider the possibility of helping them to quit or reduce smoking. Applicable NOC labels include Risk Control: Tobacco Use and Knowledge: Substance Use Control.

NURSING INTERVENTIONS FOR RESPIRATORY WELLNESS

For all older adults, nursing interventions to promote respiratory wellness focus on preventing respiratory infections and protecting from secondhand smoke. Nursing interventions for older adults who smoke focus on cessation. The following Nursing Interventions Classification labels are pertinent to these goals: Environmental Risk Protection, Health Education, Immunization/Vaccination Management, Infection Control, Infection Protection, Referral, and Smoking Cessation Assistance.

Promoting Respiratory Wellness

For all older adults, disease prevention and health promotion interventions related to respiratory function include pneumonia and influenza vaccinations and education about the importance of avoiding environmental tobacco smoke. These interventions are discussed in the following sections and summarized in Boxes 21-4 and 21-5. In addition, numerous educational materials are available for use in disease prevention and health promotion interventions, and many of these are available in languages other than English.

Wellness Opportunity

Nurses promote self-care behaviors by encouraging older adults to use patient teaching materials, which are available from such agencies as American Cancer Society; American Lung Association; Office on Smoking and Health, CDC; and the Lung Association of Canada among others.

See **ONLINE LEARNING ACTIVITY 21-4:**
HEALTH PROMOTION RESOURCES
at **http://thepoint.lww.com/Miller8e.**

Preventing Lower Respiratory Infections

Interventions to prevent pneumonia and influenza are particularly important because about 85% of deaths due to these diseases were among people aged 65 and older (National Center for Health Statistics, 2016). Moreover, pneumonia and influenza are the only diseases of all the leading causes of death in older adults that can be prevented through immunizations and without major investment of time, money, and motivation. The influenza and pneumococcal vaccines are safe and well tolerated in older adults, and studies indicate that these measures reduce morbidity and mortality and decrease hospitalization admission rates for respiratory infections and COPD (Walters, Tang, Poole, et al., 2017).

Current evidence-based guidelines recommend that older adults receive a series of two types of pneumococcal vaccinations, designated as 13-valent pneumococcal conjugate vaccine (PCV13) and 23-valent pneumococcal polysaccharide vaccine (PPSV23) (Fabel, Horton, & Shealy, 2016). Because these recommendations have been revised several times since the first guidelines were published in 1997, it is imperative to teach older adults about the importance of discussing their immunization status with their primary care practitioner.

Many institutional settings have standing orders for influenza and pneumonia vaccinations, and nurses play a primary role in implementing this health promotion intervention in community, residential, and institutional settings. In addition, all health care workers should receive annual influenza

Box 21-5 Health Promotion Teaching About Respiratory Problems

Factors That Increase the Risk for Pneumonia and Influenza

- Diabetes or any chronic lung, heart, or kidney disease
- Hospitalization within the past year for heart or lung diseases
- Severe anemia or a debilitating condition
- Confinement to bed or very limited mobility
- Residence in a nursing home or other group living setting
- Immunosuppressive medications

Preventing Respiratory Infection

- Wash your hands frequently with an antibacterial soap or hand sanitizer.
- Avoid hand-to-mouth and hand-to-eye contact.
- Avoid inhaling air that has been contaminated with particles from the cough or sneeze of someone with an infection.
- Avoid crowds during the influenza season.
- Be sure that influenza and pneumonia vaccinations are up-to-date.

Information About Influenza Vaccinations

- New vaccinations are developed every year, based on information about the strains of viruses that are most likely to affect people during the influenza season.
- Vaccines are made from inactivated viruses and, therefore, should have few or no side effects.
- People who are allergic to eggs and egg products should NOT receive influenza immunizations.
- Immunizations do not offer immediate protection because there is a 2- to 3-week delay in developing an antibody response.

- Every year, the manufacturers of the influenza vaccine provide recommendations as to the best time for administering the vaccine for optimal effectiveness. The best time is during the late fall, but the exact time period will vary slightly from year to year.
- Vaccines are not 100% effective, but they are helpful for most older people.
- Influenza immunizations provide protection against the most serious viruses but not against all types of respiratory infections.
- The duration of effectiveness of vaccinations may be shorter than 6 months in some older people; therefore, one vaccination might not protect the person through the entire season.
- Medicare and many other health insurance programs pay for influenza shots.

Information About Pneumonia Vaccinations

- Pneumonia vaccinations are recommended for people older than 65 years of age.
- Pneumonia vaccinations were considered one-time-only immunizations, but current guidelines recommend a series of two types.
- It is important to talk with your primary care practitioner to make sure your immunization status is up to date.
- Side effects, if they occur, are not serious and will subside within a few days.
- Common side effects include a slight fever accompanied by pain, redness, or tenderness at the injection site.
- Pneumonia vaccinations are covered by Medicare and other health insurance.

---

vaccinations to prevent transmission, thereby indirectly reducing mortality from influenza in the older population. Box 21-5 summarizes current information about influenza and pneumonia immunizations, along with information about risk factors for these illnesses.

See ONLINE LEARNING ACTIVITY 21-5: HEALTH DISPARITIES IN IMMUNIZATIONS at http://thepoint.lww.com/Miller8e.

Diversity Note

Estimated pneumococcal vaccination rates for people aged 65 and older in 2015 were 68% for non-Hispanic whites, 41.3% for Hispanics, and 50% for non-Hispanic blacks (National Center for Health Statistics, 2016).

Interventions to prevent pneumonia and other lower respiratory tract infections are an important aspect of health promotion for older adults. For example, assuring the provision of good oral hygiene, including measures to prevent plaque accumulation, is an evidence-based nursing intervention for preventing pneumonia, especially aspiration pneumonia (O'Connor, 2016). Additional nursing interventions for preventing lower respiratory infections include meticulous attention to handwashing and optimal positioning and turning of patients who have limited mobility.

Eliminating the Risk From Smoking

Smoking is the single most important preventable cause of disease and death in the United States and therefore should be a major target of disease prevention activities for all people who smoke tobacco. Because older smokers are likely to have smoking-related functional consequences, smoking cessation will address secondary or tertiary prevention rather than primary prevention. Smoking cessation is widely recognized as a cost-effective and evidence-based health promotion activity that should be a priority for health care professionals (Schauer, Wheaton, Malarcher, et al., 2016).

Educational interventions for older smokers begin by addressing attitudes that influence health-related behaviors. For example, if an older person expresses an "I'm-too-old-to-change" attitude, an initial step is to explore the older adult's understanding of his or her ability to change behavioral patterns. Older adults may be motivated to quit smoking because of changes in their health status. Information about models of behavior change (discussed in Chapter 5) is applicable to helping smokers quit. In 2015, the National Cancer Institute established a website with resources specifically for helping older adults quit smoking. Online Learning Activity 21-6 provides links to this website and other resources related to quitting smoking.

Another commonly expressed belief that nurses can address through health education is "It's too late to do any good." When nurses encounter this type of attitude, they can emphasize that the substantial health benefits derived from quitting smoking are both immediate and long term. Benefits from smoking cessation for people of any age include improved quality of life, decreased susceptibility to smoking-related illnesses (e.g., heart disease and cancer), and a more rapid recovery from illnesses that usually are exacerbated by smoking.

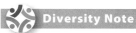

Wellness Opportunity

Nurses support wellness in older adults by communicating that old age is not an inevitable barrier to changing health-related behaviors: It's never too late to quit.

Diversity Note

The Centers for Disease Control provides educational materials addressing specific groups, including Asian Americans; African Americans; Hispanics; American Indians/Alaska Natives; and Lesbian, Gay, Bisexual, and Transgender (available at www.cdc.gov).

Guidelines emphasize the importance of nurses and other health care providers initiating the topic of tobacco dependence and routinely identifying and intervening with all tobacco users, including older adult, at every opportunity. Additional points of evidence-based guidelines are as follows:

- Tobacco dependence is a chronic disease that may require repeated interventions; however, effective treatments can significantly increase rates of long-term abstinence.
- Individual, group, and telephone counseling methods are effective; problem solving and social support as part of treatment are especially effective counseling interventions.
- Nicotine-based medications that reliably increase long-term smoking abstinence are nicotine gum, inhaler, lozenge, patch, and nasal spray.
- Non-nicotine medications that are effective for smoking cessation include sustained-release bupropion (Wellbutrin™) and varenicline (Chantix™); however, the Food and Drug Administration has issued warnings about serious cardiovascular and neuropsychiatric symptoms that can occur with varenicline.
- Counseling and medication are effective for treating tobacco dependence, but the combination of these methods is more effective than either alone.

(Centers for Disease Control and Prevention, 2016c; Lindson-Hawley, Hartmann-Boyce, Fanshawe, et al., 2016; Scholz, Santos, Buzo, et al., 2016).

Nonpharmacologic interventions that are effective for smoking cessation include exercise, guided imagery, breathing techniques, positive self-talk, journaling, integration of rewards, and identification of habit breakers for events that trigger smoking (Jackson, 2016). Box 21-6 can be used as a guide to teaching

---

Box 21-6 Health Promotion Teaching About Cigarette Smoking

Attitudes About Smoking

- Stopping smoking at any age is more beneficial than continuing to smoke.
- Many of the harmful effects of smoking are reversed once the smoker quits.
- Although some of the effects of past smoking are irreversible, all of the harmful effects of future smoking can be avoided by quitting now.
- Smoking is a major risk factor for many cancers, including those of the lung, head, stomach, kidney, and pancreas.
- Smoking is a major risk factor for lung and heart disease, including high blood pressure and heart attacks.
- Passive smoking (inhaling smoke from the air) is associated with an increased risk for many diseases.

Types of Tobacco

- The lower the tar and nicotine content of cigarettes, the less harmful the effects. Many cigarettes with lower tar and nicotine levels, however, have additional chemical additives that can be harmful.
- Pipe and cigar smokers are at a higher risk for chronic lung disease than nonsmokers, just as cigarette smokers are.
- The harmful effects of tobacco use on the mouth and upper respiratory tract are equal for all types of tobacco, including smokeless tobacco. All smokers have the same risk for developing cancer of the mouth and upper respiratory tract. Snuff, chewing tobacco, and smokeless tobacco contain nicotine and many other harmful chemicals. The only advantage of smokeless tobacco is that it does not affect other people nearby.

Approaches to Quitting

- Any reduction in present tobacco use is better than maintaining the current level. The negative effects of smoking are directly proportional to the number of cigarettes inhaled.
- Various forms of prescription and over-the-counter nicotine substitutes (e.g., gum, skin patches, and nasal sprays) are available and may be helpful, especially when used in conjunction with counseling and self-help techniques.
- Besides nicotine substitutes, some non-nicotine prescription medications and over-the-counter products may be effective as a component of a smoking cessation program.
- People who are trying to quit smoking should discuss their goals with a health care professional to identify the methods that may be most effective.
- Many self-help programs are available for support and education regarding quitting smoking.
- Information about group programs can be obtained on the Internet or by calling the local office of any of the following organizations: American Lung Association, American Heart Association, or American Cancer Society.

Nonpharmacologic Practices to Help Quit Smoking

- Exercise, music, imagery, massage, meditation, affirmations, deep breathing, stress reduction, social support, or individual or group counseling.

older adults about quitting smoking. Nurses also can emphasize that health insurance programs such as Medicare cover the cost of counseling and other interventions for smoking cessation.

Technology to Promote Wellness in Older Adults

Nurses can teach about technologic solutions to support smoking cessation. The following websites provide interactive web-based programs to help individuals implement a personal smoking cessation plan:

- American Lung Association, www.quitterinyou.org
- Be Tobacco Free, http://smokefree.gov
- UCanQuit2 for veterans, www.ucanquit2.org

 GLOBAL PERSPECTIVE

Nurses in China are strongly encouraged to actively support smoking cessation interventions, including recommending smoke-free home environments to support quit attempts (Sarna, Bialous, Zou, et al., 2016).

Screening for Lung Cancer in Smokers

In addition to addressing smoking cessation, health promotion interventions for smokers should address lung cancer screening. In 2015, the Centers for Medicare & Medicaid Services began covering screening for lung cancer with low-dose computer tomography. Based on evidence that screening for lung cancer reduces lung cancer mortality by 20%, the U. S. Preventive Services Task Force recommends annual screening for lung cancer in individuals between the ages of 55 and 80 who meet the following criteria: 30-pack-per-year

smoking history and either currently smoke or quit smoking within the past 15 years (van der Aalst, Ten Haaf, & de Koning, 2016). Nurses play important roles in encouraging older smokers to discuss the benefits and risks of this relatively new screening test with their primary care practitioners (Lowenstein, Richards, Leal, et al., 2016).

 See ONLINE LEARNING ACTIVITY 21-6: HELPING OLDER ADULTS QUIT SMOKING at http://thepoint.lww.com/Miller8e.

EVALUATING EFFECTIVENESS OF NURSING INTERVENTIONS

Measuring the effectiveness of interventions for the nursing diagnosis of Ineffective Breathing Pattern is based on a reassessment of subjective indicators such as ease of breathing and objective indicators such as lung sounds and respiratory rate and rhythm. An indicator of successful health education interventions for older adults with Ineffective Breathing Pattern is that they can accurately identify factors that can be addressed to improve their respiratory function. Interventions for the nursing diagnosis of Risk for Infection can be documented on a record of the person's history of immunizations for pneumonia and influenza. For older adults who smoke, effectiveness of interventions is measured by the person's increased knowledge about the detrimental effects of smoking and by his or her willingness to develop a plan to stop smoking. Long-term effectiveness would be evaluated by the person's successful participation in the smoking cessation program.

Unfolding Case Study

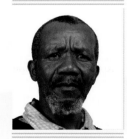

Four Oaks/shutterstock.com

Part 2: Mr. R. at 77 Years of Age

Mr. R. is now 77 years old and attends the senior center with his wife three times a week for meal and social programs. During your weekly senior wellness clinic, he comes to have his blood pressure checked and says that he is thinking about quitting smoking, but that his son just quit and gained a lot of weight and had a lot of trouble sleeping. He's not sure if quitting smoking is worth the effort, especially because his son has been so miserable since he quit. Also, at his age, it probably won't do any good to quit now, he says.

THINKING POINTS

- What further questions would you ask to assess Mr. R.'s readiness to discuss quitting smoking?
- What health promotion teaching would you do?

- What would your response be if you determine that Mr. R. is not ready to consider quitting smoking?

Part 2: Mr. R. at 77 Years of Age (Continued)

QSEN APPLICATION

QSEN Competency	Knowledge/Skill/Attitude	Learning Activity Related to Mr. R.
Patient-centered care	(K) Integrate understanding of multiple dimensions of patient-centered care	Elicit additional information about Mr. R.'s fears of quitting smoking and being too old to benefit
	(K) Examine common barriers to active involvement in patients in their own health care processes	Ask about previous personal experiences with quitting smoking
	(A) Value seeing health care situations "through patients' eyes"	Using pertinent information from Box 21-6, teach Mr. R. about quitting smoking
Teamwork and collaboration	(K) Recognize contributions of other individuals and groups in helping patient achieve health goals	Encourage Mr. R. to use resources for quitting smoking (e.g., from National Quit Smoking Program)
Evidence-based practice	(S) Locate evidence reports related to clinical practice topics and guidelines	Read guidelines and teaching tools for health care professionals to help patients quit smoking from Agency for Healthcare Research and Quality (www.ahrq.gov)

Unfolding Case Study

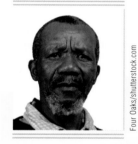

Four Oaks/shutterstock.com

Part 3: Mr. R. at 83 Years of Age

Mr. R. is now 83 years old and recently moved into an assisted living complex where you are employed as the nurse. When he comes in for his flu shot, he asks you how he can get some nicotine gum because he has heard that this is a good way to cut down on cigarettes. Now that he lives in the assisted living complex, he can't smoke in the dining room, and he'd like to chew nicotine gum before and after he eats. He admits that he smokes a pack of cigarettes every day but denies having experienced any bad effects from smoking. Mr. R. sees his doctor for COPD and takes Flovent, two puffs twice a day, and Serevent, two puffs twice a day.

NURSING ASSESSMENT

You begin your nursing assessment by exploring Mr. R.'s attitudes about smoking and ascertaining his knowledge about the harmful effects of cigarette smoking. Mr. R. says he thought about quitting smoking many times but never actually tried to quit because his wife smoked even more than he did until she died a few months ago. He felt it would be too hard to quit as long as she was smoking two packs per day. He also states that he's heard a lot about passive smoking and he figured it wasn't worth trying to quit as long as he was around his wife's cigarette smoke. He states that he's been smoking for 40 years, and if he hasn't gotten lung cancer by now, he's not going to get it at his age. To comply with the rules in the assisted living facility, Mr. R. says he plans to chew nicotine gum when he can't smoke cigarettes, but he sees no reason to quit.

In assessing Mr. R.'s knowledge about the effects of cigarette smoking, you determine that he is aware of some of the harmful effects of passive smoking but has very little information about the detrimental effects of cigarette smoking. He relates that his wife died of lung cancer, but he attributes her death to a history of breast cancer, which she had 10 years before the lung cancer. Mr. R. has no knowledge about cigarette smoking as a risk factor for cardiovascular disease, nor does he realize that his hypertension poses an additional risk. Mr. R. reports that he has experienced no ill effects from cigarette smoking, but when you ask about his history of respiratory infections, he admits he had pneumonia 3 years ago. He says that he received a pneumonia shot, so he doesn't have to worry about getting pneumonia again, and that he has had bronchitis several times, but now that he won't be out shoveling snow, he doesn't worry about getting any lung infections either.

(continued)

Part 3: Mr. R. at 83 Years of Age *(Continued)*

NURSING DIAGNOSIS

Based on the assessment findings, an appropriate nursing diagnosis would be Ineffective Health Maintenance, related to insufficient knowledge about the effects of tobacco use and self-help resources. Some of Mr. R.'s statements reflect a lack of accurate information about the harmful effects of cigarette smoking, particularly regarding risks for respiratory infections and impaired cardiovascular function. Other statements probably reflect an intellectualization of his continued smoking. Your intuition tells you that, with some education and support, he may be willing to quit smoking.

NURSING CARE PLAN FOR MR. R.

Expected Outcome	Nursing Interventions	Nursing Evaluation
Mr. R. will increase his knowledge about the harmful effects of cigarette smoking	• Give Mr. R. brochures and illustrations provided by the Office on Smoking and Health and use them to discuss the effects of cigarette smoking • Use brochures from the American Heart Association to discuss the risk factors for cardiovascular disease • Discuss cigarette smoking as a risk factor for respiratory infections • Give Mr. R. a copy of Box 21-6 and discuss the immediate and long-term benefits of quitting smoking	• Mr. R. will verbalize correct information about the risks of cigarette smoking • Mr. R. will describe the benefits derived from quitting smoking
Mr. R. will be knowledgeable about techniques for quitting smoking	• Using information from the American Lung Association, discuss some of the strategies for quitting smoking (e.g., quitting "cold turkey," using nicotine substitutes, participating in self-help groups)	• Mr. R. will describe the advantages and disadvantages of the various methods of quitting smoking
Mr. R. will quit smoking	• Identify the method Mr. R. prefers for quitting smoking • Emphasize the importance of nutrition, exercise, and adequate fluid intake • Agree on realistic goals for smoking cessation • Discuss supportive resources. Set up weekly appointments at the senior wellness clinic for support and further discussions	• Mr. R. will report that he has stopped or significantly reduced his smoking

THINKING POINTS

- How would you assess Mr. R.'s readiness and motivation to quit smoking?
- What health education approach would you take with Mr. R.?
- What additional interventions or health education points would you use for Mr. R.?

QSEN APPLICATION

QSEN Competency	Knowledge/Skill/Attitude	Learning Activity Related to Mr. R.
Patient-centered care	(K) Integrate understanding of multiple dimensions of patient-centered care (S) Elicit patient values, preferences, and expressed needs (A) Value seeing health care situations "through patients' eyes"	Explore Mr. R.'s attitudes about smoking and assess his knowledge about harmful effects of smoking Discuss realistic goals for quitting smoking as an important intervention for promoting health

QSEN APPLICATION (Continued)

QSEN Competency	Knowledge/Skill/Attitude	Learning Activity Related to Mr. R.
Teamwork and collaboration	(K) Recognize contributions of other individuals and groups in helping patient achieve health goals	Use information from Box 21-6 to discuss ways of quitting smoking
	(S) Integrate the contributions of others who play a role in helping patient achieve health goals	Facilitate the use of Internet resources and support groups pertinent to quitting smoking
Evidence-based practice	(S) Base individualized care plan on patient values, clinical expertise, and evidence	Use educational materials from the American Heart Association, the American Lung Association, and the Office on Smoking and Health to teach about detrimental effects of smoking and beneficial effects of quitting

Chapter Highlights

Age-Related Changes That Affect Respiratory Function (Table 21-1)

- Upper airway changes (e.g., calcification of cartilage)
- Increased anteroposterior diameter
- Chest wall stiffness, weakened muscles
- Alveoli enlarged and have thinner walls
- Alterations in lung volumes and airflow
- Decreased compensatory response to hypercapnia and hypoxia

Risk Factors That Affect Respiratory Wellness (Box 21-1)

- Tobacco use
- Secondhand smoke and other environmental factors
- Occupational hazards

Functional Consequences Affecting Respiratory Wellness (Table 21-1)

- Mouth breathing, diminished cough reflex, less efficient gag reflex
- Increased use of accessory muscles, increased energy expended for breathing
- Diminished efficiency of gas exchange, decreased PaO_2 levels
- Decreased vital capacity, slight decrease in overall efficiency
- Increased susceptibility to lower respiratory infections
- Pneumonia in older adults

Pathologic Condition Affecting Respiratory Function: COPD

- COPD: a group of diseases that cause chronic airflow obstruction and breathing-related problems

Nursing Assessment of Respiratory Function (Boxes 21-2 and 21-3)

- Overall respiratory function
- Detection of lower respiratory infections

- Tobacco use and attitudes regarding smoking
- Identification of age-related variations

Nursing Diagnosis

- Health-Seeking Behaviors
- Ineffective Breathing Pattern
- Risk for Infection

Planning for Wellness Outcomes

- Vital Signs, Respiratory Status: Airway Patency, and Respiratory Status: Ventilation
- Immune Status, Immunization Behavior, and Community Risk Control
- Knowledge: Health Behaviors
- Risk Control: Tobacco Use and Knowledge: Substance Use Control

Nursing Interventions for Respiratory Wellness (Boxes 21-4 and 21-5)

- Promoting respiratory wellness
- Preventing lower respiratory infections
- Eliminating the risk from smoking
- Screening for lung cancer in smokers

Evaluating Effectiveness of Nursing Interventions

- Ease of breathing
- Up-to-date status for pneumonia immunization
- Influenza immunization every year
- For older adults who smoke: active participation in smoking cessation behaviors

Critical Thinking Exercises

1. What will a healthy, nonsmoking, 83-year-old person experience in his or her daily life with regard to respiratory function?
2. What would you include in a health education program, designed for older adults, on the prevention of pneumonia and influenza?

3. How would you address the following statement made by a 71-year-old person: "I've lived this long and don't have lung cancer; why should I start worrying now?"

4. Find the names, addresses, and phone numbers of local agencies that would be appropriate resources for someone interested in quitting smoking. Contact at least one of these organizations to find out specific information about support groups, written materials, and other resources.

 For more information about the topics discussed in this chapter, be sure to check out the interactive Online Learning Activities and other helpful resources at http://thepoint.lww.com/Miller8e.

REFERENCES

American Cancer Society. (2016a). Key statistics for lung cancer. Available at www.cancer.org

American Cancer Society. (2016b). Study confirms there is no safe level of smoking. Available at www.cancer.org

Awan, K. H., & Patil, S. (2016). Association of smokeless tobacco with oral cancer – evidence from South Asian studies: A systematic review. *Journal of the College of Physicians and Surgeons – Pakistan, 26,* 775–780.

Bal Ozkaptan, B., & Kapucu, S. (2016). Home nursing care with the self-care model improves self-efficacy of patients with chronic obstructive pulmonary disease. *Japanese Journal of Nursing Science, 13,* 365–377.

Bastian, L., Gray, K., DeRycke, E., et al. (2016). Differences in active and passive smoking exposures and lung cancer incidence between veterans and non-veterans in the Women's Health Initiative. *The Gerontologist, 56,* S102–S111.

Benowitz, N. L., & Burbank, A. D. (2016). Cardiovascular toxicity of nicotine: Implications for electronic cigarette use. *Trends in Cardiovascular Medicine, 26,* 515–523.

Brandenberger, C., & Muhlfeld, C. (2016). Mechanisms of lung aging. *Cell & Tissue Research, 367,* 469–480.

Bucheli, J. R., Manshad, A., Ehrhart, M. D., et al. (2016). Association of passive smoking with pre-diabetes risk in a predominantly Hispanic population. *Journal of Investigative Medicine, 65,* 328–332.

Campos, M. W., Serebrisky, D., & Castaldelli-Maia, J. M. (2016). Smoking and cognition. *Current Drug Abuse Reviews,* 2016 Aug 3. doi: 10.2174/1874473709660803101633.

Centers for Disease Control and Prevention. (2016a). Current cigarette smoking among adults in the United States. Available at www.cdc.gov.

Centers for Disease Control and Prevention. (2016b). Health effects of secondhand smoke. Available at www.cdc.gov.

Centers for Disease Control and Prevention. (2016c). Cessation materials for state tobacco control programs. Available at www.cdc.gov.

Chen, K. H., Liu, C. Y., Shyu, Y. I., et al. (2016). Living with chronic obstructive pulmonary disease: The process of self-managing chronic obstructive pulmonary disease. *The Journal of Nursing Research, 24,* 262–271.

Dixit, S., Pletcher, M. J., Vittinghoff, E., et al. (2016). Secondhand smoke and atrial fibrillation: Data from the Health eHeart Study. *Heart Rhythm, 13,* 3–9.

Ebihara, S., Sekiya, H., Miyaga, M., et al. (2016). Dysphagia, dystussia, and aspiration pneumonia in elderly people. *Journal of Thoracic Disease, 8,* 632–639.

Fabel, P. H., Horton, E. C., & Shealy, K. (2016). What are the latest recommendations for pneumococcal vaccines? *Journal of the American Association of Physician Assistants, 29,* 13–14.

Global Initiative for Chronic Obstructive Lung Disease. (2016). Global strategies for the diagnosis, management, and prevention of chronic obstructive pulmonary disease. Available at www.goldcopd.org.

Goncalves, M. T., Mitchell, T. J., & Lord, J. M. (2016). Immune ageing and susceptibility to Streptococcus pneumoniae. *Biogerontology, 17,* 449–465.

Hattab, Y., Albassan, S., Balaan, M., et al. (2016). Chronic obstructive pulmonary disease. *Critical Care Nurses Quarterly, 39,* 124–130.

Herdman, T., & Kamitsura, S. (Eds). (2018). *NANDA International Nursing Diagnoses Definitions and Classification, 2018–2020* (11th ed., pp. 34–44). New York: Thieme Publishers.

Hollaar, V., van der Wierink, C., van der Putten, G. J., et al. (2016). Defining characteristics and risk indicators for diagnosing nursing home-acquired pneumonia and aspiration pneumonia in nursing home residents, using the electronically-modified Delphi method. *BioMed Central Geriatrics, 16.* doi: 10.1186/s12877-016-0231-4.

Inoue-Choi, M., Liao, L. M., Reyes-Guzman, C., et al. (2017). Association of long-term, low-intensity smoking with all-cause and cause-specific mortality in the National Institutes of Health-AARP Diet and Health Study. *Journal of the American Medical Association, Internal Medicine, 177,* 87–95.

Jackson, C. (2016). Smoking cessation. In B. Dossey & L. Keegan (Eds.), *Holistic nursing: A handbook for practice* (7th ed., pp. 819–844). Boston, MA: Jones & Bartlett.

Kanzigg, L. A., & Hunt, L. (2016). Oral health and hospital-acquired pneumonia in elderly patients: A review of the literature. *Journal of Dental Hygiene, 90,* Suppl 1, 15–21.

Kentson, M., Todt, K., Skargren, E., et al. (2016). Factors associated with experience of fatigue, and functional limitations due to fatigue in patients with stable COPD. *Therapeutic Advances in Respiratory Disease, 10,* 410–424.

Lahoussse, L., Ziere, G., Verlinden, V. J., et al. (2016). Risk of frailty in elderly with COPD: A population-based study. *Journals of Gerontology: Biological Sciences and Medical Sciences, 71,* 689–695.

Lee, S. H., Hong, J. Y., Lee, J. U., et al. (2016). Association between exposure to environmental tobacco smoke at the workplace and risk for developing a colorectal adenoma: A cross-sectional study. *Annals of Coloproctology, 32,* 51–57.

Lindson-Hawley, N., Hartmann-Boyce, J., Fanshawe, T. R., et al. (2016). Interventions to reduce harm from continued tobacco use. *Cochrane Database of Systematic reviews,* 2016 Oct 13. doi: 10.CD005231.

Lorbergs, A. L., O'Connor, G. T., Zhou, Y., et al. (2017). Severity of kyphosis and decline in lung function: The Framingham Study. *Journals of Gerontology: Biological Sciences and Medical Sciences, 72,* 689–694.

Lowenstein, L., Richards, V., Leal, V., et al. (2016). A brief measure of smokers' knowledge of lung cancer screening with low-dose computed tomography. *Preventive Medicine Reports, 4,* 351–356.

Malas, M., van der Tempel, J., Schwartz, R., et al. (2016). Electronic cigarettes for smoking cessation: A systematic review. *Nicotine & Tobacco Research, 18,* 1926–1936.

McCormick-Ricket, I., Canterbury, M., Ghaffar, A., et al. (2016). Measuring the effect of environmental tobacco smoke on lung function: Results from a small observational investigation of acute exposure. *Journal of Occupational and Environmental Medicine, 58,* 1028–1033.

McEldaney, J., Kuchel, G., Zhou, X., et al. (2016). T-cell immunity to influenza in older adults: A pathophysiological framework for development of more effective vaccines. *Frontiers in Immunology, 7.* doi: 10.3389/fimmu.2016.00041.

National Center for Health Statistics. (2016). *Health, United States, 2015.* Washington DC: U. S. Government Printing Office.

O'Connor, L. J. (2016). Oral health care. In M. Boltz, E. Capezuti, T. Fulmer, & D. Zwicker (Eds), *Evidence-Based Geriatric Nursing Protocols for Best Practice,* pp. 103–109. New York: Springer Publishing.

O'Malley, P. A. (2017). Safety and efficacy of electronic cigarettes: Update for the clinical nurse specialist. *Clinical Nurse Specialist, 31,* 17–19.

Ordonez-Mena, J., Schottker, B., Mons, U., et al. (2016). Quantification of the smoking-associated cancer risk with rate advancement periods: meta-analysis of individual participant data from cohorts of the CHANCES consortium. *BioMed Central Medicine, 14*. doi: 10.1186/s12916-016-0607-5.

Ortega, O., Sakwinska, O., Combremont, S., et al. (2016). High prevalence of colonization of oral cavity by respiratory pathogens in frail older patients with oropharyngeal dysphagia. *Neurogastroenterology & Motility, 27*, 1804–1816.

Registered Nurses Association of Ontario (RNAO). (2010). Nursing care of dyspnea: The 6th vital sign in individuals with chronic obstructive pulmonary disease. Toronto, ON: RNAO. Document and related resources available at www.rnao.ca.

Saensom, D., Merchant, A. T., Wara-Aswapati, N., et al. (2016). Oral health and ventilator-associated pneumonia among critically ill patients: A prospective study. *Oral Disease, 22*, 709–714.

Salloum, R. G., Getz, K. R., Tan, A. S., et al. (2016). Use of electronic cigarettes among cancer survivors in the U. S. *American Journal of Preventive Medicine, 51*, 762–766.

Sarna, L., Bialous, S. A., Zou, X. N., et al. (2016). Helping smokers quit: Behaviours and attitudes of Chinese registered nurses. *Journal of Advances in Nursing, 72*, 107–117.

Schauer, G. L., Wheaton, A., Malarcher, A., et al. (2016). Health-care provider screening and advice for smoking cessation among smokers with and without COPD: 2009-2010 National Adult Tobacco Survey. *Chest, 149*, 676–684.

Scholz, J., Santos, P., Buzo, C., et al. (2016). Effects of aging on the effectiveness of smoking cessation medication. *Oncotarget, 7*, 30032–30039.

Schroff, P., Hitchcock, J., Schumann, C., et al. (2016). Pulmonary rehabilitation improves outcomes in chronic obstructive pulmonary disease independent of disease burden. *Annals of the American Thoracic Society, 14*, 26–32.

Sinha, D. N., Abdulkader, R. S., & Gupta, P. C. (2016). Smokeless tobacco-associated cancers: A systematic review and meta-analysis of Indian studies. *International Journal of Cancer, 138*, 1368–1379.

Takizawa, C., Gemmell, E., Kenworthy, J., et al. (2016). A systematic review of the prevalence of oropharyngeal dysphagia in stroke, Parsinson's disease, Alzheimer's disease, head injury, and pneumonia. *Dysphagia, 31*, 434–441.

Toda, N., & Okamura, T. (2016). Cigarette smoking impairs nitric oxide-mediated cerebral blood flow increase: Implications for Alzheimer's disease. *Journal of Pharmacological Sciences, 131*, 223–232.

Torres-Sanchez, I., Valenza, M. C., Cabrera-Martos, I., et al. (2016). Effects of an exercise intervention in frail older patients with chronic obstructive pulmonary disease hospitalized due to an exacerbation: A randomized controlled trial. *COPD, 14*, 37–42.

van der Aalst, C. M., Ten Haaf, K., & de Koning, H. J. (2016). Lung cancer screening: Latest developments and unanswered questions. *Lancet Respiratory Medicine, 4*, 749–761.

Vaz Fragoso, C. A., McAvay, G., Van Ness, P., et al. (2016). Aging-related considerations when evaluating the forced expiratory volume in 1 second (FEV1) over time. *Journals of Gerontology: Biological Sciences and Medical Sciences, 71*, 929–934.

Vidyassagaran, A. L., Siddigi, K., & Kanaan, M. (2016). Use of smokeless tobacco and risk of cardiovascular disease: A systematic review and meta-analysis. *European Journal of Preventive Cardiology, 23*, 1970–1981.

Walters, J. A., Tang, J. N., Poole, P., et al. (2017). Pneumococcal vaccines for preventing pneumonia in chronic obstructive pulmonary disease. *Cochrane Database of Systematic Reviews, 2017* Jan 24; 1:CD001390. doi: 10.1002/14651858.CD001390.pub4.

Yang, C., Wang, X., Huang, C. H., et al. (2016). Passive smoking and risk of colorectal cancer: A meta-analysis of observational studies. *Asia Pacific Journal of Public Health, 28*, 394–403.

chapter 22

Safe Mobility

LEARNING OBJECTIVES

After reading this chapter, you will be able to:

1. Delineate age-related changes that affect mobility and safety.

2. Identify risk factors that increase the risk for osteoporosis and influence the safety and mobility of older adults.

3. Discuss the following functional consequences: diminished musculoskeletal function, increased susceptibility to fractures, and increased susceptibility to falls.

4. Discuss the psychosocial and long-term consequences of falls, fractures, and osteoporosis.

5. Conduct a nursing assessment of musculoskeletal performance and risks for falls and osteoporosis.

6. Identify interventions directed toward safe mobility and the elimination of risks for falls and osteoporosis.

KEY TERMS

body sway	fragility fracture
bone density	osteoarthritis
fall risk assessment tools	osteopenia
fall risk–increasing drugs	osteoporosis
fear of falling	sarcopenia

Mobility is one of the most important aspects of physiologic function because it is essential for maintaining independence and because serious consequences occur when falls occur. For older adults, mobility is influenced by age-related changes to some extent, but risk factors play a much larger role. Because of the many risks that affect mobility, falls and fractures are an unfortunately common occurrence in old age. Older adults, then, have the dual challenge of maintaining mobility skills and avoiding falls and fractures. For these reasons, safety is an integral aspect of mobility.

AGE-RELATED CHANGES THAT AFFECT MOBILITY AND SAFETY

The bones, joints, and muscles are the body structures most closely associated with mobility, but many additional functional aspects are involved in *safe* mobility. Neurologic function, for example, influences all facets of musculoskeletal performance, and sensory function influences the ability to interact safely with the environment. In the musculoskeletal system, osteoporosis is the age-related change that has the most significant overall impact, has been studied the most, and is most amenable to interventions aimed at prevention and management.

Bones

Bones provide the framework for the entire musculoskeletal system and function with other systems to facilitate movement. Additional functions of bone in the human body include storing calcium, producing blood cells, and supporting and protecting body organs and tissues. Bone is composed of an outer layer, called cortical or compact bone, and an inner, spongy meshwork, called trabecular or cancellous bone. The proportion of cortical to trabecular components varies according to bone type. Long bones, such as the radius and femur, are composed of as much as 90% cortical cells, whereas flat and vertebral bones are composed primarily of trabecular cells. Both cortical and trabecular bone components are affected by age-related changes, but the rate and impact of age-related changes differ in the two types of bones.

Promoting Musculoskeletal Wellness in Older Adults

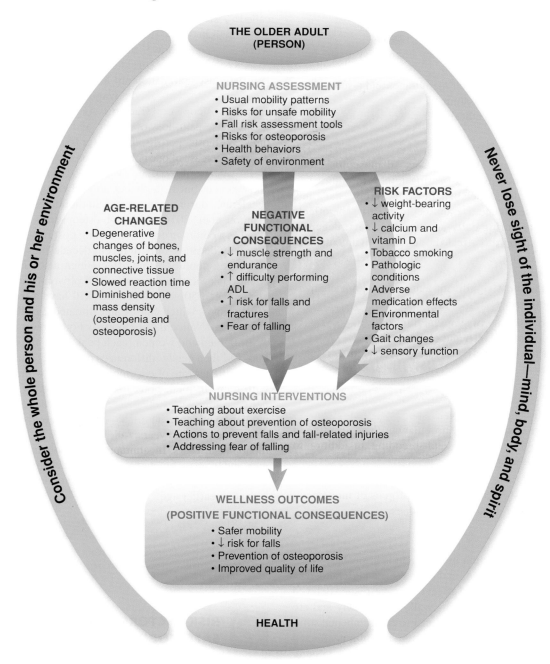

THE OLDER ADULT (PERSON)

Consider the whole person and his or her environment

Never lose sight of the individual—mind, body, and spirit

NURSING ASSESSMENT
- Usual mobility patterns
- Risks for unsafe mobility
- Fall risk assessment tools
- Risks for osteoporosis
- Health behaviors
- Safety of environment

AGE-RELATED CHANGES
- Degenerative changes of bones, muscles, joints, and connective tissue
- Slowed reaction time
- Diminished bone mass density (osteopenia and osteoporosis)

NEGATIVE FUNCTIONAL CONSEQUENCES
- ↓ muscle strength and endurance
- ↑ difficulty performing ADL
- ↑ risk for falls and fractures
- Fear of falling

RISK FACTORS
- ↓ weight-bearing activity
- ↓ calcium and vitamin D
- Tobacco smoking
- Pathologic conditions
- Adverse medication effects
- Environmental factors
- Gait changes
- ↓ sensory function

NURSING INTERVENTIONS
- Teaching about exercise
- Teaching about prevention of osteoporosis
- Actions to prevent falls and fall-related injuries
- Addressing fear of falling

WELLNESS OUTCOMES (POSITIVE FUNCTIONAL CONSEQUENCES)
- Safer mobility
- ↓ risk for falls
- Prevention of osteoporosis
- Improved quality of life

HEALTH

Bone growth reaches maturity in early adulthood, but bone remodeling continues throughout one's lifetime. The following age-related changes affect this remodeling process in all older adults:

- Increased bone resorption (i.e., breakdown of bone that is necessary for remodeling)
- Diminished calcium absorption
- Increased serum parathyroid hormone
- Impaired regulation of osteoblast activity

- Impaired bone formation secondary to reduced osteoblastic production of bone matrix
- Fewer functional marrow cells resulting from replacement of marrow with fat cells
- Decreased estrogen in women and testosterone in men

Muscles

Skeletal muscles, which are controlled by motor neurons, directly affect all activities of daily living (ADLs).

Age-related changes that have the greatest impact on muscle function include:

- Decreased size and number of muscle fibers
- Loss of motor neurons
- Replacement of muscle tissue by connective tissue and, eventually, by fat tissue
- Deterioration of muscle cell membranes and a subsequent escape of fluid and potassium
- Diminished protein synthesis

Joints and Connective Tissue

Numerous age-related changes affect all musculoskeletal joints, including non–weight-bearing joints. In contrast to the bones or muscles, which benefit from exercise, the joints are harmed by continued use and begin to show the effects of wear and tear during early adulthood. In fact, degenerative processes begin to affect the tendons, ligaments, and synovial fluid during early adulthood, even before skeletal maturity is reached.

Some of the most significant age-related joint changes include the following:

- Diminished viscosity of synovial fluid
- Degeneration of collagen and elastin cells
- Fragmentation of fibrous structures in connective tissue
- Outgrowths of cartilaginous clusters because of continuous wear and tear
- Formation of scar tissue and areas of calcification in the joint capsules and connective tissue
- Degenerative changes in the articular cartilage resulting in extensive fraying, cracking, and shredding, in addition to a pitted and thinned surface

Consequences of these changes include impaired flexion and extension, diminished protection from forces of movement, and degeneration of the underlying bones.

Nervous System

Diminished muscle function in older adults is strongly influenced by age-related changes in the central and peripheral nervous system. For example, an effect of the age-related delayed reaction time is that older adults walk more slowly and are less able to respond in a timely manner to environmental stimuli. Maintenance of balance in an upright position is affected by the following age-related changes of the nervous system: altered visual abilities, a slower righting reflex, impaired proprioception, and diminished vibratory and positioning sensations in the lower extremities. In addition, age-related changes in postural control cause an increase in **body sway**, which is a measure of the motion of the body while standing.

OSTEOPENIA AND OSTEOPOROSIS

Loss of bone mass affects all adults as they age; however, the extent to which it occurs is affected by many variables. **Bone density** (i.e., the amount of calcium and other minerals in a bone segment) is routinely evaluated in older adults. Bone density is scored according to standard deviations (SD) below that of healthy 30-year-old adults of the same race and sex, called a *T-score*. A normal T-score is between −1 and +1. When a T-score is between −1 and −2.5, the diagnosis is **osteopenia**; when a T-score is lower than this, the diagnosis is **osteoporosis**. Osteoporosis is considered a "silent disease" because it is usually asymptomatic until a fracture occurs with little or no trauma, which is called a **fragility fracture** (it can also be called an osteoporotic fracture). As osteoporosis progresses, it can cause pain, loss of height, and increased risk of fractures. With osteoporosis, the risk for fracture doubles for each T-score decrease of one point (Geusens & van den Berg, 2016).

Prevalence of osteoporosis increases with age in both men and women, but it begins at an earlier age in women and accelerates during menopause (Stathopoulos, Zoubos, Papaioannou, et al., 2016). Although osteoporosis has been recognized as a common condition among postmenopausal women for many decades, only in recent decades has it been recognized as a condition that affects men also. This increased attention is warranted because 50% of women and up to 25% of men aged 50 years and older will have a fracture due to osteoporosis, which causes an estimated 2 million fractures every year (National Osteoporosis Foundation, 2016).

Both men and women reach peak bone mass during their mid-30s, then gender differences begin to account for the relatively higher rate of osteoporosis among women compared with men. In men, bone loss occurs steadily at about 1% per year after peak bone mass has been reached. In contrast, women experience an annual rate of bone loss of up to 7% during menopausal years, followed by 1% to 2% during postmenopausal years. In summary, osteoporosis occurs in both men and women, but women have a much greater percentage of bone loss over their lifetime and experience greater bone loss at an earlier age.

> **◈ Diversity Note**
>
> Because of osteoporotic changes, women have a higher incidence of fractures than men at any given age (Shanbhogue, Brixen, & Hansen, 2016).

 RISK FACTORS THAT AFFECT SAFE MOBILITY

Risk factors affect overall musculoskeletal function and safe mobility, with additional risk factors contributing to increased incidence of osteoporosis, fractures, and falls. Health promotion interventions can alleviate many risks and prevent the serious functional consequences associated with falls and fractures.

Risk Factors That Affect Overall Musculoskeletal Function

Low level of physical activity (i.e., lack of exercise) is the most commonly occurring risk in all older adults, ranging from healthy older adults to those who are frail or seriously ill. This is particularly pertinent to health promotion because interventions to improve physical activity in older adults have extensive benefits, not only for improving overall musculoskeletal function and preventing falls and fractures but also for many other aspects of functioning, as discussed in Chapter 5 as a focus of health promotion.

Nutritional deficits are important risk factors for diminished overall musculoskeletal performance and risk for falls and fractures. Adequate dietary intake of calcium is strongly associated not only with prevention of fractures but also with healthy overall musculoskeletal function. Protein and vitamin D deficiencies are associated with **sarcopenia** (i.e., age-related loss of muscle mass) and increased risk for frailty and falls (Bruyere, Cavalier, Buckinx, et al., 2017; Oh, Jeon, Reid Storm, et al., 2017).

Wellness Opportunity

Many lifestyle, environmental, and other modifiable factors can be addressed to improve overall musculoskeletal function and prevent falls and fractures in older adults.

Risk Factors for Osteoporosis and Fragility Fractures

In addition to risks that affect overall musculoskeletal function, some conditions increase the risk for osteoporosis and fragility fractures, as listed in Box 22-1. Although some risk

---

 Box 22-1 Risk Factors for Osteoporosis and Fragility Fractures

Factors That Increase the Risk for Osteoporosis

- Age 65 or 70 years or older for women and men, respectively
- Inadequate physical activity, especially weight-bearing and muscle-strengthening exercises
- Family history of osteoporosis or fragility fracture
- Low calcium intake, both past and current
- Vitamin D deficiency
- Hormonal deficiency
- Cigarette smoking (active or passive)
- Excessive alcohol intake
- Pathologic conditions (e.g., endocrine disorders, inflammatory conditions, malabsorption syndromes)
- Medications (e.g., corticosteroids, anticonvulsants, anticoagulants, aromatase inhibitors, selective serotonin reuptake inhibitors, proton pump inhibitors)

Risk Factors for Fragility Fracture, in Addition to Risks for Osteoporosis

- Postmenopausal status for women
- 75 years or older for men
- Female sex
- Previous fragility fracture
- Undertreatment of osteoporosis
- Low body mass index
- Falls
- Rheumatoid arthritis

Unfolding Case Study

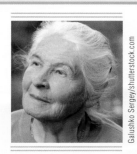

Galushko Sergey/shutterstock.com

Part 1: Ms. M. at 61 Years of Age

Ms. M. is 61 years old and works as the secretary in the Senior Circle of Care program where you conduct health screening and educational programs. This senior wellness program is sponsored by one of the nonprofit hospitals in Minneapolis, Minnesota. Ms. M.'s responsibilities include finding and organizing health education materials under the direction of the nurses. You often go to lunch with her and discuss social and health-related topics. Ms. M. has always been inquisitive about health-related concerns, and one day she asks your advice about osteoporosis. She says that both she and her mother, who is 83 years old, have been receiving flyers about getting a bone density test and that her mother asked if she would go with her so that they could both be tested. You know from past conversations that Ms. M.'s mother fractured her wrist when she was in her 60s, but otherwise is relatively healthy. Ms. M. is fairly healthy, although she admits that she "could stand to lose a little weight and get more exercise." You also know from previous discussions that Ms. M. had been using hormonal replacement therapy for several years but discontinued this last year. In your work as a wellness nurse, you have developed and presented several health education programs about osteoporosis so you are familiar with recent literature on osteoporosis.

THINKING POINTS

- Based on what you know about Ms. M., what would you tell her about her risk factors for osteoporosis?
- Based on what you know about Ms. M.'s mother, what additional information would you want to know before advising her about a test for her mother?

- What suggestions would you make to help Ms. M. become more knowledgeable about osteoporosis?

factors, such as age, ethnicity, and family history, cannot be changed, other conditions can be addressed through health promotion interventions. Current emphasis is on modifiable risk factors, including low level of weight-bearing activity, cigarette smoking, excessive alcohol consumption, and nutritional deficits. For example, a low serum level of vitamin D, a condition that can be readily treated, is associated with increased risk for osteoporosis and fractures (Gorter, Krijnen, & Schipper, 2016; Malgo, Appleman-Dijkstra, Termaat, et al., 2016). When medications or pathologic conditions are a primary underlying cause, the condition is referred to as secondary osteoporosis. Osteoporosis in up to 30% of postmenopausal women and 50% of men may have an underlying, and potentially treatable, cause (Sheu & Diamond, 2016). Guidelines recommend that older adults with risk factors, including the medications listed in Box 22-1, be monitored more frequently and treated (as appropriate) for osteoporosis (Hant & Bolster, 2016).

In recent years, there is increasing attention on identifying risks for fragility fractures and preventing fall-related injuries. In particular, a major focus of hospital quality and safety initiatives is the prevention of serious injuries that result from in-hospital falls in medical and postsurgical patients. Conditions that increase the risk for fragility fractures are listed in Box 22-1. It is imperative to consider that a combination of risk factors significantly increases the risk for fragility fractures.

Diversity Note

Analysis of 4301 falls in men and women aged 60 and over concluded that risk factors varied by sex. For women, frailty and incontinence were associated with increased risk for falls; for men, older age, higher levels of depressive symptoms, and inability to perform a standing balance test were associated with increased risk for falls (Gale, Cooper, & Sayer, 2016).

▶ RISK FACTORS FOR FALLS

Falling is unfortunately very common among older adults and it has been the focus of much attention in the United States and many other countries for decades. More than a half century ago, an article titled "On the Natural History of Falls in Old Age" began with the following declaration: "The liability of old people to tumble and often to injure themselves is such a commonplace of experience that it has been tacitly accepted as an inevitable aspect of aging, and thereby deprived of the exercise of curiosity" (Sheldon, 1960, p. 1685). In recent years, geriatricians and gerontologists have challenged this view that falls are a normal consequence of aging or are accidental or random events. There is now wide agreement that falls and mobility problems result from multiple, diverse, and interacting risk factors. The current clinical approach is to identify the most likely causes and contributing conditions and to plan interventions to prevent

falls. Current emphasis also is on reducing the harm when falls do occur.

Numerous studies have been published about risks for falls, with increasing attention to risks associated with different settings, such as acute care, long-term care, and community-based residences. A consistent research finding across all settings is that falls are the result of a combination of risk factors, rather than any one condition. Moreover, the risk for falls increases in proportion to the number of fall risk factors. An additional focus is on preventing serious fall-related injuries, such as fractures and traumatic brain injury, which occur in one out of five falls (Centers for Disease Control and Prevention, 2016). Risk factors for falls can be categorized according to their origin as intrinsic or extrinsic, as discussed in the following sections and summarized in Box 22-2.

Box 22-2 Risk Factors for Falls

Pathologic Conditions and Functional Impairments

- Age-related conditions (e.g., nocturia, osteoporosis, gait changes, postural hypotension, sensory deficits)
- Cardiovascular diseases (e.g., arrhythmias or myocardial infarction)
- Respiratory diseases (e.g., chronic obstructive pulmonary disease)
- Neurologic disorders (e.g., parkinsonism, cerebrovascular accident)
- Metabolic disturbances (e.g., dehydration, electrolyte imbalances)
- Musculoskeletal problems (e.g., osteoarthritis)
- Transient ischemic attack
- Vision impairments (e.g., cataracts, glaucoma, macular degeneration)
- Cognitive impairments (e.g., dementia, confusion)
- Psychosocial factors (e.g., depression, anxiety, agitation)

***Adverse Effects of Prescription
or Over-the-Counter Medications***

- Anticholinergics
- Anticonvulsants
- Antidepressants
- Antihistamines
- Antihypertensives
- Antipsychotics
- Benzodiazepines
- Diuretics
- Insulin and oral hypoglycemics
- Narcotics
- Sedative hypnotics
- Systemic glucocorticoids

Environmental Factors

- Inadequate lighting
- Lack of handrails on stairs
- Slippery floors
- Throw rugs
- Clutter, cords, or other objects in the walking path
- Unfamiliar environments
- Highly polished floors
- Improper height of beds, chairs, or toilets
- Physical restraints

Intrinsic Conditions

Older adults commonly experience conditions that increase the risk for falls including all the following: nocturia, sleep problems, gait changes, orthostatic hypotension, decreased muscle strength, and central nervous system changes. In addition, vision impairment is an independent risk for falls in older adults because of its effects on mobility, balance, safety, fear of falling, and ability to perform daily activities. In general, commonly occurring pathologic conditions can increase the risk for falls in older adults in all of the following ways:

- Pathologic conditions can cause functional impairments that affect vision, balance, or mobility.
- Pathologic conditions may be treated with medications that create risks for falling.
- Chronic conditions often interfere with optimal exercise and other health practices that are important in promoting safe mobility.

Depression and cognitive impairments can increase the risk for falls, especially in combination with other risk factors. For example, both dementia and depression diminish one's awareness of the environment and can interfere with the ability to process information about environmental stimuli. Depressed older adults are at increased risk for falls secondary to gait changes, adverse medication effects, and a diminished ability to concentrate on and respond to environmental factors. Considering these possible associations, it is not surprising that most falls resulting in injuries occur in people who have functional impairments and multiple, chronic medical problems.

Adverse Effects of Medications

For decades, numerous studies have identified an association between adverse effects of prescription and over-the-counter medications and increased risk for falls. The term fall risk–increasing drugs refers to medications that are strongly associated with increased risk for recurrent falls. Medications containing anticholinergic ingredients have been consistently identified as fall risk–increasing drugs (Marcum, Wirtz, Pettinger, et al., 2016). It is important to recognize that many nonprescription products for sleep, colds and allergies contain diphenhydramine, which has strong anticholinergic effects that can impair psychomotor skills necessary for safe mobility. Polypharmacy (discussed in Chapter 8) has been associated with an increased risk of recurrent and injurious falls, with current emphasis on the use of two or more fall risk–increasing drugs rather than the overall number of drugs (Zia, Kamaruzzaman, & Tan, 2016).

In addition to identifying medications associated with increased risk for falls, it is important to recognize adverse medication effects associated with fall-related injuries. For example, anticoagulant medications, which are commonly used for stroke prevention, increase the risk for serious bleeding if a fall occurs. Some medications that are likely to increase the risk for falls are listed in Box 22-2.

Environmental Factors

Some environmental hazards were discussed in Chapter 7 in relation to safety, but additional environmental influences must be considered specifically in relation to falls. In health care settings, for example, falls are most likely to occur in the bedroom and bathroom. In the bedroom, most falls occur while the person is getting in or out of bed, and some falls are related to climbing over siderails or footboards. In the bathroom, falls generally occur while transferring on or off toilet seats or while hurrying to urinate or defecate. In community settings, most falls occur in the home, particularly in stairways, bedrooms, and living rooms. Environmental hazards that increase the risk for falls in homes include clutter, poor lighting, and lack of handrails on stairs or grab bars in bathrooms.

Physical Restraints

A physical restraint is any device, method, or equipment that immobilizes or reduces the ability of the patient to move his or her arms, legs, body, or head freely. Examples of physical restraints are belts, hand mitts, soft wrist or leg restraints, certain types of chairs, and full siderails in certain circumstances. Prior to the 1990s, the use of physical restraints in health care settings was viewed as a protective mechanism for preventing falls, reducing staff workload, and shielding an institution from liability. In recent decades, however, there has been mounting evidence that the use of physical restraints is not effective for fall prevention and in fact is associated with substantial risk of serious injury or fatality (Bradas, Sandhu, & Mion, 2016). Currently, the use of physical restraints is an indicator of quality of care in health care settings, and health care organizations are implementing major initiatives to limit or eliminate the use of any restrictive devices. Agencies that have promoted evidence-based recommendations related to reduction of restraints include the American Nurses Association, the American Geriatrics Society, the British Geriatrics Society, the U.S. Food and Drug Administration (FDA), the Centers for Medicare and Medicaid Services (CMS), and the Joint Commission (previously known as the Joint Commission on Accreditation of Healthcare Organizations).

 Interprofessional Collaboration

Reducing the use of restraints in health care settings requires a comprehensive interprofessional approach that includes staff education, organizational strategies, and interventions to improve physical and cognitive function of patients (Bradas, Sandhu, & Mion, 2016). In addition to the fall-prevention interventions discussed in this chapter, interventions for management of behaviors caused by dementia and delirium are pertinent to restraint reduction, as discussed in Chapter 14. Ethical considerations related to physical restraints are discussed in Chapter 9.

Unfolding Case Study

Part 2: Ms. M. at 67 Years of Age

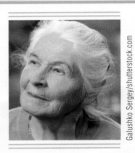

Galushko Sergey/shutterstock.com

Ms. M. is now 67 years old and has retired from her secretarial job. She attends weekly social and lunch gatherings at the local senior center, where you are the wellness nurse. One day she comes to the center with a cast on her left wrist and reports that she fractured her wrist when she slipped and fell on ice in her driveway. Ms. M. stopped taking hormonal therapy several years ago because she had been taking it for 10 years and was concerned about long-term effects. You also know that she takes medications for arthritis, hypertension, and depression and that she self-monitors her blood pressure. In the past 10 years, she has gradually gained "a little weight every year" and her current height/weight is 5'3"/175 pounds, which is a BMI of 31. She participates in the weekly "mall walkers" exercise program but rarely exercises independently. She says that "my housework is enough exercise" and that the weekly group exercise activity is "as much as my arthritis will tolerate." She lives in a small one-floor house. Although Ms. M. says she is not really concerned about sustaining any more fractures because she views the recent fall as a "fluke of bad winter luck," she makes an appointment to talk with you. During the appointment, she reports that she is a "little concerned about osteoporosis."

THINKING POINTS

- What risk factors for osteoporosis can you identify from what you already know about Ms. M.?
- What risk factors for falls and fall-related injuries can you identify from what you already know about Ms. M.?
- Can you identify any factors that reduce her risk for falls or fractures?

- What additional information about Ms. M. would be helpful in identifying additional risks for osteoporosis?
- What additional information would be helpful in identifying additional risks for falls and fractures?

QSEN APPLICATION

QSEN Competency	Knowledge/Skill/Attitude	Application to Ms. M. at 67 Years
Patient-centered care	(K) Integrate understanding of multiple dimensions of patient-centered care	Identify Ms. M.'s risks for fractures
	(K) Describe strategies to empower patients in all aspects of the health care process	Identify positive aspects of Ms. M.'s lifestyle so you can build on these when teaching about health promotion strategies
	(K) Examine common barriers to active involvement of patients in their own health care processes	Address Ms. M.'s lack of knowledge about osteoporosis and prevention of fragility fractures
Evidence-based practice	(K) Describe how the strength and relevance of available evidence influence the choice of intervention	Apply evidence-based information from Box 22-1 to assess risks for osteoporosis and fragility fractures and teach Ms. M. about prevention of fragility fractures
	(S) Base individualized care plan on patient values, clinical expertise, and evidence	

 GLOBAL PERSPECTIVE

The World Health Organization considers the use of physical restraints a human rights issue. Physical restraints are rarely used in geriatric care settings in the United Kingdom; however, this practice is common in many countries. In Spain a major initiative using "dementia champions" was successful in reducing the use of restraints through staff education (Muniz, Gomez, Curto, et al., 2016).

 FUNCTIONAL CONSEQUENCES AFFECTING MUSCULOSKELETAL WELLNESS

Older adults can partially compensate for age-related changes that affect overall musculoskeletal function through health promotion interventions, such as good nutrition and physical activity. The functional consequences of osteoporosis, however, are quite serious, as are the functional consequences that result from the many risk factors that contribute to falls and fractures in older adults. As with many other aspects of function in older adulthood, cumulative and interacting effects of risk factors rather than age-related changes most significantly affect function and quality of life.

Effects on Overall Musculoskeletal Function

Muscle strength, endurance, and coordination are affected to some extent by age-related changes, even in the absence of risk factors. Beginning around the age of 40 years, muscle strength declines gradually, resulting in an overall decrease of 30% to 50% by the age of 80 years, with a greater decline in muscle strength in the lower extremities than in the upper extremities. In addition, a person's current level of activity and lifelong patterns of exercise can influence muscle strength at any age. Muscle endurance and coordination diminish as a result of age-related changes in the muscles and central nervous system. Because of these changes, older adults experience muscle fatigue after shorter periods of exercise compared with their younger counterparts.

Joint function begins to decline during early adulthood and progresses gradually to cause the following changes in range of motion:

- Decreased range of motion in the upper arms
- Decreased lower back flexion
- Decreased external rotation of the hip
- Decreased hip and knee flexion
- Decreased dorsiflexion of the foot

These changes result in slowed performance of daily activities, such as writing, eating, grooming, and putting shoes and socks on; difficulty climbing stairs and curbs; and an overall diminished ability to respond to environmental stimuli.

Gait changes, which differ in men and women, are one of the more noticeable functional consequences that occur after the age of 75 years. Older women develop a narrower standing and walking gait and bowlegged-type changes that affect the lower extremities and alter the angle of the hip. Older men develop a wider walking and standing gait, characterized by less arm swing, a shorter stride, decreased steppage height, and a more flexed position of the head and trunk than when they were younger. The overall impact of these changes is that older men and women have a slower walking speed and spend more time in the support phase of gait than in the swing phase. It is important to note that any significant gait changes that occur are not due to aging alone but are consequences of other conditions, such as osteoarthritis or neurologic disorders (e.g., dementia, Parkinson disease).

Susceptibility to Falls and Fractures

The combination of age-related changes and multiple interacting risk factors doubly jeopardizes older adults by increasing the probability of both falls and fractures. Fractures are not unique to older adults, but they differ in many respects from those that occur in younger populations. First, fragility fractures occur with little or no trauma, for example, from an impact that is no more severe than that which results from falling to the floor from a standing position. Second, the risk of fractures increases in direct relation to age. Third, fractures and fall-related injuries in older adults are likely to have serious and long-term consequences affecting level of functioning, quality of life, and morbidity and mortality. For example, hip fractures are associated with significant functional decline, long-term disability, permanent admissions to long-term care facilities, and high mortality rates during the first year postfracture (Meehan, Hommel, Hertz, et al., 2016).

Fear of Falling

Since the early 1990s, there has been increasing attention to **fear of falling**, which is excessive anxiety about falling that leads to activity avoidance and decline in functioning. Up to three-fourths of older adults in long-term care and community settings express fear of falling, with increased prevalence associated with the following characteristics:

- Female sex
- Older age
- History of falls
- History of stroke or hip fracture
- Hearing or vision impairment
- Impaired functioning, particularly regarding balance and gait status
- Dependency in activities of daily living
- Poor self-rated health
- Symptoms of depression
- Use of seven or more medications

(Goh, Nadarajah, Hamzah, et al. 2016; Hoang, Jullamate, Piphatvanitcha, et al., 2016; Malini, Lourenco, & Lopes, 2016; Moriera Bde, Dos Anjos, Pereira, et al., 2016; Palagyi, Ng, Rogers, et al., 2016). Functional consequences of fear of falling include increased dependency, activity restrictions, functional decline, social isolation, and increased risk for falling. In addition, fear of falling, which is associated with poorer function recovery after a hip fracture, is a modifiable condition that can be addressed to improve functional outcomes (Auais, Alvarado, Curcio, et al., 2016; Bower, Wetherell, Petkus, et al., 2016).

Diversity Note

A study of community-dwelling Mexican Americans between the ages of 72 and 96 found that those who did not speak English or did not understand spoken English had a higher rate of fear of falling than their English-speaking counterparts (James, Conatser, Karabulut, et al., 2016).

Wellness Opportunity

Nurses respect older adults' autonomy and involve them in decisions by creatively finding ways to ensure safety while also allowing as much freedom of movement as possible.

PATHOLOGIC CONDITION AFFECTING MUSCULOSKELETAL FUNCTION: OSTEOARTHRITIS

Osteoarthritis is a degenerative inflammatory disease affecting joints and attached muscles, tendons, and ligaments; it is characterized by pain, swelling, and limited movement in joints. A leading cause of disability in the United States, osteoarthritis affects older adults disproportionately. Osteoarthritis is a complex disease process that results from the interplay of risk factors such as genetics, obesity, and age-related changes. Current research emphasizes the importance of addressing osteoporosis and osteoarthritis as treatable conditions that increase the risk for falls and fractures (Geusens & van den Bergh, 2016).

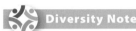
Diversity Note

Whites and African Americans have similar rates of osteoarthritis, but African Americans have a higher rate of osteoarthritis-related activity limitation.

Because self-care is an important aspect of managing osteoarthritis, nurses focus on health education interventions. Nurses can encourage participation in self-management programs, which are effective for managing pain and preventing disability associated with osteoarthritis (Baruth, Wilcox, McClenaghan, et al., 2016). In addition, nurses can teach people with osteoarthritis about the following evidence-based self-care practices:

- Participate in a variety of aerobic, resistance, and strengthening exercise programs (e.g., yoga, aquatherapy, tai chi)
- Avoid high-impact activities
- Wear sturdy, shock-absorbing shoes
- Pace activities with rest periods
- Maintain ideal weight
- Use orthotics, supports, brace, or shoe inserts as appropriate
- Use canes, walkers, and other assistive devices as appropriate to relieve weight-bearing joints, improve balance, or achieve independent functioning
- Use moist heat and analgesics for pain

Care plans for managing osteoarthritis are most effective when they are based on an interdisciplinary approach that includes medicine, nursing, and rehabilitation therapies. Nurses emphasize the importance of obtaining regular medical care for ongoing evaluation and management as the condition progresses and as new treatments are developed. An important nursing role is facilitating referrals to physical and occupational therapists to improve muscle strength and promote safe and independent functioning. Online Learning Activity 22-1 provides links to reliable sources of information about physical activity and self-management interventions for people with arthritis.

See ONLINE LEARNING ACTIVITY 22-1: ADDITIONAL INFORMATION ABOUT SELF-MANAGEMENT FOR PEOPLE WITH ARTHRITIS at http://thepoint.lww.com/Miller8e.

Wellness Opportunity

Older adults with osteoarthritis need to engage in self-care activities, including making responsible decisions about promoting optimal comfort and functioning.

NURSING ASSESSMENT OF MUSCULOSKELETAL FUNCTION

Nursing assessment of musculoskeletal function focuses on identifying risks for falls, fractures, and osteoporosis, with attention to those factors that can be modified or alleviated through nursing interventions. Nurses can use a fall risk assessment tool to identify older adults who might benefit from appropriate preventive interventions.

Assessing Musculoskeletal Performance

Assessment of overall musculoskeletal performance begins with observation of the person's mobility and activities. In addition to watching the person walk, it is especially important to observe the person getting up from a chair. The Timed Up and Go (TUG) test is an evidence-based and simple-to-use tool for assessing gait speed and balance that has been widely used since the early 1990s in the United States and other countries to identify older adults who may be at increased risk for fractures (Chun, Cho, Yang, et al., 2017). This test is a reliable measure of gait speed, as well as an indicator of fall risk and ability to safely perform ADLs. The TUG, which is illustrated in Figure 22-1, can be administered in 5 minutes or less and it can be used repeatedly to identify declines or improvements over time. Higher scores (i.e., longer time to complete the tasks) are associated with increased risk for falls. A score of 12 seconds or more is the most evidence-based measure to determine risk of future falls in community settings (Lusardi, Fritz, Middleton, et al., 2017). One review of studies cites the mean performance score increasing from 8.6 seconds for "apparently healthy" older adults aged 65 to 75 to 17.2 seconds for those aged 85 and over (Benavent-Caballer, Sendin-Magdalena, Lison, et al., 2016). Before administering this test, it is important to explain and demonstrate the procedure and have the person wear regular footwear and use usual assistive devices.

See ONLINE LEARNING ACTIVITY 22-2: VIDEO AND ADDITIONAL RESOURCES RELATED TO THE TIMED UP AND GO AND OTHER ASSESSMENT TOOLS at http://thepoint.lww.com/Miller8e.

Assessment information also is obtained by asking questions about the person's ability to perform ADLs, as

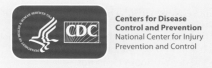

Patient: _____   Date: _____   Time: _____   AM/PM

The Timed Up and Go (TUG) Test

Purpose: To assess mobility

Equipment: A stopwatch

Directions: Patients wear their regular footwear and can use a walking aid if needed. Begin by having the patient sit back in a standard arm chair and identify a line 3 meters or 10 feet away on the floor.

> **Instructions to the patient:**
> When I say **"Go,"** I want you to:
> 1. Stand up from the chair
> 2. Walk to the line on the floor at your normal pace
> 3. Turn
> 4. Walk back to the chair at your normal pace
> 5. Sit down again

On the word **"Go"** begin timing.

Stop timing after patient has sat back down and record.

Time: _____ **seconds**

An older adult who takes ≥12 seconds to complete the TUG is at high risk for falling.

> Observe the patient's postural stability, gait, stride length, and sway.
>
> **Circle all that apply:** ■ Slow tentative pace ■ Loss of balance ■ Short strides ■ Little or no arm swing ■ Steadying self on walls ■ Shuffling ■ En bloc turning ■ Not using assistive device properly
>
> Notes:

For relevant articles, go to: **www.cdc.gov/injury/STEADI**

Centers for Disease Control and Prevention National Center for Injury Prevention and Control

STEADI Stopping Elderly Accidents, Deaths & Injuries

FIGURE 22-1 The Timed Up and Go (TUG) test. (Reprinted from the CDC; http://www.cdc.gov/homeandrecreationalsafety/pdf/steadi/timed_up_and_go_test.pdf.)

discussed in Chapter 7. When limitations are identified, it is important to find out whether the older adult is using assistive devices to improve safety, mobility, balance, independence, or overall function. If the person is not using such devices—and may benefit from them—it is important to assess the person's knowledge about the availability of such devices. It also is important to assess the person's attitude

about using assistive devices because attitudes are likely to influence the acceptability of using recommended aids.

In addition to experiencing minor changes in performing ADLs, older adults experience diminished height and changes in posture. Older adults may or may not be concerned about or aware of a loss of height; however, a loss of about 2 to 4 cm per decade is normal, owing to osteoporosis and other age-related changes. Including a question about the person's usual height and any noticeable loss of height will give the nurse an opportunity to assess the older adult's awareness of this change. Although the functional consequences of decreased height are minimal, older people who never were very tall may experience increased difficulty performing activities that depend on height. In these situations, they may find that it is safer and more effective to use assistive devices, such as long-handled reachers. They may also need encouragement to rearrange cupboards so that the most frequently used items are accessible. Another assessment implication of decreased height is that the pants legs of older adult's clothing may be too long, especially if the person also has lost weight. Therefore, nurses observe whether the length of pants legs increases the risk for falls because this risk can be alleviated through relatively simple interventions. Box 22-3 summarizes guidelines for assessing overall musculoskeletal performance in older adults.

Identifying Risks for Osteoporosis

Nurses assess risks for osteoporosis (listed in Box 22-1) in all older adults, with emphasis on factors that can be addressed through health promotion interventions, such as adequate intake of calcium and vitamin D and participation in regular weight-bearing exercise. Nurses also identify modifiable risk factors, such as smoking and drinking excessive amounts of alcohol, that can be alleviated through lifestyle interventions. Nurses obtain much of the information regarding risks for osteoporosis during an overall assessment or health history, and they consider this information in relation to mobility and safety. See Box 22-3 for assessment questions and considerations relating to osteoporosis.

Wellness Opportunity

From a wellness perspective, nurses ask older adults to identify enjoyable ways of engaging in physical activities that improve strength and balance.

Identifying Risks for Falls and Injury

Identifying fall risks is an essential and interprofessional aspect of health care for all older adults because it is imperative to initiate preventive interventions. The best assessment information is obtained by observing the

---

Box 22-3 Guidelines for Assessing Overall Musculoskeletal Function and Risks for Falls, Osteoporosis, and Fragility Fractures

Questions to Assess Overall Musculoskeletal Performance

- Do you have any trouble performing your usual activities because of joint limitations?
- Do you have any pain or discomfort in your joints?
- Do you ever feel like you are losing your balance?
- Do you have any trouble walking or getting around?
- Do you use any assistive devices (e.g., a walker, quad cane, or reaching devices) to help you do things?

Questions to Assess Risks for Osteoporosis and Fragility Fractures

Questions to Ask All Older Adults

- Do you know of any blood relatives who have had osteoporosis or who have sustained fractures late in life?
- Have you sustained any fractures during your adult years? (If yes, ask additional questions regarding age at the time, type, location, circumstances, treatment, and so on.)
- What is your usual intake of foods high in calcium and vitamin D and do you take any supplements?
- Have you ever had your bone density measured?
  - ◆ Do you take any medications for prevention or management of osteoporosis?
- If you have osteoporosis have you ever talked with your primary care practitioner about prevention of fractures?

Questions to Assess Risk for Falls and Fear of Falling

- Have you had any falls in the past few years? (If yes, ask additional questions about the circumstances and ask about pertinent risk factors as summarized in Box 22-2.)
- Do you have any concerns about falling? (If yes, ask additional questions about specific fears, such as *What do you think might happen if you were to fall?*)
  - ◆ Do you take any precautions to prevent falls?

- Are there any activities you would like to do, but do not do, because of any difficulty moving or getting around? (If yes, ask about specific activities, such as shopping, using public transportation, etc.)
- Are there any activities you would like to do, but do not do, because you are afraid of falling? (If yes, ask about specific activities, such as going up or down stairs, taking a bath or shower, etc.)

Observations Regarding Overall Musculoskeletal Performance

- Measure and record the person's present height and stated peak height.
- Observe the individual's walking and gait pattern.
- Use the Timed Up and Go test (Figure 22-1).

Information From the Overall Assessment That Is Also Useful in Assessing Musculoskeletal Function

- Observe and document a functional assessment, as described in Chapter 7.
- How much exercise does the person get on a regular basis? In particular, how much weight-bearing exercise?
- Does the person smoke cigarettes?
- How much alcohol does the person consume?
- What is the person's usual daily intake of calcium and vitamin D?
- Does the person have any medical conditions that are associated with falls or osteoporosis (as summarized in Boxes 22-1 and 22-2)?
- Is the person taking any prescription or over-the-counter medications that might create risks for falls?
- Does the person have postural hypotension?
- Is the person moderately or seriously visually impaired?
- Does the person have any cognitive impairments or other psychosocial impairments (e.g., depression) that diminish his or her attention to the environment or interfere with the ability to respond to environmental stimuli?

person in his or her environment and paying attention to the person's awareness of and attention to unsafe conditions. Observations also provide information about adaptive behaviors that otherwise might not be acknowledged. For example, a person might state that he or she has no difficulty with stair climbing, but observations might reveal that the person performs this activity in a highly unsafe manner. When nurses do not have the opportunity to observe home environments directly, they can observe the person in the immediate environment and ask the person or caregivers about the older adult's ability to function safely in that setting. They can also consider referrals to home care agencies for home assessment as part of the discharge plan.

Another important aspect of assessing the environment in any setting is identifying the factors that are likely to cause serious injury if a fall does occur. For example, stationary objects such as bathroom sinks or heavy wooden furniture can cause serious head injuries if someone falls near the object. The guidelines summarized in Chapter 7 can be used to assess the safety of any environment and can be applied to all older adults, particularly those who have intrinsic risk factors for falls.

Important assessment information can be obtained simply by asking all older adults about any falls they have experienced during the past year. Box 22-3 includes assessment questions that are applicable to older adults who are independent or relatively independent.

Wellness Opportunity

Whenever possible, nurses actively involve the older adult and family members in identifying environmental factors that either support or create risks for safe mobility.

Many **fall risk assessment tools** are used to identify people who are at risk for falls so that preventive measures can be implemented. In addition to using the TUG (as already discussed), nurses can informally assess gait and balance by observing the person's usual walking pattern, paying particular attention to any gait or balance unsteadiness or unusual patterns. If any abnormalities are noted, nurses can facilitate referrals for further evaluation by a physical therapist. Evidence-based fall risk assessment tools, such as the Hendrich II Fall Risk Model (Figure 22-2), are widely used in health care settings to identify and document patients who have increased risks for falls. Online Learning Activity 22-3 provides additional information and links to fall risk assessment tools that are commonly used by nurses in various settings. Assessment questions aimed at identifying fear of falling and related negative functional consequences are included in Box 22-3.

Although fall risk assessment tools are useful in identifying people who are at high risk for falls, they do not address the underlying conditions. When older adults have several risk factors or have already had fall-related injuries, a comprehensive fall assessment should be performed in a multidisciplinary setting, such as a geriatric assessment program. A comprehensive fall assessment addresses all the following: mental status, nutrition, environment, medications, pathologic conditions, functional assessment, usual footwear, and a complete physical examination (including visual acuity, musculoskeletal function, neurologic function, and cardiovascular status).

Assessing Fear of Falling and Falls Risk Awareness

Because fear of falling (not just actually falling) has negative functional consequences, nurses include at least one question about fear of falling in any assessment of falls and fall risk. If the older person expresses a fear of falling, it is important to ask additional questions in relation to specific activities that may be associated with fear of falling. If the older person relies on family or other caregivers for assistance, it is important to assess caregiver concerns and observations. The Falls Efficacy Scale is an evidence-based tool that has been used since 1990 to measure fear of falling. The Falls Efficacy Scale-International is currently used in community settings in Europe and North America to identify concerns about falling in the context of engaging in usual activities (Figueirdo & Santos, 2017; Greenberg, Sullivan-Marx, Sommers, et al., 2016). This tool is recommended by the Hartford Institute for Geriatric Nursing, as described in Online Learning Activity 22-3.

It is important to recognize that fear of falling, which is associated with negative functional consequences, differs from self-awareness of risk for falls, which is a characteristic that can be protective. For example, the Falls Risk Awareness Questionnaire has been used in acute care settings to help patients identify their risks for falls so targeted fall-prevention interventions can be implemented (Sitzer, 2016). In community settings, self-assessment of risks for falls is an important and integral part of fall-prevention programs, as discussed in the section on Interventions in Community-Based Settings.

See **ONLINE LEARNING ACTIVITY 22-3: ADDITIONAL INFORMATION ABOUT FALL RISK ASSESSMENT TOOLS at http://thepoint.lww.com/Miller8e.**

Wellness Opportunity

Nurses can use the nursing diagnosis Readiness for Enhanced Self-Health Management for healthy older adults who are willing to explore opportunities for improving musculoskeletal function and preventing falls and fractures.

Hendrich II Fall Risk Model

RISK FACTOR	RISK POINTS	SCORE
Confusion/Disorientation/Impulsivity	4	
Symptomatic Depression	2	
Altered Elimination	1	
Dizziness/Vertigo	1	
Gender (Male)	1	
Any Administered Antiepileptics (Anticonvulsants): (Carbamazepine, Divalproex Sodium, Ethotoin, Ethosuximide, Felbamate, Fosphenytoin, Gabapentin, Lamotrigine, Mephenytoin, Methsuximide, Phenobarbital, Phenytoin, Primidone, Topiramate, Trimethadione, Valproic Acid)[1]	2	
Any Administered Benzodiazepines[2]: (Alprazolam, Chloridiazepoxide, Clonazepam, Clorazepate Dipotassium, Diazepam, Flurazepam, Halazepam,[3] Lorazepam, Midozolam, Oxazepam, Temazepam, Triazolam)	1	
Get-Up-and-Go Test: "Rising from a Chair" If unable to assess, monitor for change in activity level, assess other risk factors, document both on patient chart with date and time.		
Ability to Rise in Single Movement—No Loss of Balance With Steps	0	
Pushes Up, Successful in One Attempt	1	
Multiple Attempts Successful	3	
Unable to Rise Without Assistance During Test If unable to assess, document this on the patient chart with the date and time.	4	
(A Score of 5 or Greater = High Risk)	**TOTAL SCORE**	

On-going Medication Review Updates:

[1] Levetiracetam (Keppra) was not assessed during the original resreach conducted to create the Hendrich Fall Risk Model. As an antieptileptic, levetiracetam does have a side effect of somnolence and dizziness, which contributes to its fall risk and should be scored (effective June 2010).

[2] The study did not include the effect of benzodiazepine-like drugs since they were not on the market at the time. However, due to their similarity in drug structure, mechanism of action, and drug effects, they should also be scored (effective January 2010).

[3] Halazepam was included in the study but is no longer available in the United States (effective June 2010).

FIGURE 22-2 The Hendrich II Fall Risk Model, a fall risk assessment tool recommended by the Hartford Institute for Geriatric Nursing. (© Ann Hendrich, Inc. Used with permission.)

Unfolding Case Study

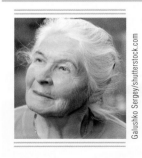

Part 3: Ms. M. at 74 Years of Age

Ms. M. is now 74 years old and goes to the senior center three or four times weekly for lunch. You have been the wellness nurse at the center for several years and are quite familiar with Ms. M. because she frequently attends your weekly healthy aging class. After your recent class on "Keeping Your Bones Healthy and Moving Well," she made an appointment to see you. She tells you that she has significantly cut down on her exercise because she experienced pain in one knee about a month ago after she took a long walk in the park with her dog. She talked with her doctor about this and was told to start taking ibuprofen, but she has not started taking it because she is not sure how much to take and

Galushko Sergey/shutterstock.com

Part 3: Ms. M. at 74 Years of Age *(Continued)*

her knee does not bother her except when she takes a long walk. She used to take her dog for daily walks, but now she ties him out and stays indoors. Current prescription medications are enalapril 5 mg twice daily, and hydrochlorothiazide 25 mg daily. She also takes a multiple vitamin daily and acetaminophen 1000 mg every 6 hours as needed. She continues to live in her one-floor house and is independent in doing all of her household chores. She also is responsible for all year-round outdoor maintenance activities, including mowing the lawn, raking leaves, and shoveling snow.

THINKING POINTS

- What assessment questions from Box 22-3 would you ask Ms. M. at this time?
- Would you use any information from Box 22-1 or Box 22-2 at this time?

- What myths or misunderstandings related to mobility and exercise might be influencing Ms. M.?
- Would you take any steps to assess Ms. M.'s home environment for fall risks?

NURSING DIAGNOSIS

Impaired Physical Mobility is a nursing diagnosis that is applicable when the assessment identifies limitations in mobility of an older adult. This diagnosis is defined as "limitation in independent, purposeful movement of the body or of one or more extremities" (Herdman & Kamitsuru, 2018, p. 219). Related factors common in older adults include arthritis, depression, chronic pain, fractured hip, and neurologic disorders (e.g., dementia or Parkinson disease). The nursing diagnosis of Risk for Falls is applicable for older adults who have a history of or risks for falls. Related factors common in older adults include all those factors listed in Box 22-2. If older adults have a diagnosis of osteoporosis or a history of fractures and their risks for falls and fractures are not being addressed, the nursing diagnosis of Ineffective Health Maintenance would be applicable because the focus is on secondary prevention.

PLANNING FOR WELLNESS OUTCOMES

When planning care for older adults who are at risk for osteoporosis, nurses identify wellness outcomes that focus on primary and secondary prevention. In these situations, any of the following Nursing Outcomes Classification (NOC) terms might be pertinent: Health Promoting Behavior, Knowledge: Health Promotion, Risk Control, or Risk Detection.

Nursing goals for an older adult with a nursing diagnosis of Impaired Physical Mobility focus on restoring functional abilities, preventing further loss of function, and preventing falls and injuries. NOC terminology applicable to an older adult with this nursing diagnosis includes Ambulation, Balance, Endurance, Mobility, or Activity Tolerance.

Care of older adults with a nursing diagnosis of Risk for Falls focuses on preventing the occurrence of falls and fall-related injuries by implementing fall-prevention programs. The following NOC terminology would be applicable with regard to safety and fall prevention: Fall Prevention Behavior, Falls Occurrence, Knowledge: Fall Prevention, Risk Detection, Safe Home Environment, and Safe Health Care Environment.

Wellness Opportunity

Wellness outcomes that address the body–mind–spirit interrelatedness for people who are afraid of falling include Anxiety Self-Control, Coping, Fear Self-Control, and Quality of Life.

NURSING INTERVENTIONS FOR MUSCULOSKELETAL WELLNESS

Nurses have numerous opportunities to promote musculoskeletal wellness because most older adults can benefit from learning about health promotion interventions for improved musculoskeletal function and prevention of osteoporosis, falls, and fractures. Thus, interventions focus not only on direct actions to prevent falls but also on teaching about eliminating or addressing risks. Some Nursing Interventions Classification terminologies that would be applicable to the interventions discussed in the following sections include Environmental Management: Safety, Exercise Promotion, Fall Prevention, Health Education, Risk Identification, and Teaching: Individual.

Promoting Healthy Musculoskeletal Function

Engaging in physical activity is a major health promotion intervention for compensating for age-related changes that affect musculoskeletal function. Positive effects of exercise include improved functioning, increased bone strength, and prevention of falls and disability. Flexibility exercises can improve range of motion, and weight-bearing exercise is an essential intervention for osteoporosis. Moderate aerobic exercise can prevent loss of muscle mass in older adults and is especially important for those who are intentionally trying to lose weight. Thus, an important nursing intervention is to help older adults identify ways in which they can incorporate physical activity as a daily health promoting practice, as discussed in Chapter 5.

In recent years, there has been increasing attention to holistic types of exercise that address balance, mobility, and the mind–body connection. Tai chi, which is a traditional Chinese martial art and a mind–body exercise that involves focused attention and a series of fluid and continuous movements, has been used in Asian countries for centuries and is now widely available in Western countries. Many studies and systematic reviews have confirmed the following beneficial effects of tai chi related to musculoskeletal function (Hwang, Chen, Lee-Hseih, et al., 2016; Jones, Starcher, Eicher, et al., 2016; Li, Harmer, & Fitzgerald, 2016):

- Improved balance and neuromuscular coordination
- Increased muscle strength, flexibility, and endurance
- Improved postural stability
- Decreased risk of falls and fractures
- Reduced fear of falling

In addition to being beneficial for overall musculoskeletal function, tai chi has been identified as an effective intervention for chronic conditions, including osteoarthritis, Parkinson disease, and peripheral neuropathy (Ballard, Arce-Esquivel, Haas, et al., 2016; Choi, 2016; Kwok, Choi, & Chan, 2016; Wang, Schmid, Iversen, et al., 2016).

Yoga is another body–mind therapy that is effective for improving balance and mobility, and reducing fear of falls in older adults (Nick, Petramfar, Ghodsbin, et al., 2016; Youkhana, Dean, Wolff, et al., 2016). One longitudinal study found that a 12-minute daily yoga regimen improved bone mineral density in the spines and femurs of participants (Lu, Rosner, Chang, et al., 2016). Recent studies identify dancing as a safe, feasible, and enjoyable intervention for improving balance and preventing falls in older adults, including those with Parkinson disease (Filar-Mierzwa, Dlugosz, Marchewka, et al., 2016; Zafar, Bozzorg, & Hackney, 2016).

See ONLINE LEARNING ACTIVITY 22-4: RESOURCES FOR HEALTH PROMOTION MATERIALS RELATED TO MUSCULOSKELETAL WELLNESS at http://thepoint.lww.com/Miller8e.

Wellness Opportunity

Walking, dancing, swimming, tai chi, and bicycle riding are examples of wellness interventions that are enjoyable and have positive effects on the body, mind, and spirit.

Teaching About Osteoporosis

Interventions for prevention and treatment of osteoporosis need to be an integral part of fracture prevention regimens for older adults, particularly in health care settings where a major focus of care is on chronic conditions (e.g., home care and long-term care settings). Although primary care practitioners are responsible for diagnosing and treating osteoporosis, nurses are responsible for health education about osteoporosis interventions and prevention of fractures. Because awareness about osteoporosis in men is just beginning to develop, nurses have a particular responsibility for teaching older men about screening for osteoporosis. It also is important to focus health education on older adults who already have had fractures because secondary prevention measures are often overlooked. See Online Learning Activity 22-5 for additional information about prevention and treatment of osteoporosis, including health education materials for multicultural communities.

Health education includes information about risk factors with emphasis on developing a plan to address the modifiable risk factors. Nurses can encourage older adults with risk factors to ask their primary care practitioner about screening tests and interventions. All adults can benefit from lifestyle interventions for osteoporosis, and teaching about these self-care activities is well within the realm of nursing responsibilities. Important self-care interventions for osteoporosis include daily weight-bearing activities, quitting smoking, and limiting alcohol intake.

Wellness Opportunity

Promoting self-care practices to prevent osteoporosis is particularly important when teaching older adults who have a history of falls or fractures.

Nurses can also teach older adults and their caregivers about the importance of adequate intake of calcium and vitamin D. A registered dietitian, if available, can evaluate a food journal to determine the usual intake of calcium and vitamin D. If intake does not provide at least 1000 to 1200 mg of calcium and 800 to 2000 IU of vitamin D, then health teaching focuses either on increasing dietary intake to the recommended amount or on taking a daily supplement. In long-term care facilities, all care plans should include a review of nutritional interventions for osteoporosis, particularly in relation to preventing fractures. Nurses can take the lead in involving dietitians and primary care providers in developing and implementing appropriate preventive interventions. Box 22-4 summarizes health promotion information that can be used as a guide for teaching older adults about osteoporosis.

Until recently, medical interventions for osteoporosis focused primarily on women, but there is increasing attention to safe and effective pharmacologic treatments for men. This is warranted because osteoporosis in underrecognized and undertreated in men, and more men than women die every year as a consequence of hip fractures (Alejandro & Constantinescu, 2017). A major goal of pharmacologic interventions for osteoporosis is prevention of fragility fractures, which are associated with serious consequences, including chronic pain, decreased quality of life, and

Box 22-4 Health Promotion Teaching About Osteoporosis

Health Promotion Interventions for Early Detection and Treatment

- Review risk factors for osteoporosis as summarized in Box 22-1.
- Plan interventions for modifiable risk factors using Boxes 22-1 and 22-3 as guides.
- Encourage discussion with the primary care provider about bone density tests.
- Encourage discussion with the primary care provider about medical interventions for osteoporosis if risk factors are present.
- Encourage discussion with the primary care provider about prevention of fractures if osteoporosis is diagnosed.

Lifestyle Interventions

- Implement weight-bearing exercise regimen for one-half hour daily.
- Engage in activities such as yoga, swimming, massage, acupressure, and tai chi.
- Wear supportive shoes.
- Discontinue cigarette smoking.
- Maintain ideal body weight.
- Avoid excessive alcohol intake

Nutritional Interventions

- A daily intake of at least 1000 mg of calcium from food sources is recommended, rather than using calcium supplements that may have adverse effects.
- Foods that are high in calcium include milk, cheese, yogurt, custard, ice cream, raisins, tofu, canned salmon or sardines, and broccoli and other dark green vegetables.
    - If a higher dose of calcium is required, e.g., for osteoporosis, this should be under the direction of a primary care practitioner.
- Provide adequate dietary intake of vitamin D and use supplement if needed to assure daily intake of at least 800 to 1000 IU vitamin D.
    - People with low serum vitamin D levels may require higher daily doses, which should be taken under the direction of a primary care practitioner.

significant morbidity and mortality. In recent years, many types of medications have been approved for prevention of fragility fractures, which are in addition to the menopausal hormonal therapy that was widely used until the mid-1990s. The following pharmaceutical agents are used for treatment of osteoporosis and prevention of fragility fractures in older adults with risk factors:

- Bisphosphonates: alendronate (Fosamax), ibandronate (Boniva), risedronate (Actonel), zoledronic acid (Zometa)
- Calcitonin
- Denosumab (Xgeva, Prolia)
- Estrogen (e.g., Premarin)
- Raloxifene (Evista)
- Parathyroid hormone (e.g., Teriparatide)

Because these medications are associated with various adverse effects, it is imperative to advise older adults to discuss the benefits and risks with their primary care practitioners so they can make informed decisions about this important preventive intervention.

Current emphasis also is on secondary prevention for older adults who have already had fractures. The International Osteoporosis Foundation supports the use of Fracture Liaison Services as a cost-effective and evidence-based model of coordinated services to prevent subsequent fractures through multifaceted interventions for osteoporosis (Cosman, Nicpon, & Nieves, 2016; Osuna, Ruppe, & Tabatabai, 2017; Yong, Masucci, Hoch, et al., 2016). Roles for nurses in these programs include risk identification, patient teaching, and care coordination.

In summary, there is sound evidence that pharmacologic treatment of osteoporosis can improve bone density, reduce the rate of bone loss, and decrease the risk for fragility fractures, including hip fracture. Pharmacologic treatment is just one component of a comprehensive management plan that must also include nutritional intake of calcium and vitamin D, physical activity to maintain musculoskeletal function and reduce the risk for falls, and patient education regarding osteoporosis and fall prevention. Use Online Learning Activity 22-5 for current evidence-based information related to osteoporosis and other aspects of musculoskeletal wellness.

See ONLINE LEARNING ACTIVITY 22-5: **ADDITIONAL INFORMATION ABOUT OSTEOPOROSIS** at http://thepoint.lww.com/Miller8e.

A Student's Perspective

This past week, I chose to do the water aerobics with the older adults at the health and fitness center. I was encouraged by the vitality and general zest for life that these older women showed. I was enlightened by their sense of pride in their health and level of activity. I left with the impression that this group activity was something that each of them attributed her good health to. I also noted that they got more out of this activity than just physical exercise. The social connection that these women had was truly admirable. They were constantly encouraging each other and me during the class. They also used the time just to connect with each other and discuss normal life events.

My take-away lesson from this experience was the importance of having opportunities like this for older adults to exercise their muscles as well as their social personalities. Older adults are often portrayed as socially inferior in today's popular culture, but I felt these older women were living truly balanced lives, maybe more so than me in some respects. I think that often I find myself so busy that I do not take time to invest myself in more meaningful relationships—something that these people are obviously benefiting from.

Clint H.

Unfolding Case Study

Part 4: Ms. M. at 79 Years of Age

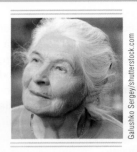

Galushko Sergey/shutterstock.com

Recall that you are the nurse at the wellness program where Ms. M., now 79 years old, regularly attends your health education programs. Based on additional assessment information, you know that Ms. M. does not take any calcium or vitamin D supplements because she drinks milk twice daily and believes that this should be sufficient. She stopped having menstrual periods when she was 50 years old and began hormonal therapy a few years later. She stopped taking estrogen when she was in her mid-60s because she began "hearing too many bad things about estrogen." Ms. M. fractured her wrist 4 years ago when she reached her arms out to diminish the impact of a fall. At that time, orthopedic surgeon said that her x-rays showed that her "bones were a little thin but not bad for her age." She has not had any further x-rays or any bone density tests and says her primary care practitioner has never brought up the subject of osteoporosis because "I guess he's too worried about my heart problems to be concerned about my bones." Although she fell once when she was raking leaves last fall and tripped over a small tree stump, she has had no serious fall-related injuries since she fractured her wrist. She does not smoke and drinks alcohol only on major social occasions. When you assessed her blood pressure, you found that her blood pressure while standing was 146/86 mm Hg and while reclining was 128/78 mm Hg. Her record of self-monitored blood pressure readings indicates that her usual blood pressure is around 134/82 mm Hg. Her vision is adequate, but she has stopped driving at night and is being monitored by her ophthalmologist for progression of bilateral cataracts. Her eye doctor told her that she is likely to need cataract surgery sometime during the next 2 to 3 years.

THINKING POINTS

- What further assessment information would you want to have?
- What health promotion interventions would you advise for Ms. M.? Specifically, what health teaching would you do with regard to further assessment, lifestyle interventions, nutrition and nutritional supplements, and pharmacologic interventions?

- What educational materials would you use for Ms. M.?
- What follow-up health promotion would you consider for Ms. M.? Specifically, how would you work with Ms. M. to develop lifelong health promotion interventions?

QSEN APPLICATION

QSEN Competency	Knowledge/Skill/Attitude	Application to Ms. M. at 79 Years
Patient-centered care	(K) Integrate understanding of multiple dimensions of patient-centered care	Use information in Boxes 22-2 and 22-3 to identify conditions that increase the risk for falls and fractures
	(K) Describe strategies to empower patients in all aspects of the health care process	
	(S) Elicit patient values, preferences, and expressed needs	
	Use effective communication skills to explore Ms. M.'s willingness to address risks	
Evidence-based practice	(K) Describe how the strength and relevance of available evidence influence the choice of intervention	Use Online Learning Activities 22-4 and 22-5 to find additional evidence-based information related to management of osteoporosis and prevention of fractures
	(S) Read original research and evidence reports related to clinical practice	Teach Ms. M. about evidence-based interventions for osteoporosis as summarized in Box 22-4
	(A) Value evidence-based practice as integral to determining the best clinical practice	

PREVENTING FALLS AND FALL-RELATED INJURIES

Prevention of falls and fall-related injuries requires interprofessional implementation of multifaceted interventions addressing contributing factors. Interventions need to be individualized to address risk factors within each situation; in addition, they vary according to setting. This topic is discussed in relation to type of setting and also in relation to risks for individual older adults.

Interventions in Health Care Settings

In 2008, the CMS identified falls and trauma (e.g., fractures, dislocations, intracranial injuries) as hospital-acquired conditions that would not be covered if they occurred in a health care facility that received Medicare or Medicaid. This led to major efforts to prevent the occurrence of falls and serious fall-related injuries in all health care settings. Fall-prevention interventions in health care settings are influenced by organizational factors as well as direct nursing care. Nurses have key roles in all aspects of these programs. As succinctly stated in best-practice guidelines, "Effective fall-prevention programs in acute care hospitals are championed by nurses using one or more approaches in collaboration with interprofessional teams" (Gray-Miceli & Quigley, 2016).

Key aspects of fall-prevention programs in health care settings are the identification of people who are at risk for falls and fall-related injuries and the consistent implementation of preventive actions by all staff. Health-care institutions establish policies and practices that typically include a visual communication tool and guidelines for interventions. As an example, Online Learning Activity 22-6 provides a link to an article by Hefner, McAlearney, Mansfield, et al. (2016), which describes the Falls Wheel program. The article illustrates a visual communication tool that allows for patient categorization according to fall risk and fall-related injury simultaneously. Implementation of this Falls Wheel program was effective in reducing falls with harm by almost 50% in an acute care setting during the year-long implementation period. Interventions, such as the ones listed in Box 22-5, were listed for each risk category on the wheel, and staff education was a major component of the Falls Wheel program. Numerous evidence-based resources and toolkits describing comprehensive fall-prevention programs are available from major organizations such as the Agency for Healthcare Research and Quality, the Joint Commission, and the U. S. Department of Veterans Affairs Center for Patient Safety. Education of patients, long-term care residents, and families is recommended as an essential part of fall-prevention programs (Opsahl, Ebright, Cangany, et al., 2017; Schoberer, Breimaier, Mandl, et al., 2016.

Box 22-5 A Fall-Prevention Program for Older Adults Being Cared for in Hospitals or Nursing Homes

Identification of Patients/Residents Who Are at Risk for Falling

- Use a nursing judgment and a fall risk assessment tool to identify any risks for falling and fall-related injuries (e.g., medications, osteoporosis, medical conditions, history of falls, impaired cognition, diminished alertness, impaired mobility, age 75 years or older).
- Document the risk factors on the designated fall assessment guide.
- Use a multidisciplinary approach to address any risk factors for falls, osteoporosis, or fall-related injuries.
- Frequently reassess the risks for falls and fall-related injuries at predetermined times (e.g., every shift, every day, whenever there is a change in the patient's/resident's functional status).
- Use color-coded items (e.g., brightly colored stickers for the chart, a brightly colored wrist band, and signs near the person's bed and outside the room) to identify those who are included in the fall-prevention program.

Education of the Staff, Patient/Resident, and Family

- Instruct the patient or resident and family about the fall-prevention program and provide written information about preventing falls and obtaining help if falls occur.
- Provide staff education about the fall-prevention program and the risk factors for falls, especially those factors that the staff influences (e.g., use of restraints, selection of footwear).

- Use posters and fliers to heighten staff awareness of the fall-prevention program.

Interventions to Be Implemented for All High-Risk Patients/Residents

- Keep the call light within reach at all times.
  - ◆ Respond quickly to calls for assistance
  - ◆ Assess toileting needs at frequent intervals
- Make sure that ambulatory patients wear sturdy, nonslip footwear when out of bed.
- Offer assistance with activities of daily living and try to anticipate the person's needs before help is needed.
- Encourage the person to call for help when needed.
- Assure close monitoring and frequent checks for all patients/residents who cannot be relied on to call for help.
- Make sure the bed is in the lowest position possible and the wheels are locked.
- Carefully and frequently assess the environment for factors that increase the risk for either falls or fall-related injuries; address all modifiable risk factors.
- Consider the use of a movement-detection device.
- Adhere to institutional policies about use of physical restraints, including bedrails.
- If appropriate, orient the person to person, place, and time every shift and as needed.
- Document fall-prevention interventions on the person's chart.

See ONLINE LEARNING ACTIVITY 22-6: ARTICLE DESCRIBING THE FALLS WHEEL PROGRAM at http://thepoint.lww.com/Miller8e.

Interventions in Community Settings

In community settings, national and local organizations are addressing the prevention of falls and fall-related injuries as a major public health concern. In 2014, the Centers for Disease Control and Prevention developed the Stopping Elderly Accidents, Deaths & Injuries (STEADI) initiative to encourage all health care providers to routinely incorporate fall prevention in their usual care. Effective fall-prevention programs in community settings include the following components: assessments of risks, functional status, and environmental safety; strength and balance exercises; medication review; vision interventions; home safety modifications; and teaching of adults, families, and caregivers (Bamgbade & Dearmon, 2016; Yount, 2016). Box 22-6 summarizes evidence-based recommendations related to preventing falls in older adults who live in independent settings.

Addressing Intrinsic Risk Factors

Because any gait and balance impairment increases the risk for falls, interventions that improve mobility are likely to be beneficial in preventing falls. Interventions for improving mobility are implemented primarily by rehabilitation therapists, nurses, and nursing staff, often through an interdisciplinary approach. Teaching about the proper use of mobility aids and other assistive devices (Figure 22-3) is an important part of fall-prevention programs. Nurses are responsible for raising questions about whether an older adult may benefit from the use of mobility aids or assistive devices and facilitating a referral to a physical therapist for evaluation and teaching. In community settings, nurses can teach older adults and their caregivers about the availability of various mobility aids, transfer assistance devices, and other aids that might improve safety. Nurses can suggest that older adults seek professional help with selecting appropriate mobility aids and assistive devices. Home health care equipment supplies have therapists or staff members who can provide advice and assist with processing insurance claims. When mobility aids are prescribed, nursing responsibilities include making sure that the aids are accessible, encouraging the person to use the aids, and facilitating referrals for reassessment if questions arise about the safety or effectiveness of the mobility aids.

Because proper footwear is essential to prevent slips and falls, nurses can advise older adults about wearing nonslip footwear both indoors and outdoors. It is especially important to advise older adults to wear slip-resistant, supportive, low-heeled footwear in wet, icy, or snowy conditions. Nurses also can help older adults explore resources for assistance with removal of ice and snow from walkways. For example, a local office on aging or other organization may provide snow removal or outdoor maintenance services at little or no cost for older adults.

In recent years, fall-prevention literature has emphasized the effectiveness of various exercise routines as an

---

Box 22-6 Evidence-Based Practice: Preventing Falls in Older Adults in Community Settings

Statement of the Problem

- About 30% of community-dwelling older adults fall each year.
- Many studies in recent years have identified evidence-based interventions that are effective for reducing falls, risks for falls, and fall-related injuries.

Recommendations for Screening and Assessment

- Ask older adults if they have had a fall during the past year.
- Find out details about circumstances of each fall.
- Ask about gait and balance problems.
- Perform simple test for gait and balance (e.g., Timed Get Up and Go).
- Arrange for multifactorial fall risk assessment including comprehensive physical examination, functional assessment, environmental assessment, medical history, and medication review.

Evidence-Based Fall-Prevention Interventions

- Implementation of interventions for individual fall risks identified during multifactorial assessment.
- Participation in a multiple component group or home-based exercise program that includes balance, strength, and gait-training exercises.
- Optimal management of all medical conditions, especially cardiac arrhythmias and postural hypotension.

- Modification of prescription medication regimens, including gradual withdrawal of psychotropic medication.
- Treatment of vision impairment: cataract surgery as needed, not using multifocal lenses while walking.
- Management of foot problems and footwear.
- Vitamin D supplementation for people with lower serum vitamin D levels.
- Home safety assessment and modification, which is particularly effective for people who are visually impaired and when delivered by an occupational therapist.

Recommendations for Nursing Interventions

- Facilitate implementation of applicable evidence-based interventions.
- Teach about recommended level of physical activity for older adults: 2.5 hours of moderate-intensity or 1.25 hours of vigorous-intensity aerobic physical activity every week, plus muscle-strengthening activities twice weekly, and balance training 3 or more days per week for those with risks for falls.
- Teach about self-care actions, including using appropriate assistive devices and safety measures (e.g., antislip shoe devices in icy conditions).

Source: American Geriatrics Society and British Geriatrics Society (2010); Gillespie, Robertson, Gillespie, et al. (2012); U.S. Preventive Services Task Force (2012).

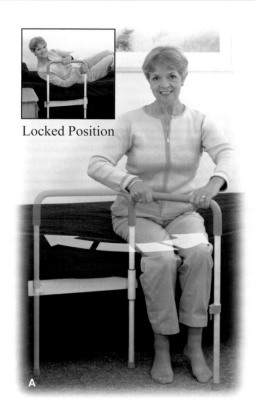

Locked Position

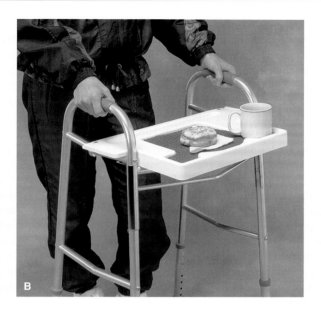

FIGURE 22-3 The use of assistive devices can help reduce the risk of falls. (**A**) Transfer assistive devices are used to facilitate safer transfer in and out of beds. (**B**) Walkers are available in various styles with wheels, brakes, baskets, seats, and other features to improve safety and mobility. Photographs reprinted with permission from ActiveForever.com.)

intervention for reducing intrinsic fall risk. An important role for nurses is to identify those older adults who may benefit from gait and balance training programs and to facilitate referrals for physical therapy when appropriate. In addition to being recommended for older adults who are at risk for or have experienced falls, physical therapy for strength and gait training is recommended for management of sarcopenia (Dhillon & Hasni, 2017). Nurses are also responsible for encouraging adequate and consistent follow-through with recommended exercise programs. In long-term care settings, nurses generally oversee restorative nursing programs in which nursing assistants help residents with walking and other exercise regimens established by physical therapists. These restorative nursing routines are essential aspects of fall-prevention programs. Group physical activity programs that include resistance and balance exercises are effective for improving musculoskeletal function and preventing fragility fractures in community and long-term care settings (Hassan, Hewitt, Keogh, et al., 2016; Huovinen, Ivaska, Kiviranta, et al., 2016). Many programs incorporate exercises aimed specifically at improving gait, balance, ankle strength, or other aspects of fall prevention.

Comprehensive fall-prevention programs include multidisciplinary interventions for specific risks, including pharmacists for addressing medication effects or neurologists for addressing pathologic conditions. If a multidisciplinary team is not available for a comprehensive approach, nurses have essential roles in identifying appropriate professional resources and facilitating referrals for these services.

Addressing Extrinsic Risk Factors

Interventions for addressing extrinsic risk factors, such as environmental conditions and use of restraints, are applicable for older adults in any setting. Patients who are at risk for falls should receive referrals for home assessments when they are discharged from hospitals. The safety assessment guidelines provided in Chapter 7 can help with planning interventions that may eliminate or reduce environmental risks. In addition, environmental modifications to improve a person's vision, as discussed in Chapter 17, are applicable to fall prevention.

> **Wellness Opportunity**
>
> Fall-prevention interventions that address the person–environment relationship can be as simple and effective as involving older adults in decisions about removing or replacing slippery throw rugs.

Using Monitoring Devices in Health Care Settings

Monitoring devices can be useful in alerting staff to potentially unsafe patient/resident movement; however, concerns have been raised about the overuse and negative consequences of some types of devices. All monitoring devices contain a mechanism for transmitting a signal to a remote location (e.g., a nursing station) when activated by certain levels of patient/resident movement. Some devices, such as a pad, are applied to the bed or chair, whereas others are attached to the person's clothing. Less restrictive devices are programmed specifically for the person's movement in a confined environment, such as his or her room. Alarm-type devices emit a loud signal and are associated with negative consequences, including disruptive noise, activity restrictions for the patient, and a false sense of security for staff.

Most movement-detection devices were originally designed for institutional use, but simplified monitoring and signal systems have now been developed for home use by family caregivers. In home settings, a simple auditory room-monitoring device (i.e., a "baby room monitor") may be useful when caregivers need to detect the sound of someone moving around in another room. A major limitation of any movement-detection device is that its effectiveness depends on the timely response of someone who is able to prevent the fall. These devices are not useful for people living alone or for people without responsible and responsive caregivers.

Providing Assistance in Independent Settings

For people living alone and at risk for falls, it is important to consider interventions for summoning help in a timely manner if falls occur. Many types of personal emergency response systems are available and these involve the use of a small portable transmitter that is worn on the person's body or clothing. Figure 22-4 illustrates one example of a commonly used personal emergency response system. When the person falls, he or she can summon help by using the transmitter to signal a receiver unit attached to the telephone. In turn, a call is automatically made to the personal emergency response system provider, who then checks in with the person on a speakerphone system and calls the local emergency response team or a contact person, such as a neighbor or family member if the person needs help. Some of these devices are set up so that a monitoring call is made to the person once a day if the person does not push a reset button or otherwise notify the company that he or she is well.

The effectiveness of personal emergency response system depends on the ability of the fallen person to signal for help and on the availability of a helping person. A major limitation of such devices is that cognitively impaired people may not be able to learn to use them. Hospitals, home care agencies, and local offices on aging provide information about local personal emergency response system programs, and information about national programs is available on the Internet. Cordless phones, especially if preprogrammed for emergency help and placed within reach where someone might fall, can also be used for obtaining help.

Technology to Promote Wellness in Older Adults

Nurses have taken strong leadership roles in developing and testing an automated in-home fall risk assessment and detection sensor for predicting gait changes and preventing falls. A technology-based sensor system that involves sensors, a depth camera, and Doppler radar has been used in a senior living facility to alert nursing staff to potential falls. After several years of development and testing, nursing studies indicate that this type of monitoring has the potential to alert nursing staff to increased fall risk so timely interventions can be implemented to prevent falls (Phillips, DeRoche, Rantz, et al., 2017; Rantz, Skubic, Abbott, et al., 2015). Although this technology is not yet widely available, nurses can teach older adults and their caregivers to explore products for fall detection and prevention at websites sponsored by nonprofit organizations such AARP (www.aarp.org).

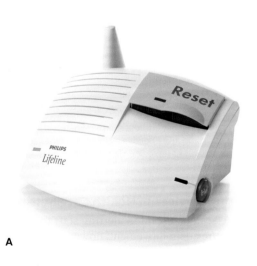

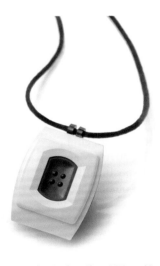

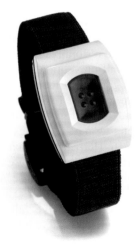

A   **B**   **C**

FIGURE 22-4 Example of a personal emergency response system receiver with (**A**) white "box," (**B**) necklace, and (**C**) bracelet. (Used with permission from Philips Respironics.)

Preventing Fall-Related Injuries

When falls cannot be prevented, interventions are directed toward reducing the risk of fractures and other serious fall-related injuries. Two interventions for preventing fall-related injuries that should be used for people who are at risk for falls are (1) to implement evidence-based measures for osteoporosis (discussed previously) and (2) to adapt the environment as much as possible to reduce the risk for fall-related injuries. Heavy furniture that is in a pathway where a fall is likely to occur can be moved out of the way or replaced with items that would move easily if the person falls into them. Also, hard edges of sinks and built-in cabinets can be padded. Particular attention should be paid to padding hard edges of bathroom cabinets and either padding or removing swinging shower doors. Using a bed that can be adjusted to a very low position can reduce the risk of injury from falling out of bed. Soft mats can be placed near beds and in other locations where people are likely to fall, but caution must be used so that these pads do not become fall risks.

Finally, it is imperative to recognize that restraints do not necessarily reduce the risk for falls and are associated with more serious fall-related injuries, as already discussed. In recent years, federal regulations have mandated that health care institutions develop policies for restraint reduction or restraint-free care. Evidence-based guidelines emphasize the need for individualized care plans to prevent falls and for education of patients, family members, and all caregiving staff members about the concept of restraint-free care as well as fall-prevention measures.

Wellness Opportunity

Health promotion interventions need to be broad and include precautions to minimize the risk of injury if falls do occur.

Addressing Fear of Falling

Any interventions that reduce the risk of falls are also likely to reduce a person's fear of falling, but some people may need additional interventions to address this problem. For example, nurses can address fear of falling in the same way they address other fears: encourage the expression of feelings and provide education and reassurance about interventions that are being implemented as part of an individualized fall-prevention care plan. Health promotion interventions focused on nutrition and increased physical activity can reduce fear of falling (Kapan, Luger, Haider, et al., 2017). Family members and caregivers should be included in nursing interventions and health education to address fear of falling. For people living alone, a personal emergency response system may be reassuring and at least alleviate the fear of being helpless if a fall occurs.

Wellness Opportunity

Nurses address body–mind–spirit interrelatedness by talking with older adults about ways to diminish their fear of falling and about ways to improve their safety.

Promoting Caregiver Wellness

In home and community settings, preventing falls and fall-related injuries are major responsibilities for caregivers of people who have risks for falls or a history of falls. This responsibility can significantly increase the stress for families as they try to balance the desire of the older adult to have privacy and independence against the risk of the person falling and incurring significant, or even fatal, injuries. Nurses working in home care settings often address this issue and weigh the responsibility to respect autonomy versus the responsibility to assure safety. Information in Chapters 9 and 10 is applicable to ethical issues when working with caregivers to address these questions.

In clinical settings, nurses can address caregiver stress related to their concerns about falls by arranging for a multidisciplinary approach to risk assessment and interventions for preventing falls and fall-related injuries. These assessments are available at outpatient geriatric assessment programs and through skilled home care agencies for people who are homebound. Nurses also can teach caregivers about fall-prevention strategies and resources for additional information, as described in Box 22-7.

EVALUATING EFFECTIVENESS OF NURSING INTERVENTIONS

Nursing care for older adults with impaired musculoskeletal function is evaluated by the degree to which the person achieves and maintains the highest possible level of independence and safe mobility. Nursing care of older adults who are at high risk for osteoporosis is evaluated according to the degree to which the older adult incorporates preventive measures in his or her daily life. For example, older adults might begin a regimen of three half-hour periods of weight-bearing exercise weekly. The nursing care of older adults who are at high risk for falls and fall-related injuries is evaluated according to the extent to which falls and serious injuries are prevented. Nurses cannot, of course, measure the number of falls that do not occur, but they can measure the risk factors that have been addressed in the care plan. Evaluation of these risk factors is facilitated by careful documentation of interventions, such as environmental modifications and fall-prevention programs.

Box 22-7 Caregiver Wellness

Family caregivers often experience stress because their older relative desires to remain independent even though he or she is at risk for falls, has already had a fall, or even is a "frequent faller." In these situations caregivers weigh the right of the older adult to take risks versus the need for safety and protection. When faced with this situation, it is important to use professional resources for promoting as safe and independent functioning as possible for the older person and peace of mind for concerned relatives. Implementing some strategies that promote safety and prevent injuries and thereby help to relieve caregiver stress follow.

Strategies for Preventing Falls and Fall-Related Injuries in Home Settings

Interventions to Reduce the Risk for Falls

- Obtain a comprehensive fall risk assessment to identify and address risks related to medical conditions, medication effects, and functional limitations.
- Obtain ophthalmologic evaluation to assure optimal visual function (e.g., cataract surgery may improve safety).
- Arrange for a home visit by a physical therapist or other qualified professional to identify and address environmental risks.
- Modify the home for safety by installing grab bars, handrails, good lighting, and other appropriate modifications for safe and independent mobility.

Actions to Promote Safe and Independent Functioning

- Arrange for occupational and physical therapy evaluations and recommendations for assistive devices, home modification for safety, and therapeutic exercises.
- Encourage frequent participation in enjoyable and beneficial physical activity programs, such as dancing, tai chi, water exercises.
- Encourage the person to engage in home-based physical activity by using videos, Wii Fit, and simple exercise equipment; consider doing these activities with them.

Actions to Assure Timely Response for Assistance

- Arrange for personal emergency response system.
- Place cordless phones in strategic locations in the home.
- Encourage the person to keep a cell phone handy at all times.
- If the person has memory problems, frequently remind him about the importance of calling for help when needed.

Resources for Information About Fall Prevention in Home Settings

- Centers for Disease Control and Prevention:www.cdc.gov/HomeandRecreactionalSafety/Falls/Index.html
- Fall Prevention Center of Excellence: www.stopfalls.org
- National Center for Patient Safety Falls Toolkit: www.patientsafety.va.gov/Safey/Topics/fallstoolkit/index.html
- National Resource Center for Safe Aging: www.safeaging.org

Unfolding Case Study

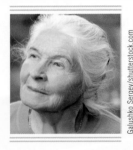

Galushko Sergey/shutterstock.com

Part 5: Ms. M. at 89 Years of Age

Ms. M. is now 89 years old and has been admitted to the hospital for heart failure. Additional diagnoses include arthritis, osteoporosis, recurrent depression, early-stage dementia, and history of fractured wrist at age 75 and fractured hip 3 years ago. Current medications include furosemide (Lasix), 40 mg twice daily; enalapril (Vasotec), 10 mg twice daily; alendronate (Fosamax) 70 mg; Os-Cal with D; and sertraline (Zoloft), 50 mg at bedtime. Ms. M. lives alone in an assisted-living facility, where she receives help with her medications and goes to the dining room for meals. You are the nurse on the acute care floor assigned to her care on the day of admission.

NURSING ASSESSMENT

During your initial nursing assessment, Ms. M. is quiet and withdrawn. When you ask about her living situation, she says she moved to the assisted-living facility after the hospitalization and rehabilitation for her fractured hip. At the time of the injury, she had been living alone. She had fallen while making her way to the bathroom at night and remained lying on the floor until her daughter came to visit her the next morning. During the past year, Ms. M. reports that she has fallen twice in the assisted-living facility, but that she has been able to call for help and has not had any serious injuries. You determine that Ms. M. will need help in ambulating to the bathroom and that she should be supervised whenever she gets out of bed.

Ms. M. confides that she is worried that she will have to move to the nursing home section of her facility if she falls again. She is very depressed about her lack of energy and her hospitalization for heart failure. A mental status assessment indicates that Ms. M. is alert and oriented but that her short-term memory is impaired. She has a great deal of difficulty with abstract ideas, such as learning to use the call button. You check her vital signs, which are within normal range, with no evidence of postural hypotension.

NURSING DIAGNOSIS

In addition to the nursing diagnoses related to Ms. M.'s medical condition, you identify a nursing diagnosis of Risk for Falls. Related factors include a history of falls and fractures, weakness, diuretic and cardiovascular medications, depression, and impaired cognition. You are concerned about preventing falls during her hospitalization.

Part 5: Ms. M. at 89 Years of Age *(Continued)*

NURSING CARE PLAN FOR MS. M.

Expected Outcome	Nursing Interventions	Nursing Evaluation
Ms. M. will ambulate safely and avoid falls during her hospitalization	• Identify Ms. M. as a participant in the fall-prevention program by using an orange wrist bracelet, posting a Fall Alert sign near her bed, and placing an orange Fall Alert sticker on her chart • Provide Ms. M. with a brochure that explains the fall-prevention program • Reassess fall risks every shift and document these on the Fall Assessment form included in Ms. M.'s chart • Talk with Ms. M.'s physician about a referral for physical therapy • Keep the call light button within her reach and review instructions for its use every shift • Assess benefits and risks of using bedrails, and discuss these with Ms. M. and her family • Make sure that the bed is in the lowest possible position with the wheels locked • Use a movement-detection bed pad and explain to Ms. M. that the purpose of the pad is to ensure that the staff knows when she needs to get out of bed • Every 2 hours, when Ms. M. is awake, the nursing staff will ask her if she needs to go to the bathroom	• Ms. M. will receive assistance with ambulation every time she is out of bed • Ms. M. will not fall during her hospitalization

THINKING POINTS

• If you were the nurse on the acute care floor where Ms. M. was a patient, what concerns would you address in a discharge plan? Would you identify any additional nursing diagnoses related to safe mobility and musculoskeletal function? What additional nursing interventions would you plan to supplement this care plan that is focused on preventing falls during Ms. M.'s hospitalization?

• If you were a nurse in the assisted-living facility where Ms. M. lives, what concerns would you have about her care? How would you address these concerns in a care plan?

QSEN APPLICATION

QSEN Competency	Knowledge/Skill/Attitude	Application to Ms. M. at 89 Years
Patient-centered care	(K) Integrate understanding of multiple dimensions of patient-centered care (K) Examine common barriers to active involvement of patients in their own health care processes (S) Elicit patient values, preferences, and expressed needs (S) Provide patient-centered care with sensitivity and respect for diversity of the human experience (S) Communicate care provided and needed at each transition in care. (A) Value seeing health care situations "through patients' eyes"	Use fall risk assessment tool and additional assessment information from Box 22-3 to develop fall-prevention interventions based on identified needs Use effective communication skills to explore psychosocial factors that influence Ms. M.'s current health situation Identify interventions to assure continuity of care when Ms. M. is discharged

(continued)

QSEN APPLICATION (Continued)

QSEN Competency	Knowledge/Skill/Attitude	Application to Ms. M. at 89 Years
Teamwork and collaboration	(K) Describe scopes of practice and role of health care team members	Facilitate referral for physical therapy to address fall risks
	(K) Recognize contributions of other individuals and groups in helping patient achieve health goals	Facilitate referral for social worker to address psychosocial needs
	(S) Integrate the contributions of others who play a role in helping patient achieve health goals	Talk with primary care practitioner and social worker about a referral for comprehensive geriatric assessment services for assessing fall risk and mental status, either during hospitalization or after Ms. M. is discharged

Chapter Highlights

Age-Related Changes That Affect Mobility and Safety

- Degenerative changes in bones, muscles, joints, and connective tissue
- Central nervous system changes: slowed reaction time, body sway
- Diminished bone density (i.e., osteopenia and osteoporosis)

Risk Factors That Affect Safe Mobility

- Risk factors for impaired musculoskeletal function: physical inactivity, nutritional deficits
- Risk factors for osteoporosis and fractures: lack of weight-bearing activity, increased age, tobacco smoking, excessive alcohol consumption, certain medications (e.g., corticosteroids) (Box 22-1)
- Risk factors for falls: intrinsic conditions, adverse medication effects, environmental factors, physical restraints (Box 22-2)

Functional Consequences Affecting Musculoskeletal Wellness

- Diminished muscle strength, endurance, and coordination
- Increased difficulty performing ADLs
- Increased susceptibility to falls, fractures, and fall-related injuries
- Fear of falling

Pathologic Condition Affecting Musculoskeletal Wellness: Osteoarthritis

- Osteoarthritis is a degenerative inflammatory disease that is a leading cause of disability in the United States
- Self-management is an important focus of nursing care

Nursing Assessment of Musculoskeletal Function (Box 22-3)

- Assessing overall musculoskeletal performance (Figure 22-1)
- Identifying risks for osteoporosis
- Assessing for safety of the environment
- Using fall risk assessment tools (Figure 22-2)

Nursing Diagnosis

- Wellness nursing diagnosis: Readiness for Enhanced Self-Health Management
- Related to fall risks: Impaired Physical Mobility, Risk for Falls, Ineffective Health Maintenance

Planning for Wellness Outcomes

- Balance, Endurance, Mobility, Activity Tolerance
- Risk Control, Risk Detection
- Fall-Prevention Behavior
- Safe Home Environment, Safe Health Care Environment

Nursing Interventions for Musculoskeletal Wellness

- Promoting healthy musculoskeletal function
- Teaching about osteoporosis (Box 22-4)

Preventing Falls and Fall-Related Injuries

- Interventions in health care settings (Box 22-5)
- Interventions in community settings (Box 22-6)
- Using monitoring devices in health care settings and personal emergency response systems in home settings (Figure 22-4)
- Preventing fall-related injuries
- Addressing fear of falling
- Promoting caregiver wellness (Box 22-7)

Evaluating Effectiveness of Nursing Interventions

- Maintenance of highest level of safe mobility
- Incorporation of preventive measures in daily life to ensure safety and prevent osteoporosis
- Expressed feelings of safety and improved quality of life

Critical Thinking Exercises

1. Identify factors that increase or reduce the risk for osteoporosis.
2. Describe how each of the following age-related changes or risk factors might increase an older person's risk for falls and fractures: nocturia, osteoporosis, medications, altered gait, pathologic conditions, sensory impairments, cognitive impairments, functional impairments, slowed reaction time.
3. Describe the environmental factors that you would assess, in both home and institutional settings, to identify potential risks for falls.
4. Describe how you would design and implement a fall-prevention program in a long-term care facility.
5. How would you deal with a daughter who demanded that restraints be used whenever her 84-year-old mother, who is a patient on your acute care floor, is sitting in a chair?
6. What information would you include in health education about osteoporosis?
7. Use the internet to find information about fall-prevention products that you might use in clinical practice.

 For more information about topics discussed in this chapter, be sure to check out the interactive Online Learning Activities and other helpful resources at http://thepoint.lww.com/Miller8e.

REFERENCES

Alejandro, P. & Constantinescu, F. (2017). A review of osteoporosis in the older adult. *Clinics in Geriatric Medicine, 33*, 27–40.

American Geriatrics Society and British Geriatrics Society. (2010). AGS/BGS Clinical Practice Guideline: Prevention of falls in older persons. Available at www.ahrq.gov, guidelines summary NGC-9165.

Auais, M., Alvarado, B. E., Curcio, C. L., et al. (2016). Fear of falling as a risk factor for mobility disability in older people at five diverse sites of the IMIAS study. *Archives of Gerontology & Geriatrics, 66*, 147–153.

Ballard, J. E., Arce-Esquivel, A. A., Haas, B. K., et al. (2016). Tai chi exercise on muscle strength and function in peripheral neuropathy patients: 2578 Board #101. *Medicine and Science in Sports and Exercise, 48*(5 Suppl 1), 715.

Bamgbade, S., & Dearmon, V. (2016). Fall prevention for older adults receiving home healthcare. *Home Healthcare Now, 34*, 68–75.

Baruth, M., Wilcox, S., McClenaghan, B., et al. (2016). Clinically meaningful changes in functional performance resulting from self-directed interventions in individuals with arthritis. *Public Health, 133*, 116–123.

Benavent-Caballer, V., Sendin-Magdalena, A., Lison, J. F., et al. (2016). Physical factors underlying the time "Up and Go" test in older adults. *Geriatric Nursing, 37*, 122–127.

Bower, E. S., Wetherell, J. L., Petkus, A., et al. (2016). Fear of falling after hip fracture: Prevalence, course, and relationship with one-year functional recover. *American Journal of Geriatric Psychiatry, 24*, 1228–1236.

Bradas, C., Sandhu, S., & Mion, L. (2016). Physical restraints and side rails in acute and critical care settings. In M. Boltz, E. Capezuti, T. Fulmer, & D. Zwicker (Eds.), *Evidence-based practice protocols for best practice* (5th ed., pp. 381–394). New York: Springer Publishing Co.

Bruyere, O., Cavalier, E., Buckinx, E., et al. (2017). Relevance of vitamin D in the pathogenesis and therapy of frailty. *Current Opinion in Clinical Nutrition and Metabolic Care, 20*, 26–29.

Centers for Disease Control. (2016). STEADI (Stopping Elderly Accidents, Deaths & Injuries): Materials for Health Care Providers. Available at www.cdc.gov

Choi, H. J. (2016). Effects of therapeutic tai chi on functional fitness and activities of daily living in patients with Parkinson disease. *Journal of Exercise and Rehabilitation, 12*, 499–503.

Chun, S. H., Cho, B., Yang, H. K., et al. (2017). Performance on physical function tests and the risk of fractures and admissions: Findings from a national health screening of 557,648 community-dwelling older adults. *Archives of Gerontology and Geriatrics, 68*, 174–180.

Cosman, F., Nicpon, K., & Nieves, J. W. (2016). Results of a fracture liaison service on hip fracture patients in an open healthcare system. *Aging Clinical and Experimental Research, 29*, 331–334.

Dhillon, R. J., & Hasni, S. (2017). Pathogenesis and management of sarcopenia. *Clinics in Geriatric Medicine, 33*, 17–26.

Figueiredo, D., & Santos, S. (2017). Cross-cultural validation of the Falls Efficacy Scale-International (FES-I) in Portuguese community-dwelling older adults. *Archives of Gerontology & Geriatrics, 68*, 168–173.

Filar-Mierzwa, K., Dlugosz, M., Marchewka, A., et al. (2016). The effect of dance therapy on the balance of women over 60 years of age: The influence of dance therapy for the elderly. *Journal of Women and Aging, 23*, 1–8.

Gale, C. R., Cooper, C., & Aihie Sayer, A. (2016). Prevalence and risk factors for falls in older men and women: The English Longitudinal Study of Ageing. *Age & Ageing, 45*, 789–794.

Geusens, P. P., & van den Bergh, J. (2016). Osteoporosis and osteoarthritis: Shared mechanisms and epidemiology. *Current Opinion in Rheumatology, 28*, 97–103.

Gillelspie, L. D., Robertson, M. C., Gilespie, W. J., et al. (2012). Interventions for preventing falls in older people living in the community (Review). The Cochrane Database of Systematic Reviews. Doi: 10.1002/14651858.CD007614.pub3

Goh, H. T., Nadarajah, M., Hamzah, N. B., et al. (2016). Falls and fear of falling after stroke: A case-control study. *P M & R: The Journal of Injury, Function, and Rehabilitation, 8*, 1173–1180.

Gorter, E. A., Krijnen, P., & Schipper, I. B. (2016). Vitamin D deficiency in adult fracture patients: Prevalence and risk factors. *European Journal of Trauma and Emergency Surgery, 42*, 369–378.

Gray-Miceli, D., & Quigley, P. A. (2016). Preventing falls in acute care. In M. Boltz, E. Capezuti, T. Fulmer, & D. Zwicker (Eds.), *Evidence-based practice protocols for best practice* (5th ed., pp. 283–309). New York: Springer Publishing Co.

Greenberg, S. A., Sullivan-Marx, E., Sommers, M. L., et al. (2016). Measuring fear of falling among high-risk, urban, community-dwelling older adults. *Geriatric Nursing, 37*, 489–495.

Hant, F. N., & Bolster, M. B. (2016). Drugs that may harm bone: mitigating the risk. *Cleveland Clinic Medical Journal, 83*, 281–288.

Hassan, B., Hewitt, J., Keogh, J., et al. (2016). Impact of resistance training on sarcopenia in nursing care facilities: A pilot study. *Geriatric Nursing, 37*, 116–121.

Hefner, J., McAlearney, A. S., Mansfield, J., et al. (2015). A Falls Wheel in a large academic medical center: An intervention to reduce patient falls with harm. *Journal for Healthcare Quality, 37*, 374–380.

Herdman, T., & Kamitsura, S. (Eds). (2018). *NANDA International Nursing Diagnoses Definitions and Classification, 2018–2020* (11th ed., pp. 34–44). New York: Thieme Publishers.

Hoang, O. T., Jullamate, P., Piphatvanitcha, N., et al. (2016). Factors related to fear of falling among community-dwelling older adults. *Journal of Clinical Nursing, 26,* 68–76.

Huovinen, V., Ivaska, K. K., Kiviranta, R., et al. (2016). Bone mineral density is increased after 16-week resistance training intervention in elderly women with decreased muscle strength. *European Journal of Endocrinology, 175,* 571–582.

Hwang, H. F., Chen, S., J., Lee-Hsieh, J., et al. (2016). Effects of home-based tai chi and lower extremity training and self-practice on falls and function outcomes in older fallers from the emergency department: A randomized controlled trial. *Journal of the American Geriatrics Society, 64,* 518–525.

James, E. G., Conatser, P., Karabulut, M., et al. (2016). Mobility limitations and fear of falling in non-English speaking older Mexican-Americans. *Ethnicity & Health,* 2016 Oct 14.

Jones, D. L., Starcher, R. W., Eicher, J. L., et al. (2016). Adoption of a Tai Chi intervention, Tai Ji Quan: Moving for Better Balance, for fall prevention by rural faith-based organizations, 2013-2014. *Public Health Research, Practice and Policy, 13,* 160083. doi: 10.5888/pcd13.160083.

Kapan, A., Luger, E., Haider, S., et al. (2017). Fear of falling reduced by lay led home-based program in frail community-dwelling older adults: A randomized controlled trial. *Archives of Gerontology & Geriatrics, 68,* 25–32.

Kwok, J. Y., Choi, K. C., & Chan, H. Y. (2016). Effects of mind-body exercises on the physiological and psychosocial well-being of individuals with Parkinson's disease: A systematic review and meta-analysis. *Complementary Therapies in Medicine, 29,* 121–131.

Li, F., Harmer, P., & Fitzgerald, K. (2016). Implementing an evidence-based fall prevention intervention in community senior centers. *American Journal of Public Health, 106,* 2026–2031.

Lu, Y. H., Rosner, B., Chang, G., et al. (2016). Twelve-minute daily yoga regimen reverses osteoporotic bone loss. *Topics in Geriatric Rehabilitation, 32,* 81–87.

Lusardi, M., Fritz, S., Middleton, A., et al. (2017). Determining risk of falls in community dwelling older adults: A systematic review and meta-analysis using posttest probability. *Journal of Geriatric Physical Therapy, 40,* 1–34.

Malgo, F., Appleman-Dijkstra, N. M., Termaat, M. F., et al. (2016). High prevalence of secondary fractures for bone fragility in patients with a recent fracture independently of BMD. *Archives of Osteoporosis, 11*:12. doi: 10.1007/s11657-016-0258-3.

Malini, F. M., Lourenco, R. A., & Lopes, C. S. (2016). Prevalence of fear of falling in older adults, and its associations with clinical, functional and psychosocial factors: the Frailty in Brazilian Older People-Rio de Janeiro study. *Geriatrics and Gerontology International, 16,* 336–344.

Marcum, Z. A., Wirtz, H. S., Pettinger, M., et al. (2016). Anticholinergic medication use and falls in postmenopausal women: findings from the Women's Health Initiative cohort study. *BioMed Central Geriatrics, 16*:76. doi: 10.1186/s12877-016-0251-0.

Meehan, A., Hommel, A., Hertz, K., et al. (2016). Care of the older adult with fragility hip fracture. In M. Boltz, E. Capezuti, T. Fulmer, & D. Zwicker (Eds), *Evidence-based geriatric nursing protocols for best practice* (5th ed., pp. 591–617). New York: Springer Publishing.

Moreira Bde, S., Dos Anjos, D. M., Pereira, D. S., et al. (2016). The geriatric depression scale and the timed up and go test predict fear of falling in community-dwelling elderly women with type 2 diabetes mellitus: A cross-sectional study. *BioMed Central Geriatrics,* 2016 Mar 3. doi: 10.1186/s12877-016-0234-1.

Muniz, R., Gomez, S., Curto, D., et al. (2016). Reducing physical restraints in nursing homes: A report from Maria Wolff and Sanitas. *Journal of the American Medical Directors Association, 17,* 633–639/

National Osteoporosis Foundation. (2016). Debunking the Myths. Available at www.nof.org.

Nick, N., Petramfar, P., Ghodsbin, F., et al. (2016). The effect of yoga on balance and fear of falling in older adults. *P M & R: The Journal of Injury, Function, and Rehabilitation, 8,* 145–151.

Oh, C., Jeon, B. H., Reid-Storm, S. H., et al. (2017). The most effective factors to offset sarcopenia and obesity in the older Korean: physical activity, vitamin D, and protein intake. *Nutrition, 33,* 169–173.

Opsahl, A., Ebright, P., Cangany, M., et al. (2017). Outcomes of adding patient and family education to fall prevention bundled interventions. *Journal of Nursing Care Quality, 32,* 252–258.

Osuna, P. M., Ruppe, M. D., & Tabatabai, L. S. (2017). Fracture liaison services: Multidisciplinary approaches to secondary fracture prevention.*Endocrine Practice, 23,* 199–206.

Palagyi, A., Ng, J. Q., Rogers, K., et al. (2016). Fear of falling and physical function in older adults with cataract: Exploring the role of vision as a moderator. *Geriatrics and Gerontology International,* Dec 4 [Epub] doi: 10.1111/ggi.12930.

Phillips, L., DeRoche, C., Rantz, M., et al. (2017). Using embedded sensors in independent living to predict gait changes and falls. *Western Journal of Nursing Research, 39,* 78–94.

Rantz, M., Skubic, M., Abbott, C., et al. (2015). Automated in-home fall risk assessment and detection sensor system for elders. *Gerontologist, 55,* S78–S87.

Schoberer, D., Breimaier, H., Mandl, M., et al. (2016). Involving the consumers: An exploration of users' and caregivers' needs and expectations on a fall prevention brochure: A qualitative study. *Geriatric Nursing, 37,* 207–214.

Shanbhogue, V. V., Brixen, K., & Hansen, S. (2016). Age- and sex-related changes in bone microarchitecture and estimated strength: A three-year prospective study using HRpQCT. *Journal of Bone & Mineral Research, 31,* 1541–1549.

Sheldon, J. H. (1960). On the natural history of falls in old age. *British Medical Journal, 2,* 1685–1690.

Sheu, A., & Diamond, T. (2016). Secondary osteoporosis. *Australian Prescriber, 39,* 85–87.

Sitzer, V. (2016). Development of an automated self-assessment of fall risk questionnaire for hospitalized patients. *Journal of Nursing Care Quality, 31,* 46–53.

Stathopoulos, K. D., Zoubos, A. B., Papaioannou, N. A., et al. (2016). Differences of bone mineral mass, volumetric bone mineral density, geometrical and structural parameters and derived strength of the tibia between premenopausal and postmenopausal women of different age groups. *Journal of Musculoskeletal and Neuronal Interactions, 16,* 113–121.

U. S. Preventive Services Task Force. (2012). Prevention of falls in community-dwelling older adults: U. S. Preventive Services Task Force Recommendation Statement. *Annals of Internal Medicine, 157*(3), 197–204.

Wang, C., Schmid, C. H., Iversen, M. D., et al. (2016). Comparative effectiveness of tai chi versus physical therapy for knee osteoarthritis: A randomized trial. *Annals of Internal Medicine, 165,* 77–86.

Yong, J. H., Masucci, L., Hoch, J. S., et al. (2016). Cost-effectiveness of a fracture liaison service: A real-world evaluation after 6 years of service provision. *Osteoporosis International, 27,* 231–240.

Youkhana, S., Dean, C. M., Wolff, M., et al. (2016). Yoga-based exercise improves balance and mobility in people aged 60 and over: A systematic review and meta-analysis. *Age & Ageing, 45,* 21–29.

Yount, J. (2016). Strength in Numbers: A community education program to prevent falls in older adults. *Home Healthcare Now, 34,* 369–373.

Zafar, M., Bozzorg, A., & Hackney, M. E. (2016). Adapted tango improves aspects of participation in older adults versus individuals with Parkinson's disease. *Disability Rehabilitation,* Oct 21 [Epub]. doi: 10.1080/09638288.2016.1226405.

Zia, A., Kamaruzzaman, S. B., & Tan, M. P. (2016). The consumption of two or more fall risk-increasing drugs rather than polypharmacy is associated with falls. *Geriatrics and Gerontology International,* Jan 28. doi: 10.1111/ggi.12741.

Integumentary Function

For many people, and particularly for older adults, skin is the most visible indicator of the combined effects of biologic aging, lifestyle, and environment. Thus, the skin, hair, and nails have not only physiologic functions but also many social functions. In addition to its crucial function of protection of underlying structures, the skin directly affects all the following processes:

- Thermoregulation
- Excretion of metabolic wastes
- Synthesis of vitamin D
- Maintenance of fluid and electrolyte balance
- Sensations of pain, touch, pressure, temperature, and vibration

The social functions of the skin include facilitating communication and serving as an indicator of race, gender, work status, and other personal characteristics.

Hair serves to protect underlying organs, primarily the skin, from injury and adverse temperatures. In addition, in social contexts, the length and style of one's hair can reflect certain characteristics such as age, gender, and personality. Although hair is one of the most visible manifestations of aging, hair color can easily be altered if gray is viewed as an undesirable indicator of age. Like the skin and hair, nails have both a physiologic and social capacity. Physiologically, nails protect the underlying tissue from injury. In social contexts, nails can reflect personal characteristics such as grooming and occupational activities.

AGE-RELATED CHANGES THAT AFFECT THE INTEGUMENTARY SYSTEM

The skin is the largest, as well as the most visible body organ. Structurally, the skin comprises three layers: the epidermis, the dermis, and the subcutaneous tissue. Hair, nails, and sweat glands are also parts of the integumentary system. In addition to age-related changes, genetics, lifestyle, and environmental factors exert a significant effect on the integumentary system and have a cumulative effect in older adults.

Epidermis

The epidermis is the relatively impermeable outer layer of skin that serves as a barrier, preventing both the loss of body

Promoting Skin Wellness in Older Adults

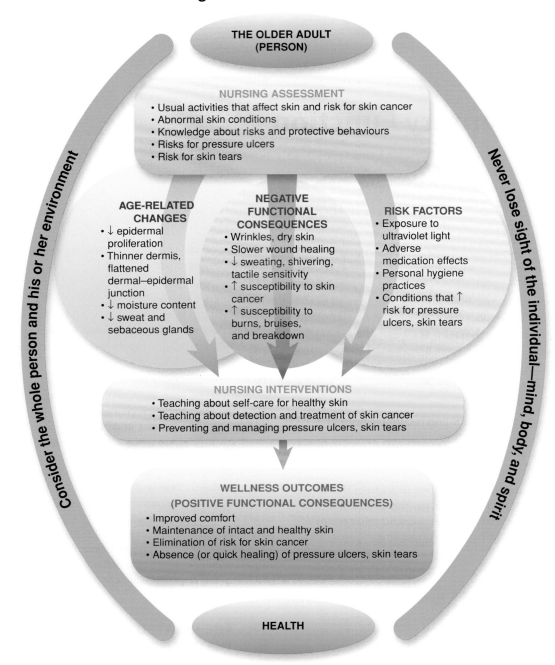

THE OLDER ADULT (PERSON)

NURSING ASSESSMENT
- Usual activities that affect skin and risk for skin cancer
- Abnormal skin conditions
- Knowledge about risks and protective behaviours
- Risks for pressure ulcers
- Risk for skin tears

AGE-RELATED CHANGES
- ↓ epidermal proliferation
- Thinner dermis, flattened dermal–epidermal junction
- ↓ moisture content
- ↓ sweat and sebaceous glands

NEGATIVE FUNCTIONAL CONSEQUENCES
- Wrinkles, dry skin
- Slower wound healing
- ↓ sweating, shivering, tactile sensitivity
- ↑ susceptibility to skin cancer
- ↑ susceptibility to burns, bruises, and breakdown

RISK FACTORS
- Exposure to ultraviolet light
- Adverse medication effects
- Personal hygiene practices
- Conditions that ↑ risk for pressure ulcers, skin tears

NURSING INTERVENTIONS
- Teaching about self-care for healthy skin
- Teaching about detection and treatment of skin cancer
- Preventing and managing pressure ulcers, skin tears

WELLNESS OUTCOMES
(POSITIVE FUNCTIONAL CONSEQUENCES)
- Improved comfort
- Maintenance of intact and healthy skin
- Elimination of risk for skin cancer
- Absence (or quick healing) of pressure ulcers, skin tears

HEALTH

Consider the whole person and his or her environment

Never lose sight of the individual—mind, body, and spirit

fluids and the entry of substances from the environment. Layers of cells in the epidermis undergo a continual cycle of regeneration, cornification, and shedding. Epidermal cells develop in the innermost layer of the epidermis and continually migrate to the surface of the skin where they are shed. With increasing age, these cells become larger and more variable in shape, and the rate of epidermal turnover gradually decreases.

Melanocytes are epidermal cells that give the skin its color and provide a protective barrier against ultraviolet radiation. Beginning around the age of 25 years, the number of active melanocytes decreases by 18% to 20% each decade. With increased age, the number of Langerhans cells, which serve as macrophages, also decreases in both sun-exposed and sun-protected skin; the decrease ranges from 50% to 70% in sun-exposed skin. Another age-related change is a decrease in the moisture content of the outer epidermal layer.

Papillae give the skin its texture and connect the epidermis to the underlying dermis at the dermal–epidermal junction. With increased age, the papillae retract, causing a flattening of the dermal–epidermal junction and diminishing the surface area between the epidermis and dermis. This age-related change slows the transfer of nutrients and oxygen between the dermis and epidermis.

Dermis

The primary functions of the dermis include temperature regulation, sensory perception, and nourishment for all skin layers. Components of the dermis function in the following ways:

- Collagen: constitutes 80% of the dermis and provides elasticity and tensile strength to prevent tearing and over-stretching
- Elastin: maintains skin tension to allow stretching in response to movement
- Dermal ground substance: determines skin turgor and elastic properties due to its water-binding capacity
- Blood vessels in the deep plexus: facilitate efficient thermoregulation
- Blood vessels in the superficial plexus: supply nutrients to the epidermal layer
- Cutaneous nerves: receive and transmit sensory information regarding pain, pressure, temperature, and deep and light touch

The following age-related changes begin in early adulthood and progress gradually: Dermal thickness diminishes, elastin increases in quantity and decreases in quality, dermal vascular bed decreases, and fibroblasts and mast cells decrease. These age-related changes cause atrophy of the hair bulbs and sweat and sebaceous glands.

Subcutaneous Tissue and Cutaneous Nerves

The subcutis is the inner layer of fat tissue that serves the following functions: protection of underlying tissues, storage of calories, insulation of the body, and regulation of heat loss. With increased age, some areas of subcutaneous tissue atrophy and other areas hypertrophy, with the overall effect being a gradual increase in the proportion of body fat during older adulthood. This increased body fat is more pronounced in women than in men and is most noticeable in the waists of men and the thighs of women. Age-related changes also affect the cutaneous nerves responsible for sensations of pressure, vibration, and light touch.

Sweat and Sebaceous Glands

Eccrine and apocrine sweat glands originate in the dermal layer and are most abundant in the palms of the hands, soles of the feet, and axillae. Eccrine glands, which are important for thermoregulation, open directly onto the skin surface and are most abundant on the palms, soles, and forehead. Apocrine glands are larger than eccrine glands and open into hair follicles, primarily in the axillae and genital area. The sole function of these glands is to produce secretions,

which create a distinctive body odor. Both eccrine and apocrine glands decrease in number and functional ability with increased age.

Sebaceous glands, which continually secrete sebum, are present in the dermal skin layer over every part of the body except the palms of the hands and the soles of the feet. Functionally, sebum prevents the loss of water and inhibits bacterial and fungal growth. The secretion of sebum begins to diminish during the third decade, with women having a greater decline than men.

Nails

The rate of nail growth is influenced by many factors including age, climate, state of health, circulation to and around the nails, and activity of the fingers and toes. Nail growth begins to slow in early adulthood, with a gradual decrease of 30% to 50% during a normal life span. Nails of older adults gradually become thinner, fragile, brittle, and more prone to splitting. In appearance, the older nail is dull, opaque, longitudinally striated, and yellow or gray, with decreased lunula size.

Hair

Hair color and distribution change to some degree in all older adults, with the most noticeable changes being graying and thinning. Hair distribution is also affected by age-related changes, with patches of coarse terminal hair developing over the upper lip and lower face in older women and in the ears, nares, and eyebrows of older men. Another age-related change is a progressive loss of body hair, initially in the trunk, then in the pubic area and axillae.

 ## RISK FACTORS THAT AFFECT SKIN WELLNESS

The risk factors that influence the skin and hair of older adults include heredity, lifestyle and environmental factors, and adverse medication effects. Lifestyle and environmental factors have a cumulative effect that manifests more fully during later adulthood, but it is important to identify the risk factors that nurses can address through health education. Nutritional deficiencies increase the risk for pathologic conditions affecting the integumentary system (e.g., dermatitis, alopecia). Nutritional factors also are a significant risk for pressure injuries, as discussed in the section on pathologic conditions affecting the skin.

Genetic Influences

Heredity plays an important role in the development of skin and hair changes. People with fair skin, light hair, and light eyes are more sensitive to the effects of ultraviolet radiation than people with dark skin, as evidenced by the fact that skin cancers are common in light-skinned people of northern European ancestry but rare in African Americans.

Health Behaviors and Environmental Influences

Tobacco smoking, sun exposure, air pollution, and alcohol abuse are the health behaviors and environmental factors that studies have identified as risks for skin aging (Humbert, Dreno, Krutmann, et al., 2016; Krutmann, Bouloc, Sore, et al., 2016). Sun exposure and tobacco smoking, which are the risks most closely associated with skin cancer, are the ones that can readily be addressed through health promotion interventions. In addition, because the water content of the stratum corneum is influenced by relative humidity, xerosis (dry skin) is exacerbated when the relative humidity is below 30%.

Sociocultural Influences

Cultural factors, societal attitudes, and advertising trends influence hygiene and skin care practices. People in industrialized societies place a high value on frequent bathing and the use of commercial products for hygienic and cosmetic purposes. Although most of the personal practices associated with these values are desirable or harmless in younger adults, they may adversely affect older adults. For example, frequent bathing with harsh deodorant soaps may cause or exacerbate dry skin problems in an older person.

> ### Wellness Opportunity
>
> From a holistic nursing perspective, nonjudgmentally consider the influence of cultural and societal attitudes on personal care practices and address any factors that negatively affect self-esteem.

Medication Effects

Common adverse medication effects involving the skin include pruritus, dermatoses, and photosensitivity reactions. Less common adverse medication effects on the skin and hair include alopecia and pigmentation changes of the skin or hair. Cytotoxic agents are the type of drug most commonly associated with hair loss, but other drugs that can cause alopecia include anticoagulants, nonsteroidal anti-inflammatory agents, and cardiovascular medications.

Dermatoses, or rashes, are the most frequently cited adverse effect of medications, and they can be caused by virtually any medication. Although drug-related skin eruptions (also called fixed-drug eruptions) vary widely in their manifestations, maculopapular eruptions are the most common reactions. Drug-related dermatoses can occur from 1 day to 4 weeks after initiating or discontinuing the causative medication. The following medications have been identified as causes of adverse cutaneous reactions: aspirin and other nonsteroidal anti-inflammatory drugs, barbiturates, carbamazepine, tetracyclines, sulfamethoxazole, and metformin (less commonly) (Steber, Perkins, & Harris, 2016; Walters & Woessner, 2016). In addition, ophthalmic medications, such as those prescribed for glaucoma or post-cataract surgery, can cause periorbital dermatitis (Grey & Warshaw, 2016).

Photosensitivity is an adverse medication effect that causes an intensified response to ultraviolet radiation. The inflammatory reaction is initially distributed over sun-exposed areas, but it may spread to nonexposed areas and persist even after the medication is discontinued. Photosensitivity may begin during a seasonal exposure to bright sunlight or during a vacation in an unusually hot climate. Medications commonly associated with photosensitivity reactions include antimicrobials, hydrochlorothiazide, nonsteroidal anti-inflammatory drugs, and cardiovascular drugs (Monteiro, Rato, & Martins, 2016; Zuba, Koronowska, Osmola-Mankowska, et al., 2016).

In addition to causing adverse effects, medications can indirectly cause skin problems by exacerbating age-related changes. For example, fluid loss from diuretics can exacerbate xerosis and cause further discomfort or skin problems for the older adult. Another example of the combined effects of aging and medications is that older adults taking anticoagulants are likely to bruise easily, and bruising may become extensive.

 ## FUNCTIONAL CONSEQUENCES AFFECTING SKIN WELLNESS

Age-related changes and risk factors negatively affect many functions of the skin including thermoregulation, tactile sensitivity, and wound healing. Age-related changes do not interfere with the protective function of the nails; however, the nails in older persons are brittle and more likely to split. People who hold negative attitudes about aging may experience psychosocial consequences when changes in the appearance of the skin and hair become visible indicators of aging.

Delayed Wound Healing and Increased Susceptibility to Skin Problems

The regeneration of healthy skin takes twice as long for an 80-year-old as for a 30-year-old person. In perfectly intact skin, this slowed regeneration has no noticeable effects. When skin integrity is compromised; however, this age-related change contributes to delayed wound healing, even for superficial wounds. The consequences of age-related changes that affect the healing of deep wounds include an increased risk for postoperative wound disruption, decreased tensile strength of healing wounds, and increased risk of secondary infections.

Age-related changes in all layers of the skin combine with the effects of long-term exposure to the sun and other risk factors to increase the susceptibility of older adults to many types of problems (e.g., skin tears, pressure injuries, stasis dermatitis), as delineated in Table 23-1 and described in the section on pathologic conditions affecting skin. In addition, the age-related diminished immune function increases older adults' susceptibility to skin cancers and other pathologic conditions.

TABLE 23-1 Functional Consequences Affecting Skin and Appendages

Age-Related Change	Consequence
Decreased rate of epidermal proliferation	Delayed wound healing; increased susceptibility to infection
Flattened dermal–epidermal junction; thinning of dermis; degenerative changes of collagen; increased quantity, but decreased quality, of elastin	Decreased resiliency; increased susceptibility to injury, bruising, mechanical stress, ultraviolet radiation, and blister formation
Reductions in dermal blood supply and the number of melanocytes and Langerhans cells	Decreased intensity of tanning; irregular pigmentation; increased susceptibility to skin cancer; diminished dermal clearance, absorption, and immunologic response
Reductions in eccrine sweat, subcutaneous fat, and dermal blood supply	Decreased sweating and shivering; increased susceptibility to hypothermia or hyperthermia
Decreased moisture content	Dry skin; discomfort
Decreased number of Meissner and Pacinian corpuscles	Diminished tactile sensitivity; increased susceptibility to burns
Slowed nail growth	Increased susceptibility to cracking and injury; delayed healing
Changes in hair color, quantity, and distribution	Negative impact on self-esteem in proportion to negative attitudes

 GLOBAL PERSPECTIVE

Worldwide, more older adults in developing countries than developed countries die from cellulitis and other skin infections, whereas more older adults in developed countries than in developing countries die from skin cancer. This may be explained in part by, in developing countries, larger proportions of fair-skinned people and the cultural emphasis on outdoor activities and indoor tanning services (Blume-Peytavi, Kottner, Sterry, et al., 2016).

Photoaging

Photoaging is the term used to describe skin changes that occur because of exposure to ultraviolet radiation, even at levels that do not cause any detectable sunburn. These changes are sometimes viewed as premature aging; however, they are biologically distinct processes that occur independently and are superimposed on normal aging changes. Studies indicate that sun exposure accounts for up to 90% of visible skin aging (Keaney, 2016). One reason for the misconception that photoaging is an age-related change is that the cumulative effects of ultraviolet radiation may not be evident until later adulthood. Common characteristics of photoaging are as follows:

- Coarse, leathery, and ruddy or yellowed appearance
- Deep wrinkles, particularly on the face and neck
- Pathologic lesions and seborrheic and actinic keratoses
- Thickened epidermis
- Enlarged sebaceous glands
- Marked loss of elasticity
- Dilated and tortuous blood vessels
- Numerous freckles

 Diversity Note

Photoaging in darkly pigmented skin presents as uneven pigmentation (Vashi, Maymone, & Kundu, 2016).

Comfort and Sensation

Dry skin is one of the most universal complaints of older adults, affecting up to 85% of noninstitutionalized older people. Age-related changes, such as diminished output of sebum and eccrine sweat, contribute to a decrease in the moisture content of the skin. Risk factors that may contribute to dry skin include stress, smoking, sun exposure, dry environments, excessive perspiration, adverse medication reactions, excessive use of soap, and certain medical conditions (e.g., hypothyroidism).

Tactile sensitivity begins to decline around the age of 20 years, eventually causing older adults to have a diminished and less intense response to cutaneous sensations. This decline is attributable, at least in part, to age-related changes in Pacinian and Meissner corpuscles, which are the skin receptors that respond to vibration. Other contributing factors include lower body temperature and functional alterations in the central nervous system. Functionally, older adults are more susceptible to scald burns because of their diminished ability to feel dangerously hot water temperatures.

Thermoregulation is also affected by age-related reductions in eccrine sweat, subcutaneous fat, and dermal blood supply. These age-related changes interfere with sweating, shivering, peripheral vasoconstriction and vasodilation, and insulation against adverse environmental temperatures. Thus, older adults are more at risk for the development of hypothermia and heat-related illnesses, as discussed in Chapter 25.

Cosmetic Effects

The overall cosmetic effect of age-related skin changes is that the skin looks paler, thinner, and more translucent and is irregularly pigmented. Age-related changes that cause these cosmetic effects include decreased melanocytes and diminished dermal circulation. Additional indicators of age-related skin changes include sagging and wrinkling, which are caused by age-related changes in the epidermis and dermis, particularly those affecting collagen. Decreased subcutaneous tissue contributes to sagging skin, particularly over the upper arms, by allowing gravity to pull the skin downward. Various skin growths and lesions that are common in older adults are described in the section on Nursing Assessment.

Although these changes in appearance are gradual and do not interfere significantly with physiologic function, the psychosocial consequences of these changes can be significant because of the social value placed on personal appearance and negative attitudes that may be held about growing old. Regardless of age, one's physical appearance has been shown to be an important determinant of self-perception, and modern societies associate attractiveness with young-looking skin.

Wellness Opportunity

Nurses can promote positive attitudes about aging by challenging societal perspectives that associate beauty only with youth.

Because of the high visibility of the face and neck, any signs of increased age that are prominent around the eyes and mouth may be particularly bothersome to the person who wants to avoid visible indications of age. Characteristic signs of advanced age that are evident around the eyes include increased pigmentation, crow's-feet wrinkles, and fat and fluid accumulation in the upper lid and under the eye. Also, because of diminished skin elasticity and the loss and shifting of subcutaneous fat, the neck skin sags, and a double chin may develop. Table 23-1 summarizes the functional consequences resulting from age-related changes of the skin, hair, nails, and glands.

PATHOLOGIC CONDITION AFFECTING SKIN: SKIN CANCER

A serious functional consequence of the age-related skin changes and long-term sun exposure is the increased incidence of skin cancers in older adults. Skin cancer, which is classified as melanoma or non-melanoma skin cancer, is by far the most common type of cancer diagnosed in westernized countries. Incidence of all types of skin cancer has been steadily increasing at the rate of 3% or more per year for three decades, with exponential increases among older adults (John, Trakatelli, Gehring, et al., 2016; Paddock, Lu, Bandera, et al., 2016; Tripp, Watson, Balk, et al., 2016). Studies indicate that approximately 90% of non-melanoma skin cancer are attributable to excessive sun exposure (Griffin, Ali, & Lear, 2016). Occupational sun exposure is identified as a risk for skin cancer in veterans, farmers, and outdoor construction workers (Sena, Girko, de Carvalho, et al., 2016; Yoon, Phibbs, Chow, et al., 2016). Immunosuppression is an additional factor that increases the risk for skin cancer.

Non-melanoma skin cancers that are common in older adults are basal cell carcinoma and squamous cell carcinoma. **Basal cell carcinoma**, which is the most common type, occurs most often on the head and neck (Figure 23-1A).

If diagnosed and treated during its early stage, the cure rate for basal cell carcinoma is close to 100%; however, if left untreated, it invades the surrounding tissue. **Squamous cell carcinoma** occurs most commonly on the head, neck, forearms, and dorsal hands (Figure 23-1B). Squamous cell skin cancer accounts for 20% of non-melanoma skin cancers and is a deadly threat because of its ability to metastasize to any part of the body (Burton, Ashack, & Khachemoune, 2016).

Melanoma, which originates in the melanocytes, is the most serious type of skin cancer, accounting for 90% of all skin cancer deaths, with disproportionately higher mortality rates for older adults (Aubuchon, Bolt, Janssen-Heijnen, et al., 2017; Weiss, Han, Darvishian, et al., 2016). Moreover, early detection and treatment are imperative for improving the outcomes of all types of skin cancer, and nurses have an essential role in assessing and teaching older adults about skin cancer, as discussed in the sections on nursing assessment and nursing interventions (also, see Figure 23-1C).

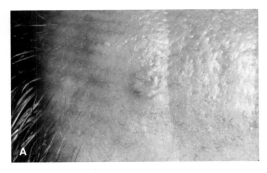

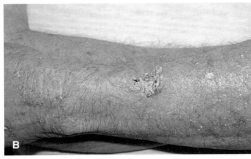

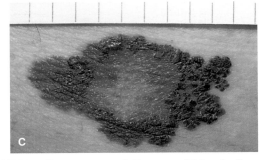

FIGURE 23-1 Common types of skin cancer: (**A**) basal cell carcinoma; (**B**) squamous cell carcinoma; (**C**) melanoma. (A and C: Reprinted with permission from Rosenthal, T. C., Williams, M. E., & Naughton, B. J. (2007). *Office care geriatrics.* Philadelphia, PA: Lippincott Williams & Wilkins; and B: from Goodheart, H. P. (2003). *Goodheart's photoguide of common skin disorders.* (2nd ed.) Philadelphia, PA: Lippincott Williams & Wilkins.)

Nurses also need to consider risk factors in their assessments and address them in health promotion. Advanced age increases the risk for all types of skin lesions including skin cancers. Exposure to ultraviolet rays, including those from tanning booths, is a risk factor that is highly associated with skin cancers and that is most amenable to protective measures. Other risks for melanoma include family history, fair skin, sunburn susceptibility, and number of severe sunburns.

Diversity Note

Melanoma is more common in men and light-skinned people, with significant and disproportionately high increases among older adults in recent decades (Olazagasti-Lourido, Ma, Lohse, et al., 2016; Wang, Zhao, & Ma, 2016). Survival rates for melanoma are highest for women and non-Hispanic whites (Crocetti, Fancelli, Manneschi, et al., 2016; Dawes, Tsai, Gittleman, et al., 2016).

Wellness Opportunity

Nurses promote self-care for wellness by teaching older adults to use a mirror and examine their skin for suspicious changes once a month.

PATHOLOGIC CONDITION AFFECTING SKIN: SKIN TEARS

Skin tears are wounds caused by shear, friction, or blunt force causing a separation of skin layers. A systematic review identified the most prevalent risk factor as older age, followed by impaired mobility, falls and accidental injuries, previous skin tears, cognitive impairment, dependence in transfers (Strazzieri-Pulido, Peres, Campanili, et al., 2017). The International Skin Tear Advisory Panel developed and validated a classification system describing skin tears as follows:

- Type 1, no skin loss: linear or flap tear that can be repositioned to cover the wound bed
- Type 2, partial flap loss (i.e., separation of the epidermis from the dermis): skin cannot be repositioned to cover the wound bed
- Type 3, total flap loss (i.e., separation of both the epidermis and dermis from the underlying structure): total loss of skin, exposing entire wound bed

(LeBlanc, Baranoski, Holloway, et al., 2013).

Skin tears are recognized as a serious problem because they are associated with significant functional consequences such as pain, functional impairment, and increased length of stay in hospitals and long-term care facilities. Current evidence-based guidelines emphasize the following goals of treatment: treat the cause, implement prevention protocol, provide for moist wound healing, avoid trauma, protect surrounding skin, manage exudate, avoid infection, and control pain (LeBlanc, Baranoski, Christensen, et al., 2016). Twice-daily skin moisturizing is recommended as a component of

a prevention program in long-term care facilities (LeBlanc, Kozell, Martins, et al., 2016). The International Skin Tears Advisory Panel provides up-to-date and evidence-based information about prevention, prediction, assessment, and treatment of skin tears (see Online Learning Activity 23-1).

See **ONLINE LEARNING ACTIVITY 23-1:** **EVIDENCE-BASED INFORMATION ABOUT SKIN TEARS** at http://thepoint.lww.com/Miller8e.

PATHOLOGIC CONDITION AFFECTING SKIN: PRESSURE INJURY

During the four decades since pressure ulcers (also called pressure sores) were first described in medical literature, major organizations have revised definitions of this unique type of pathologic skin problem several times. Most recently, in 2016, the National Pressure Ulcer Advisory Panel (NPUAP) adopted a change in terminology and revised the definitions, as discussed in the section on Staging Systems. In keeping with current guidelines published by the NPUAP, the term *pressure injury* is used in this text, except when quoting a reference that uses the term pressure ulcer. The Centers for Medicare and Medicaid Services (CMS) and other major agencies are in the process of updating their terminology to be consistent with the NPUAP terminology; however, in the interim, both terms are used interchangeably.

The NPUAP (2016) defines a **pressure injury** as "localized damage to the skin and underlying soft tissue usually over a bony prominence or under a medical or other device." The injury can present as intact skin or an open ulcer and may be painful. The injury occurs as a result of intense and/or prolonged pressure or pressure in combination with shear. Figure 23-2 illustrates areas of the body that are most susceptible to development of pressure injury, with sacrum/coccyx and heel being the first and second most common sites.

Pressure Injury Staging System

Staging systems have been used since 1975 to describe the extent of tissue damage to classify pressure ulcers according to anatomic depth of soft-tissue damage. Staging systems have been widely used in the United States and other countries and have been reviewed and updated periodically. In 2016, an NPUAP-appointed task force engaged in a comprehensive process to review and update the staging system based on extensive review of literature and input that included researchers, clinical experts, and a global interdisciplinary expert collaboration (Edsberg, Black, Goldberg, et al., 2016). The **Pressure Injury Staging System** that currently is recommended in the United States is described and illustrated in Table 23-2. This Staging System with updated terminology and definitions has been adopted and endorsed by major national and international organizations, including The Joint Commission, the National Database of Nursing Quality Indicators, the Canadian Association of

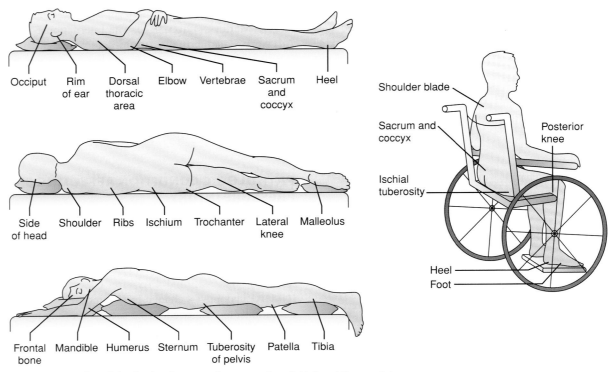

Occiput Rim of ear Dorsal thoracic area Elbow Vertebrae Sacrum and coccyx Heel

Side of head Shoulder Ribs Ischium Trochanter Lateral knee Malleolus

Frontal bone Mandible Humerus Sternum Tuberosity of pelvis Patella Tibia

Shoulder blade Sacrum and coccyx Ischial tuberosity Posterior knee Heel Foot

FIGURE 23-2 The risk for the development of pressure ulcers is higher at these points.

TABLE 23-2 NPUAP Pressure Injury Staging System

Stage 1 Pressure Injury: Nonblanchable erythema of intact skin
Intact skin with a localized area of nonblanchable erythema, which may appear differently in darkly pigmented skin. Presence of blanchable erythema or changes in sensation, temperature, or firmness may precede visual changes. Color changes do not include purple or maroon discoloration; these may indicate deep tissue pressure injury.

Stage 2 Pressure Injury: Partial-thickness skin loss with exposed dermis
Partial-thickness loss of skin with exposed dermis. The wound bed is viable, pink or red, moist, and may also present as an intact or ruptured serum-filled blister. Adipose is not visible and deeper tissues are not visible. Granulation tissue, slough and eschar are not present. These injuries commonly result from adverse microclimate and shear in the skin over the pelvis and shear in the heel. This stage should not be used to describe moisture associated skin damage including incontinence associated dermatitis, intertriginous dermatitis, medical adhesive related skin injury, or traumatic wounds (skin tears, burns, abrasions).

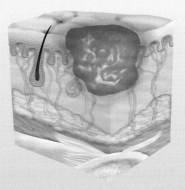

TABLE 23-2 NPUAP Pressure Injury Staging System *(Continued)*

Stage 3 Pressure Injury: Full-thickness skin loss

Full-thickness loss of skin, in which adipose is visible in the ulcer and granulation tissue and epibole (i.e., rolled wound edges) are often present. Slough and/or eschar may be visible. The depth of tissue damage varies by anatomical location; areas of significant adiposity can develop deep wounds. Undermining and tunneling may occur. Fascia, muscle, tendon, ligament, cartilage and/or bone are not exposed. If slough or eschar obscures the extent of tissue loss this is an Unstageable Pressure Injury.

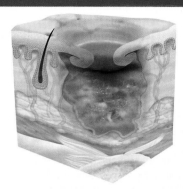

Stage 4 Pressure Injury: Full-thickness skin and tissue loss

Full-thickness skin and tissue loss with exposed or directly palpable fascia, muscle, tendon, ligament, cartilage or bone in the ulcer. Slough and/or eschar may be visible. Epibole, undermining and/or tunneling often occur. Depth varies by anatomical location. If slough or eschar obscures the extent of tissue loss this is an unstageable pressure injury.

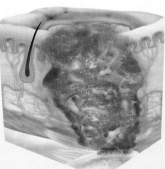

Unstageable Pressure Injury: Obscured full-thickness skin and tissue loss

Full-thickness skin and tissue loss in which the extent of tissue damage within the ulcer cannot be confirmed because it is obscured by slough or eschar. If slough or eschar is removed, a Stage 3 or Stage 4 pressure injury will be revealed. Stable eschar (i.e., dry, adherent, intact without erythema or fluctuance) on the heel or ischemic limb should not be softened or removed.

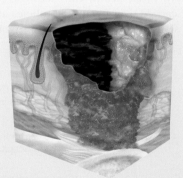

Deep Tissue Pressure Injury: Persistent nonblanchable deep red, maroon or purple discoloration

Intact or nonintact skin with localized area of persistent nonblanchable deep red, maroon, purple discoloration or epidermal separation revealing a dark wound bed or blood filled blister. Pain and temperature change often precede skin color changes. Discoloration may appear differently in darkly pigmented skin. This injury results from intense and/or prolonged pressure and shear forces at the bone–muscle interface. The wound may evolve rapidly to reveal the actual extent of tissue injury, or may resolve without tissue loss. If necrotic tissue, subcutaneous tissue, granulation tissue, fascia, muscle, or other underlying structures are visible, this indicates a full-thickness pressure injury (Unstageable, Stage 3, or Stage 4). Do not use deep tissue pressure injury to describe vascular, traumatic, neuropathic, or dermatologic conditions.

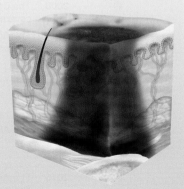

Figures from Edsberg, L., Black, J. M., Goldberg, M., et al. (2016). Revised National Pressure Ulcer Advisory Panel Pressure Injury Staging System. *Wound Ostomy Continence Nursing,* 2016, *43*(6), 1–13. *"Text and Photos used with permission from the National Pressure Ulcer Advisory Panel, November 11, 2016."*

Enterostomal Nurses Association, and the Pan Pacific Pressure Injury Alliance of Australia.

Once a pressure ulcer is identified according to the defined stages, it must be frequently reassessed to evaluate the effectiveness of interventions. Since 1996, the NPUAP has encouraged the use of a standardized tool for assessing changes in pressure ulcers called the Pressure Ulcer Scale for Healing (PUSH) tool. The PUSH tool scores pressure ulcers according to size, exudates, and tissue type, with changes in the PUSH score over time indicating the progression or regression of the pressure ulcer.

Although the term "reverse staging" has been used to describe the progression of a later-stage pressure ulcer to a healed stage, the NPUAP has advised against this practice because it does not accurately reflect the pathophysiologic processes that occur. The NPUAP provides many educational resources related to the staging classification and the PUSH tool. The tool includes quick reference guides in English and other languages (see Online Learning Activity 23-2).

Pressure Injuries as a Measure of Safety and Quality of Care

Since the early 2000s, there has been increasing attention to pressure injuries as a major safety and quality-of-care concern in all health care settings. Major initiatives that have carried over to current policies and practices in health care settings are summarized in Figure 23-3. Nurses have consistently provided strong leadership in addressing this important issue through organizations such as the American Nurses Association, the National Pressure Ulcer Advisory Panel (NPUAP), and the Wound, Ostomy, and Continence Nurses Association.

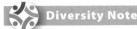 **Diversity Note**

Analysis of data related to pressure ulcers across the skin pigmentation spectrum shows that persons with darkly pigmented skin have a higher incidence of serious pressure ulcers but a lower incidence of superficial tissue damage. Evidence-based guidelines emphasize the importance of assessing darkly pigmented skin for changes in color and sensation, particularly over bony prominences (Ayello & Sibbald, 2016).

Functional Consequences

Pressure injuries are associated with many serious functional consequences, including pain, loss of function, and decreased quality of life. The NPUAP emphasizes the important role of nurses in assessing and intervening for pain in patients with pressure injuries. Pain is common in patients with pressure injuries and has been described with all the following terms: sore, sharp, burning, throbbing, stabbing, and stinging (Kim, Ahh, Lynn, et al., 2016). Additional functional consequences of hospital-acquired pressure injuries are increased length of stay and increased mortality (Pittman, Beeson, Terry, et al., 2016).

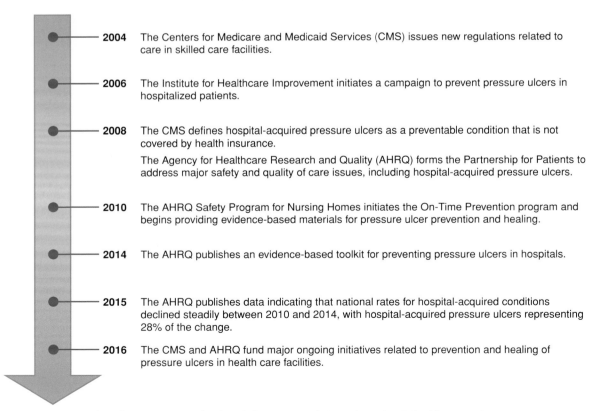

FIGURE 23-3 Timeline of major initiatives that have led to current policies and practices in health care settings.

Risk Identification

Identification of patients who are at risk for developing pressure injuries is a major focus of nursing care. Evidence-based tools are used to identify and rate risk factors for pressure injury development. In the United States, the Braden Scale is the most consistently validated and widely used tool for identifying the risk for pressure injury (Miller, Frankenfield, Lehman, et al., 2016). As illustrated in Figure 23-4, the Braden Scale has 6 categories of risk, with a cumulative score of 18 or less representing a higher risk. Current guidelines recommend that clinicians consider not only the total Braden Scale score but also address any low subscale scores (Ayello & Sibbald, 2016). Additional information about risk identification, nursing assessment, and interventions for prevention is summarized in Box 23-1.

Evidence-Based Practice for Pressure Ulcers

Financial and quality-of-care implications related to pressure ulcers have led to an abundance of information about interventions for preventing and healing pressure ulcers, as summarized in Box 23-1. Although much progress has been made in identifying interventions for preventing and

BRADEN SCALE FOR PREDICTING PRESSURE SORE RISK

Patient's Name _____   Evaluator's Name _____   Date of Assessment

SENSORY PERCEPTION Ability to respond meaningfully to pressure-related discomfort	**1. Completely Limited** Unresponsive (does not moan, flinch, or grasp) to painful stimuli, due to diminished level of consciousness or sedation. OR limited ability to feel pain over most of body.	**2. Very Limited** Responds only to painful stimuli. Cannot communicate discomfort except by moaning or restlessness. OR Has a sensory impairment which limits the ability to feel pain or discomfort over 1/2 of body.	**3. Slightly Limited** Responds to verbal commands, but cannot always communicate discomfort or the need to be turned. OR Has some sensory impairment which limits ability to feel pain or discomfort in 1 or 2 extremities.	**4. No Impairment** Responds to verbal commands. Has no sensory deficit which would limit ability to feel or voice pain or discomfort.
MOISTURE Degree to which skin is exposed to moisture	**1. Constantly Moist** Skin is kept moist almost constantly by perspiration, urine, etc. Dampness is detected every time patient is moved or turned.	**2. Very Moist** Skin is often, but not always moist. Linen must be changed at least once a shift.	**3. Occasionally Moist:** Skin is occasionally moist, requiring an extra linen change approximately once a day.	**4. Rarely Moist** Skin is usually dry, linen only requires changing at routine intervals.
ACTIVITY Degree of physical activity	**1. Bedfast** Confined to bed.	**2. Chairfast** Ability to walk severely limited or nonexistent. Cannot bear own weight and/or must be assisted into chair or wheelchair.	**3. Walks Occasionally** Walks occasionally during day, but for very short distances, with or without assistance. Spends majority of each shift in bed or chair.	**4. Walks Frequently** Walks outside room at least twice a day and inside room at least once every two hours during waking hours.
MOBILITY Ability to change and control body position	**1. Completely Immobile** Does not make even slight changes in body or extremity position without assistance.	**2. Very Limited** Makes occasional slight changes in body or extremity position but unable to make frequent or significant changes independently.	**3. Slightly Limited** Makes frequent though slight changes in body or extremity position independently.	**4. No Limitation** Makes major and frequent changes in position without assistance.
NUTRITION Usual food intake pattern	**1. Very Poor** Never eats a complete meal. Rarely eats more than 1/2 of any food offered. Eats 2 servings or less of protein (meat or dairy products) per day. Takes fluids poorly. Does not take a liquid dietary supplement. OR Is NPO and/or maintained on clear liquids or IV's for more than 5 days.	**2. Probably Inadequate** Rarely eats a complete meal and generally eats only about 1/2 of any food offered. Protein intake includes only 3 servings of meat or dairy products per day. Occasionally will take a dietary supplement. OR Receives less than optimum amount of liquid diet or tube feeding.	**3. Adequate** Eats over half of most meals. Eats a total of 4 servings of protein (meat, dairy products) per day. Occasionally will refuse a meal, but will usually take a supplement when offered. OR Is on a tube feeding or TPN regimen which probably meets most of nutritional needs.	**4. Excellent** Eats most of every meal. Never refuses a meal. Usually eats a total of 4 or more servings of meat and dairy products. Occasionally eats between meals. Does not require supplementation.
FRICTION & SHEAR	**1. Problem** Requires moderate to maximum assistance in moving. Complete lifting without sliding against sheets is impossible. Frequently slides down in bed or chair, requiring frequent repositioning with maximum assistance. Spasticity, contractures or agitation leads to almost constant friction.	**2. Potential Problem** Moves feebly or requires minimum assistance. During a move skin probably slides to some extent against sheets, chair, restraints, or other devices. Maintains relatively good position in chair or bed most of the time but occasionally slides down.	**3. No Apparent Problem** Moves in bed and in chair independently and has sufficient muscle strength to lift up completely during move. Maintains good position in bed or chair.	

Total Score

FIGURE 23-4 The Braden Scale is a widely used screening tool to identify people at risk for pressure ulcers. Scores = 15–18, at risk; 13–14, moderate risk; 10–12, high risk; less than 9, very high risk. (Reprinted with permission from Braden, B., & Bergstrom, N. (1988). Permission to use this tool should be sought at www.bradenscale.com.)

E·B·P Box 23-1 Evidence-Based Practice: Prevention of Pressure Injuries

Overview

- A pressure injury is localized damage to the skin and underlying soft tissue, usually over a bony prominence or related to a medical or other device.
- Pressure injuries are caused by a combination of intense and/or prolonged pressure in combination with shear.
- Soft tissue tolerance is affected by microclimate, nutrition, perfusion, comorbidities, and condition of the soft tissue.
- Hospital-acquired pressure injuries are considered a preventable condition and an indicator of safety and quality of care.

Risk Identification and Nursing Assessment

- Perform a head-to-toe skin assessment at the following times: on admission to a health care facility or home care service, whenever a patient's condition changes, and according to acuity status:
  - Acute care: every shift
  - Long-term care: weekly for 4 weeks, then quarterly
  - Home care: every nurse visit
- Pay particular attention to all the following skin areas:
  - All bony prominences (Figure 23-2)
  - Under medical devices (e.g., catheters, oxygen, tubing, face masks, braces)
- Ask patients about pain or discomfort over bony prominences or related to medical devices
- Identify risk factors using a validated and reliable tool, such as the Braden Scale (Figure 23-3)
- Consider immobility, malnutrition, and incontinence as major high risk factors
- Assess additional parameters in patients with darkly pigmented skin: changes in skin tone, temperature, tissue consistency compared with surrounding skin
- Consider the following conditions that are associated with increased risk for pressure injury: diabetes, obesity, cardiovascular disease, hip fracture, critical illness, any condition that compromises circulation or nutrition and hydration status
- Consider the following additional factors in surgical patients: length of time in surgery, number of hypotensive episodes, low-core body temperature during surgery

Recommendations Related to Nutritional Status

- Assess nutritional status using a valid and reliable tool, such as the Mini-Nutritional Assessment (see Chapter 18)

- Consider hospitalized patients to be at risk for undernutrition or malnutrition associated with frailty, diagnoses, or NPO status
- Refer patients with nutritional risks for pressure ulcers and those who have pressure injuries to a registered dietician
- Assure optimal nutritional intake (discussed in Chapter 18)
- Incorporate recommendations from registered dietician into care plan
- Assess body weight at appropriate intervals and document changes

Recommendations for Skin Care

- Cleanse the skin promptly after episodes of incontinence or exposure to moisture or wetness
- Use skin cleansers that are pH balanced for the skin
- Use skin moisturizer daily

Recommendations Related to Overall Care

- Avoid positioning on an area of erythema or pressure injury
- Reposition all individuals at risk for pressure injury, unless contraindicated
- Establish a repositioning plan that considers all the following:
  - Individual's level of immobility, body size, weight
  - Exposure to moisture (e.g., incontinence, drainage)
  - Positioning in relation to medical devices
- Base schedule for repositioning on support surface in use and on tolerance of the skin for pressure
- Consider lengthening the night-time intervals between repositioning to allow for uninterrupted sleep
- Use pressure redistribution surfaces and support surfaces to protect vulnerable areas
- Use protective foam or breathable dressings under medical devices
- Use heel offloading devices or foam dressings to protect heels

Cultural Considerations Related to Interventions

- Consider that products for wound care may contain animal-based collagen and discuss with patients who may have cultural conflicts.
- Examples of animal-derived products that may conflict with the patient's ideology or cultural background are porcine products for Jewish or Muslim patients, and bovine products for Hindu patients.

Source: Ahn, Cowan, Garvan, et al., 2016; Ayello & Sibbald, 2016; Lachenbruch, Ribble, Emmons, et al., 2016; National Pressure Ulcer Advisory Panel, 2016; Neloska, Damevska, Nikolchev, et al., 2016; Rao, Preston, Strauss, et al., 2016.

---

healing pressure ulcers, research is ongoing and recommendations continue to develop. For example, repositioning is consistently identified as an effective measure; however, the long-standing criterion of turning patients every 2 hours has been replaced with the recommendation to individualize repositioning schedules based on the patient's condition, care goals, vulnerable skin areas, and type of support surface being used (Ayello & Sibbald, 2016). Because research is ongoing and plentiful, nurses can keep up-to-date on evidence-based recommendations by exploring information in the resources described in Online Learning Activity 23-2.

 See **ONLINE LEARNING ACTIVITY 23-2: CASE STUDY AND EVIDENCE-BASED INFORMATION RELATED TO PRESSURE ULCERS** at **http://thepoint.lww.com/Miller8e.**

 NURSING ASSESSMENT OF SKIN

Because the skin is the largest and most visible organ of the body, it is relatively easy to identify problems that affect it. In addition, the integumentary system provides clues to other areas of physiologic and psychosocial function, such as nutrition, hydration, and personal care. Nurses collect information about the skin, hair, and nails during an assessment interview and through physical examination procedures. Opportunities for direct examination also arise during routine nursing care activities, such as assisting with personal care or listening to the lung and heart sounds. Assessment of the skin, hair, and nails can also provide information to validate or raise questions about other areas of function. For example, the observation that an older man has a beard of several days' growth, when combined with assessment information about his overall function, may support conclusions about the need for assistance with personal care activities.

Identifying Opportunities for Health Promotion

Assessment questions identify the person's perception of problems, risk factors that may contribute to skin problems, and any personal care behaviors that influence hair and skin status. Assessing these aspects of skin care can help identify opportunities for health education about risk factors and healthy skin care practices. Older adults may initiate a discussion about age spots or other noticeable skin changes, and they are usually very receptive to information about skin and hair care. Information about medications and other risk factors, which is obtained as part of the overall assessment, is incorporated into the skin assessment. Likewise, other pertinent information obtained during a comprehensive assessment, such as information about fluid intake, nutritional status, and mobility and safety, is applicable to the assessment of the skin. Box 23-2 summarizes assessment questions related to the skin and nails.

Observing Skin, Hair, and Nails

Close inspection of the skin in a warm, private, and well-lit environment is an essential component of skin assessment. Examination of the skin is particularly important because older adults may focus on cosmetic conditions, such as skin tags, instead of questioning more serious conditions such as skin cancer. Assessment observations of skin include all the following: color, turgor, dryness, overall condition, bruises,

and any growths or pathologic conditions. Cultural variations also are noted. For example, skin changes may be difficult to assess in people with dark pigmentation.

The common occurrence of various skin lesions complicates the assessment of skin in older adults. Although most of these changes are harmless, some are cancerous or precancerous. An important aspect of health promotion is to reassure the older adult about the harmless changes and to encourage medical evaluation of the questionable ones. In general, the following characteristics of a skin lesion warrant medical evaluation:

- Redness
- Swelling
- Dark pigmentation
- Moisture or drainage
- Pain or discomfort
- Raised or irregular edges around a flat center

In addition, any lesion that undergoes change, or any sore that does not heal within a reasonable time, requires further evaluation. Evaluation is also indicated when, because of its location, a mole or other skin lesion is subject to frequent rubbing or irritation.

Document all the following characteristics of any skin lesions: size, shape, color, location, macular (flat) versus papular (raised), superficial versus penetrating, discrete versus diffuse borders, and the presence or absence of inflammation, redness, or discharge. Terminology related to various skin lesions in older adults is confusing, and many terms are used interchangeably. Table 23-3 describes some of the terms used for skin lesions that are common in older adults; some of these lesions are shown in Figure 23-5.

Nursing assessment of the skin, hair, and nails can provide clues to a broad spectrum of physiologic functioning, particularly in combination with additional assessment information. For example, brown-stained fingertips are an indication of cigarette use, and feces under the fingernails and around the cuticle may be a clue to constipation. In some circumstances, toenails provide clues to mobility difficulties, particularly when extremely long nails curl under the toes. Observations of the skin may provide the only objective evidence of serious functional problems that the older person might not otherwise acknowledge. For example, multiple bruises, particularly in various stages of healing, may be a significant clue to falls, alcoholism, self-neglect, or physical abuse. Observation and documentation of these signs are particularly important when neglect or abuse is suspected as described in Chapter 10 for detailed description of elder abuse.

In assessing the skin for clues to the broader aspects of function, keep in mind that some of the usual manifestations may be altered in older adults. For example, skin turgor on the hands or arms is an indication of hydration status; however, this is not necessarily a reliable indicator in frail older adults. Also, age-related changes make it difficult to assess patterns of wound using the same standards that are applied to younger adults.

Box 23-2 Interview Questions for Assessing the Integument

Questions to Assess Risk Factors and Skin Problems

- Do you have any concerns about or trouble with your skin?
- Do you have any problems with rashes, itching, swelling, or dry skin?
- Do you have any sores that will not heal?
- Do you bruise easily?
- Have you been treated for skin cancer or any other skin problems?
- How much time do you spend in the sun?
- Do you spend time in tanning booths?
- Do you do anything to protect yourself from the effects of the sun?

Questions to Assess Personal Care Practices

- How do you manage your bathing?
- How often do you take a bath or shower?
- What temperature water do you use?
- Do you use soap every time you bathe?
- What kind of soap do you use?
- Do you use any kind of skin lotion, creams, or ointments? What kind do you use and how frequently do you use it? Where do you apply it?
- Do you have any problems with your fingernails or toenails?
- Do you get or need any help with nail care?

TABLE 23-3 Common Skin Lesions in Older Adults

Common Term(s)	Description
Age spots, liver spots, senile freckles	Pale to dark brown macules, occurring most frequently on exposed areas
Actinic keratosis, solar keratosis	Red, yellow, brown, or flesh-colored papules or plaques; gritty texture; surrounded by erythema; *premalignant*
Senile purpura	Areas of brown or bluish discoloration that look like bruising
Seborrheic keratosis	Brown or black papules or plaques with sharp edges and a waxy or wart-like texture; appearing most frequently on trunk and face
Sebaceous hyperplasia	Yellowish, doughnut-shaped elevations; common on face, particularly in men
Senile angiomas, cherry or ruby angiomas, telangiectasia	Bright, ruby red, pinpoint, superficial elevations of small blood vessels
Spider angiomas	Tiny, red papules with radiating arms; *may indicate a pathologic condition*
Venous stars	Bluish, irregular, sometimes spider-shaped lesions, appearing mainly on the legs or the chest
Venous lakes, benign venous angiomas	Bluish papules with sharp borders, appearing mainly on the lips or the ears
Acrochordons, skin tags	Flesh-colored, pedunculated, or stalk-like lesions
Corns, calluses	Hard masses of keratin caused by repeated pressure or irritation
Xanthelasma	Fatty deposits, usually around the eyes; *may be related to a pathologic condition*, particularly if large or numerous

Observations of the hair, skin, and nails also can provide clues to self-care abilities and aspects of psychosocial function. For example, poor personal grooming may be indicative of functional limitations or psychosocial influences such as lack of motivation or awareness due to depression or dementia. The use of unusually deep hues of hair coloring or facial cosmetics may indicate impaired color perception. Box 23-3 summarizes nursing observations pertaining to the integumentary system.

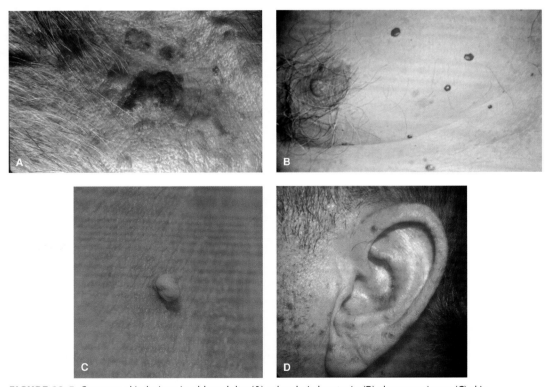

FIGURE 23-5 Common skin lesions in older adults: (**A**) seborrheic keratosis; (**B**) cherry angioma; (**C**) skin tag; (**D**) venous lakes or benign venous angiomas. (A and D: Reprinted with permission from Rosenthal, T. C., Williams, M. E., & Naughton, B. J. (2007). *Office care geriatrics*. Philadelphia, PA: Lippincott Williams & Wilkins; **B:** Reprinted with permission from Weber, J., & Kelley, J. (2002). *Health assessment in nursing* (2nd ed.). Philadelphia, PA: Lippincott Williams & Wilkins; **C:** Reprinted with permission from Edwards, L., & Lynch, P.L. (2011). *Genital dermatology atlas*. (2nd ed.) Philadelphia, PA: Lippincott Williams & Wilkins.)

Box 23-3 Observations Regarding the Integument

Examination of the Skin

- What is the color?
- Are there any areas of irregular pigmentation?
- Are there any areas of sunburn or tan?
- Are there areas that are discolored in any way?
- Are there any indications of poor circulation, particularly in the extremities (e.g., varicosities, or areas of red, blue, or brown discoloration indicative of chronic stasis problems in the lower extremities)?
- What is the skin temperature?
- Is there a marked difference between the temperature of the extremities and that of the rest of the body?
- How does the skin feel in terms of moisture? Is it dry? Clammy? Oily?
- What is the skin's texture? Is it smooth or rough?
- Does the skin look tissue-paper thin?
- What is the turgor of the abdominal skin?
- Are scars present? (If so, describe their location and appearance.) Are there any signs of falling or physical abuse?
- Are any of the lesions described in Table 23-3 present?

Examination of the Hair and Nails

- What are the color, texture, and general condition of the hair?
- What is the distribution pattern of the hair?
- Is there any evidence of dandruff, scaling, or other problems with the hair?
- What are the color, length, cleanliness, and general condition of the toenails and fingernails?
- What are the color and general condition of the nail beds of the toes and fingers?

Personal Care Practices

- What is the person's overall appearance with regard to grooming and attention to personal attractiveness?
- If grooming is poor, does the person express concern about this or provide an explanation?
- Are there any psychosocial factors that influence personal care practices (e.g., is the person socially isolated or overburdened with caregiving responsibilities and, therefore, inattentive to personal care)?
- Are any of the following signs of neglect evident: presence of a body odor; unkempt, uncut, or matted hair; unusually long and unkempt fingernails or toenails; patches of brown crust on the skin; bruises; or any pathologic skin conditions?

Unfolding Case Study

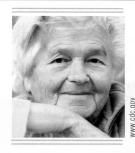

www.cdc.gov

Part 1: Ms. S. at 84 Years of Age

Ms. S. is an 84-year-old white woman who lives in her own home on the coast of Florida. She is quite active and healthy and enjoys golfing and "beach-combing." She attends the local senior center, where you are the wellness nurse. The local chapter of the American Cancer Society is cosponsoring a skin cancer screening day at the senior center, and you have been asked to prepare a health education program titled "Checking Your Skin for Serious Changes." You are also assisting the dermatologist with the screening examinations. Ms. S. attends the health education part of your program and says she is not sure if she can stay for the screening. She just has one "age spot," and she knows it is not serious because she has "had a couple skin cancers removed, and this one looks different." You look at the questionable spot, and you assess it as a brown, raised plaque with a gritty texture, about 1 cm in diameter.

THINKING POINTS

- What additional assessment information would you want to obtain from Ms. S.?

- How would you use Table 23-3 and Boxes 23-2 and 23-3 in your assessment?
- What advice would you give Ms. S. about her skin?

QSEN APPLICATION

QSEN Competency	Knowledge/Skill/Attitude	Application to Ms. S. When She Is 84 Years of Age
Evidence-based practice	(K) Describe how the strength and relevance of available evidence influence the choice of intervention	Apply evidence-based information in Table 23-3 and Boxes 23-2 and 23-3 when you assess Ms. S. and teach her about the importance of participating in the health education program that includes a screening performed by a dermatologist
	(S) Base individualized care plan on patient values, clinical expertise, and evidence	
	(A) Value evidence-based practice as integral to determining the best clinical practice	

(continued)

QSEN APPLICATION *(Continued)*

QSEN Competency	Knowledge/Skill/Attitude	Application to Ms. S. When She Is 84 Years of Age
Teamwork and collaboration	(K) Recognize contributions of other individuals and groups in helping patient achieve health goals	Assume leadership role in coordinating plans for dermatologist to provide screenings for skin cancer during health education program
	(S) Integrate the contributions of others who play a role in helping patient achieve health goals	

NURSING DIAGNOSIS

When older adults have any skin breakdown nurses can use the nursing diagnosis of Impaired Skin Integrity, defined as "altered epidermis and/or dermis" (Herdman & Kamitsuru, 2018, p. 406). When older adults have any risk factors for skin tears or pressure ulcers, nurses can use the nursing diagnosis of Risk for Impaired Skin Integrity, which is defined as "vulnerable to alteration in epidermis and/or dermis, which may compromise health" (Herdman & Kamitsuru, 2018, p. 407). Related factors that commonly affect older adults include frailty, incontinence, limited mobility, nutritional deficits, or a combination of these factors.

If the older adult has any skin lesion that requires medical evaluation, the nursing diagnosis of Ineffective Health Maintenance might be applicable. This is defined as the "inability to identify, manage, and/or seek out help to maintain well-being" (Herdman & Kamitsuru, 2018, p. 150). This nursing diagnosis also might be pertinent for older adults who do not use protective measures when they are exposed to ultraviolet radiation from sunlight or tanning beds.

Wellness Opportunity

Nurses can use the wellness nursing diagnosis Readiness for Enhanced Knowledge: Skin Care for older adults who are interested in learning how to address risks for conditions such as dry skin and skin cancer.

PLANNING FOR WELLNESS OUTCOMES

When older adults have conditions that affect skin comfort or integrity, nurses identify wellness outcomes as an essential part of the nursing process. Similarly, when they have risks for conditions that can cause skin problems (e.g., skin cancer or pressure ulcers), nursing goals focus on prevention.

Wellness Opportunity

Nurses promote wellness when they plan outcomes to address skin comfort and the prevention of skin cancer.

For healthy older adults with risk factors (e.g., history of skin cancer) or minor skin problems (e.g., xerosis), applicable Nursing Outcomes Classification (NOC) terminology includes Comfort Level, Tissue Integrity: Skin and Mucous Membranes, Knowledge: Health Behavior, Health Seeking Behavior, Nutritional Status, Risk Control: Cancer, and Risk Control: Sun Exposure.

For older adults with pressure ulcers or other types of wounds or skin breakdown, NOC terms include Impaired Skin Integrity, Wound Healing: Primary Intention, and Wound

Healing: Secondary Intention. Outcomes are achieved through interventions discussed in the following section.

NURSING INTERVENTIONS FOR SKIN WELLNESS

Nurses have many opportunities for promoting wellness with regard to comfort, self-esteem, and maintenance of a healthy integumentary system. Nursing interventions for healthy older adults focus on promoting self-responsibility for identifying and seeking further evaluation for harmful or questionable lesions. This is especially important for older adults with a history of melanoma because of the high rate of recurrence and the effectiveness of skin self-examination in identifying this lesion at an early stage (Coups, Manne, Stapleton, et al., 2016). Interventions for physically compromised older adults focus on maintaining intact skin and managing pressure ulcers. The following Nursing Interventions Classification terminologies can be used to document interventions: Hair Care, Health Education, Health Screening, Nutrition Therapy, Positioning, Pressure Management, Pressure Ulcer Prevention, Pruritus Management, Risk Identification, Self-Esteem Enhancement, Skin Surveillance, and Wound Care.

Promoting Healthy Skin

Because one's overall health significantly affects the condition of the skin, maintenance of optimal nutrition and hydration is an important intervention in the skin care of older adults. Health promotion interventions also address

Box 23-4 Health Promotion Teaching About Skin Care for Older Adults

Maintaining Healthy Skin

- Include adequate amounts of fluid in the daily diet.
- Use humidifiers to maintain environmental humidity levels of 40% to 60%.
- Apply moisturizing lotions twice daily or as needed.
- Use moisturizing lotions immediately after bathing, when the skin is still moist.
- Avoid massaging over bony prominences when applying lotions.
- Avoid skin care products that contain perfumes or isopropyl alcohol.
- Avoid multiple-ingredient preparations because unnecessary additives may cause allergic responses.
- Inspect skin monthly for suspicious-looking changes.

Personal Care Practices

- When bathing or showering, use soap sparingly or use a mild, unscented soap (e.g., Dove, Tone, Basis, Aveeno).
- Maintain water temperatures for bathing at about 90° to 100°F.
- Rinse well after using soap. Whirlpool baths stimulate circulation, but moderate temperatures should be maintained.
- Apply moisturizing products after bathing, rather than using them in the bath water, to minimize the risk for falls on oily surfaces and to maximize the benefits of the emollient.
- Use emollient products containing petrolatum or mineral oil (e.g., Keri, Eucerin, Aquaphor, Vanicream, Vaseline).
- If you use bath oils, take extra safety precautions to prevent slipping.

- If moisturizing products are applied to the feet, wear nonskid slippers or socks before walking.
- Dry your skin thoroughly, particularly between your toes and in other areas where your skin rubs together.
- When drying your skin, use gentle, patting motions rather than harsh, rubbing motions.
- Obtain regular podiatric care.

Preventing Sun Damage and Skin Cancers

- Wear wide-brimmed hats, sun visors, sunglasses, and light-colored clothing when exposed to the sun.
- Wear clothing made of cotton, rather than polyester fabrics, because ultraviolet rays can penetrate polyester.
- Apply sunscreen products liberally beginning 1 hour before sun exposure and reapplying at frequent intervals.
- Use sunscreen lotions with an SPF of 30. Avoid exposure to the sun between 10:00 AM and 4:00 PM.
- Protect yourself from ultraviolet rays even on cloudy days and when you are in the water (lake, pool, ocean).
- Artificial tanning booths use ultraviolet type A rays, which have been found to cause damage and increase the risk for skin cancers.

Preventing Injury From Abrasive Forces

- Do not use starch, bleach, or strong detergents when laundering clothing or linens.
- Use soft terry or cotton washcloths.
- If waterproof pads are necessary, make sure that an adequate amount of soft, absorbent material is placed near the body.

---

environmental factors and personal care practices that influence the condition of the skin. Box 23-4 can be used as a guide to teaching older adults, or caregivers of dependent older adults, about skin health. In hospitals and long-term care facilities, there is increasing evidence to support the effectiveness and cost- and time-saving method of using prepackaged disposable bathing products instead of the traditional bed bath (Gillis, Tency, Roelant, et al., 2016; Noddeskou, Hemmingsen, & Hordam, 2016).

Although questions have also been raised about the safety and efficacy of sunscreens, recent Food and Drug Administration regulatory guidelines emphasize the following:

All sunscreening agents must be tested and meet requirements for claims about effectiveness.

- Claims for broad-spectrum agents must protect from both ultraviolet A and ultraviolet B rays.
- Claims for reduction of skin cancer and skin aging can be made only with an SPF between 15 and 50.
- Claims of "waterproof," "sweatproof," or "sunblocks" are not permitted because they overemphasize the product's efficacy.
- Claims of "water resistant" need to be substantiated by tests for 40 or 80 minutes.
- Acceptable forms of sunscreen include oils, gels, sprays, creams, pastes, butters, and ointment; forms that are *not* acceptable include wipes, powders, shampoos, towelettes, and body washes.

This information can be incorporated in health education about use of sunscreens to protect older adults from skin cancer and other skin changes. Online Learning Activity 23-3 lists resources for teaching older adults about prevention of skin cancer.

 See ONLINE LEARNING ACTIVITY 23-3: RESOURCES FOR INFORMATION ABOUT SKIN CANCER at http://thepoint.lww.com/Miller8e.

Preventing Skin Wrinkles

The best methods of preventing skin lesions and wrinkles are avoiding too much exposure to sunlight and using a sunscreen and other protective measures (as summarized in Box 23-4) when exposure to sunlight is unavoidable. Topical products containing alpha- or beta-hydroxy acids may be beneficial in reversing wrinkles and promoting the regression of solar keratoses. Be alert to the possibility that older adults might develop an allergic or sensitivity reaction to some of the ingredients in topical products. Information about the harmful effects of sunlight should be included in health education about the maintenance of healthy skin and prevention of undesirable cosmetic and pathologic skin changes. Also, encourage people who are concerned about wrinkles and dry skin to discuss medical interventions with their primary care provider.

Preventing Dry Skin

Petrolatum and other emollients are effective in alleviating dry skin discomfort, because they moisturize and lubricate the skin. The effectiveness of an emollient is based on its ability to prevent water evaporation, so the beneficial effects will be enhanced when it is applied to skin that already has some degree of moisture. Thus, an emollient agent is most effective when it is applied to moist skin immediately after bathing. See Box 23-4 for information on the use of emollients and other interventions designed to prevent or care for dry skin in older adults.

Detecting and Treating Harmful Skin Lesions

Early detection and treatment of cancerous or precancerous skin lesions are key factors in preventing serious functional consequences, because the cure rate for most skin cancers approaches 100% with early excision. The nurse's role is to detect any suspicious-looking lesions and to encourage or facilitate further evaluation. Encourage all older adults to use the following guide to identify any skin changes that require further evaluation:

- **A**symmetric shape: irregular or different-looking sides
- **B**order that is irregular: ragged, notched, blurred, irregular
- **C**olor change: different shades, uneven distribution
- **D**iameter: larger than a quarter of an inch (6 mm), increasing

If older adults or their caregivers have avoided medical evaluation because of fears about cancer, provide reassurance about the high cure rate and the minimal chance of long-term problems if early treatment is initiated. Similarly, if they have ignored suspicious changes because

Unfolding Case Study

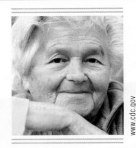

www.cdc.gov

Part 2: Ms. S. at 86 Years of Age

Ms. S. is 86 years old and continues to attend the senior center in Florida where you are responsible for presenting a health education program titled "Maintaining Healthy Skin." You plan to emphasize the importance of self-care techniques such as checking for skin changes. Ms. S. is very interested in attending the program and tells you she will be bringing her 80-year-old sister, who also lives in Florida. Ms. S. worries about her sister because she uses a wheelchair and is very frail. You know that several of the participants at the senior program use wheelchairs, and you plan to include health education about preventing pressure ulcers.

THINKING POINTS

- Outline your health education points for a half-hour program including specific points about preventing pressure ulcers.
- How would you use Table 23-2 and Box 23-4 in your program?

- Find additional information that you would consider using as educational materials for this program.

QSEN APPLICATION

QSEN Competency	Knowledge/Skill/Attitude	Application to Ms. S. When She Is 86 Years of Age
Evidence-based practice	(K) Describe how the strength and relevance of available evidence influence the choice of intervention	Use Table 23-2 and Box 23-4 for evidence-based information in the health education program
	(S) Base individualized care plan on patient values, clinical expertise, and evidence	
	(A) Value evidence-based practice as integral to determining the best clinical practice	

they attribute them to "normal aging," teach about the importance of further evaluation. Box 23-4 includes health promotion information about the prevention and early detection of skin cancer.

EVALUATING EFFECTIVENESS OF NURSING INTERVENTIONS

Nursing care for older adults with dry or itching skin is evaluated by determining the degree to which the interventions alleviate the person's complaints. It may take several weeks for older adults to feel the full effects of skin care interventions because of an age-related delay in dermal response to external stimuli. Also, there is a great deal of individual variation among older adults in their response to interventions. Thus, it may be necessary to evaluate the effects of one type of soap or lotion for several weeks before trying a different brand if the problem does not resolve. Because environmental humidity affects skin comfort, environmental conditions may also influence the evaluation of interventions.

The effectiveness of interventions for older adults at risk for skin breakdown is measured by the absence of skin tears or pressure ulcers. The effectiveness of interventions for pressure ulcers is determined by the rate of healing and prevention of complications such as osteomyelitis. Because significant cost and quality-of-life issues are associated with pressure ulcers, preventing skin breakdown can have far-reaching positive consequences for older adults who are at risk for developing pressure ulcers.

Unfolding Case Study

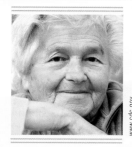

www.cdc.gov

Part 3: Ms. S. at 92 Years of Age

Ms. S. is now 92 years old and lives in an assisted-living facility in Florida. She ambulates with a walker and needs assistance with meals, medications, and personal care. Three months ago, her doctor prescribed hydrochlorothiazide 25 mg every morning for isolated systolic hypertension. She has a history of arthritis but does not take any medication for it. Ms. S. attends your monthly nursing clinic for health education and blood pressure monitoring. When she comes to see you in January, she complains of dry skin and discomfort.

NURSING ASSESSMENT

You interview Ms. S. about her personal care practices and find out that she soaks in the tub in lukewarm water three times weekly and enjoys using bath salts and perfumed skin lotions. She spends much of her leisure time outdoors on the patio or in the air-conditioned solarium. She does not use sunscreens because she thinks they are unnecessary and too oily. She states that she has not had sunburn for several years and that she has built up a good tolerance to the sun. She does not wear sunglasses or sun hats. She reports that she has had three skin cancers removed in the past 10 years, one from her cheek, one from her arm, and one from her ear lobe. She says she does not worry about recurrent skin cancer because she no longer swims outside or sits by the swimming pool. Also, because she does not get sunburned, she believes she is not at risk for skin cancer.

Inspection of Ms. S.'s skin reveals dry, wrinkled skin on her face and arms, and unevenly tanned skin on her face, neck, and extremities. She has many age spots over the exposed skin areas but no suspicious-looking lesions. Ms. S. has blue eyes and fair skin.

NURSING DIAGNOSIS

Your nursing diagnosis is Ineffective Health Maintenance related to excessive sunlight exposure and insufficient knowledge of the effects of ultraviolet light. Evidence for this diagnosis comes from her misconceptions about risk factors for skin cancer and other skin problems. Also, you identify her lack of knowledge about the potential photosensitivity reactions associated with use of hydrochlorothiazide as a factor that contributes to Ineffective Health Maintenance.

(continued)

Part 3: Ms. S. at 92 Years of Age (Continued)

NURSING CARE PLAN FOR MS. S.

Expected Outcome	Nursing Interventions	Nursing Evaluation
Ms. S.'s discomfort from dry skin will be alleviated	● Discuss and describe age-related skin changes ● Discuss risk factors that contribute to skin discomfort (e.g., bath salts, perfumed lotions, unprotected exposure to sunlight) ● Use Box 23-4 to teach Ms. S. about skin care practices directed toward alleviating dry skin	● Ms. S. will report that she no longer experiences skin discomfort and dryness
Ms. S.'s knowledge about risk factors for skin cancer will increase	● Discuss the relationship between skin cancer and exposure to ultraviolet rays ● Explain that any exposure to ultraviolet rays is a risk factor for skin cancer ● Emphasize that a history of skin cancer increases the chance of recurrent skin cancer	● Ms. S. will verbalize an awareness of the risk factors for skin cancer
The factors that increase Ms. S.'s risk of skin problems and skin cancer will be eliminated	● Inform Ms. S. that hydrochlorothiazide may increase the risk for photosensitivity, making protective measures increasingly important ● Use Box 23-4 as a guide for discussing measures to avoid sun damage ● Emphasize the importance of using sunscreens and wearing wide-brimmed hats when in the solarium or outside	● Ms. S. will use measures to reduce the risk for skin cancer and sun damage

THINKING POINTS

● What risk factors would you address in your care plan?

● How would you promote Ms. S.'s personal responsibility for skin care, including addressing risks for skin cancer?

QSEN APPLICATION: MS. S. WHEN SHE IS 92 YEARS OF AGE

QSEN Competency	Knowledge/Skill/Attitude	Application to Ms. S.
Patient-centered care	(K) Integrate understanding of multiple dimensions of patient-centered care	Identify the conditions that are likely to cause dry skin and increase the risk for skin problems
	(K) Describe strategies to empower patients in all aspects of the health care process	Provide accurate information to dispel myths and misunderstanding and improve Ms. S.'s knowledge about risks for skin cancer
	(K) Examine nursing roles in assuring coordination, integration, and continuity of care	Recognize the important health promotion role of nurses in teaching about self-care actions to prevent skin dryness and cancer
Evidence-based practice	(S) Base individualized care plan on patient values, clinical expertise, and evidence	Apply evidence-based guidelines summarized in Box 23-4 to teach about measures to prevent sun damage
	(A) Value evidence-based practice as integral to determining the best clinical practice	

Chapter Highlights

Age-Related Changes That Affect Skin Wellness (Table 23-1)

- Thinner dermis, flattened dermal–epidermal junction
- Diminished moisture content
- Decreased dermal blood supply
- Fewer sweat and sebaceous glands
- Nails become thinner, fragile, brittle, prone to splitting
- Changes in patterns of hair distribution

Risks Factors That Affect Skin Wellness

- Genetic factors (hair color and distribution, skin cancer)
- Smoking, sun exposure, stress
- Personal hygiene practices
- Adverse medication effects
- Factors that increase the risk for skin breakdown

Functional Consequences Affecting Skin Wellness (Table 23-1)

- Delayed wound healing
- Increased susceptibility to skin problems (skin cancer, breakdown, pressure ulcers)
- Xerosis (dry skin), discomfort
- Irregular pigmentation and other cosmetic changes
- Decreased tactile sensitivity, increased susceptibility to burns
- Diminished sweating and shivering, increased susceptibility to hypothermia and heat-related conditions

Pathologic Condition Affecting Skin: Skin Cancer (Figure 23-1)

- Non-melanoma: basal cell carcinoma, squamous cell carcinoma
- Melanoma

Pathologic Condition Affecting Skin: Skin Tears

- Skin tears are wounds caused by shear, friction, or blunt force causing a separation of skin layers

Pathologic Condition Affecting Skin: Pressure Injury

- Risk is higher at points illustrated in Figure 23-2
- Pressure injuries are an important measure of safety and quality of care (Figure 23-3)
- Pressure injuries are associated with serious functional consequences
- The Braden Scale (Figure 23-4) is an evidence-based tool for identifying risks for pressure injuries
- The Pressure Injury Staging System (Table 23-1) is an evidence-based guide for assessing pressure injuries
- Evidence-based practice guidelines (Box 23-1) address multifaceted interventions for prevention and care

Nursing Assessment of Skin (Table 23-3; Boxes 23-2 and 23-3)

- Abnormal skin conditions
- Personal care practices
- Skin lesions common in older adults (Table 23-3; Figure 23-5)

Nursing Diagnosis

- Readiness for Enhanced Knowledge: Skin
- Impaired Skin Integrity (or Risk for)
- Ineffective Health Maintenance

Planning for Wellness Outcomes

- Comfort Level
- Tissue Integrity: Skin and Mucous Membranes
- Nutritional Status
- Risk Control: Cancer
- Wound Healing

Nursing Interventions for Skin Wellness (Box 23-4)

- Health promotion teaching about healthy skin
- Preventing skin wrinkles
- Preventing dry skin
- Detecting and treating suspect skin changes

Evaluating Effectiveness of Nursing Interventions

- Alleviation of complaints (e.g., dryness)
- Evaluation of suspect skin changes
- Absence of pressure ulcers in high-risk older adults
- Wound healing

Critical Thinking Exercises

1. What changes would a healthy 85-year-old person notice with regard to his or her skin, hair, and nails?
2. Describe the questions you would ask and the observations you would make to assess the skin, hair, and nails of an 82-year-old person.
3. Describe at least eight skin lesions that are normal and three skin lesions that require further evaluation.
4. You are asked to give a 20-minute presentation on "Maintaining Healthy Skin" at a senior center. Outline the content of your health education program.
5. What would you teach the family caregivers of a 74-year-old woman who sits in a wheelchair for 14 hours a day with regard to the prevention of pressure ulcers?

For more information about the topics discussed in this chapter, be sure to check out the interactive Online Learning Activities and other helpful resources at http://thepoint.lww.com/Miller8e.

REFERENCES

Ahn, H., Cowan, L., Garvan, C., et al. (2016). Risk factors for pressures including suspected deep tissue injury in nursing home facility residents: Analysis of National Minimum Data Set 3.0. *Advances in Skin & Wound Care, 29,* 178–189.

Aubuchon, M., Bolt, L., Janssen-Heijnen, M., et al. (2017). Epidemiology, management and survival outcomes of primary cutaneous melanoma: A ten-year overview. *Acta Chirugica Belgica, 17,* 29–35.

Ayello, E. A., & Sibbald, R. G. (2016). Preventing pressure ulcers and skin tears. In M. Boltz., E. Capezuti., T. Fulmer., et al. (Eds.) *Evidence-based practice protocols for best practice* (5th ed., pp. 395–415). New York: Springer Publishing Co.

Blume-Peytavi, U., Kottner, J., Sterry, W., et al. (2016). Age-associated skin conditions and diseases: Current perspectives and future options. *The Gerontologist, 56,* S 230–S242.

Burton, K. A., Achack, K. A., & Khachemoune, A. (2016). Cutaneous squamous cell carcinoma: A review of high-risk and metastatic disease. *American Journal of Dermatology, 17,* 491–508.

Coups, E., Manne, S., Stapleton, J., et al. (2016). Skin self-examination behaviors among individuals diagnosed with melanoma. *Melanoma Research, 26,* 71–76.

Crocetti, E., Fancelli, L., Manneschi, G., et al. (2016). Melanoma survival: sex does matter, but we don't know how. *European Journal of Cancer Research, 25,* 404–409.

Dawes, S. M., Tsai, S., Glttleman, H., et al. (2016). Racial disparities in melanoma survival. *Journal of the American Academy of Dermatology, 75,* 983–991.

Edsberg, L., Black, J. M., Goldberg, M., et al. (2016). Revised National Pressure Ulcer Advisory Panel Pressure Injury Staging System. *Wound Ostomy & Continence Nursing, 43*(6), 1–13.

Gillis, K., Tency, I., Roelant, E., et al. (2016). Skin hydration in nursing home residents using disposable bed baths. *Geriatric Nursing, 37,* 175–179.

Grey, K. R., & Warshaw, E. M. (2016). Allergic contact dermatitis to ophthalmic medications: A review of relevant allergens and alternative testing methods. *Dermatitis, 27*(6), 333–347.

Griffin, L. L., Ali, F. R., & Lear, J. T. (2016). Non-melanoma skin cancer. *Clinical Medicine (London) 16,* 62–65.

Herdman, T., & Kamitsura, S. (Eds). (2018). *NANDA International Nursing Diagnoses Definitions and Classification, 2018–2020* (11th ed., pp. 34–44). New York: Thieme Publishers.

Humbert, P., Dreno, B., Krutmann, J., et al. (2016). Recommendations for managing cutaneous disorders associated with advancing age. *Clinical Interventions in Aging, 11,* 141–148.

John, S., M., Trakatelli, M., Gehring, R., et al. (2016). Consensus report: Recognizing non-melanoma skin cancer, including actinic keratosis, as an occupational disease – A call to action. *Journal of the European Academy of Dermatology and Venerealogy, 30*(3), 38–45.

Keaney, T. C. (2016). Aging in the male face: Intrinsic and extrinsic factors. *Dermatologic Surgery, 42,* 797–803.

Kim, J., Ahn, H., Lynn, D., et al. (2016). Building a biopsychosocial conceptual framework to explore pressure ulcer pain. *Healthcare, 4*(1). doi: 10.3390/healthcare40100007.

Krutmann, J., Boulot, A., Sore, G., et al. (2016). The skin aging exposome. *Journal of Dermatological Science.* doi: 10.1016/j.jdermsci.2016.09.015.

Lachenbruch, C., Ribble, D., Emmons, K., et al. (2016). Pressure ulcer risk in the incontinent patient: Analysis of incontinence and hospital-acquired pressure ulcers from the International Pressure Ulcer Prevalence Survey. *Journal of Wound, Ostomy, and Continence Nursing, 43*(3), 235–241.

LeBlanc, K., Baranoski, S., Christensen, D., et al. (2016). The art of dressing selection: A consensus statement on skin tears and best practice. *Advances in Skin & Wound Care, 29,* 32–45.

LeBlanc, K., Baranoski, S., Holloway, S., et al. (2013). Validation of a new classification system for skin tears. *Advances in Skin & Wound Care, 26*(6), 263–266.

LeBlanc, K., Kozell, K., Martins, L., et al. (2016). Is twice-daily skin moisturizing more effective than routine care in the prevention of skin tears in the elderly population? *Journal of Wound, Ostomy, and Continence Nursing, 43,* 17–22.

Miller, N., Frankenfield, D., Lehman, E., et al. (2016). Predicting pressure ulcer development in clinical practice. *Journal of Wound, Ostomy, and Continence Nursing, 43,* 133–139.

Monteiro, A. F., Rato, M., & Martins, C. (2016). Drug-induced photosensitivity: Photoallergic and phototoxic reactions. *Clinical Dermatology, 34,* 571–581.

National Pressure Ulcer Advisory Panel. (2016). NPUAP pressure injury stages. Retrieved from www.npuap.org.

Neloska, L., Damevska, K., Nikolchev, A., et al. (2016). The association between malnutrition and pressure ulcers in elderly long-term care facility. *Open Access Macedonian Journal of Medical Sciences, 4,* 423–427.

Noddeskou, L. H., Hemmingsen, L. E., & Hordam, B. (2016). Elderly patients' and nurses' assessment of traditional bed bath compared to prepacked single units – randomized controlled trial. *Scandanavian Journal of Caring Sciences, 29,* 347–352.

Olazagasti Lourido, J. M., Ma, J. E., Lohse, C. M.et al. (2016). Increasing incidence of melanoma in the elderly: An epidemiological study in Olmsted County, Minnesota. *Mayo Clinic Proceedings.* doi: 10.1016/j.mayocp.2016.06.028.

Paddock, L. E., Lu, S. E., Bandera, E., et al. (2016). Skin self-examination and long-term melanoma survival. *Melanoma Research, 26,* 401–408.

Pittman, J., Beeson, T., Terry, C., et al. (2016). Unavoidable pressure ulcers. *Journal of Wound Ostomy and Continence Nursing, 43,* 32–38.

Rao, A., Preston, A., Strauss, R., et al. (2016). Risk factors associated with pressure ulcer formation in critically ill cardiac surgery patients. *Journal of Wound Ostomy and Continence Nursing, 43,* 242–247.

Sena, J., Girao, R., J., de Carbalho., S., M., et al. (2016). Occupational skin cancer: Systematic review. *Revista da Associacao Medica Brasileira, 62,* 280–286.

Steber, C. J., Perkins, S. L., Harris, K. B. (2016). Metformin-induced fixed-drug eruption confirmed by multiple exposures. *American Journal of Case Reports, 17,* 231–234.

Strazzieri-Pulido, K. C., Peres, G. R., Campanili, T. C., et al. (2017). Incidence of skin tears and risk factors: A systematic literature review. *Journal of Wound Ostomy and Continence Nursing, 44,* 29–33.

Tripp, M. K., Watson, M., Balk, S., et al. (2016). State of the science on prevention and screening to reduce melanoma incidence and mortality: The time is now. *CA: A Cancer Journal for Clinicians, 66,* 460–480.

Vashi, N., de Castro Maymone, M. B., & Kundu, R. (2016). Aging differences in ethnic skin. *Journal of Clinical Aesthetic Dermatology, 9,* 31–38.

Walters, K. M. & Woessner, K. M. (2016). An overview of nonsteroidal anti-inflammatory drug reactions. *Immunology & Allergy Clinics of North America, 36,* 625–641.

Wang, Y., Zhao, Y., & Ma, S. (2016). Racial differences in six major subtypes of melanoma: Descriptive epidemiology. *BioMed Central Cancer, 16,* 691.

Weiss, S. A., Han, J., Darvishian, F., et al. (2016). Impact of aging on host immune response and survival in melanoma: An analysis of 3 patient cohorts. *Journal of Translational Medicine, 14* (1), 299.

Yoon, J., Phibbs, C. S., Chow, A., et al. (2016). Costs of keratinocyte carcinoma (Nonmelanoma skin cancer) and actinic keratosis treatment in Veterans Health Administration. *Dermatologic Surgery, 42,* 104101047.

Zuba, E. B., Koronowska, S., Osmola-Mankowska, A., et al. (2016). Drug-induced photosensitivity. *Acta Dermatovenerol Croatia, 24*(1), 55–64.

chapter 24

Sleep and Rest

the many ways in which sleep influences and is influenced by one's health status, little was known about this essential aspect of health until recently. The establishment of sleep disorders centers during the 1970s paved the way for major advances in research and clinical practice related to all aspects of sleep as a health issue. As knowledge about the effects of sleep on health has increased, researchers, clinicians, and policy makers are addressing concerns about sleep as an essential component of wellness. In particular, there is much attention to sleep and sleep disorders as a major factor that affects not only one's quality of life but also one's risks for disease and death. Currently the National Healthy Sleep Awareness Project and *Healthy People 2020* are two of the major national initiatives that address sleep health as a public health concern for people of all ages. Because sleep patterns of older adults are affected by age-related changes and risk factors, nurses are called upon to address sleep issues as an essential component of wellness-focused care.

AGE-RELATED CHANGES THAT AFFECT SLEEP AND REST

A half century of sleep research has provided a strong base of information about age-related changes in sleep patterns, as well as the many sleep disorders that affect older adults. Sleep patterns of older adults are affected by complex relationships among a wide range of physiologic, environmental, and psychosocial factors. This section describes age-related changes in sleep characteristics, and the next section discusses risk factors that often affect sleep in older adults.

Sleep Quantity and Quality

Sleep efficiency, which is the percentage of time asleep during the time in bed, begins to decline even in healthy adults after the age of 50. This diminished sleep efficiency is

Approximately one-third of a person's lifetime is spent in sleep, during which time many metabolic processes decelerate, production of growth hormone increases, tissue repair and protein synthesis accelerate, and cognitive and emotional information is processed. Despite

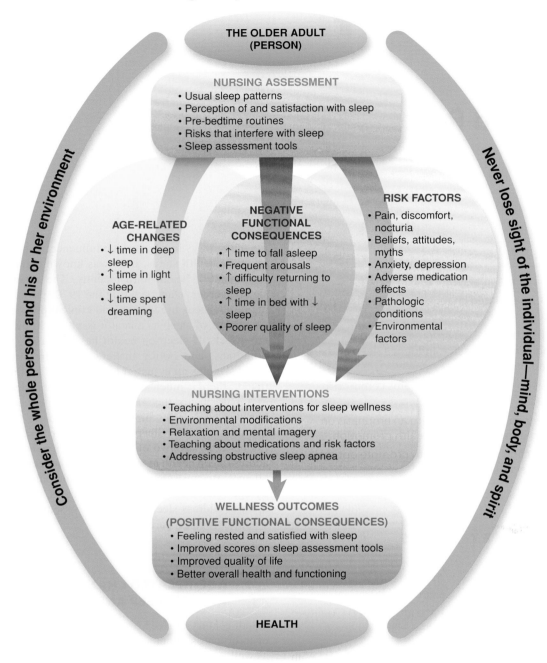

Promoting Sleep Wellness in Older Adults

THE OLDER ADULT (PERSON)

NURSING ASSESSMENT
- Usual sleep patterns
- Perception of and satisfaction with sleep
- Pre-bedtime routines
- Risks that interfere with sleep
- Sleep assessment tools

AGE-RELATED CHANGES
- ↓ time in deep sleep
- ↑ time in light sleep
- ↓ time spent dreaming

NEGATIVE FUNCTIONAL CONSEQUENCES
- ↑ time to fall asleep
- Frequent arousals
- ↑ difficulty returning to sleep
- ↑ time in bed with ↓ sleep
- Poorer quality of sleep

RISK FACTORS
- Pain, discomfort, nocturia
- Beliefs, attitudes, myths
- Anxiety, depression
- Adverse medication effects
- Pathologic conditions
- Environmental factors

NURSING INTERVENTIONS
- Teaching about interventions for sleep wellness
- Environmental modifications
- Relaxation and mental imagery
- Teaching about medications and risk factors
- Addressing obstructive sleep apnea

WELLNESS OUTCOMES
(POSITIVE FUNCTIONAL CONSEQUENCES)
- Feeling rested and satisfied with sleep
- Improved scores on sleep assessment tools
- Improved quality of life
- Better overall health and functioning

HEALTH

Consider the whole person and his or her environment

Never lose sight of the individual—mind, body, and spirit

attributed both to prolonged sleep latency, which is the time required to fall asleep, and to an increased number of awakenings during the night. Nocturnal sleep patterns are described in terms of sleep cycles, which are made up of **sleep stages**. Sleep stages are classified according to the presence of rapid eye movements (REMs) or the absence of this characteristic (non-REM). In adults, a cycle typically begins with stage I non-REM (lightest sleep), progresses through stage IV (deepest sleep), recurs in reverse order, and is followed by REM

sleep (dream stage). As the cycle repeats during the night, non-REM length decreases and REM increases so more time is spent in dream stage. During the non-REM stages, hormones are released, muscles relax, body systems slow, and essential restorative functions take place.

In addition to the presence of REMs, REM sleep is characterized by the following physiologic changes: flaccid muscles, increased gastric acid secretions, increased cerebral blood flow, fluctuating blood pressure and thermoregulation,

TABLE 24-1 Age-Related Changes in Sleep

Sleep Characteristics	Healthy Older Adults (vs. Healthy Younger Adults)
Non-REM	Gradual increase in length of light sleep stages with less time in deep sleep More frequent shifts in and out of light sleep
REM (dream stage)	Shorter episodes Begins earlier in the night Less intense
Sleep initiation	Longer time to fall asleep
Sleep maintenance	More frequent arousals
Sleep efficiency	Reduced amount of sleep during time in bed, more time in napping to compensate
Sleep schedule	Shift in nocturnal sleep phase to earlier bedtime and wakening

Non-REM, non–rapid eye movement; REM, rapid eye movement.

and increased rate and irregular rhythm of pulse and respirations. These physiologic alterations can exacerbate some medical problems. For example, increased gastric acid secretion during REM sleep may precipitate gastrointestinal pain for people with peptic ulcer disease. Likewise, people with chronic obstructive pulmonary disease may experience dyspnea or even a respiratory crisis because of decreased oxygen saturation during REM periods.

With increasing age, the length of the lightest sleep stage increases gradually, resulting in more frequent shifts in and out of lighter sleep stages during older adulthood. Similarly, although the number of episodes of REM sleep does not change significantly, the episodes are shorter, resulting in proportionately less time spent in REM. Table 24-1 summarizes the usual adult sleep cycle and typical age-related changes in sleep patterns.

Circadian Rhythm

Sleep patterns are determined, in part, by an individual's **circadian rhythm**, also known as a *biologic clock*. Body functions that have a circadian pattern include thermoregulation, sleep–wake cycles, and secretion of many hormones, including cortisol and melatonin. The sleep–wake circadian rhythm generally causes adults to become sleepy between 10 PM and midnight and to awaken feeling rested between 6 AM and 8 AM. With increasing age, **advanced sleep phase** occurs, causing older adults to become sleepy earlier in the evening and to awaken earlier in the morning. Age-related alterations in circadian rhythm affect sleep quantity and quality, and these disturbances are likely to be exacerbated by lack of exposure to bright light.

▶ RISK FACTORS THAT CAN AFFECT SLEEP

This section provides an overview of risk factors that commonly occur in older adults and lead to the common complaint of sleep problems, which are discussed in the section on Functional Consequences. Pain, dementia, and delirium are risk factors that are common in older adults and are discussed in Chapters 28 and 14.

Psychosocial Factors

Anxiety and worry are associated with difficulty falling asleep, frequent arousals during the night, and difficulty returning to sleep. Lack of information about age-related sleep changes can cause anxiety and excessive worry about sleep. Health education interventions discussed later in this chapter can be used to teach about actions to improve sleep. When anxiety and worry is associated with other causes, nurses can teach about stress-reduction interventions, as discussed in the section on Nursing Interventions for Sleep Wellness.

Older adults with few or no interesting activities, work demands, social responsibilities, or environmental stimuli may find it particularly difficult to establish healthy sleeping patterns. Socially isolated older adults may stay in bed for long periods because of boredom, lack of motivation, difficulty concentrating, or a desire to withdraw from stressful situations. Similarly, if an older adult spends all of his or her time in the same room, the lack of differentiation between space for waking and sleeping activities may interfere with sleep patterns. Interventions discussed in Chapter 12 (Psychosocial Wellness) can be used to address this risk.

Environmental Conditions

Noise and many other environmental conditions can significantly influence sleep patterns, particularly for patients in acute care settings. Studies of hospitalized patients confirm that noise in general and staff conversations in particular are a major source of disrupted sleep and contribute significantly to diminished sleep quantity and quality (Dobing, Frolova, McAlister, et al., 2016; Gathecha, Rios, Buenaver, et al., 2016). Studies also show a positive relationship between improved sleep and the implementation of relatively simple environmental interventions in acute care settings, such as using white noise, calming music, and daytime bright light exposure (Farokhnezhad Afshar, Bahramnezhad, Asgari, et al., 2016; Dubose & Hadi, 2016).

Environmental conditions can be problematic for people who live in institutional settings or with other people as in the following examples:

- Lack of privacy and sleeping in close proximity to others
- Uncomfortably low or high temperatures (often due to inadequate heating or cooling systems)
- Excessive light in bedrooms, patient/resident rooms, and hallways
- Insufficient exposure to bright light during the day, leading to diminished production of melatonin
- Hot and humid conditions, especially for menopausal women who experience more nighttime hot flashes when the air is hot and humid

Needs and schedules of others in long-term care facilities or home settings can influence sleep of older adults. For example, in institutional settings, the time for awakening patients or residents is often based on the most efficient use of nursing and dietary time, and patients/residents are expected to adjust their sleep routines accordingly. Similarly, dependent older adults in home settings may have to adjust their sleep routines to the schedule of family caregivers who have work responsibilities. In home settings, older adults who are caregivers may have their sleep interrupted by dependent family members who require care during the night. In some households, both the person with dementia and the family caregivers may be experiencing significant and nightly sleep disruptions.

Pathologic Conditions

Pathologic conditions interfere with sleep and increase the risk for sleep-related disorders for many reasons, as delineated in Table 24-2. In addition to these conditions that can interfere with sleep, sleep disorders are pathologic conditions that are characterized by disturbed sleep, as discussed in the section on Pathologic Conditions Affecting Sleep. Nocturia (discussed in Chapter 19) is common in older adults and is a

topic that is receiving much attention in relation to sleep disorders and sleep quality (Duffy, Scheuermaier, & Loughlin, 2016; Kim, Moon, & Kim, 2016).

Wellness Opportunity

Nurses promote wellness by identifying subtle risk factors, such as chronic pain and discomfort, that are often overlooked and that can be addressed through many types of holistic interventions.

Effects of Bioactive Substances

Adverse effects of medications and other bioactive substances can interfere with sleep in a number of ways. Prescription medications that can cause disturbed sleep include steroids, antidepressants, aminophylline preparations, thyroid extracts, antiarrhythmic medications, and centrally acting antihypertensives. These effects are not unique to older adults; however, adverse effects of medication are more likely to occur in older adults, as discussed in detail in Chapter 8.

Caffeine can affect all aspects of sleep quality and quantity, especially by being associated with difficulty staying asleep (Chaudhary, Grandner, Jackson, et al., 2016). Although low doses of nicotine can have relaxing and sedative effects, higher doses interfere with sleep because of nicotine's stimulant effect as well as its effects on respiration. Alcoholic beverages initially induce drowsiness but also suppress REM sleep and cause frequent awakenings, resulting in less total sleep and more daytime sleepiness. People who abstain from alcohol after long-term abuse may experience insomnia for a few years after withdrawing from it. Alcohol and other central nervous system depressants can exacerbate sleep disorders and lead to additional detrimental effects. Table 24-3

TABLE 24-2 Pathophysiologic Factors Affecting Sleep	
Risk Factor	**Sleep Alteration**
Arthritis	Chronic pain and discomfort that interfere with sleep
COPD	Awakening as a result of apnea and respiratory distress
Nocturia	Sleep disruptions due to needing to use the bathroom
Diabetes mellitus	Awakening secondary to nocturia or poorly controlled blood glucose levels; increased incidence of OSA
Gastrointestinal disorders, ulcers	Nocturnal pain secondary to increased gastric secretions during REM sleep
Hypertension	Early morning awakening
Hyperthyroidism	Increased difficulty falling asleep
Nocturnal angina	Awakening without perception of pain, especially during REM sleep
PLMS, RLS	Awakening caused by recurrent involuntary leg movements
Malignancies	Increased incidence of RLS
Chronic kidney disease	Increase incidence of PLMS, RLS, and OSA
Parkinsonism	Increased time awake; decreased amount of sleep
Dementia	Alterations of all sleep stages
Delirium	Increased somnolence *or* inability to sleep

COPD, chronic obstructive pulmonary disease; OSA, obstructive sleep apnea; PLMS, periodic limb movements in sleep; REM, rapid eye movement; RLS, restless legs syndrome.

TABLE 24-3 The Effect of Various Medications and Chemicals on Sleep	
Medication or Chemical	**Sleep Alteration**
Alcohol	Suppression of REM sleep, early morning awakening
Alcohol or hypnotic withdrawal	Sleep disturbances, nightmares
Anticholinergics	Hyperreflexia, overactivity, muscle twitching
Barbiturates	Suppression of REM sleep, nightmares; hallucinations, paradoxical responses
Benzodiazepines	Awakening secondary to apnea
Beta-blockers	Nightmares
Corticosteroids	Restlessness, sleep disturbances
Diuretics	Awakening for nocturia, sleep apnea secondary to alkalosis
Theophylline, levodopa, isoproterenol, phenytoin	Interference with sleep onset and sleep stages
Antidepressants	PLMS, suppression of REM sleep

PLMS, periodic limb movements in sleep; REM, rapid eye movement.

summarizes the effects of various medications and chemicals on sleep in older adults.

See **ONLINE LEARNING ACTIVITY 24-1: RESOURCES FOR MORE INFORMATION ABOUT SLEEP** at http://thepoint.lww.com/Miller8e.

FUNCTIONAL CONSEQUENCES AFFECTING SLEEP WELLNESS

The overall functional consequences of age-related changes in sleep are insufficient, inefficient, and poor quality sleep, as summarized in Table 24-1. In addition, the high prevalence of risk factors that can interfere with sleep increases the vulnerability of older adults to sleep disorders and complaints. Common sleep complaints of older adults include daytime sleepiness, difficulty falling asleep, and frequent arousals during the night. Studies indicate that significant sleep problems affect 25% to 30% of the adult population, with 65% to 74% of adults in the United States reporting difficulties with sleep at least a few times a week (Liu, Wheaton, Chapman, et al., 2016; National Center on Sleep Disorders Research, 2011). Poor sleep is associated with increased risk for all the following serious health consequences: stroke, cancer, obesity, diabetes, cardiovascular diseases, cognitive impairments, metabolic syndrome, substance abuse, accidental injuries, and all-cause mortality (Grandner, Alfonso-Miller, Fernandez-Mendoza, et al., 2016; Grossman, 2016; Lo, Groeger, Cheng, et al., 2016). Depression is strongly associated with sleep problems, but it is difficult to determine if it is a cause or effect of sleep problems (Chang, Pan, Kawachi, et al., 2016; Leggett, Burgard, & Zivin, 2016).

Diversity Note

A national survey of adults in the United States found that the prevalence of poor sleep patterns was highest among Native Hawaiians/Pacific Islanders, blacks, and American Indian/Alaska Natives, compared with Asians, Hispanics, and whites (Liu, Wheaton, Chapman, et al., 2016).

PATHOLOGIC CONDITIONS AFFECTING SLEEP: SLEEP DISORDERS

Sleep disorders are receiving much attention as a major health-related concern, particularly in relation to the increasing research identifying serious negative health consequences of these disorders. Increasingly, sleep disorders are being addressed in relation to risks for other medical conditions and as a quality-of-life issue.

Excessive Sleepiness

Excessive sleepiness (i.e., the inability to maintain alertness or vigilance because of hypersomnolence) is a hallmark symptom associated with sleep disorders. Excessive sleepiness differs from fatigue, which manifests as difficulty sustaining a high level of physical performance (Dean, Klimpt, Morris, et al., 2016). An evidence-based geriatric nursing protocol for best practice emphasizes that excessive sleepiness should not be dismissed as an insignificant condition; rather, it should be evaluated by health care providers because it can have significant health effects (Dean, Klimpt, Morris, et al., 2016). This evidence-based protocol for nursing practice is summarized in Box 24-1.

Insomnia

Insomnia is a chronic or transient sleep disorder characterized by a complaint of poor sleep quality or difficulty initiating or maintaining sleep that causes daytime impairment. Chronic insomnia is negatively associated with all aspects of well-being in older adults (Abell, Shipley, Ferrie, et al., 2016). In addition to the risk factors related to difficulty sleeping (discussed earlier in this chapter), excessive anxiety about one's ability to sleep is a factor that contributes to chronic insomnia. There is increasing evidence to support nonpharmacologic approaches, such as cognitive-behavioral therapy, rather than hypnotic medications for management of insomnia (Qaseem, Kansagara, Forciea, et al., 2016) (refer to Evidence-Based Practice Box 24-1).

Obstructive Sleep Apnea

Obstructive sleep apnea (also called sleep disordered breathing) is a sleep disorder that has been the focus of much research and clinical attention since 1988, when the U.S. Congress established the National Commission on Sleep Disorders Research. Primary manifestation of OSA are (1) the involuntary cessation of airflow for 10 seconds or longer (i.e., apnea) and (2) the occurrence of more than five to eight of these episodes per hour. This condition occurs because the muscles responsible for holding the throat open relax during sleep and block the passage of air. Symptoms of OSA include daytime fatigue, morning headaches, diminished mental acuity, and loud snoring punctuated by brief periods of silence. OSA is not exclusively a condition of older adults, but it is strongly associated with increased age, with a prevalence of 20% to 40% of older adults in the general population (McMillan & Morrell, 2016). Recent studies also have identified higher risk for OSA in people who live in neighborhoods with a low walking environment, particularly for men and obese individuals; this is consistent with reduced risk with greater physical activity (Billings, Johnson, Simonelli, et al., 2016).

OSA is a major focus of researchers and clinicians because of the mounting evidence that it leads to serious consequences, and even death, when it is undiagnosed and untreated. Strong evidence links OSA to increased risk for all the following: stroke, hypertension, diabetes, depression, heart failure, atrial fibrillation, and cognitive impairment (BaHammam, Kendzerska, Gupta, et al., 2016; Bauters, Rietzschel, Hertegonne, et al., 2016; Kerner & Roose, 2016;

Box 24-1 Evidence-Based Practice: Excessive Sleepiness

Overview

- Healthy older adults experience the following changes in sleep: decreased deep sleep stages, longer time until sleep onset, and stage 1 sleep, and decreased sleep efficiency
- Factors common in older adults that cause or contribute to the excessive sleepiness include all the following: age-related changes in chronobiology, sleep disorders, psychological disorders (e.g., anxiety, depression), chronic illness symptoms (e.g., pain), adverse effects of medications, and environmental factors
- In older adults, the most common sleep disorders causing excessive sleepiness are OSA, insomnia, and RLS
- Consequences of excessive sleepiness are decreased alertness, delayed reaction time, and diminished cognitive performance.

Sleep Disturbances During Hospitalization

- Because 22% to 61% of hospitalized patients experience sleep disturbances, routine care should include interventions to assess and improve sleep.

Recommendations for Nursing Assessment

- Daytime sleepiness is often viewed falsely as normal or unpreventable in older adults; this misperception reduces the likelihood that this condition will be appropriately evaluated and treated.
- Obtain a sleep history, based on information from both the patient and family members, including information about sleep patterns and sleep-related behaviors.
- Use the ESS as a valid and reliable tool for identifying excessive sleepiness
- Use the STOP-BANG tool for identifying risks for OSA: **S**noring, **T**ired, **O**bserved gaps in breathing, blood **P**ressure high, **B**MI more than 35, **A**ge over 50, **N**eck circumference greater than 40 cm, and **G**ender male.
- Assess sleep history and consider primary and secondary causes of excessive sleepiness.

- When possible, observe patients for snoring, apnea during sleep, excessive leg movements during sleep, and difficulty staying awake during normal daytime activities.

Recommendations for Patient Teaching

Teach older adults and caregivers about the following sleep-promoting measures:

- Use the bed only for sleeping or sex.
- Develop consistent and rest-promoting bedtime routines and maintain the same schedule daily.
- If awakened during the night, avoid looking at the clock.
- Avoid or limit naps to 10–15 minutes.
- Sleep in a cool, quiet environment.
- Avoid the following before bedtime: caffeine, nicotine, alcohol, large meals, exercise, emotionally charged activities.
- If you cannot fall asleep after 15 or 20 minutes, go to another room and engage in a quiet activity until you are sleepy again.

Recommendations for Care

- Work with primary care practitioners to ensure optimal management of medical conditions, psychological disorders, and symptoms that interfere with sleep.
- Teach patients and families about lifestyle measures for improving sleep among all family members.
- Incorporate sleep-hygiene measures and ongoing treatment of existing sleep disorders into the plan of care for older adults in all settings.
- Work with prescribing practitioners to review and, if appropriate, adjust medications that can cause drowsiness or sleep impairment.
- Suggest referral to a sleep specialist for moderate or severe sleepiness or a clinical profile consistent with major sleep disorders.

Adapted from Dean, G. E., Klimpt, M. L., Morris, J. L., & Chasens, E. R. (2016). Excessive sleepiness. In M. Boltz, E. Capezuti, T. Fulmer, & D. Zwicker (Eds.), *Evidence-based geriatric nursing protocols for best practice* (5th ed., pp. 431–442). New York: Springer Publishing Company.

Khayat & Pleister, 2016). Studies also confirm that treatment of OSA is clearly associated with positive health benefits such as all the following:

- Improved control of atrial fibrillation (Nalliah, Sanders, & Kalman, 2016)
- Decreased cardiovascular and all-cause mortality (Fu, Xia, Yi, et al., 2016)
- Improved glycemic control and insulin resistance in patients with type 2 diabetes (Martinez-Ceron, Barquiel, Bezos, et al., 2016)
- Decreased 6-month readmissions after discharge in patients with heart failure (Sharma, Mather, Gupta, et al., 2016)
- Reduced blood pressure in patients with hypertension (Maeder, Schoch, & Rickli, 2016)
- Improved quality of life, increased energy, better concentration (Giunta, Salifu, & McFarlane, 2016)

Because of the link between OSA and serious medical conditions, health care professionals need to identify signs and symptoms and initiate referrals for further evaluation, as discussed in the section on Teaching about Management of Sleep Disorders.

Sleep-Related Movement Disorders

In recent years, researchers and clinicians have focused on two movement disorders that occur during sleep and are strongly associated with disturbed sleep patterns: restless legs syndrome (RLS) and periodic limb movements during sleep (PLMS). The conditions have overlapping and similar manifestations and frequently coexist, making it difficult to distinguish between them. Increased age is a risk factor for both RLS and PLMS, and symptoms may increase over time.

Restless legs syndrome, also known as *Willis–Ekbom disease*, is a sensorimotor condition characterized by the following symptoms:

- An almost irresistible urge to move the legs (or other body parts), usually accompanied or caused by unpleasant sensations, which are often described as itchy, crawling, burning, or creepy
- Onset of symptoms occurs or worsens during rest or inactivity
- Symptoms are relieved by movement, such as walking or stretching
- Symptoms are worse in the evening or occur only at night

An additional characteristic is that the symptoms are not due to another condition, such as leg cramps, fibromyalgia, arthritis, or positional discomfort. Symptoms of RLS can interfere with both initiating and maintaining sleep; during waking hours, RLS disrupts periods of rest and relaxation. Risk factors for RLS include diabetes, iron deficiency, chronic renal failure, and adverse effects of medications (e.g., most antidepressants, antipsychotic agents, and possibly antihistamines). RLS often occurs early during the course of Parkinson disease and worsens gradually, causing significant sleep disturbances (Moccia, Erro, Picillo, et al., 2016). Nurses can teach older adults with symptoms of RLS about the importance of obtaining an evaluation for medication management of RLS. In addition, the following health promotion interventions may alleviate symptoms:

- Moderate amounts of regular exercise, such as walking or using a stationary bike
- Stress reduction techniques, such as yoga or meditation
- Gentle massage of legs
- Soaking in warm bath
- Avoiding alcohol and excessive caffeine
- Quitting smoking (if applicable)

Periodic limb movements during sleep, also known as *nocturnal myoclonus,* is the occurrence of brief muscle contractions, spaced at intervals of about 20 to 40 seconds, that cause leg jerks, or rhythmic movements of muscles in the foot or leg. They may occur several times to more than 200 times nightly, with increased occurrence during the first half of the night. PLMS can contribute to complaints of insomnia, frequent arousals, and increased daytime sleepiness. Risks for PLMS include RLS, anxiety, depression, cardiovascular disease, and cerebrovascular disease, particularly post-stroke (Haba-Rubio, Marti-Soler, Marques-Vidal, et al., 2016; Moro, Goparaju, Castillo, et al., 2016; Woo, Lee, Hwang, et al., 2017).

Diversity Note

Women have at least a 40% increased risk for developing insomnia and twice the risk for RLS compared to men (Guidozzi, 2015). Studies indicate that the direct relationship between age and poor sleep is more consistent in women (Madrid-Valero, Martinez-Selva, Ribeiro do Couto, et al., 2017).

Diversity Note

A large multi-ethnic study found that blacks, Hispanics, and Asians had a higher prevalence of sleep disorders and were less likely to be diagnosed compared with whites. The authors of this study suggest that these factors may contribute to health disparities (Chen, Wang, Zee, et al., 2015).

See **ONLINE LEARNING ACTIVITY CHECKPOINT 24-2: LEARNING MORE ABOUT OBSTRUCTIVE SLEEP APNEA** at **http://thepoint.lww.com/Miller8e.**

 NURSING ASSESSMENT OF SLEEP

Identifying Opportunities for Health Promotion

In recent years, nurses and other health care professionals have recognized the importance of assessing sleep as an essential aspect of wellness and quality of life. Nurses assess sleep patterns to determine the adequacy of the person's usual sleep and rest pattern and to identify factors that either contribute to or interfere with the quality and quantity of sleep. Goals of nursing assessment are (1) to identify health-promoting behaviors that can be encouraged and (2) to identify conditions that interfere with sleep so these can be addressed. Many of the contributing factors are addressed through educational interventions, such as teaching about self-care interventions to promote sleep. Box 24-2 provides guidelines for

---

 Box 24-2 Guidelines for Assessing Sleep and Rest

Questions to Assess the Perception of Quality and Adequacy of Sleep

- On a scale of 1–10, with 10 as the highest, how would you rate your sleep?
- When you awaken in the morning, do you feel like you are rested?
- Do you feel drowsy or sleepy during the day or early evening?
- Does fatigue interfere with your desired daytime activity level?

Questions to Assess Nighttime Sleep Pattern

- Where do you sleep at night (e.g., bed, couch, recliner chair)?
- How long does it usually take to fall asleep after you get into bed?
- Do you think you lie awake too long before falling asleep?
- After you fall asleep, how many times do you wake up during the night?
- What kinds of things disturb your sleep during the night (e.g., getting up to urinate; activities of roommates or other people in the setting; environmental factors, such as noise or lighting)?
- If changes in living arrangements have occurred in the past few months: Has your sleep pattern changed since … (e.g., since you came to this nursing home; since your spouse passed away)?

Questions to Identify Opportunities for Health Education

- What is your usual time for getting into bed?
- Describe your usual activities during the daytime and evening.
- What factors help you fall asleep (e.g., food or drink, relaxation strategies, environmental influences)?
- What conditions interfere with good sleep (e.g., pain, discomfort, anxiety, depression)?
- Do you take any medicines to help you sleep?
- Do you take medicines to help you stay awake during the day?
- Do you drink alcoholic or caffeinated beverages, or take medicines that contain alcohol or caffeine during the late afternoon or evening? (If yes, how much and what kind?)
- Do you smoke or use nicotine products? (If yes, what kind and how much?)
- Are you aware, or has anyone told you, that you snore or stop breathing during your sleep?
- Do your legs kick or jump involuntarily while you sleep?

Unfolding Case Study

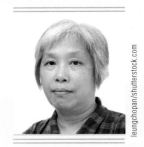

Part 1: Mrs. Z. at 66 Years of Age

Mrs. Z. is 66 years old and recently retired from her job as office manager for a law firm. She considers herself to be in good health, although she has had hypertension for 20 years and osteoarthritis for the past several years. She self-monitors her blood pressure and takes atenolol, 50 mg daily. She occasionally takes an over-the-counter analgesic medication when her arthritis pain bothers her. She just started going to the local senior center once a week for lunch and social and educational activities. During one of your weekly senior wellness clinics, Mrs. Z. comes to talk with you about her difficulty sleeping. She reports that since she has retired, she often wakes up several times during the night and has difficulty returning to sleep. She used to sleep an average of 7 to 8 hours nightly and could easily return to sleep if she woke up during the night. Now she is lucky if she gets 6 hours of sleep because she lies in bed for several hours when she wakes during the night. She used to go to bed between 10 and 11 PM and get up promptly between 6:30 and 7 AM. Now that she is retired, she goes to bed around 11 PM, but stays in bed until 10 AM.

THINKING POINTS

- What age-related changes may be contributing to Mrs. Z.'s dissatisfaction with her sleep?
- What risk factors might be contributing to Mrs. Z.'s dissatisfaction with her sleep?

- What further assessment information would you need to obtain, and how would you obtain it?

---

nursing assessment of independent older adults and caregivers of dependent older adults about sleep and rest patterns.

In addition to obtaining information from older adults and their caregivers, nurses observe behavioral indicators of sleep and rest patterns. This is especially important when objective observations are contrary to subjective complaints. For example, older adults may complain of not sleeping at all, but when observed by caregivers, they may appear to be sleeping during the entire night. By contrast, older adults who deny any problems sleeping may nap frequently and readily fall asleep during daytime activities. Observations also are essential for identifying key signs of OSA, such as snoring and breaks in breathing patterns.

> **Wellness Opportunity**
>
> Be aware of opportunities to help older adults identify self-care measures to improve sleep quantity and quality, rather than view this as an inevitable consequence of aging.

Evidence-Based Assessment Tools

Older adults can use evidence-based sleep assessment tools for self-assessment or for self-reporting to health care professionals. Two easy-to-use and readily available tools that have been tested for validity and reliability are the **Pittsburgh Sleep Quality Index (PSQI)** and the **Epworth Sleepiness Scale (ESS)**. The PSQI assesses sleep quality and patterns over the past month, and the ESS focuses on daytime sleepiness over the past week. A recent systematic review and meta-analysis found that the PSQI showed strong reliability and validity (Mollayeva, Thurairajah, Burton, et al., 2016).

Online Learning Activity 24-3 provides links to additional information about and illustration of these tools.

 See ONLINE LEARNING ACTIVITY 24-3: TOOLS FOR ASSESSING SLEEP IN OLDER ADULTS at http://thepoint.lww.com/Miller8e.

NURSING DIAGNOSIS

When healthy older adults are interested in learning self-care activities to improve their sleep pattern, the nursing diagnosis of Readiness for Enhanced Sleep is applicable. This wellness nursing diagnosis is defined as "A pattern of natural, periodic suspension of relative consciousness to provide rest and sustain a desired lifestyle, which can be strengthened" (Herdman & Kamitsuru, 2018, p. 215). Nursing diagnoses pertinent to older adults who have sleep problems (or risks for) include (Risk for) Insomnia, (Risk for) Sleep Deprivation, and (Risk for) Disturbed Sleep Pattern.

> **Wellness Opportunity**
>
> Nurses can be alert to opportunities to include the wellness nursing diagnosis of Readiness for Enhanced Sleep for older adults who are willing to explore interventions that improve their sleep patterns in any setting.

PLANNING FOR WELLNESS OUTCOMES

When older adults experience sleep disturbances or have risk factors that affect sleep patterns, nurses identify wellness outcomes as an essential part of the nursing process. Nursing Outcomes Classification (NOC) terms that most directly relate to interventions to enhance sleep or address sleep problems in older adults are Sleep, Rest, Health Promoting Behavior, Comfort Status: Environment, Personal Well-Being, Anxiety Level, Knowledge: Health Behavior, and Pain: Disruptive Effects.

> **Wellness Opportunity**
>
> Quality of Life is a wellness outcome that may be achieved when nursing interventions are directed toward enhancing sleep.

NURSING INTERVENTIONS FOR SLEEP WELLNESS

Nursing interventions to promote sleep wellness for older adults include health education and direct interventions, such as environmental modifications and comfort and relaxation strategies. In particular, studies support the use of progressive muscle relaxation exercises as an intervention to improve sleep quality, even in hospitalized patients (Alparslan, Orsal, & Unsal, 2016). It is important to adapt these interventions to the individual needs of older adults in various settings. For example, in community settings the focus is on teaching older adults and their caregivers about self-care interventions that can improve sleep patterns. In long-term care settings, the focus is on interventions that can be implemented routinely to improve sleep patterns of residents. In acute-care settings, there is increasing emphasis on the importance of identifying and addressing sleep apnea as an integral component of care, particularly for patients with cardiovascular and respiratory diseases (Konikkara, Tavella, Wiles, et al., 2016; Sharma, Chowdhury, Tang, et al., 2016). Similarly,

there is increasing emphasis on addressing sleep disorders as an integral component of rehabilitation following stroke or cardiovascular events (Fox, Purucker, Holzhacker, et al., 2016; Hermann & Bassetti, 2016).

The following pertinent Nursing Interventions Classification terminologies are appropriate for documentation of interventions: Sleep Enhancement, Anxiety Reduction, Exercise Promotion, Music Therapy, Risk Identification, Environmental Management: Comfort, Pain Management, Relaxation Therapy, and Self-Efficacy Enhancement.

Teaching Older Adults About Interventions for Sleep Wellness

Increasingly, nonpharmacologic interventions for improving sleep are being emphasized as safe and effective alternatives to medications, which can have many adverse effects (see the section on Educating Older Adults about Medications and Sleep). Box 24-3 summarizes current research conclusions about nonpharmacologic interventions for improving sleep.

An important aspect of health promotion is to teach older adults about normal age-related changes and help them identify risk factors that can affect their sleep, as described in Tables 24-1 and 24-2. When contributing factors are identified, help older adults plan interventions to address risks such as stress and chronic pain or discomfort. In addition, use information in Box 24-4 to teach about self-care actions (sometimes called *sleep hygiene*) for promoting sleep wellness. If older adults are not familiar with relaxation techniques, give them a copy of Box 24-5 and teach them about deep breathing, progressive relaxation, and mental imagery. Encourage older adults to use audio devices with automatic

---

Box 24-3   Evidence-Based Practice: Research Conclusions About Nonpharmacologic Interventions to Improve Sleep

- Meditation, mindfulness, and mindfulness-based stress reduction are consistently identified as effective interventions for improving sleep (Dentico, Ferrarelli, Riedner, et al., 2016; Gallegos, Moynihan, & Pigeon, 2016; Maruthai, Nagendra, Sasidharan, et al., 2016).
- Daily moderate physical activity improves sleep for older adults (Karimi, Soroush, Towhidi, et al., 2016; Kredlow, Capozzoli, Hearon, et al., 2015; Scholtens, van Munster, & van Kempen, 2016).
- Participation in aquatic exercise twice weekly for 1 hour has been found to improve sleep efficiency in older adults with mild sleep impairments (Chen, Fox, Ku, et al., 2016).
- Muscle relaxation techniques (e.g., progressive muscle relaxation, autogenic training) improve sleep, particularly when stress is a contributing condition (Alparslan, Orsal, & Unsal, 2016).
- Many studies and evidence-based guidelines find strong support for cognitive behavioral treatment for insomnia (e.g., Alessi, Martin, Fiorentino, et al., 2016; Brasure, Fuchs, MacDonald, et al., 2016; Brenes, Danhauer, Lyles, et al., 2016; Morin, Beaulieu-Bonneau, Belanger, et al., 2016).
- Studies find good support for the use of yoga and tai chi (body–mind interventions) in improving sleep (Du, Dong, Zhang, et al., 2016).

- Acupuncture may be effective for sleep disorders, particularly if chronic pain is an influencing factor (Hayhoe, 2017; Lee & Lim, 2016; Shergis, Ni, Jackson, et al., 2016).
- Acupressure, which can be used as a self-care intervention, can be effective for improving sleep quality (Hmwe, Subramaniam, & Tan, 2016; Zeng, Liu, Wang, et al., 2016).
- Listening to soothing music is effective for improving sleep quality (Andrews, 2016; Wang, Chair, Wong, et al., 2016).
- White noise is recommended for improving sleep in the coronary care unit (Farokhnezhad Afshar, Bahramnezhad, Asgari, et al., 2016).
- Melatonin, a sleep-regulating hormone produced by the pineal gland, can be effective in managing circadian sleep disorders and jet lag (Cardinali, Golombek, Rosenstein, et al., 2016).
- Melatonin and bright light therapy should be first-line treatments for people with dementia and sleep disorders (Ooms & Ju, 2016).
- Aromatherapy with lavender essential oil may be helpful for promoting sleep (Karadag, Samancioglu, Ozden, et al., 2017).
- Massage therapy is beneficial for improving sleep in older adults (McFeeters, Pront, Cuthbertson, et al., 2016).
- Daily, 30-minute foot baths with water at 40° C were effective in improving sleep quality in residents of a long-term care facility (Kim, Lee, & Sohng, 2016).

Box 24-4 Health Promotion Teaching About Sleep

Actions to Take

- Establish a bedtime ritual that is effective for you, and try to follow it every night.
- Maintain the same daily schedule for waking, resting, and sleeping.
- Take a warm, relaxing bath in the afternoon or early evening.
- After 1:00 PM, avoid foods, beverages, and medications that contain caffeine or stimulants (e.g., tea, cocoa, coffee, chocolate, sugar, refined carbohydrates, and some over-the-counter pain relievers and cold preparations).
- Prebedtime foods that promote sleep include milk (warm), chamomile tea, and a light snack of complex carbohydrates (e.g., whole grains).
- Use one or more of the following relaxation methods: imagery, meditation, deep breathing, progressive relaxation, soothing music, body or foot massage, rocking in a chair, reading nonstimulating materials, or watching nonstimulating television.
- Perform daily moderate aerobic exercise, preferably before the late afternoon, but avoid vigorous exercise in the evening.
- Assure adequate intake of the following nutrients: zinc, calcium, magnesium, manganese, vitamin C, and vitamin B complex.

Actions to Avoid

- Do not drink alcohol before bedtime because it may cause early morning awakening. If you use alcohol, use only in small amounts.

- Do not smoke cigarettes in the evening because nicotine is a stimulant.
- If your bedtime is temporarily changed, try to keep your waking time as close to the usual time as possible, and avoid staying in bed beyond your usual waking time.
- Do not use your bed for reading or other activities not associated with sleeping.
- If you awaken during the night and cannot return to sleep, get out of bed after 30 minutes and engage in a nonstimulating activity, such as reading, in another room.
- Arise at your usual time, even if you have not slept well.

Complementary and Alternative Care Practices

- Yoga, tai chi, meditation, imagery, aromatherapy, massage, soothing music, relaxation techniques, and a warm bath or warm footbath may be effective in promoting sleep.
- Melatonin, a sleep-regulating hormone, can be effective in improving sleep, but it can interact with other medications and also can cause daytime sleepiness.

Special Precautions

- Although widely promoted as sleep aids, herbs should be used with caution in older adults because of their possible adverse effects.
- Inform your health care professionals about any use of herbs, aromatherapy, or other complementary and alternative care practices.

shutoffs to listen to soothing music or provide instructions for deep breathing, guided imagery, or relaxation exercises.

See ONLINE LEARNING ACTIVITY 24-4: JOURNAL ARTICLE AND ADDITIONAL RESOURCES FOR EVIDENCE-BASED INTERVENTIONS at http://thepoint.lww.com/Miller8e.

Wellness Opportunity

Health education about sleep is particularly important in community and long-term care settings because nurses have more opportunities to focus on quality-of-life issues.

Improving Sleep for Older Adults in Institutional Settings

Older adults in acute and long-term care settings have a high prevalence of sleep disturbances, and these disturbances can lead to serious and detrimental health consequences, as already delineated. Nurses who work evening or night shifts have many opportunities to engage in direct care activities that promote good nighttime sleep, which are in addition to environmental interventions discussed in the next section.

For older adults in any setting, nursing responsibilities include addressing factors that interfere with sleep, ensuring the most comfortable environment possible, and individualizing

Box 24-5 Relaxation and Mental Imagery Techniques that Promote Sleep

Deep Breathing

- Focus your attention on your breathing; extend your belly and draw in a deep breath as you count.
- Hold your breath for three or four counts.
- Exhale completely.
- Repeat this pattern, focusing your total attention on breathing.
- Phrases, such as "I am sleepy," or counting may be repeated during each exhalation to help keep your attention focused on breathing.

Progressive Relaxation

- Start by focusing your attention on the muscles in your toes.
- Flex or tense these muscles, and then relax them.
- Repeat two or three times.

- Focus your attention on the muscles in your foot.
- Flex or tense, then relax these muscles, two or three times.
- Repeat this process, progressively focusing on different muscle groups and proceeding from your feet to your head.

Mental Imagery

- Begin with deep breathing exercises to relax yourself.
- Focus your attention on a serene and peaceful scene, visualize the setting, and imagine the sounds (e.g., a beach with waves gently washing ashore).
- Imagine yourself in the setting, lying relaxed, enjoying the environment.
- Keep your attention focused on the scene.
- Imagine repetitive motions, such as waves on the beach or sheep jumping over a fence.

care plans so that they incorporate personal preferences for optimal sleep conditions. The following relatively simple nursing actions can improve sleep in hospitalized patients: supporting the person's usual sleeping schedule and routines, providing assistance with personal care and comfortable positioning, providing comfort measures (e.g., warm beverage, a brief massage, maintaining a quiet environment with minimal lighting).

If dementia or depression interferes with sleep onset, a helpful intervention is to simply stay with the older person to provide reassurance until the person is able to fall asleep. In addition, relief of pain, anxiety, and physical discomfort are nursing responsibilities that can affect the sleep of older adults. Older adults who are cognitively impaired may not request analgesics but may give nonverbal cues that pain is interfering with sleep, as discussed in Chapter 28. Be alert to this possibility and assess for chronic or acute pain, and recognize that an analgesic taken 30 minutes before bedtime may help induce sleep in people with chronic pain or discomfort.

Because daytime activities influence sleep patterns, care plans in long-term care settings should incorporate appropriate types and amounts of activities in each older adult's daily routine. Also, residents should be exposed to adequate bright lights during the day. Evening and nighttime routines need to be based on a comprehensive assessment of the needs of the older adult and consider any conflicting needs. For example, for some older adults, the need for an uninterrupted night's sleep may outweigh the potential benefits of being awakened for nighttime care tasks. In many situations, the needs can be addressed during the person's usual waking time, rather than performing the tasks on a rigid schedule designed for the convenience of staff.

Modifying the Environment to Promote Sleep

Environmental modifications are among the simplest and most effective interventions to improve sleep, especially in institutional settings. For example, simple actions such as closing bedroom doors and adjusting bedroom lighting can improve sleep. Elimination of unnecessary staff-initiated noise, especially conversations at the nursing station, is another helpful intervention for patients/residents located near the center of nursing activity. In long-term care settings, nurses can document preferences for bedtime routines that promote sleep on each resident's care plan and assure that these measures are carried out by nursing staff. In long-term care settings where residents share rooms, decisions about room assignments should take into consideration the compatibility of individual needs. Once room assignments have been made, roommate behaviors that interfere with sleep can be addressed by a room change, if necessary.

If a noisy environment contributes to sleeping difficulties, and the noise cannot be controlled or eliminated, the older person may wish to use earplugs. People who live alone, however, should be cautioned about the danger of blocking out protective noises, such as that of a smoke alarm. If environmental noise cannot be eliminated, it can be masked by white noise (e.g., using a fan, air conditioner, soft music, or recordings of white noise). In addition to addressing noise in the environment, interventions address temperature in the sleeping area. The nighttime room temperature should be comfortable, and is usually slightly lower than during the day. In cooler environments, the older adult should wear a nightcap to prevent loss of heat through the head.

Educating Older Adults About Medications and Sleep

Hypnotics may be effective for short-term management of sleep disorders, especially in temporary circumstances, such as in acute care settings; however, the adverse effects of most hypnotics can outweigh their advantages. Benzodiazepines (e.g., flurazepam [Dalmane], triazolam [Halcion], temazepam [Restoril]) were the most commonly prescribed sleep medication for older adults until the early 1990s. This class of drugs is not commonly used for insomnia because of concerns about adverse effects, including dependency with subsequent withdrawal and rebound symptoms. Nonbenzodiazepine agents (e.g., zolpidem [Ambien], zaleplon [Sonata], eszopiclone [Lunesta], and ramelteon [Rozerem]) have been available since 1993, but recent studies indicate that these drugs may be associated with infrequent but serious adverse effects, such as cognitive and behavioral changes (Asnis, Thomas, & Henderson, 2016; Lai, 2016; Wilt, MacDonald, Brasure, et al., 2016). In addition, older adults often use over-the-counter medications, such as diphenhydramine and other antihistamines, for their sedating effects; however, there is little evidence that they are effective for improving sleep when used for more than several days and they are associated with serious adverse effects because of their strong anticholinergic actions. Box 24-6

Box 24-6 Health Promotion Teaching About Medications and Sleep

- Older adults are more susceptible than younger adults to the adverse effects of many prescription sleeping medications, including benzodiazepines (e.g., flurazepam, triazolam, and temazepam).
- Over-the-counter sleeping preparations usually contain diphenhydramine and can have adverse effects, such as confusion, constipation, or blurred vision, either alone or in combination with other medications.
- Sleeping medications, even over-the-counter ones, are likely to have adverse effects that interfere with daytime function and with the quality of nighttime sleep.
- Many hypnotic medications are not effective for long-term use because of increasing tolerance, which may develop within the first week and usually develops after a month of regular use.
- Sleep medications can interfere with the dream stage of sleep and cause a rebound effect, characterized by nightmares and excessive dreaming, after they are discontinued.
- Alcohol is likely to cause nightmares and awakenings during the latter part of the night.
- Medications that can interfere with sleep include steroids, diuretics, theophylline, anticonvulsants, decongestants, and thyroid hormone.
- Combining a sleeping medication with any other medication can be harmful or even fatal.

summarizes pertinent teaching points that nurses can use to educate older adults and their caregivers about the effects of alcohol, medications, and certain chemicals on sleep.

Nurses have important roles in correcting misperceptions about sleep and teaching older adults about nonpharmacologic ways of improving sleep.

Teaching About Management of Sleep Disorders

Evidence-based guidelines emphasize the important role that nurses have in identifying and referring patients for sleep disorders because they have many opportunities to observe patients' sleep patterns and assess their patients' perceptions of sleep (Dean, Klimpt, Morris, et al., 2016). Teaching about interventions for OSA is an important nursing responsibility because of the serious health consequences that develop when the condition is not adequately treated. This is especially important because the disorder affects so many older adults and is associated with serious health consequences, as discussed earlier in this chapter.

Many types of interventions are available for treating OSA, so obtaining a comprehensive evaluation and treatment at a sleep disorders clinic should be considered. The "gold standard" for treating OSA is continuous positive airway pressure (CPAP) therapy, which is effective in improving symptoms and preventing serious complications. Although CPAP adherence is an essential first-line treatment for OSA, there is a high rate of nonadherence, which nurses can address by encouraging older adults to explore other treatment options (Rotenberg, Murariu, & Pang, 2016). Although most people who use CPAP equipment do so independently in their homes, older adults in hospitals and long-term care settings may need assistance with managing their nightly treatments. Figure 24-1 illustrates an older adult using a CPAP machine.

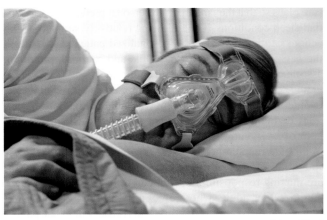

FIGURE 24-1 A continuous positive airway pressure machine. (Used with permission from Philips Respironics.)

Nurses promote sleep wellness for older adults who experience sleep problems by teaching about the importance of having any sleep disorder evaluated by a knowledgeable professional.

 Technology to Promote Wellness in Older Adults

Technology is widely used for assessment and management of OSA in nonclinical settings, as exemplified in the following studies:

- Home sleep apnea testing is an alternative to polysomnography in a sleep clinic, with demonstrated feasibility and accuracy (Boulos, Elias, Wan, et al., 2017; Cairns, Sarmeiento, & Bogan, 2017).
- Apps for smartphones and mobile devices are used to improve self-monitoring of CPAP use in home settings (Isetta, Torres, Gonzalez, et al., 2017).
- Teleconsultation via video conferencing is used to facilitate accessibility for CPAP education and follow-up (Bruyneel, 2016).

Nurses can encourage older adults to explore technology-based resources for assessment and management of OSA at websites such as the National Sleep Foundation (www.sleepfoundation.org). In 2015, the National Sleep Foundation formed a Sleep Technology Council to provide evidence-based information about sleep technology products.

Unfolding Case Study

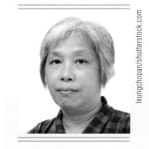

leungchopan/shutterstock.com

Part 1: Mrs. Z. at 66 Years of Age *(Continued)*

Mrs. Z. returns for further discussion of her sleep problem after filling out the PSQI based on her experiences during the past month. In addition, she has followed your instructions to keep a "sleep log" describing her daily activities, including exercise, and the effect of these activities on her sleep. Per your request, she has documented the types of foods and beverages she consumes regularly. You review the assessment information with her and find out that when she is home she spends most of her time reading or doing crossword puzzles. She attends the senior center weekly, plays bridge two evenings a week, and goes to lunch with friends a few times every week. She enjoys gardening during the summer but has no other interest in physical activities.

Part 1: Mrs. Z. at 66 Years of Age *(Continued)*

She avoids exercise because she is afraid that physical activity "will get the old arthritis all stirred up." On further questioning, she estimates that when she worked, she walked about one half mile daily. She drinks about "a pot" of coffee daily and has coffee and cookies at bridge games. She enjoys a glass of wine in the evenings. When she wakes up during the night, she usually gets up and goes to the bathroom, then returns to bed and lies there "thinking" until she returns to sleep. Her sleep log reflects that she often stays awake for as long as 2 hours before returning to sleep. She says she's heard that melatonin is good for insomnia and asks your opinion about trying it.

THINKING POINTS

- What myths and misunderstandings about sleep would you address?
- What risk factors might you address through health education?
- Because you can see Mrs. Z. weekly at the wellness clinic, you can develop a long-term teaching plan.

- How would you establish priorities for immediate and long-term goals?
- What information from Boxes 24-4 through 24-6 would you use for health education with Mrs. Z.?

EVALUATING EFFECTIVENESS OF NURSING INTERVENTIONS

The effectiveness of interventions for the nursing diagnosis of disturbed sleep pattern or for the wellness diagnosis of Readiness for Enhanced Sleep can be measured subjectively or objectively. A subjective measurement would be that the older adult reports that he or she feels rested and refreshed upon awakening in the morning. If a sleep assessment tool is used during the initial assessment, it can be used again for a reassessment after interventions have been implemented. An example of an objective measurement would be that the older adult can sleep for 6 to 8 hours at night with only brief interruptions, and that the person looks and acts rested during the day.

Unfolding Case Study

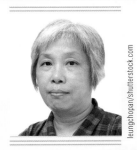

leungchopan/shutterstock.com

Part 2: Mrs. Z. at 79 Years of Age

Mrs. Z. is now 79 years old and is being admitted to a long-term care facility for skilled care after a total hip replacement. Her diagnoses include osteoarthritis and osteoporosis. After a few weeks in the facility, she plans to return to her ranch-style home where she lives with her husband. Before surgery, she was independent in her activities of daily living, and she expects to regain her independence and walk with a walker. The hospital transfer form has orders for acetaminophen 1000 mg every 8 hours and zolpidem tartrate 5 mg at bedtime as needed.

NURSING ASSESSMENT

During the admission interview, you ask Mrs. Z. about her sleep patterns. She states that for the past few years, she has been awakened frequently at night by her hip pain and other arthritic discomforts. In addition, she reports that she would usually get up three or four times during the night to go to the bathroom. When questioned further, she explains that the pain and discomfort would wake her, and so she would go to the bathroom because she wanted to move around, not because she felt an urge to urinate that often. Although her doctor had prescribed medications for pain, she did not take them regularly because she was concerned about adverse effects. During her 1-week hospitalization, she had taken a sleeping pill several times as well as Tylenol with codeine. Mrs. Z. expresses anxiety about sleeping in the long-term care facility because she says that the noise in the hospital was very disruptive to her sleep. She reports that she feels rested in the morning if she gets at least 6 hours of sleep during the 8 hours she spends in bed. During her hospitalization, she never felt rested in the morning and was unable to sleep for 6 hours except when she took sleeping pills. Mrs. Z. says that listening to relaxing music helps her to fall asleep.

(continued)

Part 2: Mrs. Z. at 79 Years of Age (Continued)

NURSING DIAGNOSIS

In addition to nursing diagnoses related to Mrs. Z.'s osteoarthritis and hip surgery, you identify a nursing diagnosis of Disturbed Sleep Pattern. Related factors are pain, age-related changes, and environmental conditions. You decide that you will not list nocturia as an associated factor because Mrs. Z. does not feel an urge to void during the night. Rather, she wakes up with pain and then goes to the bathroom. You decide to list age-related changes as a related factor because it is important for Mrs. Z. to understand that, even though she may not awaken with pain, she may awaken because of age-related changes.

NURSING CARE PLAN FOR MRS. Z.

Expected Outcome	Nursing Interventions	Nursing Evaluation
Mrs. Z. will identify factors that influence her sleep pattern	• Describe age-related changes in sleep patterns • Discuss the important role of pain-relieving measures in promoting good sleep	• Mrs. Z. will be able to describe the age-related changes and other conditions that affect her sleeping pattern
Mrs. Z. will consistently obtain 6 hours of sleep nightly without the aid of sleeping medications	• Administer Tylenol as ordered and evaluate its effectiveness in controlling Mrs. Z.'s pain • Explain that sleeping medications should be avoided, except for periodic use in short-term situations • Assign Mrs. Z. to a room that is not close to the nursing station • Make sure Mrs. Z.'s door is closed at night • Encourage Mrs. Z. to play quiet music at bedtime • Give Mrs. Z. a copy of Boxes 24-5 and 24-6 and discuss additional nonpharmacologic methods for promoting sleep	• Mrs. Z. will report that she is not awakened by pain • Mrs. Z. will report that she feels rested upon awakening in the morning

THINKING POINTS

- What additional assessment information pertinent to Mrs. Z.'s sleep patterns would you like to have, and how would you obtain this information?
- What additional nursing interventions would you include in the care plan to address Mrs. Z.'s disturbed sleep pattern? Would you use any of the information in Box 24-4 or give her a copy of it?

- What concerns specifically related to sleep would you have about Mrs. Z. after she is discharged from the skilled nursing facility to her own home? How would you address these concerns in your health promotion interventions?

QSEN APPLICATION

QSEN Competency	Knowledge/Skill/Attitude	Application to Mrs. Z. When She Is 79 Years of Age
Patient-centered care	(K) Integrate understanding of multiple dimensions of patient-centered care	Identify pre-existing conditions as well as immediate risks that can affect Mrs. Z.'s sleep
	(K) Describe strategies to empower patients in all aspects of the health care process	Teach Mrs. Z. about normal sleep changes and risk factors so she feels more control over her sleep
	(K) Examine nursing roles in assuring coordination, integration, and continuity of care	Recognize that it is important to address sleep concerns as part of a comprehensive care plan in long-term care settings
	(S) Communicate care provided and needed at each transition in care	Teach Mrs. Z. about interventions she can use at home after being discharged
	(A) Value seeing health care situations "through patients' eyes"	

Chapter Highlights

Age-Related Changes That Affect Sleep and Rest (Table 24-1)

- Diminished sleep efficiency
- Alterations in sleep cycles and stages
- Shifts in circadian rhythm

Risk Factors That Can Affect Sleep (Tables 24-2 and 24-3)

- Psychosocial factors: beliefs, attitudes, anxiety, depression, boredom
- Environmental factors: noise, light, lack of privacy
- Pathologic conditions and functional impairment (e.g., pain and discomfort, medication effects, physiologic disorders)
- RLS and PLMS

Functional Consequences Affecting Sleep Wellness

- Longer time needed to fall asleep
- Frequent arousals during the night
- More time in bed to achieve same quantity of sleep
- Diminished quality of sleep (less dreaming and deep sleep)

Pathologic Condition Affecting Sleep: Sleep Disorders

- Excessive sleepiness (Box 24-1)
- OSA

Nursing Assessment of Sleep (Box 24-2)

- Perception of quantity and quality of sleep
- Factors that affect sleep
- Usual sleep pattern and behaviors that affect it
- Actual sleep pattern (observed in institutional settings)
- Evidence-based assessment tools: PSQI and ESS

Nursing Diagnosis

- Readiness for Enhanced Sleep
- Disturbed Sleep Pattern

Planning for Wellness Outcomes

- Sleep
- Rest
- Comfort level
- Personal well-being

Nursing Interventions for Sleep Wellness (Boxes 24-3 Through 24-6)

- Teaching about interventions to promote healthy sleep patterns
- Modifying the environment
- Individualizing care in institutional settings
- Explaining relaxation and mental imagery techniques
- Teaching about medications that affect sleep
- Addressing OSA

Evaluating Effectiveness of Nursing Interventions

- Expressed feelings of being rested upon awakening
- Improved score on sleep assessment tool
- Observations that the person is sleeping at night

Critical Thinking Exercises

1. What is an older adult likely to experience with regard to sleep and rest patterns? How would you explain these changes to an older adult?
2. Identify three specific factors in each of the following categories that might interfere with sleep: environmental influences, physiologic disturbances, and psychosocial factors.
3. How would you assess an 82-year-old person who comes to the nursing clinic at the senior wellness center complaining of feeling tired all the time and not getting enough sleep?
4. What would you include in a half-hour presentation on "Tips for Good Sleep" for participants in a senior wellness program at a community-based center?
5. What information about sleep and rest would you include in an in-service program for evening and night shift nursing assistants employed in a long-term care facility?

 For more information about the topics discussed in this chapter, be sure to check out the interactive Online Learning Activities and other helpful resources at http://thepoint.lww.com/Miller8e.

REFERENCES

Abell, J. G., Shipley, M. J., Ferrie, J. E., et al. (2016). Association of chronic insomnia symptoms and recurrent extreme sleep duration over 10 years with well-being in older adults: A cohort study. *BMJ Open, 6,* e009501.

Alessi, C., Martin, J. L., Fiorentino, L., et al., (2016). Cognitive behavioral therapy for insomnia in older Veterans using nonclinical sleep coaches: Randomized controlled trial. *Journal of the American Geriatrics Society, 64,* 1830–1838.

Alparslan, G. B., Orsal, Ö., & Unsal, A. (2016). Assessment of sleep quality and effects of relaxation exercise on sleep quality in patients hospitalized in internal medicine services in a university hospital. *Holistic Nursing Practice, 30*(3), 155–165.

Andrews, L. (2016). Music for insomnia in adults. *Clinical Nursing Specialist, 30,* 198–199.

Asnis, G. M., Thomas, M., & Henderson, M. A. (2015). Pharmacotherapy treatment options for insomnia: A primer for clinicians. *International Journal of Molecular Sciences, 17,* 50.

BaHammam, A. S., Kendzerska, T., Gupta, R., et al. (2016). Comorbid depression in obstructive sleep apnea: An under-recognized association. *Sleep and Breathing, 20,* 447–456.

Bauters, F., Rietzschel, E. R., Hertegonne, K. B., et al. (2016). The link between obstructive sleep apnea and cardiovascular disease. *Current Atherosclerosis Reports, 18*(1), 1.

Billings, M. E., Johnson, D. A., Simonelli, G., et al. (2016). Neighborhood walking environment and activity level are associated with obstructive sleep apnea: The multi-ethnic study of atherosclerosis. *Chest, 150*(5):1042–1049.

Boulos, M., Elias, S., Wan, A., et al. (2017). Unattended hospital and home sleep apnea testing following cerebrovascular events. *Journal of Stroke and Cerebrovascular Disease, 26*, 143–149.

Brasure, M., Fuchs, E., MacDonald, R., et al. (2016). Psychological and behavioral interventions for managing insomnia disorder: An evidence report for a clinical practice guidelines by the American College of Physicians. *Annals of Internal Medicine, 165*, 113–124.

Brenes, G. A., Danhauer, S. C., Lyles, M. F., et al. (2016). Effects of telephone-delivered cognitive-behavioral therapy and nondirective supportive therapy on sleep, health-related quality of life, and disability. *American Journal of Geriatric Psychiatry, 24*, 846–854.

Bruyneel, M. (2016). Technical developments and clinical use of telemedicine in sleep medicine. *Journal of Clinical Medicine, 5*, 116.

Cairns, A., Sarmiento, K., & Bogan, R. (2017). Utility of home sleep apnea testing in high-risk veterans. *Sleep & Breathing.* doi: 10.1007/s11325-017-1467-8.

Cardinali, D. P., Golombek, D. A., Rosenstein, R. E., et al. (2016). Assessing the efficacy of melatonin to curtail benzodiazepine/Z drug abuse. *Pharmacology Research, 109*, 12–23.

Chang, S. C., Pan, A., Kawachi, I., et al. (2016). Risk factors for late-life depression: A prospective cohort study among older women. *Preventive Medicine, 91*, 144–151.

Chaudhary, N. S., Grandner, M. A., Jackson, N. J., et al. (2016). Caffeine consumption, insomnia, and sleep duration: Results from a nationally representative sample. *Nutrition, 32*, 1193–1199.

Chen, L. J., Fox, K. R., Ku, P. W., et al. (2016). Effects of aquatic exercise in older adults with mild sleep impairment: A randomized controlled trial. *International Journal of Behavioral Medicine, 23*, 501–506.

Chen, X., Wang, R., Zee, P., et al. (2015). Racial/ethnic differences in sleep disturbances: The multi-ethnic study of atherosclerosis (MESA). *Sleep, 38*, 877–888.

Dean, G. E., Klimpt, M. L., Morris, J. L. et al. (2016). Excessive sleepiness. In M. Boltz, E. Capezuti, T. Fulmer, & D. Zwicker (Eds.), *Evidence-based geriatric nursing protocols for best practice* (5th ed., pp. 431–442). New York: Springer Publishing Company.

Dentico, D., Ferrarelli, F., Riedner, B. A., et al., (2016). Short meditation trainings enhance non-REM sleep low-frequency oscillations. *PLoS One, 11*(2), e0148961.

Dobing, S., Frolova, M., McAlister, F., et al. (2016). Sleep quality and factors influencing self-reported sleep duration and quality in the general internal medicine inpatient population. *PLOS ONE, 11*(6), doi: 10.1371/journal.pone.0156735.

Du, S., Dong, J., Zhang, H., et al. (2015). Taichi exercise for self-rated sleep quality in older people: A systematic review and meta-analysis. *International Journal of Nursing Studies, 52*, 368–379.

DuBose, J. R., & Hadi, K. (2016). Improving inpatient environments to support patient sleep. *International Journal of Quality Health Care, 28*(5):540–553.

Duffy, J. F., Scheuermaier, K., & Loughlin, K. R. (2016). Age-related sleep disruption and reduction in the circadian rhythm of urine output: Contribution to Nocturia? *Current Aging Science, 9*(1), 34–43.

Farokhnezhad Afshar, P., Bahramnezhad, F., Asgari, P., et al. (2015). Effect of white noise on sleep in patients admitted to a coronary care. *Journal of Caring Sciences, 5*(2), 103–109.

Fox, H., Purucker, H. C., Holzhacker, I., et al. (2016). Prevalence of sleep-disordered breathing and patient characteristics in a coronary artery disease cohort undergoing cardiovascular rehabilitation. *Sleep-disordered breathing and cardiovascular rehabilitation, 36*, 421–429.

Fu, Y., Xia, Y., Yi, H., et al. (2016). Meta-analysis of all-cause and cardiovascular mortality in obstructive sleep apnea with or without continuous positive airway pressure treatment. *Sleep & Breathing, 21*, 181–189.

Gallegos, A. M., Moynihan, J., & Pigeon, W. R. (2016). A secondary analysis of sleep quality changes in older adults from a randomized

trial of an MBSR program. *Journal of Applied Gerontology,* Aug 10. doi: 10.1177/073464816663554.

Gathecha, E., Rios, R., Buenaver, L. F., et al. (2016). Pilot study aiming to support sleep quality and duration during hospitalizations. *Journal of Hospital Medicine, 11*, 467–472.

Giunta, J., Salifu, M. O., & McFarlane, S. I. (2016). Sleep disorders and cardio-renal disease: Implications for minority populations. *Epidemiology, 6*(3). doi: 10.4172/2161-1165.1000e120.

Grandner, M. A., Alfonso-Miller, P., Fernandez-Mendoza, J., et al. (2016). Sleep: Important considerations for the prevention of cardiovascular disease.*Current Opinion in Cardiology, 31*, 551–561.

Grossman, E. S. (2016). Enduring sleep complaints predict health problems: A six-year follow-up of the survey of health and retirement in Europe. *Aging & Mental Health,* Aug 2: 1–9. doi: 10.1080/13607863.2016.1209735.

Guidozzi, F. (2016). Gender differences in sleep in older men and women. *Climacteric, 18*, 715–721.

Haba-Rubio, J., Marti-Soler, H., Marques-Vidal, P., et al. (2016). Prevalence and determinants of periodic limb movements in the general population. *Annals of Neurology, 79*, 464–474.

Hayhoe, S. (2017). Insomnia: Can acupuncture help? *Pain Management, 7*(1):49–57.

Herdman, T., & Kamitsura, S. (Eds). (2018). *NANDA International Nursing Diagnoses Definitions and Classification, 2018–2020* (11th ed., pp. 34–44). New York: Thieme Publishers.

Hermann, D. M., & Bassetti, C. L. (2016). Role of sleep-disordered breathing and sleep-wake disturbances for stroke and stroke recovery. *Neurology, 87*(13), 1407–1416.

Hmwe, N. T., Subramaniam, P., & Tan, L. P. (2016). Effectiveness of acupressure in promoting sleep quality: A systematic review of randomized controlled trials. *Holistic Nursing Practice, 30*, 283–293.

Isetta, V., Torres, M., Gonzalez, K., et al. (2017). A new mHealth application to support treatment of sleep apnea patients. *Journal of Telemedicine & Telecare, 23*, 14–18.

Karadag, E., Samancioglu, S., Ozden, D., et al. (2017). Effects of aromatherapy on sleep quality and anxiety of patients. *Nursing in Critical Care, 22*, 105–112.

Karimi, S., Souroush, A., Towhidi, et al. (2016). Surveying the effects of an exercise program on the sleep quality of elderly males. *Clinical Interventions in Aging, 11*, 997–1002.

Kerner, N. A., & Roose, S. P. (2016). Obstructive sleep apnea is linked to depression and cognitive impairment: Evidence and potential mechanisms. *American Journal of Geriatric Psychiatry, 24*, 496–508.

Khayat, R., & Pleister, A. (2016). Consequences of obstructive sleep apnea: Cardiovascular risk of obstructive sleep apnea and whether continuous positive airway pressure reduces that risk. *Sleep Medicine Clinics, 11*, 273–286.

Kim, H. J., Lee, Y., & Sohng, K. Y. (2016). The effects of footbath on sleep among older adults in nursing home: A quasi-experimental study. *Complementary Therapies in Medicine, 26*, 40–46.

Kim, J. W., Moon, Y. T., & Kim, K. D. (2016). Nocturia: The circadian voiding disorder. *Investigative and Clinical Urology, 57*(3), 165–173.

Konikkara, J., Tavella, R., Wiles, L., et al. (2016). Early recognition of obstructive sleep apnea in patients hospitalized with COPD exacerbation is associated with reduced readmission. *Hospital Practice, 44*, 41–47.

Kredlow, M. A., Capozzoli, M. C., Hearon, B. A., et al. (2015). The effects of physical activity on sleep: A meta-analytic review. *Journal of Behavioral Medicine, 38*, 427–449.

Lai, S. W. (2016). Risks and benefits of zolpidem use in Taiwan; A narrative review. *BioMedicine, 6*(2), 8.

Lee, S. H., & Lim, S. M. (2016). Acupuncture for insomnia after stroke: A systematic review and meta-analysis. *BMC Complementary and Alternative Medicine, 16*, 228.

Leggett, A., Burgard, S., & Zivin, K. (2016). The impact of sleep disturbance on the association between stressful life events and depressive symptoms. *Journals of Gerontology: Psychological Sciences and Social Sciences, 71*, 118–128.

Liu, Y., Wheaton, A., Chapman, D., et al. (2016). Prevalence of healthy sleep duration among adults – United States, 2014. *Centers for Disease Control and Prevention, Morbidity and Mortality Weekly Report, 65*, 137–140.

Lo, J. C., Groeger, J. A., Cheng, G. H., et al. (2016). Self-reported sleep duration and cognitive performance in older adults: A systematic review and meta-analysis. *Sleep Medicine, 17*, 87–98.

Madrid-Valero, J. J., Martinez-Selva, J. M., Ribeiro do Couto, B., et al. (2017). Age and gender effects on the prevalence of poor sleep quality in the adult population. *Gaceta Sanitaria, 31*, 18–22.

Maeder, M. T., Schoch, O. D., & Rickli, H. (2016). A clinical approach to obstructive sleep apnea as a risk factor for cardiovascular disease. *Vascular Health and Risk Management, 12*, 85–103.

Martinez-Ceron, E., Barquiel, B., Bezos, A., M., et al. (2016). Effect of continuous positive pressure on glycemic control in patients with obstructive sleep apnea and type 2 diabetes: A randomized clinical trial. *American Journal of Respiratory Critical Care Medicine, 194*, 476–485.

Maruthai, N., Nagendra, R. P., Sasidharan, A., et al. (2016). Senior Vipassana Meditation practitioners exhibit distinct REM sleep organization from that of novice meditators and health controls. *International Review of Psychiatry, 28*, 279–287.

McFeeters, S., Pront, K. M., Cuthbertson, L., et al. (2016). Massage, a complementary therapy effectively promoting the health and well-being of older people in residential care settings: A review of the literature. *International Journal of Older People Nursing, 11*, 266–283.

McMillan, A., & Morrell, M., J. (2016). Sleep disordered breathing at the extremes of age: The elderly. *Breathe, 12*, 50–60.

Moccia, M., Erro, R., Picillo, M., et al. (2016). A four-year longitudinal study on restless legs syndrome in Parkinson disease. *Sleep, 39*, 405–412.

Mollayeva, T., Thurairajah, P., Burton, K., et al. (2016). The Pittsburgh sleep quality index as a screening tool for sleep dysfunction in clinical and non-clinical samples: A systematic review and meta-analysis. *Sleep Medicine Review, 25*, 52–73.

Morin, C. M., Beaulieu-Bonneau, S., Belanger, L., et al. (2016). Cognitive-behavior therapy singly and combined with medication for persistent insomnia: Impact on psychological and daytime functioning. *Behavior Research and Therapy, 87*, 109–116.

Moro, M., Goparaju, B., Castillo, J., et al. (2016). Periodic limb movements of sleep: Empirical and theoretical evidence supporting objective at-home monitoring. *Nature and Science of Sleep, 8*, 277–289.

Nalliah, C. J., Sanders, P., & Kalman, J. M. (2016). Obstructive sleep apnea treatment and atrial fibrillation: A need for definitive evidence. *Journal of Cardiovascular Electrophysiology, 27*, 1001–1010.

National Center on Sleep Disorders Research. (2011). *National Institutes of Health Sleep Disorders Research Plan. NIH Publication No. 11-7820.* Washington, DC: U.S. Department of Health and Human Services.

Ooms, S., & Ju, Y. E. (2016). Treatment of sleep disorders in dementia. *Current Treatment Option in Neurology, 18*, 40.

Qaseem, A., Kansagara, D., Forciea, M. A., et al. (2016). Management of chronic insomnia disorder in adults: A clinical practice guideline from the American College of Physicians. *Annals of Internal Medicine, 165*, 125–133.

Rotenberg, B., Murariu, D., & Pang, K. P. (2016). Trends in CPAP adherence over twenty years of data collection: A flattened curve. *Journal of Otolaryngology – Head and Neck Surgery, 45*, 43.

Scholtens, R. M., van Munster, B. C., van Kempen, M. F., et al. (2016). Physiological melatonin levels in healthy older people: A systematic review. *Journal of Psychosomatic Research, 86*, 20–27.

Sharma, S., Chowdhury, A., Tang, L., et al. (2016). Hospitalized patients at high risk for obstructive sleep apnea have more rapid response system events and interventions is associated with reduced events. *PLoS One, 11*, e0153790.

Sharma, S., Mather, P., Gupta, A., et al. (2016). Effect of early intervention with positive airway pressure therapy for sleep disordered breathing on six-month readmission rates in hospitalized patients with heart failure. *American Journal of Cardiology, 117*, 940–945.

Shergis, J. L., Ni, X., Jackson, M. L., et al. (2016). A systematic review of acupuncture for sleep quality in people with insomnia. *Complementary Therapies in Medicine, 26*, 11–20.

Wang, Q., Chair, S. Y., Wong, E. M., et al. (2016). The effects of music intervention on sleep quality in community-dwelling elderly. *Journal of Complementary and Alternative Medicine, 22*, 576–584.

Wilt, T. J., MacDonald, R., Brasure, M., et al. (2016). Pharmacologic treatment of insomnia disorder: An evidence report for a clinical practice guideline by the American College of Physicians. *Annals of Internal Medicine, 165*, 103–112.

Woo, H. G., Lee, D., Hwang, K. J., et al. (2017). Post-stroke restless leg syndrome and periodic limb movements in sleep. *Acta Neurological Scandinavia, 135*(2):204–210 .

Zeng, H., Liu, M., Wang, P., et al. (2016). The effects of acupressure training on sleep quality and cognitive function in older adults: A 1-year randomized controlled trial. *Research in Nursing and Health, 39*, 328–336.

Thermoregulation

After reading this chapter, you will be able to:

1. Describe age-related changes that affect an older adult's normal body temperature, febrile response to illness, and response to hot and cold environmental temperatures.

2. Identify risk factors that affect thermoregulation in older adults and increase the potential for hypothermia or heat-related illness.

3. Assess the following aspects of thermoregulation: baseline temperature, risks for altered thermoregulation, hypothermia, heat-related illness, and febrile response to illness.

4. Discuss the functional consequences of altered thermoregulation in older adults.

5. Implement health promotion interventions for preventing hypothermia and heat-related illness in older adults.

KEY TERMS

accidental hypothermia	heat-related illness
acclimatize	hypothermia
heat exhaustion	hyperthermia
heat stroke	thermoregulation

The primary function of thermoregulation is to maintain a stable core body temperature in a wide range of environmental temperatures. In the presence of infections, thermoregulation also assists in maintaining homeostasis. Under normal circumstances, the core body temperature is maintained at 97°F (36.1°C) to 99°F (37.2°C) through complex physiologic mechanisms governing heat production

and dissipation. Because older adults experience age-related changes and additional risk factors that affect thermoregulation, they are vulnerable to **hypothermia**, an abnormally low body temperature, and **hyperthermia**, an abnormally elevated body temperature, for example, from heat stroke, fever, or similar conditions. The term **heat-related illness** is used in this chapter when hyperthermia occurs in response to hot environmental temperatures, in contrast to when it is related to pathophysiologic causes. This chapter focuses on nursing assessment and interventions related to altered thermoregulation in older adults.

 AGE-RELATED CHANGES THAT AFFECT THERMOREGULATION

With increased age, subtle alterations in thermoregulation occur, and these become important considerations in caring for healthy, as well as frail, older adults. **Thermoregulation** is a complex adaptive response that involves many internal and external influences. Internal conditions that affect thermoregulation include metabolic rate, pathologic processes, muscle activity, peripheral blood flow, amount of subcutaneous fat, central nervous system function, the temperature of the blood flowing through the hypothalamus, and effects of medications and other bioactive substances. External influences on thermoregulation include environmental temperature, humidity level, airflow, and the type and amount of clothing and covering used. The following sections address these factors in relation to the ability of older adults to respond to environmental temperatures and in relation to normal body temperature.

Response to Cold Temperatures

In cold environmental temperatures, the body normally initiates physiologic mechanisms to prevent loss of body heat and increase heat production. At the same time, individuals usually initiate protective behaviors to warm the body and protect themselves from adversely cold temperatures.

Promoting Healthy Thermoregulation in Older Adults

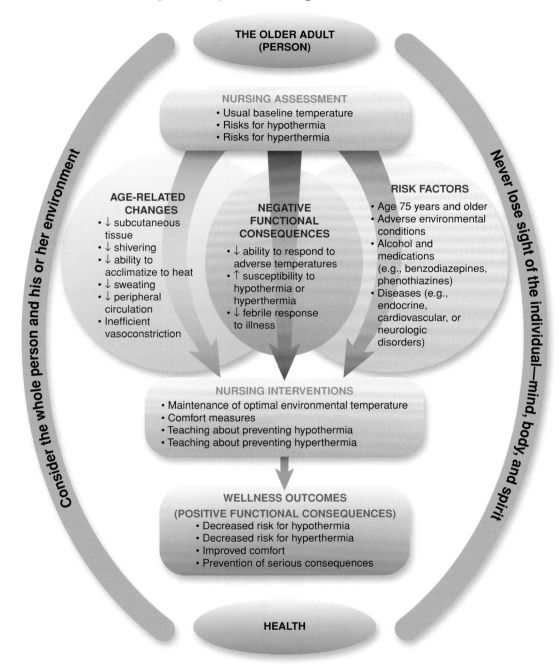

THE OLDER ADULT
(PERSON)

NURSING ASSESSMENT
• Usual baseline temperature
• Risks for hypothermia
• Risks for hyperthermia

Consider the whole person and his or her environment

Never lose sight of the individual—mind, body, and spirit

AGE-RELATED
CHANGES
• ↓ subcutaneous tissue
• ↓ shivering
• ↓ ability to acclimatize to heat
• ↓ sweating
• ↓ peripheral circulation
• Inefficient vasoconstriction

NEGATIVE
FUNCTIONAL
CONSEQUENCES
• ↓ ability to respond to adverse temperatures
• ↑ susceptibility to hypothermia or hyperthermia
• ↓ febrile response to illness

RISK FACTORS
• Age 75 years and older
• Adverse environmental conditions
• Alcohol and medications (e.g., benzodiazepines, phenothiazines)
• Diseases (e.g., endocrine, cardiovascular, or neurologic disorders)

NURSING INTERVENTIONS
• Maintenance of optimal environmental temperature
• Comfort measures
• Teaching about preventing hypothermia
• Teaching about preventing hyperthermia

WELLNESS OUTCOMES
(POSITIVE FUNCTIONAL CONSEQUENCES)
• Decreased risk for hypothermia
• Decreased risk for hyperthermia
• Improved comfort
• Prevention of serious consequences

HEALTH

Physiologic mechanisms that are protective in response to cold environments include shivering, muscle contraction, increased heart rate, peripheral vasoconstriction, dilation of the blood vessels in the muscles, insulation of deeper tissues by subcutaneous fat, and release of thyroxine and corticosteroid by the pituitary gland. Voluntary protective actions that people commonly initiate in cold temperatures include seeking shelter, ingesting warm fluids, wearing warm clothing or covering, and increasing activity to stimulate circulation.

The following age-related changes are likely to interfere with an older person's ability to respond to cold temperatures:

● Inefficient vasoconstriction
● Decreased cardiac output
● Decreased muscle mass
● Diminished peripheral circulation
● Decreased subcutaneous tissue
● Delayed and diminished shivering

These changes begin during the fifth decade, with cumulative effects being experienced during the seventh or eighth decade. The overall outcome of these changes is a dulled perception of cold and a concomitant lack of stimulus to initiate protective actions, such as adding more clothing or raising the environmental temperature.

Response to Hot Temperatures

In hot environmental temperatures, or when metabolic heat production is high, the normal mechanisms for heat dissipation are the production of sweat to facilitate evaporation and the dilation of peripheral blood vessels to facilitate heat radiation. When exposed to hot climates or engaged in strenuous activity daily for 7 to 14 days, healthy adults are able to **acclimatize** (i.e., gradually increase their metabolic efficiency to adapt to higher temperatures).

The older person's ability to acclimatize and respond to heat stress is altered by the following age-related changes:

- Higher threshold for the onset of sweating
- Diminished response when sweating occurs
- Dulled sensation of warm environments
- Renal and cardiovascular changes
- Diminished thirst sensation, which can lead to inadequate fluid intake

The overall effect of these changes is that even healthy older adults are more susceptible to heat-related illnesses because they are less able to adapt to hot environments.

Normal Body Temperature and Febrile Response to Illness

The long-standing norm for body temperature has been 98.6°F (37°C); however, studies indicate normal core body temperature in older adults begins to decrease between the ages of 40 and 50 years (Neff, Hoffmann, Zeiss, et al., 2016). An elevated temperature, or fever, is the body's protective response to pathologic conditions, such as cancer, infection, dehydration, or connective tissue disease. This protective response is blunted in older adults because of age-related changes involving thermoregulation and the immune system. Implications for nursing care related to normal body temperature and febrile response to illness are discussed in the sections on functional consequences and assessment.

 ### RISK FACTORS THAT AFFECT THERMOREGULATION

Increased age is a risk factor for both hypothermia and heat-related illnesses, which are likely to occur even in moderately cold or hot environments. In addition, pathophysiologic disorders, adverse medication reactions, and socioeconomic conditions increase the risk for serious consequences related to altered thermoregulation.

Conditions That Increase the Risk for Hypothermia

The risk for hypothermia is increased by conditions that decrease heat production (e.g., inactivity, malnutrition, endocrine disorders, neuromuscular conditions), increase heat loss (e.g., burns, vasodilation), or affect the normal thermoregulatory process (pathologic conditions of the central nervous system). Medical disorders that predispose to hypothermia include stroke, sepsis, dementia, malnutrition, multiple sclerosis, renal failure, Parkinson disease, and endocrine disorders (Cheshire, 2016). Medications and alcohol can predispose a person to hypothermia by suppressing shivering, inducing vasodilation, or affecting the central nervous system. Excessive use of alcohol can increase the risk for hypothermia by dulling sensory perceptions and interfering with cognitive skills necessary for initiating protective behaviors. Medications and other conditions that increase the risk for hypothermia are listed in Box 25-1.

Conditions That Increase the Risk for Heat-Related Illness

The risk for heat-related illness is increased by physiologic alterations that increase internal heat production (e.g., hyperthyroidism) or interfere with the ability to respond to heat stress (e.g., cardiovascular disease, fluid or electrolyte

---

 Box 25-1 Risk Factors for Hypothermia or Heat-Related Illness in Older Adults

Risks for Hypothermia and Heat-Related Illness

- Age 75+ years
- Adverse environmental temperatures
- Pathophysiologic alterations
- Socioeconomic conditions related to poor housing

Risks for Hypothermia

- Alcohol, especially excessive amounts
- Stroke
- Dementia
- Diabetic ketoacidosis
- Endocrine disorders (e.g., hypothyroidism, hypoadrenalism)
- Malnutrition
- Parkinson disease
- Renal failure
- Medications: opioids, antipsychotics, barbiturates, benzodiazepines, and tricyclic antidepressants

Risks for Heat-Related Illness

- Alcohol and alcohol withdrawal
- Dehydration
- Diabetic ketoacidosis
- Hyperthyroidism
- Excessive exercise or even moderate exercise in hot and humid environments
- Medications: diuretics, cardiovascular agents, and anticholinergic agents (including antihistamines, phenothiazines, tricyclic antidepressants)

imbalance). Recent researchers have focused on the effects of diabetes as a risk for heat stress, particularly in people with poor glycemic control or complications, such as neuropathy (Kenny, Sigal, & McGinn, 2016). In addition, medical disorders, such as cardiovascular disease and Parkinson disease, can worsen the severity of heat-related illness and decrease the chance of full recovery.

Medications can predispose to heat-related illness by increasing diuresis (e.g., diuretics), increasing heat production (e.g., salicylate intoxication), or interfering with sweating (e.g., anticholinergics) or peripheral vasodilation (e.g., beta-adrenergic blocking agents). A study comparing adverse medication reactions in older adults during heat waves and normal summers implicated the following medications: diuretics, serotonic antidepressants, angiotensin-converting enzyme inhibitors, and proton pump inhibitors (Sommet, Durrieu, Lapeyre-Mestre, et al., 2012). Alcohol increases the risk for heat-related illness by inducing diuresis, and excessive alcohol can increase the risk by increasing heat production. Another drug-related risk factor for hyperthermia is the recreational use of stimulants, such as heroin, cocaine, amphetamine, or methamphetamine (Cheshire, 2016).

Environmental and Socioeconomic Influences

Environmental temperatures—especially in combination with low socioeconomic indicators—can increase the vulnerability of older adults, particularly those older than 75 years, to hypothermia or heat-related illness. Recent journal articles are addressing concerns about the effects of climate change with regard to the increasing prevalence of hospitalizations for illnesses associated with extremes in both hot and cold environmental temperatures (Rhoades, Gruber, & Horton, 2017). For example, studies indicate that a distinct form of chronic kidney disease is linked to recurrent heat exposure and "may represent one of the first epidemics due to global warming" (Glaser, Lemery, Rajagopalan, et al., 2016, p. 1472).

All people who live in geographic areas with extreme temperature variations are especially vulnerable to the effects of adverse environmental temperatures; however, frail older adults often develop hypothermia or heat-related conditions even in moderately hot or cold climates because of additional interacting conditions. For example, heat-related illness can be precipitated in older adults by moderate exercise in moderately hot and humid weather. Insufficient fluid intake is another contributing condition, and this is likely to occur if older adults rely solely on their sensation of thirst, which is decreased due to age-related changes.

In addition to the obvious influence of hot or cold temperatures, homelessness, substandard living conditions, and diets deficient in protein and calories are conditions associated with both hypothermia and heat-related illness. Heat waves are especially hazardous for older adults living in environments with poor ventilation and high levels of humidity and air pollutants. Blacks and older adults are at increased risk of heat-related illnesses during heat waves, as

are those with any of the following risk factors: living alone, urban living, chronic heart disease, lack of participation in social activities at least weekly, and lack of air conditioning, especially in bedrooms (Cheshire, 2016; Gronlund, Zanobetti, Wellenius, et al., 2016; Lee, Lee, & Park, 2016; Zhang, Nitschke, Krackowizer, et al., 2017).

Social isolation is a factor that increases the risk for progression of heat-related illness or hypothermia because people rarely are able to self-report these conditions. Thus, they may not receive help in a timely manner. Older adults who live alone and have dementia may be at increased risk if they do not have the cognitive skills to adjust the thermostat and wear proper clothing or the ability to recognize the symptoms and call for help in a timely manner. Additional risk factors are summarized in Box 25-1.

Behaviors Based on Lack of Knowledge

Lack of knowledge about age-related vulnerability to hypothermia and heat-related illness may create risks secondary to inadequate protective measures. For example, when the use of air conditioning or heating is curtailed as a cost-saving measure, younger adults may be able to adjust to the moderately hot or cool temperature, whereas older adults may develop hypothermia or a heat-related illness under the same circumstances. If older adults and their caregivers are not aware of the age-related increased vulnerability to heat- and cold-related illnesses, they may not take appropriate protective measures, such as removing or adding clothing.

In the presence of infection or other pathophysiologic alterations, lack of knowledge about normal temperature in older adults may result in undetected illnesses. For example, caregivers and health care professionals may falsely assume that no infection is present if there is no fever. Similarly, if they believe that the baseline temperature for all adults is 98.6°F (37°C), they may not recognize an elevated temperature in someone whose baseline temperature is lower than this.

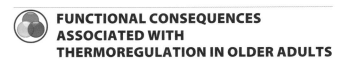

FUNCTIONAL CONSEQUENCES ASSOCIATED WITH THERMOREGULATION IN OLDER ADULTS

A healthy older adult in a comfortable environment will experience few, if any, functional consequences of altered thermoregulation. In the presence of any risk factor, however, hypothermia or heat-related illness may develop in an older adult. Even moderately adverse environmental temperatures can precipitate hypothermia or heat-related illness in an older adult, especially in the presence of additional predisposing factors, such as certain medications or pathologic conditions. For older adults in whom hypothermia or heat-related illness develops, the risk of subsequent morbidity or mortality from this condition is greater than that for their younger counterparts. For example, a recent systematic review and meta-analysis of epidemiologic evidence found that a 1°C increase in temperature was associated with increased risk for cardiovascular and respiratory illness and death, and a 1°C decrease in temperature was associated with increased respiratory and cardiovascular death rates and increased risk for respiratory illness. Moreover, this same review of over 16 million elderly case events concludes that for older adults, temperature is associated with an increased risk across every cause-specific indicator of mortality and most morbidity outcomes (Bunker, Wildenhain, Vandenbergh, et al., 2016). Another recent study concluded that the higher mortality rates due to hot temperatures predominantly occurred within 3 days, whereas those related to cold temperatures could persist for several weeks (Bao, Wang, Yu, et al., 2016).

In the United States, hypothermia and heat-related illness usually are seasonal hazards that occur during cold spells and heat waves. A review of Medicare beneficiaries found that hyperthermia accounted for more hospital visits, but hypothermia caused higher mortality rates and resulted in higher rates of admission and longer hospital stays (Noe, Jin, & Wolkin, 2012). A review of almost 10,000 heat- or cold-related deaths of U. S. residents between 2006 and 2010 found that the highest death rates occurred in people aged 85 and older, with the second highest rate among those aged 75 to 84, as illustrated in Figure 25-1 (Berko, Ingram, Saha, et al., 2014).

 GLOBAL PERSPECTIVE

Many countries are addressing concerns about the effects of climate change as a risk for increased morbidity and mortality, particularly in relation to the current unprecedented rate of population aging worldwide. (Bunker, Wildenhain, & Vandenbergh, 2016).

Altered Response to Cold Environments

Increased age is associated with an increased vulnerability to hypothermia because most older adults are less aware of a low core body temperature, less efficient in their physiologic response to cold, and less apt to take corrective actions when necessary. A low environmental temperature usually contributes to hypothermia, and the term **accidental hypothermia** is used when low environmental temperature is the primary cause of the condition. Even in normal environmental temperatures, however, the condition can result from serious alterations in homeostasis, such as can occur with anesthesia or endocrine or neurologic disorders. Accidental hypothermia can occur in older adults as a consequence of exposure to moderately cool temperatures, and may affect as many as 10% of older adults living in areas affected by cold climates (e.g., parts of Spain, China, Canada, Great Britain, and the United States).

In the early stages of hypothermia, the older adult probably will not shiver or complain of feeling cold. In the absence of any protective measures, hypothermia will progress, clouding mental function. The effects of impaired thermoregulation are cumulative, and hypothermia progresses rapidly after the core body temperature falls to 93.2°F (33.9°C). The age-related diminished ability of the kidney to conserve water and the common occurrence of inadequate fluid intake in older adults exacerbate the effects of hypothermia. If the process is not reversed, death from hypothermia will result from the myocardial effects of seriously impaired thermoregulation. Table 25-1 indicates the physiologic effects of hypothermia according to stages from mild to severe.

Altered Response to Hot Environments

Functional consequences that affect an older adult's ability to respond to hot environments include delayed and diminished sweating and inaccurate perception of environmental

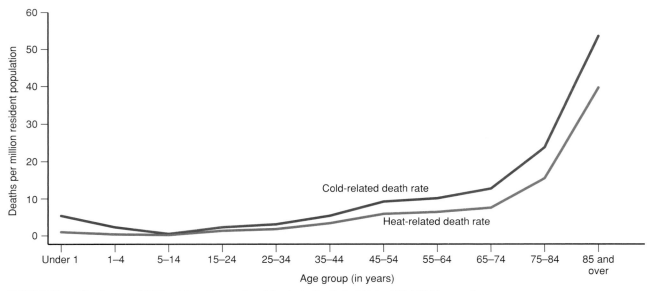

FIGURE 25-1 Distribution of 9992 cold- and heat-related deaths in the United States 2006–2010 according to age. Adapted from Centers for Disease Control and Prevention/National Vital Statistics System, 2006-2010. Available at https://www.cdc.gov/nchs/data/nhsr/nhsr076.pdf

TABLE 25-1 Physiologic Effects of Hypothermia According to Stages from Mild to Severe

Body System	Mild Hypothermia	Moderate Hypothermia	Severe Hypothermia
Neurologic	↓ dexterity ↓ muscle control Difficulty in speaking Amnesia Confusion	Nearly unconscious Coma No voluntary movement	No response to pain
Musculoskeletal	Shivering that cannot be controlled	No shivering	No shivering
Skin	Pale Cool Flushed	Pale Cyanotic	Cyanotic
Cardiovascular	Tachycardia	Dysrhythmias Hypotension	Severe hypotension Asystole
Renal	Diuresis	↓ output	No output
Respiratory	Tachypnea	↓ respiratory rate	Pulmonary edema
Vascular	Vasoconstriction		
Gastrointestinal	↓ motility ↓ liver function	↓ motility	Ischemic pancreatitis Ileus Gastric ulcers

Source: Davis, R. A. (2012). The big chill: Accidental hypothermia. *American Journal of Nursing,* 112(1), 41.

temperatures. Because of these functional consequences, the older adult is more likely to have heat-related illnesses, including heat exhaustion and heat stroke. **Heat exhaustion** is a condition that develops gradually from depletion of fluid, sodium, or both. It can occur in active or immobilized older people who are dehydrated or underhydrated and exposed to hot environments. **Heat stroke** is an even more serious condition that is likely to occur in active older adults because of a combination of age-related thermoregulatory changes and risk factors, such as overexertion and warm environments. Heat stroke can also occur in immobilized older adults in hot environments, either as a progression of untreated heat exhaustion or as a result of a combination of risk factors. The underlying mechanism in heat stroke is an inability to balance the rates of heat production and dissipation. This balance depends primarily on sweating and cardiac output.

In hot environments, the effects of altered thermoregulation are cumulative, and heat-related illnesses progress rapidly after the body temperature reaches 105.8°F (40.6°C). If fluid volume is not adequate to meet the requirements for effective sweating, then heat-related illness will progress even more rapidly. If heat-related illness is not reversed, death will result from respiratory depression.

Altered Thermoregulatory Response to Illness

Age-related changes in the thermoregulatory centers of the hypothalamus diminish the older adult's febrile response to illness and infections. Thus, infections are likely to be undetected until they progress and manifest as a functional decline or change in mental status. Older adults with infections may have a normal or even lower than normal temperature, but when their temperature is compared with their baseline temperature, at least a slight elevation is evident. A nursing implication of this is that even a subtle temperature elevation from baseline may be a significant indicator of an underlying disease that requires medical attention.

Altered Perception of Environmental Temperatures

Older adults often report feeling chilly or cold, even in very warm environments, and they generally prefer environmental temperatures that are at least 75°F (23.9°C). Inaccurate perceptions of environmental temperatures are associated with pathophysiologic conditions, such as dementia, thyroid disorders, or cardiovascular inefficiency, rather than with age-related changes alone.

Psychosocial Consequences of Altered Thermoregulation

Psychosocial consequences are associated with hypothermia, heat-related illness, or diminished fever response. If hypothermia or heat-related illness is overlooked, or if interventions are not initiated at an early stage, the condition

Unfolding Case Study

Part 1: Mrs. T. at 76 Years of Age

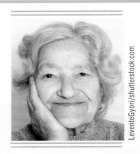

Mrs. T. is 76 years old and lives alone in a large farmhouse in a rural county in central Ohio. She has lived on this 20-acre farm for 49 years and has been a widow for 2 years. She has four children and eight grandchildren, but they all live in other states. Mrs. T. has been able to manage her farm with a part-time farmhand who comes a couple of times a week to help feed the several dozen chickens and collect eggs. When her farmhand doesn't come, she manages the chores by herself. She has hypertension and type 2 diabetes, and manages reasonably well medically. She adheres to her diabetic diet and takes her medications daily. She sends her farmhand to the city once weekly for groceries and drives to the nearby church on Sundays. Once a month she attends the county senior center, where you are the nurse. It is the middle of July, and summer in Ohio this year has been unusually hot and humid. A drought and heat wave are predicted for central Ohio and you are planning to present a health education program called "Hot Tips for Surviving the Summer." You are particularly concerned about Mrs. T. and several other participants who live in isolated areas and have little contact with others.

THINKING POINTS

- What factors increase the risk of Mrs. T. developing a heat-related illness? Which ones would you discuss in your health education program?

- In your health education program, how would you explain heat-related illnesses and the associated signs and symptoms?

QSEN APPLICATION

QSEN Competency	Knowledge/Skill/Attitude	Application to Mrs. T.
Patient-centered care	(K) Describe how diverse backgrounds function as a source of values	When planning the educational program identify aspects of rural living that increase the risks for heat-related illnesses
	(S) Elicit patient values, preferences, and expressed needs	During the educational program, elicit information from Mrs. T. about ways in which she can reduce the risks for heat-related illnesses
	(S) Provide patient-centered care with sensitivity and respect for diversity of the human experience	
	(A) Value seeing health care situations "through patients' eyes"	

may progress to the point of impairing cognitive function. Likewise, if a diminished or delayed febrile response to an infection is not recognized, a treatable condition may be overlooked and treatment may unintentionally be delayed or denied. Untreated infections are likely to progress in severity and, in older adults, may manifest primarily as a functional decline, such as impaired cognition.

NURSING ASSESSMENT OF THERMOREGULATION

Nursing assessment of thermoregulation addresses the older person's baseline body temperature, any risk factors for altered thermoregulation, manifestations of hypothermia or heat-related illness, and febrile response to illness. Assessment information is essential for planning health education

interventions for primary prevention of heat- and cold-related conditions and for timely interventions to prevent serious or irreversible effects. Assessment information is also important in detecting infections at an early stage. Nurses obtain much of the pertinent information about risk factors as part of the overall assessment; they also obtain information by observing the environment, measuring the person's body temperature, and interviewing the older adult and the caregivers of dependent older adults.

Assessing Baseline Temperature

Body temperature measurements show a diurnal fluctuation of 1°F to 2°F, with lower temperatures during sleeping and greater fluctuations during periods of fever-inducing illness. Because older adults normally have a lower body temperature and may have a diminished febrile response to infection, it is especially important to determine the person's usual temperature, as well as to characterize the usual pattern of diurnal variation. Because many types of thermometers are now available, it is important to document the method used for assessing temperature. Also, when assessing for hypothermia, it is advisable to use several methods and to make sure that the thermometers are able to detect low body temperatures.

Nurses can encourage older adults in home settings to establish a baseline by recording their temperature at different times of the day for several days when they are feeling well. Doing this seasonally by people who live in fluctuating climates and annually by those who live in stable climates provides a reference point when symptoms of illness or functional decline occur. In long-term care settings baseline temperature data, including normal fluctuations, should be documented on the chart. Box 25-2 summarizes the principles underlying nursing assessment of thermoregulation in older adults.

Identifying Risk Factors for Altered Thermoregulation

Anyone older than 75 years is at risk for altered thermoregulation, as are older adults who have one or more of the risk factors listed in Box 25-1. Because many of the risk factors for altered thermoregulation are modifiable, it is important to identify those that can be addressed through health promotion interventions. Information about medications and pathologic disorders is obtained during the overall assessment, and it is important to identify any conditions that predispose the person to hypothermia or heat-related illness. In addition to assessing for risks for hypothermia or heat-related illnesses, recognize that a low baseline body temperature is a risk for undetected fever. It is important to document the person's baseline temperature and note this as a risk factor for both hypothermia and undetected febrile conditions if temperature is below 98°F (36.7°C).

Most nurses do not have the opportunity to observe and assess the older adult's home environment, but they can ask pertinent questions and listen for clues to detect environmental risk factors. For example, older adults who live alone and express concern about keeping the house warm in winter should be considered to be at risk for hypothermia. Likewise, older adults who live in poor housing conditions, or with family members who keep the house at low temperatures during winter months, should be considered to be at risk for hypothermia. Older adults who live in poorly ventilated houses without air conditioning should be considered to be at risk for heat-related illness during heat waves. Interview

---

 Box 25-2 Guidelines for Assessing Thermoregulation

Principles of Temperature Assessment

- Document the person's baseline body temperature and its diurnal and seasonal variations.
- Assume that even a small elevation above the baseline temperature can be an indicator of the presence of a pathologic process.
- Document actual temperature and deviations from the baseline, rather than using such terminology as "afebrile."
- Carefully follow all the standard procedures for accurate temperature measurement. Use a thermometer that registers temperatures lower than 95°F (35°C).
- Consider the influence of temperature-altering medications when evaluating a temperature reading (e.g., medications that mask a fever).
- Do not assume that an infection will necessarily be accompanied by an elevated temperature.
- Remember that, in the presence of an infection, a decline in function or change in mental status may be an earlier and more accurate indicator of illness than an alteration in temperature.
- Do not assume that an older adult will initiate compensatory behaviors or complain of discomfort when exposed to adverse environmental temperatures.

Questions to Assess Risk Factors for Hypothermia or Heat-Related Illness

- Do you have any particular health problems that occur in hot or cold weather?
- Are you able to keep your house or room at a comfortable temperature in both summer and winter months?
- What do you do to cope with hot temperatures in the summer?
- Do you have any difficulty paying your utility bills?

- What forms of protection against the cold do you use in the winter months (e.g., electric blanket, supplemental sources of heat)?
- Have you ever received medical care for exposure to heat or cold?
- Have you ever fallen and not been able to get up or get help?

Observations to Assess Risk Factors for Hypothermia or Heat-Related Illness

- Does the older person live in a house where the temperature is kept below 70°F (21.1°C) during the winter?
- Does the person drink alcohol or take temperature-altering medications (see Box 25-1)?
- Does the person live alone? If so, what is the frequency of outside contacts?
- Does the person have any pathologic conditions that predispose him or her to hypothermia (e.g., endocrine, neurologic, or cardiovascular disorders)?
- Is the person's fluid and nutritional intake adequate?
- Does the person have postural hypotension? (See Chapter 20, Table 20-2 and Boxes 20-1 and 20-2 for assessment criteria relating to postural hypotension.)
- Is the person immobilized or sedentary? Is the person's judgment impaired because of dementia, depression, or other psychosocial disorders?
- Does the person live in a poorly ventilated dwelling without air conditioning?
- Are atmospheric conditions very hot, humid, or polluted?
- Does the person engage in active exercise during hot weather?
- Does the person have any chronic illness that predisposes him or her to heat-related illness?
- Is the person at risk for hyponatremia or hypokalemia because of medications or chronic illnesses?

questions aimed at identifying risk factors for altered thermoregulation are listed in Box 25-2.

Assessing for Hypothermia

Hypothermia is best detected by measuring core body temperature with a thermometer that registers below 95°F (35°C). Even in environmental temperatures of 68°F (20°C) or 69°F (20.6°C), an older person may become hypothermic, especially if other risk factors, such as immobility or hypothermia-inducing medications, are present. Early signs of hypothermia are subtle, and the most objective assessment tool is a comparison of the person's body temperature with their usual baseline temperature. Cool skin in unexposed areas, such as the abdomen and buttocks, is a distinguishing characteristic of hypothermia. It is important to recognize that older adults may not shiver or complain of feeling cold. As untreated hypothermia progresses, additional signs may include lethargy, slurred speech, mental changes, impaired gait, puffiness of the face, slowed or irregular pulse, low blood pressure, slowed tendon reflexes, and slow, shallow respirations. Severe stages of hypothermia are characterized by muscular rigidity, diminished urinary function, and a progression of all other manifestations to the point of stupor and coma. The skin will feel very cool and, contrary to what might be expected, the color of the skin will be pink. Also contrary to what might be expected, a hypothermic person may not shiver, particularly if the body temperature is below 90°F (32.2°C).

See ONLINE LEARNING ACTIVITY 25-1: ARTICLE ABOUT ACCIDENTAL HYPOTHERMIA at http://thepoint.lww.com/Miller8e.

Assessing for Heat-Related Illness

Manifestations of heat-related illnesses range from mild headache to life-threatening respiratory and cardiovascular disturbances. In the early stages of heat-related illness, the person will feel weak and lethargic and may complain of headache, nausea, and loss of appetite. The skin will be warm and dry, and the sweating response may be absent, especially if the person's fluid intake is low. As the heat-related condition progresses, these manifestations will be exacerbated, and the following signs will become evident: dizziness, dyspnea, tachycardia, vomiting, diarrhea, muscle cramps, chest pain, mental impairment, and a wide pulse pressure.

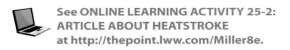

See ONLINE LEARNING ACTIVITY 25-2: ARTICLE ABOUT HEATSTROKE at http://thepoint.lww.com/Miller8e.

Assessing the Older Adult's Febrile Response to Illness

Because the manifestations of delayed or diminished febrile response to infections are likely to be very subtle, nurses assess for any temperature changes from the person's baseline as well as for additional signs of illness, such as a decline in function or change in mental status. Nurses also should examine assumptions about thermoregulation that may apply to younger adults but not to older adults. For example, the expectation that pneumonia is accompanied by an elevated temperature is not necessarily applicable to older adults, as discussed in Chapter 21. Thus, nurses need to be particularly vigilant about subtle temperature changes and other manifestations of fever. A more reliable indicator of elevated temperature in older adults would be an increase of 2°F (1°C) above the person's baseline. See Box 25-2 for a summary of some of these considerations.

NURSING DIAGNOSIS

Pertinent nursing diagnoses related to thermoregulation are Hypothermia (i.e., body temperature below normal range), Hyperthermia (i.e., body temperature elevated above normal range), and Ineffective Thermoregulation (i.e., temperature fluctuation between hypothermia and hyperthermia). In addition, the nursing diagnosis of Risk for Ineffective Thermoregulation is applicable when the person has risk factors for hypothermia or heat-related illness. For example, an 85-year-old woman with diabetes, dehydration, low body mass index, who is taking a diuretic, an antipsychotic, and an oral hypoglycemic would have risk factors for both hypothermia and heat-related illness. Related factors that are common in older adults include immobility, advanced age, medication effects, adverse environmental conditions, and acute and chronic illnesses. For older adults living alone, social isolation may be a related factor that increases the risk for experiencing more serious consequences if hypothermia or heat-related illness occurs.

PLANNING FOR WELLNESS OUTCOMES

When caring for older adults with risks for hypothermia or heat-related illness, nurses identify wellness outcomes as an essential component of the nursing process. Nurses can use the following Nursing Outcomes Classification terminologies in their care plans addressing risks for altered thermoregulation: Health Promoting Behavior, Hydration, Knowledge: Health Behavior, Knowledge: Personal Safety, Risk Detection, Risk Control, Safe Home Environment, Thermoregulation, and Vital Signs: Body Temperature.

Outcomes vary depending on the setting. In acute care settings, nurses are more likely to focus on outcomes that pertain to the patient's immediate physical condition (e.g., Hydration, Thermoregulation, and Vital Signs: Body Temperature). A focus of nursing care in long-term care settings is early detection of infections. In home and other community settings, nurses might be able to provide group or individual health education for older adults who are at risk for development of hypothermia or heat-related illness, especially during times of extreme weather conditions. In these situations, nurses focus more on teaching about self-care and environmental modifications to prevent hypothermia or heat-related illness.

> ### Wellness Opportunity
>
> Nurses promote wellness when their care plans include health-promoting behaviors to prevent hypothermia and heat-related illness.

NURSING INTERVENTIONS TO PROMOTE HEALTHY THERMOREGULATION

Health promotion interventions to address altered thermoregulation are directed toward primary prevention of hypothermia and heat-related illness. Health promotion interventions also address early detection of altered thermoregulation and prompt initiation of interventions to restore thermal balance and to prevent detrimental effects. Comfort interventions are initiated to promote well-being in older adults. Nurses can use the following Nursing Interventions Classification terminologies to document interventions: Temperature Regulation, Hypothermia Treatment, Hyperthermia Treatment, Environmental Management, Health Education, Risk Identification, Surveillance, and Teaching: Individual (or Group).

Addressing Risk Factors

Maintenance of an environmental temperature of around 75°F (23.9°C) is the single most important intervention to prevent hypothermia or heat-related illness. In addition, relative humidity can be altered to minimize the discomfort and detrimental effects associated with extremely warm or cool environments. With comfortable indoor temperatures, the ideal humidity is between 40% and 50%, although an acceptable range is between 20% and 70%. Older adults can be encouraged to humidify the air in their homes during the dry winter months by using humidifiers, either alone or with their heating systems. Simpler measures, such as keeping pans of water on heating vents or using a vaporizer near the bed at night, may be appropriate if a humidifier is unavailable.

An intervention for older adults at risk for hypothermia or heat-related illnesses is to teach about government- and community-sponsored programs that provide assistance for addressing needs related to weather-related risks. For example, the federally sponsored Low Income Home Energy Assistance Program (LIHEAP) provides financial assistance for heating bills in many areas of the United States where cold winters are the norm. Other government-sponsored programs provide financial assistance, such as low-interest loans, for home winterization and modernization measures to protect against adverse weather conditions. Older people and their family caregivers can be encouraged to obtain information about these programs through their local Area Agency on Aging.

> ### Wellness Opportunity
>
> Nurses promote wellness for socially isolated older adults by identifying ways of developing a system of social contact, such as a friendly phone call program, that ensures daily contact during periods of adversely hot or cold weather.

Promoting Healthy Thermoregulation

In cool environmental temperatures, interventions to prevent hypothermia include using adequate clothing and covering, especially for the hands, feet, and head because these areas of the body have the heaviest concentration of nerve endings that are sensitive to heat loss. Nurses can encourage older adults to wear caps, thermal socks, and several layers of warm clothing when appropriate. Electric blankets used during the night are a relatively inexpensive form of protection in cool environments, but proper safety precautions must be taken. Space heaters often are used to provide intense heat in a small area, but they can create serious fire and safety hazards. In addition to environmental considerations, special attention must be directed toward ensuring adequate nutrition, including fluid intake, and assuring that all medical conditions are optimally managed.

During heat waves, heat-related illness can affect older adults living in their own homes or in long-term care settings that are not air-conditioned. In long-term care facilities without air conditioning, nurses need to ensure that all residents have adequate fluid intakes. Nurses also must observe for early signs of heat-related illness, especially in residents who are immobile or who have medical problems, such as endocrine or circulatory disorders, that predispose them to heat-related illness. If only parts of the facility are air-conditioned, nurses can encourage residents to spend time in those areas

Box 25-3 Health Promotion Teaching About Hypothermia and Heat-Related Illness

Environmental and Personal Protection Considerations for Preventing Hypothermia

- Maintain a constant room temperature as close to 75°F (23.9°C) as possible, with a minimum temperature of 70°F (21.1°C).
- Use a reliable, clearly marked thermometer to measure room temperature.
- Wear close-knit, but not tight, undergarments to prevent heat loss; wear several layers of clothing.
- Wear a hat and gloves when outdoors; wear a nightcap and socks for sleeping.
- Wear extra clothing in the early morning when your body metabolism is at its lowest point.
- Use flannel bedsheets or sheet blankets.
- Use an electric blanket set on a low temperature.
- Take advantage of programs that offer assistance with utility bills and home weatherization.

Environmental and Personal Protection Action to Prevent Heat-Related Illnesses

- Maintain room temperatures below 85°F (29.4°C).
- If your residence is not air-conditioned, use fans to circulate the air and cool the environment.
- During hot weather, spend time in public air-conditioned settings, such as libraries or shopping malls.
- Drink extra noncaffeinated, nonalcoholic liquids, even if you don't feel thirsty.
- Wear loose-fitting, lightweight, light-colored, cotton clothing.
- Wear a hat or use an umbrella to protect yourself against sun and heat when you are outside.

- Avoid outdoor activities during the hottest time of the day (i.e., between 10:00 AM and 2:00 PM); perform them during the cooler hours of the morning or evening.
- Place an ice pack or cold, wet towels on your body, especially on the head, the groin area, and armpits. Take cool (about 75°F [23.9°C]) baths or showers several times daily during heat waves, but do not use soap every time.

Health Promotion Actions for Maintaining Optimal Body Temperature

- Maintain adequate fluid intake by drinking 8 to 10 glasses of noncaffeinated, nonalcoholic liquid daily.
- Do not rely on your thirst sensation as an indicator of the need for fluid.
- Eat small, frequent meals rather than heavy meals.
- Avoid drinking caffeinated beverages, such as cola and coffee.
- Avoid drinking alcohol.
- In cold weather, engage in moderate physical exercise and indoor activities to increase circulation and heat production.

Preventive Measures and Additional Approaches

- Know your normal temperature in the morning and in the evening.
- Be aware of seasonal variations in your baseline temperature.
- Obtain pneumonia and influenza immunizations (as discussed in Chapter 21).
- Maintain good nutrition, especially adequate protein
- Engage in physical activity, but avoid exertion during hot weather, and use protective clothing during cold weather

and can provide assistance for residents who have mobility limitations. Nurses working in long-term care facilities need to be proactive in establishing and implementing facility-wide practices to protect residents during heat waves (Kunze & Leistner, 2016).

Nurses can teach older adults living in community settings about measures to cool the environment, such as those summarized in Box 25-3. Older adults may be reluctant to use fans or air conditioners because of a desire to save money on utility bills; however, if they understand the health risks associated with heat-related illness, they may use these appliances judiciously. If the home setting cannot be cooled adequately during heat waves, encourage older adults to spend time in air-conditioned public places. Additional self-care actions to prevent heat-related illness during heat waves include the provision of adequate fluids and the avoidance of heavy meals and strenuous exercise. Box 25-3, which summarizes interventions for the prevention of heat-related illness, can be used as a patient education tool for older adults.

GLOBAL PERSPECTIVE

Based on recommendations of the World Health Organization beginning in 2008, governments in European and Asian countries

have developed "heat-health action plans" that include early warning systems, timely public and medical advice, and public policies that promote improved housing and urban planning. More recently, countries also are advocating for the development of cold wave prevention plans to reduce mortality attributable to low temperatures.

Promoting Caregiver Wellness

Caregivers of older adults who have risks for hypothermia or heat-related illness may benefit from the health promotion resources that are listed in Online Learning Activity 25-3. For example, caregivers may be interested in finding out about programs for assistance with utility bills or home modifications for improved energy efficiency and comfort. Use the information in Box 25-3 to teach about strategies for preventing hypothermia and heat-related illnesses. In addition, it is important to encourage caregivers to establish a plan for at least daily communication with socially isolated older adults, especially during heat waves or cold spells.

 See ONLINE LEARNING ACTIVITY 25-3: RESOURCES FOR HEALTH PROMOTION at http://thepoint.lww.com/Miller8e.

Unfolding Case Study

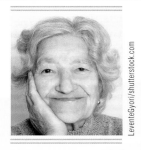

Part 1: Mrs. T. at 76 Years of Age *(Continued)*

Recall that Mrs. T. is 76 years old and a participant at the county senior center where you will be presenting a health education program.

THINKING POINTS

- How would you incorporate assessment information into your health education program?
- How would you use information from Box 25-3 to teach about preventing heat-related illnesses?

- What specific suggestions would you make about early detection of heat-related illnesses to the participants at this rural senior center?
- How would you find health education materials to use for your program?

EVALUATING EFFECTIVENESS OF NURSING INTERVENTIONS

Nurses evaluate care of older adults diagnosed with risk for hypothermia/heat-related illness or ineffective thermoregulation according to the extent to which the risks are eliminated. It is not always possible to know whether risk factors were eliminated, but nurses can evaluate the effectiveness of their teaching by asking for feedback from older adults and their caregivers. Nurses also can suggest referrals for resources and ask the older adult about his or her intent to follow through. For example, if housing and financial factors increase the risk of hypothermia and heat-related illnesses, nurses can refer the older adult to a program such as LIHEAP and document the person's response to this information. When nurses teach about preventing hypothermia and heat-related illnesses, effectiveness is evaluated on the basis of the person's ability to describe ways of decreasing the risk factors for hypothermia or heat-related illnesses.

Unfolding Case Study

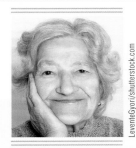

Part 2: Mrs. T. at 87 Years of Age

Mrs. T. is now 87 years old and continues to live alone in her own home in a rural area of central Ohio. She has a history of hypertension and diabetic retinopathy, and was recently hospitalized for uncontrolled diabetes. Upon discharge from the hospital in November, she was referred to the Visiting Nurses Association for teaching about insulin administration and monitoring of her diabetic care.

NURSING ASSESSMENT

During your initial visit, you observe that Mrs. T.'s house is poorly maintained and has no insulation or other weatherization. Mrs. T. tells you that she has lived in this house for 60 years and that, in recent years, she has had difficulty keeping up with maintenance because of her poor eyesight and limited income. She has few social contacts, but her daughter visits her every other week and a neighbor visits weekly and brings her groceries. About once a month, friends pick her up and take her to church. Your assessment reveals that although Mrs. T. has difficulty preparing meals because of her poor eyesight, she is independent in all other activities of daily living.

During your initial visit, you identify several risk factors for hypothermia, so during subsequent visits you follow up with further assessment. You learn that Mrs. T. was taken to the emergency department in January 2 years ago to be treated for hypothermia.

(continued)

NURSING ASSESSMENT *(Continued)*

She recalls that her daughter had come for her usual visit and had found her in a very weak and confused state. Her description of the situation is that "they just warmed me up at the hospital and sent me home again. I could have done that myself if my daughter would have just let me be." It is apparent that she did not consider her condition to be of particular concern. In the winter, she keeps her utility bills low by using a small, portable heater in the living room during the day and moving it into the bedroom at night. Mrs. T. keeps her thermostat at 65°F (18.3°C) during the day and 60°F (15.6°C) at night. A neighbor told her that the county office on aging had a program to assist with utility bills, but she is embarrassed to ask her daughter to drive her to the county office to apply for this "welfare help."

NURSING DIAGNOSIS

In addition to addressing the nursing diagnoses related to Mrs. T.'s diabetes, you identify a nursing diagnosis of Hypothermia. Related factors include advanced age, diabetes, social isolation, poor housing conditions, low environmental temperatures, and a history of hypothermia.

NURSING CARE PLAN FOR MRS. T.

Expected Outcome	Nursing Interventions	Nursing Evaluation
Mrs. T.'s knowledge about risk factors for hypothermia will be increased	• Discuss risk factors for hypothermia, with emphasis on Mrs. T.'s diabetes, social isolation, environmental conditions, and history of hypothermia	• Mrs. T. will be able to state at least four factors that place her at risk for hypothermia
Mrs. T.'s knowledge about ways of preventing hypothermia will be increased	• Use Box 25-2 to discuss interventions to prevent hypothermia and to explore ways of applying these interventions to Mrs. T.'s situation	• Mrs. T. will implement strategies aimed at reducing her risk of hypothermia
The risk factor of low temperatures in Mrs. T.'s house will be eliminated	• Inform Mrs. T. about LIHEAP and explain that she may qualify for assistance with utility bills as well as help with weatherization • Emphasize that LIHEAP is an important health-related program aimed at preventing hypothermia in older adults • Ask Mrs. T.'s permission to arrange for a home assessment by a LIHEAP staff person	• Mrs. T. will accept assistance from the LIHEAP program • Mrs. T. will have her house weatherized • Mrs. T. will keep her thermostat at 70°F (21.1°C) during the winter
The risk factor of social isolation will be eliminated	• Suggest home-delivered meals to Mrs. T. as a means of providing prepared meals and daily contact • Emphasize that one of the purposes of such programs is to ensure that socially isolated older adults have daily contact with someone who can monitor their well-being • Ask Mrs. T. for permission to contact her daughter to suggest that she call her mother daily during cold spells to make sure she is okay	• Mrs. T. will accept home-delivered meals • Mrs. T.'s daughter will phone daily during cold spells

THINKING POINTS

• How would you address Mrs. T.'s perception that hypothermia does not have serious health-related implications?

• What additional interventions might you consider to address Mrs. T.'s risk of hypothermia?

Part 2: Mrs. T. at 87 Years of Age *(Continued)*

QSEN APPLICATION

QSEN Competency	Knowledge/Skill/Attitude	Application to Mrs. T. When She Is 87 Years Old
Patient-centered care	(K) Describe strategies to empower patients in all aspects of the health care process	Identify misinformation and lack of information that interfere with the use of available resources
	(K) Examine common barriers to active involvement in patients	Recognize that Mrs. T. values her independence and emphasize that prevention of hypothermia is an important way to maintain health and autonomy
	(S) Elicit patient values, preferences, and expressed needs	
	(A) Value seeing health care situations "through patients' eyes"	
Teamwork and collaboration	(K) Recognize contributions of other individuals and groups in helping patient achieve health goals	Provide information about community resources and obtain permission to facilitate a referral for LIHEAP assistance
	(S) Integrate the contributions of others who play a role in helping patient achieve health goals	Obtain permission to involve Mrs. T.'s daughter in the care plan

Chapter Highlights

Age-Related Changes That Affect Thermoregulation

- Inefficient vasoconstriction
- Decreased cardiac output
- Diminished subcutaneous tissue and muscle mass
- Decreased peripheral circulation
- Delayed and diminished shivering
- Diminished ability to acclimatize to heat

Risk Factors That Affect Thermoregulation (Box 25-1)

- Environmental factors (e.g., temperatures, humidity)
- Socioeconomic and housing factors (e.g., poor ventilation, inadequate heat, lack of air conditioning)
- Insufficient knowledge about altered thermoregulation
- Medications and alcohol
- Chronic and acute conditions (e.g., infections; cardiovascular, endocrine, and neurologic conditions)
- Inactivity
- Social isolation

Functional Consequences Affecting Thermoregulation in Older Adults

- Compromised ability to respond to hot or cold environments
- Increased susceptibility to hypothermia and heat-related illness
- Lower baseline temperature
- Diminished febrile response to infections
- Dulled perception of environmental temperatures

Nursing Assessment of Thermoregulation (Box 25-2)

- Establish baseline temperature, including diurnal variations
- Identify risks for hypothermia or heat-related illness
- Observe for additional manifestations of infections

Nursing Diagnosis

- Hypothermia
- Hyperthermia
- Ineffective Thermoregulation
- Risk for Ineffective Thermoregulation
- Readiness for Enhanced Knowledge: Prevention of Hypothermia (or Hyperthermia)

Planning for Wellness Outcomes

- Health Promoting Behaviors
- Knowledge: Personal Safety
- Risk Detection
- Risk Control
- Safe Home Environment
- Thermoregulation

Nursing Interventions to Promote Healthy Thermoregulation (Box 25-3)

- Maintaining healthy environmental conditions
- Teaching about measures to protect from hypothermia
- Teaching about measures to prevent heat-related illness
- Promoting caregiver wellness

Evaluating Effectiveness of Nursing Interventions

- Evidence that risk factors are eliminated
- Feedback about improved knowledge regarding prevention of hypothermia and heat-related illness
- Feedback about referrals for community resources

Critical Thinking Exercises

1. Describe four major functional consequences that an older adult is likely to experience with regard to thermoregulation. How would you explain these changes to an older adult?
2. Explain how each of the following factors might affect an older person's thermoregulation: medications, pathologic conditions, environmental conditions, socioeconomic factors, and lack of knowledge.
3. What would you include in an assessment of thermoregulation in an older adult?
4. What would you teach older adults about hypothermia and its prevention?
5. What would you teach older adults about heat-related illnesses and their prevention?
6. Find appropriate health education materials on the internet to use in teaching older adults about hypothermia and heat-related illnesses.

For more information about the topics discussed in this chapter, be sure to check out the interactive Online Learning Activities and other helpful resources at http://thepoint.lww.com/Miller8e.

REFERENCES

Bao, J., Wang, Z., Yu, C., et al. (2016). The influence of temperature on mortality and its lag effect: A study in four Chinese cities with different latitudes. *BioMed Central Public Health, 16,* 375.

Berko, J., Ingram, D. D., Saha, S., & Parker, J. D. (2014). *Deaths attributed to heat, cold, and other weather events in the United States, 2006-2010. National Health Statistics Reports Number, 76.* Hyattsville, MD: National Center for Health Statistics.

Bunker, A., Wildenhain, J., Vandenbergh, A., et al. (2016). Effects of air temperature on climate-sensitive mortality and morbidity outcomes in the elderly: A systematic review and meta-analysis of epidemiological evidence. *EBioMedicine, 6,* 258–268.

Cheshire, W. P. (2016). Thermoregulatory disorders and illness related to heat and cold stress. *Autonomic Neuroscience: Basic and Clinical, 196,* 91–104.

Glaser, J., Lemery, J., Rajagopalan, D., et al. (2016). Climate change and the emergent epidemic of CKD from heat stress in rural communities: The case for heat stress neuropathy. *Clinical Journal of the American Society of Nephrologists, 11,* 1472–1483.

Gronlund, O. J., Zanobetti, A., Wellenius, G. A. et al. (2016). Vulnerability to renal, heat and respiratory hospitalizations during extreme heat among U. S. elderly. *Climate Change, 136,* 631–645.

Kenny, G., Sigal, R., & McGinn, R. (2016). Body temperature regulation in diabetes. *Temperature, 3*(1), 119–145.

Kunze, M., & Leistner, L. (2016). Community action plan for extreme heat waves. *Geriatric Nursing, 37,* 326–328.

Lee, W., K., Lee, H. A., & Park, H. (2016). Modifying effect of heat waves on the relationship between temperature an d mortality. *Journal of the Korean Medical Sciences, 31,* 702–708.

Neff, L., M., Hoffman, M. E., Zeiss, D. M., et al. (2016). Cory body temperature is lower in postmenopausal women than premenopausal women: Potential implications for energy metabolism and midlife weight gain. *Cardiovascular Endocrinology, 5*(4), 151–154.

Noe, R. S., Jin, J. O., & Wolkin, A. F. (2012). Exposure to natural cold and heat: Hypothermia and hyperthermia Medicare claims, United States, 2004–2005. *American Journal of Public Health, 102*(4), e11–e18.

Rhoades, J., Gruber, J., & Horton, B. (2017). Developing an in-depth understanding of elderly adult's vulnerability to climate change. *Gerontologist,* [Epub Feb 3 2017] doi: 10.1093/geront/gnw167.

Sommet, A., Durrieu, B., Lapeyre-Mestre, M., et al. (2012). A comparative study of adverse drug reactions during two heat waves that occurred in France in 2003 and 2006. *Pharmacoepidemiology and Drug Safety, 21*(3), 285–288.

Zhang, Y., Nitschke, M., Krackowizer, A., et al. (2017). Risk factors for deaths during the 2009 heat wave in Adelaide, Australia: A matched case-control study. *International Journal of Biometeorology, 61*(1), 35–47.

Sexual Function

Because sexual function in older adults encompasses many physiologic and psychosocial aspects of sexuality and intimate relationships, this chapter's perspective is broad. Although sexual function is not a dominant focus of gerontological nursing care in most situations, it is a core component of quality of life that does not necessarily diminish in importance during older adulthood. Thus, in situations in which quality of life is a focus of nursing care, an essential nursing responsibility is assessing sexual function and implementing interventions to promote sexual wellness.

AGE-RELATED CHANGES THAT AFFECT SEXUAL FUNCTION

Loss of reproductive ability at the onset of menopause in women is an age-related change in sexual function that is clearly delineated. Additional and more subtle age-related changes in sexual function include diminished reproductive abilities in older men and alterations in both male and female responses to sexual stimulation. Older adults generally can compensate for any age-related changes in their response to sexual stimulation; however, when risk factors are present, they may experience additional changes in sexual function. This section focuses on age-related changes affecting physiologic aspects of sexual function. The wide range of commonly occurring risk factors are discussed in the Risk Factors and Pathologic Conditions sections.

Changes Affecting Older Women

Beginning around the fifth decade of life, the frequency of ovulation diminishes and menstrual cycles become shorter and irregular. **Menopause** is the normal age-related physiologic process that indicates the loss of reproductive ability in women. The average age of naturally occurring menopause is 52 years, but onset can vary widely from 40 to 58 years (North American Menopause Society, 2016). Menopause also can occur prematurely due to surgery, radiation, or chemotherapy that affects the reproductive organs.

Promoting Sexual Wellness in Older Adults

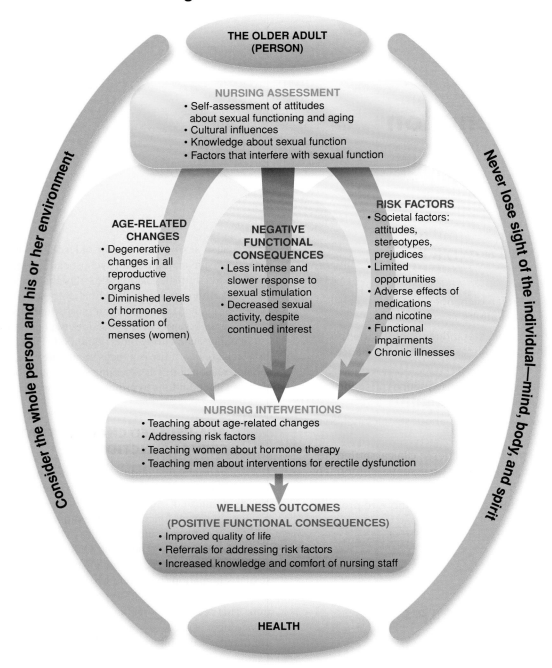

In addition to affecting reproductive ability, menopause influences other aspects of sexual function and quality of life, primarily because of the accompanying decline in endogenous estrogen levels. Although endogenous estrogen levels decline in all postmenopausal women, the effects of this decline are influenced by factors such as the following: length of time since onset of menopause; production of hormones by the adrenal cortex; and body weight, with higher body fat being positively correlated with higher levels of estrogen.

Between 75% and 80% of all menopausal women experience **vasomotor symptoms**, which is the term used to describe a constellation of symptoms that includes hot flashes (also called hot flushes), night sweats, fatigue, and sleep disturbances (Tepper, Brooks, Randolph, et al., 2016). A hot flash, which in one of the most common bothersome symptoms, is characterized by the sudden onset of heat, perspiration, and flushing that spreads from the head to trunk. Symptoms last from 1 to 5 minutes and may be accompanied by chills, nausea, anxiety, palpitations, and clamminess.

Although the severity of symptoms varies significantly, hot flashes can cause embarrassment, sleep disruptions, significant discomfort, and interruptions in activities, including sexual activities. Trajectories of hot flashes vary significantly with regard to onset, severity, and length of time they are experienced; however, these symptoms may last for a decade or longer (Tepper, Brooks, Randolph, et al., 2016).

Diminished estrogen levels can directly affect sexual function for older women in all the following ways: sexual organs atrophy, vaginal secretions diminish, labia lose their fullness, the amount of pubic hair decreases, and breasts become more pendulous and have less mammary tissue. In addition to these effects on sexual function and quality of life, estrogen deficiency affects nonreproductive tissues, including skin, brain, bone, colon, muscle, and the entire cardiovascular system (Thornton, 2016). Consequently, decreased estrogen is associated with increased risk for osteoporosis and other pathologic conditions, such as cardiovascular disease. In addition, menopausal hormonal changes have been identified as a risk factor for depressive symptoms, with increasing prevalence associated with longer time in menopause and increased experiences of stressful life events (Almeida, Marsh, Flicker, et al., 2016; Gordon, Rubinow, Eisenlohr-Moul, et al., 2016; Hickey, Schoenaker, Joffe, et al., 2016).

Diversity Note

A large longitudinal study of a multiracial/ethnic cohort of women transitioning through menopause indicated that menopausal vasomotor symptoms in black women were more likely to begin later and be more persistent and severe relative to white women (Tepper, Brooks, Randolph, et al., 2016). Studies have found a low prevalence of vasomotor symptoms among Japanese women, which may be related to low rates of obesity (Yokota, Makita, Hirasawa, et al., 2016).

Changes Affecting Older Men

Male reproductive function depends on the secretion of testosterone and other hormones, the production and release of sperm, and the motility of sperm through the urethra. All male reproductive organs undergo age-related degenerative changes and production of viable sperm gradually diminishes. However, these changes affect men to varying degrees, with some men never losing their reproductive abilities.

The term **andropause** (or *male menopause*) was first used in the mid-1940s to describe the age-related decline in testosterone in men that begins around the age of 30 years and is analogous to the age-related decline in estrogen in women. Although studies confirm that serum testosterone decreases about 1% to 1.5% per year as a normal age-related change in men, not all men experience symptoms of decreased testosterone. The term **late-onset hypogonadism** (also called *androgen deficiency in the older male* or *testosterone deficiency syndrome*) is used to describe a condition in which a man has a low testosterone level and several or more of the following manifestations:

- Loss of muscle tissue and strength
- Osteoporotic fracture
- Diminished facial, axillary, and pubic hair
- Mood changes
- Sleep disturbances
- Fatigue
- Hot flashes
- Decreased libido
- Erectile dysfunction

Recent studies suggest that low serum testosterone levels are associated with many pathologic conditions, such as diabetes, obesity, osteoporosis, and cardiovascular disease. However, it is unknown whether the relationship between pathologic conditions and low testosterone levels is bidirectional, causative, or simply concurrent (Corona, Maseroli, Rastrelli, et al., 2016; Dimopoulou , Ceausu, Depypere, et al., 2016).

RISK FACTORS THAT AFFECT SEXUAL FUNCTION

Many types of risk factors can affect sexual function and expressions of sexuality, ranging from individual physical, functional, and psychosocial factors to broader societal and cultural influences. Although many of these risks affect people at any age, older adults are likely to experience several or more risks and some risks are unique to older adults. This section provides an overview of risk factors that occur most commonly in older adults.

Sociocultural Influences

Because personal attitudes about sexuality are shaped by societal influences, it is important to consider the societal context of attitudes about sexuality, particularly with regard to women and older adults. Strict Victorian standards of morality that began in the 1800s in Europe and North America strongly influenced older cohorts of Americans. According to Victorian standards, masturbation, homosexual activity, public displays of affection, and sex with anyone except a marital partner were totally taboo. Women's sexuality was a particular target of negative attitudes and hysterectomies were viewed as an appropriate treatment for women's sexual problems.

During the mid-1950s, the "Kinsey Report" brought public attention to previously taboo topics, such as orgasm, masturbation, premarital sex, and marital infidelity. After this major turning point in perspectives on female sexuality, attitudes about sexuality changed significantly; however, it is important to recognize that women who are in their 80s or 90s today may lack accurate information about sexuality and, at the same time, they may resist attempts to discuss topics that they consider taboo.

Another sociocultural factor that influences perspective on sexuality and aging is the strong association in Western societies between sexual attractiveness and physical attributes in very gender-specific and stereotypical ways. Because these images contrast sharply with typical portrayals of older adults as physically unattractive, they foster a false perception that older adults have lost the interest in or capacity for sexual activity. This can become a self-fulfilling prophecy if older adults believe this stereotype. Even if older adults do not believe these stereotypes, they may be embarrassed to acknowledge their sexual desires and activities for fear of being considered abnormal.

In stark contrast to the "sexless senior" stereotype, the recent proliferation of media attention to pharmacologic and medical therapies for improving sexual function in older men and women may be establishing countermyths. These countermyths can create false expectations and lead to self-perceptions of inadequacy. Health care professionals need to address myths and misunderstandings by providing accurate sexual information that enables older adults to set positive and realistic expectations that can lead to self-acceptance related to both the possibilities and limitations of their situations (Atallah, 2016).

In addition to being affected by myths and stereotypes, older adults who are lesbian, gay, bisexual, and transgender (LGBT) usually have long-term experiences of prejudice and misinformation related to their sexual orientation and identity. Even though attitudes have changed in recent years—and are continuing to change—older adults in these diverse groups of sexual minorities have experienced decades of stigma and discrimination and they are more likely than younger generations to be secretive about their sexual orientation or identity. In addition, the disproportionately high death rate among younger gay men when **human immuno-deficiency virus (HIV)** was at its peak (1987–1996) continues to exert a strong influence on social networks and personal lives of current cohorts of older gay men.

 Global Perspective

In Spain, attitudes about sexuality are strongly influenced by the Catholic religion, which teaches that the sole purpose of sexual intercourse is procreation within marriage. In this sociocultural environment, older women may limit their expressions of sexuality, despite their continued desire (Palacios-Cena, Martínez-Piedrola, & Pérez-de-Heredia, et al., 2016).

Wellness Opportunity

Nurses can holistically address sexual wellness by being nonjudgmental about choices of close personal relationships and expressions of sexuality.

Social Circumstances

Availability of a satisfactory partner is a major factor that influences opportunities for sexual activities during older

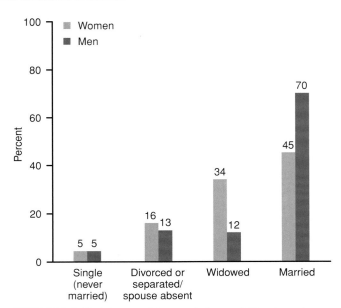

FIGURE 26-1 Marital status of the population aged 65 and over, by age group and sex, percent distribution, 2010. *Note:* Married includes married, spouse present; married, spouse absent; and separated. These data refer to the civilian noninstitutionalized population. (Adapted from U.S. Census Bureau, Current Population Survey, Annual Social and Economic Supplement, 2015.)

adulthood, and this is especially true for older heterosexual women whose husbands are deceased or in poor health. Although higher levels of sexual interest and activity are reported by men at any age compared with women at a similar age, this gender difference widens during older adulthood. This is partly attributable to the fact that women outnumber men in older age groups, with a sex ratio of 127.2 women for every 100 men at age 65 and 192.2 women for every 100 men at age 85 (Administration on Aging, 2016). Similarly, the proportion of married women also decreases with increasing age, as illustrated in Figure 26-1.

Privacy is generally considered a requisite for sexual activity, and adults who live in their own homes are usually able to arrange for this. However, older adults who live in institutions, group settings, or family homes may find it difficult or impossible to arrange for privacy, especially if their sexual needs are ignored or considered abnormal or even morally deviant. Even if some privacy is possible in institutional settings, additional constraints include the inability to lock doors and ensure total privacy, negative attitudes of staff and families about sexual interactions, and institutional policies that do not allow a resident to freely engage in sexual relationships. For example, residents of long-term care facilities may find that staff "report" their sexual activities to supervisors or families, even when the people involved are capable of making independent decisions.

Wellness Opportunity

Nurses in long-term care settings need to create opportunities for privacy if a resident desires this.

Adverse Effects of Medication, Alcohol, and Nicotine

Since the 1980s, adverse effects of medication have been recognized as a major cause of erectile dysfunction in men. Slag and colleagues (1983) found that 34% of 1180 male patients in a medical clinic were impotent, and 25% of the 188 subjects who subsequently underwent further evaluation were found to have medication-induced erectile dysfunction. In recent years, there has been increasing attention to sexual adverse effects of medications as a major factor that influences quality of life and adherence to prescribed regimens in both men and women.

Specific adverse medication effects that interfere with sexual function in men include a decreased or absent libido; difficulty obtaining or maintaining an erection; dry, premature, or retrograde ejaculation; and inability to achieve orgasm. Women may experience the following medication-induced limitations in sexual function: diminished vaginal lubrication, decreased or absent libido, and inability to achieve orgasm. Box 26-1 lists some of the medications that are commonly associated with sexual dysfunction. These effects usually disappear when the medication is discontinued, and occasionally the effects will disappear if the dose is decreased.

Because alcohol depresses the central nervous system, it can interfere with sexual function. Although alcohol can decrease inhibitions and heighten sensual and sexual interest in social settings, excessive amounts can depress the central nervous system and interfere with sexual performance. Moderate amounts of alcohol normally do not interfere with sexual performance; however, in combination with other risk factors, such as medications or pathologic conditions, even small amounts of alcohol may be detrimental to the sexual performance of older adults.

Cigarette smoking was first identified as a cause of erectile dysfunction in the mid-1980s, and recent studies have confirmed that smoking increases the risk for sexual dysfunction in both men and women (Bolat, Akdeniz, Ozkaya, et al., 2016; Choi, Shin, Lee, et al., 2015). Nicotine interferes with circulation to the sexual organs and accentuates the effects of other risk factors, such as diabetes, hypertension, and vascular disease. In addition, cigarette smoking is associated with earlier onset of menopause and longer duration of hot flashes (Smith, Gallicchio, Miller, et al., 2016; Yang, Suh, Kim, et al., 2015).

Effects of Chronic Conditions

Chronic conditions that have consistently been identified as having detrimental effects on sexual wellness in men and women include pain, cancer, diabetes, depression, and cardiovascular disease. Increasingly, much attention is being paid to the common occurrence of sexual dysfunction in people with type 2 diabetes. Of particular importance for health promotion, studies indicate that risk of sexual dysfunction in people with diabetes can be reduced with a Mediterranean diet and good glycemic control (Binmoammar, Hassounah, Alsaad, et al., 2016; Maiorino, Bellastella, Caputo, et al., 2016).

Cardiovascular disease (e.g., heart failure, coronary artery disease) is strongly associated with many aspects of sexual dysfunction, including decreased libido, inhibited performance, diminished pleasure, and decreased frequency of sexual activities. Sexual function is affected not only by the physical manifestations of coronary heart disease (e.g., angina and reduced levels of activity) and adverse effects of medications but also by psychological factors that commonly occur in people with cardiovascular disease. For example, even when no physiologic basis exists for abstaining from sexual intercourse after a myocardial infarction, sexual activity is often limited or absent because of fatigue, depression, diminished sexual desire, and fears and anxiety of the person or the sexual partner.

Although chronic conditions create risks for sexual dysfunction, it is imperative to avoid generalizations and assumptions. For example, a study of women aged 45 to 60 found that the main risk factors associated with sexual dysfunction in the women with multimorbidity (i.e., the presence of two or more chronic conditions in the same person) were anxiety, lack of physical activity, and no sexual intercourse during the past month (Valadares, Lui-Filho, Costa-Paiva, et al., 2016).

Gender-Specific Conditions

Prostatic hyperplasia (also called *benign prostatic hypertrophy*) is a common pathologic condition in which the prostate gland gradually enlarges and affects the urinary tract and sexual function. Men with prostatic hyperplasia often experience erectile dysfunction, ejaculatory dysfunction, and urinary incontinence, which can interfere with enjoyment of sexual activities. After surgical treatment (i.e., prostatectomy) only 5% to 16% of men obtain the quality of erection that they had prior to surgery, even with newer surgical techniques intended to reduce adverse effects (Emanu, Avildsen, & Nelson, 2016).

 Box 26-1 Medications That Can Interfere With Sexual Function

Angiotensin-converting enzyme inhibitors
Alpha-adrenergic blockers or agonists
Antidepressants
Antiepileptics
Antihistamines
Antiparkinson agents
Antipsychotics
Benzodiazepines
Beta-blockers
Calcium channel blockers
Diuretics
Dopamine agonists
Histamine H_2 antagonists
Monoamine oxidase inhibitors
Nonsteroidal anti-inflammatory drugs
Alcohol, nicotine, recreational drugs

Prostatic hypertrophy also affects urinary function, as discussed in Chapter 19.

Sexual function in older women can be affected by their increased susceptibility to inflammations, such as urethritis and vaginitis because of the thinning of the vaginal tissue and the decreased acidity and quantity of vaginal secretions. These conditions can occur after intercourse and cause urinary urgency and burning that persists for several days. They also can interfere with enjoyment of sexual intercourse. Since 2014, the term **genitourinary syndrome of menopause (GSM)** is being used as a medically more comprehensive term for the constellation of signs and symptoms involving changes to the external female genitalia, vagina, urethra, and bladder that are caused by hormonal changes (North American Menopause Society, 2016). Manifestations of genitourinary syndrome of menopause include all the following:

- Vaginal or vulvar dryness
- Vaginal or vulvar itching, irritation, or burning
- Decreased lubrication
- Dyspareunia or discomfort with intercourse
- Dysuria
- Urinary urgency
- Recurrent urinary tract infections

(North American Menopause Society, 2016; Sophocles, 2016). At least half of postmenopausal women experience symptoms of GSM, with 60% of those experiencing moderate or severe symptoms (Iglesia, 2016; Pinkerton, Bushmakin, Abraham, et al., 2016). Symptoms of GSM have substantial negative consequences on sexual function and interpersonal relationships. Health care professionals are encouraged to ask postmenopausal women about these symptoms and emphasize that symptoms can successfully be managed with over-the-counter lubricants and moisturizers or with prescription medications (Edwards & Panay, 2016).

Functional Impairments

Functional impairments associated with chronic conditions can interfere with enjoyment of sexual activity in many ways, as in the following examples:

- Chronic obstructive pulmonary disease may cause hypoxia and severe shortness of breath in response to the high physiologic demands of sexual activity.
- Arthritis and other musculoskeletal disorders are likely to be associated with pain, stiffness, muscle spasms, and limited flexibility.
- Urinary incontinence can interfere with satisfying sexual relationships in people of any age, but this condition is more common in older adults.
- Medical conditions and adverse medication effects can have physiologic effects that interfere with all phases of sexual function.

Functional limitations increase with advancing age and are likely to combine with other risk factors to interfere with sexual function. In addition to direct effects of functional limitations, people with visible disabilities are often misperceived as unable to engage in sexual activities. As with other stigma and stereotypes, these perceptions can have a negative effect on one's overall sexual self-concept and also on sexual function and relationships. This is particularly relevant to older adults who live in institutional settings because attitudes of the staff members and other residents can affect the residents' expressions of sexuality.

Sensory impairments can also interfere with sexual function because sensory stimulation is an important part of sexual pleasure and intimate communication. For example, an older adult with impaired hearing may find it difficult or impossible to carry on the intimate conversations that are often a part of sexual interactions. Similarly, hearing impairments can interfere with professional efforts to assess and counsel older adults on this sensitive topic. Likewise, impairments affecting vision, smell, or touch can interfere with some of the usual sensual stimulation associated with sexual activities.

Attitudes and Behaviors of Families and Caregivers

In addition to societal influences, the attitudes and behaviors of family members and caregivers can affect sexual wellness of older adults, particularly for those who are dependent on others for their care. In institutional settings, attitudes of staff members can significantly affect the way in which residents express or repress their sexual needs. In general, sexual needs of residents are ignored, except when staff observe expressions of sexuality that are deemed inappropriate. For example, older adults who desire sexual relationships and intimacy outside of traditional heterosexual marriages often experience discrimination.

Although much progress has been made in social acceptance of LGBT people, health care professionals may convey judgmental attitudes. Since 2015, the Centers for Medicare and Medicaid has mandated that all health care programs that receive federal funds establish nondiscrimination protections for people who identify as LGBT. These protections extend to older adults receiving services in institutional and community-based settings, including nursing homes.

A common concern in long-term care settings is that family members are often involved with decisions about a resident's sexual expressions, even when the resident is competent. This occurs either because the staff initiate the contact with the family or the family requests assistance from the facility in setting boundaries on the resident's expressions of sexuality. Even in assisted living facilities—which are designed to promote autonomy and independence—staff and administrators often attempt to limit or prevent resident's expressions of sexuality and intimacy to avoid conflicts with families (Barmon, Burgess, Bender, et al., 2017). When residents of long-term care facilities are cognitively impaired or diagnosed with dementia, additional conflicts arise, as discussed in the next section.

Effects of Dementia on Sexual Expressions

When older adults are cognitively impaired, issues related to sexual expression are compounded by concerns about competency, decision making, the personal meaning of behaviors, and whether the behavior arises from dementia. People with dementia often experience a loss of sexual desire; however, **inappropriate sexual behaviors** (also called hypersexuality or disinhibited behavior) also occur in people with dementia. Inappropriate sexual behaviors include masturbation in public places, exposing oneself, sexual talk, physically intimate touching or grabbing, or getting into bed with someone. It is important to recognize that acts that may be perceived as sexual in origin may in fact be expressions of unmet needs or manifestations of pain, discomfort, or anxiety. Sometimes, the behaviors are normal but they become problematic because of the context or the environment. For example, masturbating or disrobing in public places is considered sexually inappropriate behaviors, but these actions may be due to dementia-related disinhibition. Another important consideration is that normal expressions of an older adult's personal needs may be deemed inappropriate by observers, including health care professionals, who are judgmental or biased. Nursing management of inappropriate sexual behavior is discussed in Chapter 14.

For people in residential or long-term care settings questions may arise about the ability of the person with dementia to make decisions about intimate relationships and sexual expressions. This is particularly problematic with regard to nonmarital or other nontraditional relationships. It also raises questions related to sexual abuse—for example, with regard to the person's ability to engage willingly in physical sexual interactions, even with one's spouse. These decisions are complex and should take into account not only the effect on the spouse or partners but also whether sexual interactions could be beneficial or positive for the person with dementia. Most importantly, assessment of capacity to consent needs to be based on a multifaceted assessment of the individual, including consideration of his or her values and interpersonal relationships. Nurses can use information in Box 26-2 as a guide for assessing an older adult's capacity to consent to physical sexual interactions. In situations involving questions about capacity to consent, nurses need to initiate a referral for an interprofessional comprehensive evaluation. Residential and long-term care facilities should have policies and procedures describing a process for this comprehensive evaluation, including a description of professionals who would participate. Nursing supervisors and nursing staff are key members of such committees, which also would typically include any of the following professionals: social workers, care managers, medical personnel, and mental health professionals.

 See ONLINE LEARNING ACTIVITY 26-1: EVIDENCE-BASED INFORMATION ABOUT ISSUES REGARDING SEXUALITY at http://thepoint.lww.com/Miller8e.

 Box 26-2 Guide for Assessing an Older Adult's Capacity to Consent to Physical Sexual Interactions

Does the person understand ALL of the following:
- That the act is sexual in nature?
- That one's body is private?
- That they have the right to say "no" to any unwanted sexual actions?
- That engagement in certain sexual acts may involve health risks?

Does the person have the ability to express choices about relationships?

Are the sexual interactions enjoyable, pleasurable, or positive in other ways?

Are there indicators of negative effects of the relationship?

Are there indicators of negative consequences of the sexual interactions?

Has the person expressed regret after previously engaging in similar sexual interactions?

Is the relationship consistent with the person's values and personal history?

Source: Miller, C. A. (2017). *Elder abuse and nursing: What nurses need to know and can do.* Used with permission, Springer Publishing Company.

 ## FUNCTIONAL CONSEQUENCES AFFECTING SEXUAL WELLNESS

Sexual function involves reproduction, response to sexual stimulation, and interest and participation in sexual activity. Although reproductive aspects of sexual function typically are less important in later life, sexual well-being is an important component of overall quality of life throughout older adulthood. Although age-related changes directly affect reproduction, other aspects of sexuality are affected more directly by risk factors. In addition, because sexual dysfunctions commonly occur in older men and women as a consequence of risk factors, these are discussed in this section.

Response to Sexual Stimulation

The Masters and Johnson (1966) investigation has been widely recognized as the landmark study of human physiologic response to sexual stimulation. This classic study of 694 adults in a laboratory setting identified four phases of physiologic response to sexual stimulation in men and women. An analysis of data on older subjects led to the following conclusions:

- Older adults maintain their ability to respond to sexual stimulation, but their response is slower and less intense.
- Regularly engaging in sexual activity helps older adults respond to sexual stimulation.
- Any major changes in response to sexual stimulation are associated with risk factors rather than aging, per se.

Although older adults were greatly underrepresented in this study, the findings of Masters and Johnson have been widely accepted as the knowledge base about age-related changes in physiologic response to sexual stimulation. Normal age-related changes in male and female responses to sexual stimulation and the associated consequences are discussed in the following sections and summarized in Table 26-1. In recent years, there has been increasing emphasis on multifactorial factors that influence all aspects of sexuality, with emphasis on sexual wellness as an essential component of quality of life and positive subjective well-being for older adults (Lee, Vanhoutte, Nazroo, et al., 2016). Studies indicate that older adults in positive relationships continue to enjoy sexual quality of life because they have acquired skills and strategies to buffer age-related declines (Forbes, Eaton, & Krueger, 2017).

Sexual Interest and Activity

During the 1940s and 1950s, the Kinsey surveys first brought information about sexual behaviors of older adults to public attention by concluding that the frequency of sexual activity gradually declines with increasing age but sexual interest and competence do not necessarily decline. Sexual interest, attitudes, activity, and satisfaction are a continuation of lifelong patterns, and they remain stable in older adulthood unless risk factors interfere with sexual function. As discussed in the Risk Factors section, conditions that commonly affect sexual interest and activity in older adults include social circumstances, poor health, pathologic conditions, adverse medication effects, and influences of family and caregivers. The sexual needs and interest of older adults, including residents of long-term care

facilities, do not necessarily decrease, but their opportunities for sexual activity are often limited.

In recent decades, studies of sexuality and aging have focused on broader aspects, such as affection, friendships, and intimacy. For older adults, these aspects of sexual function may become more important as the number of opportunities for sexual activities diminishes. For example, one of the first studies addressing sexual behaviors found that the most common sexual activities in a sample of 202 adults aged 80 to 102 years were touching and caressing without sexual intercourse (Bretschneider & McCoy, 1988). Additional components of sexuality that are especially important for older adults include kissing, hugging, intimacy, fantasy, masturbation, oral sex, loving words, physical closeness, and expressions of affection (Lochlainn & Kenny, 2013). As stated in evidence-based guidelines for nurses, "Despite the negative stereotypes, sexual identity and the need for intimacy do not disappear with increasing age, and older adults do not morph into celibate, asexual beings" (Steinke, 2016, p. 166).

In summary, older adults do not lose their interest in or capacity for sexual activity because of age-related changes, but risk factors such as misinformation, social circumstances, pathologic conditions, environmental constraints, and adverse medication effects commonly interfere with sexual function. A normal consequence of aging, however, is that the response of older men and women to sexual stimulation is slower, less intense, and of shorter duration. As one 79-year-old man reported, "It's like sparklers, not fireworks."

TABLE 26-1 Functional Consequences for Response to Sexual Stimulation

Phase	Changes in Female Response	Changes in Male Response
Excitement phase	Breasts not as engorged	Longer time required to attain erection
	Sexual flush diminished	Less firm erection
	Delayed or diminished vaginal lubrication	Longer maintenance of erection before ejaculation
	Decreased expansion of vaginal wall	Increased difficulty regaining an erection if lost
	Decreased vasocongestion of labia	Reduced scrotal and testicular vasocongestion
Plateau phase	Decreased areolar engorgement	Diminished nipple turgidity and sexual flush
	Less intense sexual flush	Less intense muscle tension
	Less intense myotonia	Slower penile erectile response
	Decreased vasocongestion of labia	Delayed and diminished testicular elevation
	Reduced Bartholin gland secretions	Fewer rectal sphincter contractions
	Slower/less marked uterine elevation	Diminution of ejaculatory expulsion force by about 50%
Orgasmic phase	Fewer rectal sphincter contractions	Absent or diminished sense of ejaculatory inevitability
	Decreased number and intensity of orgasmic contractions	Fewer and less intense ejaculatory contractions
Resolution phase	Slower loss of nipple erection	Slower loss of nipple erection
	Quicker return to pre-excitement stage	Longer refractory period
		Rapid penile detumescence and testicular descent

It is important to recognize that many interacting physical and psychosocial factors affect sexual wellness in a unique way for each older adult.

Sexual Dysfunction in Men and Women

Erectile dysfunction, defined as the inability to achieve or maintain an erection sufficient for satisfactory sexual function, is the most common sexual dysfunction affecting older men. Until the early 1990s, this condition was called *impotence*, but the National Institutes of Health proposed this change in terminology to reflect the broader understanding of erectile dysfunction as a complex condition associated with many interacting factors. Although erectile dysfunction is not the only type of male sexual dysfunction, it is the one that has been studied the most and has received the most public attention since 1998 because of the availability of medications, such as sildenafil (Viagra), and the widespread publicity about these medications that continues today. Other types of male sexual dysfunction include problems with ejaculation and diminished desire. Men at any age are likely to experience erectile dysfunction, but the incidence increases gradually with increasing age. It is currently viewed as a complex disease associated with multiple interacting factors, as discussed in the Risk Factors section.

In recent years, health care practitioners and pharmaceutical companies have started addressing **female sexual dysfunction**, similar to the way in which erectile dysfunction has been addressed since the early 1990s. Female sexual dysfunction includes disorders that affect sexual desire (including motivation and physical drive), sexual arousal, orgasm, or pain during or after sexual activities (i.e., dyspareunia or vaginismus). In addition to interpersonal sociocultural influences, conditions that increase the risk for female sexual dysfunction include the following: diabetes, decreased estrogen, cardiovascular disease, cigarette smoking, alcohol consumption, urinary incontinence, pelvic floor disorders, anxiety, depression, and adverse medication effects (Caruso, Rapisarda, & Cianci, 2016; Nazapour, Simbar, & Tehrani, 2016).

See ONLINE LEARNING ACTIVITY 26-2: INFORMATION ABOUT SEXUAL PROBLEMS IN OLDER MEN AND WOMEN at http://thepoint.lww.com/Miller8e.

PATHOLOGIC CONDITION AFFECTING SEXUAL WELLNESS: SEXUALLY TRANSMITTED DISEASES

In recent years, the incidence of sexually transmitted diseases among adults aged 55 years and older has been increasing significantly, and rates of screening and testing are disproportionately low (Tillman & Mark, 2016). Rates of sexually transmitted diseases are higher in men, particularly in those who are recently widowed and using a phosphodiesterase type 5 inhibitor, such as Viagra (Brandon, 2016). Reasons for increasing incidence of sexually transmitted diseases

Unfolding Case Study

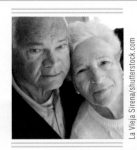

La Vieja Sirena/shutterstock.com

Part 1: Mr. and Mrs. J. at 73 and 71 Years of Age

You are the "wellness nurse" at the senior center where Mr. and Mrs. J. come for the meal program and social interaction. Mr. J. is 73 years old and has hypertension and a history of a heart attack. He takes diltiazem (Cardizem), 300 mg daily; furosemide (Lasix), 20 mg daily; and propranolol (Inderal), 80 mg three times daily. Mrs. J., who is 71 years old, describes herself as generally healthy, but with a history of depression and some arthritis. She takes ibuprofen 400 mg twice daily, and sertraline (Zoloft), 50 mg daily. During your nursing clinics, Mr. J. and several other men have asked you about the drug that is advertised on television for men who have trouble satisfying their partners. The senior center director also has noticed an increased interest in this topic and has asked that you plan a group health information session called "Sexuality and Aging."

THINKING POINTS

- Develop a plan for teaching older adults about the normal changes in sexual function that they are likely to experience.
- What risk factors would you discuss in relation to sexuality and aging?

- What educational materials would you use?
- What teaching would you do about interventions?

such as syphilis, chlamydia, and HIV among adults age 55 and older are multifaceted and include the following:

- Increasing availability and use of phosphodiesterase type 5 inhibitors among men
- Increased numbers of older adults who are healthy and physically and socially active
- Increased availability of senior living communities and internet dating sites
- Altered tissue integrity and immune function associated with aging
- Decreased fear of pregnancy and subsequent decrease in condom use
- Lack of health education regarding sexually transmitted diseases
- Delay in diagnosis and treatment because of lack of screening
- Misperception that HIV risk is low in older adults

(DeMarco, Brennan-Ing, Sprague, et al., 2017; Spadt & Kusturiss, 2016).

Another factor that contributes to the increased incidence of sexually transmitted diseases in older adults that is particularly relevant for health education is the fact that older adults with risk behaviors (e.g., not using condoms, frequent nonmonogamous sexual interactions) tend to underestimate their risk for, and lack information about, sexually transmitted infections (Syme, Cohn, & Barnack-Tavlaris, 2016; Tuddenham, Page, Chaulk, et al., 2016).

Health care practitioners who provide care to older adults are increasingly aware of the need to address HIV as a sexually transmitted infection that is becoming more common among older adults. The effectiveness of antiretroviral therapy since the late 1980s has enabled many HIV-infected people to live longer with this condition, which is now considered a chronic disease, before it progresses to/acquired immunodeficiency syndrome (AIDS). As a result of the use of highly effective antiretroviral treatments during the past two decades, fewer than one-third of the people who have been diagnosed and treated will die from conditions traditionally associated with HIV infection.

Statistics about HIV generally define "older adult" as someone aged 50 years and older based on the Centers for Disease Control and Prevention (CDC) demographic distribution of cases on a bell curve (with an average age of around 30 years). In 2013, 25% of all Americans diagnosed with HIV infection were aged 55 and older, and 6% were aged 65 and older (CDC, 2015). The diagnosis of HIV for people at any age is always accompanied by major health-related issues, but some issues are more unique to older adults. For example, HIV-infected older adults have higher rates of certain cancers, renal disease, and cardiovascular disease (Karpiak & Havlik, 2017). Although nurses in gerontological care settings are not expected to be experts in all aspects of HIV, they are expected to holistically assess and address the complex needs of older adults with this condition, and, perhaps first and foremost, communicate a nonjudgmental approach

---

Box 26-3 Issues Associated With HIV in Older Adults

Issues Related to Diagnosis and Progression

- Older adults have the same risk factors as younger people but tend to be less aware of risks.
- Older adults are likely to be diagnosed later in the course of the infection. Later diagnoses can occur for the following reasons: health care providers may not test for HIV infection, older people may not consider themselves to be at risk, older adults may attribute symptoms to normal aging or pathologic conditions other than HIV.
- Older adults have a shorter interval before progression to AIDS, particularly if HIV was diagnosed after the age of 60 years.
- HIV-positive older adults are at increased risk for dying due to AIDS or other conditions.

Associated Medical Concerns

- Older adults with HIV are likely to be dealing with commonly occurring comorbidities, such as cardiovascular disease and some cancers (e.g., lung, leukemia, melanoma, and all areas of the gastrointestinal tract).
- Dementia and cognitive impairment occurs more frequently in older HIV patients.
  - Older adults have a diminished and delayed immune response to treatments.
  - Metabolism of antiretroviral medications is altered in older adults and this may lead to liver toxicity and other adverse effects.
  - Common adverse effects of antiretroviral therapy include osteoporosis, pancreatitis, lipid disorders, peripheral neuropathy, and high serum levels of lactic acid.

Associated Psychosocial Issues

- Older adults with HIV have high rates of depression.
- Older adults are more likely to have less social support due to ageism, living alone, perceived stigma, and nondisclosure of HIV status.
- Caregivers of people with HIV experience significant levels of stress, which is exacerbated by associated factors such as stigma, uncertainty, depression, social isolation, and impaired cognitive function.

---

in all interactions with people who have risks for, or a diagnosis of, HIV. Box 26-3 summarizes issues related to HIV that are most relevant to gerontological nursing.

Diversity Note

Blacks/African Americans and Hispanics/Latinos have higher rates of HIV infection diagnosis compared with whites, and this disparity is greater among those who are 50 years or older (Centers for Disease Control, 2015).

An important assessment consideration is that HIV may initially manifest as a nonspecific viral illness with signs and symptoms similar to seasonal flu or mononucleosis. These early manifestations may subside after several weeks, and HIV antibodies will appear in the blood between 3 and 6 weeks after the initial infection. If appropriate treatment is initiated in a timely manner, people with HIV can expect to live a near normal life expectancy, although they are likely to experience additional health issues, as summarized in Box 26-3.

Treatment of HIV generally includes a combination of antiretroviral agents and other types of medications to control disease progression. The pharmacologic regimen requires close monitoring for therapeutic and adverse effects. Adherence is a common problem for people with HIV, for various reasons including cost of medications and adverse effects, making these issues important aspects of assessing older adults with HIV.

Nurses have important responsibilities with regard to promoting wellness for older adults with HIV, including addressing related psychosocial needs. In addition to addressing medical conditions related to HIV, nursing interventions address psychosocial aspects for the person with HIV and his or her caregivers. For example, the assessment and intervention guidelines for depression discussed in Chapter 15, including those related to suicide, are applicable for older adults with HIV. In addition, consider the cultural needs by suggesting resources specific for people who identify as LGBT or other minorities (e.g., black), as discussed in Chapter 2.

Teaching about safe sex is a nursing responsibility that is often overlooked when caring for older adults, but it is particularly important with regard to preventing and managing HIV. Older adults need to recognize that safe sex practices are imperative for anyone who has sex with someone other than a long-term partner who is 100% monogamous. Nurses also need to teach about early detection of sexually transmitted infections and encourage appropriate testing for anyone with risk factors. Recognize that older men and women are less likely than younger adults to have received information about sexually transmitted diseases or the use of condoms for protection. They also are likely to have less experience with multiple partners, and they may need information about how to discuss safe sex practices with partners (Brandon, 2016). Nurses can incorporate information about safe sex in their health education about sexual activity for older adults, as discussed in the section on nursing interventions and summarized in Box 26-6 later in this chapter.

See ONLINE LEARNING ACTIVITY 26-3: INFORMATION ABOUT OLDER ADULTS AND HIV at http://thepoint.lww.com/Miller8e.

NURSING ASSESSMENT OF SEXUAL FUNCTION

Nurses do not necessarily include sexual function in every assessment, but it is an essential aspect when addressing quality-of-life issues that affect day-to-day function. Thus, assessment of sexual function is especially important in home care and long-term care settings (e.g., group homes, nursing facilities, and assisted-living facilities). In rehabilitation settings, assessment of sexual function can be included as an essential activity of daily living of all patients, regardless of factors such as marital status or sexual orientation (Milspaw, Brandon, & Sher, 2016). Sexual function is often neglected in nursing assessments because of the high degree of privacy associated with sexual function and the stereotype of the "sexless senior" that is prevalent in U.S. society. In addition, gender or generational differences between the health professional and the older person may interfere with an assessment of sexual function. Although all of these factors may explain why sexual function in older adults is so often overlooked, they do not justify its exclusion.

Self-Assessment of Attitudes About Sexual Function and Aging

Because of the private nature of sexual function and associated emotional responses and cultural factors, nurses are often uncomfortable discussing this topic. Additional discomfort occurs because nurses are not confident in dealing with concerns about human sexuality as an integral part of their nursing practice. They are even less comfortable initiating this topic with older adults or with people who are not in a traditional marital relationship. Thus, an assessment of personal attitudes about sexuality and aging is a prerequisite to addressing sexual wellness. Box 26-4 lists some of the questions nurses can use to examine their own attitudes toward the sexual function of older adults. Some questions are specific to adults in long-term care facilities because of the dominant role of nurses in addressing sexual function as a quality-of-life issue for residents.

Wellness Opportunity

Nurses should take time for self-assessment to increase their comfort with, openness to, and sensitivity about issues related to sexual wellness for older adults.

Significant cultural differences between the nurse and the older adult may increase the difficulty of discussing sexual function. Box 26-5 summarizes some cultural aspects of sexual function that may be applicable to nursing assessment. Nurses may also be uncomfortable discussing sexual function with older adults who are in a nontraditional relationship, such as LGBT. Thus, an important aspect of self-assessment is to identify attitudes toward nontraditional sexual activities because these attitudes can influence the assessment and care of people who do not conform to the nurse's or societal expectations. When assessing sexual function, establish a trusting relationship, have an awareness of gay and lesbian culture and other nontraditional sexual relationships, and communicate a nonjudgmental attitude by using appropriate or gender-neutral terminology. For example, the word *partner* includes a spouse as well as a same-sex relationship and asking about someone who is a *confidant* is

Box 26-4 Assessing Personal Attitudes Toward Sexuality and Aging

What Do I Believe About Sexuality and Aging?

- Do I hold the misconception that older people, especially unmarried ones, are no longer interested in or capable of sexual activities?
- Do I believe the subtle messages that inaccurately associate sexual activities only with youth and attractiveness?
- Do I hold age-specific standards regarding sexual activity and romantic relationships? (e.g., Do I think it is okay for young adults to kiss or hold hands, but inappropriate or "cute" for older people to do this?)

What Do I Believe About the Nurse's Role With Regard to the Sexual Function of Older Adults?

- Do I base my nursing practice on the misconception that sexual function is strictly a private matter that health professionals should not address?
- Do I view sexual function as an activity of daily living that should be included in a comprehensive assessment of long-term care needs of older adults?
- Do I feel more comfortable discussing sexual function with people who are of the same gender and age range as myself, but very uncomfortable in discussing this matter with people who are old enough to be my parents or grandparents?
- Do I avoid discussion of sexual function with older adults because I believe they are not interested in sexual activity or are uncomfortable discussing this topic?
- Do I avoid discussing sexual function with older adults who are not in traditional marital relationships?

- What beliefs do I hold about the assessment of sexual function based on the age of the person? For example, do I think sexual function should be assessed in sexually active teenagers who are at risk for unwanted pregnancy, but not older people?
- Am I comfortable incorporating health education about safe sex practices with older adults?

What Is My Attitude About Various Expressions of Sexual Activity?

- How do I view sexual activity and romantic relationships between unmarried people, or between people of the same gender?
- How do I view masturbation?
- Do my views about masturbation or sexual activity between unmarried or same-gender people influence my assessment of and interventions for people who engage in these activities?
- Am I tolerant and nonjudgmental toward people whose views and practices are nontraditional or different from mine?

For Nurses in Settings Where Long-Term Needs Are Addressed

- How do I feel about the rights of residents to engage in sexual activity in private, either with themselves or people of their own choosing?
- Do I try to ensure privacy for those residents who desire it?
- If I am aware of the sexual activities of a resident, do I think that I should inform the administrator, a family member, or another "responsible adult?"

broader than asking about marital status. Also, recognize that since 2015 same-sex marriage has been legally recognized throughout the United States; however, LGBT couples in long-term committed relationships may choose not to marry for a variety of reasons. When addressing an older adult

who has acknowledged that he or she identifies as LGBT, nurses can ask in a nonjudgmental manner about the terminology that person prefers in reference to his or her partner or spouse. Terminology related to people who identify as LGBT is delineated in Box 26-5.

Box 26-5 Cultural Considerations: Cultural Aspects of Sexual Function

Expressions of Sexuality and Intimacy

- In some cultures, direct eye contact, especially between a man and woman, is interpreted as an expression of intimacy.
- In some cultures, it is taboo for a man to be alone with a woman other than his wife.
- Touching another person (particularly of the opposite sex) is considered taboo in many cultures.
- In some cultures, heterosexual men and women commonly hold hands with another person of the same gender.
- Not all cultures value sexual equality between men and women.
- Homosexuality is accepted in some cultures but is considered taboo or is kept secret among family members in others.

Assessment Considerations

- In some cultures, it is considered taboo for postmenopausal women to have their breasts or vagina examined, even by a health care provider.
- Menopausal manifestations may vary in different cultural groups (e.g., Japanese women may not experience hot flashes).

Terms Describing Sexual Orientation (i.e., One's Sexual and Romantic Attraction)

- *Heterosexual:* sexual attraction to people of the opposite sex
- *Bisexual:* sexual attraction to both men and women
- *Homosexual:* sexual attraction to people of the same sex; the term applies to both men and women and is associated more with biologic aspects rather than with lifestyle characteristics
- *Gay:* the term that is associated with lifestyle characteristics of men who feel romantically attracted to other men
- *Lesbian:* the term that is associated with lifestyle characteristics of women who feel romantically attracted to other women

Terms Describing Sexual Identity (i.e., a Combination of Biologic Characteristics and Social Roles)

- *Transgender:* people whose gender identity, gender expression, or behavior do not conform to that typically associated with the sex to which they were assigned at birth
- *Female-to-male* or *male-to-female transgenders* may be preparing for or recovering from sexual reassignment surgery, or they may be using long-term hormonal therapy as a nonsurgical option

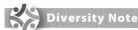

Diversity Note

It is important to recognize that transgender adults may choose to transition during older adulthood for the following reasons: no longer being constrained by job or family considerations; individual maturation factors associated with increasing self-acceptance and personal perception of successful aging; and changing societal attitudes and expanded resources and supports (Fabbre, 2017).

Assessing Sexual Function in Older Adults

Two goals of assessing sexual function in older adults are to provide an opportunity for the older adult to discuss any concerns related to sexual function and to identify risk factors, including lack of information and risk-taking behaviors. Although the extent of the assessment varies according to individual circumstances, it minimally includes questions about the gynecologic aspects for women and genitourinary aspects for men. Incorporate these questions into a routine assessment of overall function and then ask an additional open-ended question about sexual interest and activities. When problems or risk factors are identified, obtain enough additional information to suggest appropriate resources for further evaluation. Box 26-6 summarizes guidelines for assessing sexual function in older adults. In addition, nurses have important roles in teaching about screening for and prevention of sexually transmitted infections.

The Hartford Institute for Geriatric Nursing recommends that nurses use the PLISSIT assessment model as a routine nursing assessment for older adults. The four components of this model are as follows:

- Obtaining *Permission* from the client to initiate sexual discussion
- Providing *Limited Information* about sexual function
- Giving *Specific Suggestions* for the individual to proceed with sexual relations
- Providing *Intensive Therapy* surrounding the issues of sexuality for the client

Online Learning Activity 26-4 provides additional information demonstrating the application of this tool in a clinical setting.

See ONLINE LEARNING ACTIVITY 26-4: EVIDENCE-BASED TOOL FOR ASSESSING SEXUALITY FOR OLDER ADULTS at http://thepoint.lww.com/Miller8e.

NURSING DIAGNOSIS

When nurses identify risks that interfere with sexual function, or when older adults express an interest in discussing sexual function, the appropriate nursing diagnosis is Ineffective Sexuality Pattern, defined as "expressions of concern regarding own sexuality" (Herdman & Kamitsura, 2018, p. 306). Related factors commonly identified in older adults include medication effects; endocrine diseases (e.g.,

diabetes); cardiovascular diseases; genitourinary conditions; functional impairments secondary to chronic conditions (e.g., limited range of motion as a result of arthritis); psychosocial circumstances (e.g., lack of a partner); and myths and misunderstandings about age-related changes. The case example at the end of this chapter addresses this nursing diagnosis.

Wellness Opportunity

The nursing diagnosis of Readiness for Enhanced Knowledge: Sexual Function would be applicable to older adults who express an interest in learning about the effects of aging or risk factors on sexual wellness.

PLANNING FOR WELLNESS OUTCOMES

Increased knowledge about sexual functioning is an expected outcome for older adults who lack accurate information about age-related changes and risk factors. An outcome for residents of long-term care facilities would be Client Satisfaction: Protection of Rights. For a long-term care resident who is LGBT, an applicable outcome would be Client Satisfaction: Cultural Needs Fulfillment. Nurses can use the following additional Nursing Outcomes Classification terminologies in care plans to promote sexual wellness for older adults: Body Image, Knowledge: Sexual Functioning, Personal Well-Being, Self-Esteem, and Psychosocial Adjustment: Life Change.

Wellness Opportunity

Quality of Life is a wellness outcome for older adults who achieve more satisfying relationships through a variety of expressions of intimacy.

NURSING INTERVENTIONS TO PROMOTE HEALTHY SEXUAL FUNCTION

Nurses have many opportunities to teach older adults about healthy sexual function as an important aspect of quality of life, particularly in community and long-term care settings. Teaching about age-related changes and risk factors is especially important for gerontological nurses because many older adults, as well as family and caregivers, hold stereotypes or have little accurate information about sexuality and aging. For documentation in care plans, use the following Nursing Interventions Classification terminologies: Body Image Enhancement, Energy Management, Health Education, Patient Rights Protection, Sexual Counseling, Self-Esteem Enhancement, Teaching: Sexuality, and Teaching: Safe Sex.

Teaching Older Adults About Sexual Wellness

Unlike sex therapists or primary health care providers, nurses are not expected to provide sex education or direct

Box 26-6 Guidelines for Assessing Sexual Function in Older Adults

Interview Atmosphere and Communication Techniques

- Ensure both privacy and comfort.
- Be nonjudgmental and matter-of-fact in verbal and nonverbal communication.
- If feasible, sit face-to-face in chairs, rather than conducting the interview while the person being interviewed is in bed.
- If feasible, allow the person being interviewed to wear usual daytime clothing, rather than a hospital gown.

Initiation and Discussion of the Topic

- Begin by acknowledging feelings of discomfort and by stating the reason for discussing this topic (e.g., "I know that sexuality is a private matter and people are often uncomfortable discussing this topic. However, as a nurse, I consider sexuality to be an aspect of health and well-being, and it may have a significant bearing on your overall care.").
- Include statements that address stereotypes and require a response from the older adult (e.g., "Our society tends to view old people as being uninterested in sex, but for most older people, this is not true. Many older people are less sexually active than when they were younger, but this is not because of age-related changes. Have you experienced any changes in your sexual activities in the past few years?").
- Initiate the topic near the end of a comprehensive assessment interview, and begin with questions about the physiologic aspects of male or female function, such as those that follow.
- Incorporate at least one question to assess the appropriateness of including information about safe sex practices in your health teaching (e.g., "If you have sex with partners other than someone who is in a long-term monogamous relationship with you, what precautions do you take?").

Interview Questions to Assess Male Sexual Function

- Have you ever had prostate problems or related surgery? Have you ever been told that you have or had an enlarged prostate?
- How often do you undergo a complete medical examination? When was your last complete physical examination done?
- Do you ever experience dribbling of urine or have problems holding your water?
- Do you have any trouble initiating the stream of urine?
- After you have urinated (passed water), do you still feel like you haven't emptied your bladder completely?
- Do you have to get up during the night to empty your bladder? If so, how many times?
- Have you ever noticed any blood in your urine?
- Do you ever have any discharge from your penis?
- Do you have any sores, lumps, ulcers, irritations, or areas of inflammation on your penis or scrotum?
- Do you have any trouble with erection or ejaculation?

Interview Questions to Assess Female Sexual Function

- How many children, if any, have you had? How many pregnancies?
- At what ages did your menstrual periods begin and end?
- Have you ever had a Pap (Papanicolaou) test? When was your most recent Pap test and gynecologic examination?
- Have you ever had a mammogram? When was the most recent one?
- Have you ever been taught to examine your breasts for lumps?
- Do you examine your breasts for lumps? How often?
- Have you noticed any changes in your breasts? Do you ever have any discharge from your nipples?
- Do you have any burning, itching, or irritation in the vaginal area?
- Do you ever have any vaginal discharge or bleeding?
- Do you have any difficulties with sexual intercourse?

Principles for Assessing Sexual Interest and Activities

- If the older adult makes a clear statement that this topic is irrelevant, do not insist on further questions. If the older adult responds to questions, however, do not discontinue the interview because of your own discomfort.
- Do not assume that an assessment of sexual function is irrelevant to unmarried people.
- For both married and unmarried older adults, use open-ended questions to elicit information about intimate relationships (e.g., "Is there anything you would like to ask or discuss about intimate relationships?").
- For a married person, open-ended questions may be asked about the partner's influence on sexual activities (e.g., "Has your husband experienced any changes in his health that have affected your sexual activities?").
- Listen for statements that reflect myths, a negative self-image, or self-fulfilling prophecies, such as "Of course I stopped being interested in sex after menopause," or "I can't have an erection because I have prostate trouble."
- If risk factors, such as certain medications or pathologic conditions, have been identified earlier in the interview, ask additional questions, such as "Have you had any difficulties with sexual activities since your heart attack?" or "Do you have any questions about the possible effects of diabetes on sexual activity?"
- Emphasize the clinical reason for the questions ("Sometimes certain illnesses or medications interfere with sexual function, and we want to identify any problems you might be having in this area.").
- Use open-ended questions that allow for either closure of the topic or a further discussion of issues ("Is there anything you would like to discuss with regard to your sexual relationships?").

interventions; however, nurses are expected to address sexual function as a quality-of-life concern. Evidence-based nursing guidelines state that "the most important intervention to improving sexuality among the older adult population is education" (Steinke, 2016, p. 170). Health education about sexual wellness for older adults includes the following information:

- Acknowledgment that sexual function is within the usual realm of health promotion for older adults, especially in long-term care settings

- Effects of age-related changes on sexual function
- Risk factors that cause or contribute to problems with sexual function
- Resources for addressing identified problems and risk factors
- Protection from sexually transmitted infections

In addition, nurses in long-term care settings often need to address attitudes of the staff members, families, and residents by providing accurate information and modeling nonjudgmental behaviors.

Box 26-7 Health Education About Sexual Activity for Older People

Facts True for Both Older Men and Older Women

- Older people remain fully capable of enjoying orgasm, but their response to sexual stimulation usually is slower, less intense, and of shorter duration. Increasing the amount and diversity of sexual stimulation and experimenting with different positions can compensate for these changes and increase sexual enjoyment.
- The "use it or lose it" principle applies to sexual activity.
- Sexual problems in older people occur for the same reasons they occur in younger people. That is, they may be related to illness or disability, medications or alcohol, or psychological and relationship factors. A cause of sexual problems that is unique to older people is the self-fulfilling prophecy of the "sexless senior" stereotype.
- The following habits enhance sexual enjoyment: exercising regularly, avoiding or limiting consumption of alcohol, maintaining optimal health and nutrition, using hearing aids and corrective lenses as needed, and engaging in sexual activities when you are relaxed and your energy level is at its peak.
- If you experience problems with sexual function, seek advice from a professional who is skilled in working with older people. Medical help can be obtained from a urologist, gynecologist, or other medical specialist. If there is no medical basis for the problem, a sex therapist or marriage counselor might be helpful.
- If you engage in sexual activity with anyone other than your long-term monogamous partner, protect yourself from sexually transmitted infections and talk with your health care practitioner about being tested periodically.

Facts Specific to Older Men

- Periodic difficulties with erection and ejaculation do not necessarily indicate that you are impotent.
- After you've reached orgasm, it may be 1 or 2 days before you are able to reach full orgasm again.
- Many new treatment options are available for treating erectile dysfunction (impotence). If your health care provider cannot provide up-to-date information about these options, ask for a referral for an appropriate evaluation and discussion of various options.

Facts Specific to Older Women

- Using a water-soluble lubricant will compensate for decreased vaginal lubrication. Do *not* use petroleum jelly because it is not a very effective lubricant for this purpose and can predispose you to infection.
- Estrogen is beneficial in preventing some problems with sexual function, but the relative risks and benefits of such therapy should be considered and discussed thoroughly with your primary care provider.
- You may have vaginal irritation or urinary tract infections, especially after sexual intercourse, because of age-related thinning of the vaginal wall. Such problems may be avoided by the following interventions:
  - Drink plenty of fluids.
  - Use an estrogen cream or vaginal lubricant.
  - Maintain good hygiene in the vaginal area.
  - If you have a male partner, have him thrust his penis downward, toward the back of your vagina.
  - Empty your bladder before and after intercourse.

It is important to use excellent communication skills and ensure privacy and confidentiality when teaching older adults or caregivers about age-related changes and risk factors that affect sexual function. Use an approach that is open, respectful, nonjudgmental, and gender neutral. Box 26-7 is a teaching tool written in nontechnical terms that can be used for health education of older adults. As with many other aspects of health education, emphasize that major changes in sexual function are not due to age-related changes alone, which are summarized in Table 26-1. Use Online Learning Activity 26-5 to explore resources for reliable information about sexuality and aging.

See ONLINE LEARNING ACTIVITY 26-5: RESOURCES FOR HEALTH PROMOTION at http://thepoint.lww.com/Miller8e.

Wellness Opportunity

Nurses promote personal responsibility for sexual wellness by suggesting sources of accurate information that older adults can use.

Addressing Risk Factors

If an older adult with significant changes in sexual function also has a pathologic condition, takes a medication, or uses any substance that might be a contributing factor, provide information about the potential influence of these risk factors. This is particularly important when the older person inaccurately attributes sexual problems to aging rather than to a manageable and reversible risk factor. For example, an older man may attribute a problem with attaining an erection to age-related changes, when, in fact, he has diabetes and takes an antihypertensive medication that is associated with erectile dysfunction. Use Box 26-1 to identify some of the medications that can interfere with sexual function. When a potential relationship between a risk factor and sexual problems is identified, suggest that the older adult seek professional advice. A complete medical evaluation by a primary care provider who is knowledgeable about the sexual problems of older adults is a good starting point. When a review of medications identifies adverse effects that contribute to sexual dysfunction, alternative drugs or reduced doses may resolve the problem. For example, people with hypertension are less likely to have sexual dysfunction when treated with calcium channel blockers, angiotensin-converting enzyme inhibitors, or peripheral alpha-adrenergic receptor blockers. After medical problems are addressed, a mental health professional may be an appropriate resource if problems with sexual function persist.

Arthritis is one of the most common pathologic conditions affecting older adults, and in many cases, it is self-managed with little or no medical supervision. Often, the symptoms are not severe enough to motivate the older adult to seek medical

Box 26-8 Health Education About Sexual Activity for People With Arthritis

The pain, fatigue, and joint limitations of arthritis may interfere with, but do not have to curtail, your enjoyment of sexual activity. In fact, sexual activity can be beneficial to you because it stimulates the release of cortisone, adrenalin, and other chemicals that are natural pain relievers. The following actions may enhance your sexual enjoyment and minimize the effects of arthritis:

- Engage in sexual activity when you feel least fatigued and most relaxed.
- Use analgesic medications and other methods of pain relief before engaging in sexual activity.
- Use relaxation techniques before engaging in sexual activity. Relaxation techniques that may be helpful for arthritis include warm baths or showers and the application of hot packs to the affected joints.
- Maintain optimal health through good nutrition and a proper balance of rest and activity.
- Experiment with different sexual positions and use pillows for comfort and support.
- Increase the time spent in foreplay.
- Use a vibrator if your ability to massage is limited by arthritis.
- Use a water-soluble jelly for vaginal lubrication.

Box 26-9 Health Education About Sexual Activity for People With Cardiovascular Disease

- Participation in a medically supervised exercise program can reduce oxygen requirements during sexual activity and improve the quality of your sex life.
- The typical energy expenditure for sexual intercourse is equivalent to that used for climbing two flights of steps.
- Do not engage in sexual activity in extremely hot and humid environments.
- Wait 3 hours after consuming alcohol or a large meal before initiating sexual activity.
- Engage in sexual activity when your energy is at its peak and you are feeling rested and relaxed.
- Avoid sexual activity during times of intense emotional stress.
- Avoid engaging in sexual activity with a partner with whom you are uncomfortable (e.g., an extramarital partner).
- Experiment with different positions to find one that is least demanding of your energy.
- Consider using nitroglycerin, if ordered by your primary care provider, as needed before sexual activity.
- Know that many types of oral medications for erectile dysfunction can cause serious (even fatal) interactions with nitrates.
- Consult your primary care provider if you experience chest pain during or after sexual activity, or breathlessness or heart palpitations persisting for 15 minutes after orgasm.

evaluation and treatment, but they may interfere with sexual activities. In such cases, nurses can use Box 26-8 to teach about self-care interventions that may be effective in improving the quality of sexual activities for the older adult with arthritis. Nurses can also suggest that older adults who have arthritis obtain pamphlets from local chapters of the Arthritis Foundation (see resources in Online Learning Activity 26-6).

Another pathologic condition often associated with sexual dysfunction is coronary artery disease, particularly in those who have had myocardial infarctions or who have undergone coronary artery bypass surgery. Nurses have important—but often overlooked—roles in providing information about sexual concerns for their partners in all health care settings, including at discharge from acute care. Studies indicate that patients with cardiovascular conditions expect their health care providers to initiate discussions about sexual activity (Steinke, Johansen, Dusenbury, 2016). For example, fear and anxiety are major barriers to resumption of sexual activity after myocardial infarctions, and nurses and other health care professionals could effectively address these barriers through health education (Zeydi, Sharafkhani, Armat, et al., 2016). Nurses can encourage older adults to discuss concerns about sexual activity with their cardiology professional or primary care practitioner and can provide health education using the general guidelines outlined in Box 26-9. Nurses also can inform older adults that the American Heart Association has a free booklet that provides advice about sexual activity for patients with common cardiovascular conditions (see resources in Online Learning Activity 26-6).

Online Learning Activity 26-6 provides a link to an article about practical approaches and evidence-based guidelines

that nurses can use to address sexual function in patients with cardiovascular disease. Case examples illustrate application of information to patients with angina pectoris, myocardial infarction, coronary artery bypass grafting, implanted cardioverter defibrillator, and heart failure. Overall principles discussed in this article can be applied to assessment and health education related to other aspects of sexual function for older adults.

See ONLINE LEARNING ACTIVITY 26-6: ARTICLE WITH CASE SCENARIOS ABOUT COUNSELING PATIENTS WITH CARDIOVASCULAR DISEASE at http://thepoint.lww.com/Miller8e.

Promoting Sexual Wellness in Long-Term Care Settings

Responsibilities of nurses in long-term care settings to address sexual needs differ from those responsibilities of nurses in acute care or home settings in the following ways:

- Intense medical needs of patients in acute care settings take precedence over sexual needs.
- The short duration of stay in acute care settings is not conducive to addressing long-term sexual needs of patients.
- Because of the high degree of privacy and autonomy for people in their own homes, home care nurses are not routinely concerned about sexual needs.

Residents in long-term care facilities, however, usually are not acutely ill, are planning to stay in the facility for a long time, and do depend on the nursing staff to ensure the privacy necessary to meet their personal needs. Thus, the nurse in long-term care facilities must address the sexual needs of residents as an integral part of the overall care plan.

Staff education is an important part of addressing the sexual needs of older adults in long-term care facilities because staff members need to know about all aspects of sexuality and aging, including the lifelong interest in and need for sexual activity and intimate relationships. Audiovisual materials can be used to stimulate discussion about the unique aspects of meeting sexual needs in institutional settings and about the responsibilities and limitations of staff members. Nurses generally participate in such in-services as part of the interdisciplinary team, which also includes social service and administrative staff. Presenters and discussion leaders should be nonjudgmental and matter-of-fact so that they model the most effective approach for addressing this sensitive topic.

When the ability of a cognitively impaired resident to give informed consent is questionable, an interdisciplinary team can assess competence to participate in an intimate relationship. Emphasis should be placed on the Residents' Rights bill, as defined by the federal government in the 1987 Nursing Home Reform Law. Sexual needs of residents of long-term care facilities are protected through the rights to:

- Self-determination
- Participation in their own care
- Independence in making personal decisions
- Reasonable accommodation of their needs and preferences
- Privacy and unrestricted communication with any person of their choice
- Immediate access by their relatives and others, subject to reasonable restriction with the resident's permission

In addition to educating staff members about the sexual needs and rights of residents, nurses are responsible for ensuring privacy for those residents who desire it. If a resident does not have a private room, staff members try to provide privacy, while still respecting the rights of any roommates. Sometimes, the role of the nurse will be that of a negotiator, assisting residents in reaching mutually acceptable agreements about privacy and shared space.

Wellness Opportunity

Nurses respect autonomy by working with other staff members to assess the ability of someone with dementia to make decisions about expressions of sexuality.

Teaching Women About Interventions

Hormonal therapy refers to the use of estrogen alone or with progestogen for symptoms of natural or surgically induced menopause. Use of **menopausal hormonal therapy (MHT)** (also called hormonal replacement therapy) has a long and controversial history, beginning in the 1940s when it was a common medical intervention to alleviate vasomotor symptoms associated with menopause. During the early 2000s, results of the Women's Health Initiative and other major studies raised questions about the safety of MHT. Consequently, many women who had been taking MHT for years discontinued these medications, and fewer women initiated this intervention. Currently, major organizations such as the North American Menopause Society and international consensus groups periodically update their recommendations based on evolving evidence. Consistently, recommendations emphasize the importance of basing decisions about MHT on an individualized assessment of the person's risks and benefits by a knowledgeable health care practitioner. For all older women, interventions that may be beneficial and without controversy are those that emphasize a healthy lifestyle (e.g., regular exercise, stress management, nutritious food, healthy weight, and no smoking). In addition, women can be encouraged to use lubricants, moisturizers, or prescription estrogen cream for vaginal dryness. Because these recommendations change frequently based on evolving evidence, it is important to keep up to date on current recommendations through reliable resources listed in Online Learning Activity 26-6.

Teaching Men About Interventions

Testosterone therapy has gained increasing attention in recent years, with prescriptions for various forms of testosterone tripling in the last decade in the United States (Hackett, 2016). Although earlier studies indicated that testosterone replacement therapy was associated with increased risk for prostate cancer and cardiovascular disease, more recent studies (including meta-analyses) have questioned these findings and indicate that increased testosterones levels are associated with reduced mortality as well as overall health benefits, such as increased lean body mass and reduced total cholesterol (Guo, Gu, Liu, et al., 2016; Hassan & Barkin, 2016; Khera, 2016). The most consistent conclusion of recent studies is that treatment decisions should be individualized, based on a multifaceted approach, and include full discussion of potential benefits and risks (Hackett, 2016; Nian, Ding, Hu, et al., 2017). Nurses have important roles in encouraging older men to seek a comprehensive evaluation of signs and symptoms that may be associated with late-onset hypogonadism so informed decisions can be made about treatment approaches.

Interventions for erectile dysfunction have been available for several decades, but until recently, these interventions were not widely used, in part because men did not seek help for this condition. The recent explosion of media attention related to medications and other interventions has brought much attention to this topic and erectile dysfunction is now commonly recognized as a treatable condition. Sildenafil (Viagra) is the most commonly used drug of this type, called oral phosphodiesterase-5 inhibitors, and additional drugs in this class are vardenafil (Levitra), tadalafil (Cialis), and avanafil (Stendra). These medications are prescribed either as needed or on a regular dosing schedule depending on the onset and duration of action of each one. Common adverse effects include headache, flushing, indigestion, dizziness, and nasal congestion. These medications are contraindicated for men taking nitrate medications because they can cause serious and even fatal adverse effects.

In addition to the oral agents that are widely publicized, several types of semi-rigid or inflatable penile prostheses, such as the vacuum erection device, are used as safe and effective treatments for erectile dysfunction. Some of these devices require a surgical procedure, but some can be self-administered. Another pharmacologic approach is the administration of a vasoactive drug, such as prostaglandin E1 (Alprostadil), as an intracavernosal injection, a topical cream, or an intraurethral suppository. In recent years, penile rehabilitation programs have evolved as a common treatment for erectile dysfunction following prostatectomy; however, patients have difficulty maintaining compliance with this treatment during the 18 to 24 months required for effectiveness (Emanu, Avildsen, & Nelson, 2016; Matthew, 2016). Recent studies also indicate that pelvic floor muscle exercises, which are described in Chapter 19, may be effective for some types of male sexual dysfunction (Kirages & Johnson, 2016). Nurses do not need to be familiar with the details of these procedures, but they need to know enough about interventions to suggest that men discuss their options with a physician. Also, nurses can teach about roles of specialists, such as physical therapists for pelvic floor muscle rehabilitation.

Another nursing responsibility is to discuss interventions to address risk factors that cause or contribute to sexual dysfunction. Risk factors that are within the realm of health education include obesity, smoking cessation, glucose control, and treatment of hyperlipidemia

(Rubin & Goldstein, 2016). In addition, it is important to suggest that men have their medications reviewed by prescribing practitioners in relation to potential causes of erectile dysfunction. Psychotherapy and behavioral therapy are primary or adjunctive treatment options to address the psychosocial issues that may be contributing to erectile dysfunction. Decisions about appropriate treatment options must be based on a comprehensive evaluation by a urologist or a primary care provider who is knowledgeable about erectile dysfunction and sexual health issues. The primary responsibility of nurses is to keep current on the types of interventions that are available and to teach about the importance of seeking help for erectile dysfunction.

EVALUATING EFFECTIVENESS OF NURSING INTERVENTIONS

Nursing care for older adults with the diagnosis of Ineffective Sexuality Pattern is evaluated by the degree to which risk factors are eliminated, particularly through the provision of accurate information. For example, older adults may verbalize an improved understanding of the age-related changes that affect their response to sexual stimulation. In turn, this information can alleviate anxiety about sexual performance and improve quality of life. Interventions to alleviate risk factors, such as medical conditions or adverse medication/chemical effects, would be considered successful if the older adult follows through with a referral to an appropriate resource. One measure of successful intervention in long-term care settings would be that staff members increase their understanding of the sexual needs of older adults and are more comfortable allowing appropriate sexual expressions by the residents.

Unfolding Case Study

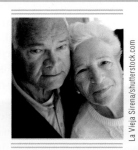
La Vieja Sirena/shutterstock.com

Part 2: Mr. and Mrs. J. at 75 and 73 Years of Age

Mr. and Mrs. J. are now 75 and 73 years old, respectively, and they have moved to an assisted-living facility where you are the nurse. Their health conditions have not changed significantly in the past 2 years, with the exception of Mrs. J. having more difficulty walking because of her arthritis. Mr. and Mrs. J. recently moved to the facility because they needed help with transportation and wanted to live in a place where they had fewer responsibilities and more time to enjoy life. During one of their appointments, Mrs. J. becomes tearful and says she has been disappointed in their move from their own home. She says, "Now we have the time to enjoy our life together, but we seem to be in each other's way all the time. When we lived in our own home, we were so busy with the yard and the housekeeping and all the daily chores, we never had time to think about what we enjoy together. Now I don't have to cook meals and worry about getting to the grocery store, but we aren't enjoying the time we have together."

Part 2: Mr. and Mrs. J. at 75 and 73 Years of Age *(Continued)*

NURSING ASSESSMENT

On further discussion, Mrs. J. acknowledges that she talked with her husband about having more "intimate time and resuming sexual activities that have decreased in the past few years because we were always so tired and never seemed to have much time." In reply, Mr. J. stated that "We're probably too old to do those things, and old people shouldn't expect to have the fun in bed that we used to have." Mrs. J. says she used to believe that, but recently she's been talking with some of the other women in the assisted-living facility who seem to be enjoying sexual activities. Mr. and Mrs. J. relate that they had a good sexual relationship until Mr. J.'s heart attack 5 years ago. After that, he lost interest in sexual activities, even though he was told he could resume all his usual activities except for very strenuous activity, such as shoveling snow. Mrs. J. says she masturbates occasionally, but she doesn't find that very satisfying. Mrs. J. expresses concern about being comfortable in the sexual position they used previously because her arthritis has gotten worse in the past few years.

NURSING DIAGNOSIS

You address Ineffective Sexuality Patterns as your nursing diagnosis for Mr. and Mrs. J. Related factors include myths and lack of information about the age-related changes and risk factors that influence sexual function. Potential risk factors that you identify are Mr. J.'s medications and his lack of information about sexual function after a heart attack.

NURSING CARE PLAN FOR MR. AND MRS. J.

Expected Outcome	Nursing Evaluation	Nursing Interventions
Mr. and Mrs. J.'s knowledge about age-related changes and risk factors that affect sexual function will be increased	• Use Box 26-7 as a basis for discussion of sexual function in later adulthood	• Mr. and Mrs. J. will verbalize correct information about sexual function in older adulthood
The risk factors associated with Mr. J.'s heart attack and medication regimen will be addressed	• Explain that many medications for heart problems and high blood pressure are associated with problems with sexual function • Use Box 26-9 as a basis for discussing sexual activity as it relates to people with heart problems • Encourage Mr. J. to talk with his primary care provider about his medication regimen and about his heart condition. Suggest that he inquire whether a different medication would effectively treat his high blood pressure without interfering with sexual function	• Mr. J. will agree to talk with his primary care provider about the potential relationship between his medications and heart condition and his lack of sexual activity
The risk factors associated with Mrs. J.'s arthritis will be addressed	• Use Box 26-8 to discuss sexual activity as it relates to people with arthritis	• Mrs. J. will identify ways to increase her comfort during sexual activities

THINKING POINTS

- What risk factors are likely to influence Mrs. J.'s enjoyment of sexual activity?
- What risk factors are likely to affect Mr. J.'s enjoyment of sexual activity?
- What health education would you provide for Mrs. J., and what patient teaching tools would you use?
- What health education would you provide for Mr. J., and what patient teaching tools would you use?

(continued)

Part 2: Mr. and Mrs. J. at 75 and 73 Years of Age *(Continued)*

QSEN APPLICATION

QSEN Competency	Knowledge/Skill/Attitude	Application to Mr. & Mrs. J. When They Are 75 and 73 Years Old
Patient-centered care	(K) Integrate understanding of multiple dimensions of patient-centered care (K) Describe strategies to empower patients in all aspects of the health care process (K) Discuss principles of effective communication (S) Elicit patient values, preferences, and expressed needs (S) Provide patient-centered care with sensitivity and respect for diversity of the human experience (S) Assess own level of communication skill in encounters with patients and families	• Base care plan on an assessment of individual needs of both Mr. and Mrs. J. • Provide information about age-related changes and risk factors that affect sexual function as an intervention for empowering Mr. and Mrs. J. toward resolution of their sexual issues • Assess your own attitudes related to sexuality in older adults, so you can effectively discuss this topic with Mr. and Mrs. J. • Communicate a nonjudgmental and open attitude when discussing this sensitive topic
Evidence-based practice	(S) Base individualized care plan on patient values, clinical expertise, and evidence (S) Read original research and evidence reports related to clinical practice (A) Value evidence-based practice as integral to determining the best clinical practice.	Stay current on the topic of sexual function in older adults by exploring the resources listed in Online Learning Activities 26-1 and 26-6

Chapter Highlights

Age-Related Changes That Affect Sexual Wellness

- Diminished levels of hormones and degenerative changes of reproductive organs in both men and women
- Women: cessation of menses, onset of menopause, loss of reproductive ability
- Men: Low testosterone (i.e., andropause), gradual decline but not total loss of reproductive ability

Risk Factors That Affect Sexual Wellness

- Societal influences, especially on attitudes, stereotypes, and prejudices
- Effects of attitudes and behaviors of families and caregivers, especially on dependent older adults
- Limited opportunities for sexual activity (lower ratio of men to women, health conditions)
- Adverse effects of medication, alcohol, and nicotine (Box 26-1)
- Chronic conditions
- Gender-specific conditions
- Functional impairments
- Dementia (Box 26-2)

Functional Consequences Affecting Sexual Wellness

- Reproductive ability: ceases in women, diminishes in men
- Response to sexual stimulation: slower and less intense (Table 26-1)
- Sexual interest and activity: maintenance of interest and capacity in most older adults, but diminished sexual activity due to risk factors
- Male and female sexual dysfunction

Pathologic Condition Affecting Sexual Wellness: Human Immunodeficiency Virus

- Increasing numbers of adults aged 50 years and older have HIV
- Health-related concerns associated with HIV in older adults (Box 26-3)
- Risk factors differ for older adults (less likely to be tested or to practice safe sex)
- Nurses have important roles in identifying new cases of HIV, assessing risks for sexually transmitted infections, and assessing treatment issues (i.e., adverse effects, drug interactions)
- Nurses need to teach about safe sex practices

Nursing Assessment of Sexual Function

- Self-assessment of attitudes about sexual function and aging (Box 26-4)
- Assessment of cultural influences (Box 26-5)
- General principles of and specific interview questions for nursing assessment (Box 26-6)
- Using the PLISSIT assessment model

Nursing Diagnosis

- Readiness for Enhanced Knowledge: Sexual Functioning
- Ineffective Sexuality Pattern

Planning for Wellness Outcomes

- For residents in long-term care facilities: Client Satisfaction, Protection of Rights, Cultural Needs Fulfillment
- Body Image
- Personal Well-Being
- Self-Esteem
- Sexual Functioning

Nursing Interventions to Promote Sexual Wellness (Boxes 26-7 Through 26-9)

- Teaching older adults about sexual wellness: age-related changes and risk factors
- Addressing risk factors: teaching about sexual activity for people with arthritis or cardiovascular disease
- Promoting sexual wellness in long-term care facilities: staff education, protection of rights, ensuring privacy
- Teaching women about interventions for the effects of menopause and men about interventions for erectile dysfunction

Evaluating Effectiveness of Nursing Interventions

- Provision of accurate information to dispel myths and misconceptions
- Improved quality of life
- Referrals to health care professionals for addressing risk factors
- Increased knowledge and comfort of staff in long-term care facilities

Critical Thinking Exercises

1. Describe the attitudinal risk factors on the parts of society, older adults, and health care providers that can interfere with healthy sexual function in older adults.
2. Summarize the functional consequences that are likely to affect sexual function in healthy older men and women.
3. What are the responsibilities of nurses in each of the following settings related to assessment of sexual function in older adults: community setting, acute care facility, and long-term care facility?
4. Describe the assessment and health education approaches you might use for a 73-year-old married man who confides that he has difficulty making his wife "happy in bed."

5. Spend a few minutes answering all the questions included in Box 26-3, Assessing Personal Attitudes Toward Sexuality and Aging. What did you learn about yourself?

 For more information about the topics discussed in this chapter, be sure to check out the interactive Online Learning Activities and other helpful resources at http://thepoint.lww.com/Miller8e.

REFERENCES

Administration on Aging. (2016). *A profile of older Americans: 2015.* Washington DC: U. S. Department of Health and Human Services.

Almeida, O. P., Marsh, K., Flicker, L., et al. (2016). Depressive symptoms in midlife: The role of reproductive stage. *Menopause: The Journal of the North American Menopause Society, 23,* 669–675.

Atallah, S. (2016). Cultural aspects in sexual function and dysfunction in the geriatric population. *Topics in Geriatric Rehabilitation, 32,* 156–166.

Barmon, C., Burgess, E. O., Bender, A. A., et al. (2017). Understanding sexual freedom and autonomy in assisted living: Discourse of residents' rights among staff and administrators. *Journals of Gerontology: Psychological Sciences and Social Sciences, 72,* 457–467.

Binmoammar, T. A., Hassounah, S., Alsaad, S., et al. (2016). The impact of poor glycaemic control on the prevalence of erectile dysfunction in men with type 2 diabetes mellitus: A systematic review. *Journal of the Royal Society of Medicine, Open,* Feb 12; 7(3): 2054270415622602. Doi: 10.1177/2054270415622602.

Bolat, M. S., Akdeniz, E., Ozkaya, S., et al. (2016). Smoking and lower urinary tract symptoms. *Urology Journal, 12,* 2447–2451.

Brandon, M. (2016). Psychosocial aspects of sexuality with aging. *Topics in Geriatric Rehabilitation, 32,* 151–155.

Bretschneider, J. G., & McCoy, N. L. (1988). Sexual interest and behavior in healthy 80- to 100-year olds. *Archives of Sexual Behavior, 17,* 109–129.

Caruso, S., Rapisarda, A. M., & Cianci, S. (2016). Sexuality in menopausal women. *Current Opinion in Psychiatry, 29,* 323–330.

Centers for Disease Control and Prevention (CDC). (2015). *National HIV Prevention Progress Report.* Available at www.cdc.gov.

Choi, J., Shin, D. W., Lee, S., et al. (2015). Dose-response relationship between cigarette smoking and female sexual dysfunction. *Obstetrics & Gynecology Science, 58,* 302–308.

Corona, G., Maseroli, E., Rastrelli, G., et al. (2016). Is late-onset hypogonadotropic hypogonadism a specific age-dependent disease, or merely an epiphenomenon caused by accumulating disease-burden? *Minerva Endocrinology, 41,* 196–210.

DeMarco, R. F., Brennan-Ing, M., Sprague, C., et al. (2017). Ageism, aging and HIV: Community responses to prevention, treatment, care and support. *Interdisciplinary Topics in Gerontology and Geriatrics, 42,* 234–239.

Dimopoulou, C., Ceausu, I., Depypere, H., et al. (2016). EMAS Position statement: Testosterone replacement therapy in the aging male. *Maturitas, 84,* 94–99.

Edwards, D., & Panay, N. (2016). Treating vulvovaginal atrophy/ genitourinary syndrome of menopause: How important is vaginal lubricant and moisturizer composition? *Climacteric, 2,* 151–161.

Emanu, J. C., Avildsen, I. K., & Nelson, C. J. (2016). Erectile dysfunction after radical prostatectomy: prevalence, medical treatments, and psychosocial interventions. *Current Opinion in Supportive and Palliative Care, 10,* 102–107.

Fabbre, V. D. (2017). Agency and social forces in the life course: The case of gender transitions in later life. *Journals of Gerontology: Psychological Sciences and Social Sciences, 72,* 479–487.

Forbes, M. K., Eaton, N. R., & Krueger, R. F. (2017). Sexual quality of life and aging: A prospective study of a nationally representative sample. *Journal of Sex Research, 54,* 137–148.

Gordon, J., Rubinow, D., Eisenlohr-Moul, T., et al. (2016). Estradiol variability, stressful life events, and the emergence of depressive symptomatology during the menopausal transition. *Menopause: The Journal of the North American Menopause Society, 23,* 357–366.

Guo, C., Gu, W., Liu, X., et al. (2016). Efficacy and safety of testosterone replacement therapy in men with hypogonadism: A meta-analysis study of placebo-controlled trials. *Experimental and Therapeutic Medicine, 11,* 853–863.

Hackett, G. (2016). An update on the role of testosterone replacement therapy in the management of hypogonadism. *Therapeutic Advances in Urology, 8*(21), 147–160.

Hassan, J., & Barkin, J. (2016). Testosterone deficiency syndrome: benefits, risks, and realities associated with testosterone replacement therapy. *Canadian Journal of Urology, 23* (Supplement 1), 20–26.

Herdman, T., & Kamitsura, S. (Eds). (2018). *NANDA International Nursing Diagnoses Definitions and Classification, 2018–2020* (11th ed., pp. 34–44). New York: Thieme Publishers.

Hickey, M., Schoenaker, D., Jaffe, J., et al. (2016). Depressive symptoms across the menopause transition: Findings from a large population-based cohort study. *Menopause: The Journal of the North American Menopause Society, 23,* 1287–1293.

Iglesia, C. (2016). What's new in the world of postmenopausal sex? *Current Opinion in Obstetrics and Gynecology, 28,* 449–454.

Karpiak, S. E., & Havlik, R. (2017). Are HIV-infected older adults aging differently? *Interdisciplinary topics in Gerontology and Geriatrics, 42,* 11–27.

Khera, M. (2016). Male hormones and men's quality of life. *Current Opinion in Urology, 26,* 152–157.

Kirages, D., & Johnson, E. (2106). Pelvic floor muscle rehabilitation to improve sexual function in geriatric men. *Topics in Geriatric Rehabilitation, 32,* 174–182.

Lee, D., Vanhoutte, B., Nazroo, J., et al. (2016). Sexual health and positive subjective well-being in partnered older men and women. *Journal of Gerontology: Psychological Sciences and Social Sciences, 71,* 698–710.

Lochlainn, M. N., & Kenny, R. A. (2013). Sexual activity and aging. *Journal of the American Medical Directors Association, 14*(8), 565–572.

Maiorino, M. I., Bellastella, G., Caputo, M., et al. (2016). Effects of Mediterranean diet in sexual function in people with newly diagnosed type 2 diabetes: the MEDITA trial. *Journal of Diabetes Complications, 30,* 1519–1524.

Masters, W. H., & Johnson, V. E. (1966). *Human sexual response.* Boston, MA: Little, Brown and company.

Matthew, A. (2016). Core principles of sexual health treatments in cancer for men. *Current Opinion in Supportive and Palliative Care, 10,* 38–43.

Milspaw, A., Brandon, K., & Sher, T. (2016). Including sexual function in patient evaluation in the rehabilitation setting. *Topics in Geriatric Rehabilitation, 32,* 221–228.

Nazarpour, S., Simbar, M., & Tehrani, F. R. (2016). Factors affecting sexual function in menopause: A review article. *Taiwanese Journal of Obstetrics & Gynecology, 55,* 480–487.

Nian, Y., Ding, M., Hu, S., et al. (2017). Testosterone replacement therapy improves health-related quality of life for patients with late-onset hypogonadism: A meta-analysis of randomized controlled trials. *Andrologia, 49.* Doi: 10.1111/and.12630. [Epub 2016 Jul 8.]

North American Menopause Society. (2016). *Clinical care recommendations: Menopause.* Available at www.nams.org.

Palacios-Cena, D., Martínez-Piedrola, R. M., Pérez-de-Heredia, M, et al. (2016). Expressing sexuality in nursing homes. The experience of older women: A qualitative study. *Geriatric Nursing, 37,* 470–477.

Pinkerton, J., Bushmakin, A., Abraham, L., et al. (2016). Most bothersome symptom in women with genitourinary syndrome of menopause as a moderator of treatment effects. *Menopause: The Journal of the North American Menopause Society, 23,* 1092–1101.

Rubin, R., & Goldstein, I. (2016). Medical management of sexual dysfunction in the aging male. *Topics in Geriatric Rehabilitation, 32,* 167–173.

Slag, M., Morley, J. E., Elson, M. K., et al. (1983). Impotence in medical clinic patients. *Journal of the American Medical Association, 249,* 1736–1740.

Smith, R. L., Gallicchio, L., Miller, S. R., et al. (2016). Risk factors for extended duration and timing of peak severity of hot flashes. *PLOS ONE, 1,* e0155079.

Sophocles, M. E. (2016). Medical management of age-related hormonal changes that affect sexual function. *Topics in Geriatric Rehabilitation, 32,* 188–192.

Spadt, S. K., & Kusturiss, E. (2016). Female sexual function and aging. *Topics in Geriatric Rehabilitation, 32,* 193–198.

Steinke, E. E., (2016). Issues regarding sexuality. In M. Boltz, E. Capezuti, T. Fulmer, & D. Zwicker (Eds), *Evidence-based geriatric nursing protocols for best practice,* pp. 165–178. New York: Springer Publishing.

Steinke, E. E., Johansen, P. P., & Dusenbury, W. (2016). When the topic turns to sex: Case scenarios in sexual counseling and cardiovascular disease. *Journal of Cardiopulmonary Rehabilitation and Prevention, 36,* 145–156.

Syme, M. L., Cohn, T. J., & Barnack-Tavlaris, J. (2017). A comparison of actual and perceived sexual risk among older adults. *Journal of Sex Research, 54,* 149–160.

Tepper, P. G., Brooks, M. M., Randolph, J. F. Jr., et al. (2016). Characterizing the trajectories of vasomotor symptoms across the menopausal transition. *Menopause: The Journal of the North American Menopause Society, 23,* 1067–1074.

Thornton, M. (2016). Human skin: a mirror for estrogen action? *Menopause: The Journal of the North American Menopause Society, 23,* 119–120.

Tillman, J., L., & Mark, H. D. (2016). HIV and STI testing in older adults: An integrative review. *Journal of Clinical Nursing, 24,* 15–16.

Tuddenham, S. A., Page, K., Chaulk, P., et al. (2016). Patients fifty years and older attending two sexually transmitted disease clinics in Baltimore, Maryland. *International Journal of STD and AIDS, 28,* 330–344.

Valadares, A., Lui-Filho, J., Costa-Paiva, L., et al. (2016). Middle-aged female sexual dysfunction and multimorbidity: A population-based study. *Menopause: The Journal of the North American Menopause Society, 23,* 304–310.

Yang, H. J., Suh, P., Kim, S., et al. (2016). Effects of smoking on menopausal age: Results from Korea National Health and Nutrition Examination Survey, 2007 to 2012. *Journal of Prevention and Public Health, 48,* 216–224.

Yokota, M., Makita, K., Hirasawa, A., et al. (2016). Symptoms and effects of physical factors in Japanese middle-aged women. *Menopause: The Journal of the North American Menopause Society, 23,* 974–983.

Zeydi, A., Sharafkhani, M., Armat, M., et al. (2016). Women's sexual issues after myocardial infarction. *Dimensions of Critical Care Nursing, 35,* 285–203.

part 5

Promoting Wellness During Illness and Transitions in Care

Unfolding Patient Stories: Henry Williams · Part 2

Recall from Part 4 Henry Williams, who has chronic obstructive pulmonary disease (COPD). He recently received pulmonary rehabilitation after another hospitalization for an acute exacerbation of COPD. Following rehab, he moved to an assisted living apartment with his wife, Ertha, who has problems with memory and confusion. How can the nurse help Henry and Ertha transition to assisted living? What health-promoting, self-care behaviors can the nurse recommend to help the couple maintain an optimal level of independence and wellness? Describe how a holistic nursing plan of care for Henry's COPD can change when he is hospitalized with an acute exacerbation of COPD. Explain how the nurse can promote effective transitions in care.

Care for Henry and other patients in a realistic virtual environment: **v*Sim*** *for Nursing* (thepoint. lww.com/vSimGerontology). Practice documenting these patients' care in DocuCare (thepoint.lww.com/ DocuCareEHR).

Unfolding Patient Stories: Julia Morales and Lucy Grey · Part 3

Recall from Parts 1 and 2 Julia Morales, who made the decision supported by her partner, Lucy, to stop treatment for lung cancer. How would the nurse introduce and explain hospice care as an option for Julia? How can the nurse collaborate with the interprofessional team to promote dignified end-of-life care? What steps would the nurse take to assure that Julia's and Lucy's decisions about treatment are respected by all health care team members?

Care for Julia, Lucy, and other patients in a realistic virtual environment: **v*Sim*** *for Nursing* (thepoint. lww.com/vSimGerontology). Practice documenting these patients' care in DocuCare (thepoint.lww.com/ DocuCareEHR).

chapter 27

Caring for Older Adults During Illness

Several factors differentiate care of older adults from that of other populations and add to the challenge of promoting wellness. Foremost among these is the reality that most older adults—and all of those whom nurses care for in acute and long-term care settings—are coping with several or even many pathologic conditions that threaten their wellness. Despite the effects of pathologic conditions, however, nurses can identify numerous opportunities to promote wellness by addressing the whole person in addition to focusing on pathologic conditions and functional limitations. This chapter describes characteristics of illness in older adults and discusses an approach to holistic care that is applicable for older adults who have chronic or progressively declining conditions. Concepts related to wellness during illness are applied to nursing care for older adults who have cancer, diabetes, and heart failure. In addition, roles of nursing in providing care and comfort are discussed in the context of palliative care. Needs of caregivers of older adults are also addressed in this chapter. Lastly, roles of nursing in relation to transitional care (introduced in Chapter 6) are illustrated through the Transitional Care Unfolding Case Study that continues in Chapters 28 and 29.

SCOPE AND CHARACTERISTICS OF ILLNESS IN OLDER ADULTS

Older adults commonly have several chronic conditions that accumulate and affect their daily functioning and quality of life. Consequently, they typically receive health care on a continuing basis for chronic conditions and periodically for acute episodes. During periods of stable chronic conditions, self-care (also called self-management) is an essential component of health care, as discussed in Chapter 5 and throughout this book. Thus, the health of older adults often fluctuates unpredictably and is usually affected by multiple interacting conditions. Even when acute conditions are the primary focus of care, as in hospital settings, nurses need to consider the interplay between chronic and acute conditions.

The combined and cumulative effects of aging and disease make it more difficult for an older adult to maintain and return to an optimal level of independence. The cumulative effects of these interacting forces can lead to a "yo-yoing" effect: The person experiences cycles of ups and downs in health, and after each cycle fails to return to the height of the previous cycle. With diminishing resiliency during subsequent cycles, the yo-yo eventually loses its ability to bounce back. For example, older adults with heart failure may be hospitalized intermittently when their condition becomes unstable. Promoting wellness during illness involves holistically addressing the changing needs of older adults as they progress through these cycles of ups and downs. Examples of wellness-oriented interventions include building on the person's strengths, supporting self-care actions, and strengthening and supporting the person's resources for care.

Because older adults are likely to require skilled nursing services after hospitalizations, each spell of illness may involve several transitions in care requiring nurses to address issues related to continuity of care. In addition, ongoing interprofessional collaboration is necessary to ensure that the person regains independent function and maintains as much quality of life as possible. Eventually, these conditions can lead to placement in a long-term care facility, particularly if the older adult does not have adequate support for managing care at home. As conditions progress, older adults may face the challenges of dying. Thus, nurses have key roles not only in addressing immediate issues, but also in assuring that older adults benefit from interprofessional collaboration and effective transitions in care during all phases of illness.

> ### ⬤ Wellness Opportunity
>
> By attending to the body–mind–spirit interconnectedness of older adults, nurses can identify opportunities to provide physical comfort and support emotional and spiritual growth even in situations involving inevitable physical decline.

Multimorbidity

In recent years, there has been increasing recognition of the complexity of caring for older adults who have **multimorbidity**, which is a combination of chronic and acute conditions. Prevalence estimates for multimorbidity among older populations range from 55% to 98% (Collerton, Jagger, Yadegarfar, et al., 2016). For example, the majority of older adults hospitalized with heart failure have concurrent conditions, such as cognitive impairment, depression, and sleep apnea, that contribute to poor health outcomes if they are not addressed (Stewart, Riegal, Ahamed, et al., 2016). Effects of multimorbidity include shorter life expectancy, increased functional dependency, poorer quality of life, and increased use of acute and long-term care services. Since 2012, the American Geriatrics Society has emphasized the following guiding principles of care that are pertinent to roles of nurses in promoting wellness during illness (American Geriatrics Society, 2012):

- Elicit and incorporate patient preferences during the medical decision-making process.
- Assure that education and assessments are ongoing, multifaceted, individualized, and delivered using a variety of methods, settings, and health care professionals.
- Assure that individualized care plans are developed and implemented by interdisciplinary health care teams, with

coordination of care to include family, friends, and paid caregivers across all sites of care, including the home.
- Interpret and apply medical literature specifically to older adults with multimorbidity, with consideration of the degree to which the evidence base applies to the individual.
- Frame clinical management decisions within the context of risks, burdens, benefits, and prognosis (e.g., remaining life expectancy, functional status, quality of life).
- Choose therapies (including medications) that optimize benefit, minimize harm, and enhance quality of life.

These guiding principles are especially important in relation to the roles of nurses as advocates, coordinators of care, and communicators with patients, families, caregivers, physicians, and other professionals.

Atypical Presentation

Atypical presentation (i.e., signs and symptoms of a disease differ from what is expected because they are altered, subtle, absent, or nonspecific) is common in older adults. For example, infections, such as pneumonia or urinary tract infection, in older adults may present atypically through falls, changes in behavior or functioning, and vague physical manifestations (e.g., increased fatigue or loss of appetite). Another aspect of atypical presentation is that usual manifestations of an infection, such as elevated temperature or specific complaints of pain or discomfort, may be absent or manifest in unusual ways, such as in behavioral changes in people with dementia. In addition, adverse medication effects may present atypically, as discussed in Chapter 8. Atypical presentation of disease is especially common in people who are cognitively impaired or older than 85 years. A major nursing responsibility is to maintain a heightened awareness of the potential for atypical presentations in older adults and explore all potential underlying causes of signs and symptoms in these patients.

Geriatric Syndromes

The term **geriatric syndromes** refers to conditions that do not fit a specific disease category but have a significant negative effect on the older person's level of functioning and quality of life. Although definitions of geriatric syndromes vary, experts agree that these conditions are highly prevalent and caused by the interplay among several risk factors and underlying conditions. Moreover, they often coexist and lead to frailty and functional decline. A study identified the most commonly occurring geriatric syndromes in hospitalized older adults discharged to skilled nursing facilities as falls, nutritional problems, incontinence, and depression (Bell, Vasilevskis, Saraf, et al., 2016). Conditions discussed in this textbook that are considered geriatric syndromes include all of the following:

- Adverse medication effects: Chapter 8
- Elder abuse: Chapter 10
- Dementia and delirium: Chapter 14
- Depression: Chapter 15
- Hearing loss: Chapter 16

- Visual impairment: Chapter 17
- Malnutrition: Chapter 18
- Urinary incontinence: Chapter 19
- Falls and osteoporosis: Chapter 22
- Pressure ulcers: Chapter 23
- Sleep disturbances: Chapter 24
- Pain: Chapter 28

Frailty

Since the early 2000s, frailty has been discussed in geriatric literature as a syndrome characterized by three or more of the following:

- Unintentional weight loss of more than 10 pounds in the previous year
- Self-reported exhaustion
- Weakness (as measured by grip strength)
- Slow walking speed
- Low level of physical activity

(Fried, Tangen, Walston, et al., 2001). Frailty is strongly associated with clinically relevant negative health outcomes, including falls, disability, dehydration, cognitive decline, hospitalization, admission for long-term care, and death (McCrow, Morton, Travers, et al., 2016; Roppolo, Mulasso, Gobbens, et al., 2015). Currently, frailty is considered a public health priority because interventions to address risk factors can reduce negative health-related outcomes (Cesari, Prince, Thiyagarajan, et al., 2016). A longitudinal study of persons aged 65 and older in the United States found higher rates of frailty associated with the following characteristics: older age, female sex, lower income, racial and ethnic minorities, and residents of supportive housing (Bandeen-Roche, Seplaki, Huang, et al., 2015). Geriatric experts recommend that all persons over 70 years old and those with significant weight loss related to chronic disease be screened for frailty, so interventions can be implemented to prevent negative consequences (Satake & Arai, 2017). Studies also indicate that older adults with diabetes and heart failure should be assessed for frailty because these conditions are strongly associated with the incidence and serious consequences of frailty (Cobo, Vazquez, Reviriego, et al., 2016; Jang, 2016; Vidan, Blaya-Novakova, Sanchez, et al., 2016).

 GLOBAL PERSPECTIVE

In Italy, a study of 210 older adults ±73 found that physical frailty is closely linked to a significant worsening of psychosocial factors, including depressive symptoms, social isolation, and feelings of loneliness (Mulasso, Roppolo, Giannotta, et al., 2016).

Roles of Nurses in Addressing Multimorbidity, Atypical Presentations, and Frailty

A common characteristic of multimorbidity, atypical presentations, and frailty is that all these conditions require both coordination of care and interprofessional collaboration. In all settings, nurses are the linchpins of coordination and collaboration, as discussed in Chapter 5 and illustrated in the case example that unfolds across Chapters 27 through 29. Another common characteristic is that all contributing factors need to be identified through a comprehensive geriatric assessment. With regard to frailty, the current emphasis is on primary prevention in older adults who are identified as having risk factors and on secondary prevention in older adults who already are frail. Nurses can address frailty through health promotion interventions related to nutrition, physical activity, medication management, and self-management of chronic conditions. For example, nurses can teach older adults about the importance of dietary intake of protein and monounsaturated fatty acids in preventing frailty (Sandoval-Insausti, Perez-Tasigchana, Lopez-Garcia, et al., 2016).

 GLOBAL PERSPECTIVE

In Japan, a 10-year frailty-prevention initiative involving health education and comprehensive geriatric assessments resulted in improved functional health of older long-term care residents and extended life expectancy at age 70 years among community-dwelling older adults (Shinkai, Yoshida, Taniguchi, et al., 2016).

See ONLINE LEARNING ACTIVITY 27-1: ADDITIONAL INFORMATION ABOUT CHARACTERISTICS OF ILLNESS IN OLDER ADULTS at http://thepoint.lww.com/Miller8e.

CONNECTING THE CONCEPTS OF WELLNESS, AGING, AND ILLNESS

The concepts of wellness and aging are readily connected when discussing older adults who are healthy, functional, and satisfied with their lives. However, the greater challenge is to apply the concept of wellness to the nursing care of people who are functionally impaired or are seriously ill or dying. In these circumstances, it is imperative to view wellness in the broader context of the body–mind–spirit interrelationship as well as one's relationships with self, others, and all that is sacred to the individual. Thus, when caring for older adults who are ill, nurses have unique opportunities to promote wellness by addressing needs related not only to physical comfort, health, and function but also to emotional comfort and spiritual well-being, as in the following examples:

- Helping older adults identifies personal strengths that are not dependent on their physical health and functioning (e.g., emotional, interpersonal, and spiritual qualities), then identifying strategies that build on or improve these personal characteristics
- Supporting and promoting interpersonal relationships that can improve the older adult's health, functioning, and quality of life

TABLE 27-1 Nursing Outcomes Classifications (NOCs) and Nursing Interventions Classifications (NICs) for Promoting Wellness in Older Adults During Illness

Type of Needs	NOC	NIC
Psychosocial needs	Anxiety Level, Coping, Decision Making, Fear Level, Participation in Health Care Decisions, Personal Autonomy, Personal Well-Being, Self-Direction of Care, Self-Esteem, Social Involvement, Stress Level, Suffering Severity	Anxiety Reduction, Counseling, Coping Enhancement, Decision-Making Support, Emotional Support, Patient Rights Protection, Resiliency Promotion, Support Group, Simple Guided Imagery, Touch
Comfort needs	Comfort Level, Pain Control, Pain: Disruptive Effects, Sleep, Symptom Control, Thermoregulation	Pain Management, Positioning, Simple Massage, Temperature Regulation, Therapeutic Touch
Health promotion needs	Fall Prevention Behavior; Health Promoting Behavior; Immunization Behavior; Knowledge: Diet, Disease Process, Health Behavior, Health Resources, Illness Care, Medication; Nutritional Status; Physical Fitness; Risk Control; Risk Detection; Self-Care Status; Safe Home Environment	Anticipatory Guidance, Environmental Management: Comfort/Safety, Exercise Promotion, Fall Prevention, Health Education, Immunization Management, Nutrition Management, Risk Identification, Self-Responsibility Facilitation, Simple Relaxation Therapy, Skin Surveillance, Sleep Enhancement, Surveillance: Safety
Spiritual needs	Hope, Spiritual Health	Active Listening, Forgiveness Facilitation, Guilt Work Facilitation, Hope Instillation, Presence, Reminiscence Therapy, Religious Ritual Enhancement, Self-Awareness Enhancement, Spiritual Growth Facilitation, Spiritual Support
Quality-of-life needs	Leisure Participation, Personal Well-Being, Quality of Life	Animal-Assisted Therapy, Aromatherapy, Family Involvement Promotion, Humor, Music Therapy

- Helping older adults identifies realistic goals for quality of life, which can be identified in any situation when wellness is conceptualized in the context of the body–mind–spirit interrelationship
- Facilitating the use of new relationships and resources, and strengthening the support resources that already are in place for older adults, their families, and caregivers
- Identifying ways of supporting wellness for families and caregivers of dependent older adults

In addition to holistically addressing needs of older adults during illness, nursing interventions focus on promoting personal responsibility for health because self-care is essential for achieving optimal health in people who have chronic illnesses. Nurses can help older adults identify ways to assume personal responsibility, even when they depend on others for care. Because personal responsibility for health—with regard to both overall wellness and specific chronic conditions—often requires that a person address health-related behaviors, nurses can apply principles of behavior change as discussed in Chapter 5.

Self-efficacy is another aspect of health promotion that is particularly important for older adults who self-manage care for one or more chronic conditions. Nurses have numerous opportunities to address self-efficacy, for example, by providing positive feedback about progress older adults are making toward managing a complex medication routine. Challenging ageist attitudes and communicating confidence in an older adult's ability to learn and apply new information is another intervention for improving self-efficacy.

Even when illnesses compromise the health, functioning, and quality of life of older adults, nurses can usually identify wellness-oriented outcomes and interventions if they use a holistic perspective. For example, nurses can suggest that older adults who have difficulty engaging in outdoor walking or exercises that require good balance and mobility explore other options in group settings, such as aquatic exercise or tai chi programs. Programs such as these are available in most communities and they can provide additional positive outcomes, such as increased socialization. Table 27-1 lists examples of Nursing Outcomes Classification (NOC) and Nursing Interventions Classification (NIC) labels related to psychosocial, comfort, health promotion, and spiritual needs. Nurses can incorporate these outcomes and interventions into care plans in conjunction with addressing the needs that are directly related to the primary health conditions.

A Student's Perspective

I learned a lot from my interview this past week. The woman I spoke with has gone through a lot of hardships in her life— and is still going through hardships—but she continues to move forward despite setbacks. She is suffering from physical ailments, but her faith in God keeps her head above water. This woman was open to questioning and insightful with her answers. For being a quiet woman, she has a lot of inner strength.

For a while after she was diagnosed with multiple sclerosis, she suffered depression and lost five dress sizes unintentionally. She also became fatigued and withdrawn. This was in line with how it has been shown that physical ailments can cause stress in a person and that this in turn can cause other physical ailments. This is a first-hand experience of how depression can cause more than just sad feelings. Once she accepted her fate, she gained back two dress sizes and is holding there, which she is content with.

Her daughter has also been diagnosed with multiple sclerosis, which is a blessing and burden at the same time. Her daughter has been diagnosed at a much younger age and has more serious problems with it, causing her to be periodically hospitalized. It is difficult for a mother to watch her daughter go through this, but it's a blessing that she has someone to share the experience with.

As stated earlier, her faith in God keeps her head above water. She still has her bouts with frustration, but she believes that God only gives what we can handle and that he is always there for her. Her strength is encouraging to the people around her. I know it has given me strength.

Anita M.

APPLYING WELLNESS CONCEPTS IN SPECIFIC PATHOLOGIC OR CHRONIC CONDITIONS

All clinically oriented chapters in this text discuss ways in which nurses promote wellness in relation to usual aspects of functioning and some common chronic conditions of older adults. The content in the next sections is not intended to address pathophysiologic conditions in-depth; rather the intent is to focus on ways in which nurses can promote wellness in older adults who have cancer, diabetes, or heart failure. These three conditions are discussed within the framework of the Functional Consequences Theory to illustrate the application of wellness concepts within the context of health promotion.

Promoting Wellness for Older Adults With Cancer

Because cancer requires the passage of time before it reaches the stage of being a diagnosable disease, older adults experience higher rates of cancer. The median age of cancer diagnosis is 66 years, with 25% of new cases being diagnosed in people aged 65 to 74, and 28% in those aged 75 and older (National Cancer Institute, 2015). Despite overall decline in cancer death rates during the past two decades, cancer is the leading cause of death among adults aged 40 to 79 years, with the most common types of cancer that lead to death in men and women aged 60 and older being lung and bronchus, colorectal, pancreas, and prostate (men) and breast (women) (Seigel, Miller, & Jemal, 2016).

Decisions about screening and treatment of cancer in older adults can be complicated for several reasons. First, older adults have been underrepresented in clinical trials, so there are fewer evidence-based guidelines about recommendations. Second, they are likely to have coexisting conditions that increase their susceptibility to adverse effects of treatments. Third, decisions about screening and treatment may be influenced by ageism. Such decisions should be based on a comprehensive geriatric assessment that considers all the following: overall health and functioning, effects of concomitant conditions, life expectancy, potential benefits versus harms, and the individual's values and preferences

(Dale, Chow, & Sajid, 2016; Denewet, DeBreucker, Luce, et al., 2016). Nursing guidelines for cancer care of older adults recommend that nurses use appropriate tools to assess functional status, risk for falls, emotional and cognitive status, and medication evaluation (Overcash, 2016).

Diversity Note

Significant racial disparities exist in many aspects of cancer detection, treatment, and survival. For instance, among Medicare-insured patients, blacks are less likely than whites to receive standard therapies for lung, breast, colorectal, and prostate cancers. Another example is that even though black women have lower rates of breast cancer than white women, they have higher mortality rates (Siegel, Miller, & Jemal, 2016).

Nursing Assessment

From a health promotion perspective, nurses assess older adults to identify their knowledge and attitudes about screening for the types of cancer most likely to develop. For example, skin cancer is one of the most commonly occurring types and it can be readily detected through self-examination. Thus, it is important to assess the older adult's knowledge about age-related skin changes and interventions for preventing cancer, as discussed in Chapter 23. When caring for an older adult who has cancer, nurses promote wellness by identifying psychosocial aspects, such as the meaning of cancer for the individual, coping strengths and supports, and the person's ability to participate in decisions about screening and care.

Wellness Nursing Diagnoses and Wellness Outcomes

Readiness for Enhanced Knowledge is a wellness nursing diagnosis applicable for older adults who are interested in learning about screening and prevention of cancer. For older adults who have been diagnosed with cancer, this diagnosis would be applicable for those who are interested in learning more about holistically oriented resources such as palliative care or hospice services.

Two NOCs applicable to prevention and early detection of cancer are Health Promoting Behavior and Knowledge: Health Behavior. Outcomes that are pertinent to holistically caring for older adults with cancer include Comfort, Coping, and Quality of Life.

Nursing Interventions

Cancer is an important focus of health promotion efforts because more than half of all cancer deaths could be prevented through healthy lifestyle choices (American Cancer Society, n.d.). Health promotion interventions focus on teaching older adults about primary prevention and early detection of cancer, as discussed in Chapter 5. Nurses can encourage older adults and surrogate decision makers to discuss cancer detection and treatment options with their primary care providers with an emphasis on quality of life. In addition, emphasize that decisions should be made in conjunction with a comprehensive geriatric assessment that considers overall functioning, patient and caregiver goals, and the effects of other conditions (Burhenn, McCarthy, Begue, et al., 2016).

For older adults already diagnosed with cancer, nurses address all aspects of pain and comfort (see Chapter 28). Also, because people with cancer commonly use complementary and alternative therapies, nurses can encourage them to discuss these therapies with their primary care practitioner and obtain information from reliable sources (e.g., the National Cancer Institute and the National Center for Complementary and Alternative Medicine). In addition, encourage the use of self-care practices, such as yoga, guided imagery, and meditation, to alleviate symptoms associated with cancer and cancer treatments. Additional wellness-oriented nursing interventions include offering hope, support, and encouragement, and considering referrals for hospice and palliative care. Online Learning Activity 27-2 provides additional information about nursing assessment and interventions related to cancer in older adults.

Diversity Note

The American Cancer Society's Circle of Life program provides excellent culturally specific health education resources about prevention of cancer for American Indian and Alaska Native communities. These resources can be accessed at http://www.cancer.org/circleoflife.

See ONLINE LEARNING ACTIVITY 27-2: RESOURCES FOR ADDITIONAL INFORMATION ABOUT PROMOTING WELLNESS IN OLDER ADULTS WITH CANCER at http://thepoint.lww.com/Miller8e.

Wellness Opportunity

Nurses can promote personal responsibility for wellness by teaching older adults about screening and preventive actions they can take.

Promoting Wellness for Older Adults With Diabetes Mellitus

Diabetes mellitus is one of the most common chronic conditions in the United States, with the highest prevalence (25.9%) among adults aged 65 years or older (American Diabetes Association, 2016a). Declining beta-cell function and increased insulin resistance (glucose intolerance) are age-related changes that increase the risk for developing diabetes. Risk factors for diabetes include obesity, hypertension, family history, physical inactivity, high levels of triglycerides, and low levels of high-density lipoproteins. Serious consequences of diabetes include renal failure,

retinopathy, neuropathy, cognitive decline, persistent pain, lower extremity amputations, and cardiovascular diseases, including stroke, hypertension, myocardial infarction, and coronary artery disease. Moreover, older adults with diabetes are at greater risk for depression, premature death, functional disability, and coexisting illnesses (American Diabetes Association, 2016d). Current emphasis is on effective management of diabetes as an intervention for preventing multimorbidity and conditions such as cardiovascular disease depression (American Diabetes Association, 2016b; Jones, Clay, Ovalle, et al., 2016).

Diversity Note

Age-adjusted rates of diagnosed diabetes by race are as follows: Native American and Alaskan Natives, 15.9%; blacks, 13.2%; Hispanics, 12.8%; Asian Americans, 9.0%; and whites, 7.6% (Centers for Disease Control and Prevention, 2014).

Disease management and nursing care related to diabetes are complicated by the common occurrence of concomitant conditions in older adults. For example, infections can affect the optimal doses of insulin and hypoglycemic agents, and chronic arthritis or periodic flare-ups of gout are likely to affect the older adult's level of activity. Another complicating factor is that older adults are likely to be taking medications (e.g., corticosteroids) that can lead to disease instability. Self-management of diabetes is affected by conditions that occur more commonly in older adults (e.g., dementia, functional limitations) and by situational circumstances, such as dependence on others or financial constraints that affect ability to purchase medications and appropriate foods.

Nursing Assessment

Although nurses are not expected to diagnose diabetes, they are expected to know about variations in diagnostic indicators that are specific to older adults. For example, the renal threshold for glucose increases in older adults, so glycosuria may not be an accurate indicator. The American Diabetes Association Standards of Medical Care states that any one of the following four conditions is a diagnostic indicator for diabetes:

- Glycosylated hemoglobin (HbA_{1c}) of 6.5% or more
- Fasting blood glucose of 126 mg/dL or more (8-hour fast)
- Symptoms of hyperglycemia (e.g., polyuria, polydipsia, weight loss) and a random (i.e., anytime during the day) blood glucose of 200 mg/dL or more
- Two-hour blood glucose value during oral glucose tolerance test 200 mg/dL or more with glucose load of 75 g

(American Diabetes Association, 2016c).

The HbA_{1c} is routinely used to monitor glucose control in people with diabetes, with the target goal being 7% or less. In recent years, there has been increasing consensus that reasonable target goals for older adults based on their health status are as follows:

- <7.5% for healthy older adults
- <8% for patients with multimorbidity or moderate functional or cognitive impairments
- <8.5% for those with poor health, limited life expectancy, or moderate to severe functional or cognitive impairments

(American Diabetes Association, 2016d). A major consideration for glycemic goals in older adults is to achieve optimal control without recurrent episodes of hypoglycemia.

In addition to the usual nursing assessment parameters for diabetes, a holistic nursing approach for older adults addresses related issues, such as the meaning of the condition, the influence of ageist attitudes that affect management, and socioeconomic and cultural influences. Box 27-1 summarizes some questions that are more specific to assessment of diabetes in older adults from a wellness perspective.

Wellness Nursing Diagnoses and Wellness Outcomes

Readiness for Enhanced Knowledge is a wellness nursing diagnosis applicable for older adults who are interested in learning about diabetes, particularly regarding improved understanding of how this condition affects their health. Nurses can use the wellness nursing diagnosis of Readiness for Enhanced Self-Care when they care for older adults who are interested in improving personal responsibility

for management of their condition, including preventing complications.

NOC terms that would be pertinent to promoting wellness in older adults with diabetes include Diabetes Self-Management, Blood Glucose Level, Health Promoting Behavior, Knowledge: Diabetes Management, and Self-Care Status.

Nursing Interventions

Diabetes self-management education is widely recognized as an essential evidence-based intervention for all people with diabetes (Powers, Bardsley, Cypress, et al., 2016). The following topics are included in self-management education: monitoring, nutritional therapy, medications, physical activity, foot care, vision assessment, signs and symptoms of hyperglycemia and hypoglycemia, and management of associated medical conditions (e.g., hypertension, hyperlipidemia, renal function). When caring for older adults with diabetes, nurses often need to address conditions that make self-management more difficult, such as involving and teaching caregivers and compensating for memory deficits. Older adults with diabetes may benefit from referrals for community-based services, including home-delivered meals, assistance with grocery shopping or meal preparation, participation in group meal programs, transportation to appointments, and assistance with medication management or glucose monitoring. An intervention for older adults with limited mobility is to consider referrals for aquatherapy classes as a way of engaging in safe and enjoyable physical activity. Online Learning Activity 27-3 provides links to health promotion information about diabetes self-management, including materials for culturally diverse groups.

Box 27-1 Assessment Guidelines for Older Adults With Diabetes

Considerations About the Meaning of Diabetes

- What terminology is appropriate for discussing the condition (e.g., older adults may refer to diabetes as "sugar")?
- What is the person's understanding of diabetes?

Considerations for Disease Management

- What is the person's understanding of personal responsibility for managing diabetes?
- Socioeconomic influences: Who does grocery shopping and meal preparation? What foods are included in the usual meal pattern? What is the usual "budget" for food? Where does the person eat meals?
- What cultural factors affect health beliefs, disease management, food preparation, eating patterns, and health-related behaviors, such as exercise?
- What concomitant conditions affect the older adult's self-care abilities?

Considerations Regarding the Influence of Ageist Attitudes

- Do ageist attitudes (of the older adult, caregiver, or health care professionals) interfere with setting wellness-oriented goals? (e.g., "I've been eating donuts for breakfast all my life, why should I worry about that now at my age?")
- Does the older adult (or do others) inaccurately associate a sense of hopelessness with his or her condition because of advanced age? (e.g., "At my age, I can't do anything about my sugar levels.")

GLOBAL PERSPECTIVE

In the Netherlands, self-care is the cornerstone of diabetes care and involves health care professionals as well as the person's social network, community organizations, and information technologies. Nurses deliver most of the care, and patients and providers establish individualized written treatment plans describing goals and planned activities, including lifestyle changes (Wensing, Koetsen-ruijter, Rogers, et al., 2014).

See ONLINE LEARNING ACTIVITY 27-3: RESOURCES FOR ADDITIONAL INFORMATION ABOUT HEALTH PROMOTION FOR OLDER ADULTS WITH DIABETES at http://thepoint.lww.com/Miller8e.

Wellness Opportunity

Nurses can teach all older adults about actions they can take to prevent diabetes by using resources, such as the tools adapted from the Diabetes Prevention Program, which are available from the National Diabetes Education Program at www.ndep.nih.gov.

Promoting Wellness for Older Adults With Heart Failure

Heart failure is a complex and multisystem syndrome caused by cardiac muscle dysfunction and characterized by ventricular dilation and/or hypertrophy, venous congestion, and inadequate oxygen delivery. This condition is of particular concern for gerontological health care practitioners for the following reasons:

- It is the most common cause of hospital admissions for older adults.
- Evidence-based literature demonstrates that at least half of admissions or readmissions are deemed preventable.
- The prevalence of heart failure increases with age, with more than 75% of those affected being older than 65.
- The downward trajectory of heart failure can be delayed through health promotion measures.
- Nurses are among the health care professionals who are in key position to assess, intervene, and teach about self-care.

(Schipper, 2016).

Older adults with heart failure are at increased risk for serious conditions such as arrhythmias, hypotension, falls, sleep disorders, drug interactions, and adverse medication effects. Because of consequences such as these—which make it a major source of chronic disability, increased mortality, and impaired quality of life—heart failure in older adults has emerged as a major focus of health promotion interventions. Even with optimal treatment, heart failure is a life-limiting condition, characterized by periods of stability interspersed with exacerbations, which will eventually require palliative care and hospice services (Glogowska, Simmonds, McLachlan, et al., 2016; Lewin & Schaefer, 2017).

In recent years, there has been increasing attention to establishing transitional care programs as "the new norm" for improving quality of care and reducing readmission rates for patients with heart failure, with essential roles for nurses (Albert, Barnason, Deswal, et al., 2015; Kansagara, Chiovaro, Kagen, et al., 2016). Part I of the unfolding case that begins in this chapter illustrates the roles of nurses in promoting wellness for Mr. B soon after he has been diagnosed as having heart failure. As Mr. B's condition progresses and the case unfolds through Chapter 29, scenarios illustrate roles of nurses in promoting wellness through all stages of illness.

Diversity Note

Blacks have the highest risk for heart failure and a greater 5-year mortality rate compared with whites (Yancy, Jessup, Bozkurt, et al., 2013).

Nursing Assessment

Nurses assess for signs and symptoms of heart failure in older adults using the same assessment techniques that apply to adults of any age. However, older adults are more likely to have concomitant conditions that can affect the assessment.

For example, because older adults with significant mobility limitations may not experience dyspnea on exertion if their activity level is minimal, nurses need to consider other limiting factors when they assess the effects of heart failure on respirations. It is important to ask very direct questions about specific symptoms because early symptoms may be attributed to aging or chronic conditions.

Another assessment consideration is that older adults with heart failure are likely to have some degree of chronic renal failure, which often fluctuates within an abnormal range. Thus, nurses need to identify and document the older adult's usual indicators of renal function (i.e., ranges of blood urea nitrogen and creatinine that are typical for that individual). It is also important to assess for electrolyte imbalances and adverse medication effects, which commonly are associated with diminished renal function, as discussed in Chapter 8.

In addition to assessing signs and symptoms of heart failure, nurses assess risk factors, paying particular attention to those that can be addressed through health promotion interventions. Factors that increase the risk for heart failure include hypertension, coronary artery disease, myocardial infarction, family history of heart failure, hyperthyroidism, diabetes, smoking, and obesity. Even though older adults may have long-term patterns of behavior that affect disease management (e.g., smoking, inadequate physical activity, or high-sodium diets), nurses need to assess attitudes about changing these behaviors so that they can address this in health promotion teaching. Additional wellness-focused assessment considerations that are important for older adults who have heart failure are outlined in Box 27-2.

 Box 27-2 Assessment Guidelines for Older Adults With Heart Failure

Considerations About the Meaning of Heart Failure

- What is the older adult's understanding of heart failure?
- What terminology is appropriate for discussing the condition? Does the term failure cause anxiety or fear?
- What personal experiences or those of significant others are influencing the older adult's response to cardiovascular disease? (e.g., How life-threatening does the person perceive this to be?)

Considerations Regarding the Influence of Ageist Attitudes

- Do ageist attitudes interfere with health promotion interventions? (e.g., Do health care providers avoid teaching about smoking cessation because they think the person is too old to quit or to benefit from quitting?)

Considerations Regarding Disease Management

- Does the older adult have questions or fears about engaging in therapeutic or enjoyable activities (e.g., exercise, swimming, sexual relationships)? If so, would he or she benefit from health education about this?
- Do socioeconomic factors affect disease management (e.g., limited income that interferes with ability to purchase needed medications or healthy foods)?

Wellness Nursing Diagnoses and Wellness Outcomes

Nurses can use the wellness nursing diagnosis of Readiness for Enhanced Therapeutic Regimen Management to promote increased personal responsibility for management of heart failure and prevention of hospitalizations and other complications. The wellness nursing diagnosis of Readiness for Enhanced Fluid Balance is applicable when older adults with heart failure are interested in learning about actions they can take to improve and maintain fluid and electrolyte balance.

Outcomes that are pertinent to promoting wellness in older adults with heart failure include Cardiac Disease Self-Management, Energy Conservation, Health Promoting Behavior, and Knowledge: Cardiac Disease Management.

Nursing Interventions

A key nursing intervention for older adults with heart failure is teaching about self-care because even with expert clinicians, patients are responsible for implementing interventions, recognizing and addressing symptoms, and making appropriate decisions about seeking medical care. In addition to focusing on usual interventions directed toward disease management, wellness-oriented care plans for older adults with heart failure focus on teaching about actions the person can take to achieve the best possible level of functioning and quality of life despite the chronic condition. For example, nurses can teach older adults about planning appropriate rest and energy management techniques to achieve optimum quality of life with limited energy. From a holistic perspective, nurses also need to address psychosocial consequences associated with heart failure, such as fear, anxiety, loneliness, and depression (discussed in Chapters 12, 13, and 15). Similarly, when older adults with heart failure experience distressing symptoms such as pain or dyspnea, a referral for palliative care may be appropriate. The unfolding case that begins at the end of this chapter illustrates roles of nurses in addressing the needs of an older adult as his heart failure progresses. At all stages, nurses have key roles in assuring effective transitional care, as discussed in the care plans.

GLOBAL PERSPECTIVE

In Italy, a prospective, randomized, controlled trial of heart failure patients, older than 70 years, found that those who participated in a 6-month cardiac rehabilitation program that included exercise training had fewer hospitalizations and improved functional abilities and perceived quality of life (Antonicelli, Spazzafumo, Scalvini, et al., 2016).

See **ONLINE LEARNING ACTIVITY 27-4: ADDITIONAL INFORMATION ABOUT HEALTH PROMOTION FOR OLDER ADULTS WITH HEART FAILURE** at http://thepoint.lww.com/Miller8e.

Wellness Opportunity

Because stress-reduction activities are especially important when older adults have chronic conditions, such as heart failure, nurses can suggest relaxation and health promotion activities such as deep breathing, meditation, and guided imagery.

HOLISTICALLY CARING FOR OLDER ADULTS WHO ARE SERIOUSLY ILL: FOCUSING ON CARE AND COMFORT

Care and comfort are core components of all nursing, but they become even more important when a cure is not feasible. Equating aging with inability to cure is both inaccurate and unjust. Similarly, it is a disservice to older adults to focus only on curing disease when treatments are more detrimental or risky than the underlying conditions. Caring for older adults often involves a combination of caring and curing, with the emphasis shifting away from curing and more toward caring as disease conditions accumulate and progress. Moreover, because of the complexity of illness in older adults, rarely is there a clearly defined "turning point" when the focus changes from cure to care. Thus, goals of care may fluctuate or include a combination of curing one condition while simultaneously providing care and comfort for other conditions. Increasingly, geriatricians, gerontologists, ethicists, and gerontological nurses are challenged to identify ways to improve *quality* of life for people whose *quantity* of life is limited.

The emergence and expansion of palliative care programs in recent years provide a framework for promoting wellness during serious illness, and this model is increasingly used to address the complex and cumulative effects of incurable conditions. The National Consensus Project for Quality Palliative Care (2013) described the characteristics of palliative care as follows:

- Palliative care is both a philosophy of care and an organized system for achieving the best possible quality of life for patients and their family caregivers.
- Recipients of care are patients and their families facing problems associated with a broad range of persistent, life-threatening, or recurring conditions that adversely affect their daily functioning or will predictably reduce life expectancy (e.g., frailty, acute stroke, malignancies, dementia, and other neurodegenerative conditions).
- Goals are to prevent and relieve suffering, enhance quality of life, optimize function, assist with decision making, and provide opportunities for personal growth.
- Ideally, palliative care is initiated early in the course of an illness and concurrently with curative or disease-modifying treatment.

Palliative care models are based on an interprofessional team approach, with nurses assuming essential roles. These models are particularly applicable to holistically addressing the needs of older adults because of the emphasis on quality of life during serious or life-limiting illness. For example, emphasis is placed on respecting individual preferences, sharing caring moments, promoting self-directed care, and honoring the intrinsic worth and uniqueness of each person.

Palliative care services were initially developed within hospice services. Now, in addition to remaining an integral component of hospice programs, these programs are widely available outside of hospice programs. The 2010 Patient Protection and Affordable Care Act supports the development of palliative care services in all Medicare-certified settings, with the goal of lowering cost of care and improving health care outcomes. By 2014, two thirds of US hospitals with 50 or more beds and 90% of those with 200 beds or more provided palliative care services (Dumanovsky, Augustin, Rogers, et al., 2016). Despite the importance and availability of palliative care, these services are underutilized, with one study finding that only 39% of eligible patients in 33 US hospitals were referred for palliative care (Szekendi, Vaughn, Lai, et al., 2016). This chapter focuses on palliative care for older adults with chronic declining conditions, and Chapter 29 discusses palliative care as a component of hospice and end-of-life care.

Although the terms palliative care and hospice are commonly used interchangeably, the programs differ in significant ways, as summarized in Box 27-3. Differences related to prognosis and use of curative treatments are particularly important because families, older adults, and even health care professionals tend to narrowly and inaccurately associate palliative care with hospice services and end-of-life care. Another common misconception is that palliative care and hospice programs focus primarily on patients with cancer;

however, these services are available throughout the continuum of many progressive declining conditions. For example, palliative care services can be embedded in other specialty clinics such geriatrics, heart failure, kidney failure, and liver failure (Dahlin, 2016). In recent years, there also has been increasing attention to palliative care for people with dementia, as demonstrated by the goal of the U.S. National Plan to Address Alzheimer's disease to provide palliative care throughout the trajectory of the disease by 2018 (Alzheimer's Association National Plan Care and Support Milestone Workgroup, 2016). Because palliative care is strongly associated with hospice or end-of-life care, the term "supportive care" is more acceptable to professionals, patients, and families, and it is replacing the term palliative care in oncology and other health care settings (Chou, Gaysynsky, & Persoskie, 2016; Hui & Bruera, 2016).

Nurses have an important responsibility to recognize the appropriateness of a referral for palliative care and to initiate discussion of this option with older adults and their families. Nurses can use information in Box 27-4 as a guide to identifying the conditions that would prompt consideration of a referral for hospice or palliative care. When discussing palliative care services with older adults or their families, emphasize that although these services are provided within all hospice programs, they also are available outside of hospice programs, and they have a broader range of admission criteria. Palliative care for patients with heart failure

---

Box 27-3 Comparison of Characteristics of Hospice and Palliative Care

Similarities

Both hospice and palliative care programs:
- Provide care across all settings, including homes and community settings, for patients with serious or life-limiting illnesses
- Focus on person-centered care to address physical comfort and psychosocial and spiritual well-being of the person and all caregivers
- Use pharmacologic and nonpharmacologic therapies and complementary modalities, for comprehensive symptom management
- Provide education and support for families and all support people, including health care professionals
- Are covered by Medicare, Medicaid, and other health insurance programs

Differences

- Hospice services are based on a diagnosis of a life-limiting illness with a prognosis of 6 months or less
- Palliative care can be provided ongoing or intermittently during the course of a serious or life-limiting illness without regard to length of prognosis
- Palliative care can include disease-treatment and life-sustaining measures

---

Box 27-4 Conditions That Would Prompt Nurses to Consider a Referral for Hospice or Palliative Care

Examples of symptoms that can be addressed through palliative care or hospice:
- Pain
- Anorexia
- Dyspnea
- Frailty
- Functional dependency
- Significant weight loss
- Behavioral manifestations of dementia or depression

Examples of circumstances that may warrant a referral for palliative care or hospice:
- Frequent hospitalizations for unstable conditions
- Emotional distress related to serious illness
- Family support needs related to caregiving for person with serious illness
- Decisions about discontinuing life-sustaining treatments (e.g., dialysis, artificial nutrition, and hydration)
- Ethical dilemmas about care or decision-making capacity

Examples of diagnoses that may qualify a person for palliative care or hospice:
- Cancer
- Dementia
- Heart failure
- Chronic lung disease
- Parkinson disease
- End-stage liver disease
- End-stage renal disease

Box 27-5 Evidence-Based Practice: Family Caregiving

Overview

- Family caregivers are a key link in providing safe and effective transitional care as older adults move across care settings.
- Increased caregiver strain is associated with lack of preparedness for the role, caring for someone with dementia, and poor-quality relationships between caregiver and care recipient.
- Helping caregivers with the role-acquisition process is a critical nursing function that facilitates good transitional care

Components of Nursing Assessment

Context of caregiving:
- Relationship between caregiver and care recipient
- Caregiver roles and responsibilities
- Physical environment
- Actual financial resources and potential support resources
- Cultural background of those involved

Caregiver's perception of health and functioning of care recipient:
- Activities that caregiver needs help with
- Presence of cognitive impairment or behavioral problems
- Presence of mobility limitations

Caregiver's skills, abilities, and knowledge to provide care

Quality of family relationships

Indicators of problems with quality of care or signs of elder mistreatment

Caregiver's physical and mental health status:
- Self-rated health
- Health conditions and symptoms (e.g., anxiety, depression, caregiver stress)

- Rewards of caregiving
- Self-care activities

Recommended Assessment Tool

- Modified Caregiver Strain Index (see Figure 27-1)

Strategies for Nursing Care

Identify content and skills needed to increase caregiver's preparedness
- Information about the care needed
- Coaching about caregiving role

Partner with caregiver to identify strategies for addressing issues and concerns

Generate strategies for issues and concerns that caregiver identifies as priorities

Assist the caregiver in identifying strengths in the situations

Assist the caregiver in finding and using resources

Help caregiver incorporate self-care strategies

Use an interprofessional approach by involving a team of health care professionals

Source: Messecar, D. C. (2016). Family caregiving. In M. Boltz, E. Capezuti, T. Fulmer, & D. Zwicker (Eds.), *Evidence-based geriatric nursing protocols for best practice* (pp. 137–163). New York: Springer Publishing.

---

is of particular interest with dual goals of preventing hospitalizations and improving quality of care. Nurses can obtain more information about palliative care programs by exploring the resources listed in Online Learning Activity 27-5.

See ONLINE LEARNING ACTIVITY 27-5: ARTICLE AND RESOURCES FOR ADDITIONAL INFORMATION ABOUT PALLIATIVE CARE at http://thepoint.lww.com/Miller8e.

ADDRESSING NEEDS OF FAMILIES AND CAREGIVERS

During periods of illness—whether acute, chronic, or declining—the importance of relationships increases in proportion to the need not only for physical care and practical assistance but also for emotional and spiritual care. Thus, when nurses care for older adults during illness, families and caregivers are an integral focus of care because the multifaceted needs of dependent older adults cannot be met without a strong support system. Nurses have crucial roles not only in supporting caregiver wellness but also in working with families and caregivers to assure effective transitions of care for older adults with complex or unstable conditions, as summarized in the evidence-based geriatric nursing protocol

for the best practice related to family caregiving (Messecar, 2016). In most health care settings, the extent to which nurses can address caregiver needs is limited by time constraints and the need to focus on the immediate and complex needs of the older adult. Despite these limitations, however, nurses can use the Modified Caregiver Strain Index (Figure 27-1) to identify families who may benefit from more in-depth assessment and follow-up. Box 27-5 summarizes evidence-based information about nursing assessment and interventions related to family caregiving. Table 27-2 lists NOC and NIC terms that are pertinent to promoting wellness for caregivers. Supplemental materials related to this topic, including resources for family caregivers, are provided in Online Learning Activity 27-6.

See ONLINE LEARNING ACTIVITY 27-6: ADDITIONAL INFORMATION ABOUT FAMILY CAREGIVING AND LINKS TO RESOURCES FOR CAREGIVERS at http://thepoint.lww.com/Miller8e.

SPOTLIGHT ON TRANSITIONAL CARE

As presented in Chapter 6, transitional care is a major focus of health care for older adults who require care across different settings during the course of illness. The following

Directions: Here is a list of things that other caregivers have found to be difficult. Please put a checkmark in the columns that apply to you. We have included some examples that are common caregiver experiences to help you think about each item. Your situation may be slightly different, but the item could still apply.

	Yes, On a Regular Basis = 2	Yes, Sometimes = 1	No = 0
My sleep is disturbed (For example, the person I care for is in and out of bed or wanders around at night)			
Caregiving is inconvenient (For example: helping takes so much time or it's a long drive over to help)			
Caregiving is a physical strain (For example: lifting in or out of a chair; effort or concentration is required)			
Caregiving is confining (For example: helping restricts free time or I cannot go visiting)			
There have been family adjustments (For example: helping has disrupted my routine; there is no privacy)			
There have been changes in personal plans (For example: I had to turn down a job; I could not go on a vacation)			
There have been other demands on my time (For example: other family members need me)			
There have been emotional adjustments (For example: severe arguments about caregiving)			
Some behavior is upsetting (For example: incontinence; the person cared for has trouble remembering things; or the person I care for accuses people of taking things)			
It is upsetting to find the person I care for has changed so much from his/her former self (For example: he/she is a different person than he/she used to be)			
There have been work adjustments (For example: I have to take time off for caregiving duties)			
Caregiving is a financial strain			
I feel completely overwhelmed (For example: I worry about the person I care for; I have concerns about how I will manage)			

[Sum responses for "Yes, on a regular basis" (2 pts each) and "yes, sometimes" (1 pt each)]   Total Score =

FIGURE 27-1 Modified Caregiver Strain Index. (From Thornton, M., & Travis, S. S. (2003). Analysis of the reliability of the Modified Caregiver Strain Index. *The Journals of Gerontology: Psychological Sciences and Social Sciences, 58*(2), S129. © Copyright The Gerontological Society of America. Reproduced by permission of the publisher.)

TABLE 27-2 Nursing Outcomes Classifications (NOCs) and Nursing Interventions Classifications (NICs) for Promoting Wellness in Caregivers

Type of Needs	NOC	NIC
Needs related to caregiver role	Caregiver Adaptation to Patient Institutionalization, Caregiver Emotional Health, Caregiver Endurance Potential, Caregiver Home Care Readiness, Caregiver Lifestyle Disruption, Caregiver–Patient Relationship, Caregiver Performance: Direct/Indirect Care, Caregiver Physical Health, Caregiver Stressors, Caregiver Well-Being	Caregiver Support, Case Management, Counseling, Energy Management, Family Support, Family Integrity Promotion, Resiliency Promotion, Role Enhancement, Self-Awareness Enhancement, Support Group
Needs related to using resources and managing care	Information Processing, Knowledge: Health Resources, Participation in Health Care Decisions, Role Performance	Decision-Making Support, Health Education, Health System Guidance, Referral, Respite Care, Support System Enhancement, Teaching: Individual, Telephone Consultation
Psychosocial needs	Anxiety Level, Coping, Decision Making, Depression Level, Family Coping, Family Resiliency, Fear Level, Grief Resolution, Loneliness Severity, Self-Esteem, Stress Level	Active Listening, Anticipatory Guidance, Anxiety Reduction, Cognitive Restructuring, Coping Enhancement, Emotional Support, Grief Work Facilitation, Mood Management, Presence, Simple Guided Imagery
Spiritual and quality-of-life needs	Hope, Leisure Participation, Quality of Life, Sleep, Social Involvement, Social Support, Spiritual Health	Forgiveness Facilitation, Guilt Work Facilitation, Hope Instillation, Humor, Sleep Enhancement, Spiritual Support

case example illustrates the role of a nurse who is providing transitional care for Maria Lopez, an older adult with several chronic conditions. The case continues to unfold in Chapters 28 and 29 as a way of underscoring the roles of nurses in assuring continuity of care for Maria Lopez as her condition changes.

Transitional Care Unfolding Case Study

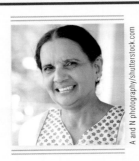

A and N photography/shutterstock.com

Part I: Maria Lopez as She is Discharged from Hospital to Home

Background Information: Maria Lopez

Maria Lopez immigrated from Mexico to a rural area of Texas 22 years ago with her husband and their four children, who ranged in age from 10 to 16 years old at that time. Her husband was a hardworking agricultural worker until he died after a brief illness from lung cancer 4 years ago. Maria developed a social network with other immigrants who attended the Saint Joseph Catholic Church, where Spanish was the primary language. The children attended the local public schools and soon became fluent in English. The family spoke Spanish at home, and although Maria could understand English phrases, she was more comfortable with Spanish. Besides, Maria had little need to learn English because all her friends spoke Spanish. After attending the local high school, the Lopez children went to the nearby community college and eventually attended college.

When Maria was 60 years old, she was diagnosed with type 2 diabetes and hypertension, and she had chronic pain from osteoarthritis. In addition, her body mass index (BMI) had gradually been increasing, and by the age of 68 it was 35. By the time Maria became a widow at age 64, her children had all married, and three lived in other states. Her oldest son, Carlos, lived 2 hours away by car. Until recently, Maria attended daily mass at Saint Joseph Catholic Church and was active with the Altar & Rosary Society at the church. During the past several months, however, Maria has become increasingly homebound because her breathing becomes labored when she walks, and her feet are constantly swollen.

When Carlos and his sisters have called their mother recently, she has reported that everything is fine; however, they shared with each other their concerns about her health because she sounds short of breath when they talk with her. Also, when they ask about her usual activities at Saint Joseph, she admits that she has not been attending but is vague about the reason.

Part I: Maria Lopez at 68 Years of Age *(Continued)*

Carlos visits and is concerned about the decline in his mother's health since he saw her 6 weeks ago. He asks his mother about her health because he sees that her feet are swollen and she has difficulty breathing when she walks from one room to another. In response to his inquiries, Maria tells him that her close friend, who is a curandera (i.e., a traditional healer), has advised her to use an herbal preparation for her breathing. Although the preparation hasn't yet improved her breathing, her feet are no longer swollen in the mornings—only in the afternoons and evenings. The curandera has also been treating her diabetes. For the past month Maria has been cutting her metformin dose in half because the curandera assured her that she will get better if she keeps taking the herbs, so Maria figures she can halve her medication dose without any negative effects. Maria has canceled her doctor appointments at the Senior Health Center because she trusts the curandera's guidance and doesn't think she needs advice from a physician.

Background Information: San Christos Hospital

Last year San Christos Hospital began an aggressive campaign to reduce readmissions for heart failure because the Centers for Medicare & Medicaid had identified this issue as a major concern related to quality of care and cost of care. After studying various models of transitional care, San Christos Hospital developed a nurse-led program called Safe, Coordinated, and Effective Discharges (SCED). During the first 3 years of the program, all patients who were admitted with the diagnosis of heart failure were automatically admitted to the SCED program. The mainstay of the program was a SCED nurse (i.e., a registered nurse who had received additional training in care management) who was available on day and evening shifts. Responsibilities of the SCED nurse included components delineated in Box 6-6.

Nurse Jessica: SCED Nurse at San Christos Hospital

Nurse Jessica, the SCED nurse at San Christos Hospital, is notified of the admitting diagnosis of heart failure for Maria Lopez and extracts the following pertinent information from the chart:

> *Patient admitted yesterday with the following diagnoses: obesity, heart failure, hypertension (BP 196/108), and uncontrolled type 2 diabetes (A1C 8.4). Her son brought her to the emergency department stating she had become progressively more homebound due to difficulty breathing and swollen feet. He also expressed concerns that she seemed depressed and had not been taking her medications for diabetes and hypertension properly. He had not seen her for 6 weeks and was "stunned" at the decline in her condition.*

Nurse Jessica uses her bilingual skills when she meets with Maria Lopez. In Spanish, she introduces herself and addresses the patient as "Señora Lopez" before proceeding to explain her role. Nurse Jessica emphasizes that she is working with the doctor and all team members to assure that Maria's health improves during the hospitalization and that she is able to return home and manage her conditions with support from health care professionals. Nurse Jessica asks about Señora Lopez's family and other support resources, and gains permission to involve Carlos in discussions about her current and ongoing care.

Nurse Jessica works with all of Maria's other care providers during the course of Maria's hospitalization and documents the SCED transitional care plan (see Table 27-3). In addition, Nurse Jessica performs a medication reconciliation on admission and again at discharge (see Chapter 8 for a description of medication reconciliation). Nurse Jessica prepares a discharge packet of information and reviews all the information with Señora Lopez. She includes educational materials written in Spanish, which she has obtained from resources such as those listed in Online Learning Activities 27-3 and 27-4. Discharge papers include information about a follow-up medical appointment with her primary care practitioner, as well as contact information about home care services that will be provided by the San Christos Care-at-Home Program.

(continued)

Part I: Maria Lopez at 68 Years of Age *(Continued)*

Plans also include all of the following postdischarge components:

- Nurse Jessica will call Señora Lopez at the following postdischarge intervals: second day, 2 weeks, 4 weeks.
- Nurse Jessica will call Carlos at the following postdischarge intervals: 1, 2, and 4 weeks.
- During phone calls, Nurse Jessica will discuss all of the following topics with Señora Lopez and Carlos: management of medical conditions, questions about treatment plans or medical conditions, coordination of care with the curandera, and the effectiveness of all follow-up services (e.g., home care services).
- A discharge summary and pertinent information from the patient's health record will be provided to all health care professionals involved with follow-up.
- Patient will receive skilled nursing care from the San Christos Care-at-Home Program.

I P C

THINKING POINTS

- How does the care provided by Nurse Jessica differ from usual hospital care?
- How does Nurse Jessica work with other professionals to implement this transitional care plan?
- What additional actions could Nurse Jessica incorporate in this plan, particularly regarding health literacy and culturally appropriate care? (Refer also to Chapters 2 and 5.)
- Explore the resources in Online Learning Activities 27-3 and 27-4, and find ones that you would use for Maria Lopez if you were Nurse Jessica.

TABLE 27-3 Key Issues, Planned Interventions, and Expected Outcomes for Effective Transitional Care for Maria Lopez

Issues	Nursing Interventions	Outcome
Knowledge deficit: heart failure	Teach patient and family all of the following: • Signs and symptoms of heart failure • Medication management • Self-management interventions (e.g., monitoring weight) • Sodium restriction	Patient will be able to manage heart failure at home.
Knowledge deficit: type 2 diabetes	Teach patient and family all of the following: • Factors that affect blood glucose (e.g., diet, physical activity, infections) • Medication management • Self-monitoring with glucometer	Patient's A1C level will be 7.4 or less in 3 months.
Knowledge deficit: hypertension	Teach patient and family all of the following: • Medication management • Self-monitoring	Patient's blood pressure will be maintained at 140/85 or under.

Poor management of chronic conditions	• During hospitalization:
	  • Provide educational materials in Spanish
	  • Use teach-back method to ensure understanding of content
	  • Focus on essential information
	  • Provide for ongoing teaching
	• Refer for skilled nursing follow-up at home through San Christos Care-at-Home Program.
	• When patient is no longer homebound, refer to classes on diabetes and healthy aging at San Christos Senior Center.
		Patient will be able to manage chronic conditions with ongoing support and assistance from community-based resources.

Limited health literacy; Spanish as primary language	• Bilingual nursing staff deliver all health education in Spanish language. • For patient teaching, nurses who do not speak Spanish will request translation service, which is available through hospital Community Services Office.	Patient will receive educational materials matched to her level of understanding and language skills.
Lack of coordination between curandera and other health care providers	• Use nonjudgmental approach to elicit information about herbal treatments recommended by curandera. • Have pharmacist review all nonprescription medications for potential adverse effects or interactions with prescribed medications. • Ask patient if curandera can be included in discussions about treatment plans. • Encourage patient to talk with all health care providers about treatments recommended by curandera.	Patient will be able to safely and effectively incorporate remedies recommended by her curandera with prescribed treatment plan directed by her primary care practitioner.

Chapter Highlights

Characteristics of Illness in Older Adults

- Older adults commonly have several chronic conditions, resulting in cycles of ups and downs in health that eventually can lead to death.
- Assessment of illness in older adults is complicated because conditions may manifest as atypical presentations
- The term *geriatric syndrome* refers to conditions that do not fit a specific disease category but have a significant negative effect on the older person's level of functioning and quality of life.
- Older adults with multiple pathologic conditions may experience frailty.
- Nurses play important roles in addressing multimorbidity, atypical presentation, and frailty through ensuring coordination of care and interprofessional collaboration.

Connecting the Concepts of Wellness, Aging, and Illness

- A holistic perspective enables nurses to identify ways of promoting wellness by addressing needs related to physical health and functioning and emotional and spiritual well-being.
- An important aspect of wellness is promoting personal responsibility for health through self-care measures and management of chronic conditions.
- Nurses challenge ageist attitudes and provide health education to foster behavior change when appropriate.
- Many NIC and NOC terms are applicable in care plans that address psychosocial, comfort, health promotion, and spiritual needs (Table 27-1).

Applying Wellness Concepts in Specific Pathologic or Chronic Conditions

- Nurses connect the concepts of wellness, aging, and illness by addressing needs within the broader context of the body–mind–spirit interrelationship.
- Nursing interventions to promote wellness during illness focus on promoting personal responsibility and fostering self-efficacy.

Promoting Wellness for Older Adults With Cancer

- Older adults are disproportionately affected by cancer, they are less likely to be screened for cancer, and they are diagnosed at a later stage.
- From a health promotion perspective, nurses assess older adults to identify their knowledge and attitudes about screening for the types of cancer that they are most likely to develop.
- Nurses holistically address the needs of older adults already diagnosed with cancer.
- Nurses can teach older adults about primary prevention interventions and about screening recommendations (Box 27-1).

Promoting Wellness for Older Adults With Diabetes

- Diabetes is common among older adults, with the highest prevalence among Native American and Alaskan Natives, blacks, and Hispanics.
- Disease management and nursing care related to diabetes are complicated by the common occurrence of concomitant conditions and by the increased vulnerability of older adults to complications.
- In addition to usual assessment parameters, nurses identify ageist attitudes and the meaning of diabetes (Box 27-2).
- Care plans for older adults with diabetes include all the usual interventions and additional teaching points (e.g., teaching caregivers, referring for community-based services, and appropriate ways of engaging in physical activity).

Promoting Wellness for Older Adults With Heart Failure

- Heart failure is the leading cause of hospitalizations and readmissions among older adults in the United States, with more than half of these admissions being potentially preventable with effective self-care.
- In addition to assessing all the usual signs and symptoms of heart failure, nurses assess effects of other conditions, risk factors that can be addressed through health promotion, and other aspects that are specific to older adults (e.g., the effects of ageist attitudes).
- In addition to all the usual teaching points, wellness-oriented care plans focus on teaching about actions the person can take to achieve the best possible level of functioning and quality of life, despite the effects of heart failure.

Holistically Caring for Older Adults Who Are Ill: Focusing on Caring and Comforting

- Palliative care is a widely available model of care that comprehensively addresses the needs of patients with serious or life-limiting illnesses through a person-centered approach that also focuses on the needs of families and caregivers.
- Palliative care is a part of hospice care, but it also is provided outside of hospice (Box 27-4)
- Nurses have important roles in suggesting referrals for palliative care and talking with older adults and their families about the scope of these services.

Addressing Needs of Families and Caregivers

- Nurses promote caregiver well-being by identifying and addressing issues related to the multiple and sometimes overwhelming needs of caregivers (Box 27-5; Figure 27-1).
- Many NIC and NOC terms are applicable in care plans that address caregivers with regard to role performance; use of resources and management of care; and psychosocial, spiritual, and quality-of-life needs (Table 27-2).

Spotlight on Transitional Care

- The Transitional Care Unfolding Case Study describes how Nurse Jessica implements a model of transitional care for an older adult who is discharged from an acute care setting.

Critical Thinking Exercises

1. Identify an older person (in your personal life or clinical experience) who has recently been hospitalized and address the following in relation to that person:
   - How many different conditions (e.g., acute and chronic illness, functional limitations, support resources, psychosocial factors, or environmental factors) affected how the person was able to adapt to the hospitalization?
   - How did these factors affect the outcome for the person (e.g., longer hospitalization, increased dependency on others, discharge plans)?
   - Select two NOC and NIC terms from Table 27-1 that you could apply to a care plan to promote wellness for this person.

2. Think about your expectations for older adults who are affected by multiple interacting conditions and identify any ageist attitudes or assumptions that are likely to affect your care.

3. Find information about local resources for palliative care and prepare yourself to teach older adults and their families about this service.

4. Identify a situation in your personal life or clinical experience that requires caregiving assistance from a family member at least once weekly and address the following in relation to this situation:
   - What benefits (rewards) and stresses are caregivers likely to experience?
   - Select two NOC and NIC terms from Table 27-2 that you could apply to a care plan to address the needs of the caregiver.

 For more information about topics discussed in this chapter, be sure to check out the interactive Online Learning Activities and other helpful resources at http://thepoint.lww.com/Miller8e.

REFERENCES

Albert, N. M., Barnason, S. B., Deswal, A., et al. (2015). Transitions of care in heart failure: A scientific statement from the American Heart Association. *Circulation Heart Failure, 8,* 384–409.

Alzheimer's Association National Plan Care and Support Milestone Workgroup. (2016). Report on milestones for care and support under the U.S. National Plan to address Alzheimer's disease. *Alzheimer's & Dementia, 12,* 334–369.

American Cancer Society. (n.d.). *Stay healthy.* Available at www.cancer.org. Accessed on May 15, 2016.

American Diabetes Association. (2016a). *Statistics about diabetes.* Available at www.diabetes.org. Accessed on May 17, 2016.

American Diabetes Association (2016b). Cardiovascular disease and risk management. Standards of medical care in diabetes: 2016. *Diabetes Care, 39* (Suppl 1), S60–S71.

American Diabetes Association. (2016c). Classification and diagnosis of diabetes. Standards of medical care in diabetes: 2016. *Diabetes Care, 39* (Suppl 1), S13–S22.

American Diabetes Association. (2016d). Older adults. Standards of medical care in diabetes: 2016. *Diabetes Care, 39* (Suppl 1), S81–S85.

American Geriatrics Society. (2012). Guiding principles for care of older adults with multimorbidity: An approach for clinicians. *Journal of the American Geriatrics Society.* doi:10.1111/j.1532–5415.2012.04188.x.

Antoniclli, R., Spazzafumo, L., Scalvini, S., et al. (2016). Exercise: a new "drug" for elderly patients with chronic heart failure. *Aging, 8*(3), 1–13. Available at www.impactaging.com.

Bandeen-Roche, K., Seplaki, C. L., Huang, J., et al. (2015). Frailty in older adults: A nationally representative profile in the United States. *Journals of Gerontology A Biological Sciences and Medical Sciences, 70,* 1427–1434.

Bell, S. P., Vasilevskis, E. E., Saraf, A. A., et al., (2016). Geriatric syndromes in hospitalized older adults discharged to skilled nursing facilities. *Journal of the American Geriatrics Society.* doi.10.1011/jgs.14035.

Burhenn, P. S., McCarthy, A. L., Beque, A., et al. (2016). Geriatric assessment in daily oncology for nurses and allied health care professionals: Opinion paper of the Nursing and Allied Health Interest Group of the International Society of Geriatric Oncology (SIOG). *Journal of Geriatric Oncology, 7,* 315–324.

Centers for Disease Control and Prevention. (2014). *National diabetes statistics report: Estimates of diabetes and its burden in the United States.* Available at www.cdc.gov/diabetes. Accessed on May 17, 2016.

Cesari, M., Prince, M., Thiyagarajan, J. A., et al. (2016). Frailty: An emerging public health priority. *Journal of the American Medical Directors Association, 17*(3), 188–192.

Chou, W. S., Gaysynsky, A., & Persoskie, A. (2016). Health literacy and communication in palliative care. In E. Wittenberg, B. Ferrell, J. Goldsmith, et al. (Eds.), *Textbook of palliative care communication* (pp. 90–101). Oxford: Oxford University Press.

Cobo, A., Vazquez, L. A., Reviriego, J., et al. (2016). Impact of frailty in older patients with diabetes mellitus: A review. *Endocrinology and Nutrition, 63*(6), 291–303.

Collerton, J., Jagger, C., Yadegarfar, M. E., et al. (2016). Deconstructing complex multimorbidity in the very old: Findings from the Newcastle 85+ study. *Biomedical Research International, 2016.* doi: 10.1155.2016/8745670.

Dahlin, C. (2016). Palliative care models. In M. Boltz, E. Capezuti, T. Fulmer, & D. Zwicker (Eds.), *Evidence-based practice protocols for best practice* (5th ed., pp. 651–667). New York: Springer Publishing Co.

Dale, W., Chow, S., & Sajid, S. (2016). Socioeconomic considerations and shared-care models of cancer care for older adults. *Clinics in Geriatric Medicine, 32,* 35–44.

Denewet, N., DeBraucker, S., Luce, S., et al. (2016). Comprehensive geriatric assessment and comorbidities predict survival in geriatric oncology. *Acta Clinical Belgium, 71,* 206–213. [Epub ahead of print]

Dumonovsky, T., Augustin, R., Rogers, M., et al. (2015). The growth of palliative care in U. S. Hospitals: A status report. *Journal of Palliative Medicine, 19*(1), 8–15.

Fried, L. P., Tangen, C. P., Walston, J., et al. (2001). Frailty in older adults: Evidence for a phenotype. *The Journals of Gerontology: Biological Sciences and Medical Sciences, 56*(3), M146–M156.

Glogowska, M., Simmonds, R., McLachlan, S., et al. (2016). "Sometimes we can't fix things": A qualitative study of health care professionals' perceptions of end of life care for patients with heart failure. *BioMed Central Palliative Care, 15,* 3.

Hui, D., & Bruera, E. (2016). Integrating palliative care into the trajectory of cancer care. *Nature Reviews Clinical Oncology, 13,* 159–171.

Jang, H. C. (2016). Sarcopenia, frailty, and diabetes in older adults. *Diabetes and Metabolism Journal, 40*(3), 182–189. [Epub ahead of print]

Jones, L. C., Clay, O. J., Ovalle, F., et al. (2016). Correlates of depressive symptoms in older adults with diabetes. *Journal of Diabetes Research, 2016.* doi: 10.1155/2016/8702730.

Kansagara, D., Chiovaro, J. C., Kagen, D., et al. (2016). So many options, where do we start? An overview of care transitions literature. *Journal of Hospital Medicine, 11,* 221–230.

Lewin, W. H., & Schaefer, K. G. (2017). Integrating palliative care into routine care of patients with heart failure: Models for clinical collaboration. *Heart Failure Review.* doi: 10.1007/s10741–017–9599–2.

McCrow, J., Morton, M., Travers, C., et al. (2016). Associations between dehydration, cognitive impairment, and frailty in older hospitalized patients. *Journal of Gerontological Nursing, 42*(5), 19–27.

Messecar, D. C. (2016). Family caregiving. In M. Boltz, E. Capezuti, T. Fulmer, & D. Zwicker (Eds.), *Evidence-based practice protocols for best practice* (5th ed., pp. 137–163). New York: Springer Publishing Co.

Mulasso, A., Roppolo, M., Giannotta, F., et al. (2016). Associations of frailty and psychosocial factors with autonomy in daily activities: A cross-sectional study in Italian community-dwelling older adults. *Clinical Interventions in Aging, 11,* 37–45.

National Cancer Institute. (2015). Percent of new cancers by age group: All cancer sites. Available at www.nih.nci.gov. Accessed May 15, 2016.

Overcash, J. (2016). Cancer assessment and intervention strategies. In M. Boltz, E. Capezuti, T. Fulmer, & D. Zwicker (Eds.), *Evidence-based practice protocols for best practice* (5th ed., pp. 525–535). New York: Springer Publishing Co.

Powers, M. A., Bardsley, J., Cypress, M., et al. (2016). Diabetes self-management education and support in Type 2 diabetes: A joint position statement of the American Diabetes Association, the American Association of Diabetes Educators, and the Academy of Nutrition and Dietetics. *Clinical Diabetes, 34,* 70–80.

Roppolo, M., Mulasso, A., Gobbens, R. J., et al (2015). A comparison between uni- and multidimensional frailty measures: Prevalence, functional status, and relationship with disability. *Clinical Interventions in Aging, 10,* 1669–1678.

Sandoval-Insausti H, Perez-Tasigchana RF, Lopez-Garcia E, et al. (2016). Macronutrients intake and incident frailty in older adults: A prospective cohort study. *Journals of Gerontology: Medical Sciences, 71*(10), 1329–1334. [Epub ahead of print]

Satake, S., & Arai, H. (2017). Implications of frailty screening in clinical practice. *Current Opinion in Clinical Nutrition, 20,* 4–10.

Schipper, J. E. (2016). Fluid overload: Identifying and managing heart failure patients at risk of hospital readmission. In M. Boltz, E. Capezuti, T. Fulmer, & D. Zwicker (Eds.), *Evidence-based practice protocols for best practice* (5th ed., pp. 503–524). New York: Springer Publishing Co.

Seigel, R., Miller, K., & Jemal, A. (2016). Cancer statistics, 2016. *Cancer Journal, 66,* 7–30.

Shinkai, S., Yoshida, H., Taniguchi, Y., et al. (2016). Public health approach to preventing frailty in the community and its effects on healthy aging in Japan. *Geriatrics and Gerontology International, 16*(Suppl 1), 87–97.

Stewart, S., Riegel, B., Boyd, C., et al. (2016). Establishing a pragmatic framework to optimise health outcomes in heart failure and multimorbidity (ARISE-HF): A multidisciplinary position statement. *International Journal of Cardiology, 212,* 1–10.

Szekendi, M. K., Vaughn, J., Lai, A. et al. (2016). The prevalence of inpatients at 33 U. S. hospitals appropriate for and receiving referrals to palliative care. *Journal of Palliative Medicine, 19,* 360–372.

The National Consensus Project for Quality Palliative Care. (2013). *Clinical practice guidelines for quality palliative care.* Available at www.nationalconsensusproject.org. Accessed on October 10, 2013.

Vidan, M. T., Blaya-Novakova, V., Sanchez, E., et al. (2016). Prevalence and prognostic impact of frailty and its components in non-dependent elderly patients with heart failure. *European Journal of Heart Failure, 18*(7), 869–875. [Epub ahead of print]

Wensing, M., Koetsenruijter, J., Roger, S., et al. (2014). Emerging trends in diabetes care practice and policy in the Netherlands: A key informant study. *BioMed Central Research Notes, 7,* 693.

Yancy, C. W., Jessup, M., Bozkurt, B., et al. (2013). 2013 AACF/AHA guideline for the management of heart failure: A report of the American College of Cardiology Foundation/American Heart Association Task Force on Practice Guidelines. *Journal of the American College of Cardiology, 62*(16), e147–e239.

chapter 28

Caring for Older Adults Experiencing Pain

LEARNING OBJECTIVES

After reading this chapter, you will be able to:

1. Differentiate between types of pain: nociceptive, acute, persistent, cancer.
2. Discuss unique aspects of pain in older adults, including prevalence, causes, and complexities of assessment and management.
3. Examine and dispel commonly held misconceptions about pain in older adults.
4. Discuss cultural aspects of pain.
5. Apply evidence-based guidelines for assessment and management of pain in older adults who are cognitively impaired.
6. Describe principles of analgesic medication use in older adults.
7. Discuss evidence-based nursing interventions for managing pain in older adults.

KEY TERMS

acute pain	opioid analgesics
addiction	opioid abuse and misuse
adjuvant analgesics	
cancer pain	pain
dependence	pain intensity
neuropathic pain	persistent pain
nociception	tolerance
nonopioid analgesics	WHO pain relief ladder

Pain is a biopsychosocial phenomenon with multiple dimensions, including sensory, cognitive, emotional, developmental, behavioral, spiritual, and cultural influences. Pain is very common among older adults, and nursing assessment and management is complicated by factors such as age-related changes, impaired mental status, and concomitant conditions. In addition, knowledge and attitudes of care providers can enhance or interfere with accurate assessment and effective management of pain, particularly with regard to older adults. This chapter provides an overview of pain and discusses assessment and management of pain, emphasizing aspects that are most pertinent to care of older adults. The Transitional Care Unfolding case study, which continues from Chapter 27, illustrates roles of nurses in addressing Maria Lopez's pain, with particular attention to ways in which nurses address continuity of care and interprofessional collaboration.

DEFINITIONS AND TYPES OF PAIN

Pain is an unpleasant sensory and subjective experience associated with actual or potential injury. The subjective quality of pain is defined as whatever the experiencing person says it is, existing whenever she or he says it does (McCaffery, 1968). Objectively, pain is a physiologic process that occurs in response to a noxious stimulus. Because pain is multifaceted, there are many ways of classifying it. The following sections describe commonly used classifications according to underlying mechanisms (i.e., nociceptive and neuropathic) and duration (i.e., acute and persistent). Cancer pain is also described because of its unique characteristics and its common occurrence in older adults.

Nociceptive and Neuropathic Pain

Nociception, which is the physiologic process that leads to the perception of a noxious stimulus as being painful, involves four processes: transduction, transmission, perception, and modulation (Figure 28-1). *Transduction* involves the activation of primary nociceptive fibers (i.e., the primary afferent neurons throughout the body) when tissue damage occurs from any of the following sources: mechanical

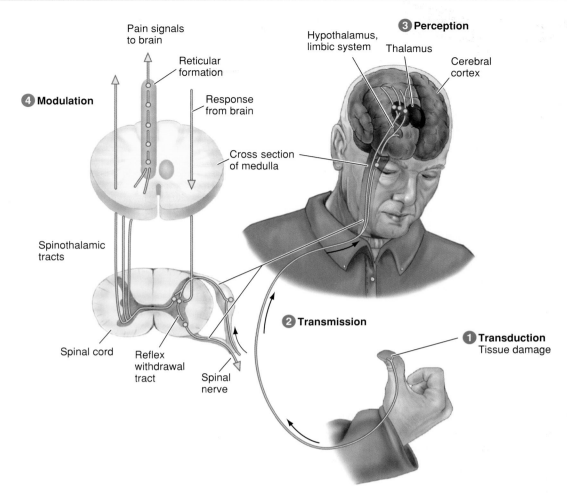

FIGURE 28-1 Processes involved in the physiology of pain. (Adapted with permission from Karch, A.M. (2011). *Focus on nursing pharmacology* (5th ed.). Philadelphia, PA: Lippincott Williams & Wilkins.)

(e.g., surgery, trauma, tumor), thermal (e.g., burn, extreme cold), or chemical (e.g., toxin, chemotherapy). Excitatory compounds are released through local tissues, immune cells, or nerve endings, and include serotonin, bradykinin, histamine, substance P, and prostaglandins. These physiologic processes set off an action potential, which is the second phase of nociception, called *transmission*. During transmission, information passes through the dorsal root ganglia to the spinal cord, and then continues through multiple ascending pathways to the brainstem. Effectiveness of analgesic medications is based on their ability to modify specific aspects of transduction and transmission.

Perception, the third process of nociception, is the point at which pain is consciously experienced. Sensory, emotional, and cognitive areas of the brain are involved in the perception of pain. Effectiveness of cognitive-behavioral therapies and other body–mind modalities is related to this aspect of nociception. The final process of nociception, *modulation,* refers to the physiologic responses to painful stimuli, which involves both the central and peripheral nervous systems and many neurochemicals, including serotonin, norepinephrine,

and endogenous opioids. Effectiveness of antidepressants for relief of pain is associated with their effects on serotonin and norepinephrine.

Neuropathic pain is caused by an abnormal processing of sensory stimuli by the central or peripheral nervous system (i.e., damage to or dysfunction that affects any part of the central or autonomic nervous systems). In contrast to nociceptive pain, which is triggered by an immediate noxious stimulus, neuropathic pain can occur in the absence of immediate tissue damage or inflammation. Also in contrast to nociceptive pain, which serves to warn and protect from further injury, neuropathic pain serves no useful purpose (Pasero & Portenoy, 2011).

Neuropathic pain involves complex responses of many peripheral and central mechanisms. Peripheral mechanisms are activated by actual or potential tissue damage due to mechanical, thermal, or chemical stimuli, as described in the section on nociceptive pain. In addition, viruses, infections, ischemia, metabolic disease (e.g., diabetes), nutritional deficiencies, and neurologic diseases can activate peripheral pain mechanisms. Abnormalities in processing information

TABLE 28-1 Comparison of Nociceptive and Neuropathic Pain		
Characteristic	**Nociceptive Pain**	**Neuropathic Pain**
Underlying mechanism	*Normal* processing of noxious stimuli in response to actual or potential tissue injury or inflammation	*Abnormal* processing of sensory input sustained by damage to or dysfunction of the nervous system
Physiologic processes	Transduction, transmission, perception, modulation	Sensitization due to abnormal peripheral and central processing of noxious stimuli
Subtypes and examples according to origin	Somatic: skin, bone, joint, connective tissue, mucous membranes, subcutaneous tissue (e.g., burn, bruise, arthritis, tendonitis, fibromyalgia, myofascial pain) Visceral: gastrointestinal, urinary tract, or other internal organs due to blockage, pressure, or infection (e.g., tumors, cholecystitis, kidney stones)	Central pain from injury to or dysfunction of the central nervous system (e.g., poststroke pain, multiple sclerosis, spinal cord injury) Peripheral mononeuropathy results in pain along nerve pathway (e.g., nerve root compression or trigeminal neuralgia) Peripheral polyneuropathy results in pain along the distribution of many peripheral nerves (e.g., trigeminal neuropathy, postherpetic neuralgia, phantom limb, diabetic neuropathy, chronic postsurgical pain)
Common descriptors	Somatic: aching, deep, throbbing, dull, sharp, tender, gnawing, pressure Visceral: cramping, squeezing, shooting, pressure	Burning, shooting, knife-like, tingling, pins and needles
Sensory symptoms	Not common except hypersensitivity in immediate area of injury	Numbness, tingling, pricking, hypersensitive to touch
Distribution	Proximal radiation common	Distal radiation common
Motor symptoms	Weakness due to pain experience	Neurologic-associated weakness if motor nerves are involved

during transduction and transmission combine with dysfunctions in central mechanisms to cause sensitization, which leads to increasingly stronger responses in the pain transmission pathway. When this occurs, pain is experienced with little or no stimulus. Table 28-1 compares characteristics of nociceptive and neuropathic pain and lists examples of types.

 See ONLINE LEARNING ACTIVITY 28-1: EVIDENCE-BASED INFORMATION ABOUT NOCICEPTIVE VERSUS NEUROPATHIC PAIN IN OLDER ADULTS at http://thepoint.lww.com/Miller8e.

Acute and Persistent Pain

Although the term persistent (also called chronic) pain describes the length of time the pain is experienced, there is increasing evidence that this type of pain has additional unique characteristics. Whereas acute pain has a sudden onset and is linked to a specific event, injury, or illness, persistent pain develops when the central nervous system continues to process pain signals as though new injuries were occurring.

Acute pain is sharp and immediate pain caused by an injury to tissue or triggered by physiologic malfunction or severe illness. It is the normal, predictable physiologic response to an adverse chemical, thermal, or mechanical stimulus, and its purpose is to lead to the resolution of the causative agent or event. Common causes of acute pain include burns, trauma, medical or surgical procedures, or medical conditions, such as cancer or postherpetic neuralgia. Acute pain is generally

time limited and responds effectively to anti-inflammatory and opioid medications as well as other approaches.

Persistent pain lasts longer than 3 to 6 months or beyond the expected time of healing from the initial causative event. National data indicate that prevalence of persistent pain has been steadily increasing among all demographic groups, with people age 65 and over consistently reporting the highest rates (Institute of Medicine [IOM], 2011). The IOM (2011) summarized the following conclusions about persistent pain:

- Persistent pain represents a pathologic transition from acute pain.
- Causes of persistent pain include underlying pathologic process, injury, medical treatment, surgical interventions, inflammations, and neuropathic pain.
- The cause of persistent pain is not always identifiable.
- In most cases, persistent pain should be considered a disease in its own right.
- Persistent pain can affect every aspect of a person's life.
- Management of persistent pain requires biopsychosocial approach that addresses physiologic, psychological, social, emotional, and spiritual aspects of the person.

Physiologically, the perception of persistent pain involves multiple neurotransmitters and receptors at many sites of the autonomic and central nervous system. Although the phenomenon is not well understood, there is increasing evidence that persistent pain begins with an acute nociceptive process that at some point combines with neuropathic characteristics to develop into persistent pain. One focus of research is on dysregulation of descending pathways that in turn lad to "pain chronification" (Ingvar, 2015; Ossipov, Morimra, &

Porreca, 2014). Research such as this is relevant to developing innovative and multimodal interventions for management of persistent pain. A clinically relevant implication of this research is that nurses need to assure timely and adequate management of acute pain, for example, during postsurgical care. It also is imperative to address postsurgical pain, which affects 5% to 10% of patients 1 year after surgery, in outpatient settings for up to 6 months after surgery (Katz, Weinrib, Fashier, et al., 2015). Another implication is that nurses can encourage older adults to explore a variety of evidence-based interventions, as discussed in the section on Nonpharmacologic Interventions for Managing Pain.

 See ONLINE LEARNING ACTIVITY 28-2: CASE STUDY VIDEOS ON ACUTE PAIN AND CHRONIC PAIN at http://thepoint.lww.com/Miller8e.

Cancer Pain

Cancer pain is a complex phenomenon caused by the cancer itself, concomitant disease, or adverse effects of treatments (e.g., surgery, radiation, or chemotherapy). Cancer pain can be acute, persistent, nociceptive, neuropathic, or—as is most often the case—a combination of these types. Pain is caused directly by the cancer and indirectly by effects of the cancer, such as compression due to tumor infiltration and neuropathy from chemotherapy. Studies have documented high prevalence rates of cancer pain as in the following examples (IOM, 2011):

- Multiple myeloma (100%)
- Metastatic or advanced-stage disease (64%)
- During anticancer treatment (59%)
- Breast cancer (58%)
- Lung cancer (56%), colorectal cancer (41%)

Because half of all cancers occur in people age 65 or older, addressing cancer pain is particularly pertinent when caring for older adults.

UNIQUE ASPECTS OF PAIN IN OLDER ADULTS

Despite much evidence that many aspects of pain differ in older adults, research on pain in older adults lags behind other areas of pain research. There is widespread agreement, however, that pain is underdetected and poorly managed in older adults (Horgas, Yoon, & Grall, 2016). Nursing assessment and management of pain are challenging not only because of age-related changes but also because of coexisting conditions, such as dementia, delirium, surgery, or acute or chronic illness, that affect many older adults. Additional complicating factors include lack of evidence-based guidelines, misconceptions and misinformation, and the presence of several types and locations of pain (e.g., neuropathic pain plus acute pain, pain at more than one site, acute pain superimposed on persistent pain, cancer pain combined with persistent pain). This section provides an overview of unique aspects of pain in older adults, and the assessment and interventions sections address specific aspects of pain in older adults who are cognitively impaired.

Age-Related Changes

Although many processes involved with pain perception can be altered by age-related changes in neurologic mechanisms, little is known about the functional consequences of these changes in older adults. Whereas some studies indicate that older adults have a diminished response to noxious stimuli, numerous studies also find that they are more vulnerable to experiencing severe or persistent pain and have diminished ability to tolerate severe pain (IOM, 2011). A recent review of studies concluded that "ageing seems to make the individual more vulnerable to suffering from pain, which is in line with clinical findings of increased pain prevalence in the elderly" (Defrin, Amanzio, de Tommaso, et al., 2015, p. 1398).

Age-related changes in pharmacokinetics and pharmacodynamics, as discussed in Chapter 8, can affect analgesic medications in older adults and increase the risk for adverse effects. Even this aspect, however, is variable, because studies have found no age-related difference in appropriate doses of postoperative morphine, particularly when doses were normalized according to body weight (Pasero & McCaffery, 2011a). A guiding principle with regard to pain in older adults is to consider the person's age as one of the many variables that can influence assessment and management.

Prevalence and Causes

Pain is common in older adults, with up to 76% of older adults living in independent settings and from 83% to 93% of nursing home residents experiencing persistent pain (Horgas, Yoon, & Grall, 2016). Musculoskeletal conditions such as arthritis are the most common cause of persistent pain in older adults, with pain often being experienced at multiple sites. Cancer is another condition that disproportionately affects older adults and is a common cause of pain. Studies also indicate that pain is highly prevalent among people with dementia, whether they live in home or long-term care settings (de Tommaso, Arendt-Nielsen, Defrin, et al., 2016).

 FUNCTIONAL CONSEQUENCES OF PAIN IN OLDER ADULTS

Pain is associated with numerous immediate and long-term consequences, and older adults are particularly vulnerable because pain is often superimposed on other undesirable conditions. An important functional consequence of acute pain, especially if it is undertreated, is the increased risk of developing persistent pain. Additional functional consequences commonly experienced by older adults include the following:

- Diminished physical function to the point of disability
- Psychosocial effects: fatigue, anxiety, depression

- Increased risk for falls
- Sleep disturbances
- Weight loss
- Increased dependency
- Increased loneliness and fatigue
- Diminished quality of life
- Decreased life expectancy
- Increased risk for cardiovascular disease

(Marshall, Litwack-Harrison, Cawthon, et al., 2016; Morales-Espinoza, Kostov, Salami, et al., 2016; Rapo-Pylkko, Haanpaa, & Lilra, 2016). Overall, any degree of pain diminishes one's quality of life and causes suffering not only for the person who experiences pain but also for those who live with and care about that person.

 GLOBAL PERSPECTIVE

The Global Burden of Disease study emphasizes that "chronic pain is clearly the most important current and future cause of morbidity and disability across the world, with large recent increases in both the number of individuals affected and years lost to disability, coupled with static or rising prevalence rates" (Rice, Smith, & Blyth, 2016, p. 792).

CULTURAL ASPECTS OF PAIN

Cultural factors can significantly influence the way people experience, express, and manage their pain, as illustrated by the examples and associated nursing implications in Box 28-1. As with all aspects of culturally appropriate care, it is imperative to be aware of different expressions of pain commonly used by cultural groups, while at the same time avoiding stereotypes and basing care on characteristics of each person as an individual. In addition, it is imperative to recognize cultural influences on the development of plans for management of chronic pain. Cross-cultural studies indicate that Western-centric pain management plans promote self-management of chronic pain, including active coping strategies; however, non-Western cultural groups may prefer passive, symptom-focused management strategies (Brady, Veljanova, & Chipchase, 2016).

 Diversity Note

A study of Hispanic and non-Hispanic white older adults with chronic musculoskeletal pain found that providers' language competencies and inclusion of family members in discussions were key elements in decisions about pain management plans, particularly for Spanish-speaking patients. Another finding was that non-Hispanic whites solicited advice from friends who had formal medical training, whereas Hispanic participants typically turned to friends who had knowledge about home remedies (Riffin, Pillemer, Reid, et al., 2015).

It also is important to recognize disparities and diversities in pain prevalence and management, as in the following examples, which are particularly relevant to care of older adults:

- Patients age 65 or older receive inadequate doses—or even no doses—of analgesic medications for cancer or postoperative pain.
- Racial and ethnic minorities are at high risk for receiving inadequate pain relief.
- Women are more likely than men to be undertreated for pain.
- People with low health literacy or low English proficiency, particularly recent immigrants, report greater pain.
- Higher pain rates are strongly associated with lower income and level of education.
- Across all groups, women consistently report a higher prevalence of persistent pain than men.
- Fears, concerns, and misconceptions about analgesic types and doses affect prescribing behaviors and therapeutic adherence by older adults and their caregivers.
- Older adults commonly fear negative consequences of analgesics. A common, but misconceived, fear is that of addiction.
- Pain descriptions may be misunderstood by patients who speak another language.
- Some cultural groups may believe that people should be able to manage pain without professional help.
- Some cultural groups may view "complaining" about pain, even to a health care professional, as inappropriate behavior.

(IOM, 2011; Noreika, Bobb, & Coyne, 2016; Pasero & McCaffery, 2011b).

The first step in assessing and managing pain in older adults is to recognize the influences of personal biases, attitudes, experiences, misconceptions, and lack of information about assessment and management. For example, studies using vignettes found that assessment and management of pain by nurses are influenced by their personal experiences of pain and also by their perceived acceptability of the patient's lifestyle (Pasero & McCaffery, 2011b). Another study found that health care providers underestimated pain in female patients and were more likely to recommend analgesics for male patients and psychological treatment for female patients (Schafer, Prkachin, Kaseweter, et al., 2016). Personal factors that influence assessment and management of pain in older adults can be addressed by self-assessment and by keeping up-to-date on evidence-based guidelines, as reviewed in the following sections.

 ## NURSING ASSESSMENT OF PAIN IN OLDER ADULTS

An accurate assessment of pain is based on recognizing the unique way in which each individual experiences and expresses pain, as described in the classic definition of pain being whatever the person experiencing it says it is (McCaffery, 1968). Despite the simplicity of this definition,

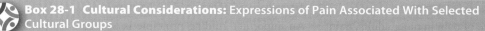

Box 28-1 Cultural Considerations: Expressions of Pain Associated With Selected Cultural Groups

Group	Assessment and Intervention Considerations	Nursing Implications
African Americans	May believe as part of their spiritual and religious foundation that pain and suffering are inevitable and must be endured; this belief may contribute to a higher pain tolerance. May believe that pain and suffering can be relieved by prayers and the laying on of hands; if pain persists it may be due to lack of faith	Teach about effectiveness of analgesics as an intervention for pain. Encourage the use of religious practices as an additional intervention rather than a solitary intervention
Amish	Are reluctant to express pain and physical discomfort	Identify subtle and nonverbal signs of pain or discomfort and offer analgesics accordingly
Arabs	Pain is regarded as unpleasant and something to be controlled; however, they may be reluctant to express pain with professionals	Recognize that family members may request analgesics on behalf of the patient
Chinese	Tend to describe pain in terms of diverse body symptoms rather than specific or localized (e.g., "dull" or "diffuse" rather than "stabbing"). May explain pain as imbalance between yin and yang. Interventions include oils, massage, warmth, relaxation, aspirin, and sleeping on the affected area	Recognize the variation in reports of pain. Support interventions as adjuvants to analgesic medications.
Filipinos	May appear stoic due to their belief that pain is part of living an honorable life and part of the process of spiritual purification while still on earth. May be viewed as an opportunity to reach fuller spiritual life or to atone for past transgressions. May rely on religious or spiritual practices for pain management	Observe for signs of pain and discomfort
Haitians	Pain is described as *doule,* but Haitians may be vague about the location because they believe that the whole body is affected. Injections are the preferred method for medication administration, followed by elixirs, tablets, and capsules	Acknowledge that the whole body is affected, but ask the person to identify specific points. Consider cultural preferences regarding medication administration
Hindu	A fatalistic attitude about illness is common, and is associated with their religious beliefs of *karma*. Thus, they may be stoic and not express pain. Pain is attributed to God's will, the wrath of God, or a punishment from God that is to be borne with courage. Asian Indian Hindus may prefer herbal remedies	Pay particular attention to nonverbal indicators of pain and ask about the meaning of their pain
Japanese	Bearing pain is considered a virtue and a matter of family honor. *Itami* is the word for pain. Because addiction is a strong taboo, patients may be reluctant to accept pain medication	Encourage the expression of pain as an important component of accurate assessment. Consider the use of regularly scheduled medications rather than a patient-controlled approach
Jewish	Verbalization of pain is acceptable and common. Individuals want to know the cause of the pain, which is just as important as obtaining relief	Talk with patients about causes of pain
Mexican	Pain is perceived as a necessary part of life, and enduring pain is often seen as a sign of strength. Pain is viewed as the will of God and the type and amount of pain a person experiences are divinely predetermined	Ask about the person's experience of pain and pay particular attention to nonverbal indicators of pain
Puerto Ricans	May be outspoken in expressing pain (e.g., *Ay!* is a verbal moaning of *dolor*). May prefer oral or intravenous analgesics rather than injections or rectal medications. May use heat, herbal teas, and prayer for pain management	Use appropriate pain assessment tools; do not judge pain expression as an exaggeration

Source: Purnell, L. D. (2014). *Guide to culturally competent health care* (3rd ed.). Philadelphia, PA: F.A. Davis.

assessment of pain is very complex, even when people can describe their pain. When a person's level of cognition is impaired or when communication barriers exist, assessment of pain is even more challenging (as discussed in the next section). Additional complications are associated with the common occurrence of concomitant conditions in older adults. As emphasized by a recent nursing study, the decision-making process for assessing and managing pain requires that nurses and all health care professionals engage in an ongoing process of using intuition and experiences to "build a picture" of the patient (Dowding, Lichtner, Allcock, et al., 2016).

Identifying Common Misconceptions

Despite the common occurrence of pain in older adults, pain should never be viewed as a normal part of aging. When health care professionals view pain as a part of life and a natural consequence of the aging process, older adults may experience frustration when they perceive this as a dismissive attitude (Collis & Waterfield, 2015). In addition, this misconception can affect assessment and management of pain in older adults, causing serious negative consequences affecting functioning and quality of life. Evidence-based information about pain in older adults is becoming increasingly available to dispel misconceptions and guide health care professionals in assessment and management. For example, recent studies provide evidence-based tools for assessing pain in nonverbal patients, as discussed in the section on Assessment in Older Adults Who Are Cognitively Impaired. Thus, an initial step in assessing pain is to identify misconceptions, such as the ones delineated in Box 28-2. An associated step is to keep up-to-date on evidence-based guidelines related to pain in older adults by using the resources delineated in Online Learning Activity 28-3.

See ONLINE LEARNING ACTIVITY 28-3: EVIDENCE-BASED INFORMATION ABOUT NURSING ASSESSMENT AND MANAGEMENT OF PAIN IN OLDER ADULTS at http://thepoint.lww.com/Miller8e.

Box 28-2 Misconceptions That Can Affect Assessment and Management of Pain

Misconceptions Commonly Held by Health Care Professionals

- Older adults have a high pain tolerance.
- People with dementia do not experience pain.
- People who are sleeping are not experiencing pain.
- People who can be distracted from pain usually do not have severe pain.
- Opioids should not be used for older adults or for people with a history of substance abuse
- Elevated vital signs are a reliable indicator of pain intensity.
- Behavioral manifestations are more reliable than patients' self-reports.

Concerns Commonly Held by Older Adults and Their Caregivers

- Desire to avoid a diagnosis that is serious, untreatable, or life-threatening
- Fears related to addiction to or adverse effects of analgesics
- Concern about being perceived as a complainer
- Desire to maintain stoicism or avoid expression of feelings that may be perceived as a weakness
- Perceptions about pain being an atonement or punishment that should not be addressed by analgesics or other medical interventions
- Belief that morphine and strong analgesics are used only for terminal situations
- Stigma associated with opioids and other prescription analgesics

Obtaining Information About Pain

An important guiding principle is to assess for pain during initial contacts with patients, at frequent intervals, whenever the person's condition changes, and as an essential and ongoing component of pain management interventions. During an initial contact and whenever pain is of recent onset, a comprehensive assessment, as described in this section, is imperative. A less comprehensive but comparative assessment needs to be conducted at appropriate intervals after analgesics and other pain management interventions have been administered and whenever pain management interventions are changed. For example, in acute care settings, effectiveness of analgesics should be assessed 30 to 60 minutes after administration. A reassessment typically includes questions about pain intensity and length of time the intervention was effective.

Because a patient's self-report about pain is considered the "gold standard" for pain assessment, begin by asking about the person's experience of pain. Allow older adults enough time to process the information and respond, and recognize that they may refer to pain by words such as *burning, discomfort, aching, soreness,* or *hurting.* Another effective strategy is to ask older adults to describe how pain affects their daily life or quality of life. For example, ask if pain or discomfort prevents them from participating in activities they would like to do.

Essential assessment information also is obtained by observing for nonverbal indicators of pain, such as facial expressions, body movements, or decreased activity. Information also can be elicited from family members and caregivers when additional input would be helpful, particularly if the older adult is not a reliable reporter for any reason. If the person's level of functioning has changed recently, find out if pain or discomfort is a contributing factor.

Pain rating scales are used to assess **pain intensity**, which is the subjective determination of the strength, concentration, or force of the pain. Because pain intensity is an easily measured indicator that can be used to assess changes at different times, it is often referred to as the "fifth vital sign." Pain rating scales are routinely used to provide a standardized measure of pain that can be documented at appropriate intervals as an integral part of assessment and reassessment. The Numerical Rating Scale (NRS) is widely used; however, the Verbal Descriptor Scale (VDS) is the one recommended for use with older adults (see Figure 28-2). The VDS is a reliable and valid measure of pain intensity; moreover, studies identify it as the easiest to use for and most preferred by older adults (Horgas, Yoon, & Grall, 2016). This scale, which can be used with the NRS, uses a continuum of verbal cues ranging from no pain to the worst pain possible. It is imperative to supplement information from these tools with documentation of broader aspects, such as self-reports and nursing observations.

Nursing assessment of pain focuses on information about the older adult's experience of acute, persistent, and intermittent pain, including characteristics of different types. When

Pain intensity scales

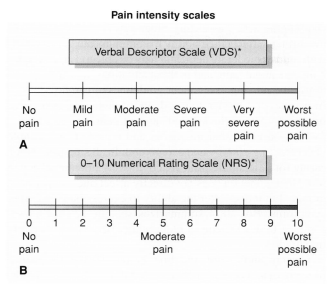

* If used as a graphic rating scale, a 10-cm baseline is recommended.

FIGURE 28-2 Examples of pain rating scales: **A.** Verbal Description Scale. **B.** Numerical Rating Scale.

patients experience more than one type of pain, or if it is present in different locations, letters or other marks can be used to distinguish sites and descriptors. Pain assessment also addresses the person's experiences with and concerns about analgesics or other interventions. Box 28-3 can be used as a guide for assessing these components of pain. An important aspect of documenting or discussing patient experiences of pain is avoiding the phrase "complains of pain" because this is associated with a negative attitude toward patients and may reflect a desire that patients cope better or talk less about their pain. Rather, it is more appropriate and objective to state that patients "report pain" when documenting information about a patient's experience of pain (Pasero & McCaffery, 2011b).

Another aspect of pain assessment is using open-ended questions to identify the person's expectations for relief, as well as the meaning he or she associates with the pain. Personal goals for pain management may be based on the degree to which pain affects daily functioning and quality of life, and on the person's desire to avoid adverse effects of management. Nurses can ask questions such as the following to assess pain management goals and potential interventions,

 Box 28-3 Questions to Assess Pain in Older Adults

Initial questions to ascertain need for further assessment:
- Are you experiencing pain, discomfort, aching, right now?
- Do you have more than one type of pain?
- Have you had this before or is this new? (If pain has been present before, ask about how it differs, what makes it better or worse, and other questions.)
- Describe the pain in your own words.

If the person acknowledges having pain, use a pain rating scale and document location(s) on this figure.

Ask about the following characteristics for each type of pain reported:
- Frequency
- Duration
- Precipitating factors
- Alleviating factors
- Variations, such as changes in intensity
- Previous medical evaluation
- Usual management strategies (pharmacologic and nonpharmacologic)

Ask about effects of pain on functioning and quality of life:
- Daily activities (sleep, eating, appetite, ability to get around, level of independence, driving, and so forth)
- Level of physical activity for functioning or enjoyment
- Relationships with other (e.g., social interactions, family activities)
- Emotions (e.g., anger, happiness, irritability, mood)
- Cognitive abilities (e.g., concentration, thinking)
- Participation in enjoyable activities (e.g., hobbies, travel)

Assess the following aspects of analgesic history:
- Current and past use of analgesics
- Names, doses, and effectiveness of prescription and nonprescription analgesics
- Experiences with adverse effects
- Analgesics taken on set schedule or as needed
- Use of analgesics during previous 24 hours and influence of these on pain rating scale and other assessment information

Assess concerns about, or fear of, adverse effects, including addiction.

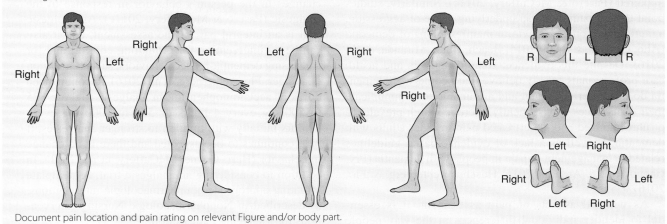

Document pain location and pain rating on relevant Figure and/or body part.

which are particularly applicable with regard to persistent pain:

- Does the person expect to be free of pain or is a certain level of pain acceptable?
- What level of functioning is the person expecting to attain?
- Is the person interested in self-management interventions, such as a physical activity program?
- Is the person concerned about adverse effects of medications?
- Would a referral to a pain management practitioner be helpful?
- Is it appropriate to consider a referral for physical or occupational therapy?
- Is the person interested in information about complementary and alternative medicine (CAM) practices or practitioners (e.g., reiki, relaxation, guided imagery, acupuncture)?

In addition to asking assessment questions, observe and document pertinent physical assessment findings, such as vital signs; overall appearance; nonverbal indicators; level of functioning; and skin color, temperature, and integrity. For example, observe whether the person limits or avoids a particular activity because of pain or discomfort. In addition, observe the person's verbal and nonverbal expressions of emotional responses to pain and incorporate pertinent information in the assessment.

 GLOBAL PERSPECTIVE

In the Netherlands, primary care nurses used comprehensive geriatric assessments to successfully identify pain in older adults and improve access to tailored pain management. Nurses were proactive in initiating and implementing pain action plans that consisted of actions or agreements related to continuity of care (Muntinga, Jansen, Schellevis, et al., 2016).

Pain in Older Adults Who Are Cognitively Impaired

Studies indicate that the pain transmission process is unaltered in people who have dementia; however, the cognitive processing and interpretation of the pain stimulus may be impaired (Pasero & McCaffery, 2011c). Similarly, studies point toward pain being an underlying cause of aggression, agitation, and other behavioral manifestations of dementia (Ahn, Garvan, & Lyon, 2015; Beach, Huck, Miranda, et al., 2016). Despite this evidence, some caregivers and health care professionals falsely believe that people with dementia do not experience pain and are unable to communicate their experiences. Consequently, there is a high prevalence of unrecognized and undertreated pain in older adults with dementia, as well as a lack of evidence-based guidelines related to management of pain in people with dementia (Fry, Chenoweth, & Arendts, 2016; Husebo, Achterberg, & Flo, 2016).

As with all aspects of pain assessment, it is essential to identify individual differences in the way people

communicate their experience. This becomes even more challenging when assessing older adults whose cognitive impairment affects their ability to communicate. Older adults with mild to moderate dementia may be able to verbally communicate about pain, and in these situations, it is appropriate to use the nursing assessment guidelines already discussed. In people with moderate or advanced dementia, disruptive behaviors may be the key indicator of pain, and assessment focuses on nonverbal indicators and reports from reliable observers (e.g., family and caregivers). In all situations when caring for older adults who are cognitively impaired, keep in mind that dementia does not directly affect one's experience of pain, but it does alter the ability to express pain and other symptoms. Box 28-4 summarizes specific actions nurses can take to assess pain in older adults who are cognitively impaired.

Current studies and guidelines emphasize the importance of using evidence-based observational tools for older adults who are cognitively impaired or have communication limitations (Malara, DeBiase, Bettarini, et al., 2016). The Pain Assessment in Advanced Dementia (PAINAD) and the Pain Assessment Checklist for Seniors with Limited Ability to Communicate (PACSLAC) are two commonly used assessment tools with a strong base of evidence (Ellis-Smith, Evans, Bone, et al., 2016). More recently, a shorter version of PACSLAC, called the PACSLAC-II, was developed and tested as a reliable tool that is particularly useful and valid for discriminating between pain and nonpain states in long-term care residents. Moreover, nurses in long-term care settings preferred the PACSLAC-II because of its shorter length and its ability to facilitate documentation and greater efficiency in pain management (see Figure 28-3) (Chan, Hadjistavropoulos, Williams, et al., 2014). Online Learning Activity 28-4 provides additional information about and links to evidence-based information about commonly used tools for pain assessment in people with dementia.

If assessment findings indicate that the person with dementia is likely to be experiencing pain, it is important to do all of the following: assume pain is present, initiate a trial of analgesic medication, and observe changes in the person's behavior in response to the analgesic (Pasero & McCaffery, 2011c). An analgesic trial is an integral part of the assessment, and it also can be an intervention for promoting comfort and for addressing dementia-related behaviors, such as agitation (Habinger, Flo, Achterberg, et al., 2016). Recommended doses of acetaminophen for an analgesic trial are 325 to 500 mg every 4 hours or 500 to 1000 mg every 6 hours initially with titration to stronger analgesics, if pain continues to be suspected and there is no change in behavior (Herr, Coyne, McCaffery, et al., 2011). In addition to considering an analgesic trial, contemplate initiating appropriate nonpharmacologic interventions, as described in Nonpharmacologic Nursing Interventions for Managing Pain section.

Box 28-4 Assessing Pain in Older Adults Who Are Cognitively Impaired

General Principles

- Elicit as much verbal and nonverbal information directly from the person as possible.
- Compare current assessment findings with the person's baseline function, but recognize that the person's usual level of functioning may be affected by undiagnosed and undertreated pain.
- Know the person and recognize that the person's ability to communicate may fluctuate.
- For people with limited ability to communicate, use an evidence-based observational tool, such as PACSLAC-II (Figure 28-3).
- Base assessment conclusions on multiple sources of information.
- Assess the person under several types of conditions: for example, resting, active, different times of day, during activities of daily living.
- Use team approach for assessment and management of pain.

Identify Verbal Indicators of Pain

- Vocalizations such as sighing, moaning, chanting
- Repeated calling out "Help"
- Response to touching: "Ow," "Ouch," swearing or cursing
- Response to care-related activities: "Stop" or "Don't do that"
- Facial expressions, such as grimacing or furrowed brows
- Rubbing or protecting an extremity

Identify Behavioral Indicators

- Changes in behavior (e.g., aggression, agitation)
- Increased confusion, disorientation
- Diminished appetite

- Resistance to or combativeness during care activities
- Withdrawal from social activities
- Decreased participation in physical activities
- Spending more time in bed (with or without sleep)

Assess for Indicators of Underlying Causes of Pain (e.g., Conditions, Falls, Surgical Procedures)

- Skin infection: swelling, inflammation, breakdown
- Arthritis: joint swelling, guarding, limited use, diminished mobility
- Gout: joint inflammations
- Oral problems: check mouth for sores, redness, open areas
- Low back pain: gait changes, diminished level of activity, abnormal posture
- Urinary tract infection: changes in behavior, urinary frequency or incontinence

Obtain Pertinent Information from Family, Caregivers, and Reliable Sources

- Identify history of chronic conditions associated with pain (e.g., gout, arthritis, peripheral or postherpetic neuropathy)
- Observe for exacerbations of previously controlled chronic conditions
- Ask about usual manifestations of pain (e.g., wandering, agitation, withdrawal from activities)
- Find out about previous use of analgesics and nonpharmacologic interventions
- Ask about recent falls or acute problems that could cause pain (e.g., urinary tract infections, skin tears or injuries, or bacterial infections such as pneumonia), as well as chronic conditions.

 See **ONLINE LEARNING ACTIVITY 28-4: EVIDENCE-BASED INFORMATION ABOUT PAIN IN PEOPLE WITH DEMENTIA** at http://thepoint.lww.com/Miller8e.

 ## PHARMACOLOGIC INTERVENTIONS FOR MANAGING PAIN

Analgesic medications are the foundation of effective pain management and are the first intervention for acute and serious pain. Selection of the type and dose of analgesic is based on careful evaluation of many patient variables, including age, weight, concomitant conditions and medications, and concerns about actual and potential adverse effects (including drug interactions). Keep in mind that with careful analgesic selection and monitoring there is less risk of adverse effects from medications as compared with the serious risks associated with undertreatment of pain in older adults. Nurses have major responsibilities in preventing the undertreatment of pain and at the same time providing astute assessment and management of both therapeutic and adverse effects. This is particularly important when caring for older adults who are in long-term care facilities and those who have dementia.

Classifications of Analgesics

Three groups of analgesics are nonopioids, opioids, and adjuvants. Avoid using the term *narcotic* because this term is associated with substances that have the potential for abuse, such as cocaine, which actually have no analgesic properties. Instead, use the terms *nonopioid* and *opioid* analgesics rather than *nonnarcotics* and *narcotics*.

Nonopioid analgesics include acetaminophen; nonaspirin, nonsteroidal anti-inflammatory drugs (NSAIDs); and aspirin. Nonopioids act at the site of the injury to decrease pain; NSAIDs, for example, inhibit the release of prostaglandin from damaged cells. **Opioid analgesics** are natural, semisynthetic, or synthetic drugs that relieve pain by binding to multiple types of opioid receptors in the central nervous system. Because of this action, the release of neurotransmitters is blocked and the pain impulse cannot cross the synapse into the dorsal horn during transmission over the pain pathway. Examples of opioids are codeine, morphine, tramadol, fentanyl, and methadone. **Adjuvant analgesics** are medications that have a primary indication other than the treatment of pain, such as antidepressants or anticonvulsants, but relieve pain in some conditions. Adjuvants most often act on the modulation phase along the pain pathway by interfering with the reuptake of serotonin and norepinephrine, which inhibit the transmission of nociceptive impulses. All three groups

Pain Assessment Checklist for Seniors with Limited Ability to Communicate-II (PACSLAC-II)

Date of Assessment: _____ Time: _____	Check if present
Facial Expressions	
1. Grimacing	
2. Tighter face	
3. Pain expression	
4. Increased eye movement	
5. Wincing	
6. Opening mouth	
7. Creasing forehead	
8. Lowered eyebrows or frowning	
9. Raised cheeks, narrowing of the eyes or squinting	
10. Wrinkled nose and raised upper lip	
11. Eyes closing	
Verbalizations and Vocalizations	
12. Crying	
13. A specific sound for pain (e.g., 'ow', 'ouch')	
14. Moaning and groaning	
15. Grunting	
16. Gasping or breathing loudly	
Body Movements	
17. Flinching or pulling away	
18. Thrashing	
19. Refusing to move	
20. Moving slow	
21. Guarding sore area	
22. Rubbing or holding sore area	
23. Limping	
24. Clenched fist	
25. Going into foetal position	
26. Stiff or rigid	
27. Shaking or trembling	
Changes in Interpersonal Interactions	
28. Not wanting to be touched	
29. Not allowing people near	
Changes in Activity Patterns or Routines	
30. Decreased activity	
Mental Status Changes	
31. Are there mental status changes that are due to pain <u>and</u> are not explained by another condition (e.g., delirium due to medication, etc.)?	
TOTAL SCORE (Add up checkmarks)	

COPYRIGHT: The PACSLAC-II is copyrighted by Sarah Chan, Thomas Hadjistavropoulos and Shannon Fuchs-Lacelle. For permission to reproduce the PACSLAC contact thomas.hadjistavropoulos@uregina.ca who is authorised to provide permission on behalf of all copyright holders. The items of the PACSLAC-II are organized according to the assessment domain categories recommended by the American Geriatrics Society (2002) for patients with severe dementia. The developers of the PACSLAC-II specifically disclaim any liability arising directly or indirectly from use of application of the PACSLAC-II. Use of the PACSLAC-II may not be appropriate for some patients and the PACSLAC-II is not a substitute for a thorough assessment by a qualified health professional. The PACSLAC-II (like other observational pain assessment tools) is a screening tool and not a definitive indicator of pain. As such, sometimes it may fail to identify pain and other times \ it may incorrectly signal the presence of pain. The PACSALC-II should be used by qualified health care staff within the context of their broader knowledge and examination of the patient.

FIGURE 28-3 Pain assessment checklist for seniors with limited ability to communicate-II (PACSLAC-II). (Reprinted with permission from Chan, S., Hadjistavropoulos, T., Williams, J. & Lints-Martindale, A. (2014). Evidence-based development and initial validation of the pain assessment checklist for seniors with limited ability to communicate-II (PACSLAC-II). *Clinical Journal of Pain, 30*, 816–824.)

TABLE 28-2 Misconceptions and Realities About Analgesics

Misconception	Evidence-Based Reality
Daily use of nonopioids is safer than long-term use of opioids	Long-term use of NSAIDs is associated with more severe and life-threatening adverse effects, whereas the most common adverse effect of opioids is constipation, which can be addressed
Nonopioids are not effective for severe pain	Nonopioids alone rarely relieve severe pain, but they have an important role as adjuvants
Polypharmacy with different types of analgesics is unacceptable	Because different types of analgesics have unique mechanisms, it is acceptable and often recommended to use different types for specific purposes
Rectal or parenteral administration of NSAIDs reduces the risks of GI adverse effects	NSAIDs administered by any route inhibit prostaglandins, which are necessary to maintain the protective barrier in the GI tract
Administering NSAIDs with an antacid reduces the risk of GI adverse effects	Antacids may decrease the risk of GI effects, but they also decrease effectiveness of NSAIDs because they cause the drug to be released in the stomach instead of the small intestine
Taking opioids for pain relief leads to addiction	Addiction as a result of taking opioids for analgesia occurs less than 1% of the time
Opioids are not effective for all types of pain	All pain responds to opioids, but they are more effective in relieving visceral and somatic pain and less effective for neuropathic pain
Opioids should be avoided during early stages of progressive conditions to prevent the development of tolerance	Tolerance to opioids does not necessarily develop and the dose usually stabilizes if the pain is stable. There is no ceiling to opioid doses and patients develop tolerance to respiratory depression
Opioids commonly cause clinically significant respiratory depression	If opioid doses are titrated slowly and decreased when sedation occurs, respiratory depression is rare. Tolerance to respiratory effects develops within 72 hours of regular daily doses

GI, gastrointestinal; NSAID, nonsteroidal anti-inflammatory drug.
Source: Pasero, C., Portenoy, R. K., & McCaffery, M. (2011). Nonopiod analgesics. In C. Pasero & M. McCaffery (Eds.), *Pain assessment and pharmacologic management* (pp. 177–180). St. Louis, MO: Mosby Elsevier; Pasero, C., Quinn, T. W., Portenoy, R. K., et al (2011). Opioid analgesics. In C. Pasero & M. McCaffery (Eds.), *Pain assessment and pharmacologic management* (pp. 277–282). St. Louis, MO: Mosby Elsevier.

are effective in the perception phase, acting in different ways to decrease the conscious experience of pain perception.

Misconceptions and Realities About Analgesics

The many misconceptions about different analgesics may affect selection of medications for pain management. Table 28-2 identifies misconceptions and realities about analgesics that are most relevant to pain management for older adults.

Because misconceptions and lack of information can lead to fears and reluctance to take appropriate medications, it is important to teach older adults and their families about tolerance, dependence, and addiction. Medication **tolerance** is a physiologic protective mechanism that helps the body become accustomed to the medication so that adverse effects (except for constipation) gradually diminish. Tolerance is characterized by a decrease in one or more therapeutic effects of the medication (e.g., less analgesia) or its adverse effects (e.g., nausea, sedation, or respiratory depression). Tolerance to analgesia usually occurs during the first several days to 2 weeks of therapy.

Dependence is a normal physiologic response manifested by the development of withdrawal symptoms when an opioid is suddenly discontinued after being administered repeatedly for more than 2 weeks. Tapering (i.e., gradually reducing) the dose of an opioid as pain resolves usually prevents withdrawal symptoms. Dependence is not necessarily an indicator of addiction; rather, it indicates that the medication is medically necessary for managing symptoms.

In contrast to dependence and tolerance, **addiction** is a chronic disease with biologic, neurologic, and psychological characteristics, including one or more of the following in relation to a drug: craving, compulsive use, inability to control its use, and continued use even when harm occurs. In reality, addiction rarely occurs in relation to analgesic medications, whereas tolerance and dependence are normal responses that should be expected when opioids are taken for 2 to 4 weeks or longer (Pasero & McCaffery, 2011b).

The World Health Organization's Three-Step Pain Relief Ladder for Pain Management

The World Health Organization's (WHO) pain relief ladder was developed in the 1980s as a guide to managing persistent cancer pain. The **WHO pain relief ladder** continues to be used as a model for clinical practice. Nurses can apply this approach for selecting analgesics on the basis of the intensity of the pain, using analgesics from each of the three different classifications, and building on previously effective treatments. The three steps of the pain relief ladder (Figure 28-4) address different levels of pain intensity and also allow for the fact that not all people experience pain in the same way along the same trajectory. Therefore, tailoring therapeutic regimens to individual needs is the gold standard of pain management for older adults. It is important to recognize that treatment may begin at Step 2 or 3 for patients with higher levels of pain.

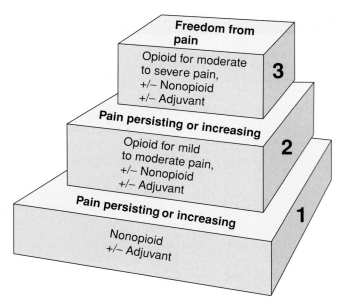

FIGURE 28-4 World Health Organization pain relief ladder. (Redrawn with permission from World Health Organization. Copyright 2005.)

Step 1 of the WHO pain relief ladder addresses mild pain (i.e., ranging from 1 to 3 out of 10 on an NRS) by recommending the use of nonopioid analgesics initially, with the addition of an adjuvant if it is deemed appropriate. Based on current recommendations, acetaminophen (Tylenol) is the first-line treatment for mild to moderate pain because it is a very effective analgesic with few side effects. Hepatotoxicity, which is the most serious adverse effect, can occur when the recommended maximum dose of 4 g/day is exceeded. Additional factors that increase the risk of hepatotoxicity include the following:

- Malnutrition or fasting
- Daily consumption of more than 2 ounces of alcohol
- Liver disease or hepatic insufficiency
- Use of other potentially hepatotoxic mediations

When calculating the daily dose of acetaminophen, consider all sources of this drug, including nonprescription combination products for conditions such as sleep and common colds. Additional adverse effects associated with high doses or long-term use of acetaminophen include increased risk of the following: hypertension, gastric effects, and renal insufficiency or failure.

The use of NSAIDs poses many serious risks for older adults including all the following: gastrointestinal bleeding, renal insufficiency or failure, decreased platelet aggregations, and even death. In 2012, the American Geriatrics Society updated its guidelines for management of persistent pain in older adults and recommended that clinicians caring for patients with moderate to severe pain, pain-related functional impairment, or diminished quality of life due to pain should consider opioid therapy if acetaminophen does not alleviate the pain. Further, the clinician should consider additional factors, "including

the potential for addiction, which is far lower in older adults" (American Geriatrics Society, 2012).

Step 2 of the WHO pain relief ladder suggests adding an opioid or opioid combination to the regimen if the pain continues to be in the mild to moderate range (e.g., it worsens from 3 to 5 of 10 on an NRS). This step *builds on* the previous one; it does not replace the use of the Step 1 nonopioid analgesics. Step 2 should also include a method of providing around-the-clock analgesia by using a breakthrough medication. For example, a patient would take acetaminophen 500 mg every 6 hours and use one tablet of Percocet (i.e., 5 mg oxycodone + 325 mg acetaminophen) every 4 hours as needed for breakthrough pain. This combination of acetaminophen and Percocet contains only half the maximum recommended dose of acetaminophen for older adults.

Step 3 interventions are considered if the pain persists or worsens (i.e., ranging from 7 to 10 on an NRS). Although both Steps 2 and 3 include the use of an opioid, different types of opioids are used in each step. Because Step 2 opioid drugs (e.g., Lortab 5/500, Tylenol #3, or Percocet) include fixed doses of acetaminophen, the extent to which these opioids can be used is limited by the recommended maximum daily dose of acetaminophen for older adults. Thus, the use of stronger opioids is the appropriate next step. Step 3 builds on Steps 1 and 2, with the continued use of nonopioids and adjuvants. Guidelines for Step 3 opioids include the following:

- Administer opioids around the clock, using a controlled-release formula to ensure a constant blood level of the analgesic medication.
- Continue to include some type of breakthrough pain medication.
- For breakthrough pain, use opioids with a short half-life so that they can be rapidly titrated for severe pain episodes.

Opioids are associated with many adverse effects, but most of these effects are dose-dependent and subside as patients develop tolerance. Constipation is the most common adverse effect, and it is the one that does not subside. Conditions that increase the risk of developing constipation include increased age, diminished mobility, gastrointestinal conditions, and medication interactions. Additional adverse effects of opioids include nausea, vomiting, sedation, and altered mental status (i.e., delirium, confusion). Interventions for preventing and addressing constipation and altered mental state are discussed in Chapters 18 and 14, respectively.

When adding analgesic medication into the wellness approach to pain management, nurses need to communicate with other members of the health care team to formulate a plan that clearly establishes and addresses the patient's pain goals, anticipated side effects, and proposed interventions for those side effects. Patients and designated family members are included as members of the decision-making team. Also, proposed interventions should be based on evidence-based guidelines (i.e., the WHO pain relief ladder) and should include nonpharmacologic interventions, when appropriate. Although nurses cannot be expected to know all the implications of all analgesics, they can become experts on frequently used drugs and keep references handy for more detailed information about additional interventions.

Special Considerations: Opioid Abuse and Misuse

Although **opioid abuse and misuse** is commonly associated with younger populations, gerontological health care professionals are raising major concerns about increasing use and misuse of prescription and illicit drugs for pain management among older adults. Analysis of national Medicare data indicates that the percentage of patients who received prescriptions for opioids more than 90 days a year increased from 4.62% in 2007 to 7.35% in 2012. Individual characteristics associated with prolonged use included older age; female gender; white race; low income; living in a lower education area; and comorbidity of drug abuse, rheumatoid arthritis, and depression (Kuo, Raji, Chen, et al., 2016). The combination of data such as these and concerns about management of persistent pain in older adults has led to major initiatives that address opioid abuse among older adults. For example, in 2016, the Gerontological Society of America joined with the Alliance for Balanced Pain Management to address the societal burden of opioid misuse (Gerontological Society of America, 2016). Also in 2016, the Centers for Disease Control and Prevention published guidelines for prescribing opioids for chronic pain, as summarized in the Evidence-Based Practice Box 28-5. Online Learning Activity 28-5 provides links to further information about appropriate use of opioids in managing chronic pain.

See ONLINE LEARNING ACTIVITY 28-5: ARTICLE ABOUT APPROPRIATE USE OF OPIOIDS IN MANAGING CHRONIC PAIN at http://thepoint.lww.com/Miller8e.

A Student's Perspective

My aging client complains periodically about pain in her shoulder. She has stated that she does not want to take anything besides aspirin when she has pain and that aspirin seems to take care of her pain. She does not take the aspirin every day. She's afraid of taking pain medications because she does not want to rely on strong medications, and she is afraid of becoming addicted. I explained to her the consequences of untreated pain and also tried to ease her fears of pain medication. She assured me that she will see her physician if the pain becomes severe when aspirin does not help her.

Thelma M.

NONPHARMACOLOGIC INTERVENTIONS FOR MANAGING PAIN

Although analgesics are essential for acute pain and in many other circumstances, nonpharmacologic interventions are a crucial component of pain management, particularly for older adults with persistent pain (Guerriero, 2017; Horgas, Yoon, & Grall, 2016). Nonpharmacologic interventions rarely have adverse effects and often have broader beneficial effects, such as relaxation, improved comfort, reduced anxiety, and improved quality of life. For example, aromatherapy with lavender oil is a relatively simple nonpharmacologic intervention that has positive effects on sleep, anxiety, and pain (O'Malley, 2017). A wellness-oriented approach to pain management for older adults involves the use of a wide variety of nonpharmacologic interventions to supplement, enhance, or diminish the need for pharmacologic interventions. This is particularly important in light of increasing concerns about misuse and abuse of opioids as well as concerns about adverse effects of pharmacologic interventions (Bruckenthal, Marino, & Snelling, 2016). Many nonpharmacologic approaches involve teaching about self-management strategies, which is an important aspect of wellness-oriented care for older adults with persistent pain. Online Learning Activity 28-6 provides information about resources for patient and caregiver teaching related to all aspects of pain management. Box 28-6 summarizes evidence-based recommendations related to nonpharmacologic approaches that may be effective for persistent pain.

See ONLINE LEARNING ACTIVITY 28-6 RESOURCES FOR PATIENT AND CAREGIVER TEACHING ABOUT PAIN, INCLUDING NONPHARMACOLOGIC APPROACHES at http://thepoint.lww.com/Miller8e.

Nonpharmacologic strategies also can be used as an adjunct to analgesic medications for acute pain. For example, physical modalities, such as application of heat or cold, are commonly used for the treatment of acute pain. Many of the interventions described in Box 28-6 for persistent pain can also be used to complement analgesic agents and decrease the need for pharmacologic interventions (Cornelius, Herr, Gordon, et al., 2017).

INTERPROFESSIONAL APPROACHES

Pain management, particularly related to persistent pain, is increasingly being recognized as a multifaceted problem that requires collaborative efforts of several professionals. This interprofessional approach develops a multidimensional care plan based on a comprehensive biopsychosocial assessment that includes physical, functional, and psychosocial components, as well

E·B·P Box 28-5 Evidence-Based Practice: Opioids for Chronic Pain Outside of Cancer, Palliative, and End-of-Life Care

Background

- An estimated 20% of patients with noncancer pain receive an opioid prescription for pain management.
- Evidence is limited to support the effectiveness of long-term opioid therapy for chronic pain outside of end-of-life care.
- Risks for long-term opioid use for chronic pain are clear and significant.
- Although some studies find moderate effectiveness for pain management in adults with chronic noncancer pain, a high percentage of patients discontinue long-term opioid use because of lack of efficacy and because of adverse events.

Recommendations for Initiating or Continuing Opioids for Chronic Pain

- Nonpharmacologic therapy and nonopioid pharmacologic therapy are preferred.
- Opioids should be considered only if expected outcomes for both pain and function are expected to outweigh the risks.
- If opioids are used, they should be combined with nonpharmacologic and nonopioid therapies.

Benefits and Harms of Opioid Therapy

- Long-term opioid therapy is associated with increased risk for all of the following: increased risk for opioid use disorder, overdose, myocardial infarction, and motor vehicle injury.
- Population groups that are at greater risk for harm include older adults; patients with sleep apnea or sleep-disordered breathing; and patients with depression, mental health conditions, or substance abuse disorders.
- Reduced renal or hepatic function can result in greater peak effect and longer duration of action.
- Age-related changes affecting medications can result in a narrow therapeutic window between safe dosages and those associated with respiratory depression and overdose.
- Older adults may be at increased risk for falls and fractures related to opioids.

Nonopioid Pharmacologic Approaches

These include:
- Acetaminophen
- NSAIDs
- Cyclooxygenase 2 (COX-2) inhibitors
- Certain anticonvulsants (e.g., gabapentin, pregabalin)
- Certain antidepressants (e.g., tricyclics, serotonin, and norepinephrine reuptake inhibitors)

- Interventional approaches, such as epidural injection for lumbar radiculopathy, can provide short-term improvement
- Topical NSAIDs are recommended for patients >75 years to treat localized osteoarthritis

Concerns About and Contraindications Related to Nonopioid Pharmacologic Approaches

- Acetaminophen should be avoided in patients with liver failure, and dose should be reduced in patients with hepatic insufficiency or a history of alcoholism.
- NSAIDs and COX-2 inhibitors are associated with gastrointestinal bleeding or perforation, as well as renal and cardiovascular risks.
- NSAIDs are associated with increased risk for stroke and heart attack, and these risks might increase with higher doses or longer use.
- NSAID use is associated with gastritis, peptic ulcer disease, and fluid retention.
- NSAIDs should be used with caution in people with hypertension, renal insufficiency, or heart failure.

Special Considerations

- Consider whether cognitive limitations might interfere with management of opioid therapy for older adults with dementia or other cognitive impairments; if so, determine whether a caregiver can responsibly comanage medication therapy.
- Recognize that caregivers may be able to divert opioids for uses other than the prescribed purpose.
- In all situations, long-term use of opioids should be reassessed every 4 months.

Nonpharmacologic Interventions for Persistent Pain

- Cognitive behavioral therapy (i.e., training in behavioral techniques to help patients modify situational factors and cognitive processes that exacerbate pain) has small positive effects on disability and catastrophic thinking
- Exercise therapy can help reduce pain and improve function for chronic low back pain, improve function and reduce pain for osteoarthritis of the knee and hip, and improve well-being, symptoms, and physical function for fibromyalgia.
- Therapies that combine exercise and mind–body approaches are more effective than a single modality.

Source: Dowell, D., Haegrich, T. M., & Chous, R. (2016, March 18). CDC Guideline for prescribing opioids for chronic pain: United States, 2016. *Morbidity and Mortality Weekly Report, 65*(1), 1–49.

---

as an assessment of risk for substance use (Marie and Arnstein, 2016). Assessments and interventions also are person-centered and culturally appropriate. The plan may include the following types of interventions, which are provided by palliative care teams:

- Management of medical conditions
- Management of mental health issues
- Analgesics
- Comfort measures
- Stress management
- Complementary and integrative modalities

- Rehabilitation therapies
- Social support
- Spiritual support

Nurses can facilitate referrals for palliative care teams, which are widely available in hospitals and hospice programs, as discussed in Chapter 27. Pain Resource Nurses are another resource that may be available in hospitals, long-term care settings, and home care settings. These nurses have participated in extensive pain-management education offered by the City of Hope.

Box 28-6 Evidence-Based Practice: Nonpharmacologic Interventions for Persistent Pain

Exercise and Physical Activity

- Individualized programs are recommended for various types of persistent pain, such as osteoarthritis.

Cognitive-Behavioral Therapy

- Some evidence of effectiveness in decreasing chronic pain and improving function and mood, including studies in nursing homes.
- Recommended for osteoarthritis if delivered by professional therapist.
- Recommended to improve motivation for self-management interventions, such as exercise and physical activity.

Transcutaneous/Percutaneous Electrical Nerve Stimulation (TENS/PENS)

- Recommended alone or in combinations with pharmacologic or nonpharmacologic strategies for pain relief and improved function.

Acupuncture

- Consistent evidence for chronic pain in back, shoulder, neck, and knee.

Massage

- Effective in some people for chronic nonmalignant pain.

Mindfulness Meditation

- One qualitative study of older adults with chronic low back pain showed improvements in pain, sleep, and quality of life.

Guided Imagery, Biofeedback, Relaxation Methods

- Some studies show effectiveness for pain relief and other benefits in older adults with chronic pain.

Tai Chi

- Limited evidence-based support.

Source: Abdulla, A., Adams, N., Bone, M., et al. (2013). Evidence-based clinical practice guidelines on management of pain in older people. *Age Ageing, 42,* i1–i57; Horgas, A. L. Yoon, S. L., & Grall, M. (2016). Pain management. In M. Boltz, E. Capezuti, T. Fulmer, & D. Zwicker (Eds.), *Evidence-based practice protocols for best practice* (5th ed., pp. 263–281). New York: Springer Publishing Co.

 GLOBAL PERSPECTIVE

The WHO has called upon clinicians and service providers worldwide to address painful musculoskeletal conditions by developing and implementing integrated, person-centered models of care. The rationale for this recommendation is that "the impact of impaired musculoskeletal health on individuals and society at all levels and all places on the planet is profound, with the magnitude of the burden of disease in terms of disability far exceeding other noncommunicable diseases" (Briggs, Cross, Hoy, et al., 2016, p. S251).

SPOTLIGHT ON TRANSITIONAL CARE

As presented in Chapter 6, transitional care is a major focus of health care for older adults who require care across different settings during the course of illness. The first transitional care models were implemented in acute care settings, and these models continue to be refined and modified based on ongoing research and clinical practice. Today, transitional care models are being implemented in other settings, including community settings. Online Learning Activity 28-7 provides access to an article describing the development and implementation of a transitional care model using faith community nursing. The Transitional Care Unfolding Case Study in this chapter describes how nurses in acute care and community settings provide transitional care for Maria Lopez. Recall that Nurse Jessica is the transitional care nurse at San Christos Hospital, and follow the case as Nurse Stephanie provides transitional care as a faith community nurse at Saint Joseph Church.

 See **ONLINE LEARNING ACTIVITY 28-7: ARTICLE ABOUT A TRANSITIONAL CARE MODEL USING FAITH COMMUNITY NURSES** at http://thepoint.lww.com/Miller8e.

Transitional Care Unfolding Case Study (continued from Chapter 27)

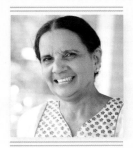 ### Part 2: Maria Lopez as She Receives Transitional Care in Her Home

Background Information: Maria Lopez

With the exception of one hospitalization for heart failure at age 73, Maria Lopez's chronic conditions have been relatively stable, with slow progression of both the diabetes and heart failure. After Maria's hospitalization, her 22-year-old granddaughter, Isabella, moved in with her and has been helping with medication management, grocery shopping, and transportation. Eighteen months ago, Maria developed a persistent cough and was diagnosed with lung cancer. Isabella accompanied her grandmother to radiation and chemotherapy appointments, and the lung cancer is now in remission. Although Maria's medical problems are stable, she experiences chronic back pain, which has been gradually worsening. During the past few months, Maria has been limiting her physical activities and no longer goes to church. Isabella reports that her grandmother seems depressed and expects Isabella to "wait on her other hand and foot." Maria is admitted to San Christos Hospital for a comprehensive geriatric assessment.

(continued)

Part 2: Maria Lopez at 76 Years of Age *(Continued)*

Background Information: San Christos Hospital and Faith Community Nurses

Following successful implementation of the nurse-led program called Safe, Coordinated, and Effective Discharges (described in Part 1 of this case in Chapter 27), Saint Joseph Catholic church asked San Christos Hospital to collaborate in developing a transitional care model for their faith community nurses. The hospital and parish adopted the faith community nurse transitional care model described by Ziebarth and Campbell (2015), and available in Online Learning Activity 28-7. Now, when members of Saint Joseph Church are admitted to San Christos Hospital, a referral is initiated for the faith community nurse to visit the parishioner in the hospital and consider the need for transitional care.

Nurse Stephanie, Faith Community Nurse at Saint Joseph Church

Three days after Maria is admitted to San Christos, Nurse Stephanie meets with Maria and Isabella and reviews the information in the hospital chart. Nurse Stephanie identifies the following information that is pertinent to providing transitional care services from the Saint Joseph faith community nursing program:

Maria Lopez was admitted to San Christos hospital for a comprehensive geriatric assessment of progressive decline in functioning and escalating persistent pain. Admitting diagnoses included osteoarthritis, hypertension, heart failure, type 2 diabetes, and lung cancer in remission. Additional diagnoses based on comprehensive geriatric assessment are depression and persistent pain. Further evaluation of Maria's persistent and progressive back pain indicated that it was due to degenerative joint disease in her vertebrae.

Maria lives in her own home with her granddaughter, Isabella, who provides assistance with all activities of daily living (ADL) and instrumental ADL. According to chart notes, the geriatric assessment team met with Isabella and Maria and discussed Isabella's concerns that her grandmother has become overly dependent because of pain. Isabella reported that she had great difficulty determining if her grandmother limited her activities because of pain, because she was depressed, or because she found satisfaction in being cared for by her granddaughter. The team discussed the probable relationship between Maria's persistent pain and her depression and withdrawal from social activities, and recommended interprofessional follow-up when Maria returns home.

Nurse Stephanie participates in a pre-discharge team conference with Maria, Isabella, and Nurse Jessica, the San Christos Hospital transitional care nurse (described in Chapter 27). The geriatric assessment team initiates referrals for the following interventions to be implemented immediately postdischarge: pain management specialist and outpatient physical and occupational therapies. The team also suggests that Nurse Stephanie provide counseling for both Maria and Isabella to address issues related to Maria's declining condition and the caregiving relationship between Maria and Isabella. Nurse Stephanie agrees to provide services through the Saint Joseph Transitional Care program and facilitate referrals for ongoing services to address the needs on a long-term basis.

In addition to the referrals initiated by the geriatric assessment team, the following interventions are planned to ensure continuity of care prior to discharge:

- Medication reconciliation, to be performed by Nurse Jessica on day of discharge and by Nurse Stephanie during first postdischarge home visit
- Written discharge instructions with information about diagnoses, treatments, and follow-up appointments (including contact information for all providers)
- Educational materials about pain management interventions
- Telephone follow-up by Nurse Jessica at the following postdischarge intervals: second day, 2 weeks, 4 weeks

Part 2: Maria Lopez at 76 Years of Age (*Continued*)

In her role as faith community transitional care nurse, Nurse Stephanie will implement the following interventions beginning 3 days postdischarge and continuing for 2 months:

- Meet Maria and Isabella at appointment with pain management specialist one week postdischarge to review pharmacologic and nonpharmacologic interventions and assure continuity of care.
- Visit Maria and Isabella 3 days postdischarge to review plan, including follow-up appointments with outpatient physical and occupational therapists.
- Reassess the situation as interventions are implemented.
- Provide ongoing recommendations for pain management strategies, with emphasis on self-management through nonpharmacologic interventions.
- Discuss additional community-based services that would be appropriate as the situation changes (e.g., adult day center for Maria, caregiver support group for Isabella, social supports through Saint Joseph Church).

THINKING POINTS

- Read the article about a transitional care model using faith community nurses and consider how this model reflects the characteristics of effective transitional care interventions delineated in Box 6-6.

- How does the nursing care for Maria Lopez and Isabella differ from usual care?
- How does Nurse Stephanie work with other professionals to implement this transitional care model?

Chapter Highlights

Definitions and Types of Pain
- Nociceptive and neuropathic pain (Figure 28-1; Table 28-1)
- Acute and persistent pain
- Cancer pain

Unique Aspects of Pain in Older Adults
- Age-related changes
- Prevalence and causes

Functional Consequences of Pain in Older Adults

Cultural Aspects of Pain (Box 28-1)

Nursing Assessment of Pain in Older Adults
- Identifying common misconceptions (Box 28-2)
- Obtaining information about pain (Figure 28-2; Box 28-3)
- Pain in older adults who are cognitively impaired (Box 28-4; Figure 28-3)

Pharmacologic Interventions for Managing Pain
- Classification of analgesics
- Misconceptions and realities about analgesics (Table 28-2)
- The WHO 3-Step Pain Relief Ladder (Figure 28-4)
- Special considerations: Opioid Abuse and Misuse (Box 28-5)

Nonpharmacologic Interventions for Managing Pain
- Nonpharmacologic interventions (Box 28-6)
- Referrals for specialized services
- Teaching about self-management strategies

Spotlight on Transitional Care
- The Transitional Care Unfolding Case Study describes how Nurse Stephanie, a faith community nurse, collaborates with an interprofessional team to assure continuity of care for an older adult in a community setting.

Critical Thinking Exercises

1. Identify an older person in your recent clinical experience who has talked with you about persistent pain, and address the following in relation to that person:
   - Which factors listed in Box 28-2 affect the person's experience of pain?
   - What assumptions from Box 28-3 are applicable to assessing pain in that person?
2. Review Box 28-6 and the section on Nonpharmacologic Interventions for Managing Pain. Develop a patient-teaching strategy to improve comfort levels in a 78-year-old woman with persistent low back pain and mild cognitive impairment.
3. Review the information about tolerance, dependence, and addiction and write a sentence for each of these concepts in terms that you could use for teaching older adults and their caregivers about medication therapy.

For more information about the topics discussed in this chapter, be sure to check out the interactive Online Learning Activities and other helpful resources at http://thepoint.lww.com/Miller8e.

REFERENCES

Ahn, H., Garvan, C., & Lyon, D. (2015). Pain and aggression in nursing home residents with dementia. *Nursing Research, 64*, 256–263.

American Geriatrics Society. (2012). *Statement on the use of opioids in the treatment of persistent pain in older adults.* Available at http//ags.org

Beach, P. A., Huck, J. T., Miranda, M. et al. (2016). Effects of Alzheimer disease on facial expression of pain. *Clinical Journal of Pain, 32*, 478–487.

Brady, B., Veljanova, I., & Chipchase, L. (2016). Are multidisciplinary interventions multicultural: A topical review of pain literature as it relates to culturally diverse patient groups. *Pain, 157*, 321–328.

Briggs, A. M., Cross, M. J., Hoy, D. G. et al., (2016). Musculoskeletal health conditions represent a global threat to healthy aging: A report for the 2015 World Health Organization World Report on Ageing and Health. *The Gerontologist, 56*, S243–S255.

Bruckenthal, P., Marino, M. A., & Snelling, L. (2016). Complementary and integrative therapies for persistent pain management in older adults. *Journal of Gerontological Nursing, 42*(12), 40–48.

Chan, S., Hadjistavropoulos, T., Williams, J. et al. (2014). Evidence-based development and initial validation of the pain assessment checklist for seniors with limited ability to communicate-II (PACSLAC-II). *Clinical Journal of Pain, 30*, 816–824.

Collis, D., & Waterfield, J. (2015). The understanding of pain by older adults who consider themselves to have aged successfully. *Musculoskeletal Care, 13*, 19–30.

Cornelius, R., Herr, K. A., Gordon, D. B., et al. (2017). Evidence-based practice guidelines: Acute pain management in older adults. *Journal of Gerontological Nursing, 43*(2), 18–27.

Defrin, R., Amanzio, M., de Tommaso, M., et al. (2015). Experimental pain processing in individuals with cognitive impairment: Current state of the science. *Pain, 156*, 1396–1408.

de Tomasso, M., Arendt-Nielsen, L., Defrin, R., et al. (2016). Pain in neurodegenerative disease: current knowledge and future perspectives. *Behavioural Neurology, 2016*, 7576292. doi: 10.1155/2016/7576292.

Dowding, D., Lichtner, V., Allcock, N., et al. (2016). Using sense-making theory to aid understanding of the recognition, assessment and management of pain in patients with dementia in acute hospital settings. *International Journal of Nursing Studies, 53*, 152–162.

Ellis-Smith, C., Evans, C., Bone, A., et al. (2016). Measures to assess commonly experienced symptoms for people with dementia in long-term care settings: A systematic review. *BioMedical Central Medicine, 14*, 38.

Fry, M., Chenoweth, L., & Arendts, G. (2016). Assessment and management of acute pain in the older person with cognitive impairment: A qualitative study. *International Emergency Nursing, 24*, 54–60.

Gerontological Society of America. (2016). From publication to practice: Addressing the societal burden of opioid misuse: Focus on a balanced approach to older adults with chronic pain. Available at www.geron.org.

Guerriero, F. (2017). Guidance on opioids prescribing for the management of persistent non-cancer pain in older adults. *World Journal of Clinical Cases, 5*(3), 73–81.

Habiger, T., Flo, E., Achterberg, W., et al. (2016). The interactive relationship between pain, psychosis, and agitation in people with dementia: Results from a cluster-randomized clinical trial. *Behavioral Neurology, 2016*, 7036415. doi:10.1155/20167036415.

Herr, K., Coyne, P. J., McCaffery, M., et al. (2011). Pain assessment in the patients unable to self-report: Position statement with clinical practice recommendations. *Pain Management Nursing, 12*(4), 230–250.

Horgas, A. L. Yoon, S. L., & Grall, M. (2016). Pain management. In M. Boltz, E. Capezuti, T. Fulmer, & D. Zwicker (Eds.), *Evidence-based practice protocols for best practice* (5th ed., pp. 263–281). New York: Springer Publishing Co.

Husebo, B. S., Achterberg, W., & Flo, E. (2016). Central nervous system drugs, 2016 May 30, [Epub ahead of print]

Ingvar, M. (2015). Learning mechanisms in pain chronification. *Pain: Journal of the International Association for the Study of Pain, 156*, S18–S23.

Institute of Medicine. (2011), *Relieving pain in America: A blueprint for transforming prevention, care, education, and research.* Washington, DC: National Academies Press.

Katz, J., Weinrib, A., Fashler, S. R., et al. (2015). The Toronto General Hospital Transitional Pain Service: development and implementation of a multidisciplinary program to prevent chronic postsurgical pain. *Journal of Pain Research, 8*, 695–702.

Kuo, Y. F., Raji, M. A., Chen, N. W., et al. (2016). Corrigendum to 'Trends in Opioid Prescriptions Among Part D Medicare Recipients from 2007 to 2012'. *The American Journal of MedicineMedicine, 130*(5), 615–616.

Malara, A., De Biase, G. A., Bettarini, F., et al. (2016). Pain assessment in elderly with behavioral and psychological symptoms of dementia. *Journal of Alzheimer's Disease, 50*, 1217–1225.

Marie, B. S., & Arnstein, P. (2016). Quality pain care for older adults in an era of suspicion and scrutiny. *Journal of Gerontological Nursing, 42*(12), 31–39.

Marshall, L. M., Litwack-Harrison, S., Cawthon, P. M., et al. (2016). A prospective study of back pain and risk of falls among community-dwelling women. *Journal of Gerontology. Series A, Biological Sciences and Medical Sciences, 71*(9):1177–1183

McCaffery, M. (1968). *Nursing practice theories related to cognition, bodily pain and man-environmental interactions.* Los Angeles, CA: UCLA Students Store.

Morales-Espinoza, E., Kostov, B., Salami, D., et al. (2016). Complexity, comorbidity, and health care costs associated with chronic widespread pain in primary care. *Pain, 157*, 818–826.

Muntinga, M. E., Jansen, A., Schellevis, G., & Nijpels, G. (2016). Expanding access to pain care for frail, older people in primary care: A cross-sectional study. *BioMed Central Nursing, 15*:26. DOI:10.1186/s12912–016–0147-S.

Noreika, D., Bobb, B., & Coyne, P. (2016). Physical pain and symptoms. In E. Wittenberg, B. R. Ferrell, J. Goldsmith, et al. (Eds.) *Textbook of palliative care communication* (pp. 263–270). New York: Oxford University Press.

O'Malley, P. A. (2017). Lavender for sleep, rest, and pain. *Clinical Nurse Specialist, 31*, 74–76.

Ossipov, M. H., Morimura, K., & Porreca, F. (2014). Descending pain modulation and chronification of pain. *Current Opinion in Supportive and Palliative Care, 8*, 143–151.

Pasero, C. & McCaffery, M. (2011a). Initiating opioid therapy. In C. Pasero & M. McCaffery (Eds.), *Pain assessment and pharmacologic management* (pp. 442–461). St. Louis, MO: Mosby Elsevier.

Pasero, C. & McCaffery, M. (2011b). Misconceptions that hamper assessment and treatment of patients who report pain. In C. Pasero & M. McCaffery (Eds.), *Pain assessment and pharmacologic management* (pp. 20–48). St. Louis, MO: Mosby Elsevier.

Pasero, C., & McCaffery, M. (2011c). Assessment tools. In C. Pasero & M. McCaffery (Eds.), *Pain assessment and pharmacologic management* (pp. 49–142). St. Louis, MO: Mosby Elsevier.

Pasero, C., & Portenoy, R. K. (2011). Neurophysiology of pain and analgesia and the pathophysiology of neuropathic pain. In C. Pasero & M. McCaffery (Eds.), *Pain assessment and pharmacologic management* (pp. 1–12). St. Louis, MO: Mosby Elsevier.

Rapo-Pylkko, S., Haanpaa, M., & Lilra, H. (2016). Chronic pain among community-dwelling elderly: A population-based clinical study. Scandinavian Journal of Primary Health Care. doi: 10.3109/02813432.2016.1160628.

Rice, A., Smith, B., & Blyth, F. (2016). Pain and the global burden of disease. *Pain, 157*, 791–796.

Riffin, C., Pillemer, K., Reid, M. C., et al (2015). Decision support preferences among Hispanic and non-Hispanic white older adults with chronic musculoskeletal pain. *Journals of Gerontology B: Psychological Sciences and Social Sciences.* doi: 10.1093/geronb/gbvo71.

Schafer, G., Prkachin, K., Kaseweter, K., et al. (2016). Health care providers' judgments in chronic pain: the influence of gender and trustworthiness. *Pain.* doi:10.1097/0000000000000536.

Zeibarth, D., & Campbell, K. (2015). A transitional care model using faith community nurses. *Journal of Christian Nursing, 33*(2), 112–118.

chapter 29

Caring for Older Adults at the End of Life

KEY TERMS

death
dignified death
end of life
hospice care
medicalization of end-of-life care
palliative sedation

As discussed in Chapter 27, gradual increases in both life expectancy and the length of time people live with chronic conditions have led to an increasing focus on care during chronic illness. Concurrently, there has been increasing attention to both quality and cost of care, particularly with regard to care during the last years of life. In addition, public advocacy about and awareness of policies and legislation related to all aspects of life and death has been growing, due in part to the ubiquitous influences of social media. Nurses and all health care providers are challenged to address issues related to end-of-life care within the context of social and political forces that are shaping public policies and health care practice. Nurses increasingly are involved with ethical decisions and clinical concerns—particularly when they care for older adults—as consumers and health care providers focus on issues related to the cost of care, treatment-related decisions, quality of life, and respect for patient wishes.

Perhaps the one constant within this broad context is that nurses can draw on their wide range of skills to promote wellness for older adults at the end of life—skills that are not dependent on outside forces but rather are dependent on knowledge. This chapter provides an overview of the broader societal context that is shaping health care services and the decisions that are made related to end-of-life care. This chapter also discusses nurses' responsibilities related to the legal and ethical issues that are prominent aspects of end-of-life care. Finally, a major intent of this chapter is to lay the foundation for nurses to provide person-centered care for older adults and their families who are facing the challenges of the end-of-life time. Because end-of-life care is complex and challenging, provision of care requires interprofessional collaboration. Thus, throughout this chapter, specialized resources are identified that nurses can use to help expand their knowledge about the associated legal, ethical, and clinical issues. The Transitional Care Unfolding Case Study at the end of the chapter (which is a continuation from Chapters 27 and 28) illustrates nurses' roles in caring for an older adult through all stages of illness, with emphasis on addressing continuity of care and interprofessional collaboration.

SOCIETAL AND HEALTH CARE PERSPECTIVES ON DEATH AND END OF LIFE

Concepts related to death, dying, and end of life have changed significantly since the early 1900s, when death was accepted as an inevitable and normal part of life. Death was a common occurrence in infants, children, and young adults, and it often occurred unexpectedly in homes or community settings due to accidents and communicable diseases. During recent decades, perspectives on death and attitudes toward dying have been changing, with wide-ranging implications for health care providers.

Medical and technologic advances that have been occurring since the middle of the 20th century have enabled health care facilities to become centers for curing disease and prolonging life. Subsequently, health care professionals began viewing death as something to be avoided because it symbolized failure. Prolonging life, even at the expense of quality, was viewed as the ultimate accomplishment: a symbol of success for patients, families, and the health care teams involved.

Death has traditionally been defined as the cessation of all biologic functions. In many situations, however, major medical and technologic developments have changed the perception of death from a clearly defined event to an evolving process. This is especially common in acute care settings in which, for example, a patient can be considered legally dead because of the absence of brain function but not be clinically dead if medical technology is used to sustain heart and lung functioning. Moreover, the broad array of life-sustaining medical interventions influences the ability to prolong life and complicates decisions about allowing the end of life to occur. The term **medicalization of end-of-life care** describes care that focuses on prolonging life through the use of medical technology rather than on interventions for comfort and quality of life.

Perspectives on Death and the End-of-Life Trajectory

For many older adults, the **end of life** may be a gradual process that is associated with the cumulative effects of chronic illness and many interacting conditions, rather than a single cause. In many cases, a major medical event, such as sepsis or a fractured hip, becomes the "tipping point" that causes the older adult to transition from a state of chronic illness to an end-of-life state in which death occurs. Nurse researchers at the Pennsylvania State University (Penrod, Hupcey, Baney, et al., 2011) described the course and duration of three end-of-life trajectories as follows:

- Expected death trajectory: steep progressive decline, often measured in clinical benchmarks, with prolonged terminal phase
- Mixed death trajectory: initial successful treatment and period of stability, followed by steep decline and short terminal phase
- Unexpected death trajectory: slow decline (i.e., periodic exacerbations with recovery never reaching former level of health), followed by extremely short terminal phase

Penrod, Hupcey, Shipley, et al. (2012) applied this concept to caregiving through the end of life; however, it can be applied to the different experiences of older adults and their caregivers across end-of-life trajectories. It is important to recognize that the early phase of these trajectories may be subtle and recognized only in retrospect, as is often the case with dementia.

Trends in Providing End-of-Life Care

Attention to cost of care as well as quality of care has received much attention in recent years, due in part to reports of national organizations such as the Institute of Medicine (IOM) and major nursing organizations. In 2014, the IOM published a landmark report on *Dying in America: Improving Quality and Honoring Individual Preferences Near the End of Life* calling for major improvements in end-of-life care based on well-documented problems and gaps in care (Institute of Medicine, 2014). This report is one of the major influences that has become a call to action for all health care providers to develop competence in addressing complex decisions and clinical aspects related to end-of-life care. As a step toward improving care and honoring individual preferences, the Centers for Medicare & Medicaid allowed reimbursement for professionals to discuss options for care during serious illness. Nursing organizations are leading the way toward improved end-of-life care through the publication of policies and educational materials to guide nursing care, as discussed in the section on nursing interventions. Major initiatives are delineated in Figure 29-1, which illustrates the interplay between societal and professional influences on the way end-of-life care is provided in the United States. Societal issues are discussed in the section on legal and ethical considerations and clinical aspects are discussed in the section on nursing interventions.

With increasing attention to both quality of care and cost of care that is unnecessary or unwanted, end-of-life care has improved in some respects but remains a major concern in many others. Comparative interviews with 622 relatives of older adults who died in 2000 and 586 relatives of older adults who died between 2011 and 2013 identified the following trends, which point to improvements and concerns:

- The unmet need for pain management decreased 9.7% (i.e., from 25.2% to 15.5%).
- There was a 14.1% increase in addressing religious and spiritual needs (i.e., from 58.3% to 72.4%).
- High rates of unmet needs for palliation of dyspnea and anxiety/depression remained.
- The overall rating of quality decreased from 56.7% in 2000 to 47.0%.

(Teno, Freedman, Kasper, et al., 2015). Currently health care organizations and policy makers are being called upon to address the unmet needs related to end of life.

Hospice and palliative care services have emerged as major resources within health care systems for providing comprehensive person-centered care to address needs of people with serious or life-limiting conditions and the needs

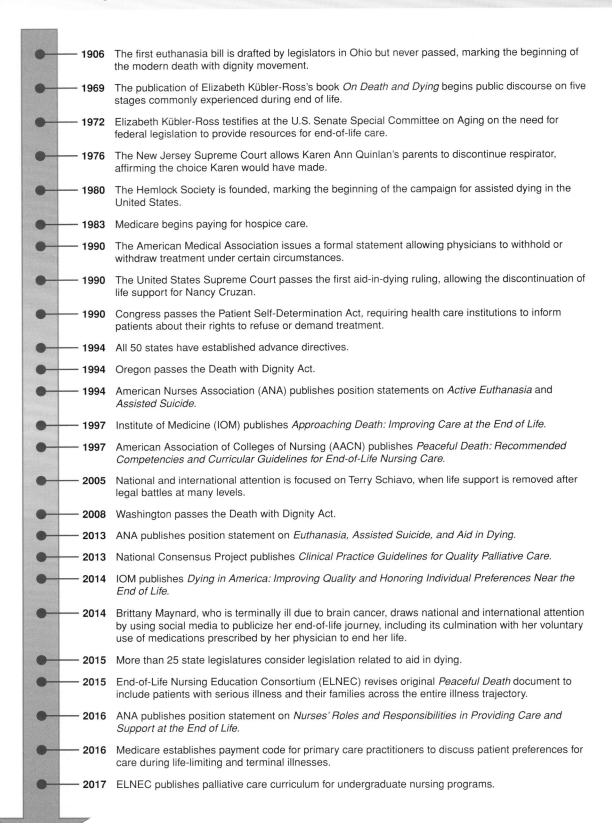

1906 The first euthanasia bill is drafted by legislators in Ohio but never passed, marking the beginning of the modern death with dignity movement.

1969 The publication of Elizabeth Kübler-Ross's book *On Death and Dying* begins public discourse on five stages commonly experienced during end of life.

1972 Elizabeth Kübler-Ross testifies at the U.S. Senate Special Committee on Aging on the need for federal legislation to provide resources for end-of-life care.

1976 The New Jersey Supreme Court allows Karen Ann Quinlan's parents to discontinue respirator, affirming the choice Karen would have made.

1980 The Hemlock Society is founded, marking the beginning of the campaign for assisted dying in the United States.

1983 Medicare begins paying for hospice care.

1990 The American Medical Association issues a formal statement allowing physicians to withhold or withdraw treatment under certain circumstances.

1990 The United States Supreme Court passes the first aid-in-dying ruling, allowing the discontinuation of life support for Nancy Cruzan.

1990 Congress passes the Patient Self-Determination Act, requiring health care institutions to inform patients about their rights to refuse or demand treatment.

1994 All 50 states have established advance directives.

1994 Oregon passes the Death with Dignity Act.

1994 American Nurses Association (ANA) publishes position statements on *Active Euthanasia* and *Assisted Suicide*.

1997 Institute of Medicine (IOM) publishes *Approaching Death: Improving Care at the End of Life*.

1997 American Association of Colleges of Nursing (AACN) publishes *Peaceful Death: Recommended Competencies and Curricular Guidelines for End-of-Life Nursing Care*.

2005 National and international attention is focused on Terry Schiavo, when life support is removed after legal battles at many levels.

2008 Washington passes the Death with Dignity Act.

2013 ANA publishes position statement on *Euthanasia, Assisted Suicide, and Aid in Dying*.

2013 National Consensus Project publishes *Clinical Practice Guidelines for Quality Palliative Care*.

2014 IOM publishes *Dying in America: Improving Quality and Honoring Individual Preferences Near the End of Life*.

2014 Brittany Maynard, who is terminally ill due to brain cancer, draws national and international attention by using social media to publicize her end-of-life journey, including its culmination with her voluntary use of medications prescribed by her physician to end her life.

2015 More than 25 state legislatures consider legislation related to aid in dying.

2015 End-of-Life Nursing Education Consortium (ELNEC) revises original *Peaceful Death* document to include patients with serious illness and their families across the entire illness trajectory.

2016 ANA publishes position statement on *Nurses' Roles and Responsibilities in Providing Care and Support at the End of Life*.

2016 Medicare establishes payment code for primary care practitioners to discuss patient preferences for care during life-limiting and terminal illnesses.

2017 ELNEC publishes palliative care curriculum for undergraduate nursing programs.

FIGURE 29-1 Landmark events that influence end-of-life care in the United States.

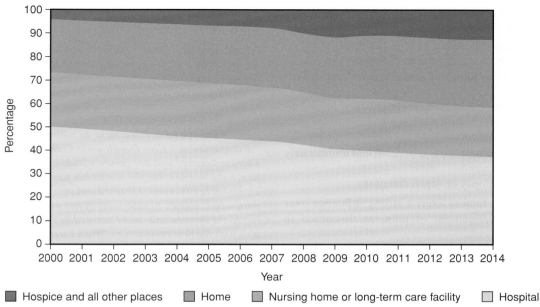

Hospice and all other places   Home   Nursing home or long-term care facility   Hospital

FIGURE 29-2 Percentage distribution of deaths by place of death: United States, 2000–2014. (Reprinted from QuickStats: Percentage Distribution of Deaths, by Place of Death—United States, 2000–2014. MMWR Morb Mortal Wkly Rep 2016;*65*:357. doi: http://dx.doi.org/10.15585/mmwr.6513a6.)

of their families. These services are credited particularly with improving the quality of care related to family experiences and patients' goal attainment (Wright, Keating, Ayanian, et al., 2016). In addition, the growth of these programs has shifted the place of death from hospitals to homes and hospices, as illustrated in Figure 29-2. Palliative care programs are discussed in Chapter 27 and hospice programs are discussed later in this chapter.

An emerging and encouraging trend is the focus of holistic nurses on "shifting the consciousness of the health care community to the importance of bringing back the goodness, compassion, peace, dignity, and release" related to the end of life (Drick, 2016). Lynn Keegan and Carole Ann Drick are two nurses who are leading a movement to implement the "Golden Room" concept to "ease the transition from life into a peaceful death" (Keegan & Drick, 2016, p. 430). The American Nurses Association is supporting this movement, with the release of a two-part continuing education videos on Conscious Living and Conscious Dying in 2016. The Conscious Dying Institute is another evolving approach to promoting a more holistic perspective on death. Based on this approach, nurses can become certified as Sacred Passage Doulas who help people who are dying view their experience as a rite of passage rather than as a medical event (Rosa & Estes, 2016).

Older Adults' Perspectives on Death and Dying

Although younger people may feel they are invincible and immune to disease or death, older adults are likely to be more aware and accepting of the inevitability of death, in part because they have experienced the deaths of family and

friends, often including those who are younger than they are. Recent studies indicate that increasing age is associated with gradually decreasing death anxiety and that a religious sense of hope is an important support for acceptance of death (Krause, Pargament, & Ironson, 2016). Despite the physical declines that are inevitable during older adulthood, older adults who develop a holistic perspective recognize that old age can present opportunities for fulfillment and self-actualization. As such, aging can be an opportunity to gain a deeper understanding of human life and "to learn to let go, take distance, re-appreciate situations, and integrate experiences into the awareness of a finite life" (Baars, 2016, p. 7). The following themes have been identified in qualitative studies of older adults with terminal cancer: adjusting to change, preserving normality, redefining normality, acknowledging the need for close relationships, having space for existential meaning-making, naming and handling decline and loss, and facing the end (Aoun, Deas, & Skett, 2016; Haug, Danbolt, Kvigne, et al., 2015). These studies underscore the importance of developing individualized nursing care plans that maintain or restore the older adult's sense of self by directly addressing end-of-life suffering and bolstering the person's sense of dignity and personhood (Aoun, Deas, & Skett, 2016).

CULTURAL ASPECTS OF DEATH AND DYING

Because cultural perspectives exert a strong influence on end-of-life experiences, all health care professionals need to be aware of their own culturally based perceptions as well as those that influence the older adults for whom they provide care. Cultural influences can affect all the following aspects of end-of-life care:

- Perceptions of a good death
- Acceptance of hospice and palliative care services
- Lines of communication about pending death and end-of-life decisions
- Expectations about medical interventions (e.g., decisions about resuscitation)
- Place where death occurs
- Practices and rituals near the end of death and immediately following death
- Decisions about autopsy or organ donations

In addition, cultural factors exert a strong influence over assessment and management of pain, as discussed in Chapter 28.

An important step in providing culturally appropriate nursing care is to periodically reflect on one's own beliefs about death, dying, and end of life. Religion and spirituality are two aspects of culture that are particularly powerful in relation to beliefs about death, dying, and end-of-life decisions. Although it may be easy to ask about a person's religious affiliation as part of a nursing assessment, the more challenging aspect of providing culturally appropriate care is identifying the person's beliefs and values that affect their care. Nurses accomplish this by asking exploratory questions with a nonjudgmental approach about customs, beliefs, and concerns about death, dying, afterlife, and end of life, as described in the section on communication. Nurses also can apply information from Chapters 2 and 13 related to aspects of culturally appropriate care.

In clinical settings, nurses are integrally involved with one of the most concrete aspects of end-of-life care: postmortem care. This care is directed by institutional policies and standards of care and is a routine aspect of nursing care. What is not routine, however, is the incorporation of end-of-life rituals, which are often culturally based and are an essential aspect of supporting families and caregivers. Box 29-1 provides information about death rituals that are commonly associated with specific groups. It also suggests interventions that nurses can apply in different situations. As with other aspects of culturally appropriate care, it is important to be aware of different practices associated with particular groups and at the same time avoid stereotypes. An effective way of addressing this issue is to inquire ahead of time about preferences of older adults, families, and caregivers, and incorporate pertinent information in the care plan.

Diversity Note

A study of Caucasian, Asian Americans, African Americans, and Hispanic Americans in California identified the following barriers to high-quality end-of-life care for multiethnic patients: financial and health insurance limitations, doctor behaviors, communication chasm, family beliefs and behaviors, health system barriers, and cultural and religious barriers (Periyakoil, Neri, & Kraemer, 2016).

A Student's Perspective

I found myself in a situation today in which I quickly recognized the importance of the lesson on cultural sensitivity in nursing. My aging client unfortunately had a significant change over the weekend, and her husband requested for her to be transported to the hospice inpatient unit. As she and I sat on her bed, she verbalized her acceptance that her disease is terminal. She wept as she voiced her heartache in telling her family of her "disappointment." Even though she is Catholic, because of her Chinese heritage and her family's Buddhist belief in "saving face," she worried that she has let her family down. While she expressed her thoughts, I listened and provided emotional support, which seemed to ease some of her grief. We transported her to the hospice unit, and I assisted in making her comfortable with the new environment. When I went out to the nurses' station to give my report, the receiving nurse's first comment to me was, "I see she is Asian and you have her religious preference documented as Catholic. Are you sure that is correct?" Because of our recent discussions and reading on cultural sensitivity, I quickly realized how we as nurses can make incorrect assumptions in categorizing individuals based on their ethnicity. I reported about my client's childhood history, her parents' belief in Buddhism, the Catholicism she was taught in school, and her long and strong Catholic faith. I found myself really understanding the importance of educating ourselves as nurses about different cultures and the effect of cultural belief systems on individualized health care. As difficult as it was for me to leave my client in a strange environment, I felt that the information I had learned and shared would enable the staff to be respectful of her beliefs, which in turn would be a positive experience for my client during her stay.

Deborah L.

CURRENT LEGAL AND ETHICAL CONCERNS

Ethical and legal questions and challenges are escalating at all levels of society as citizens, governments, institutions, and health care professionals express concerns about care and policies that directly affect end-of-life care, as discussed in the section on perspectives on end-of-life care. Similar to many other ethical issues being addressed in the United States, advocacy groups fight for rights and laws that are controversial because the issues are not clearly black or white. In addition, variations exist among the few states that have a type of death with dignity law, and several state laws are currently being challenged. Currently, federal law does not specifically protect the act of euthanasia, nor does it specifically prohibit its practice (Fink-Sammick, 2016). With the increasing attention to ethical and legal aspects of end-of-life care and decisions, it is imperative to keep up-to-date on current as well as emerging legislation. In addition, nurses need to keep up-to-date on professional codes and standards of practice, which are being revised by organizations such as the American Nurses Association and the Hospice and Palliative Nurses Association. In clinical settings,

Box 29-1 Cultural Considerations: Death Rituals Commonly Associated With Specific Groups

Group	Death Ritual	Intervention
African Americans	May respond to news of death of a loved one by falling out (i.e., sudden collapse, paralysis, and inability to see or speak)	Recognize that this is a culturally based response and not an emergency medical condition; provide support
Amish	Provide a wake-like "sitting up" during the night for seriously ill and dying family members	Arrange for privacy and accommodate family members staying overnight
Cubans	A large gathering of relatives and friends may attend the dying person and place religious artifacts around the person; candles are lit after death to illuminate the path of the spirit to the afterlife	Arrange for a gathering place close to the dying person; find electric candles if open flames are not allowed; summon clergy for religious rituals; do not move religious items
European Americans	Believe that the dying person should not be left alone	Make accommodations for family members to be present at all times
Haitians	Family members gather and pray when death is imminent and may cry uncontrollably; all family members try to be at the person's bedside at the time of death	Make accommodations for privacy, encourage family to bring in religious objects, allow families to participate in postmortem care if they desire to do so
Hindus	Priest and eldest son may perform death rites, with all male relatives assisting; women may respond with loud wailing	Provide a supportive and private environment; offer understanding of death rituals and grief behaviors
Japanese	Family members gather at the bedside at the time of death, with the eldest son having particular responsibilities at the time	Notify eldest son of pending death, identify lines of communication if eldest son is not available
Jewish	Dying person should not be left alone; death rituals vary and some are not performed on the Sabbath or holy days	Ask the closest relative specifically about postmortem practices
Koreans	Family members are expected to stay with the person who is dying and assist with care	Support family in caring for the person
Mexicans	Some, especially women, may have an ataque de nervios (i.e., the person exhibits hyperkinetic and seizure-like activity to release strong emotions) on hearing of the death of a loved one	Recognize that this is a culture-bound syndrome and treatment is usually not necessary; remain with the person, provide support, and involve family with assistance if possible
Muslim groups	The bed should be turned to face the holy city of Mecca;	
family recites prayers from the Qur'an	Facilitate positioning of the bed whenever possible, provide privacy for prayers	
Puerto Ricans	Death is perceived as a time of crisis; the head of the family (i.e., usually the oldest daughter or son) is responsible for receiving the news of death	Allow time for family to view, touch, and stay with the body before it is removed; ask if the family wants a clergy member called
Vietnamese	Flowers are avoided during illness because they are usually reserved for rites of the dead	Ask permission from the patient or family before placing flowers in a room

Source: Purnell, L. D. (2014). *Guide to culturally competent health care.* Philadelphia, PA: F. A. Davis.

nurses can rely on institutional policies and resources, such as ethics committees, to guide their care of older adults at the end of life. Online Learning Activity 29-1 provides links to helpful resources related to current legal and ethical concerns.

 See **ONLINE LEARNING ACTIVITY 29-1: RESOURCES FOR ADDITIONAL INFORMATION ABOUT LEGAL AND ETHICAL ISSUES RELATED TO END-OF-LIFE NURSING CARE** at **http://thepoint.lww.com/Miller8e.**

Shared decision making is defined as "a collaborative process that allows patients and their providers to make health care decisions together, taking into account the best scientific evidence available, as well as the patient's values and preferences" (Informed Medical Decisions Foundation, 2016). This process is consistent with providing person-centered care, and is particularly relevant to care of older adults during all phases of end-of-life care. The American Nurses Association emphasizes that "establishing goals of care for *this* patient at *this* time may provide a framework for discussion about what care should be provided" (American

Nurses Association, 2016). Additional guidelines established by the American Nurses Association (2016) related to nurses' roles in clinical decision making include the following:

- Is the goal to cure the patient or to help the patient live well with serious illness?
- Do we know that this patient is likely to die soon from this illness?
- Health care providers must acknowledge and then provide information about what is possible and what can no longer be accomplished in clear terms to the patient and family.
- Information should be shared when the health care team recognizes that the condition is terminal or that death is near.
- Once physiologic parameters have been used to frame options, then patient preferences can be elicited based on clinical realities.
- This process often involves collaboration with experts in decision making, such as ethics committees or palliative care teams.
- Providers' failure to recognize that a patient is close to death may deprive patients of the opportunities that can occur at the end of life

It is important to recognize that various terms are used to describe laws similar to the Death with Dignity Act, such as End of Life Option Act (California) or Patient Choice and Control at the End of Life Act (Vermont). Similarly, professional organizations use phrases such as "aid in dying," "patient-directed dying," "end-of-life options," and "a process intended to hasten the end of life." The terms "suicide," "euthanasia," and "assisted suicide" are considered inaccurate in the context of death with dignity laws; however, these terms continue to be used in some contexts (e.g., in other countries or in the United States by groups opposed to such laws).

Recommended clinical criteria for physician-directed dying include the following:

- Patient must be mentally competent and have an incurable condition that will likely result in death within 6 months.
- Patients must be informed of, and fully comprehend, all their end-of-life options, including discontinuing life-prolonging treatment, palliative sedation, and voluntary cessation of eating and drinking.
- All elements of informed consent must be fully documented.
- The prescribing practitioner must know that the patient's request is voluntary, rational, and enduring.

(Orentlicher, Pope, Rich, & Physician Aid-in-Dying Clinical Criteria Committee, 2016).

Nurses are challenged to address ethical issues related to decisions about patient-directed dying, and it is important to recognize that the role of nurses is not directly addressed in legislation. As more states enact a type of death with dignity act, increasing numbers of nurses will be called upon to decide if their own moral value system does or does not allow them to provide care for a patient who is choosing physician-directed death. Two alternatives to physician-assisted

dying that are legal in all 50 states are the withdrawal of life-sustaining treatment and voluntary stopping of eating and drinking (Lachman, 2015). Withdrawal of life-sustaining treatment is typically addressed through shared decision making, involving health care providers, patients, and patients' surrogate decision makers. Voluntary stopping of eating and drinking causes terminal dehydration, a condition that can be managed with palliative care measures.

Ethical considerations that nurses address in decisions related to rights of patients to direct their death are mentioned by Jannette, Bosek, and Rambur (2013) as follows:

- In the debate between beneficence and nonbeneficence, the question is whether death is seen as harmful by the patient.
- Patients seeking patient-directed death are claiming their right to die a good death in a society that tries to protect each citizen's right to life.
- The ethical principle of autonomy supports the patient's right to determine his own death, and this takes precedence over the principle of paternalism, which allows health care providers to decide what is best.

Communication strategies for discussions of assisted dying include the following:

- Use open-ended questions and statements.
- Focus on available options, such as palliative care.
- Express empathy and provide emotional support.
- Provide reassurance that the patient will not be abandoned.
- Address concerns about family and supportive others.

(Lehto, Olsen, & Chan, 2016).

Nurses can be guided by the American Nurses Association 2016 position statement on *Nurses' Roles and Responsibilities in Providing Care and Support at the End of Life* (American Nurses' Association, 2016). Online Learning Activity 29-2 provides a link to this position statement and a nursing article about discussing assisted dying with patients.

 See ONLINE LEARNING ACTIVITY 29-2: LINKS TO ANA POSITION STATEMENT AND ARTICLE WITH CASE STUDY ABOUT WHEN A PATIENT DISCUSSES ASSISTED DYING at http://thepoint.lww.com/Miller8e.

A Student's Perspective

This week, I learned that it is okay to accept that an elderly patient is ready to die and that is his/her wish. I had a patient who requested that we not perform any measures—just give him his beer with lunch, wine with dinner, and some pain medicine to make him comfortable. He stated that he has led a good life and is ready to go see God. That is really hard for me because it's my job to help people and save lives. The other aspect of that is helping people die a dignified death—it's just a really TOUGH aspect!!!

Sarah E.

HOSPICE CARE

As discussed in Chapter 27, both hospice and palliative care refer to an interdisciplinary approach to care that comprehensively addresses the needs of people with life-limiting conditions as well as their families and others who care for and care about them. All hospice programs include palliative care, but palliative care is also provided outside hospice programs. These terms are closely associated, but in the United States, criteria differ for these services. Palliative care outside of hospice is discussed in Chapter 27, and in this chapter, it is presented as an integral part of hospice and end-of-life care. Hospice care refers to a philosophy of care that seeks to support dignified dying or a good death experience for people with terminal illnesses and for their families and caregivers. The term *hospice* (from the same linguistic root as "hospitality") was first applied to specialized care for dying patients in the 1960s by physician and nurse Dame Cicely Saunders, who founded the first modern hospice—St. Christopher's—in a residential suburb of London. During a guest lecture for medical students, nurses, social workers, and chaplains at Yale University, Saunders introduced the idea of hospice care and emphasized holistic services and symptom control. This lecture sparked interest, which led to the development of hospice care as it is known today.

Hospice benefits are strongly supported by health insurance and are viewed as a cost-effective alternative to traditional medical care. As such, hospice programs treat the person, not the disease; focus on the family, not the individual; and emphasize the quality of life, not the duration. Hospice services are provided by interdisciplinary teams and include the following services: physicians; nurses; home health aides; social workers; spiritual counselors; volunteers; bereavement counselors; and speech, physical, and occupational therapists. Some programs offer additional services such as music, art, reiki, and pet therapy. These services are provided by public and private agencies in any setting, including homes, hospitals, short- or long-term residential facilities, or freestanding hospice centers.

Eligibility criteria for hospice include a physician referral and a statement that a patient has a life expectancy of 6 months or less. An important role for nurses in all settings is to encourage older adults and their families to find information about hospice even in the absence of a clearly defined "terminal" phase. Hospice programs usually arrange for exploratory meetings to discuss services and they can suggest alternative programs (e.g., palliative care) if the person is not immediately eligible.

Based on the current emphasis on improving quality of care at end of life while at the same time cutting costs of care, the Centers for Medicare & Medicaid Services initiated a new option for hospice-like services for certain enrollees in accordance with the 2010 Patient Protection and Affordable Care Act. This initiative began in 2016 and will be phased in through 5 years, allowing patients in the Medicare Care Choice Model to enroll in hospice programs while they are actively being treated for a serious illness (e.g., while receiving chemotherapy for cancer). As concerns about quality of care at the end of life continue to be addressed, additional changes in the provision of hospice care will continue to evolve. Nurses can keep up-to-date on these changes and find additional information about hospice services by exploring the resources identified in Online Learning Activity 29-3.

 See **ONLINE LEARNING ACTIVITY 29-3: ADDITIONAL RESOURCES ABOUT PROVIDING NURSING CARE AT THE END OF LIFE** at **http://thepoint.lww.com/Miller8e.**

 Diversity Note

Reviews of studies examining end-of-life care provided to ethnic/minority groups included the following: (1) hospice was most used among Whites, followed by Hispanics, and was least used by African and Asian Americans; (2) African Americans perceived a great need for hospice yet more frequently lacked knowledge; (3) African Americans preferred aggressive treatment, but care was often inconsistent with preferences (LoPresti, Dement, and Gold, 2016; Rahemi & Williams, 2016).

 GLOBAL PERSPECTIVE

The Worldwide Palliative Care Alliance describes model programs of hospice and palliative care services that are successful in diverse settings, often with limited resources. For example, programs in India and Tanzania make effective use of community health care workers, and a program in Romania is described as a beacon for training and advocacy. Model programs being implemented worldwide are described in the *Global Atlas of Palliative Care at the End of Life,* which is available at www.thewpca.org.

PROMOTING WELLNESS AT THE END OF LIFE

Wellness at the end of life is closely connected to the concept of a "good death." Core themes about what constitutes a good death include all of the following: preferences for a specific dying process, pain-free status, religiosity and spirituality, emotional well-being, quality of life, life completion, treatment preferences, dignity, presence of family, and relationship with health care providers (Meier, Gallegos, Thomas, et al., 2016). The term dignified death (also referred to as death with dignity) is appropriate for describing a good death because a recurrent theme across all professionals and consumers is the importance of maintaining dignity during the end of life. A concept analysis of death with dignity identified the most important attributes of this concept as respect for privacy, overall respect, and spiritual peace and hope (Hemati, Ashouri, Allah-Bakhshian, et al., 2016). Loss of dignity is associated with all of the following consequences: an assault on one's sense of self, feeling a diminished sense of worth, being a burden to others, loss of control over one's life, having unfinished business, worrying about the future, feeling dissatisfied with the past, and physical symptoms of fatigue and weakness (Chochinov, Johnston, McClement, et al., 2016).

Nurses and all health care providers have essential roles in assuring a dignified death through actions described in the section on nursing interventions. Studies that are most pertinent to promoting wellness for older adults at the end of life consistently identify the following aspects of dignified care:

- Being treated as an individual and with respect
- Maintaining independence, while having basic care needs met
- Maintaining physical comfort, cognitive abilities, and meaningful activities
- Being involved in decision making
- Recognizing the value of one's own life
- Having privacy and a safe environment
- Being listened to and having needs and wishes respected
- Experiencing good communication
- Feeling peaceful and ready to die
- Being in control of the dying process

(Rodriguez-Prat, Monforte-Royo, Porta-Sales, et al., 2016; Romo, Allison, Smith, et al., 2017; Romo, Dawson-Rose, Mayo, et al., 2016).

These characteristics are in accord with the "Dying Patient's Bill of Rights," a document created at a workshop on "The Terminally Ill Patient and the Helping Person" by Linda Austin (1975) to identify concretely the dignified care that dying people deserve (Box 29-2). This document

---

Box 29-2 The Dying Person's Bill of Rights

I have the right to be treated as a living human being until I die.

I have the right to maintain a sense of hopefulness, however changing its focus may be.

I have the right to express my feelings and emotions about my approaching death in my own way.

I have the right to participate in decisions concerning my care.

I have the right to expect continuing medical and nursing attention even though cure goals must be changed to comfort goals.

I have the right not to die alone.

I have the right to be free from pain.

I have the right to have my questions answered honestly.

I have the right not to be deceived.

I have the right to have help from and for my family in accepting my death.

I have the right to die in peace and with dignity.

I have the right to retain my individuality and not be judged for my decisions, which may be contrary to the beliefs of others.

I have the right to be cared for by caring, sensitive, knowledgeable people who will attempt to understand my needs and will be able to gain some satisfaction in helping me face my death.

I have the right to be cared for by those who can maintain a sense of hopefulness, however changing this might be.

I have the right to expect that the sanctity of the human body will be respected after death.

I have the right to discuss and enlarge my religious and/or spiritual experiences, whatever these may mean to others.

Source: Austin, L. (1975). Dying patient's bill of rights. In *The terminally ill patient and the helping person workshops.* Lansing, MI: Southwest Michigan Inservice Education Council

---

continues to be helpful as a guide for defining goals and interventions for individualized end-of-life care.

It is notable that Nursing Outcomes Classification (NOC) terminology of Dignified Death has been changed to Dignified Life Closure, which is consistent with the emphasis on broader aspects of quality of life at the end of life. This NOC is defined as "personal actions to maintain control when approaching end of life" and includes the following specific outcomes that are within the realm of nursing care: maintains physical independence, participates in decisions related to care, shares feelings about dying, maintains sense of control of remaining time, completes meaningful goals, shares feelings about dying, discusses spiritual concerns and experiences, exchanges affection with others, and controls treatment choices, including food and drink intake (Moorhead, Johnson, Maas, et al., 2013, p. 201). Nursing interventions to achieve these outcomes are discussed in the next section.

A Student's Perspective

When I left the nursing home today I felt better about working with people facing the certain end of their lives. Mr. F. had a really positive attitude about his inoperable brain tumor and it made me understand that I am the one who feels uncomfortable with death. He expressed that his life has meaning and that he is here for a reason. He told me about some of his goals in life: he plans to get out of the nursing home so that he can travel around the country in an RV with his wife. He seemed to imply that even if that goal never occurred, it was OK, that it was mostly something to look forward to. All of the communication with Mr. F. had a huge impact on me. It gave me a whole new perspective on how people view their lives. This man is suffering from this terrible disease, yet he still finds hope and has goals in life.

Erin H.

 ### NURSING INTERVENTIONS FOR END-OF-LIFE CARE

Despite the fact that caring for people at the end of life is one of the most challenging aspects of nursing, nurses often feel inadequate in addressing the multifaceted needs of people who are dying and their families. Since 1997, the American Association of Colleges of Nursing (AACN) has been advocating for schools of nursing to ensure that nurses are better prepared to provide quality end-of-life nursing care. During the past two decades, the End-of-Life Nursing Education Consortium (ELNEC) has grown as a partnership between the AACN and City of Hope Medical Center in Duarte, California. In 2016, the AACN Board of Directors unanimously voted to adopt CARES: Competencies and Recommendations for Educating Undergraduate Nursing Students Preparing Nurses to Care for the Seriously Ill and Their Families. This document outlines 17 competencies that need to be embedded in undergraduate curriculum to "empower future nurses to be leaders in advocating for access to quality palliative care and to compassionately promote and provide this essential care" (American Association of Colleges of Nursing, 2016). Nurses can use content in this chapter as a guide to caring for older adults at the end of life; however, it is imperative to supplement this content with in-depth information from the ELNEC, as cited in Online Learning Activity 29-3.

Communication

When caring for people at the end of life, effective communication during all interactions and phases of care is crucial for all involved, and its importance is often magnified by the complexity and uncertainty of the situation. Nurses can help people who are dying and who are involved with their care and support to express their needs by using open, honest, direct, and empathetic communication, even when they may be unsure about what to say. In all situations, presence and listening are appropriate nursing interventions. An important aspect of communication is to create and support an environment that is appropriate for the needs of the person who is dying as well as their families. Sensory components of a supportive environment include music, silence, sounds of nature, pleasant scents, conversations with loved ones, and warm blankets and other comfort items. Also, it is imperative to base all communication on the assumption that people who are dying are able to hear what is being said either to or about them. This principle applies even when the person who is dying seems unresponsive. For example, when families ask if the person is unconscious, it is usually appropriate to state, "She may not be actively responding to you, but you can assume that she is aware of your presence and your words." Box 29-3 provides examples of verbal and nonverbal communication techniques that are appropriate for end-of-life care.

Interventions for Physical Comfort

Although the end-of-life process is individualized and unpredictable, some symptoms occur commonly and require expert and timely nursing care. A systematic review of the prevalence of symptoms during the last 2 weeks of life identified the following as the most commonly occurring ones: dyspnea (56.7%), pain (52.4%), respiratory secretions (51.4%), and confusion (50.1%) (Kehl & Kowalkowski, 2013). Additional symptoms that are often addressed at the end of life include fatigue and weakness, constipation, nausea and vomiting, dehydration, and decreased appetite. Nurses can use information in Table 29-1 as a guide to nursing assessment and interventions for some commonly occurring symptoms. In addition, nurses can use information in Chapter 28 to address pain, which is a symptom that occurs frequently at the end of life and is one of the most feared symptoms associated with death.

Physical symptoms usually occur in combination, and it is not always possible to control every symptom completely.

Box 29-3 Communicating With Dying Patients and Their Families

What to Say

Tell me more about...
What questions do you have about your condition?
What are you most concerned about right now?
How are you feeling right now?
I hear your concern (worry, frustration).
How can I be helpful?
I'm here to listen and I'll do my best to help (support, alleviate discomfort).
Take your time.
Is there someone I can call to help with this? (e.g., family, religious person, medical professional)
It's okay to cry. I know this is very sad for you.
Would you prefer to be left alone?
Would you like to share some memories?

Nonverbal Communication

Maintain active presence.
Use touch purposefully.
Communicate patience and respectful waiting.
Learn to be comfortable with silence.
Allow yourself to cry and express emotions in an appropriate and supportive way.

Table 29-1 provides an overview of nursing interventions for symptom management, but end-of-life situations often require the resources of palliative care professionals. Thus, nurses have a primary responsibility for facilitating referrals for palliative care professionals who can suggest and implement interventions for difficult-to-manage symptoms, such as unrelenting pain, through interventions such as **palliative sedation**, which is commonly understood as the controlled and monitored use of nonopioid medications with the intent of reducing the patient's level of consciousness for relief of distress from intractable pain and symptoms (Hospice and Palliative Nurses Association, 2016). Nurses outside of hospice and palliative care settings usually will not be involved with clinical aspects of palliative sedation; however, all nurses need to be able to talk with patients and families about the clinical and ethical implications of this intervention. Online Learning Activity 29-4 provides links to resources for additional information about palliative sedation and management of symptoms that commonly occur at the end of life.

See **ONLINE LEARNING ACTIVITY 29-4:** **ADDITIONAL RESOURCES ABOUT PALLIATIVE SEDATION AND MANAGEMENT OF SYMPTOMS THAT COMMONLY OCCUR AT THE END OF LIFE** at http://thepoint.lww.com/Miller8e.

Spiritual Support

Spiritual care is an essential aspect of nursing care at all times and it becomes even more important at the end of life.

TABLE 29-1 Guide to Nursing Assessment and Interventions for Common Symptoms at the End of Life

Symptom	Nursing Assessment	Nursing Interventions	Pharmacologic Interventions
Fatigue (asthenia) Described as tiredness, lack of strength or endurance, or diminished concentration	Assess for associated conditions, including infection, fever, pain, depression, insomnia, anxiety, dehydration, hypoxia, medication effects	Treat underlying causes (e.g., infection, depression, malnutrition). Teach older adult to pace activities according to tolerance. Encourage physical and social activities as tolerated. Promote optimal sleep, with regular times of rest.	Corticosteroids, although generally contraindicated in older adults, may decrease fatigue in patients with cancer Treat associated conditions (e.g., with antibiotics, antidepressants)
Constipation	Assess and document abdomen and bowel elimination. If bowel movement has not occurred in more than 3 days check for an impaction.	Initiate bowel routine for anyone using opioids. Anticipate and prevent constipation with interventions described in Chapter 18.	Individualize laxative regimen based on the cause(s) of constipation, history, and preferences.
Dyspnea	Assess and document vital signs and all aspects of respirations. Overall: Assess for restlessness, anxiety, and activity tolerance.	Reassure the older adult and caregivers. Talk with older adult and caregivers about pacing rest and activities. Provide oxygen, usually at 2 to 4 L. Teach about positions that improve respiratory function, (e.g., leaning forward over a table with a pillow on top; lying on the side with head slightly elevated). Use a fan to reduce feelings of breathlessness. Teach patient to use effective breathing techniques and encourage the use of relaxation techniques.	Treat symptoms with morphine or hydromorphone, which will also relieve the breathless sensation. Use antianxiety agents or antidepressants as appropriate. Corticosteroids are used when inflammatory processes contribute to respiratory symptoms.
Nausea and vomiting	Assess for causes. Palpate abdomen and check for distention. Assess vomitus for fecal odor. Assess heartburn and nausea, which may occur after meals in squashed stomach syndrome.	Offer frequent, small meals consisting of foods preferred by the older adult. Apply damp, cool cloth to face when nauseated. Provide oral care frequently.	Metoclopramide for gastritis, partial bowel obstruction, or internal pressure on stomach from tumors. Meclizine or diphenhydramine.
Dehydration	Assess clinical signs of hydration status (e.g., skin turgor, mucous membranes). Assess vital signs: pulse, orthostatic blood pressure	Encourage fluids, ice chips, or popsicles as tolerated. Provide frequent oral care, using swabs or moistened toothettes.	Review medications with prescribing practitioner to identify those that can be discontinued.
Anorexia and cachexia	Assess for weight loss, weakness, and fatigue. Conduct physical examination for decreased fat, muscle wasting, decreased strength Assess mental status, including depression	Remove sources of unpleasant odors. Provide frequent oral care. Treat pain optimally. Provide frequent, small meals. Provide mealtime companionship. Serve meals in a place that is separate from the bed area Involve patient with meal planning Collaborate with dietitian for nutritional analysis and meal planning Encourage culturally appropriate foods.	Medications that are used to stimulate appetite, promote weight gain, and provide a sense of well-being: megestrol acetate, corticosteroids, and mirtazapine Metoclopramide is used to improve gastric motility and appetite

Despite its importance, attention to spiritual needs has been identified as an aspect of care that is often absent or inadequate during end-of-life care. Specific ways in which nurses can address spiritual needs at the end of life are described by the Hospice and Palliative Nurses Association (2010) as follows:

- Listening reflectively to the patient's and family's story with a compassionate presence

- Demonstrating empathy and the ability to journey with others in their suffering
- Recognizing and responding to spiritual distress and facilitating the discovery of meaning in the experience of illness, suffering, grief, and loss
- Eliciting key concerns with respect, including feelings of hopelessness, loss, brokenness, and other unmet spiritual and religious needs

- Identifying and responding to ethical issues and conflicts and assisting and supporting others in the application of their own values in decision making
- Creating therapeutic and healing spaces in which spiritual expression can occur
- Facilitating the use of symbol and ritual according to the needs and values of the patient and family
- Offering sensitivity, prayer, music, scripture, or other readings that are meaningful to the patient and family
- Supporting spiritual strengths of the patient and family
- Seeking additional resources as needed by the patient and family including chaplaincy or other spiritual providers

Perhaps the most easily implemented—as well as the most challenging—spiritual intervention is providing genuine presence while patients are experiencing suffering or dying. Physical needs of patients during serious illness and end of life can be intense, leaving little time for nurses to simply be present to patients and families. However, at all times while providing care, nurses can communicate compassion and focus their attention on being fully present as a nursing intervention that is "the first step into spiritual care" (du Pleussis, 2016). Another intervention that is relatively easy to implement is initiating appropriate referrals for pastoral care, hospital chaplains, faith community nurses, palliative care professionals, or other spiritual support resources. In addition, nurses can apply information in Chapters 12 and 13 in this text as a guide to nursing assessment and interventions related to spiritual care for older adults.

GLOBAL PERSPECTIVE

A pilot project in Norway demonstrated the effectiveness of specialized hospice nurses who identify and address patients' spiritual needs through interventions such as presence, active listening, communication, and physical care (Torneo, Danbolt, Kvigne, et al., 2015).

A Student's Perspective

I had a special experience with a man at the nursing and rehab center. "Mort" and I had great conversations, and he quickly became a friend. Mort was suffering from cardiovascular failure, and I knew he did not have long to live. I interviewed Mort and then wrote a paper about his life. I wrote the paper early so that I could read it to Mort before his health declined any more. I read my paper to Mort one morning, and he listened with a seeming sense of sacredness about the words being read. This was his life, and I could tell that it meant a lot to him that I wrote it all down. When I finished, Mort simply said, "I thank you … I thank you." He asked me to put the paper in a safe place so it would not get ruined. Mort and I had a special connection; he was a hero to me. The following week, I went to the clinic and found out that Mort had passed away. I am grateful that I had the opportunity to know Mort and to grow and learn from his good life. I am glad that I could serve him at this final time and help him reflect on his life.

Amy C.

Addressing Needs of the Family

Needs of family members caring for someone at the end of life are numerous and can be overwhelming. A recent study identified the following examples during interviews with family caregivers:

- Patient care challenges: pain, symptom management, safety, functional assistance
- Caregiver emotional challenges: anger, grief, being overwhelmed, feeling unappreciated
- Social support challenges: social isolation, overburden with social demands
- Financial challenges: medical expenses, loss of work, concerns about future financial security
- Health care system challenges: experiences and communication with health care professionals and organizations
- Caregiver health challenges: fatigue, neglect of own health

(Oliver, Demeris, Washington, et al., 2016). The authors of this study emphasize the need for individualized interventions to support both problem-based and emotion-based coping strategies for caregivers. Nurses have key roles in teaching families about symptom management, physical care, and resources for care. In addition, many of the interventions already discussed in this chapter address needs of the family either directly or indirectly. For example, nurses can use information about interventions in Box 29-1 and the communication techniques in Box 29-3 to teach families about supportive care. Family members may benefit from participating in care activities, or they may prefer to simply be present when care is being provided. Nurses need to continually assess needs of the family for information as well as for their desired level of involvement. At all times, nurses need to assure families it is okay for them to take a break from involvement in care or attendance, and to encourage families to address their own needs and not feel guilty about taking time for self-care activities or other responsibilities.

Also, it is important to recognize that family members' perception of quality of care during end of life is influenced as much by the care given after death as it is by the care while the patient is still alive. For example, oncology nurses who invited families to participate in or observe a "bathing and honoring practice" after the death of a loved one found that this intervention was a positive and meaningful action for supporting family members' initial grieving (Rodger, Calmes, & Grotts, 2016). In addition, because interprofessional collaboration is imperative for addressing needs of families, nurses can call on other professionals—for example, from hospice and palliative care programs. These professionals are particularly helpful when families are deciding about options for care or when desires of the patient and family are conflicting. For example, hospice professionals are experts at helping patients and families address issues related to a patient's desire to die at home.

Caring for Oneself When Providing End-of-Life Care

Nurses in all settings address a multitude of issues related to caring for older adults who are seriously or terminally ill and during the dying process. Nurses in hospice and palliative care settings generally view this work as enriching and "life-confirming" while at the same time intense and challenging (Ingebretsen & Sagbakken, 2016).

Nurses can use the following strategies to promote self-care:

- Engaging in self-reflection
- Acknowledging and expressing their own true feelings
- Acknowledging that professional grieving is normal
- Seeking group support for sharing concerns and discussing emotional issues
- Identifying with patients while simultaneously distancing themselves
- Comforting, nurturing, and being kind to themselves
- Accepting a sense of powerlessness
- Acknowledging the very important role they played
- Balancing between personal and professional dimensions
- Having opportunities for debriefing and talking with colleagues
- Attending grief support programs as needed
- Dealing with their own unfinished business related to personal or professional experiences
- Participating in funerals or memorial services for patients; and reasserting responsibilities toward self, patients, and patients' families

(Freeman, 2016; Huang, Chen, & Chiang, 2016; Ingebretsen & Sagbakken, 2016).

SPOTLIGHT ON TRANSITIONAL CARE

As presented in Chapter 6, transitional care is a major focus of health care for older adults who require care across different settings during the course of illness. Although skilled nursing facilities incorporate components of transitional care in usual discharge planning, studies suggest that there is a need for formal transitional care interventions for nursing home resident who are being discharged to home (Toles, Colon-Emeric, Asafu-Adjei, et al., 2016). The unfolding case in this chapter describes how a nurse in a skilled care facility would assure transitional care for Maria Lopez as she is discharged to home from a skilled care facility with hospice care. Online Learning Activity 29-5 provides a link to an article with a case example illustrating the nurse leader's role during transitions of care across settings for an older adult at the end of life.

 See ONLINE LEARNING ACTIVITY 29-5: ARTICLE WITH CASE EXAMPLE ILLUSTRATING NURSES' ROLES IN PROVIDING TRANSITIONAL CARE FOR AN OLDER ADULT AT THE END OF LIFE at http://thepoint.lww.com/Miller8e.

Transitional Care Unfolding Case Study (continued from Chapter 28)

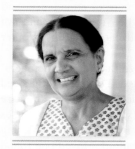

Part 3: Maria Lopez as She is Discharged from a Nursing Home to Receive Home-based Hospice Care

Maria Lopez's lung cancer has been in remission for several years. Two years ago, Isabella married and moved out of Maria's house, and another granddaughter, Regina, moved in. Regina attends the community college and is studying to become a nurse. In addition to assisting her grandmother with medications, meals, and transportation, Regina and her grandmother have developed a close relationship. Regina accompanies her grandmother to all medical appointments and has become an advocate for ensuring that the best care is provided. Last month, Maria was hospitalized for an exacerbation of heart failure, and during the hospitalization she was diagnosed with bone cancer. Maria was transferred to Holy Family Manor for skilled care, where her conditions stabilized. Maria and Regina agree to accept a referral for hospice services at home.

Nurse Juan, Nurse Coordinator for Transitional Care at Holy Family Manor

Holy Family Manor incorporates transitional care interventions into their discharge plans for all residents. Nurse Juan is the nurse care coordinator who is designated to implement the transitional care plan for Maria Lopez. Nurse Juan recognizes that it is imperative to assure good communication about decisions related to end-of-life care (refer to Chapter 9 for details). He has reviewed the advance directives with Maria and Regina and includes the written documents in discharge papers. Nurse Juan also assesses Maria's spiritual and cultural needs (refer to Chapters 2 and 13 for related information).

Part 3: Maria Lopez at 81 Years of Age (Continued)

Nurse Juan is the team leader for an interprofessional discharge conference that includes the following: Maria; Regina; Holy Family Manor staff: nurse practitioner, rehabilitation therapists, social worker, and nurse practitioner; and nurse from Our Lady of Peace Hospice program. Following the care conference Nurse Juan will oversee the implementation of a transitional care plan involving the following interventions:

- Medication reconciliation
- Written communication about Maria's preferences related to end-of-life care
- Written copy of discharge plan developed at care conference
- One day prior to discharge: meeting with Maria, Regina, and nurse from Our Lady of Peace Hospice to review plans, including follow-up services from hospice and primary care practitioner
- Ensure that Maria and Regina have contact information and written information related to Our Lady of Peace Hospice
- One week postdischarge: phone calls to Maria and Regina for feedback about care being provided through Our Lady of Peace Hospice and to address any unresolved concerns.

I P C

THINKING POINTS

- What assessment information would the team consider as they developed the discharge plan?
- How does Nurse Juan's role in providing transitional care at Holy Family Manor differ from his usual role?

- How does Nurse Juan work with other professionals to implement this plan?

Chapter Highlights

Societal and Health Care Perspectives on Death and End of Life

(Figures 29-1 and 29-2; Box 29-1)

- Concepts related to death, dying, and end of life have changed significantly as a result of demographic and health care trends (e.g., increased life expectancy, medical and technical advances).
- The end-of-life time for older adults is often a gradual process associated with cumulative effects of chronic illness and many interacting conditions.
- Cultural perspectives—of society, patients, and health care providers—exert a strong influence on all aspects of end-of-life care.
- Current emphasis is on addressing issues concerning both cost and quality of care.

Current Legal and Ethical Concerns (Box 29-2)

- Ethical and legal questions and challenges are escalating at all levels of society and health care as citizens, governments, institutions, and health care professionals address care and policies that directly and significantly affect end-of-life care.
- Nurses play important roles in promoted shared decision making related to all aspects of end-of-life care.

- Nurses are challenged to address legal and ethical issues related to decisions about patient-directed or physician-directed dying.
- Decisions about end-of-life nursing care should be based on guidelines from the American Nurses Association and the Hospice and Palliative Nurses Association.

Hospice Care

- Hospice care is a philosophy of care that seeks to support a good death experience for people with terminal illnesses and for their families and caregivers.
- Hospice benefits are strongly supported by health insurance (e.g., Medicare and Medicaid) as a cost-effective way of providing high-quality end-of-life care.

Promoting Wellness at the End of Life

- Wellness at the end of life is achieved through a dignified death, as described in the Dying Patient's Bill of Rights (Box 29-2).
- The NOC of Dignified Life Closure is applicable to promoting wellness for patients at the end of life.

Nursing Interventions for End-of-Life Care

- Nurses use verbal and nonverbal communication skills that are appropriate for addressing the complexity of end-of-life situations (Box 29-3).

- Nursing interventions address physical symptoms; however, it is not always possible to control every symptom through usual interventions (Table 29-1).
- Nurses play a major role in facilitating referrals for palliative care professionals.
- Nurses need to be knowledgeable about the clinical and ethical implications of palliative sedation.
- Nurses have numerous opportunities to provide spiritual care for patients and families as an integral part of end-of-life care.
- Nurses address the needs of families as well as their own needs for self-care.

Critical Thinking Exercises

1. Review the section on Culturally Diverse Perspectives on Death and Dying and spend a few minutes answering the questions for self-reflection.
2. Using Online Learning Activity 29-1 find information about groups who advocate both for and against Death with Dignity laws and consider which ones you agree with personally. Read the statements of the American Nurses Association and the Hospice and Palliative Nurses Association that address ethical issues related to end-of-life care and consider how you would apply these to your professional practice.
3. Using Online Learning Activity 29-2 read the article with a case study on discussing assisted dying with a patient. Consider how you would respond to a patient who requests "aid in dying."

 For more information about the topics discussed in this chapter, be sure to check out the interactive Online Learning Activities and other helpful resources at http://thepoint.lww.com/Miller8e.

REFERENCES

American Association of Colleges of Nursing. (2016). *AACN takes action to enhance end-of-life nursing care.* Press Release, February 9, 2016. Available at www.aacn.nche.edu/elnec. Accessed on July 6, 2016.

American Nurses Association. (2016). *American Nurses Association position statement: Nurses' roles and responsibilities in providing care and support at the end of life.* Available at http://nursingworld.org. Accessed on July 5, 2016.

Aoun, S., Deas, K., & Skett, K. (2016). Older people living alone at home with terminal cancer. *European Journal of Cancer Care, 25,* 356–364.

Austin, L. (1975). Dying patient's bill of rights. In *The terminally ill patient and the helping person workshops.* Lansing, MI: Southwest Michigan Inservice Education Council.

Baars, J. (2016). Aging: Learning to live a finite life. *The Gerontologist.* [Epub ahead of print] doi: 10.1093/geront/gnw089.

Chochinov, H. M., Johnston, W., McClement, S. E., et al. (2016). Dignity and distress towards the end of life across four non-cancer populations. *PLOS One, 11*(1), e0147607. doi: 10.1371/journal.pone.0147607.

Drick, C. A. (2016). Progress regarding golden rooms. E-mail communication, July 6, 2016.

du Plessis, E. (2016). Presence: A step closer to spiritual care in nursing. *Holistic Nursing Practice, 30,* 47–53.

Fink-Sammick, E. (2016). The evolution of end-of-life care: Ethical implications for case management. *Professional Case Management, 21,* 180-192.

Freeman, B. (2016). *Compassionate person-centered care for the dying.* New York: Springer Publishing Company.

Haug, S. H., Danbolt, L J., Kvigne, K., et al. (2015). How older people with incurable cancer experience daily living: A qualitative study from Norway. *Palliative and Supportive Care, 13,* 1037–1048.

Hemati, A., Ashouri, E., AllahBakhshian, M., et al. (2016). Dying with dignity: A concept analysis. *Journal of Clinical Nursing, 25,* 1218–1228.

Hospice and Palliative Nurses Association. (2010). *HPNA position statement: Spiritual care.* Available at www.hpna.org. Accessed October 7, 2013.

Hospice and Palliative Nurses Association. (2016). *HPNA position statement: Palliative sedation.* Available at www.hpna.org. Accessed October 7, 2013.

Huang, C.C., Chen, J.Y., Chiang, H.H. (2016). The transformation process in nurses caring for dying patients. *Journal of Nursing Research, 24,* 109–117.

Informed Medical Decisions Foundation. (2016). *Why shared decision making?* Available at www.informedmedicaldecisions.org. Accessed July 7, 2016.

Ingebretsen, L. P., & Sagbakke, M. (2016). Hospice nurses' emotional challenges in their encounters with the dying. *International Journal of Qualitative Studies on Health and Well-Being, 11,* 31170. doi 10:3402/qhe.v11.31170.

Institute of Medicine. (2014). *Dying in America: Improving quality and honoring individual preferences near the end of life.* Washington, DC: National Academies Press.

Jannette, J., Bosek, M. S., & Rambur, B. (2013). Advanced practice registered nurse intended actions toward patient-directed dying. *JONA's Healthcare Law, Ethics, and Regulation, 15*(2), 80–88.

Keegan, L., & Drick, C. A. (2016). Dying in peace. In Dossey, B. M & Keegan, L (Eds.), *Holistic nursing: A handbook for practice* (7th ed.). Burlington, MA: Jones & Bartlett Learning.

Kehl, K. A., & Kowalkowski, J. A. (2013). A systematic review of the prevalence of signs of impending death and symptoms in the last 2 weeks of life. *American Journal of Hospice & Palliative Care, 30*(6), 601–616.

Krause, N., Pargament, K., & Ironson, G. (2016). In the shadow of death: Religious hope as a moderator of the effects of age on death anxiety. *Journals of Gerontology: Social Sciences.* [Epub ahead of print]. doi: 10.1093/geronb/gbw039.

Lachman, V. D. (2015). Voluntary stopping of eating and drinking: An ethical alternative to physician-assisted suicide. *Medsurg Nursing, 2,* 56–59.

Lehto, R. H., Olsen, D. P., & Chan, R. R. (2016). When a patient discusses assisted dying. *Journal of Hospice and Palliative Care, 18,* 184–191.

LoPresti, M. A., Dement, F., & Gold, H. T. (2016). End-of-life care for people with cancer from ethnic minority groups: A systematic review. *American Journal of Hospice and Palliative Care, 33,* 291–305.

Meier, E. A., Gallegos, J. V., Thomas, L. P., et al. (2016). Defining a good death (successful dying): Literature review and a call for research and public dialogue. *American Journal of Geriatric Psychiatry, 24,* 261–271.

Moorhead, S., Johnson, M., Maas, M. L., et al. (Eds.). (2013). *Nursing outcomes classification (NOC).* Philadelphia, PA: Elsevier.

Oliver, D. P., Demiris, G., Washington, K. T., et al. (2016). Challenges and strategies for hospice caregivers: A qualitative analysis. *The Gerontologist.* [Epub ahed of print]. doi: 10.1093/geront/gnw054.

Orentlicher, D., Pope, T. M., & Rich, B. A.. Clinical criteria for physician aid in dying. *Journal of Palliative Medicine, 19,* 259–262.

Penrod, J., Hupcey, J. E., Baney, B., et al. (2011). End-of-life caregiving trajectories. *Clinical Nursing Research, 20*(1), 7–24.

Penrod, J., Hupcey, J. E., Shipley, P. Z., et al. (2012). A model of caregiving through the end of life: Seeking normal. *Western Journal of Nursing Research, 34*(2), 174–193.

Periyakoil, V. S., Neri, E., & Kraemer, H. (2016). Patient-reported barriers to high-quality, end-of-life care: A multiethnic, mixed-methods study. *Journal of Palliative Medicine, 19*, 373-379.

Rahemi, Z., & Williams, C. L. (2016). Older adults of underrepresented populations and their end-of-life preferences: An integrative review. *Advances in Nursing Science, 39*(4), e1–e29.

Rodgers, D., Calmes, B., & Grotts, J. (2016). Nursing care at the time of death: A bathing and honoring practice. *Oncology Nursing Forum, 43*, 363–371.

Rodriguez-Prat, A., Monforte-Royo, C., Porta-Sales, J., Escribano, X., & Balaguer, A. (2016). Patient perspectives on dignity, autonomy, and control at the end of life: Systematic review and meta-ethnography. *PLOS One.* doi: 10.1371/journal.pone.0151435.

Romo, R. D., Allison, T. A., Smith, A.K., et al. (2017). Sense of control in end-of-life decision-making. *Journal of the American Geriatrics Society, 65*(3), e70–e75.

Romo, R., Dawaon-Rose, C., Mayo, A., et al. (2016). Decision making among older adults at the end of life. *Advances in Nursing Science, 39* (4), 308–319.

Rosa, W., & Esters, T. (2016). What end-of-life care needs now. *Advances in Nursing Science, 39*(4), 333–345.

Teno, J.M., Freedman, V. A., Kasper, J. D., et al. (2015). Is care for the dying improving in the United States? *Journal of Palliative Medicine, 18*, 662–666.

Toles, M., Colon-Emeric, C., Asafu-Adjei, J., et al. (2016). Transitional care of older adults in skilled nursing facilities: A systematic review. *Geriatric Nursing, 37*, 296–301.

Tornoe, K., Danbolt, L. J., Kvigne, K., et al. (2015). A mobile hospice nurse teaching team's experience: Training care workers in spiritual and existential care for the dying – a qualitative study. *BioMed Central Palliative Care, 14*. doi: 10.1186/s12904-015-0042-y.

Wright, A. A., Keating, N. L., Ayanian, J. Z., et al. (2016). Family perspectives on aggressive cancer care near the end of life. *Journal of the American Medical Association, 315*, 284–292.

Index

Note: Page number followed by b, f, and t indicates text in box, figure, and table respectively.